MW00987744

Upcoming Titles 2009

BRAUNWALD'S HEART DISEASE COMPANIONS

THEROUX
Acute Coronary Syndromes,
2nd Ed.

OTTO *and* BONOW
Valvular Heart Disease,
3rd Ed.

MANN
Heart Failure,
2nd Ed.

TAYLOR
Atlas of Cardiac CT (Imaging Companion with DVD)

KRAMER *and* HUNDLEY
Atlas of Cardiovascular MR (Imaging Companion with DVD)

CERQUEIRA
Atlas of Nuclear Cardiology (Imaging Companion with DVD)

THOMAS
Atlas of Echocardiography (Imaging Companion with DVD)

2010

KORMOS
Mechanical Circulatory Support and Artificial Hearts

BLUMENTHAL
Prevention of Cardiovascular Disease

Published Titles

ISSA, MILLER, *and* ZIPES
Clinical Arrhythmology and Electrophysiology (2008, ISBN 9781416059981)

ANTMAN
Cardiovascular Therapeutics, 3rd Ed. (2007, ISBN 9781416033585)

BLACK *and* ELLIOTT
Hypertension (2007, ISBN 9781416030539)

CREAGER, DZAU, *and* LOSCALZO
Vascular Medicine (2006, ISBN 9780721602844)

CHIEN
Molecular Basis of Cardiovascular Disease, 2nd Ed. (2004, ISBN 9780721694283)

MANSON
Clinical Trials in Heart Disease, 2nd Ed. (2004, ISBN 9780721604084)

ST. JOHN-SUTTON *and* RUTHERFORD
Clinical Cardiovascular Imaging (2004, ISBN 9780721690681)

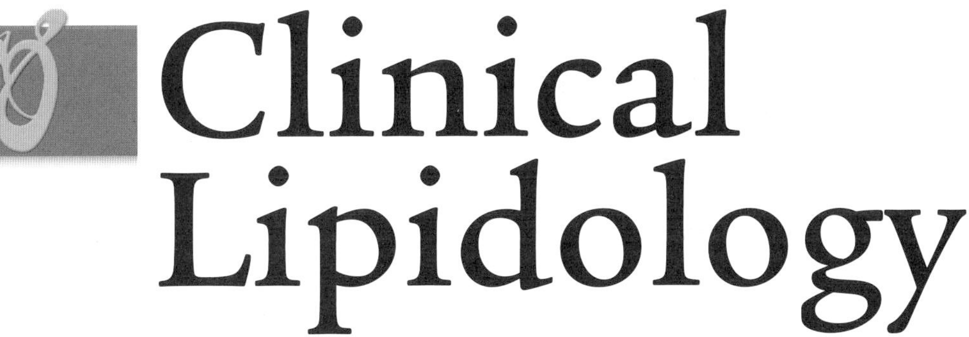

Clinical Lipidology

A Companion to Braunwald's Heart Disease

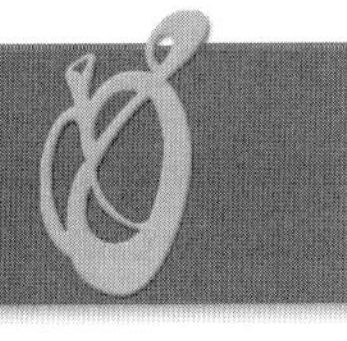

Clinical Lipidology

A Companion to Braunwald's Heart Disease

Christie M. Ballantyne, M.D.
Professor of Medicine
Chief, Section of Atherosclerosis and Vascular Medicine
Baylor College of Medicine
Houston, Texas

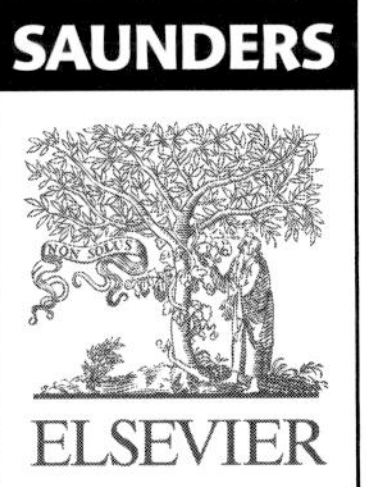

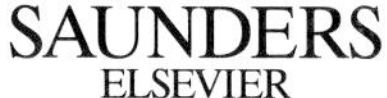

1600 John F. Kennedy Blvd.
Ste 1800
Philadelphia, PA 19103-2899

CLINICAL LIPIDOLOGY: A COMPANION TO BRAUNWALD'S HEART DISEASE
ISBN: 978-1-4160-5469-6

Notice

Knowledge and best practice in this field are constantly changing. As new research and experience broaden our knowledge, changes in practice, treatment and drug therapy may become necessary or appropriate. Readers are advised to check the most current information provided (i) on procedures featured or (ii) by the manufacturer of each product to be administered, to verify the recommended dose or formula, the method and duration of administration, and contraindications. It is the responsibility of the practitioner, relying on their own experience and knowledge of the patient, to make diagnoses, to determine dosages and the best treatment for each individual patient, and to take all appropriate safety precautions. To the fullest extent of the law, neither the Publisher nor the Authors assume any liability for any injury and/or damage to persons or property arising out of or related to any use of the material contained in this book.

The Publisher

Library of Congress Cataloging-in-Publication Data

Clinical lipidology : a companion to Braunwald's heart disease / [edited by] Christie M. Ballantyne. — 1st ed.

p. ; cm.

ISBN 978-1-4160-5469-6
1. Lipids. 2. Lipoproteins. 3. Heart—Diseases. I. Ballantyne, Christie M. II. Braunwald's heart disease.

[DNLM: 1. Lipoproteins—metabolism. 2. Cardiovascular Diseases—complications. 3. Dyslipidemias. 4. Lipid Metabolism. QY 465 C641 2009]

QP751.C55 2009

612.3'97—dc22

Executive Publisher: Natasha Andjelkovic
Editorial Assistant: Isabel Trudeau
Senior Project Manager: David Saltzberg
Design Direction: Steve Stave
Cover artwork provided by Peter Libby and Steven Lee

Printed in the U.S.A.

Last digit is the print number: 9 8 7 6 5 4 3 2 1

Acknowledgments

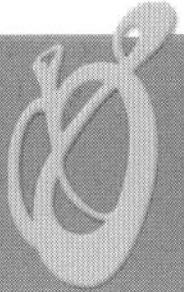

I would like to thank my family for their support during the writing of this book, since it meant time away from them: My wife, Yasmine, and my daughers, Leyla, Christina, and Katina.

I would also like to thank the individuals who inspired me to pursue academic preventive cardiology: Donald Seldin, who inspired me to teach; Jim Willerson, who was a role model for hard work and dedication to patient care; Art Beaudet, for his rigorous approach to the scientific method and critical thinking; and Tony Gotto, who was a role model as a clinician–scientist–educator–father–administrator.

I would also like to thank Kerrie Jara for her help in preparing this book.

Contributing Authors

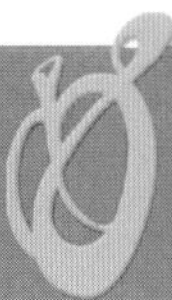

Gerd Assmann, M.D.
Institut for Klinische Chemie und Laboratoriumsmedizin, Albert-Schweitzer, Munster, Germany

Deborah Bagshaw
The Pennsylvania State University, University Park, Pennsylvania

Ashok Balasubramanyam, M.D.
Professor of Medicine, Baylor College of Medicine, Houston, Texas

Christie M. Ballantyne, M.D.
Professor of Medicine, Chief, Section of Atherosclerosis and Vascular Medicine, Baylor College of Medicine, Houston, Texas

Philip Barter, M.D., Ph.D., FRACP
The Heart Research Institute, Sydney, Australia

Harold Bays, M.D., FACP
Louisville Metabolic and Atherosclerosis Research Center (L-MARC), Louisville, Kentucky

Roger S. Blumenthal, M.D., FACC
Professor of Medicine, Director, The Johns Hopkins Ciccarone Center for the Prevention of Heart Disease, Baltimore, Maryland

H. Bryan Brewer, Jr., M.D.
Director, Washington Cardiovascular Associates; Senior Research Consultant, Lipoprotein and Atherosclerosis Research, Cardiovascular Research Institute, MedStar Research Institute, Washington, D.C.

B. Greg Brown, M.D., Ph.D.
University of Washington, Department of Medicine, Seattle, Wachington

John D. Brunzell, M.D.
Professor Emeritus, Department of Medicine, Division of Metabolism, Endocrinology and Nutrition; Clinical Director, Northwest Lipid Metabolism and Diabetes Research Laboratories; University of Washington, Seattle, Washington

Catherine Y. Campbell, M.D.
Johns Hopkins Hospital, Baltimore, Maryland

Paul L. Canner, Ph.D.
Maryland Medical Research Institute, Baltimore, Maryland

Lars A. Carlson, M.D., Ph.D., FRCP Edin
King Gustaf V Research Institute, Karolinska Institutet, Stockholm, Sweden

A. L. Catapano
Professor of Pharmacology, Department of Pharmacological Sciences, University of Milan, Milan, Italy

Tina J. Chahil, M.D.
Columbia University College of Physicians and Surgeons, Department of Medicine, Division of Preventive Medicine and Nutrition, New York, New York

Timothy S. Church, M.D., MPH, Ph.D.
Pennington Biomedical Research Center, Baton Rouge, Louisiana

David E. Cohen, M.D., Ph.D.
Director of Hepatology, Division of Gastroenterology Brigham and Women's Hospital, Harvard Medical School Director, Harvard-MIT Division of Health Sciences and Technology; Associate Professor of Medicine and Health Sciences and Technology, Harvard Medical School, Boston, Massachusetts

Michael H. Davidson, M.D., FACC
The University of Chicago Pritzker School of Medicine, Chicago, Illinois

Prakash C. Deedwania, M.D., FAHA, FACP, FACC
Veterans Administration Central California Healthcare System, University of California Fresno, Fresno, California

Jean-Pierre Després, Ph.D., FAHA
Centre de recherche de l'Hôpital Laval, Pennsylvaniavillon Marguerite-D'Youville, Québec, Canada

Sridevi Devaraj, Ph.D., DABCC
University of California Davis Medical Center, Sacramento, California

Patrick J. Devine, M.D.
Cardiology Service, Walter Reed Army Medical Center Washington, D.C.

Zahi A. Fayad, Ph.D.
Mount Sinai School of Medicine, New York, New York

Sergio Fazio, M.D., Ph.D.
Vanderbilt University Medical Center, Nashville, Tennessee

Bengt Fellstrøm, M.D., Ph.D.
Professor of Nephrology, Department of Medical Sciences, Nephrology Unit, University Hospital, Uppsala, Sweden

Peter Ganz, M.D.
University of California, San Francisco; San Francisco General Hospital, San Francisco, California

Henry N. Ginsberg, M.D.
College of Physicians and Surgeons of Columbia University, Irving Institute for Clinical and Translational Research, New York, New York

Anne Carol Goldberg, M.D., FACP, FAHA
Washington University School of Medicine, St. Louis, Missouri

Antonio M. Gotto, Jr., M.D., Dphil
Weill Cornell Medical College, New York, New York

John R. Guyton, M.D., FAHA
Duke University Medical Center, Durham, North Carolina

William S. Harris, Ph.D.
Sanford Research/USD and Sanford School of Medicine, University of South Dakota, Sioux Falls, South Dakota

Hallvard Holdaas, M.D., Ph.D.
National Hospital, Oslo, Norway

Ron C. Hoogeveen, Ph.D.
Baylor College of Medicine, Houston, Texas

Terry A. Jacobson, M.D., FACP, FAHA
Emory University School of Medicine, Atlanta, Georgia

Alan G. Jardine, BSc, M.D., FRCP
BHF Glasgow Cardiovascular Research Centre, University of Glasgow, United Kingdom

David J. A. Jenkins, M.D., Ph.D.
Department of Nutritional Sciences, Faculty of Medicine, University of Toronto, Toronto, Ontario, Canada

Ishwarlal Jialal, M.D., Ph.D.
University of California Davis Medical Center, Sacramento California

Peter H. Jones, M.D.
The Methodist Hospital, Houston, Texas

Andrea R. Josse, Bkin, MSc
Ivor Wynne Centre, Department of Kinesiology, McMaster University, Ontario, Canada

Cyril W. C. Kendall, Ph.D.
Department of Nutritional Sciences, Faculty of Medicine, University of Toronto, Toronto, Ontario, Canada

Jon A. Kobashigawa, M.D.
University of California at Los Angeles, Los Angeles, California

Marlys L. Koschinsky, B.Sc., Ph.D.
Queen's University, Kingston, Ontario, Canada

Penny M. Kris-Etherton, Ph.D., RD
The Pennsylvania State University, Department of Nutritional Sciences, University Park, Pennsylvania

Salila Kurra, M.D.
Columbia University College of Physicians and Surgeons, New York, New York

Carl J. Lavie, M.D.
Ochsner Health System, New Orleans, Louisiana

Ngoc-Anh Le, Ph.D.
Emory University School of Medicine and Atlanta Veterans Affairs Medical Center, Decatur, Georgia

Peter Libby, M.D.
Mallinckrodt Professor of Medicine, Harvard Medical School, Chief, Cardiovascular Division, Brigham and Women's Hospital, Boston, Massachusetts

MacRae F. Linton, M.D.
Vanderbilt University Medical Center, Nashville, Tennessee

Santica M. Marcovina, Ph.D., ScD
Northwest Lipid Metabolism and Diabetes Research Laboratories, Department of Medicine, University of Washington, Seattle, Washington

Patrick B. Mark, M.D.
Cardiovascular Research Centre, University of Glasgow, Glasgow, United Kingdom

Mark E. McGovern, M.D.
Miami Beach, Florida

James M. McKenney, Pharm.D.
National Clinical Research, Richmond, Virginia

C. Noel Bairey Merz, M.D.
Cedars-Sinai Medical Center, Women's Heart Center, Los Angeles, California

Michael Miller, M.D., FACC, FANA
Division of Cardiology, University of Maryland Hospital, Baltimore, Maryland

Yury I. Miller, M.D., Ph.D.
University of California, San Diego, La Jolla, California

Samia Mora, M.D., MHS
Brigham and Women's Hospital, Boston, Massachusetts

Patrick M. Moriarty, M.D.
University of Kansas Medical Center, Kansas City, Kansas

Kiran Musunuru, M.D.
Clinical Fellow, The Johns Hopkins Ciccarone Preventive Cardiology Center, Johns Hopkins University School of Medicine, Baltimore, Maryland

Kelly S. Myers, M.D.
Mount Sinai School of Medicine, New York, New York

Vijay Nambi, MBBS
Baylor College of Medicine, Houston, Texas,

Tri H. Nguyen, MSc
University of Toronto, FitzGerald Building, Toronto, Ontario, Canada

Stephen J. Nicholls, MBBS, Ph.D.
Cleveland Clinic, Cleveland, Ohio

Steven E. Nissen, M.D., MACC
Chairman, Department of Cardiovascular Medicine, Cleveland Clinic Foundation; Professor of Medicine, Cleveland Clinic Lerner School of Medicine at Case Western Reserve University, Cleveland, Ohio

G. D. Norata, Ph.D.
Department of Pharmacological Sciences, University of Milan, Milan, Italy

Melissa Ohlson, MS, RD, LD
Cleveland Clinic, Cleveland, Ohio

Chris J. Packard, DSc, FRCPath, FRCP(Gla), FRSE EurClinChem, CSci,
Glasgow Royal Infirmary, Glasgow, Scotland

F. Xavier Pi-Sunyer, M.D., MPH
St. Luke's Roosevelt Hospital Center, Columbia University, New York, New York

Donna Polk, M.D., MPH
Director of Preventive Cardiology, Hartford Hospital, Hartford, Connecticut

Henry J. Pownall, BS, MS, Ph.D.
Baylor College of Medicine, Houston, Texas

Daniel J. Rader, M.D.
University of Pennsylvania School of Medicine, Philadelphia, Pennsylvania

Robert S. Rosenson, M.D.
Professor of Medicine, Director, Lipoprotein Disorders and Clinical Atherosclerosis Research Division of Cardiovascular Medicine, University of Michigan, Ann Arbor, Michigan

James H. F. Rudd, M.D., Ph.D., MRCP
Addenbrooke's Hospital, Cambridge, United Kingdom

Joseph S. Saseen, Pharm.D., FCCP, CLS
University of Colorado Denver, Schools of Pharmacy and Medicine, Aurora, Colorado

Gregory G. Schwartz, M.D., Ph.D.
Cardiology Section, Denver VA Medical Center and University of Colorado Health Sciences Center, Denver, Colorado

Udo Seedorf, Ph.D., Dipl.-Biol.
Leibniz-Institute of Arteriosclerosis Research, Munster, Germany

Rajagopal V. Sekhar, M.D.
Translational Metabolism Unit, Division of Diabetes, Endocrinology and Metabolism, Baylor College of Medicine, Houston, Texas

Neil J. Stone M.D., MACP, FAHA, FACC
Professor of Clinical Medicine, Feinberg School of Medicine, Northwestern University, Chicago, Illinois

Allen J. Taylor, M.D., FACC, FAHA
Professor of Medicine, Chief, Cardiology Service, Walter Reed Army Medical Center, Washington, D.C.

Sotirios Tsimikas, M.D., FACC, FAHA, FSCAI
Professor of Medicine and Director of Vascular Medicine, University of California, San Diego, La Jolla, California

Krishnaswami Vijayaraghavan, M.D., FACP, FACC
Scottsdale Cardiovascular Center, Scottsdale Clinical Research Institute, CV division, Scottsdale Healthcare, Scottsdale, Arizona

David Q.-H. Wang, M.D., Ph.D.
Beth Israel Deaconess Medical Center and Harvard Medical School, Boston, Massachusetts

Nanette K. Wenger, M.D.
Emory University School of Medicine, Atlanta, Georgia

Barbara S. Wiggins, Pharm.D., CLS, FAHA
University of Virginia Health System, Charlottesville, Virginia

Peter W. F. Wilson, M.D.
Emory University School of Medicine, Cardiology and Atlanta VAMC Epidemiology and Genetics EPICORE, Atlanta, Georgia

Julia M. W. Wong, RD
Department of Nutritional Sciences, Faculty of Medicine, University of Toronto, Toronto, Ontario, Canada

Contents

Foreword

Links between lipids and cardiovascular disease emerged over the past century based on laboratory experiments and observational data in humans. For more than half a century, physicians have used cholesterol measurements for assessing the risk of future cardiovascular disease. The science of cholesterol has spawned many Nobel prizes and yielded a daunting body of basic science findings. Yet, only in the past two decades have practical tools evolved for clinical intervention on lipids. This recent burgeoning of the evidence base supporting clinical benefit has evolved to the point where most national guidelines recommend therapies that address the lipids profile. This convergence of new clinical tools and clinical trials have garnered the attention of practitioners and spurred the adoption of lipid treatments by practitioners.

Despite this progress the field of lipidology has engendered considerable ongoing controversy, confusion, and frustration. While we have good tools to manipulate low-density lipoprotein (LDL), uncertainty persists regarding how, and how far, to lower this cholesterol-carrying particle. Other prevalent lipid targets such as high-density lipoprotein (HDL) and lipoprotein (a) [Lp(a)] have proved challenging to modulate in clinically practical ways. A number of approaches to modify lipoprotein oxidation and to raise HDL levels have encountered obstacles during their clinical development.

The role of advanced lipid testing in daily practice remains uncertain. An array of tests confronts the practitioner, including lipoprotein particle number, particle size, and apolipoprotein content. How should the practicing physician adopt these specialized tests in the clinic? While many pharmacologic tools exist for manipulating aspects of the lipid profile, some prove challenging to implement in practice due to unwanted actions. Other interventions, although they may produce apparently beneficial effects on the laboratory findings, have proved elusive in terms of defining clinical benefit. So, while on the one hand we have made major advances in treating lipid disorders that undoubtedly help our patients, much opportunity remains for further inroads and the way forward requires considerable clarification.

Where can busy practitioners who want the best possible outcomes for their patients and need to keep abreast of this important, rapidly moving, but challenging field to turn for help? *Clinical Lipidology*, edited by Dr. Christie Ballantyne as part of the family of companions to *Braunwald's Heart Disease*, strives to meet this need. This text provides an authoritative and comprehensive but clinically relevent and practical compendium of contemporary lipidology. It spans the scientific foundations through practical applications to common clinical scenarios, and does not sidestep the controversial or unsolved aspects of this field. The authors have also, in the individual contributions, casted a glance to the future to lay the groundwork for rapid uptake of anticipated advances.

The individual chapters by groups of renowned experts and noted teachers provide brief but definitive tools and ready reference to guide physicians in their daily work. A number of chapters deal succinctly but authoritatively with existing and emerging biomarkers relevent to lipidology and cardiovascular risk. The chapters on intervention emphasize those that involve lifestyle change as well as pharmacologic measures. The chapters provide an evidence-based and scholarly, but balanced and accessible, approach to clinical lipidology. The editors of *Braunwald's Heart Disease* expect this unified approach to fill an important gap to enable the practitioner to diagnosis and manage lipid disorders encountered in daily clinical practice with confidence and expertise.

Peter Libby, M.D.
Robert O. Bonow, M.D.
Douglas L. Mann, M.D.
Douglas P. Zipes, M.D.
Eugene Braunwald, M.D.

Preface

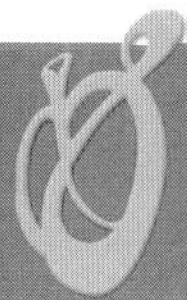

Cardiovascular disease remains the leading cause of death in industrialized societies, and the majority of events are related to atherosclerotic cardiovascular disease. However, in contrast to cancer, which is the second leading cause of death, the vast majority of cardiovascular events could be prevented if individuals were identified early in life and if preventive measures, including lifestyle modification and pharmacotherapy, were initiated. During the last quarter of a century, extraordinary developments in the field of preventive cardiology, with tremendous advances in basic science and clinical research in the area of lipids, lipoproteins, and atherosclerosis, have led to continual improvements in clinical practice. This textbook has been written for both practicing clinicians and students who are interested in effective management of lipids for the treatment and prevention of cardiovascular disease.

The textbook has been divided into three major sections: mechanisms, risk assessment, and therapy. Optimal clinical care requires understanding the basic mechanisms involving lipoprotein metabolism, genetics, and atherosclerosis, which are covered in the first section. This fundamental knowledge can be translated into clinical benefits for patients by using a systematic two-step process of screening followed by targeted interventions. The first step involves global risk assessment to identify individuals who have increased risk for developing atherosclerotic cardiovascular events, and the second step is to implement therapeutic interventions targeted to correct metabolic derangements, using both lifestyle modifications and pharmacotherapy to reduce atherothrombotic cardiovascular events. In addition to understanding the current guidelines and how to implement existing therapies optimally, it is important that physicians understand the evolving targets of therapy and in particular the principles and practices required for management of special patient populations who are high risk for atherosclerotic cardiovascular events.

This textbook has been developed to be useful for cardiologists, endocrinologists, internists, family practitioners, physician assistants, nurses, pharmacists, and other healthcare professionals who want in-depth, state-of-the-art information on the treatment of lipids and atherosclerosis. We hope that it will serve as an important resource for students and trainees. I was personally motivated to go into the field of cardiovascular disease because my father had a myocardial infarction complicated by ventricular fibrillation when I was in high school, my father's sister died of a myocardial infarction when I was in medical school, and I helped take care of my mother's brother after he suffered a large stroke complicated by expressive aphasia and hemiparesis while I was training as a cardiology fellow. We clearly now have both the knowledge and the therapies to prevent the vast majority of heart attacks and strokes that occur in our patients, and it is my greatest hope that the information in this book will be used in the successful implementation of strategies to manage lipids and other risk factors to prevent pain, suffering, and death from atherosclerotic cardiovascular disease.

Christie M. Ballantyne, M.D.

SECTION I

Basic Mechanisms

CHAPTER 1

Human Plasma Lipoprotein Metabolism

Henry J. Pownall and Antonio M. Gotto, Jr.

THE LIPOPROTEINS

Introduction

The French physician-scientist Michel Macheboeuf is acknowledged as the father of plasma lipoproteins. His seminal 1928 discovery fits the adage that science usually precedes technology, in this case by several decades. In his doctoral thesis, *Recherches sur les lipides, les stérols et les protéides du sérum et du plasma sanguinis,* Macheboeuf described horse serum lipoproteins, demonstrating the association of lipids and proteins, *ìlipido-protéidiquesî,* in plasma.[1] It is now recognized that plasma lipids are transported by lipoproteins, which are defined by the densities at which they are isolated, that is, as the high-, low-, intermediate-, and very-low-density lipoproteins (HDLs, LDLs, IDLs, and VLDLs, respectively); chylomicrons, which are intestinally derived, are composed mainly of dietary lipids and small amounts of protein. HDL appears in two subclasses, HDL_2 and HDL_3. Through a simple venipuncture, plasma lipoprotein levels, which are arguably among the most important risk factors for coronary artery disease, provide clues about the etiology of lipid disorders and about their most prominent pathologic sequela, atherosclerosis. From this window on life, a host of informative analyses has emerged. Correlations between coronary artery disease and the properties, compositions, and plasma concentrations of various analytes—lipids as well as lipoproteins—have revealed mechanisms that ultimately aided diagnosis and provided new targets for pharmacologic management of dyslipidemia and atherosclerosis.

LIPOPROTEIN PROPERTIES

The plasma lipoproteins are composed of neutral lipids, polar lipids, and specialized proteins called apolipoproteins (apos). The major neutral lipids are cholesteryl esters (CEs) and triglycerides (TGs); the polar lipids are phosphatidylcholine, sphingomyelin, and free cholesterol with small amounts of phosphatidylethanolamine and traces of other phospholipids (PLs). The compositions of the lipoproteins determine their size and structures (Table 1-1). Lipoprotein size and density are a direct function of neutral lipid content, with the largest lipoprotein particles being the least dense and having the highest ratio of neutral to polar lipids. Surface charge as revealed by agarose gel electrophoresis varies among lipoproteins according to the amount of charged lipids and the conformations of their apos. Lipoproteins have been isolated according to size, charge, and density by size exclusion chromatography, ion exchange chromatography, and ultracentrifugation, respectively, with the latter technique being used for preparative isolation.

The organization of the remainder of this chapter proceeds from our view that much of the currently unanswered lipid and lipoprotein pathologies proceed from dysregulated fatty acid metabolism, which is important in numerous diseases of public interest, including obesity, diabetes, and atherosclerosis. Although

TABLE 1-1 Properties of Human Plasma Lipoproteins

				Composition (%)					
				Core		Surface			
Class	D (nm)	d (g/mL)	Mobility	TG	CE	FC	PL	Pro	Major Apos
Chylomicrons	80–500	<0.93	α_2	86	3	2	7	2	B-48, E, A-I, A-II, A-IV, C
VLDL	30–80	0.95–1.006	Pre-β	55	12	7	18	8	B-100, C-I, C-II, C-III, E
IDL	25–35	1.006–1.019	Slow pre-β	23	29	9	19	19	B-100, E
LDL	21.6	1.019–1.063	β	6	42	8	22	22	B-100
HDL_2	10	1.063–1.125	α	5	17	5	33	40	A-I, A-II
HDL_3	7.5	1.125–1.210	α	3	13	4	25	55	A-I, A-II
Lp(a)	30	1.055–1.085	Slow pre-β	3	33	9	22	33	B-100, apo(a)

apos, apolipoproteins; D, diameter; d, density; CE, cholesteryl ester; FC, free cholesterol; HDL, high-density lipoprotein; IDL, intermediate-density lipoprotein(s); LDL, low-density lipoprotein; Lp(a), lipoprotein(a); PL, phospholipid; TG, triglyceride(s); VLDL, very-low-density lipoprotein(s).

many of the downstream effects of dysregulated fatty acid metabolism are the targets of therapy, it remains important to identify therapeutic modalities that might address underlying causes.

Nonesterified Fatty Acids

Some plasma nonesterified fatty acids (NEFAs) are derived from VLDL- and chylomicron-TG hydrolysis by lipoprotein lipase (LPL), which is attached to the capillary endothelium via proteoglycans. A small fraction of the released NEFAs is released into the plasma, particularly in the postprandial state, when rates of chylomicron-TG hydrolysis are high. Most of the liberated NEFAs transmigrate the endothelium to adipose tissue (AT), where they diffuse across the adipocyte plasma membrane and esterify glycerol-3-phosphate via the Kennedy pathway for glycerolipid synthesis. The TGs so formed associate in TG droplets that are visible under light microscopy (Fig. 1-1). The surfaces of the droplets are surrounded by a mixed monomolecular layer of PLs and by specialized proteins that are essential to normal TG storage and hydrolysis, including perilipin, Comparative Gene Identification–58 (CGI–58), and microsomal transfer pro tein (MTP)-B, a splicing variant of the canonical MTP-A that is found in liver and is associated with protein disulfide isomerase. Whereas MTB-B mediates fusion of small fat droplets into larger ones,[2] it has no direct effect on lipolysis. In contrast, perilipin and CGI–58 are important in the regulation of adipocyte lipolysis, and under fasting conditions, AT TG is a major source of plasma NEFAs.

In the absence of stimulation, perilipin on the surface of fat droplets blocks hormone-sensitive lipase

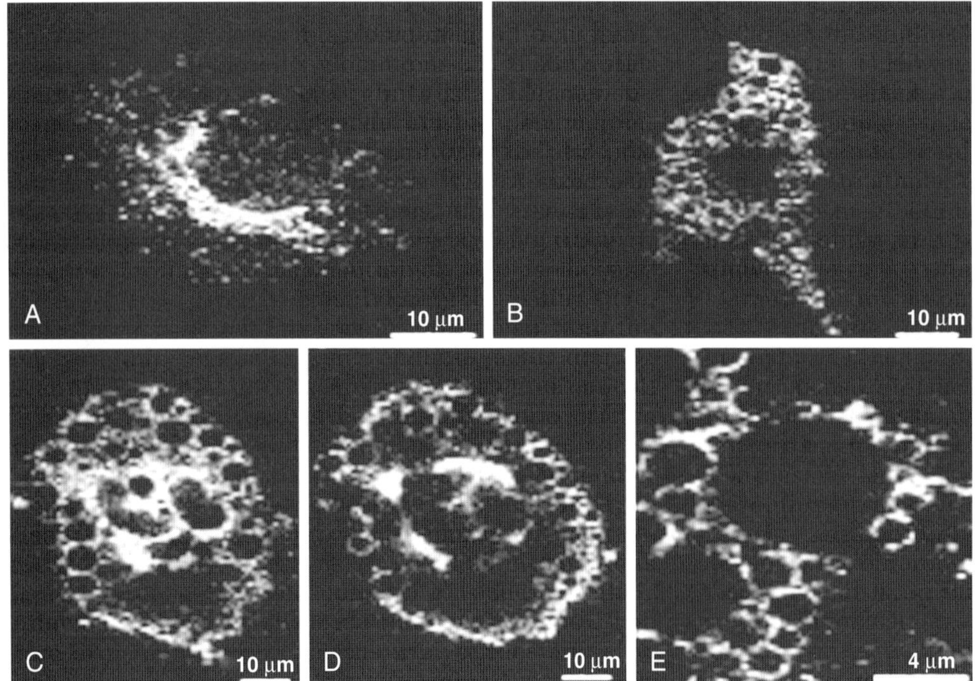

FIGURE 1-1 Confocal microscopy of MTP in 3T3-L1 cells. *A,* Fixed 3T3 cells were probed with anti-microsomal triglyceride transfer protein (MTP) followed by a second Cy3-conjugated antibody. Fluorescence occurred throughout the cell but was more profound in juxtanuclear regions. *(B–E)* Differentiated 3T3 cellsDocument1. MTP fluorescence was higher throughout compared with nondifferentiated cells and was observed around lipid droplets *(E),* especially the smaller droplets. Signals in the juxtanuclear regions remained prominent *(C, D). (From Ref. 2, with permission.)*

(HSL)–mediated hydrolysis. With β-adrenergic receptor activation, protein kinase A hyperphosphorylates perilipin, thereby rapidly altering its conformation in a way that exposes the TG to HSL. Ablation of the perilipin gene in mice is antiadipogenic and illustrates its importance in energy distribution and storage.[3] In the absence of perilipin, β-oxidation is increased and hepatic glucose production is reduced, whereas glucose tolerance and peripheral tissue insulin resistance are normal.[4] According to gene array analyses, these effects are associated with coordinated up-regulation of oxidative pathways and down-regulation of lipid biosynthesis.[5] Adipose tissue expresses another lipase, AT TG lipase,[6] which is also associated with plasma NEFAs and TGs in patients with type 2 diabetes.[7] CGI-58, a member of the subfamily hydrolase fold enzymes, activates (20-fold) adipose TG lipase, and variants of the human CGI-58 are associated with Chanarin-Dorfman syndrome, a disease characterized by ectopic fat deposition.[8] Like HSL, adipose TG lipase is essential to normal lipid metabolism in adipocytes. The combined activities of adipose TG lipase and HSL account for more than 95% of the TG hydrolase activity present in murine white AT. CGI-58 binds to perilipin A–coated lipid droplets in a manner that is dependent on the metabolic status of the adipocyte and the activity of cAMP-dependent protein kinase.[9]

The Apolipoproteins

The distribution of the apos among plasma lipoproteins (see Table 1-1) determines some of their metabolic effects. The apos, which can be classified as soluble and insoluble, are important directors of lipoprotein metabolism. The soluble apos belong to the same gene family in which the terminal exon IV codes for the region of the apo that gives it its distinguishing biologic activities. All soluble apos are exchangeable and contain extended regions of amphipathic helices that mediate binding to lipid surfaces. ApoA-I and apoC-I[10,11] are activators of cholesterol esterification via lecithin:cholesterol acyltransferase (LCAT), apoC-II stimulates LPL-mediated hydrolysis of chylomicrons and VLDL[12,13]; apoE is the ligand for the cellular uptake of IDL and chylomicron remnants.[14–16] Mechanistic links between other apos and lipid metabolism are more subtle but likely present in ways that remain to be determined. Plasma apoC-III correlates with plasma TG levels,[17,18] whereas apoA-V, which occurs at low levels in human plasma, appears to be antilipemic.[19] ApoB-100, an approximately 550-kDa nonexchangeable protein, is a major protein of VLDL, IDL, and LDL, and it contains the ligands for the cellular uptake of LDL via its receptor. Chylomicrons contain a truncated form of apoB, that is, apoB-48, which is a product of a novel mRNA editing mechanism wherein an amino acid codon is converted to a stop codon, giving an expression product that lacks the LDL receptor–binding domain.[20,21] Lipoprotein (a) [Lp (a)] is another large lipoprotein, in which the major protein, apo(a), associates with apoB via a disulfide bridge.[22]

LIPOPROTEIN PRODUCTION

Triglyceride-Rich Lipoproteins

The secreted lipoproteins VLDL and chylomicrons are assembled and secreted by hepatocytes and enterocytes in the liver and intestine, respectively. Their respective assembly is driven by the TG synthesis from endogenous and exogenous, that is, dietary, fatty acids. Thus, an important determinant of fasting plasma TG concentration is the plasma NEFA concentration that is available for hepatic uptake. Some of the NEFAs that are liberated by the hydrolysis of chylomicrons following an oral fat load are hepatically removed and used for VLDL-TG production and secretion. Insulin resistance in AT that impairs fatty acid storage also raises plasma NEFAs, which are used for VLDL production. This mechanism accounts in part for the association of diabetes and other insulin-resistant states with fasting hypertriglyceridemia (HTG) and enhanced postprandial lipemia. HTG is exacerbated by increased hepatic lipase activity, which diverts TG-derived NEFAs to the liver, where they cycle back to VLDL-TG. Although the identification of the mechanisms for protein folding is usually difficult, identification of the mechanism for VLDL assembly, which involves protein folding and the addition of specific amounts of polar and nonpolar lipids, has been much more challenging. Nevertheless, morphologic and subcellular fractionation studies of hepatocytes[23] have provided some support for a two-step model of VLDL assembly. The first step, partial lipidation of apoB with TG, CE, and PL during its translation and translocation to the lumen of the rough endoplasmic reticulum by MTP-A, yields a pre-VLDL that remains weakly associated with the endoplasmic reticulum membrane. The pre-VLDL interacts with a TG-rich particle from the smooth endoplasmic reticulum. The molecular details for this step are not known but may involve chaperones. In some hepatic cells, inadequate lipidation leads to degradation of early forms of VLDL via the ubiquitination-proteosome pathway.[24–26] Hepatic MTP-A is associated with protein disulfide isomerase, the endoplasmic reticulum retention sequence of which keeps MTP within the endoplasmic reticulum.[27] Recent studies of a splicing variant of MTP-B suggest that it is a fusogen[2] and that in hepatic cells it could mediate the fusion of pre-VLDL with TG-rich particles. This remains to be demonstrated. Studies of chylomicron assembly have been sparse, but it is presumed without much evidence to be similar to that of VLDL. As discussed later, the HTG resulting from insulin resistance in AT contributes to the complex phenotype that presents in the metabolic syndrome and obesity-linked diabetes.

Intermediate-Density Lipoproteins and Low-Density Lipoproteins

Following their entry into the plasma compartment, VLDLs are modified by LPL. VLDL, which is the major carrier of endogenous TG, contains apos B-100, E, C-I, C-II, and C-III (see Table 1-1), which are segregated during lipolysis. Hahn first reported that heparin administration released a factor that caused the clearing of human plasma.[28] This observation supported the extant view that LPL associates with capillary proteoglycans and that the main site for the uptake of the fatty acids released by LPL is peripheral tissues that are perfused via the capillary bed. In a classic citation, Korn described the properties of the clearing factor and determined that it was a lipoprotein lipase.[29] Havel and LaRosa further established the importance of LPL in lipoprotein metabolism by showing that LPL activity was stimulated by apoC-II.[30,31] Hydrolysis of TG by LPL converts VLDLs to IDLs and chylomicrons to chylomicron remnants. As expected, apoC-II and LPL deficiency are associated with severe HTG.[32] Independent of mutations in apoC-II and LPL, moderate HTG is associated with type 2 diabetes and atherosclerosis (see later discussion). Interestingly, as VLDL is hydrolyzed by LPL, the C apos, including apoC-II, transfer to HDL and lipolytic activity via LPL is arrested, leaving IDL, which is not an LPL substrate. However, in the liver, hepatic lipase, which does not require apoC-II, continues the hydrolysis of IDL to the mature apoB-100–containing product, LDL. During this step, the particle loses most of its apoE. Hepatic lipase remodels HDL through the hydrolysis of PLs and TGs, an activity that is more profound in the postprandial state.[33]

High-Density Lipoproteins

For a number of reasons, models for the structure, production, remodeling, and catabolism of HDLs have been more difficult to identify than those for the apoB-containing lipoproteins. HDLs are small and heterogeneous with respect to size and composition (see Table 1-1), so many conventional methods such as cryoelectron microscopy, x-ray crystallography, and nuclear magnetic resonance have limited value. Unlike the apoB-containing lipoproteins, all the components of HDLs are exchangeable. Thus, traditional kinetic methods cannot be used to study their turnover. Lastly, although several sources of HDL have been identified on the basis of cell studies, the quantitative importance of these sources in human HDL metabolism is not known except in cases of a natural ablation of a gene coding one of the proteins that forms HDL.

There is evidence that some HDLs are secreted, whereas others are a product of lipolysis in the plasma compartment. The human hepatic cell line, HepG2, secretes particles that have the properties of HDL and contain its major apos.[34,35] The perfusate from rat liver contains small particles that have been described as nascent HDL.[36] Studies by Patsch and Tall have shown that some HDL subclasses are formed by the lipolysis of TG-rich lipoproteins.[37,38] On the other hand, more direct studies of HDL production by human hepatocytes are needed to better understand this important process and its regulation. More recent studies have focused on the role of HDL production and remodeling in reverse cholesterol transport (RCT).

Unlike liver tissue, extrahepatic tissue can synthesize but cannot degrade cholesterol. Thus, cholesterol accumulation in macrophages, a key cell type in atherogenesis, produces a lipotoxic, pathologic state, unless there is a mechanism for its disposal; that mechanism is RCT, and HDL is its central player.[39,40] Within the context of cardiovascular disease (CVD), RCT comprises three steps: cholesterol efflux from monocyte-derived macrophages within the arterial wall, esterification and interaction with lipid transfer proteins in the plasma compartment, and selective hepatic uptake by HDL-CE by its receptor (Fig. 1-2). There are at least four mechanisms for cholesterol efflux:

- One mechanism is mediated by the microsolubilization of membrane lipids by apoA-I via its interactions with the ATP-binding cassette A1 (ABCA1) transporter, which triggers unidirectional release of cholesterol and PL, forming nascent HDL.[41–43] Tangier disease is a severe manifestation of an ABCA1 mutation in which plasma HDL-C levels are close to nil and cellular transfer of cholesterol to lipid-free apos is impaired.[44,45]
- ABCG1/G4 mediates efflux to HDL_2 and HDL_3 but not to lipid-free apoA-I.[46–48] Efflux increases with HDL-PL content. ABCG1 is highly expressed in macrophages[46–48] and might mediate efflux from macrophage–foam cells to HDL. ABCG1 might be the mechanistic link between high HDL-C and low risk of CVD.
- A third mechanism is spontaneous cholesterol desorption from the plasma membrane into the surrounding aqueous phase, where it associates with HDL. This process is driven by a cholesterol concentration gradient from high (donor) to low (acceptor); high relative levels of acceptor-sphingomyelin, which is highly cholesterophilic, increase efflux.[49–51]

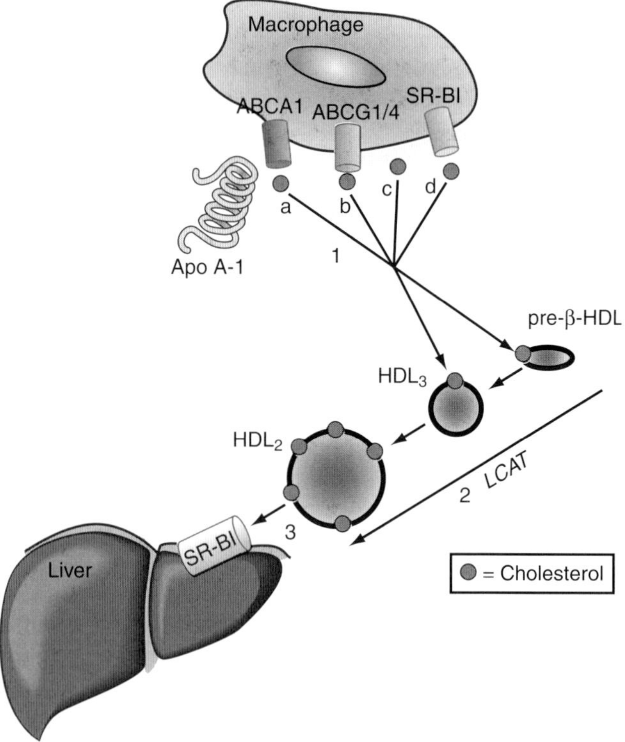

FIGURE 1-2 Cholesterol transfers from macrophages to high-density lipoprotein (HDL) via ATP-binding cassette transporter A1 (ABCA1), ABCG1/4, spontaneous transfer, and Scavenger receptor class B type I (SR-BI) *(1a–d),* and is converted to Cholesteryl ester (CE) via lecithin:cholesterol acyltransferase (LCAT) *(2).* With further cholesterol accretion and esterification, HDL grows to its mature forms from which lipids are removed by hepatic SR-BI receptors *(3).*

- Hepatic Scavenger receptor class B type I (SR-BI), which selectively removes HDL-CE, HDL-TG, and HDL-PL,[52] also mediates cholesterol efflux to HDL, a process that is dose dependent with respect to acceptor-PL content; acceptor-PL enrichment/depletion increases/decreases efflux via SR-BI; efflux is enhanced by addition of phosphatidylcholine[53] and by replacing acceptor-phosphatidylcholine with more cholesterophilic PLs such as sphingomyelin.[54–57]

Lecithin:Cholesterol Acyltransferase

After cholesterol transfer to early forms of HDL, the particle undergoes a series of remodeling reactions involving lipid transfer proteins and cholesterol esterification. Although Sperry identified a plasma cholesterol-esterifying activity in the 1930s,[58] nearly three decades elapsed before studies of families with esterification deficiency renewed interest in this process because of the emerging correlation between plasma cholesterol concentration and CVD. Studies of LCAT, which catalyzes the transfer of fatty acyl chains of phosphatidylcholine to cholesterol, prompted Glomset to propose that HDL was the vehicle for RCT, the transfer of cholesterol from peripheral tissue to the liver for disposal or recycling.[59,60] LCAT is central to RCT because it converts cholesterol to its ester, which is not as readily transferred among membranes and lipoproteins, and it converts HDL from a disc to a sphere with a core containing mostly CEs. Additional rounds of efflux to HDL and esterification produce the mature form that is eventually removed by the liver. As expected, patients with familial LCAT deficiency have very low plasma cholesteryl esters levels and an altered lipoprotein profile. The most profound effect of LCAT deficiency is corneal opacification. In a milder form of deficiency—fish eye disease—corneal opacities occur later in life and the reduction of plasma HDL-CE levels is not as profound. *In vitro* expression of variants found in LCAT deficiency and fish eye disease has revealed that the reduction in secretion and specific activity is more severe in the former.[61] Surprisingly, association of LCAT deficiency with CVD has not been firmly established, perhaps because of the small number of patients, and the studies of atherosclerosis in mice overexpressing LCAT have been contradictory.[62–66]

Lipid Transfer Proteins

Human plasma contains two proteins—cholesteryl ester transfer protein (CETP) and PL transfer protein (PLTP)—that transfer lipids among lipoproteins. Among the lipoproteins, the main donor–acceptor targets of PLTP are HDLs, which PLTP remodels into large and small particles with the concomitant dissociation of lipid-free apoA-I from HDL.[67] Studies in mice overexpressing PLTP suggest that PLTP is atherogenic because it lowers plasma HDL levels.[68] Indeed, some studies in mice have shown that systemic PLTP expression correlates positively with atherosclerotic lesion development.[69] Moreover, macrophage PLTP is an important contributor to plasma PLTP activity, and its deficiency lowers lesion development in LDL receptor–knockout mice on Western-type diet.[70,71] However, similar studies in LDL receptor–knockout mice suggest that macrophage-derived PLTP is atheroprotective.[72] These findings and the absence of natural PLTP mutants with any associated pathology in humans make it difficult to estimate the physiologic importance of PLTP.

In contrast, there is little ambiguity about the importance of CETP, and studies in humans with CETP deficiency and in mice in which the CETP gene has been inserted leave little doubt about its importance in lipid metabolism. Current evidence, particularly in patients with HTG, reveals CETP as an integrator of lipoprotein remodeling that connects the metabolism of TG-rich lipoproteins with those of HDL and LDL (Fig. 1-3). Whereas PLTP transfers mainly PLs, CETP transfers some PLs but has as its primary activity the exchange of neutral lipids—CE and TG—between lipoproteins. In normolipidemic subjects, CETP exchanges small amounts of HDL-CE for VLDL-TG, thereby producing a small increase in the TG content of HDL; effects on VLDL are small. HTG profoundly alters the effects of CETP on lipoprotein profiles, structure, and catabolism. In the presence of HTG, the high VLDL levels provide a large pool of TG for exchange with a much smaller pool of HDL- and LDL-CE so that HDL and LDL are made TG rich.[73] According to cryoelectron microscopy, enrichment of LDLs with TGs shifts their shape from oval[7] to spherical,[74,75] reduces its binding to the fibroblast LDL receptor, and lowers its stability as assessed by enhanced PLTP-mediated release of apoA-I.[76]

The Special Role of Apolipoprotein A-I in High-Density Lipoprotein Stability and Metabolism

It has long been observed that HDL is much less stable than other plasma lipoproteins. Early studies by Nichols[77] showed that the chaotrope, guanidinium chloride, triggered the release of apoA-I, but not apoA-II, TG-rich from human HDL. More recently, Mehta and colleagues[78] and Gursky[79] showed that apoA-I in native HDL

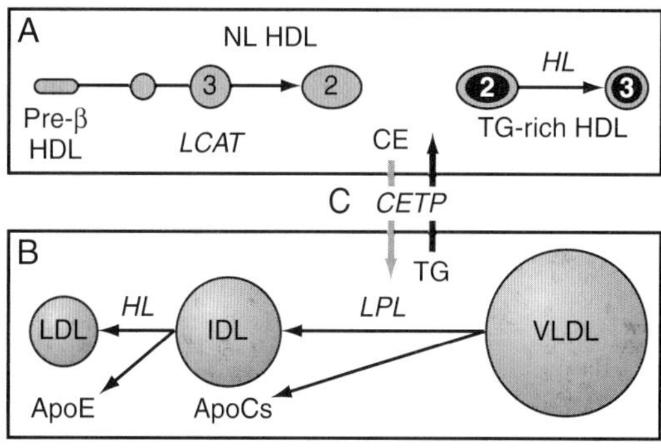

FIGURE 1-3 Formation of small, triglyceride (TG)-rich high-density lipoprotein (HDL) by the activities of cholesteryl ester transfer protein (CETP) and hepatic lipase (HL). *A,* Under normolipidemic conditions, HDL is formed via multiple cycles of phospholipid (PL) and cholesterol efflux via ABCA1 or ABCG1 followed by lecithin:cholesterol acyltransferase (LCAT)–mediated esterification that leads to a mixture of HDL_2 and HDL_3; *B,* low-density lipoprotein (LDL) is formed via lipolysis of very-low-density lipoprotein (VLDL) and intermediate-density lipoprotein (IDL) by lipoprotein lipase (LPL) and hepatic lipase (HL), during which the C and E apolipoproteins (apos) are transferred to HDL. *C,* In hypertriglyceridemia (HTG), CETP mediates the net transfer of TGs from a large pool of VLDLs to HDLs, giving TG-rich HDLs that are hydrolyzed to small, TG-rich HDLs (HDLs).

resided in a kinetic trap and that, when a mechanism for its release was provided, a large fraction of the apoA-I transferred to the aqueous phase, with the concomitant fusion of the remaining apoA-II–rich species into larger particles. The fusion product is highly stable, and treatment with guanidinium chloride does not release its remaining complement of apoA-I.[80] These studies further showed that large HDLs, including HDL_2, are more stable than small HDLs and that apoA-I and apoA-II are equally lipophilic with respect to large HDLs. Detergent perturbation,[81] LCAT,[82] CETP,[83] and especially PLTP[76] and serum opacity factor from *Streptococcus pyogenes*[84,85] also catalyze desorption of apoA-I from HDL. This effect is particularly important in cellular cholesterol efflux via ABCA1, which requires lipid-free apoA-I, and in the terminal RCT step, uptake of HDL lipids without apoA-I (see later discussion). Thus, the HDL instability first observed and characterized by physicochemical perturbations is relevant to plasma and cellular activities that alter HDL compositions *in vivo.*

Metabolic Syndrome

Metabolic syndrome (MetS) is a dyslipidemic state that is associated with a cluster of risk factors. As defined by the National Cholesterol Education Program Adult Treatment Panel III (NCEP ATP III),[86] a diagnosis of metabolic syndrome can be made if three of five conditions are found. These are HTG, low plasma HDL-C, hypertension, hyperglycemia, and a large waist circumference. Many patients with MetS eventually develop type 2 diabetes, with which it shares many characteristics, including a link with obesity. There is a growing opinion that MetS and diabetes might be better viewed as a state of dysregulated lipid metabolism with an attendant impaired rate of glucose disposal.[87,88] The morphing of diabetes and/or MetS from glucocentric to lipocentric has been driven by both clinical and basic research and according to one model should include a cluster of abnormalities that goes beyond the diagnostic criteria of NCEP ATP III (Table 1-2). As a consequence, one can narrow the search for underlying metabolic abnormalities to those that would give rise to those shown in Table 1-2. It is crucial to acknowledge that, in many cases, the abnormalities shown in Table 1-2 taken one at a time are not atherogenic, but taken together produce an atherogenic profile for which current therapies are inadequate.

TABLE 1-2	Characteristics of the Metabolic Syndrome
High plasma NEFA	Insulin resistance
Hypertriglyceridemia*	Hyperinsulinemia
Profound postprandial lipemia	Hyperglycemia*
Low HDL	Pear–apple anthropomorphism*†
No HDL_2	Low lipoprotein lipase
Small dense LDL	High hepatic lipase
Elevated CET activity	Hypertension*

*Metabolic syndrome according to National Cholesterol Education Program Adult Treatment Panel III.[86]

†Large waist circumference.

CET, cholesteryl ester transfer HDL, high-density lipoprotein; LDL, low-density lipoprotein; NEFA, nonesterified fatty acid.

Thus, one should search for treatments that address the underlying cause, thereby correcting the entire MetS cluster of abnormalities. The clustering of some of these abnormalities, for example, HTG and low HDL-C, has long been noted,[73] and it is of interest that the main therapeutic effect of gemfibrozil, a TG-lowering drug, is achieved through increased HDL-C concentrations, an indirect effect that is likely mediated by CETP.[89] CVD is increased in Japanese-American men with increased HDL levels because of a variant of CETP that does not readily exchange HDL-CE for VLDL-TG,[90] further underscoring the importance of treating the cluster of abnormalities and not just one of its components.

Two lifestyle practices—alcohol consumption and exercise—are widely viewed as cardioprotective. Regular consumption of moderate amounts of alcohol reduces CVD mortality,[91] an effect that is likely mediated by increased HDL-C and HDL-PL.[92] This occurs despite the well-known alcohol-induced inhibition of chylomicron lipolysis that leads to enhanced postprandial lipemia. Exercise has broad effects that address many of the abnormalities of MetS, including the reduction of waist circumference through weight loss. Vigorous aerobic exercise reduces plasma TG and postprandial lipemia while raising plasma HDL-C, especially the more cardioprotective fraction, HDL_2.[93] Thus, the identity of the mechanism that raises HDL-C concentrations may be more important to atheroprotection than the plasma HDL-C concentration. This view is supported by studies in mice showing that increasing SR-BI expression lowers plasma HDL-C levels while increasing RCT. Hepatic SR-BI overexpression decreases plasma HDL-C,[94–96] increases HDL-CE clearance,[95–97] and increases biliary cholesterol and its transport into bile.[94,97,98] Mice with ablated or attenuated hepatic SR-BI expression exhibit elevated plasma HDL-C and reduced selective HDL-CE clearance.[99]

Anthropomorphic Determinants of Metabolic Syndrome

Most of the MetS abnormalities shown in Table 1-2 have been cited as having a genetic component, and searches for one or more underlying atherogenic genes have been reported. On the other hand, one could postulate, based on the number of analytes involved (see Table 1-2), that MetS has a highly polygenic origin. A third hypothetical view, presented here, is that one or perhaps a few master genes that control NEFA metabolism give rise to the MetS phenotype. One of the abnormalities that could explain the occurrence of the remainder of the abnormalities is dysregulated NEFA metabolism in AT that induces systemic hyperNEFAemia. Given that circulating plasma NEFAs can rapidly enter and exit cells, plasma hyperNEFAemia could be diagnostic for systemic hyperNEFAemia, in which all tissue sites are challenged by a NEFA overload.

- In liver, the hyperNEFAemia provides the substrate needed for TG overproduction and VLDL hypersecretion that leads to HTG.
- The increased pool of VLDL is a source of additional TG that exchanges for LDL-CE and HDL-CE via CETP, thereby lowering LDL cholesterol and HDL cholesterol by reducing the CE content of LDL and HDL and forming TG-rich LDL and HDL.[73]
- The TG-rich LDL and HDL are substrates for hepatic lipase, which removes some of the TG via lipolysis, leaving small dense LDL and the smaller, less atheroprotective HDL_3 at the expense of HDL_2; both LDL and HDL are still relatively TG rich.
- Postprandial lipemia is more profound in MetS because VLDL-TG is a competitive inhibitor for chylomicron hydrolysis, and NEFAs are a product inhibitor of LPL activity.[100]
- In skeletal muscle, hyperNEFAemia is lipotoxic and its presence is associated with increased myocyte TG and reduced glucose disposal, which triggers insulin secretion that gives rise to hyperinsulinemia.[101,102]

According to this model, interventions that would address the entire MetS risk cluster would have to improve fatty acid storage in AT. The pear-to-apple anthropomorphism that is associated with MetS and revealed as increased waist circumference provides a clue to underlying causes and possible therapies.

Although obesity is associated with diabetes, insulin resistance, and CVD, this effect is depot specific.[103–108] Early studies showed a higher risk of diabetes and CVD in patients with upper body (truncal, central, abdominal, or visceral) obesity than in those with lower body (femoral-gluteal or noncentral) obesity.[109–111] Waist-to-hip circumference ratio is associated with hyperinsulinemia, impaired glucose tolerance, type 2 diabetes, and HTG[112–116] and attendant CVD.[117–122] In nondiabetic, middle-aged men, subcutaneous abdominal fat mass is a better predictor of insulin sensitivity than intraperitoneal fat mass; the sum of truncal skinfold thickness also better predicts insulin resistance than intraperitoneal, retroperitoneal, or peripheral subcutaneous fat.[123] Importantly, posterior subcutaneous abdominal fat mass better predicts insulin sensitivity than anterior subcutaneous abdominal fat mass.[125] Despite some evidence that central fat contains the underlying cause of MetS, there is other evidence that the dysregulated energy metabolism and attendant lipoatrophy in noncentral fat depots, particularly the femoral-gluteal depots, is mechanistically linked to the MetS cluster (see Table 1-2).[126–128] Thiazolidinediones, which target peroxisome-proliferator activated receptors, apparently work through depot-specific effects that improve global insulin sensitivity despite weight gain.[129–132]

High-Density Lipoprotein Therapy

Although the current RCT model is essentially a refinement of that originally described by Glomset,[60] new transporters and receptors that participate in RCT have been identified. These include cholesterol efflux via spontaneous transfer or via ABCG1, which depends on PLs. PLs are the essential cholesterophilic component of all lipoproteins, including HDL, and increased HDL-PC would be expected to increase cholesterol efflux in a way that is therapeutic.

- Reconstituted HDLs are highly cholesterophilic[133–136] and superior LCAT substrates.[137–139]
- Reconstituted HDL infusion into healthy men increases plasma PL and efflux of tissue cholesterol to small pre-β-HDL where it is esterified.[140]
- Small pre-β-HDLs cross endothelium into tissue fluid, collect free cholesterol, and transfer it to the liver, where it is converted to bile acids.[141]
- Infusion of a microemulsion of 1-palmitoyl-2-oleoyl-phosphatidylcholine (POPC) and apoA-I_{Milano}, that is, reconstituted HDL–A-I_{Milano}, produced lesion regression.[142]
- Phospholipidated HDL is more cholesterophilic than native HDL and a better cholesterol efflux acceptor.[53]
- The reaction catalyzed by serum opacity factor has some therapeutic promise; serum opacity factor transfers the CE of 100,000 HDL particles to a single particle that contains apoE while forming a PL-rich neo-HDL.[85] Hepatic clearance of the apoE-containing particles via the LDL receptor could greatly enhance RCT while the neo-HDLs, which are potential acceptors of macrophage cholesterol efflux, could initiate new RCT cycles.

Thus, discovery of new ways to increase plasma PL, particularly HDL-PL, is a promising avenue and a challenge that would complement the effects of the statin class of lipid-lowering drugs.

Acknowledgment

Henry J. Pownall is supported by grants-in-aid from the National Institutes of Health (HL-30914 and HL-56865).

REFERENCES

1. Macheboeuf M: Recherches sur les lipides, les stérols et les protéides du sérum et du plasma sanguinis: I. Entrainement des phospholipids, des sterols et des sterides par les diverses fractions au cours du fractionnement des proteides du serum. *Bull Soc Chim Biol* 1930;223:1–99.
2. Swift LL, Kakkad B, Boone C, et al: Microsomal triglyceride transfer protein expression in adipocytes: a new component in fat metabolism. *FEBS Lett* 2005;579:3183–3189.
3. Schoenborn V, Heid IM, Vollmert C, et al: The ATGL gene is associated with free fatty acids, triglycerides, and type 2 diabetes. *Diabetes* 2006;55(5):1270-1275.
4. Martinez-Botas J, Anderson JB, Tessier D, et al: Absence of perilipin results in leanness and reverses obesity in Lepr(db/db) mice. *Nat Genet* 2000;26:474–479.
5. Saha PK, Kojima H, Martinez-Botas J, et al: Metabolic adaptations in the absence of perilipin: increased beta-oxidation and decreased hepatic glucose production associated with peripheral insulin resistance but normal glucose tolerance in perilipin-null mice. *J Biol Chem* 2004;279:35150–35158.
6. Castro-Chavez F, Yechoor VK, Saha PK, et al: Coordinated upregulation of oxidative pathways and downregulation of lipid biosynthesis underlie obesity resistance in perilipin knockout mice: a microarray gene expression profile. *Diabetes* 2003;52: 2666–2674.
7. Zimmermann R, Strauss JG, Haemmerle G, et al: Fat mobilization in adipose tissue is promoted by adipose triglyceride lipase. *Science* 2004;306:1383–1386.
8. Yamaguchi T, Omatsu N, Matsushita S, Osumi T. CGI-58 interacts with perilipin and is localized to lipid droplets. Possible involvement of CGI-58 mislocalization in Chanarin-Dorfman syndrome. *J Biol Chem* 2004;279:30490–30497.

9. Subramanian V, Rothenberg A, Gomez C, et al: Perilipin A mediates the reversible binding of CGI-58 to lipid droplets in 3T3-L1 adipocytes. *J Biol Chem* 2004;279:42062–46071.
10. Fielding CJ, Shore VG, Fielding PE: A protein cofactor of lecithin:cholesterol acyltransferase. *Biochem Biophys Res Commun* 1972;46:1493–1498.
11. Soutar AK, Garner CW, Baker HN, et al: Effect of the human plasma apolipoproteins and phosphatidylcholine acyl donor on the activity of lecithin:cholesterol acyltransferase. *Biochemistry* 1975;4:3057–3064.
12. Havel RJ, Shore VG, Shore B, Bier DM: Role of specific glycopeptides of human serum lipoproteins in the activation of lipoprotein lipase. *Circ Res* 1970;27:595–600.
13. LaRosa JC, Levy RI, Herbert P, et al: A specific apoprotein activator for lipoprotein lipase. *Biochem Biophys Res Commun* 1970;41:57–62.
14. Utermann G, Jaeschke M, Menzel J: Familial hyperlipoproteinemia type III: deficiency of a specific apolipoprotein (apo E-III) in the very-low-density lipoproteins. *FEBS Lett* 1975;56:352–355.
15. Rall SC Jr, Weisgraber KH, Innerarity TL, Mahley RW: Structural basis for receptor binding heterogeneity of apolipoprotein E from type III hyperlipoproteinemic subjects. *Proc Natl Acad Sci USA* 1982;79:4696–4700.
16. Sherrill BC, Innerarity TL, Mahley RW: Rapid hepatic clearance of the canine lipoproteins containing only the E apoprotein by a high affinity receptor. Identity with the chylomicron remnant transport process. *J Biol Chem* 1980;255:1804–1807.
17. Ito Y, Azrolan N, O'Connell A, et al: Hypertriglyceridemia as a result of human apo CIII gene expression in transgenic mice. *Science* 1990;249:790–793.
18. Aalto-Setala K, Fisher EA, Chen X, et al: Mechanism of hypertriglyceridemia in human apolipoprotein (apo) CIII transgenic mice. Diminished very low-density lipoprotein fractional catabolic rate associated with increased apo CIII and reduced apo E on the particles. *J Clin Invest* 1992;90:1889–1900.
19. Pennacchio LA, Olivier M, Hubacek, et al: An apolipoprotein influencing triglycerides in humans and mice revealed by comparative sequencing. *Science* 2001;294:169–173.
20. Powell LM, Wallis SC, Pease RJ, et al: A novel form of tissue-specific RNA processing produces apolipoprotein-B48 in intestine. *Cell* 1987;50:831–840.
21. Chen S-H, Habib G, Yang C-Y, et al: Apolipoprotein B-48 is the product of a messenger RNA with an organ-specific in-frame stop codon. *Science* 1987;238:363–366.
22. McCormick SP, Ng JK, Taylor S, et al: Mutagenesis of the human apolipoprotein B gene in a yeast artificial chromosome reveals the site of attachment for apolipoprotein(a). *Proc Natl Acad Sci USA* 1995;92:10147–10151.
23. Rustaeus S, Lindberg K, Stillmark P, et al: Assembly of very low-density lipoprotein: a two-step process of apolipoprotein B core lipidation. *J Nutr* 1999;129(2S Suppl):463S–466S.
24. Dixon JL, Furukawa S, Ginsberg HN: Oleate stimulates secretion of apolipoprotein B-containing lipoproteins from Hep G2 cells by inhibiting early intracellular degradation of apolipoprotein B. *J Biol Chem* 1991;266:5080–5086.
25. Liang S, Wu X, Fisher EA, Ginsberg HN: The amino-terminal domain of apolipoprotein B does not undergo retrograde translocation from the endoplasmic reticulum to the cytosol. Proteasomal degradation of nascent apolipoprotein B begins at the carboxyl terminus of the protein, while apolipoprotein B is still in its original translocon. *J Biol Chem* 2000;275:32003–32010.
26. Zhou M, Fisher EA, Ginsberg HN: Regulated Co-translational ubiquitination of apolipoprotein B100. A new paradigm for proteasomal degradation of a secretory protein. *J Biol Chem* 1998;273:24649–24653.
27. Wetterau JR, Aggerbeck LP, Bouma ME, et al: Absence of microsomal triglyceride transfer protein in individuals with abetalipoproteinemia. *Science* 1992;258:999–1001.
28. Hahn PF: Abolishment of alimentary lipemia following injection of heparin. *Science* 1943;98:19–20.
29. Korn ED: Properties of clearing factor obtained from rat heart acetone powder. *Science* 1954;120:399–400.
30. Havel RJ, Shore VG, Shore B, Bier DM: Role of specific glycopeptides of human serum lipoproteins in the activation of lipoprotein lipase. *Circ Res* 1970;27:595–600.
31. LaRosa JC, Levy RI, Herbert P, et al: A specific apoprotein activator for lipoprotein lipase. *Biochem Biophys Res Commun* 1970;41:57–62.
32. Fojo SS, Brewer HB: Hypertriglyceridaemia due to genetic defects in lipoprotein lipase and apolipoprotein C-II. *J Intern Med* 1992;231:669–677.
33. Patsch J: Influence of lipolysis on chylomicron clearance and HDL cholesterol levels. *Eur Heart J* 1998;19(Suppl H):H2–H6.
34. Fielding CJ, Fielding PE: Cellular cholesterol efflux. *Biochim Biophys Acta* 2001;1533:175–189.
35. Thrift RN, Forte TM, Cahoon BE, Shore VG: Characterization of lipoproteins produced by the human liver cell line, Hep G2, under defined conditions. *J Lipid Res* 1986;27:236–250.
36. Chisholm JW, Burleson ER, Shelness GS, Parks JS:ApoA-I secretion from HepG2 cells: evidence for the secretion of both lipid-poor apoA-I and intracellularly assembled nascent HDL. *J Lipid Res* 2002;43:36–44.
37. Hamilton RL, Moorehouse A, Havel RJ: Isolation and properties of nascent lipoproteins from highly purified rat hepatocytic Golgi fractions. *J Lipid Res* 1991;32:529–543.
38. Tall AR, Small DM: Plasma high-density lipoproteins. *N Engl J Med* 1978;299:1232—1236.
39. Patsch JR, Gotto AM Jr, Olivercrona T, Eisenberg S: Formation of high-density lipoprotein2-like particles during lipolysis of very low-density lipoproteins in vitro. *Proc Natl Acad Sci USA* 1978;75:4519–4523.
40. Yancey PG, Bortnick AE, Kellner-Weibel G, et al: Importance of different pathways of cellular cholesterol efflux. *Arterioscler Thromb Vasc Biol* 2003;23:712–719.
41. Hara H, Yokoyama S: Interaction of free apolipoproteins with macrophages. Formation of high-density lipoprotein-like lipoproteins and reduction of cellular cholesterol. *J Biol Chem* 1991;266:3080–3086.
42. Gillotte KL, Davidson WS, Lund-Katz S, et al: Removal of cellular cholesterol by pre-beta-HDL involves plasma membrane microsolubilization. *J Lipid Res* 1998;39:1918–1928.
43. Gillotte KL, Zaiou M, Lund-Katz S, et al: Apolipoprotein-mediated plasma membrane microsolubilization. Role of lipid affinity and membrane penetration in the efflux of cellular cholesterol and phospholipid. *J Biol Chem* 1999;274:2021–2028.
44. Okuhira K, Tsujita M, Yamauchi Y, et al: Potential involvement of dissociated apoA-I in the ABCA1-dependent cellular lipid release by HDL. *J Lipid Res* 2004;45:645–652.
45. Francis GA, Knopp RH, Oram JF: Defective removal of cellular cholesterol and phospholipids by apolipoprotein A-I in Tangier Disease. *J Clin Invest* 1995;96:78–87.
46. Engel T, Lorkowski S, Lueken A, et al: The human ABCG4 gene is regulated by oxysterols and retinoids in monocyte-derived macrophages. *Biochem Biophys Res Commun* 2001;288:483–488.
47. Wang N, Lan D, Chen W, et al: ATP-binding cassette transporters G1 and G4 mediate cellular cholesterol efflux to high-density lipoproteins. *Proc Natl Acad Sci USA* 2004;101:9774–9779.
48. Nakamura K, Kennedy MA, Baldan A, et al: Expression and regulation of multiple murine ATP-binding cassette transporter G1 mRNAs/isoforms that stimulate cellular cholesterol efflux to high-density lipoprotein. *J Biol Chem* 2004;279:45980–45989.
49. Phillips MC, Johnson WJ, Rothblat GH: Mechanisms and consequences of cellular cholesterol exchange and transfer. *Biochim Biophys Acta* 1987;906:223–276.
50. Phillips MC, Gillotte KL, Haynes MP, et al: Mechanisms of high-density lipoprotein-mediated efflux of cholesterol from cell plasma membranes. *Atherosclerosis* 1998;137(Suppl):S13–S17.
51. Lund-Katz S, Laboda HM, McLean LR, Phillips MC: Influence of molecular packing and phospholipid type on rates of cholesterol exchange. *Biochemistry* 1988;27:3416–3423.
52. Acton S, Rigotti A, Landschulz KT, et al: Identification of scavenger receptor SR-BI as a high-density lipoprotein receptor. *Science* 1996;271:518–520.
53. Pownall HJ: Detergent-mediated phospholipidation of plasma lipoproteins increases HDL cholesterophilicity and cholesterol efflux via SR-BI. *Biochemistry* 2006;45:11514–11522.
54. Jian B, de la Llera-Moya M, Royer L, et al: Modification of the cholesterol efflux properties of human serum by enrichment with phospholipid. *J Lipid Res* 1997;38:734–744.
55. Niu SL, Litman BJ: Determination of membrane cholesterol partition coefficient using a lipid vesicle-cyclodextrin binary system: effect of phospholipid acyl chain unsaturation and headgroup composition. *Biophys J* 2002;83:3408–3415.
56. Pownall HJ: Detergent-mediated phospholipidation of plasma lipoproteins increases HDL cholesterophilicity and cholesterol efflux via SR-BI. *Biochemistry* 2006;45:11514–11522.

57. Yancey PG, de la Llera-Moya M, Swarnakar S, et al: High-density lipoprotein phospholipid composition is a major determinant of the bi-directional flux and net movement of cellular free cholesterol mediated by scavenger receptor BI. *J Biol Chem* 2000;275:36596–36604.
58. Sperry WM: *J Biol Chem* 1935;111:467–478.
59. Glomset JA, Parker F, Tjaden M, Williams RH: The esterification in vitro of free cholesterol in human and rat plasma. *Biochim Biophys Acta* 1962;58:398–406.
60. Glomset JA: The plasma lecithin:cholesterol acyltransferase reaction. *J Lipid Res* 1968;9:155–167.
61. Qu SJ, Fan HZ, Blanco-Vaca F, Pownall HJ: In vitro expression of natural mutants of human lecithin:cholesterol acyltransferase. *J Lipid Res* 1995;36:967–974.
62. Mehlum A, Gjernes E, Solberg LA, et al: Overexpression of human lecithin:cholesterol acyltransferase in mice offers no protection against diet-induced atherosclerosis. *APMIS* 2000;108: 336–342.
63. Mehlum A, Muri M, Hagve TA, et al: Mice overexpressing human lecithin: cholesterol acyltransferase are not protected against diet-induced atherosclerosis. *APMIS* 1997;105:861–868.
64. Berard AM, Foger B, Remaley A, et al: High plasma HDL concentrations associated with enhanced atherosclerosis in transgenic mice overexpressing lecithin-cholesteryl acyltransferase. *Nat Med* 1997;3:744–749.
65. Lambert G, Sakai N, Vaisman BL, et al: Analysis of glomerulosclerosis and atherosclerosis in lecithin:cholesterol acyltransferase-deficient mice. *J Biol Chem* 2001;276:15090–15098.
66. Furbee JW Jr, Sawyer JK, Parks JS: Lecithin:cholesterol acyltransferase deficiency increases atherosclerosis in the low-density lipoprotein receptor and apolipoprotein E knockout mice. *J Biol Chem* 2002;277:3511–3519.
67. Rao R, Albers JJ, Wolfbauer G, Pownall HJ: Molecular and macromolecular specificity of human plasma phospholipid transfer protein. *Biochemistry* 1997;36:3645–3653.
68. Ehnholm S, van Dijk KW, van't Hof B, et al: Adenovirus mediated overexpression of human phospholipid transfer protein alters plasma HDL levels in mice. *J Lipid Res* 1998;39:1248–1253.
69. Yang XP, Yan D, Qiao C, et al: Increased atherosclerotic lesions in apoE mice with plasma phospholipid transfer protein overexpression. *Arterioscler Thromb Vasc Biol* 2003;23: 1601–1607.
70. Vikstedt R, Ye D, Metso J, et al: Macrophage phospholipid transfer protein contributes significantly to total plasma phospholipid transfer activity and its deficiency leads to diminished atherosclerotic lesion development. *Arterioscler Thromb Vasc Biol* 2007;27:578—586.
71. Liu R, Hojjati MR, Devlin CM, et al. Macrophage phospholipid transfer protein deficiency and ApoE secretion: impact on mouse plasma cholesterol levels and atherosclerosis. *Arterioscler Thromb Vasc Biol* 2007;27:190–196.
72. Valenta DT, Ogier N, Bradshaw G, et al: Atheroprotective potential of macrophage-derived phospholipid transfer protein in low-density lipoprotein receptor-deficient mice is overcome by apolipoprotein AI overexpression. *Arterioscler Thromb Vasc Biol* 2006;26:1572–1578.
73. Pownall HJ, Brauchi D, Kilinc C, et al: Correlation of serum triglyceride and its reduction by omega-3 fatty acids with lipid transfer activity and the neutral lipid compositions of high-density and low-density lipoproteins. *Atherosclerosis* 1999;143:285–297.
74. Orlova EV, Sherman MB, Chiu W, et al: Three-dimensional structure of low-density lipoproteins by electron cryomicroscopy. *Proc Natl Acad Sci USA* 1999;96:8420–8425.
75. Sherman MB, Orlova EV, Decker GL, et al: Structure of triglyceride-rich human low-density lipoproteins according to cryoelectron microscopy. *Biochemistry* 2003;42:14988–14993.
76. Settasatian N, Duong M, Curtiss LK, et al: The mechanism of the remodeling of high-density lipoproteins by phospholipid transfer protein. *J Biol Chem* 2001;276:26898–26905.
77. Nichols AV, Gong EL, Blanche PJ, et al: Effects of guanidine hydrochloride on human plasma high-density lipoproteins. *Biochim Biophys Acta* 1976;446:226–239.
78. Mehta R, Gantz DL, Gursky O: Human plasma high-density lipoproteins are stabilized by kinetic factors. *J Mol Biol* 2003;328: 183–192.
79. Gursky O: Apolipoprotein structure and dynamics. *Curr Opin Lipidol* 2005;16:287–294.
80. Pownall HJ, Hosken BD, Gillard BK, et al: Speciation of Human Plasma High-Density Lipoprotein (HDL): HDL Stability and Apolipoprotein A-I Partitioning. *Biochemistry* 2007;46: 7449–7459.
81. Pownall HJ: Remodeling of human plasma lipoproteins by detergent perturbation. *Biochemistry* 2005;44:9714–9722.
82. Liang HQ, Rye KA, Barter PJ: Remodelling of reconstituted high-density lipoproteins by lecithin:cholesterol acyltransferase. *J Lipid Res* 1996;37:1962–1970.
83. Rye KA, Hime NJ, Barter PJ: Evidence that cholesteryl ester transfer protein-mediated reductions in reconstituted high-density lipoprotein size involve particle fusion. *J Biol Chem* 1997;272:3953–3960.
84. Courtney HS, Zhang YM, Frank MW, et al: Serum opacity factor, a streptococcal virulence factor that binds to apolipoproteins A-I and A-II and disrupts high-density lipoprotein structure. *J Biol Chem* 2006;281:5515–5521.
85. Gillard BK, Courtney HS, Massey JB, Pownall HJ: Serum Opacity Factor Unmasks Human Plasma High-Density Lipoprotein Instability via Selective Delipidation and Apolipoprotein A-I Desorption. *Biochemistry* 2007. 46:13170-13178. *Epub* 2007 Oct 18.
86. American Heart Association; National Heart, Lung, and Blood Institute; Grundy SM, Cleeman JI, Daniels SR, et al: Diagnosis and management of the metabolic syndrome. An American Heart Association/National Heart, Lung, and Blood Institute Scientific Statement. Executive summary. *Cardiol Rev* 2005;13:322–327.
87. McGarry JD: What if Minkowski had been ageusic? An alternative angle on diabetes. *Science* 1992;258:766–770.
88. McGarry JD: Banting lecture 2001. Dysregulation of fatty acid metabolism in the etiology of type 2 diabetes. *Diabetes* 2002;51:7–518.
89. Manninen V, Elo MO, Frick MH, et al: Lipid alterations and decline in the incidence of coronary heart disease in the Helsinki Heart Study. *JAMA* 1988;260:641–651.
90. Zhong S, Sharp DS, Grove JS, et al: Increased coronary heart disease in Japanese-American men with mutation in the cholesteryl ester transfer protein gene despite increased HDL levels. *J Clin Invest* 1996;97:2917–2923.
91. Thun MJ, Peto R, Lopez AD, et al: Alcohol consumption and mortality among middle-aged and elderly U.S. adults. *N Engl J Med* 1997;337:1705–1714.
92. Schafer C, Parlesak A, Eckoldt J, et al: Beyond HDL cholesterol increase: phospholipid enrichment and shift from HDL_3 to HDL_2 in alcohol consumers. *J Lipid Res* 2007;48:1550–1558.
93. Patsch JR, Karlin JB, Scott LW, et al: Inverse relationship between blood levels of high-density lipoprotein subfraction 2 and magnitude of postprandial lipemia. *Proc Natl Acad Sci USA* 1983;80:1449–1453.
94. Kozarsky KF, Donahee MH, Ribotti A, et al: Overexpression of the HDL receptor SR-BI alters plasma HDL and bile cholesterol levels. *Nature* 1997;387:414–417.
95. Wang N, Arai T, Ji Y, et al: Liver-specific overexpression of scavenger receptor BI decreases levels of very low-density lipoprotein ApoB, low-density lipoprotein ApoB, and high-density lipoprotein in transgenic mice. *J Biol Chem* 1998;273: 32920–32926.
96. Ueda Y, Royer L, Gong E, et al: Lower plasma levels and accelerated clearance of high-density lipoprotein (HDL) and non-HDL cholesterol in scavenger receptor class B type I transgenic mice. *J Biol Chem* 1999;274:7165–7171.
97. Ji Y, Wang N, Ramakrishnan R, et al: Hepatic scavenger receptor BI promotes rapid clearance of high-density lipoprotein free cholesterol and its transport into bile. *J Biol Chem* 1999;274:33398–33402.
98. Sehayek E, Ono JG, Shefer S, et al: Biliary cholesterol excretion: a novel mechanism that regulates dietary cholesterol absorption. *Proc Natl Acad Sci USA* 1998;95:10194–10199.
99. Varban ML, Rinninger F, Wang N, et al: Targeted mutation reveals a central role for SR-BI in hepatic selective uptake of high-density lipoprotein cholesterol. *Proc Natl Acad Sci USA* 1998;95:4619–4624.
100. Saxena U, Witte LD, Goldberg IJ: Release of endothelial cell lipoprotein lipase by plasma lipoproteins and free fatty acids. *J Biol Chem* 1989;264:4349–4355.
101. Krssak M, Petersen KF, Bergeron R, et al: Intramuscular glycogen and intramyocellular lipid utilization during prolonged exercise and recovery in man: a 13C and 1H nuclear magnetic

resonance spectroscopy study. *J Clin Endocrinol Metab* 2000;85:748–754.
102. Krssak M, Falk Petersen K, Dresner A, et al: Intramyocellular lipid concentrations are correlated with insulin sensitivity in humans: a 1H NMR spectroscopy study. *Diabetologia* 1999;42:113–116.
103. Wajchenberg BL: Subcutaneous and visceral adipose tissue: their relation to the metabolic syndrome. *Endocr Rev* 2000;21:697–738.
104. Frayn KN: Visceral fat and insulin resistance–causative or correlative? *Br J Nutr* 2000;83(Suppl 1):S71–S77.
105. Cases JA, Barzilai N: The regulation of body fat distribution and the modulation of insulin action. *Int J Obes Relat Metab Disord* 2000;24(Suppl 4):S63–S66.
106. Despres JP: Health consequences of visceral obesity. *Ann Med* 2001;33:534–541.
107. Misra A, Vikram NK: Clinical and pathophysiological consequences of abdominal adiposity and abdominal adipose tissue depots. *Nutrition* 2003;19:457–466.
108. Lebovitz HE: The relationship of obesity to the metabolic syndrome. *Int J Clin Pract* 2003;134(Suppl):18–27.
109. Garg A: Regional adiposity and insulin resistance. *J Clin Endocrinol Metab* 2004;89:4206–4210.
110. Vague J: La differenciation sexuelle: facteur determinant des formes: de l'obesite. *Presse Med* 1947;55:339–340.
111. Vague J: The degree of masculine differentiation of obesities: a factor determining predisposition to diabetes, atherosclerosis, gout, and uric calculous disease. *Am J Clin Nutr* 1956;34: 416–422.
112. Kissebah AH, Vydelingum N, Murray R, et al: Relation of body fat distribution to metabolic complications of obesity. *J Clin Endocrinol Metab* 1982;54:254–260.
113. Fujioka S, Matsuzawa Y, Tokunaga K, Tarui S: Contribution of intra-abdominal fat accumulation to the impairment of glucose and lipid metabolism in human obesity. *Metabolism* 1987;36:54–59.
114. Peiris AN, Struve MF, Mueller RA, et al: Glucose metabolism in obesity: influence of body fat distribution. *J Clin Endocrinol Metab* 1988;67:760–767.
115. Peiris AN, Hennes MI, Evans DJ, et al: Relationship of anthropometric measurements of body fat distribution to metabolic profile in premenopausal women. *Acta Med Scand* 1988;723:179–188.
116. Rimm AA, Hartz AJ, Fischer ME: A weight shape index for assessing risk of disease in 44,820 women. *J Clin Epidemiol* 1988;41:459–465.
117. Peiris AN, Sothmann MS, Hoffmann RG, et al: Adiposity, fat distribution, and cardiovascular risk. *Ann Intern Med* 1989;110:867–872.
118. Lapidus L, Bengtsson C, Larsson B, et al: Distribution of adipose tissue and risk of cardiovascular disease and death: a 12-year follow-up of participants in the population study of women in Gothenburg. *Br Med J* 1984;289:1257–1261.
119. Ohlson LO, Larsson B, Svardsudd K, et al: The influence of body fat distribution on the incidence of diabetes mellitus: 13.5 years of follow-up on the participants in the study of men born in 1913. *Diabetes* 1985;34:1055–1058.
120. Ducimetiere P, Richard J, Cambien F: The pattern of subcutaneous fat distribution in middle-aged men and the risk of coronary heart disease: the Paris Prospective Study. *Int J Obes* 1986;10:229–240.
121. Casassus P, Fontbonne A, Thibult N, et al: Upper-body fat distribution: a hyperinsulinemia-independent predictor of coronary heart disease mortality: the Paris Prospective Study. *Arterioscler Thromb* 1992;12:1387–1392.
122. Donahue RP, Bloom E, Abbott RD, et al: Central obesity and coronary heart disease in men. *Lancet* 1987;1:821–823.
123. Abate N, Garg A, Peshock RM, et al: Relationship of generalized and regional adiposity to insulin sensitivity in men. *J Clin Invest* 1995;96:88–98.
124. Misra A, Garg A, Abate N, et al: Relationship of anterior and posterior subcutaneous abdominal fat to insulin sensitivity in nondiabetic men. *Obes Res* 1997;5:93–99.
125. Balasubramanyam A, Sekhar RV, Jahoor F, et al: Pathophysiology of dyslipidemia and increased cardiovascular risk in HIV lipodystrophy: a model of "systemic steatosis". *Curr Opin Lipidol* 2004;15:59–67.
126. Sekhar RV, Jahoor F, White AC, et al: Metabolic basis of HIV-lipodystrophy syndrome. *Am J Physiol Endocrinol Metab* 2002;283:E332–E337.
127. Okura T, Nakata Y, Yamabuki K, Tanaka K: Regional body composition changes exhibit opposing effects on coronary heart disease risk factors. *Arterioscler Thromb Vasc Biol* 2004;24:923–929.
128. Lemieux I: Energy partitioning in gluteal-femoral fat. Does the metabolic fate of triglycerides affect coronary heart disease risk? *Arterioscler Thromb Vasc Biol* 2004;24:795–797.
129. Virtanen KA, Hallsten K, Parkkola R, et al: Differential effects of rosiglitazone and metformin on adipose tissue distribution and glucose uptake in type 2 diabetic subjects. *Diabetes* 2003;52:283–290.
130. Yang X, Smith U: Adipose tissue distribution and risk of metabolic disease: does thiazolidinedione-induced adipose tissue redistribution provide a clue to the answer? *Diabetologia* 2007;50:1127–1139.
131. Shadid S, Jensen MD: Effects of pioglitazone versus diet and exercise on metabolic health and fat distribution in upper body obesity. *Diabetes Care* 2003;26:3148–3152.
132. Johnson WJ, Bamberger MJ, Latta RA, et al: The bidirectional flux of cholesterol between cells and lipoproteins. Effects of phospholipid depletion of high-density lipoprotein. *J Biol Chem* 1986;261:5766–5776.
133. Johnson WJ, Bamberger MJ, Latta RA, et al: The bidirectional flux of cholesterol between cells and lipoproteins. Effects of phospholipid depletion of high-density lipoprotein. *J Biol Chem* 1986;261:5766–5776.
134. Picardo M, Massey JB, Kuhn DE, et al: Partially reassembled high-density lipoproteins. Effects on cholesterol flux, synthesis, and esterification in normal human skin fibroblasts. *Arteriosclerosis* 1986;6:434–441.
135. Davidson WS, Gillotte KL, Lund-Katz S, et al: The effect of high-density lipoprotein phospholipid acyl chain composition on the efflux of cellular free cholesterol. *J Biol Chem* 1995;270:5882–5890.
136. Matz CE, Jonas A: Micellar complexes of human apolipoprotein A-I with phosphatidylcholines and cholesterol prepared from cholate-lipid dispersions. *J Biol Chem* 1982;257: 4535–4540.
137. Matz CE, Jonas A: Reaction of human lecithin cholesterol acyltransferase with synthetic micellar complexes of apolipoprotein A-I, phosphatidylcholine, and cholesterol. *J Biol Chem* 1982;257:4541–4546.
138. Pownall HJ, Van Winkle WB, Pao Q, et al: Action of lecithin: cholesterol acyltransferase on model lipoproteins. Preparation and characterization of model nascent high-density lipoprotein. *Biochim Biophys Acta* 1982;713:494–503.
139. Chen CH, Albers JJ: Characterization of proteoliposomes containing apoprotein A-I: a new substrate for the measurement of lecithin:cholesterol acyltransferase activity. *Lipid Res* 1982;23:680–691.
140. Nanjee MN, Doran JE, Lerch PG, Miller NE: Acute effects of intravenous infusion of ApoA1/phosphatidylcholine discs on plasma lipoproteins in humans. *Arterioscler Thromb Vasc Biol* 1999;19:979–989.
141. Nanjee MN, Cooke CJ, Garvin R, et al: Intravenous apoA-I/lecithin discs increase pre-beta-HDL concentration in tissue fluid and stimulate reverse cholesterol transport in humans. *J Lipid Res* 2001;42:1586–1593.
142. Nissen SE, Tsunoda T, Tuzcu EM, et al: Effect of recombinant ApoA-I_{Milano} on coronary atherosclerosis in patients with acute coronary syndromes: a randomized controlled trial. *JAMA* 2003;290:2292–2300.

CHAPTER 2

Regulation and Clearance of Apolipoprotein B–Containing Lipoproteins

Sergio Fazio and MacRae F. Linton

INTRODUCTION

The apolipoprotein (apo)B isoforms apoB-100 and apoB-48 are derived from a single gene and play crucial roles in the metabolism of plasma lipoproteins.[1] ApoB is a nonexchangeable apoprotein that is required for the synthesis of triglyceride-rich lipoproteins in the liver (very-low-density lipoprotein [VLDL]) and intestine (chylomicrons). ApoB-100 contains 4536 amino acids and is required for the assembly of triglyceride-rich VLDL by the liver.[2] In addition, apoB-100 serves as the ligand for low-density lipoprotein (LDL) receptor–mediated clearance of LDL cholesterol particles from the blood. ApoB-48 consists of the amino terminal 2152 amino acids of apoB-100 and is essential for the formation of chylomicrons and the absorption of dietary fats in the intestine.[2,3] Elevated plasma levels of apoB-100 are a strong predictor of increased risk for cardiovascular events.[4,5] Furthermore, all the lipoproteins considered atherogenic, including LDL, intermediate-density lipoprotein (IDL), lipoprotein(a), and triglyceride-rich remnants of VLDL and chylomicrons, contain apoB as the key structural element. Therefore, understanding the molecular mechanisms regulating the biogenesis of apoB-containing lipoproteins and their clearance from plasma may provide new therapeutic targets for the prevention of coronary heart disease.

APOLIPOPROTEIN B STRUCTURE

Based on sequence analysis and computer modeling, Segrest and coworkers have proposed the model that apoB-100 has a pentapartite secondary structure (NH2-βα1-β1-α2-β2-α3-COOH), in which domains rich in amphipathic β-sheets alternate with domains rich in amphipathic α-helices.[6] The β-sheets contain critical lipid-binding domains that bind irreversibly to lipids. ApoB-48 contains only the first β-sheet of apoB-100; it is missing the second. The N-terminal βα1-domain of apoB is homologous to the lipovitellins, which are lipid transport proteins found in egg-laying species, and contain a lipid pocket used for transport of lipids.[7,8] In a previous model, Segrest and coworkers suggested that a lipid-pocket mechanism for initiation of lipoprotein particle assembly might involve the physical interaction of apoB with microsomal triglyceride transfer protein (MTP) to complete the lipid pocket.[9] MTP also shares homology with lipovitellin and from an evolutionary standpoint may be the oldest of these lipid-binding proteins.[10] However, based on a detailed analysis of the first 1000 residues of apoB using standard sequence alignment programs and computer three-dimensional homology modeling, Richardson and coworkers, including Segrest, no longer propose that MTP is required for formation of the lipid pocket.[11] Instead, they propose a hairpin-bridge lipid-pocket model in which apoB can assemble lipid delivered by MTP to form a nascent lipoprotein without requiring MTP for structural completion of the lipid pocket. In this model, salt bridges between each of four tandem charged residues (717 to 720) in the turn of the hairpin bridge and four tandem complementary residues (997 to 1000) at the C-terminus of the model lock the bridge in the closed position, allowing the formation of a bilayer within the lipid pocket.[11]

APOLIPOPROTEIN B GENE REGULATION AND EDITING

The human *aPOB* gene is located on chromosome 2 and contains 29 exons and 28 introns. Two of the exons, 26 and 29, are particularly large. Exon 26 codes for amino acids 1379 to 3903, or more than 55% of the amino acids in apoB-100.[1,12] Regulatory sequences in the region from 5 kb upstream and 1.5 kb downstream of the apoB gene direct liver-specific expression of apoB. In contrast, studies in human apoB-100 transgenic mice[13] led to the discovery that intestinal expression requires a distant enhancer located 62 to 56 kb upstream of the apoB B gene.[14] Subsequent studies have localized the intestinal enhancer to a region within 315 nucleotides 56 kb upstream of the apoB gene.[15] A number of important factors for apoB gene transcription have been identified, including C/EBP, hepatic nuclear factor–3 (HNF-3), HNF-4, and other nuclear receptors that bind the intestinal enhancer and proximal promoter.[16] Recent studies suggest that high-molecular-weight adiponectin may down-regulate apoB expression via HNF-4α,[17] and dietary induction of betaine-homocysteine S-methyltransferase appears to increase apoB mRNA and VLDL production.[18] However, there is little evidence that dietary factors modulate apoB gene expression acutely. The weight of current evidence supports the view that apoB gene expression is constitutive and that regulation of VLDL secretion is achieved primarily through cotranslation and post-translation degradation of apoB. Yet, apoB gene expression remains an active target for therapeutic intervention as evidenced by the current efforts to develop mRNA antisense to apoB as an approach to lower LDL cholesterol.[19]

Apolipoprotein B-48 Production by mRNA Editing

ApoB-48 is formed in the intestine through a unique mRNA-editing mechanism, converting codon 2153 (CAA, specifying glutamine) into a premature stop codon (UAA).[20,21] This highly specific post-transcriptional cytidine deamination targets one nucleotide (at position 6666 in the apoB cDNA) out of more than 14,000 nucleotides in the apoB transcript. The C-to-U editing of apoB mRNA is accomplished by a large multiprotein complex that consists of several factors, including two required core components, the catalytic deaminase, apoB mRNA editing enzyme (apobec)-1, and a competence factor, apobec-1 complementation factor.[22] In humans, the catalytic component of the apoB mRNA-editing complex, APOBEC-1, is highly expressed in the intestine but is absent in the liver, so essentially all the apoB produced in the intestine is apoB-48, whereas apoB-100 is produced in the liver. In contrast, APOBEC-1 is expressed in the livers of some mammals, including mice and rats, and these species therefore produce apoB-48 in the liver. Targeted deletion of apobec-1 in mice eliminates C-to-U editing of apoB mRNA but is otherwise well tolerated.[23,24] In contrast, targeted deletion of apobec-1 complementation factor, which binds to both apoB RNA and apobec-1 and thereby results in site-specific post-transcriptional editing of apoB mRNA, is embryonic lethal during the blastocyst stage (embryonic day 3.5).[25] Knockdown of the gene in hepatocytes promotes apoptosis, suggesting that apobec-1 complementation factor may play a critical role in cell survival independent of apobec-1 expression. The editing complex contains several other factors, including the inhibitory components CUG-binding protein–2, glycine-arginine-tyrosine-rich RNA–binding protein, and heterogeneous nuclear ribonucleoprotein–C1. Recent studies suggest that coordinated expression levels of the various editing components may determine the magnitude and specificity of apoB mRNA editing.[26]

ApoB mRNA editing occurs in mammals and marsupials but not in birds and is therefore a relatively late evolutionary adaptation.[22] Gene-targeting studies in mice were designed in an effort to examine the physiologic rationale for going to the trouble of editing apoB. ApoB-48 lacks the amino acids present in apoB-100 that are responsible for binding to the LDL receptor (LDLR). Therefore, chylomicrons and their remnants must rely on apoE for receptor-mediated clearance from the plasma by the LDLR or the LDLR-related protein (LRP). One hypothesis has been that apoB-48 might be required for chylomicron synthesis and secretion. In studies designed to investigate the biologic rationale for having two different isoforms of apoB, mice were created that expressed only apoB-100 or only apoB-48.[27] The difference in length of the two apoB isoforms did affect lipoprotein size, with much larger VLDL particles in apoB-100–only mice than in apoB-48–only mice on the apoE-deficient background. However, mice that expressed apoB-100 only were able to synthesize and secrete chylomicrons containing apoB-100, indicating efficient packaging and secretion of dietary lipoproteins in the intestine.[27] Furthermore, the production of lipoproteins containing only apoB-48 or apoB-100 did not appear to have an independent effect on the extent of atherosclerosis.[28] Thus, the biologic rationale and the potential evolutionary advantage for apoB editing in the intestine remain to be elucidated. Interestingly, two members of the APOBEC3 family, APOBEC3G and APOBEC3F, have been found to have potent activity against virion infectivity factor–deficient (Deltavif) human immunodeficiency virus–1 (HIV-1), whereas APOBEC3B and APOBEC3C have potent antiviral activity against simian immunodeficiency virus (SIV) but not HIV-1, suggesting that the different APOBEC3 family members function to neutralize specific lentiviruses.[29]

Mutations in the Apolipoprotein B Gene Cause Monogenic Hypercholesterolemia and Hypocholesterolemia

The fact that apoB-100 is the ligand for clearance of LDL cholesterol from blood by the LDLR led to speculation that mutant forms of apoB-100 might cause hypercholesterolemia resulting from the defective binding to the LDLR, thereby causing delayed clearance of LDL cholesterol. Metabolic studies by Vega and Grundy demonstrated that some individuals with hypercholesterolemia and normal LDLR function had LDL cholesterol exhibiting delayed clearance.[30] Subsequent *in vitro* studies demonstrated that the LDL from one of these individuals was defective in binding to LDLR on fibroblasts,[31] and a missense mutation in the apoB gene resulting in substitution of glutamine for arginine in the codon for amino acid 3500 of apoB-100 was found to be responsible for the defective binding.[32]

Familial defective apoB-100 (FDB) is an autosomal dominant disorder characterized by elevated levels of LDL cholesterol resulting from a mutation in the apoB gene that causes defective binding to the LDLR.[33] The Arg3500Gln mutation is the most common apoB gene mutation identified to cause FDB, but other less common mutations have been described. The Arg3500Gln mutation has been estimated to have arisen in Europe approximately 6500 years ago,[34] and the incidence of FDB is approximately 1 in 1000 in central Europe. The phenotype of patients with FDB includes elevated plasma levels of LDL cholesterol, tendon xanthomas, and increased risk for premature coronary artery disease, similar to the phenotype seen in heterozygous familial hypercholesterolemia (FH) caused by mutations in the LDLR.[35] The average levels of LDL cholesterol in individuals with heterozygous FDB are approximately 100 mg/dL higher than in age-matched controls but tend to be lower than in individuals with heterozygous FH.[33] In contrast to the situation in persons with FH, LDLR–mediated clearance of remnant lipoproteins is not impaired in individuals with FDB. The apoE-containing remnant lipoproteins, which depend on apoE rather than apoB-100 for LDLR-mediated clearance, are precursors of LDL. Kinetic studies support the hypothesis that LDL cholesterol levels that are lower in individuals with FDB than in those with FH are due to reduced production of LDL cholesterol[36] because of increased clearance of apoE-containing remnants.

In contrast, familial hypobetalipoproteinemia (FHβ) is an inherited disorder characterized by low levels of LDL cholesterol resulting from mutations in the apoB gene.[37] Young and colleagues first established that FHβ was due to an inherited defect in the apoB gene by demonstrating the presence of a truncated apoB-37 species in the plasma of affected members of the HJB kindred with FHβ.[38,39] In the majority of cases, FHβ is caused by nonsense or frameshift mutations that interfere with the synthesis of a full-length apoB molecule, resulting in the production of a truncated apoB species.[37] The apoB-37 allele had a 4 nucleotide deletion leading to a premature stop codon.[40] The HJB kindred had two apoB mutant alleles, and the other mutant allele produced both a truncated apoB-86 species and very low levels of the full-length apoB-100 protein through a unique mechanism of RNA polymerase stuttering on a long stretch of eight As.[41] Individuals with heterozygous FHβ have one mutant apoB allele and serum apoB and LDL cholesterol levels that are about one-third to one-fourth normal. Three members of the HJB kindred were compound heterozygotes for both mutant alleles with extremely low levels of total serum cholesterol (~30 mg/dL) and unmeasurable levels of LDL cholesterol.[38,39] Thus, compound heterozygotes or homozygotes for FHβ have severe hypocholesterolemia, which overlaps phenotypically with abetalipoproteinemia, a rare autosomal recessive condition caused by deficiency of MTP.[37,42,43] In abetalipoproteinemia, the apoB-containing lipoproteins are absent from plasma and affected individuals develop malabsorption of dietary fats, anemia with acanthocytosis, and a progressive spinocerebellar syndrome associated with peripheral neuropathy and retinitis pigmentosa.[44] These sequelae are due to malabsorption of fat-soluble vitamins and can be prevented by replacement of the fat-soluble vitamins, especially high-dose vitamin E.[45] Compound heterozygotes and homozygotes for FHβ are spared this severe phenotype if their apoB gene mutations still allow production of apoB-48.[37,43,46]

Examination of the ability of truncated apoB species to form buoyant lipoprotein particles in patients with FHβ has provided important insights into the structural requirements of apoB in lipoprotein assembly. Nonsense or frameshift mutations occurring in exons 26 to 29 have all been associated with the presence of a truncated apoB that is detectable in the plasma lipoproteins, whereas mutations in the 5′ part of the apoB gene encoding the amino terminal 30% of the apoB protein are not associated with detectable levels of a truncated apoB species in plasma.[1] Thus, in patients with FHβ with mutations predicted to yield apoB-25– and apoB-29–sized truncated proteins, no truncated apoB species are detected in plasma.[37] *In vitro* studies have shown that shorter forms of apoB, such as apoB-18, can be secreted from hepatocytes in culture, suggesting that the absence of the shorter truncated apoB species from the plasma lipoproteins *in vivo* is due to a failure to achieve adequate lipidation to form buoyant particles rather than to the inability of the short apoB species to be secreted.[1] However, apoB-31 is detected in high-density lipoprotein (HDL), and apoB-37 is found in VLDL, LDL, and HDL. In general, there is an inverse relationship between the length of the apoB species and the buoyant density of lipoproteins containing the truncated apoB species. Similarly, *in vitro* expression studies have shown an inverse relationship between length of the apoB protein and buoyant density of the lipoproteins secreted,[47] reflecting the increased number of lipid-binding regions in the longer apoB proteins.

Insights into Apolipoprotein B Expression Derived from Human Apolipoprotein B-100 Transgenic Mice

Initial efforts to develop a transgenic mouse expressing human apoB-100 made use of a cDNA/genomic minigene construct that produced transgenic mice with very low plasma levels of apoB-100.[48] Subsequently, we developed transgenic mice expressing high levels of human apoB-100 by making use of a P1 bacteriophage vector clone (p158) that contained an 80-kb insert spanning the entire 43-kb structural human apoB gene, as well as 19 kb of 5 flanking sequences and 17.5 kb of 3 flanking sequences.[13] In chow-fed hemizygous mice with more than 10 copies of the transgene, the plasma levels of human apoB were 60 to 80 mg/dL, similar to those in normolipidemic humans. In response to a high-fat diet, these human apoB-100 transgenic mice developed severe hypercholesterolemia because of the accumulation of triglyceride-rich LDL and dramatically increased atherosclerosis.[13] Normal mice express the enzyme for editing apoB in both the liver and the intestine. Interestingly, the p158 human apoB-100 transgenic mice showed robust expression of human apoB-100 with editing of 70% of the transcripts to apoB-48 in the liver but no expression of human apoB-48 in the intestine.[13] Subsequent transgenic studies using 145- and 207-kb bacterial artificial chromosomes spanning the human apoB gene indicated that appropriate expression of the apoB gene in the intestines is controlled by distant DNA sequences contained within the bacterial artificial chromosomes but absent from p158.[49,50] Interestingly, coinjection of p158 with 70 kb of apoB 5′-flanking sequences resulted in expression of the human apoB transgene in the intestine, whereas coinjection with 22 kb of apoB 3′ flanking sequences did not. These studies established that the element controlling apoB gene expression in the intestine is located more than 30 kb 5′ to the structural gene.[49] Transgenic mice created with recA-assisted restriction endonuclease cleavage-modified bacterial artificial chromosomes demonstrated that intestinal expression requires a distant enhancer located 62 to 56 kb upstream of the apoB B gene,[14] and subsequent studies localized the intestinal enhancer to a region within 315 nucleotides 56 kb upstream of the apoB gene.[15]

Unexpectedly, expression of the human apoB transgene was detected in the hearts of p158 transgenic mice,[13] an observation that was initially assumed to be an artifact but heralded the discovery that apoB-100 is normally expressed by the cardiac smooth muscle cells. Both human and mouse hearts were found to express apoB-100 and MTP and to secrete lipoproteins containing human apoB-100.[51] Unlike expression of apoB in the intestine, expression of apoB-100 by the heart does not require a distal enhancer element.[52] Metabolic labeling studies demonstrated that heart tissue from humans, human apoB transgenic mice, and normal mice secrete apoB-100–containing lipoproteins with density of LDL cholesterol.[53] Inhibition of MTP increases triglyceride accumulation in the myocardium, whereas overexpression of apoB-100 prevents fasting-induced heart triglyceride accumulation and the development of cardiomyopathy in a mouse model of diabetes.[54] Thus, lipoprotein production by the heart may allow the heart to unload excess triglycerides and may affect cardiac function by opposing the formation of cardiomyopathy.[54]

Insights into Apolipoprotein B Biology from Gene-Targeting Studies in Mice

A number of important insights into the roles of apoB in lipoprotein metabolism and developmental biology have been gleaned from studies using gene-targeting technologies to insert mutations or disrupt expression of the apoB gene. The development of mice homozygous for expression of an allele designed to produce apoB-70 using a sequence-insertion gene-targeting vector to interrupt the 3′ portion of exon 26 of the mouse *Apob* gene resulted in neurodevelopmental abnormalities, including exencephalus and hydrocephalus, and approximately 50% died in utero.[55] Genetic deletion of *Apob* proved to be lethal in utero during midgestation in homozygotes (apoB−/−).[56,57] Similarly, homozygous deficiency of MTP in gene-targeted mice also proved lethal during midgestation.[58] These results suggested critically important roles for apoB and MTP in lipoprotein synthesis in the yolk sac as a source of lipids and lipid-soluble nutrients for the developing embryo.[59,60] Interestingly, it was possible to rescue the apoB−/− mice from death in utero by crossing them with apoB transgenic mice created with the p158 clone, which lacks intestinal expression.[61] However, the HuBTg/Apob−/− mice lacked the ability to synthesize chylomicrons and therefore developed fat malabsorption and growth retardation that was most apparent during suckling.[61] The enterocytes from their small intestines were filled with lipid in the cytosol, similar to findings in patients with abetalipoproteinemia and homozygous FHβ, and two thirds of the HuBTg/Apob−/− mice died during the suckling period because of malabsorption.[61] However, HuBTg/Apob−/− mice that survived weaning were able to grow and eventually achieved normal size on a chow diet.[61] Furthermore, plasma levels of LDL cholesterol and apoB-100 in HuBTg/Apob−/− mice were similar to those in human apoB transgenic mice that synthesized chylomicrons normally (HuBTg/Apob+/+). Therefore, chylomicron secretion is not a significant determinant of the plasma levels of hepatic lipoproteins in mice on a chow diet. The introduction of point mutations in the *aPOB* gene has been used to address specific questions regarding apoB structure function. For example, by mutating candidate cysteines and making use of truncated apoB proteins, the cysteine of apoB-100 required for binding to apo(a) to form lipoprotein(a) was determined to be cysteine-4326.[62–64]

Cotranslational And Post-Translational Regulation

In general, apoB gene expression is viewed as constitutive, and acute regulation of apoB by metabolic factors is mainly post-translational. However, there is evidence to support translational regulation of apoB by insulin,[65,66] and inhibition of MTP can slow translation of apoB.[67] The molecular mechanisms for regulation of apoB mRNA translation remain incompletely understood, but there is evidence to support a role for structural properties of the 3′ and 5′ untranslated regions of apoB mRNA.[68,69] Two decades ago, pulse chase studies in cultured hepatic cell lines and primary hepatocytes demonstrated that a significant proportion of newly synthesized apoB is degraded.[70,71] Mounting evidence supports the view that regulation of the degradation of apoB is the major means for regulating the production of triglyceride-rich lipoproteins by the liver and the intestine.[72] The availability of lipids, including triglycerides, phospholipids, cholesterol, and cholesteryl esters, at the site of apoB synthesis in the endoplasmic reticulum (ER) has been shown to be a major determinant of the amount of apoB-containing lipoproteins secreted.[72,73] Thus, when an adequate supply of lipids is available, apoB is packaged into lipoproteins for secretion, but in lipid-poor states the apoB is targeted to pathways for degradation. This regulated degradation of apoB occurs by both proteasomal and nonproteasomal pathways.[72] Structural determinants of apoB influence VLDL assembly and degradation of apoB. Cell culture studies of amino terminal truncated mutants of apoB showed that the length of the apoB molecule influenced secretion and correlated with the buoyant density of the secreted VLDL particles.[47]

Unlike most secretory proteins, which are translocated efficiently into the ER lumen during translation, apoB undergoes inefficient translocation characterized by simultaneous exposure to the cytosol and ER lumen.[72] One potential explanation for this inefficient translocation is the existence of putative pause-transfer sequences (PTS) in apoB, which were proposed to interrupt translocation but not translation.[74] Alternatively, the pauses during translocation were proposed to relate to secondary structure of the apoB mRNA, resulting in cotranslational insertion of apoB into the inner leaflet of the ER.[75] Another mechanism for the inefficient translocation was proposed by Liang and colleagues, who reported that translocation efficiency of apoB-100 is dependent on the presence of a β-sheet domain between 29% and 34% of full-length apoB-100, a region of apoB that has no PTS.[76] To examine the possibility that PTS elsewhere in the N-terminal region of apoB-100 may affect translocation efficiency, cell culture studies were performed in which the cells were transfected with human apoB chimeric cDNA constructs containing PTS with and without a β-sheet and vice versa.[77] The results demonstrated that only constructs coding for a β-sheet slowed translocation, resulting in increased proteinase K sensitivity, ubiquitinylation, and increased physical interaction with Sec61α, whereas the presence of PTS had no effect.[77] These results indicate that the translocation efficiency of apoB is determined mainly by the presence of β-sheet domains. In contrast, PTS do not appear to affect translocation but may affect secretion by other mechanisms. The requirement for a β-sheet provides a potential mechanism for the regulation of apoB translocation through lipid availability involving the participation of MTP.[72]

PROTEASOMAL AND NONPROTEASOMAL DEGRADATION OF APOLIPOPROTEIN B

Triglyceride synthesis and availability for VLDL synthesis is a major regulator of proteasomal degradation of apoB.[72,78] Furthermore, specific amino acid sequences within the beta-1 domain of human apoB (amino acid segments between the carboxyl termini of apoB-34 to apoB-42 and apoB-37 to apoB-42) have been reported to promote rapid proteasomal degradation.[79] A growing body of evidence supports the concept that a lack of cotranslational lipidation of apoB directs it into these pathways for degradation as a form of quality control, preventing the exit of misfolded proteins from the ER. Inhibitors of the proteasome such as *N*-acetyl-L-leucinyl-L-leucinyl-L-norleucinal (ALLN), lactacystin, and carbobenzoxyl-leucinyl-leucinyl-norvalinal-H (MG115) can inhibit apoB degradation.[80–82] Studies of the impact of MTP inhibition on synchronized translation of apoB in HepG2 cells supported cotranslational degradation of apoB on MTP inhibition, which could be prevented by treatment with inhibitors of the proteasome.[80] ApoB targeted for proteasomal degradation is ubiquinated; moreover, the process is ATP dependent[81] and involves the cytosolic chaperones heat shock proteins (Hsp) 70 and 90.[82–84] Following inhibition of apoB degradation by proteasome inhibitors, apoB accumulates in the ER, but this secretion-incompetent apoB[80] can be secreted if new lipid synthesis is stimulated.[82] The regulation of apoB by degradation in the cytosol via the ubiquitin–proteasome pathway represented a novel mechanism for regulation of secretion of a normal mammalian protein.

An established model for the route taken for ER-associated degradation of a number of proteins entails full translocation into the ER followed by retrotranslocation into the cytosol for degradation.[72] Huang and Shelness indicated that retrograde translocation of apoB from the ER lumen to the cytosol for degradation in the proteasome appeared to be required.[85] However, a number of other studies indicate that apoB undergoes rapid cotranslational targeting to proteasomal degradation while attached to the translocon and that binding to cytosolic chaperones facilitates its extraction from the translocon for degradation in the ubiquitin–proteasome pathway.[72] Hsp90 appears to act at a step distal to Hsp70.[83] The ligases known as E3s are known to facilitate the covalent binding of ubiquitin to target proteins. Liang and coworkers have implicated the tumor autocrine motility factor receptor Gp78 as the E3 ligase involved in ubiquitinylation and proteasomal degradation of apoB.[86] A network of molecular chaperones and ER proteins has been proposed to provide quality control for the nascent apoB-VLDL particles during transit to the Golgi complex. For example, apoB has been found to be associated with Grp94, Grp78, Erp72, calreticulin, and cyclophilinB in the ER lumen and in the Golgi complex, but the chaperone-to-apoB ratio was lower in the Golgi complex. Calnexin[87] has been implicated in protecting apoB from ubiquitinylation and subsequent proteasomal degradation.[88] A proteomics approach was used to identify 99 unique proteins that were chemically cross-linked to apoB in rat liver microsomes[89]; two of the proteins identified, ferritin heavy and light chains, were shown to bind directly to apoB. Subsequent studies showed that ferritins block apoB secretion and increase ER-associated protein degradation of apoB.[90] Thus, a growing list of proteins, some previously not known to function as chaperones, have been implicated in providing quality control and facilitating the transit of apoB-VLDL particles through the secretory pathway. Interestingly, recent studies show that cotranslational degradation of proteins protects the stressed ER from protein overload.[91]

Nonproteasomal degradation of apoB has also been described but remains less well characterized than the proteasomal pathway for degradation of apoB. For example, proteasomal inhibitors do not affect apoB degradation induced by omega-3 fatty acids or insulin.[72] Omega-3 fatty acids can inhibit apoB secretion and increase apoB degradation through a nonproteasomal post-ER presecretory proteolysis pathway.[92] Treatment of hepatocytes with the iron chelator desferrioxamine, an inhibitor of iron-dependent lipid peroxidation, or vitamin E, a lipid antioxidant, reversed the omega-3–induced degradation of apoB and restored VLDL secretion, supporting a novel link between lipid peroxidation and oxidant stress with apoB-100 degradation via post-ER presecretory proteolysis.[93] Dexamethasone and choline deficiency induce degradation of apoB through nonproteasomal pathways,[72] and MTP inhibition has been reported to induce degradation of apoB through both proteasomal and nonproteasomal pathways.[94] Deficiency of phospholipid transfer protein in hepatocytes has recently been reported to decrease liver vitamin E content, increase hepatic oxidant tone, and substantially enhance reactive oxygen species (ROS)-dependent destruction of newly synthesized apoB via a post-ER process.[95] Interestingly, the LDLR has also been implicated in presecretory degradation of apoB, which is initiated in the ER and depends on the ability of the receptor to bind to apoB.[96] The ER protein ER-60, which has both proteolytic and chaperone activities, associates with apoB and has been implicated in intra-ER–mediated nonproteasomal degradation of apoB, which is inhibitable by a thiol protease inhibitor.[97] In a hamster model of insulin resistance, increased VLDL production correlates with decreased ER-60 protein, suggesting a possible mechanism for insulin resistance–induced overproduction of VLDL resulting from reduced ER-60 protein–mediated degradation of apoB.

ASSEMBLY OF APOLIPOPROTEIN B–CONTAINING LIPOPROTEINS

The assembly and secretion of VLDL by hepatocytes is a multistep process requiring apoB, MTP, and an adequate supply of lipids. The molecular mechanisms for VLDL assembly and subcellular localization for the addition of lipid remain an active area of research. As described earlier, the availability of triglyceride (and other lipids) during the synthesis of apoB-100 on the rough ER is a critical regulator of VLDL assembly. As the apoB-100 is translated, lipid is added in a process that requires MTP. The availability of adequate lipid prevents the cotranslational degradation of apoB-100. Olofsson and Boren describe the assembly of three basic particles: (1) pre-VLDL, a primordial lipoprotein that is not secreted; and (2) VLDL2, a triglyceride-poor form of VLDL that can be secreted or further lipidated to form (3) VLDL1, which is triglyceride rich.[98] Although there is evidence suggesting that triglyceride-rich particles could be formed while apoB is still attached to the translocon,[99] there is also evidence that triglyceride-poor apoB-containing lipoproteins are converted into triglyceride-rich VLDLs by rapid addition of lipid droplets in the smooth ER in what has been termed the "second step" of VLDL assembly.[100] The stimulation of triglyceride synthesis by supplementation of cells with oleic acid promotes this second step with addition of bulk lipid to form larger VLDL particles.[101] The activation of phospholipase D by ADP-ribosylation factor 1 appears to be important for formation of phosphotidylcholine, which is needed for VLDL assembly in the ER.[102] A number of studies have demonstrated that MTP is required for the early events of VLDL assembly to provide the lipid required to protect apoB from degradation[103,104]; however, *de novo* lipid synthesis and MTP are apparently not required during the later stages of VLDL assembly.[104,105] The exact subcellular location for formation of mature VLDL particles remains somewhat controversial, with some evidence supporting the formation of secretion-competent VLDL in the ER[106] but mounting evidence supports further lipidation of apoB-containing lipoproteins in post-ER compartments, including the Golgi complex, independent of MTP activity.[107–110] It seems likely that both these views may be relevant, with metabolic conditions dictating whether the triglyceride-poor VLDL is secreted directly or further lipidated to form VLDL1 in post-ER compartments.[98] The assembly process is stylized in Figure 2-1.

ApoB-containing lipoproteins have diameters as large as 200 nm in the liver and up to 1000 nm in the intestine, yet classic transport vesicles range in size from 50 to 80 nm, raising the question as to whether apoB-containing lipoproteins use the same transport system as the majority of secretory proteins or require a unique system for trafficking to the cell surface.[68] The formation of vesicles at the ER exit site depends on a GTPase known as Sar1 and a coat protein known as coatamer protein II (COPII).[98] The assembly of vesicles for ER-to-Golgi transport begins with the coating of specific areas of the ER membrane with Sar1-GTP and the Sec23/24 heterodimer.[111] Fisher and coworkers developed a cell-free system using hepatic membranes and cytosol from rat hepatoma cells to examine the exit of apoB-containing lipoproteins from the ER.[112] Using the cell-free system to reconstitute ER budding, the apoB-containing vesicles were found to contain Sec23 but to sediment at a density distinct from that of vesicles containing more typical cargo. Budding of apoB-containing vesicles required Sar1 and was inhibited by dominant negative Sar1. Treatment of rat hepatoma cells with oleic acid, which stimulates the second step of particle maturation by the addition of more lipid, did not increase the size of the apoB-containing particles in the ER or COPII-coated vesicles but did increase the size of lipoprotein particles isolated from the Golgi complex. The authors concluded that apoB exits the ER in COPII-coated vesicles but that final lipid loading occurs in a post-ER compartment.[112] In contrast, studies by Siddiqi and colleagues reported that in a cell-free system based on rat intestinal epithelial cells, COPII proteins are not required for ER budding of apoB-containing lipoproteins into prechylomicron transport vesicles but COPII proteins are required for fusion of these prechylomicron transport vesicles with the Golgi complex.[113] These studies suggest that COPII proteins are critical for the post-ER transport of apoB-containing lipoproteins in both the liver and the intestine, but the processes have distinct features that may contribute to the differences in the composition of VLDL and chylomicrons. Interestingly, Sar1b is defective in chylomicron retention disease and Anderson disease, rare recessive disorders associated with severe fat malabsorption and selective retention of chylomicron-like particles within membrane-bound compartments in the intestine.[111] Further elucidation of the roles of COPII proteins in the transport of VLDL- and chylomicron-containing vesicles may reveal new targets for drug development.

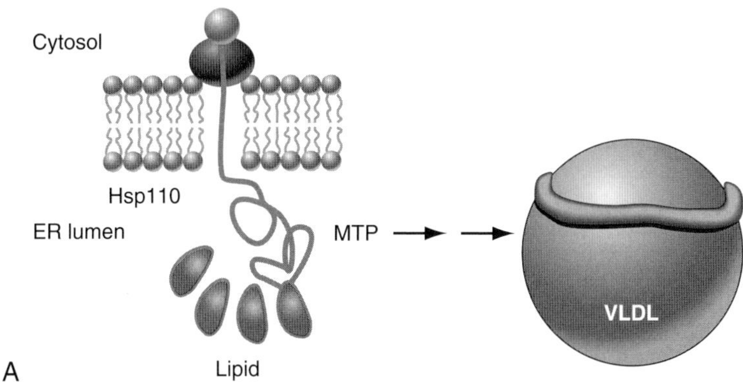

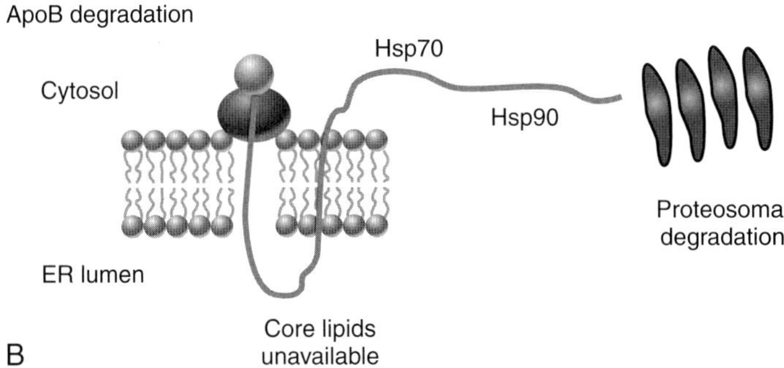

FIGURE 2-1 Lipoprotein assembly and regulation in hepatocytes. *A,* The forming apolipoprotein B (apoB-100) molecule is cotranslationally translocated, with the help of molecular chaperone heat shock protein 110 (Hsp), into the endoplasmic reticular (ER) lumen, where it gets lipidated via action of microsomal triglyceride transfer protein (MTP) to form mature very-low-density lipoprotein (VLDL). *B,* Fatty acid content of the hepatocyte influences apoB-100 degradation rates. When core lipids are not available, the carboxyl-terminal section of apoB is retranslocated to the cytosol and directed to proteasomal sites via Hsp70 and Hsp90.

PLASMA METABOLISM OF APOLIPOPROTEIN B-CONTAINING LIPOPROTEINS

The classical view of the metabolism of apoB-containing lipoproteins involves several steps that have been thoroughly investigated in humans and in experimental systems over the past 40 years.[1,98] The first step involves the secretion of mature VLDL from the liver cell in an extracellular environment that is rich in proteoglycans and receptors with high affinity for the lipoprotein. This could quickly lead to recapture of the secreted particle in a futile cycle, thereby causing hepatic steatosis. However, nature has created obstacles to the recapture of these particles in the unstirred water layer of the hepatic sinusoid. These obstacles include (1) conformational inability of the main ligand for lipoprotein trapping and uptake, apoE, to engage its receptors because of the fact that both the heparin-binding domain and the receptor-binding domain are buried in the lipid curvature; (2) enrichment of the nascent lipoprotein with apoC-III, a natural inhibitor of lipoprotein lipase (LPL); and (3) very low concentrations of LPL in the hepatic capillaries. Because of this multiple regulation system, the VLDL can exit the space of Disse and enter the circulation without significant reuptake by the hepatocyte. A similar process is at play in the intestine for the secretion of apoB-48–containing chylomicrons. Figures 2-2 and 2-3 provide a simplified schematic representation of the metabolism of triglyceride-rich lipoproteins.

The enzymes involved in the hydrolysis of plasma lipoproteins include LPL, hepatic lipase (HL), and the more recently identified endothelial lipase (EL).[114–116] LPL is bound to proteoglycans on the capillary endothelium of skeletal muscle and adipose tissue. The interaction between LPL and apoB-containing lipoproteins is significantly influenced by apoE, which has a role in slowing down the lipoprotein on the capillary bed by interacting with the proteoglycan glycocalix of the endothelial cell.[117] This hypothesis is in agreement with the observation that individuals with dysfunctional apoE or with genetic deficiency in apoE accumulate an abnormal lipoprotein, named β-VLDL, which is the result of the inability of the VLDL to interact properly with LPL in the absence of apoE.[118] The β-VLDL is also very enriched in cholesterol, suggesting that the loss of cholesterol from apoB-containing lipoproteins is also linked to an apoE–LPL interaction because the VLDL that accumulate under conditions of exclusive LPL deficiency (i.e., normal apoE levels) are not cholesterol enriched.[119] After substantial triglyceride loss induced by the interaction with LPL, the apoB-containing lipoprotein, now a remnant particle, gradually acquires the ability of being recognized by internalizing receptors in the liver and therefore can leave the plasma compartment. It is important to keep in mind that the objective of plasma lipoproteins is to redistribute triglycerides from the liver and the intestine to sites of accumulation (adipose tissue) or use (skeletal muscle) and to quickly disappear afterward to avoid unwanted accumulations in tissues such as the skin or the artery wall. It is widely believed that before the remnant lipoproteins become capable of engaging hepatic receptors such as the LDLR or the LRP1, further hydrolysis from HL is necessary.[120] HL is present only in the capillary endothelium in the liver and is responsible for hydrolysis of triglycerides and phospholipids from the remnant lipoprotein to create a particle

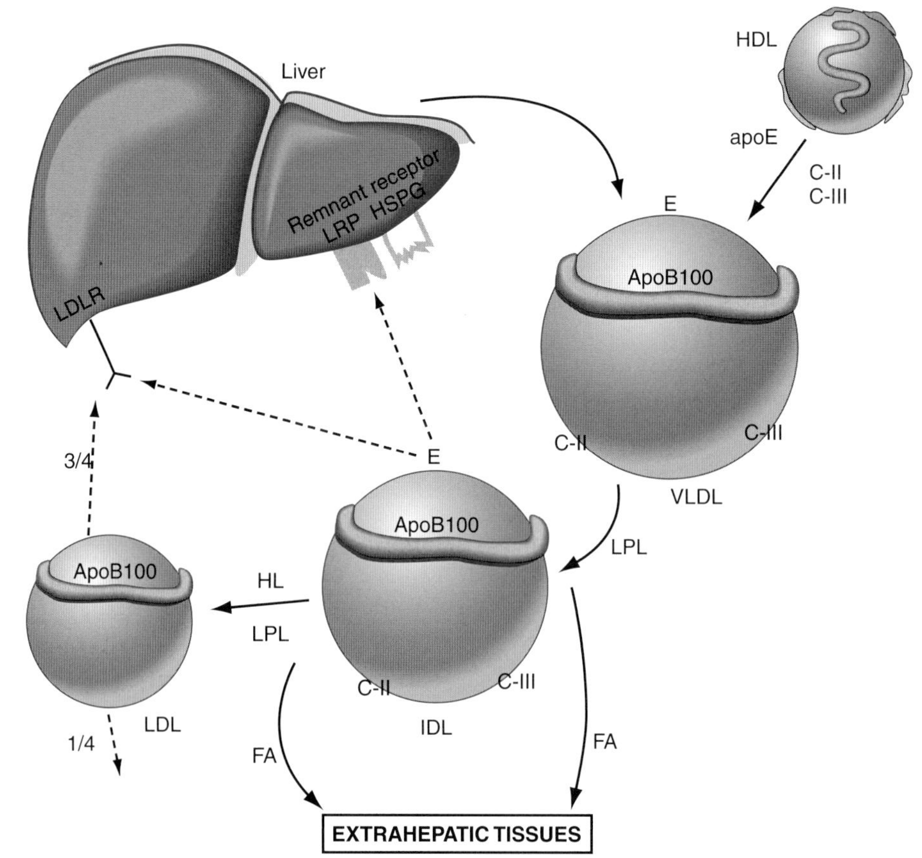

FIGURE 2-2 Metabolism of very-low-density lipoprotein (VLDL). Nascent VLDLs are lipolyzed by lipoprotein lipase (LPL) and expose critical amounts of apolipoprotein E (apoE) on their surface. This intermediate-density lipoprotein (IDL) particle can be cleared by the liver via receptor-mediated mechanisms or continue to be remodeled by LPL and by hepatic lipase (HL) to eventually produce low-density lipoprotein (LDL), an apoE-free, triglyceride (TG)-poor particle containing only apoB-100 and a load of cholesteryl esters (CEs). Interaction of the VLDL with the high-density lipoprotein (HDL) particle leads to exchange of protein (apoE and apoCs from HDL to VLDL) and lipids (CE from HDL to VLDL; TG from VLDL to HDL). HSPG, Heparan sulfate proteoglycans; LDLR, low-density lipoprotein receptor; LRP, LDLR related protein.

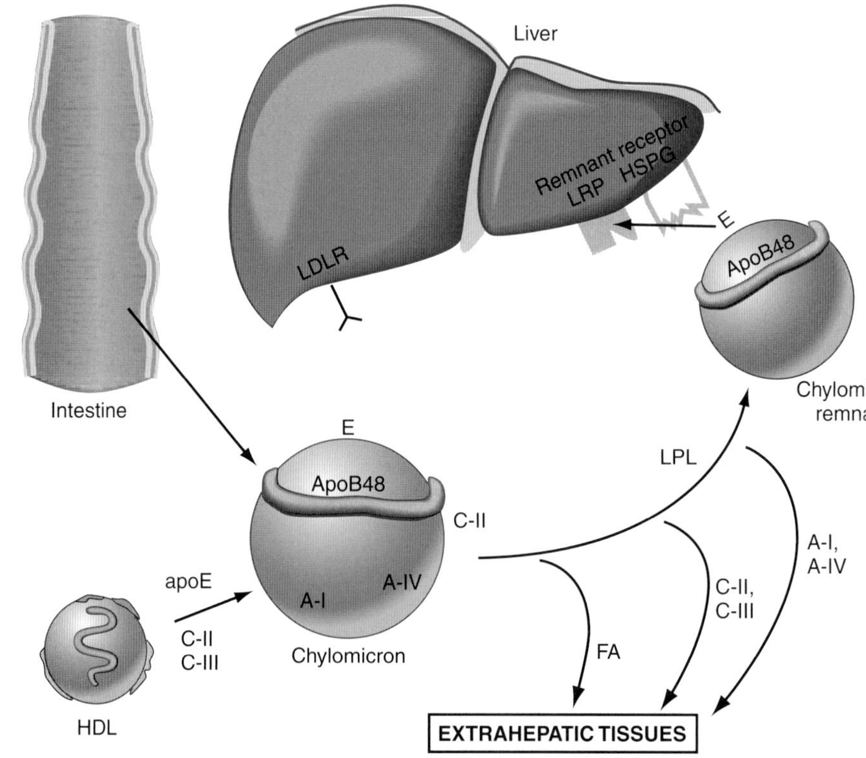

FIGURE 2-3 Metabolism of intestinal chylomicrons (CM). Production of CM starts at time of absorption of a fatty meal. Like very-low-density lipoproteins (VLDLs), CM are hydrolyzed by lipoprotein lipase (LPL) and can exchange protein and lipid material with the high-density lipoprotein (HDL). Unlike VLDL, the intermediate particle (CM remnant) will not result in the production of low-density lipoprotein (LDL) and is cleared efficiently from the liver. apo, Apolipoprotein; FA, fatty acid; LDLR, low-density lipoprotein receptor; HSPG, heparan sulfate proteoglycans; LRP, LDLR related protein.

with functional exposure of the receptor-binding domain of apoE; it therefore triggers an active uptake process by the liver and its removal from the circulation. This process is completely efficient for the remnants of apoB-48–containing lipoproteins, which in normal individuals do not contribute at all to the formation of plasma LDL. However, after HL-mediated hydrolysis, the remnants of apoB-100 lipoproteins either get promptly internalized by the liver or somehow dispose of the apoE on their surface and become LDL, the final leftover of the catabolism of VLDL. There is an obvious importance to studies directed at understanding the mechanisms by which the VLDL remnants lead to the production of LDL whereas chylomicron remnants do not. Interventions aimed at modifying catabolism of VLDL to mimic that of chylomicrons will result in reduction of plasma LDL by mechanisms complementary to that of the statins, and without loss of the essential physiologic functions (e.g., triglyceride redistribution and transport of carotenoids) of its precursor, VLDL. By consensus, the classical LDL is seen as an apoB-100–containing lipoprotein that has no apoE or other apolipoproteins, is devoid of triglycerides, and is enriched in cholesteryl esters. The only avenue for clearance from the circulation for LDL is an interaction between apoB-100 and the LDLR. ApoB-100 does not bind to LRP1 or to proteoglycans, and the interaction between apoB-100 and LDLR is about 20 times less efficient than the interaction between apoE and the same receptor.[121] In addition, one should mention that there is only one apoB-100 molecule per LDL particle, whereas there are several apoE molecules on the surface of remnant lipoproteins. The final lipase, EL, has been recently discovered as an enzyme that hydrolyzes mostly phospholipids and, to a lesser extent, triglycerides, and has an influence on HDL metabolism more than on apoB-containing lipoproteins.[122–124] The absence of EL increases HDL cholesterol by 50% in engineered mice, and inhibition of EL similarly leads to elevated levels of plasma HDL cholesterol.[125] There is evidence that EL modulates HDL cholesterol levels in human populations as well.[126] EL levels have been found to be increased in people with the metabolic syndrome and high risk of cardiovascular disease.[127] Apparently, EL is also induced by inflammation, and therefore its inhibition may be considered a target of therapy.[124] Even though the main effect of EL is thought to be on HDL metabolism, evidence has been presented on reduced levels of apoB-containing lipoproteins by expression of EL in several mouse models of dyslipidemia.[116] If observed under conditions of enzyme inhibition, this effect would reduce the interest in EL as a possible modulator of HDL cholesterol levels because increased concentrations of both HDL and apoB-containing lipoproteins are not a desirable target.

Processing of Remnant Lipoproteins

The interaction between lipoproteins and LPL has been simplistically visualized as a process whereby LPL sticks its lipophilic head into the lipoprotein particle and chews up fatty acids from core triglycerides. However, for this to occur, several mechanisms must be at play in a coordinated fashion, including the ability of the lipoprotein particle to adhere to the endothelial surface, slow down in the capillary flow and reach a halt to engage the enzyme, and then disengage after partial lipolysis. In addition, one must remember that LPL is not a transmembrane protein, so it is likely to detach from the endothelial surface after connecting with large floating particles such as the apoB-containing lipoproteins. Therefore, it is commonly understood that the system of intravascular lipoprotein hydrolysis must be significantly more complex than the model currently accepted. Several proteins, yet to be identified, might intervene in functions such as providing a platform for LPL stabilization, allowing the particle to stick to the endothelium, and maximizing the lipoprotein responsiveness to LPL action. One of these factors, as discussed earlier, is apoE. Without it, the VLDL does not undergo normal lipolysis by LPL *in vitro*, confirming the *in vivo* data that patients with dysfunctional apoE variants have inappropriate VLDL processing. Other factors include apoC-III, an inhibitor of lipolysis, and apoC-II, an LPL cofactor essential for proper lipolysis.[128] Patients with genetic deficiency of apoC-II develop a chilomicronemia syndrome similar to that of subjects homozygous for LPL deficiency.[129]

Recently discovered novel proteins have a major role in regulation of LPL activity. ApoA-V was identified as a cause for severe hypertriglyceridemia in genetically deficient mice[130] and was subsequently validated in human populations as a major modulator of triglyceride levels in plasma.[131] The fact that apoC-II–deficient subjects have massive hypertriglyceridemia despite normal expression of apoA-V (and, conversely, that apoA-V–null mice have high triglycerides with normal apoC-II levels) suggests that these two cofactors might cooperate to induce maximal LPL functionality. More recently, a protein termed glycosyl-phosphadityl-inositol-anchored, HDL-binding protein–1 (GPIHBP-1) has also been linked to triglyceride regulation.[132] Mice with the genetic deficiency of this protein develop massive hypertriglyceridemia (triglycerides >5000 mg/dL on a low-fat diet) despite normal LPL levels and normal LPL activity *in vitro*.[133] It has been proposed that GPIHBP-1 serves as a platform to stabilize LPL by binding to both LPL and chylomicrons and that it may interact with apoA-V. Moreover, a significant role for angiopoietin-like proteins 3 and 4 (angptl3 and angptl4) in lipid metabolism is currently being uncovered.[134,135] Angptl4 (fasting-induced adypocyte factor) represents the tool with which fat regulates plasma lipid metabolism, is widely expressed in the body, and is under liver X receptor (LXR) control.[136] Angptl3 is exclusively made in the liver, is less sensitive to fasting, and is under panperoxisome proliferator-activated receptor regulation.[137] The main effect of these factors on plasma lipids is mediated by the inhibition of both LPL (causing elevated triglyceride levels) and EL (causing elevated HDL cholesterol levels). It is certainly reassuring for the future of lipoprotein studies to see that an area of metabolism that had been crystallized for years in a simplified but sufficiently logical paradigm is now exposed to such turbulent growth to cause a redrawing of the basic mechanisms of LPL–VLDL interaction. Figure 2-4 provides an attempt at encompassing established and novel views of the interaction between VLDL and endothelial cell for the harmonized and regulated extraction of circulating fatty acid.

Hepatic Uptake of Remnants of Apolipoprotein B-Containing Lipoproteins

The final stages of the intravascular fate of remnant lipoproteins involve trapping in the hepatic sinusoid, binding to internalizing receptors, and removal from the circulation through cellular uptake and degradation. The trapping of remnants in the liver is a very efficient and high-capacity mechanism, a fact that

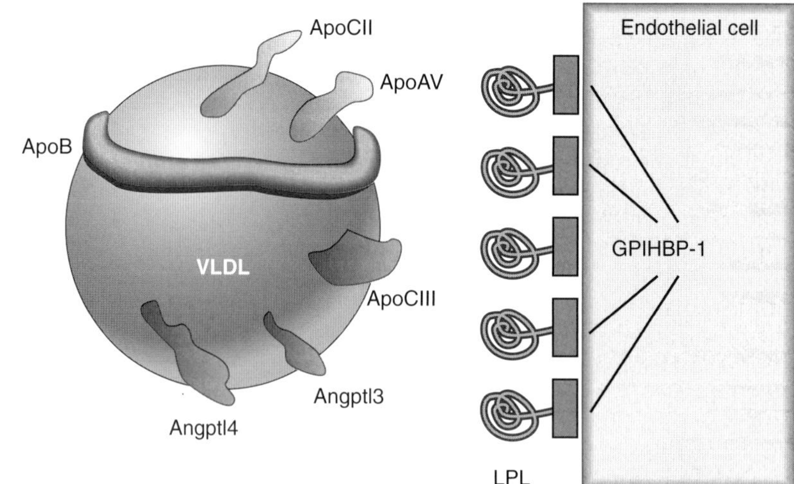

FIGURE 2-4 Novel view of the interaction between very-low-density lipoprotein (VLDL) and lipoprotein lipase (LPL) on the endothelial cell surface. LPL uses glycosyl-phosphadityl-inositol-anchored, HDL-binding protein (GPIHBP-1) as platform for function. The VLDL uses multiple surface proteins with activating and inhibitory functions to regulate rate of release of fatty acid to peripheral tissues. Apolipoprotein (apo)C-II and apoA-V are activators of lipolysis, whereas apoCIII and angptl3 and angptl4 inhibit it. Angptl4 represents a key tool for adipocytes to influence plasma triglyceride release.

explains the very fast disappearance from plasma of injected remnant lipoproteins in turnover studies. However, lipoproteins may quickly engorge the hepatic sinusoid and spill back into the circulation if trapping is not followed by active processing and uptake. This processing is normally seen as the intervention of HL on the remaining triglyceride content of the remnant, with exposure of the apoE epitopes responsible for binding to heparan sulfate proteoglycans and to receptors such as the LDLR and LRP1. In *in vitro* experiments, remnant lipoproteins bind more efficiently to the LDLR than to proteoglycans or LRP1, and therefore it is believed that under physiologic conditions, remnant clearance is regulated by this receptor.[138] However, it must not be forgotten that patients with FH, who carry genetic defects in their LDLR, show slow clearance of LDL but normal triglyceride metabolism.[139] The same has been seen in rabbit and mouse models of this human disease.[140,141] Thus, the idea of a remnant receptor has been pursued relentlessly until the discovery of LRP1, recognized by most today as a receptor contributing to the hepatic uptake of remnants under physiologic and pathologic conditions. Without LRP1 in the liver, normal mice show only minimal dyslipidemia, whereas LDLR-deficient mice develop severe chylomicronemia.[142,143] This provides support for the notion that the LDLR is capable of clearing the incoming remnants under conditions of normal load, with LRP1 acting as backup or support system when the LDLR is dysfunctional or at times of lipoprotein overload in the hepatic sinusoid (postprandial periods). What was difficult to figure out was why in *in vitro* settings, LRP1 seemed to bind with low efficiency to remnant lipoproteins, even though these particles are highly enriched in apoE (a strong ligand for LRP). Even more surprisingly, highly efficient binding was induced by the addition of extra apoE to the particle. This at first was dismissed as a sign of a possibly artifactual relationship between remnants and LRP1 but later gave rise to a fundamental discovery in lipoprotein metabolism, that of the "secretion-capture" model of remnant uptake by the liver. This model proposes the secretion of large amounts of lipid-free apoE by the hepatocyte into the sinusoid, in a "fishing net" strategy to increase the apoE concentration of incoming particles and then drag them into the cell via LRP1-mediated entry.[144] We provided final evidence of the existence of this pathway by using a bone marrow transplantation approach in mice. This method allowed us to use apoE-deficient mice and replace their hematopoietic cells with those of wild-type donors. The resulting donor macrophages were able to secrete apoE in the plasma and induce complete apoE-mediated clearance of lipoproteins and normalization of the lipid profile.[145] However, when the same experiment was repeated in apoE-negative mice also missing the LDLR, the apoE secreted by donor macrophages accumulated in high concentrations in the plasma of recipient mice but did not affect lipoprotein clearance,[146] thus suggesting that the normal clearance of apoE-containing lipoproteins in the absence of LDLR is the result of an effect attributable to the hepatic apoE involved in the secretion-capture strategy. This phenomenon can be explained either as the consequence of the hepatic sinusoid providing a tremendous additional amount of apoE to the lipoprotein so that it can engage LRP1 or as the result of a particular conformation or localization of locally produced apoE. On the contrary, the fact that the natural amount of apoE carried by the plasma lipoprotein is sufficient to activate LDLR-mediated uptake suggests that the "secretion-capture" mechanism in the liver is an alternative mode of lipoprotein uptake, in place to attenuate the consequences of genetic or environmental LDLR dysfunction. Our view of remnant uptake, under physiologic conditions, includes a major role for the LDLR and a fluctuating role for LRP1, ranging from minor (conditions of low secretion of hepatic lipid-free apoE) to prominent (conditions of high secretion of hepatic lipid-free apoE). A typical condition of low lipid-free apoE secretion occurs when the hepatocyte is actively making lipoproteins and incorporating apoE into newly assembled particles (fasting state).[147] A typical condition of high lipid-free apoE secretion occurs when the hepatocyte is idle and most apoE is routed to the secretory pathway unassociated with lipoproteins (postprandial state).[148] Insulin signaling may be involved in modulating the lipogenic state of the liver cell and regulating the receptor type most involved in remnant uptake.[68]

Because apoE modulates cellular lipid metabolism and is involved in both the assembly and secretion of VLDL as well as in the modulation of cholesterol efflux from macrophages, we studied the possibility that internalized apoE escapes lysosomal degradation and is recycled through the secretory pathway. We, and others, proceeded to establish that a significant portion (up to 60%) of apoE internalized on triglyceride-rich lipoproteins is spared degradation and is in fact recycled.[149,150] We also reported that apoE is secreted by hepatocyte cultures from apoE−/− mice transplanted with wild-type bone marrow, an obvious proof that systemic apoE is retained by the liver cell and is then resecreted.[151] Even though studies are still in progress to determine the physiologic role of this phenomenon, it is plausible that apoE recycling may be capable of augmenting the secretion-capture process by diverting to the "fishing net" the apoE ligand destined for lysosomal degradation. It is also possible that recycling apoE may serve as a sensor to gauge the rate of entry of remnant lipoproteins into the hepatocyte and inform the secretory machinery to activate corresponding rates of VLDL assembly and secretion in an effort to avoid accumulation of lipid droplets in the cell and progression toward the development of fatty liver.[152]

Finally, it has recently been proposed that heparan sulfate proteoglycans may act directly as receptors for the uptake of remnant lipoproteins. In mice engineered for the deficiency of Ndst1, the biosynthesis of heparan sulfate was reduced by 50% and the animals showed significant accumulation of cholesterol and triglycerides. Interestingly, this effect was diminished when the Ndst1 deficiency was compounded with LDLR deficiency.[153] It is possible, however, that the heparan sulfate proteoglycans are essential in docking the remnant for further processing and delivery to the internalizing receptors without being responsible directly for lipoprotein entry into the cell. Presentation of a lipoprotein to its receptor is of crucial importance, as demonstrated recently in animals lacking ARH, an adaptor protein that controls the proper positioning of the LDLR in the liver cell.[154] Hepatocytes from mice without ARH display a defect in LDL binding and uptake but show normal binding and internalization of VLDL.[155] These data suggest that the likely interaction of the VLDL with heparan sulfate proteoglycans produces a transfer of the ligand to its receptor even in a setting where the receptor has lost its ability to engage the LDL directly.[156]

EMERGING TARGETS FOR REDUCING PLASMA LEVELS OF APOLIPOPROTEIN B-CONTAINING LIPOPROTEINS

A promising area in terms of new approaches to lipid lowering is that of antisense oligonucleotide injections to target the mRNA of proteins involved in cholesterol metabolism. Although the weight of current evidence supports the view that apoB gene expression is constitutive and that regulation of VLDL secretion is achieved primarily through cotranslational and post-translational degradation, apoB gene expression remains an active target for therapeutic intervention, as evidenced by the current efforts to develop antisense to apoB mRNA as an approach to lower LDL cholesterol.[19] The initial trial in humans involving the subcutaneous injection of a 20-mer antisense oligonucleotide to apoB resulted in a 50% reduction in plasma apoB levels and a 35% reduction in LDL cholesterol, with the most common adverse event being local erythema.[157] In contrast to early studies with MTP inhibitors,[158,159] apoB inhibition does not seem to lead to malabsorption of fat or development of fatty liver. The proprotein convertase subtilisin/kexin type 9 (PCSK9) is a member of a family of proteases that is thought to promote the degradation of the LDLR. A similar antisense oligonucleotide approach is being developed to target PCSK9, with a goal of lowering LDL cholesterol by increasing LDLR upregulation.[160] In a recent animal study, a PCSK9 antisense oligonucleotide was administered to mice fed a high-fat diet for 6 weeks and resulted in 53% and 38% reductions in total cholesterol and LDL cholesterol, respectively, along with a twofold increase in hepatic LDLR protein levels.[160] Efforts to clinically develop MTP inhibitors are still under way, as evidenced by the recent report demonstrating reductions in serum levels of LDL cholesterol and apoB by 50.9% and 55.6%, respectively, in patients with homozygous FH.[161] However, treatment with the MTP inhibitor was associated with significant elevations in liver transaminases as well as the accumulation of fat in the liver, potentially limiting the safety and usefulness of the MTP inhibitor.[161] Interestingly, a recent study in mice has shown that inhibition of both MTP and liver fatty acid–binding protein is effective in lowering cholesterol without inducing fatty liver.[162] Hence a number of novel approaches for lowering apoB-containing lipoproteins are being actively pursued.

Acknowledgments

The authors are supported by grants from the NIH (HL 57986 and HL 65709 to S.F. and HL 65405 to M.L.).

REFERENCES

1. Young SG: Recent progress in understanding apolipoprotein B. *Circulation* 1990;82:1574–1594.
2. Kane JP, Havel RJ: Disorders of the biogenesis and secretion of lipoproteins containing the B apolipoproteins. In Scriver CR, Beaudet AL, Sly WS, Valle D (eds): The Metabolic Basis of Inherited Disease, 6th Ed. New York, McGraw-Hill, 1989.
3. Kane JP, Hardman DA, Paulus HE: Heterogeneity of apolipoprotein B: isolation of a new species from human chylomicrons. *Proc Natl Acad Sci USA* 1980;77:2465–2469.
4. Sniderman AD, Marcovina SM: Apolipoprotein A1 and B. *Clin Lab Med* 2006;26:733–750.
5. Walldius G, Jungner I: The apoB/apoA-I ratio: a strong, new risk factor for cardiovascular disease and a target for lipid-lowering therapy—a review of the evidence. *J Intern Med* 2006;259: 493–519.
6. Segrest JP, Jones MK, Mishra VK, et al: apoB-100 has a pentapartite structure composed of three amphipathic alpha-helical domains alternating with two amphipathic beta-strand domains. Detection by the computer program LOCATE. *Arterioscler Thromb.* 1994;14:1674–1685.
7. Baker ME: Is vitellogenin an ancestor of apolipoprotein B-100 of human low-density lipoprotein and human lipoprotein lipase? *Biochem J* 1988;255:1057–1060.
8. Shoulders CC, Narcisi TM, Read J, et al: The abetalipoproteinemia gene is a member of the vitellogenin family and encodes an alpha-helical domain. *Nat Struct Biol* 1994;1:285–286.

9. Segrest JP, Jones MK, Dashti N: N-terminal domain of apolipoprotein B has structural homology to lipovitellin and microsomal triglyceride transfer protein: a "lipid pocket" model for self-assembly of apob-containing lipoprotein particles. *J Lipid Res* 1999;40:1401–1416.
10. Shelness GS, Ledford AS: Evolution and mechanism of apolipoprotein B-containing lipoprotein assembly. *Curr Opin Lipidol* 2005;16:325–332.
11. Richardson PE, Manchekar M, Dashti N, et al: Assembly of lipoprotein particles containing apolipoprotein-B: structural model for the nascent lipoprotein particle. *Biophys J* 2005;88: 2789–2800.
12. Blackhart BD, Ludwig EM, Pierotti VR, et al: Structure of the human apolipoprotein B gene. *J Biol Chem* 1986;261: 15364–15367.
13. Linton MF, Farese RV, Chiesa G, et al: Transgenic mice expressing high plasma concentrations of human apolipoprotein B100 and lipoprotein (a). *J Clin Invest* 1993;92:3029–3037.
14. Nielsen LB, Kahn D, Duell T, et al: Apolipoprotein B gene expression in a series of human apolipoprotein B transgenic mice generated with recA-assisted restriction endonuclease cleavage-modified bacterial artificial chromosomes. An intestine-specific enhancer element is located between 54 and 62 kilobases 5′ to the structural gene. *J Biol Chem* 1998;273:21800–21807.
15. Antes TJ, Goodart SA, Huynh C, et al: Identification and characterization of a 315-base pair enhancer, located more than 55 kilobases 5′ of the apolipoprotein B gene, that confers expression in the intestine. *J Biol Chem* 2000;275:26637–26648.
16. Zannis VI, Kan HY, Kritis A, et al: Transcriptional regulatory mechanisms of the human apolipoprotein genes *in vitro* and *in vivo*. *Curr Opin Lipidol* 2001;12:181–207.
17. Neumeier M, Sigruener A, Eggenhofer E, et al: High molecular weight adiponectin reduces apolipoprotein B and E release in human hepatocytes. *Biochem Biophys Res Commun* 2007;352: 543–548.
18. Sparks JD, Collins HL, Chirieac DV, et al: Hepatic very-low-density lipoprotein and apolipoprotein B production are increased following *in vivo* induction of betaine-homocysteine S-methyltransferase. *Biochem J* 2006;395:363–371.
19. Crooke RM: Antisense oligonucleotides as therapeutics for hyperlipidaemias. *Expert Opin Biol Ther* 2005;5:907–917.
20. Chen S-H, Habib G, Yang C-Y, et al: Apolipoprotein B-48 is the product of a messenger RNA with an organ-specific in-frame stop codon. *Science* 1987;238:363–366.
21. Powell LM, Wallis SC, Pease RJ, et al: A novel form of tissue-specific RNA processing produces apolipoprotein-B48 in intestine. *Cell* 1987;50:831–840.
22. Anant S, Blanc V, Davidson NO: Molecular regulation, evolutionary, and functional adaptations associated with C to U editing of mammalian apolipoproteinB mRNA. *Prog Nucleic Acid Res Mol Biol* 2003;75:1–41.
23. Hirano K, Young SG, Farese RV Jr, et al: Targeted disruption of the mouse apobec-1 gene abolishes apolipoprotein B mRNA editing and eliminates apolipoprotein B48. *J Biol Chem* 1996;271: 9887–9890.
24. Nakamuta M, Chang BH, Zsigmond E, et al: Complete phenotypic characterization of apobec-1 knockout mice with a wild-type genetic background and a human apolipoprotein B transgenic background, and restoration of apolipoprotein B mRNA editing by somatic gene transfer of Apobec-1. *J Biol Chem* 1996;271:25981–25988.
25. Blanc V, Henderson JO, Newberry EP, et al: Targeted deletion of the murine apobec-1 complementation factor (acf) gene results in embryonic lethality. *Mol Cell Biol* 2005;25:7260–7269.
26. Chen Z, Eggerman TL, Patterson AP: ApoB mRNA editing is mediated by a coordinated modulation of multiple apoB mRNA editing enzyme components. *Am J Physiol Gastrointest Liver Physiol* 2007;292:G53–65.
27. Farese RV, Veniant MM, Cham CM, et al: Phenotypic analysis of mice expressing exclusively apolipoprotein B48 or apolipoprotein B100. *Proc Natl Acad Sci USA* 1996;93:6393–6398.
28. Veniant MM, Pierotti V, Newland D, et al: Susceptibility to atherosclerosis in mice expressing exclusively apolipoprotein B48 or apolipoprotein B100. *J Clin Invest* 1997;100:180–188.
29. Yu Q, Chen D, Konig R, et al: APOBEC3B and APOBEC3C are potent inhibitors of simian immunodeficiency virus replication. *J Biol Chem* 2004;279:53379–53386.
30. Vega GL, Grundy SM: *In vivo* evidence for reduced binding of low-density lipoproteins to receptors as a cause of primary moderate hypercholesterolemia. *J Clin Invest* 1986;78:1410–1414.
31. Innerarity TL, Weisgraber KH, Arnold KS, et al: Familial defective apolipoprotein B-100: low-density lipoproteins with abnormal receptor binding. *Proc Natl Acad Sci USA* 1987;84:6919–6923.
32. Soria LF, Ludwig EH, Clarke HRG, et al: Association between a specific apolipoprotein B mutation and familial defective apolipoprotein B-100. *Proc Natl Acad Sci USA* 1989;86:587–591.
33. Rader DJ, Cohen J, Hobbs HH: Monogenic hypercholesterolemia: new insights in pathogenesis and treatment. J Clin Invest 2003;111:1795–1803.
34. Myant NB, Forbes SA, Day IN, Gallagher J: Estimation of the age of the ancestral arginine3500→glutamine mutation in human apoB-100. *Genomics* 1997;45:78–87.
35. Myant NB: Familial defective apolipoprotein B-100: a review, including some comparisons with familial hypercholesterolaemia.[Erratum appears in Atherosclerosis 1994 105(2):253.] *Atherosclerosis* 1993;104:1–18.
36. Schaefer JR, Scharnagl H, Baumstark MW, et al: Homozygous familial defective apolipoprotein B-100. Enhanced removal of apolipoprotein E-containing VLDLs and decreased production of LDLs. *Arterioscler Thromb Vasc Biol* 1997;17:348–353.
37. Linton MF, Farese RV Jr, Young SG: Familial hypobetalipoproteinemia. *J Lipid Res* 1993;34:521–541.
38. Young SG, Bertics SJ, Curtiss LK, Witztum JL: Characterization of an abnormal species of apolipoprotein B, apolipoprotein B-37, associated with familial hypobetalipoproteinemia. *J Clin Invest* 1987;79:1831–1841.
39. Young SG, Bertics SJ, Curtiss LK, et al: Genetic analysis of a kindred with familial hypobetalipoproteinemia. Evidence for two separate gene defects: one associated with an abnormal apolipoprotein B species, apolipoprotein B-37; and a second associated with low plasma concentrations of apolipoprotein B-100. *J Clin Invest* 1987;79:1842–1851.
40. Young SG, Northey ST, McCarthy BJ: Low plasma cholesterol levels caused by a short deletion in the apolipoprotein B gene. *Science* 1988;241:591–593.
41. Linton MF, Pierotti V, Young SG: Reading-frame restoration with an apolipoprotein B gene frameshift mutation. *Proc Natl Acad Sci USA* 1992;89:11431–11435.
42. Wetterau JR, Aggerbeck LP, Bouma M-E, et al: Absence of microsomal triglyceride transfer protein in individuals with abetalipoproteinemia. *Science* 1992;258:999–1001.
43. Ross RS, Gregg RE, Law SW, et al: Homozygous hypobetalipoproteinemia: a disease distinct from abetalipoproteinemia at the molecular level. *J Clin Invest* 1988;81:590–595.
44. Scanu AM, Aggerbeck LP, Kruski AW, et al: A study of the abnormal lipoproteins in abetalipoproteinemia. *J Clin Invest* 1974;53:440–453.
45. Kayden HJ: The genetic basis of vitamin E deficiency in humans. *Nutrition* 2001;17:797–798.
46. Malloy MJ, Kane JP, Hardman DA, et al: Normotriglyceridemic abetalipoproteinemia. Absence of the B-100 apolipoprotein. *J Clin Invest* 1981;67:1441–1450.
47. Yao Z, Blackhart BD, Linton MF, et al: Expression of carboxyl-terminally truncated forms of human apolipoprotein B in rat hepatoma cells. Evidence that the length of apolipoprotein B has a major effect on the buoyant density of the secreted lipoproteins. *J Biol Chem* 1991;266:3300–3308.
48. Chiesa G, Johnson DF, Yao Z, et al: Expression of human apolipoprotein B100 in transgenic mice. Editing of human apolipoprotein B100 mRNA. *J Biol Chem* 1993;268:23747–23750.
49. Nielsen LB, McCormick SP, Pierotti V, et al: Human apolipoprotein B transgenic mice generated with 207- and 145-kilobase pair bacterial artificial chromosomes. Evidence that a distant 5′-element confers appropriate transgene expression in the intestine. *J Biol Chem* 1997;272:29752–29758.
50. McCormick SP, Ng JK, Veniant M, et al: Transgenic mice that overexpress mouse apolipoprotein B. Evidence that the DNA sequences controlling intestinal expression of the apolipoprotein B gene are distant from the structural gene. *J Biol Chem* 1996;271:11963–11970.
51. Nielsen LB, Veniant M, Boren J, et al: Genes for apolipoprotein B and microsomal triglyceride transfer protein are expressed in the heart: evidence that the heart has the capacity to synthesize and secrete lipoproteins. *Circulation* 1998;98:13–16.

52. Nielsen LB, Sullivan M, Vanni-Reyes T, et al: The DNA sequences required for apolipoprotein B expression in the heart are distinct from those required for expression in the intestine. *J MolCell Cardiol* 1999;31:695–703.
53. Boren J, Veniant MM, Young SG: Apo B100-containing lipoproteins are secreted by the heart. *J Clin Invest* 1998;101: 1197–1202.
54. Nielsen LB: Lipoprotein production by the heart: a novel pathway of triglyceride export from cardiomyocytes. *Scand J Clin Lab Invest (Suppl)* 2002;237:35–40.
55. Homanics GE, Smith TJ, Zhang SH, et al: Targeted modification of the apolipoprotein B gene results in hypobetalipoproteinemia and developmental abnormalities in mice. *Proc Natl Acad Sci USA* 1993;90:2389–2393.
56. Farese RV Jr, Ruland SL, Flynn LM, et al: Knockout of the mouse apolipoprotein B gene results in embryonic lethality in homozygotes and protection against diet-induced hypercholesterolemia in heterozygotes. *Proc Nat Acad Sci USA* 1995;92:1774–1778.
57. Huang LS, Voyiaziakis E, Markenson DF, et al: apo B gene knockout in mice results in embryonic lethality in homozygotes and neural tube defects, male infertility, and reduced HDL cholesterol ester and apo A-I transport rates in heterozygotes. *J Clin Invest* 1995;96:2152–2161.
58. Raabe M, Flynn LM, Zlot CH, et al: Knockout of the abetalipoproteinemia gene in mice: reduced lipoprotein secretion in heterozygotes and embryonic lethality in homozygotes. *Proc Nat Acad Sci USA* 1998;95:8686–8691.
59. Farese RV Jr, Cases S, Ruland SL, et al: A novel function for apolipoprotein B: lipoprotein synthesis in the yolk sac is critical for maternal-fetal lipid transport in mice. *J Lipid Res* 1996;37:347–360.
60. Terasawa Y, Cases SJ, Wong JS, et al: Apolipoprotein B-related gene expression and ultrastructural characteristics of lipoprotein secretion in mouse yolk sac during embryonic development. *J Lipid Res.* 1999;40:1967–1977.
61. Young SG, Cham CM, Pitas RE, et al: A genetic model for absent chylomicron formation: mice producing apolipoprotein B in the liver, but not in the intestine. *J Clin Invest* 1995;96:2932–2946.
62. Callow MJ, Rubin EM: Site-specific mutagenesis demonstrates that cysteine 4326 of apolipoprotein B is required for covalent linkage with apolipoprotein(a) *in vivo*. *J Biol Chem* 1995;270:23914–23917.
63. McCormick SP, Ng JK, Cham CM, et al: Transgenic mice expressing human ApoB95 and ApoB97. Evidence that sequences within the carboxyl-terminal portion of human apoB100 are important for the assembly of lipoprotein. *J Biol Chem* 1997;272:23616–23622.
64. Cheesman EJ, Sharp RJ, Zlot CH, et al: An analysis of the interaction between mouse apolipoprotein B100 and apolipoprotein(a). *J Biol Chem* 2000;275:28195–28200.
65. Sparks JD, Sparks CE: Insulin modulation of hepatic synthesis and secretion of apolipoprotein B by rat hepatocytes. *J Biol Chem* 1990;265:8854–8862.
66. Sparks JD, Zolfaghari R, Sparks CE, et al: Impaired hepatic apolipoprotein B and E translation in streptozotocin diabetic rats. *J ClinInvest* 1992;89:1418–1430.
67. Pan M, Liang JS, Fisher EA, Ginsberg HN: Inhibition of translocation of nascent apolipoprotein B across the endoplasmic reticulum membrane is associated with selective inhibition of the synthesis of apolipoprotein B. *J Biol Chem* 2000;275:27399–27405.
68. Avramoglu RK, Adeli K: Hepatic regulation of apolipoprotein B. *Rev Endocr Metabol Disord* 2004;5:293–301.
69. Pontrelli L, Sidiropoulos KG, Adeli K: Translational control of apolipoprotein B mRNA: regulation via cis elements in the 5′ and 3′ untranslated regions. *Biochemistry* 2004;43:6734–6744.
70. Boström K, Wettesten M, Borén J, et al: Pulse-chase studies of the synthesis and intracellular transport of apolipoprotein B-100 in Hep G2 cells. *J Biol Chem* 1986;261:13800–13806.
71. Borchardt RA, Davis RA: Intrahepatic assembly of very-low-density lipoproteins. Rate of transport out of the endoplasmic reticulum determines rate of secretion. *J Biol Chem* 1987;262:16394–16402.
72. Fisher EA, Ginsberg HN: Complexity in the secretory pathway: the assembly and secretion of apolipoprotein B-containing lipoproteins. *J Biol Chem* 2002;277:17377–17380.
73. Yao Z, Tran K, McLeod RS: Intracellular degradation of newly synthesized apolipoprotein B. *J Lipid Res* 1997;38:1937–1953.
74. Chuck SL, Yao Z, Blackhart BD, et al: New variation on the translocation of proteins during early biogenesis of apolipoprotein B. *Nature* 1990;346:382–385.
75. Pease RJ, Harrison GB, Scott J: Cotranslocational insertion of apolipoprotein B into the inner leaflet of the endoplasmic reticulum. *Nature* 1991;353:448–450.
76. Liang J, Wu X, Jiang H, et al:. Translocation efficiency, susceptibility to proteasomal degradation, and lipid responsiveness of apolipoprotein B are determined by the presence of beta sheet domains. *J Biol Chem* 1998;273:35216–35221.
77. Yamaguchi J, Conlon DM, Liang JJ, et al: Translocation efficiency of apolipoprotein B is determined by the presence of beta-sheet domains, not pause transfer sequences. *J Biol Chem* 2006;281:27063–27071.
78. Benoist F, Grand-Perret T: ApoB-100 secretion by HepG2 cells is regulated by the rate of triglyceride biosynthesis but not by intracellular lipid pools. *Arterioscler Thromb Vasc Biol* 1996;16:1229–1235.
79. Lapierre LR, Currie DL, Yao Z, et al: Amino acid sequences within the beta1 domain of human apolipoprotein B can mediate rapid intracellular degradation. *J Lipid Res* 2004;45:366–377.
80. Benoist F, Grand-Perret T: Co-translational degradation of apolipoprotein B100 by the proteasome is prevented by microsomal triglyceride transfer protein. Synchronized translation studies on HepG2 cells treated with an inhibitor of microsomal triglyceride transfer protein. *J Biol Chem* 1997;272:20435–20442.
81. Yeung SJ, Chen SH, Chan L: Ubiquitin-proteasome pathway mediates intracellular degradation of apolipoprotein B. *Biochemistry* 1996;35:13843–13848.
82. Fisher EA, Zhou M, Mitchell DM, et al: The degradation of apolipoprotein B100 is mediated by the ubiquitin-proteasome pathway and involves heat shock protein 70. *J Biol Chem* 1997;272:20427–20434.
83. Gusarova V, Caplan AJ, Brodsky JL, Fisher EA: Apoprotein B degradation is promoted by the molecular chaperones hsp90 and hsp70. *J Biol Chem* 2001;276:24891–24900.
84. Zhou M, Fisher EA, Ginsberg HN: Regulated Co-translational ubiquitination of apolipoprotein B100. A new paradigm for proteasomal degradation of a secretory protein. *J Biol Chem* 1998;273:24649–24653.
85. Huang XF, Shelness GS: Efficient glycosylation site utilization by intracellular apolipoprotein B. Implications for proteasomal degradation. *J Lipid Res* 1999;40:2212–2222.
86. Liang J-S, Kim T, Fang S, et al: Overexpression of the tumor autocrine motility factor receptor Gp78, a ubiquitin protein ligase, results in increased ubiquitinylation and decreased secretion of apolipoprotein B100 in HepG2 cells. *J Biol Chem* 2003;278: 23984–23988.
87. Zhang J, Herscovitz H: Nascent lipidated apolipoprotein B is transported to the Golgi as an incompletely folded intermediate as probed by its association with network of endoplasmic reticulum molecular chaperones, GRP94, ERp72, BiP, calreticulin, and cyclophilin B. *J Biol Chem* 2003;278:7459–7468.
88. Chen Y, Le Caherec F, Chuck SL: Calnexin and other factors that alter translocation affect the rapid binding of ubiquitin to apoB in the Sec61 complex. *J Biol Chem* 1998;273:11887–11894.
89. Rashid KA, Hevi S, Chen Y, et al: A proteomic approach identifies proteins in hepatocytes that bind nascent apolipoprotein B. *J Biol Chem* 2002;277:22010–22017.
90. Hevi S, Chuck SL: Ferritins can regulate the secretion of apolipoprotein B. *J Biol Chem* 1924;278:31924–31929.
91. Oyadomari S, Yun C, Fisher EA, et al: Cotranslocational degradation protects the stressed endoplasmic reticulum from protein overload. *Cell* 2006;126:727–739.
92. Fisher EA, Pan M, Chen X, et al: The triple threat to nascent apolipoprotein B. Evidence for multiple, distinct degradative pathways. *J Biol Chem* 2001;276:27855–27863.
93. Pan M, Cederbaum AI, Zhang Y-L, et al: Lipid peroxidation and oxidant stress regulate hepatic apolipoprotein B degradation and VLDL production. *J Clin Invest* 2004;113:1277–1287.
94. Cardozo C, Wu X, Pan M, et al: The inhibition of microsomal triglyceride transfer protein activity in rat hepatoma cells promotes proteasomal and nonproteasomal degradation of apoprotein b100. *Biochemistry* 2002;41:10105–10114.

95. Jiang X-C, Li Z, Liu R, et al: Phospholipid transfer protein deficiency impairs apolipoprotein-B secretion from hepatocytes by stimulating a proteolytic pathway through a relative deficiency of vitamin E and an increase in intracellular oxidants. *J Biol Chem* 2005;280:18336–18340.
96. Gillian-Daniel DL, Bates PW, Tebon A, Attie AD: Endoplasmic reticulum localization of the low-density lipoprotein receptor mediates presecretory degradation of apolipoprotein B. *Proc Nat Acad Sci USA* 2002;99:4337–4342.
97. Qiu W, Kohen-Avramoglu R, Rashid-Kolvear F, et al: Overexpression of the endoplasmic reticulum 60 protein ER-60 downregulates apoB100 secretion by inducing its intracellular degradation via a nonproteasomal pathway: evidence for an ER-60-mediated and pCMB-sensitive intracellular degradative pathway. *Biochemistry* 2004;43:4819–4831.
98. Olofsson SO, Boren J: Apolipoprotein B: a clinically important apolipoprotein which assembles atherogenic lipoproteins and promotes the development of atherosclerosis. *J Intern Med* 2005;258:395–410.
99. Mitchell DM, Zhou M, Pariyarath R, et al: Apoprotein B100 has a prolonged interaction with the translocon during which its lipidation and translocation change from dependence on the microsomal triglyceride transfer protein to independence. *Proc Nat Acad Sci USA* 1998;95:14733–14738.
100. Olofsson SO, Asp L, Boren J: The assembly and secretion of apolipoprotein B-containing lipoproteins. *Curr Opin Lipidol* 1999;10:341–346.
101. Rustaeus S, Lindberg K, Stillemark P, et al: Assembly of very-low-density lipoprotein: a two-step process of apolipoprotein B core lipidation. *J Nutr* 1999;129:463S–466S.
102. Asp L, Claesson C, Boren J, Olofsson SO: ADP-ribosylation factor 1 and its activation of phospholipase D are important for the assembly of very-low-density lipoproteins. *J Biol Chem* 2000;275:26285–26292.
103. Gordon DA, Jamil H, Sharp D, et al: Secretion of apolipoprotein B-containing lipoproteins from HeLa cells is dependent on expression of the microsomal triglyceride transfer protein and is regulated by lipid availability. *Proc Natl Acad Sci USA* 1994;91:7628–7632.
104. Gordon DA, Jamil H, Gregg RE, et al: Inhibition of the microsomal triglyceride transfer protein blocks the first step of apolipoprotein B lipoprotein assembly but not the addition of bulk core lipids in the second step. *J Biol Chem* 1996;271:33047–33053.
105. Wang Y, McLeod RS, Yao Z: Normal activity of microsomal triglyceride transfer protein is required for the oleate-induced secretion of very-low-density lipoproteins containing apolipoprotein B from McA-RH7777 cells. *J Biol Chem* 1997;272:12272–12278.
106. Yamaguchi J, Gamble MV, Conlon D, et al: The conversion of apoB100 low-density lipoprotein/high-density lipoprotein particles to apoB100 very-low-density lipoproteins in response to oleic acid occurs in the endoplasmic reticulum and not in the Golgi in McA RH7777 cells. *J Biol Chem* 2003;278:42643–42651.
107. Tran K, Thorne-Tjomsland G, DeLong CJ, et al: Intracellular assembly of very-low-density lipoproteins containing apolipoprotein B100 in rat hepatoma McA-RH7777 cells. *J Biol Chem* 2002;277:31187–31200.
108. Boström K, Borén J, Wettesten M, et al: Studies on the assembly of apo B-100-containing lipoproteins in HepG2 cells. *J Biol Chem* 1988;263:4434–4442.
109. Dixon JL, Ginsberg HN: Regulation of hepatic secretion of apolipoprotein B-containing lipoproteins: information obtained from cultured liver cells. *J Lipid Res* 1993;34:167–179.
110. Valyi-Nagy K, Harris C, Swift LL: The assembly of hepatic very-low-density lipoproteins: evidence of a role for the Golgi apparatus. *Lipids* 2002;37:879–884.
111. Shoulders CC, Stephens DJ, Jones B: The intracellular transport of chylomicrons requires the small GTPase, Sar1b. *Curr Opini Lipidol* 2004;15:191–197.
112. Gusarova V, Brodsky JL, Fisher EA: Apolipoprotein B100 exit from the endoplasmic reticulum (ER) is COPII-dependent, and its lipidation to very-low-density lipoprotein occurs post-ER. *J Biol Chem* 2003;278:48051–48058.
113. Siddiqi SA, Gorelick FS, Mahan JT, Mansbach CM 2nd: COPII proteins are required for Golgi fusion but not for endoplasmic reticulum budding of the pre-chylomicron transport vesicle. *J Cell Sci* 2003;116:415–427.
114. Bensadoun A: Lipoprotein lipase. *Annu Rev Nutr* 1991;11:217–237.
115. Kern PA: Lipoprotein lipase and hepatic lipase. *Curr Opin Lipidol* 1991;2:162–169.
116. Broedl UC, Maugeais C, Millar JS, et al: Endothelial lipase promotes the catabolism of ApoB-containing lipoproteins. *Circ Res* 2004;94:1554–1561.
117. Ehnholm C, Mahley RW, Chappell DA, et al: Role of apolipoprotein E in the lipolytic conversion of β-very-low-density lipoproteins to low-density lipoproteins in type III hyperlipoproteinemia. *Proc Natl Acad Sci USA* 1984;81:5566–5570.
118. Mahley RW, Rall SC Jr: Type III hyperlipoproteinemia (dysbetalipoproteinemia): the role of apolipoprotein E in normal and abnormal lipoprotein metabolism. In Scriver CR, Beaudet AL, Sly WS, Valle D (eds). The Metabolic Basis of Inherited Disease. *New York, McGraw-Hill,* 1995.
119. Brunzell JD: Familial lipoprotein lipase deficiency and other causes of the chylomicronemia syndrome. In Scriver CR, Beaudet AL, Sly WS, Valle D (eds). The Metabolic and Molecular Bases of Inherited Disease. *New York, McGraw Hill,* 1995.
120. Brasaemle DL, Cornely-Moss K, Bensadoun AA: Hepatic lipase treatment of chylomicron remnants increases exposure of apolipoprotein E. *J Lipid Res* 1993;34:455–465.
121. Bradley WA, Hwang S-LC, Karlin JB, et al: Low-density lipoprotein receptor binding determinants switch from apolipoprotein E to apolipoprotein B during conversion of hypertriglyceridemic very-low-density lipoprotein to low-density lipoproteins. *J Biol Chem* 1984;259:14728–14735.
122. Badellino KO, Rader DJ: The role of endothelial lipase in high-density lipoprotein metabolism. *Curr Opin Cardiol* 2004;19:392–395.
123. Broedl UC, Jin W, Fuki IV, et al: Structural basis of endothelial lipase tropism for HDL. *FASEB J* 2004;18:1891–1893.
124. Broedl UC, Jin W, Rader DJ: Endothelial lipase: a modulator of lipoprotein metabolism upregulated by inflammation. *Trends Cardiovasc Med* 2004;14:202–206.
125. Jin W, Millar JS, Broedl U, et al: Inhibition of endothelial lipase causes increased HDL cholesterol levels *in vivo*. *J Clin Invest* 2003;111:357–362.
126. deLemos AS, Wolfe ML, Long CJ, et al: Identification of genetic variants in endothelial lipase in persons with elevated high-density lipoprotein cholesterol. *Circulation* 2002;106:1321–1326.
127. Badellino KO, Wolfe ML, Reilly MP, Rader DJ: Endothelial lipase concentrations are increased in metabolic syndrome and associated with coronary atherosclerosis. *PLoS Med* 2006;3:e22 (0245–0252).
128. Carlson LA, Ballantyne D: Changing relative proportions of apolipoproteins CII and CIII of very-low-density lipoproteins in hypertriglyceridaemia. *Atherosclerosis* 1976;23:563–568.
129. Miller NE, Rao SN, Alaupovic P, et al: Familial apolipoprotein CII deficiency: plasma lipoproteins and apolipoproteins in heterozygous and homozygous subjects and the effects of plasma infusion. *Eur J Clin Invest* 1981;11:69–76.
130. Pennacchio LA, Rubin EM: Apolipoprotein A5, a newly identified gene that affects plasma triglyceride levels in humans and mice. *Arterioscler Thromb Vasc Biol* 2003;23:529–534.
131. Pennacchio LA, Olivier M, Hubacek JA, et al: Two independent apolipoprotein A5 haplotypes influence human plasma triglyceride levels. *Hum Mol Genet* 2002;11:3031–3038.
132. Young SG, Davies BS, Fong LG, et al: GPIHBP1: an endothelial cell molecule important for the lipolytic processing of chylomicrons. *Curr Opin Lipidol* 2007;18:389–396.
133. Beigneux AP, Davies BS, Gin P, et al: Glycosylphosphatidylinositol-anchored high-density lipoprotein-binding protein 1 plays a critical role in the lipolytic processing of chylomicrons. *Cell Metab* 2007;5:279–291.
134. Inaba T, Matsuda M, Shimamura M, et al: Angiopoietin-like protein 3 mediates hypertriglyceridemia induced by the liver X receptor. *J Biol Chem* 2003;278:21344–21351.
135. Mandard S, Zandbergen F, van Straten E, et al: The fasting-induced adipose factor/angiopoietin-like protein 4 is physically associated with lipoproteins and governs plasma lipid levels and adiposity. *J Biol Chem* 2006;281:934–944.
136. Koster A, Chao YB, Mosior M, et al: Transgenic angiopoietin-like (angptl)4 overexpression and targeted disruption of angptl4 and angptl3: regulation of triglyceride metabolism. *Endocrinology* 2005;146:4943–4950.

137. Ge H, Cha JY, Gopal H, et al: Differential regulation and properties of angiopoietin-like proteins 3 and 4. *J Lipid Res* 2005;46:1484–1490.
138. Hussain MM, Mahley RW, Boyles JK, et al: Chylomicron-chylomicron remnant clearance by liver and bone marrow in rabbits. Factors that modify tissue-specific uptake. *J Biol Chem* 1989;264:9571–9582.
139. Rubinsztein DC, Cohen JC, Berger GM, et al: Chylomicron remnant clearance from the plasma is normal in familial hypercholesterolemic homozygotes with defined receptor defects. *J Clin Invest* 1990;86:1306–1312.
140. Kita T, Goldstein JL, Brown MS, et al: Hepatic uptake of chylomicron remnants in WHHL rabbits: a mechanism genetically distinct from the low-density lipoprotein receptor. *Proc Natl Acad Sci USA* 1982;79:3623–3627.
141. Ishibashi S, Herz J, Maeda N, et al: The two-receptor model of lipoprotein clearance: tests of the hypothesis in "knock-out" mice lacking the low-density lipoprotein receptor, apolipoprotein E, or both proteins. *Proc Natl Acad Sci USA* 1994;91:4431–4435.
142. Rohlmann A, Gotthardt M, Hammer RE, Herz J: Inducible inactivation of hepatic LRP gene by cre-mediated recombination confirms role of LRP in clearance of chylomicron remnants. *J Clin Invest* 1998;101:689–695.
143. Willnow TE, Sheng Z, Ishibashi S, Herz J: Inhibition of hepatic chylomicron remnant uptake by gene transfer of a receptor antagonist. *Science* 1994;264:1471–1474.
144. Ji Z-S, Fazio S, Lee Y-L, Mahley RW: Secretion-capture role for apolipoprotein E in remnant lipoprotein metabolism involving cell surface heparan sulfate proteoglycans. *J Biol Chem* 1994;269:2764–2772.
145. Linton MF, Atkinson JB, Fazio S: Prevention of atherosclerosis in apoE deficient mice by bone marrow transplantation. *Science* 1995;267:1034–1037.
146. Linton MF, Hasty AH, Babaev VR, Fazio S: Hepatic ApoE expression is required for remnant lipoprotein clearance in the absence of the low-density lipoprotein receptor. *J Clin Invest* 1998;101:1726–1736.
147. Davis RA, Engelhorn SC, Pangburn SH, et al: Very-low-density lipoprotein synthesis and secretion by cultured rat hepatocytes. *J Biol Chem* 1979;254:2010–2016.
148. Fazio S, Yao Z, McCarthy BJ, Rall SC Jr: Synthesis and secretion of apolipoprotein E occur independently of synthesis and secretion of apolipoprotein B-containing lipoproteins in HepG2 cells. *J Biol Chem* 1992;267:6941–6945.
149. Fazio S, Linton MF, Hasty AH, Swift LL: Recycling of apolipoprotein E in mouse liver. *J Biol Chem* 1999;274:8247–8253.
150. Heeren J, Weber W, Beisiegel U: Intracellular processing of endocytosed triglyceride-rich lipoproteins comprises both recycling and degradation. *J Cell Sci* 1999;112(Pt 3):349–359.
151. Swift LL, Farkas MH, Major AS, et al: A recycling pathway for resecretion of internalized apolipoprotein E in liver cells. *J Biol Chem* 2001;276:22965–22970.
152. Fazio S, Linton MF, Swift LL: The cell biology and physiologic relevance of ApoE recycling. *Trends Cardiovasc Med* 2000;10:23–30.
153. MacArthur JM, Bishop JR, Stanford KI, et al: Liver heparian sulfate proteoglycans mediate clearance of triglyceride-rich lipoproteins independently of LDL receptor family members. *J Clin Invest* 2007;117:153–164.
154. Stolt PC, Bock HH: Modulation of lipoprotein receptor functions by intracellular adaptor proteins. *Cell Signal* 2006;18:1560–1571.
155. Jones C, Garuti R, Michaely P, et al: Disruption of LDL but not VLDL clearance in autosomal recessive hypercholesterolemia. *J Clin Invest* 2007;117:165–174.
156. Mahley RW, Huang Y: Atherogenic remnant lipoproteins: role for proteoglycans in trapping, transferring, and internalizing. *J Clin Invest* 2007;117:94–98.
157. Kastelein JJP, Wedel MK, Baker BF, et al: Potent reduction of apolipoprotein B and low-density lipoprotein cholesterol by short-term administration of an antisense inhibitor of apolipoprotein B. *Circulation* 2006;114:1729–1735.
158. Wetterau JR, Gregg RE, Harrity TW, et al: An MTP inhibitor that normalizes atherogenic lipoprotein levels in WHHL rabbits. *Science* 1998;282:751–754.
159. Chandler CE, Wilder DE, Pettini JL, et al: CP-346086: an MTP inhibitor that lowers plasma cholesterol and triglycerides in experimental animals and in humans. *J Lipid Res* 2003;44:1887–1901.
160. Graham MJ, Lemonidis KM, Whipple CP, et al: Antisense inhibition of proprotein convertase subtilisin/kexin type 9 reduces serum LDL in hyperlipidemic mice. *J Lipid Res* 2007;48:763–767.
161. Cuchel M, Bloedon LT, Szapary PO, et al: Inhibition of microsomal triglyceride transfer protein in familial hypercholesterolemia. *New Engl J Med* 2007;356:148–156.
162. Spann NJ, Kang S, Li AC, et al: Coordinate transcriptional repression of liver fatty acid-binding protein and microsomal triglyceride transfer protein blocks hepatic very-low-density lipoprotein secretion without hepatosteatosis. *J Biol Chem* 2006;281:33066–33077.

CHAPTER 3

Absorption and Excretion of Cholesterol and Other Sterols

David Q.-H. Wang and David E. Cohen

INTRODUCTION

Cholesterol is essential for mammalian cells, where it is utilized either as a major structural component of membranes or as a substrate for the biosynthesis of other steroids. These steroids include the sex hormones such as estradiol, progesterone, androsterone, and testosterone; adrenocortical hormones such as aldosterone and cortisone; bile acids; and vitamin D. Because it provides both dietary and reabsorbed biliary cholesterol to the body, the small intestine is a pivotal organ for cholesterol homeostasis. Indeed, by increasing dietary cholesterol, plasma cholesterol concentrations can be made to rise in most individuals. Because elevated plasma cholesterol is an important risk factor for cardiovascular diseases, numerous studies have focused on identifying cellular, physical-chemical, and genetic determinants of intestinal cholesterol absorption in humans and laboratory animals.[1]

The National Cholesterol Education Program Adult Treatment Panel III guidelines[2] along with the 2004 update and more recent American Heart Association/American College of Cardiology recommendations[3–5] have led to lower (<100 mg/dL or <70 mg/dL) targets for low-density lipoprotein (LDL) cholesterol for individuals at high risk for adverse cardiovascular events. This has resulted in a significant increase in the number of patients who require aggressive cholesterol-lowering therapy. Because the cholesterol carried in LDL is derived from both *de novo* synthesis and absorption from the diet, a better understanding of the mechanisms of intestinal cholesterol absorption should lead to novel approaches to the treatment and prevention of cardiovascular diseases.

PHYSICAL-CHEMICAL PROPERTIES AND COMPOSITIONS OF INTESTINAL LIPIDS DERIVED FROM THE DIET AND FROM BILE

Lipids are organic compounds in animals and plants that possess large aliphatic and/or aromatic hydrocarbon components. They share the common physical property of being soluble in nonpolar solvents and insoluble in water. Lipids are categorized into saponifiable and nonsaponifiable. Saponifiable lipids contain at least one ester bond, which undergoes hydrolysis in the presence of an enzyme, a strong acid, or a strong base. Hydrolysis cleaves a saponifiable lipid into two or more smaller molecules. The term *sterol* refers to any nonsaponifiable steroid alcohol with an aliphatic side chain of 8 to 10 carbon atoms and a hydroxyl group at C-3 position. The term *stenol* usually refers to sterols with one or more nuclear double bonds, whereas *stanol* refers to a saturated nucleus with no double bonds.

The ester bonds contained in saponifiable lipids confer important biologic properties related to transport across the enterocytes, which comprise the monolayer of absorptive cells that form the lining of the villi of the small intestine. For example, cholesterol is very sparingly soluble in water but has high solubility in membranes, where the steroid nucleus is embedded in the lipid bilayer and the single hydroxyl group interacts with the polar water environment. Esterification of cholesterol with a fatty acid at the C-3 position markedly decreases the polarity of the molecule. The resulting cholesteryl ester is highly insoluble in water but has increased solubility in the cores of lipoproteins. As discussed later, the enzyme-catalyzed esterification reaction plays a key role in the molecular and cellular pathways of cholesterol absorption. In contrast, nonsaponifiable lipids do not undergo hydrolysis into smaller molecules.

Lipids within the lumen of the small intestine originate from bile, from the diet, and from cells sloughed from the lining of the small intestine. In bile, bile acids, phospholipids, and cholesterol are three major lipid species, as shown in Figure 3-1. Although bile does not contain any digestive enzymes, bile acids and phospholipids play key roles in promoting digestion and its absorption by the enterocyte.

Bile acids are a family of closely related acidic sterols that are synthesized from cholesterol within the liver.[6] They comprise approximately two thirds of the solute mass of normal human bile. The common bile acids possess a steroid nucleus of four fused hydrocarbon rings with polar hydroxyl functions and an aliphatic side chain conjugated in amide linkage with glycine or taurine. Because the ionized carboxylate or sulfonate group on the side chain renders them water soluble, bile acids are classified as soluble amphiphiles. The common bile acids differ in the number and orientation of the hydroxyl groups on the steroid

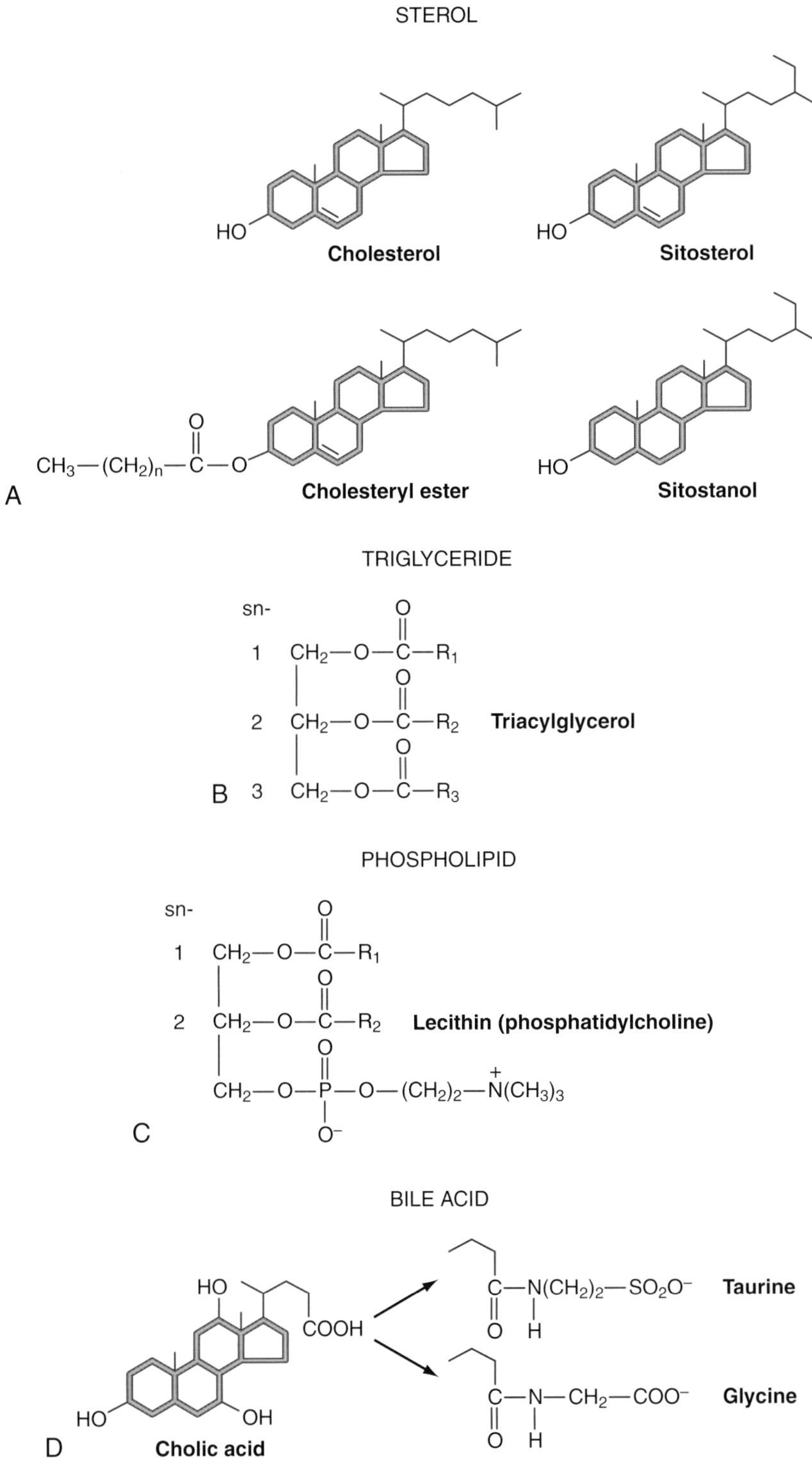

STEROL

HO Cholesterol

HO Sitosterol

A $CH_3—(CH_2)_n—C(=O)—O$ Cholesteryl ester

HO Sitostanol

TRIGLYCERIDE

B
sn-
1 $CH_2—O—C(=O)—R_1$
2 $CH_2—O—C(=O)—R_2$ Triacylglycerol
3 $CH_2—O—C(=O)—R_3$

PHOSPHOLIPID

C
sn-
1 $CH_2—O—C(=O)—R_1$
2 $CH_2—O—C(=O)—R_2$ Lecithin (phosphatidylcholine)
$CH_2—O—P(=O)(O^-)—O—(CH_2)_2—\overset{+}{N}(CH_3)_3$

BILE ACID

D
HO, HO, OH, COOH
Cholic acid

$C(=O)—N(H)(CH_2)_2—SO_2O^-$ Taurine

$C(=O)—N(H)—CH_2—COO^-$ Glycine

FIGURE 3-1 Chemical structures of common dietary and biliary lipids. *A,* Cholesterol is the most abundant steroid in animal tissues and in the intestinal lumen. Its hydroxyl group on the third carbon can react with the COOH group of a fatty acid molecule to form a cholesteryl ester. Plant sterols (e.g., β-sitosterol and β-sitostanol) are naturally occurring. Their chemical structures are very similar to cholesterol, but with structural modifications of the side chain. *B,* Triglycerides are triesters of glycerol, and each of the three OH groups of glycerol forms an ester group by reaction with the COOH group of a fatty acid to form the triacylglycerol molecule. R_1, R_2, and R_3 are fatty acids located at stereospecific number (sn)-1, sn-2 and sn-3, respectively. Monoglycerides and diglycerides contain one or two fatty acids, respectively. *C,* Phospholipids are also derivatives of glycerol and contain a phosphate ester functional group and ionic charges, as illustrated for lecithin (phosphatidylcholine), which is the major phospholipid in human bile. In general, the sn-1 position of lecithin is esterified with a saturated fatty acid and the sn-2 position is esterified with an unsaturated fatty acid. *D,* Bile acids are a family of closely related acidic sterols that are synthesized from cholesterol in the liver. The common bile acids, as represented by cholic acid, which is the primary hepatic catabolic product of cholesterol, possess a steroid nucleus of four fused hydrocarbon rings with polar hydroxyl functions and an aliphatic side chain conjugated in amide linkage with taurine or glycine.

nucleus. The hydrophilic (polar) areas of bile acids are the hydroxyl groups and conjugation side chain of either glycine or taurine, and their hydrophobic (nonpolar) area is the ringed steroid nucleus. Because of the presence of both hydrophilic and hydrophobic surfaces, bile acids are highly soluble, detergent-like amphiphilic molecules. At low concentrations in aqueous solution, bile acids exist as monomers; however, above a certain concentration, that is, when a critical micellar concentration (CMC) is exceeded, they spontaneously form negatively charged spherical aggregates called *micelles*.[6] Under normal physiologic conditions, the CMC values for common bile acids are between 1 and 20 mmol, which depends on the species of bile acids, the ionic strength and composition, and the types and concentrations of other lipids present in solution. Because bile is concentrated gradually within the biliary tree, bile acid concentrations eventually exceed their CMCs. At this point, bile acids in bile can form simple micelles. Importantly, micelles of bile acids can solubilize other types of lipids such cholesterol and phospholipids by forming mixed micelles in bile. The potency of bile acids as detergents depends critically on the distribution and orientation of hydroxyl groups around the steroid nucleus of the molecule, which is usually described as its hydrophobicity. The hydrophobicity of a bile acid can be quantified by high-performance liquid chromatography to yield a relative value that may be used to predict the biologic effects of individual bile acids.[7] The physical-chemical properties of bile acids depend on the nature and ionization state of functional groups on the side chain. In general, the glycine conjugate is more hydrophobic than the taurine conjugate. In human bile, more than 95% of bile acids are 5β,C-24 hydroxylated acidic steroids amide-linked to taurine or glycine. These conjugates are present in bile in an approximate tavrine: glycine ratio of 1:3.

The primary bile acids are hepatic catabolic products of cholesterol and are composed of cholate, with three hydroxyl groups, and chenodeoxycholate, with two hydroxyl groups. The secondary bile acids are derived from the primary bile acid species by the action of intestinal bacteria in the ileum and colon to form deoxycholate and ursodeoxycholate with two hydroxyl groups, and lithocholate with a single hydroxyl group. The most important of these reactions is 7α-dehydroxylation of primary bile acids to produce deoxycholate from cholate, and lithocholate from chenodeoxycholate. Another important secondary reaction is the 7α-dehydrogenation of chenodeoxycholate to form 7α-oxo-lithocholate. This bile acid does not accumulate in bile but is metabolized to "tertiary" bile acids by hepatic or bacterial reduction to form chenodeoxycholate (mainly in the liver) or its 7β-epimer, ursodeoxycholate (primarily by colonic bacteria).[8]

Phospholipids are derivatives of glycerol and contain a phosphate ester functional group and ionic charges (see Fig. 3-1). Approximately 10 to 20 g of biliary phospholipids enter the intestine daily, whereas the dietary contribution is only 1 to 2 g per day. The major phospholipid in human bile is lecithin (phosphatidylcholine), accounting for more than 95% of total phospholipids. Lecithin is an insoluble, swelling amphiphile with a hydrophilic, zwitterionic phosphocholine head group and hydrophobic tails consisting of two long fatty acyl chains. The remainder is composed of cephalins (phosphatidylethanolamines) and a trace amount of sphingomyelin. The phospholipids comprise 15% to 25% of total lipids in bile. Similar to all naturally occurring phospholipids, biliary lecithin is a complex mixture of molecular species. The sn-1 position is esterified by the saturated fatty acyl chains 16:0 (~75%) and 18:0 (<20%), with small amounts of monounsaturated sn-1 16:1 or 18:1 comprising the remainder. The sn-2 position is esterified by unsaturated fatty acyl species, with 18:2, 18:1, and 20:4 fatty acids predominating. The major molecular species of lecithin in human bile are 16:0 to 18:2 (40% to 60%), 16:0 to 18:1 (5% to 25%), 18:0 to 18:2 (1% to 16%), and 16:0 to 20:4 (1% to 10%). Lecithin is principally synthesized in the endoplasmic reticulum of the enterocyte from diacylglycerol by way of the cytidine diphosphate–choline pathway. Although there is a large variation in hepatic outputs of biliary bile acids, the proportion of lecithin to minor phospholipid classes in bile is essentially constant.

Cholesterol is the most abundant steroid in animal tissues and in the intestinal lumen. It is poorly soluble in an aqueous environment. Cholesterol has the cholestene nucleus with a double bond at C-5 and C-6 nucleus and a hydroxyl group on the third carbon (see Fig. 3-1). Furthermore, the aguilar methyl groups at C-10 and C-13, the hydrogen atom at C-8, and the side chain at C-17 are in β configuration. The hydrogen atoms at C-9 and C-14 are in α configuration.

The term *plant sterols* (phytosterols) refers to sterols that originate from plants, as shown in Figure 3-1. Plant sterols, which are also abundant in the intestine, are naturally occurring; their chemical structures are very similar to that of cholesterol (i.e., a Δ^5 double bond and a 3β-hydroxyl group, but with structural modifications of the side chain). Plant sterols have the same basic importance in plants as cholesterol in animals, playing critical roles in cell membrane function. Sitosterol and campesterol, which are 24-ethyl and 24-methyl analogues of cholesterol, respectively, are the most abundant plant sterols. They are consumed in the diet and may be absorbed in the intestine. However, they are usually present only at very low steady-state concentrations in human plasma. Unique sterols, such as brassicasterol and isofucosterol, may also originate from shellfish.

Triglycerides are the major source of dietary lipids and derive principally from two sources: animal fats such as butter, beef, poultry, pork, cheese, and milk fats; and vegetable oils such as corn, peanut, olive, safflower, sunflower, rapeseed, and soybean. Triglycerides are triesters of glycerol. Each of the three OH groups of glycerol forms an ester group by reaction with the COOH group of a fatty acid molecule to form the triacylglycerol molecule (see Fig. 3-1). Most dietary triglycerides contain long-chain fatty acids, including the monounsaturated oleic acid (18:1) and the saturated palmitic acid (16:0). Animal fats differ from vegetable oils in the relative amounts of saturated and unsaturated fatty acid units. The former usually contains less than 50% to 60% unsaturated fatty acid units, and the latter contains more than

80% unsaturated fatty acid units. Furthermore, triglycerides are divided into two groups: simple and complex triacylglycerol. In the former group, three molecules of the same fatty acid are esterified to glycerol. In the latter group, the three fatty acids esterified with glycerol are different. In general, naturally occurring triacylglycerols are complex triacylglycerols. In the Western diet, dietary fat constitutes as much as 50% of total calories (i.e., 100 to 160 g/day). Of the dietary fat, triglycerides contribute as much as 90% of the total calories supplies by fat. Other fats such as phospholipids yield minor numbers of calories.

SOURCES OF INTESTINAL STEROLS

Cholesterol that enters the small intestinal lumen for absorption by the enterocytes consists mainly of three sources: diet, bile, and intestinal epithelial sloughing. The average intake of cholesterol in the Western diet is approximately 300 to 500 mg/day. In the Western diet, cholesterol is a major sterol and is predominantly animal in origin. Some of dietary cholesterol exists in the esterified form. Any cholesteryl ester entering the intestine must be de-esterified by pancreatic cholesterol esterase to be absorbed. Plants and vegetables also contain a small amount of cholesterol. Plant sterols account for 20% to 25% of total dietary sterol. Therefore, the average intake of plant sterols in the Western diet constitutes approximately 75 to 170 mg/day. Although the pattern and proportions of plant sterols are broad and highly dependent on diet, β-sitosterol is an important and major plant sterol in diet.

Bile delivers 800 to 1200 mg of cholesterol per day to the intestine, and this amount is approximately two to three times the dietary intake. In bile, cholesterol is present solely in the unesterified form and accounts for up to 95% of total sterols in bile. The remaining 5% of the sterols are cholesterol precursors and dietary sterols from plant, animal, and shellfish sources. Therefore, bile provides roughly 40 to 60 mg of the noncholesterol sterols daily. The pattern and proportions of these molecules are variable and highly dependent on diet. For example, on a regular (nonshellfish) diet, the concentrations of noncholesterol sterols are less than 5%, and their pattern and proportions are cholestanol (1.5%), sitosterol (1.2%), campesterol (0.7%), lathosterol (0.6%), 24-methylene cholesterol (0.1%), stigmasterol (0.1%), brassicasterol (0.1%), and isofucosterol (0.03%). If a diet high in shellfish is consumed, shellfish sterols in bile would be increased and comprise 5% to 10% of total sterols.

The third source of intraluminal cholesterol comes from the turnover of intestinal mucosal epithelium, which provides approximately 300 mg of cholesterol per day. As discussed later, although the entire length of the small intestine has the capability to absorb cholesterol from the lumen, the major sites of absorption are the upper part of the small intestine, that is, the duodenum and proximal jejunum. Thus, since the intestinal sloughing occurs throughout the intestinal tract and cholesterol absorption seems to be confined to the very proximal small intestine, this source may not contribute significantly to cholesterol absorption.

Bacterial cell wall lipids in the human small intestine are less than 1 mg, even when abnormally colonized. Bacteria are therefore not a significant source of endogenous sterols for absorption.

MOLECULAR PHYSIOLOGY OF INTESTINAL CHOLESTEROL ABSORPTION

Intestinal absorption of cholesterol is most accurately defined as the transfer of intraluminal cholesterol into intestinal or thoracic duct lymph. By contrast, intestinal uptake of cholesterol refers to its entry from the lumen into intestinal absorptive cells. As can be inferred from this distinction, intestinal cholesterol absorption is a multistep process that is regulated by multiple genes, as shown in Figure 3-2.[1]

Intraluminal Digestion of Lipids

Lipid digestion begins in the stomach, where dietary constituents are mixed with lingual and gastric enzymes, resulting in partial fat digestion by preduodenal lipases and emulsification by peristalsis. The stomach also regulates the delivery of gastric chyme to the duodenum, where it is mixed with bile and pancreatic juice. The major lipases and proteins secreted by the pancreas into the intestinal lumen in response to a meal include carboxyl ester lipase (CEL), pancreatic triglyceride lipase, and the group 1B phospholipase A_2, as well as pancreatic lipase–related protein–1 and –2.[1] Because only unesterified cholesterol may be incorporated into bile acid–phospholipid micelles and transported to the brush border of enterocyte, a critically important step is lipase-mediated de-esterification of cholesteryl esters. However, the contribution of unesterified cholesterol (mainly biliary) to intestinal cholesterol is much greater than the dietary esterified cholesterol (<15% of dietary cholesterol). As a result, inhibition or loss of some of the pancreatic lipolytic enzyme activities would be unlikely to result in an appreciable reduction of cholesterol absorption. This may partly explain why targeted disruption of the carboxyl ester lipase (*Cel*) gene in mice has little or only a slight inhibitory effect on intestinal cholesterol absorption.[9,10] Interestingly, a lack of triglyceride hydrolytic activity in the intestinal lumen in pancreatic triglyceride lipase knockout mice reduces dietary cholesterol absorption substantially, without impairing triglyceride digestion and absorption.[11] The regulatory effects of the group 1B phospholipase A_2, as well as pancreatic lipase-related protein–1 and –2 on intestinal cholesterol absorption, have not yet been defined.

The digestion of triglycerides also begins in the stomach. The key enzymes are lingual lipase secreted by the salivary gland and gastric lipase secreted by the gastric mucosa. Humans express mainly gastric lipase, whereas rodents express primarily lingual lipase. Human gastric lipase shares many characteristics with rodent lingual lipase. Both enzymes have a pH optimum ranging from 3 to 6 and hydrolyze medium-chain triacylglycerols better than long-chain triacylglycerols.[12,13] These lipases preferentially hydrolyze fatty

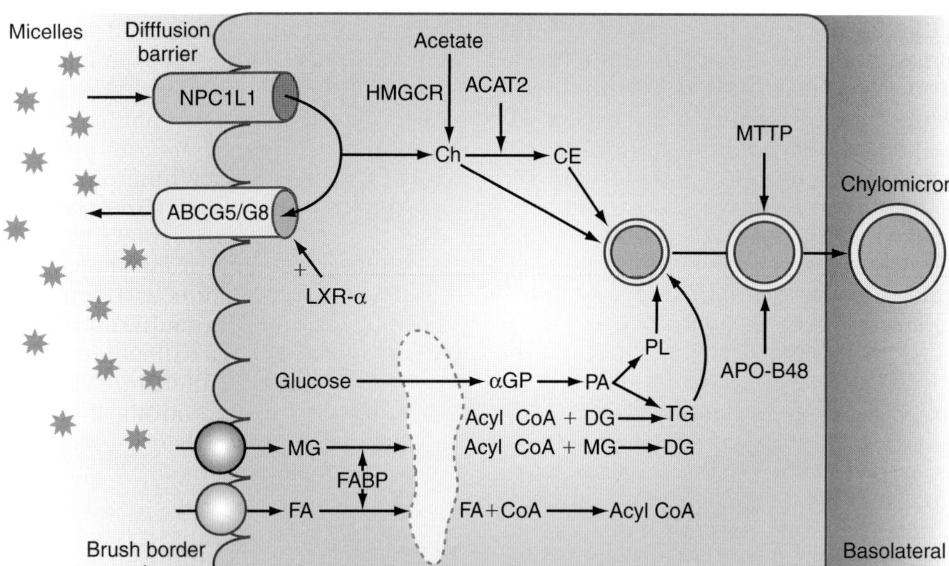

FIGURE 3-2 Within the intestinal lumen, the micellar solubilization of sterols facilitates movement through the diffusion barrier overlying the surface of the absorptive cells. In the presence of bile acids, large amounts of the sterol molecules are delivered to the aqueous-membrane interface so that the uptake rate is greatly increased. The Niemann–Pick C1–like 1 protein (NPC1L1), a newly identified sterol influx transporter, is located at the apical membrane of the enterocyte and may actively facilitate the uptake of cholesterol (Cn) by promoting the passage of sterols across the brush border membrane of the enterocyte. By contrast, ATP-binding cassette transporter G5 (ABCG5) and ABCG8 promote active efflux of cholesterol and plant sterols from the enterocyte into the intestinal lumen for excretion. Liver X receptor–alpha (LXR-α) may be essential for the up-regulation of the *ABCG5* and *ABCG8* genes in response to high dietary cholesterol. The combined regulatory effects of NPC1L1 and ABCG5 and ABCG8 play a critical role in modulating the amount of cholesterol that reaches the lymph from the intestinal lumen. Absorbed cholesterol, as well as some that is newly synthesized from acetate by 3-hydroxy-3-methylglutaryl–coenzyme A reductase (HMGCR) within the enterocyte, is esterified by acyl-coenzyme A:cholesterol acyltransferase isoform–2 (ACAT2), thereby forming cholesteryl esters (CE). Fatty acids (FA) and monoacylglycerol (MG) are taken up into enterocytes by facilitated transport. With the assistance of fatty acid–binding proteins (FABP), FA and MG are transported into the smooth endoplasmic reticulum (SER), where they are used for the synthesis of diacylglycerol (DG) and triacylglycerol (TG). Glucose is transported into the SER for the synthesis of phospholipids (PL). All of these lipids participate in the formation of chylomicrons, which also requires the synthesis of apolipoprotein B-48 (apoB-48) and the activity of microsomal triglyceride transfer protein (MTTP). As observed in lymph, the core of the secreted chylomicrons contains triglycerides and cholesteryl esters, and the surface of the particles is a monolayer containing phospholipids, mainly phosphatidylcholines, unesterified cholesterol, and apolipoproteins including apoB-48, apoA-I, and apoA-IV. Therefore, intestinal cholesterol absorption is a multistep process that is regulated by multiple genes. αGR, α-glycerophosphate; PA, phosphatidic acid.

acids at the sn-3 position to produce diacylglycerols, irrespective of the fatty acid present at that position. However, they do not hydrolyze phospholipids or cholesteryl esters.[12,14] The digestion of triglycerides by both lingual and gastric lipase in the stomach plays an important role in lipid digestion. This is evidenced by the observation that patients with cystic fibrosis can still absorb dietary triglycerides, despite a marked or complete inhibition in the secretion of pancreatic lipase.[15,16] The stomach is also the major site for the mechanical emulsification of dietary fat, which is an important prerequisite for efficient hydrolysis by pancreatic lipase. Emulsification is facilitated by the diacylglycerols and fatty acids produced as a result of the action of acid lipases in the stomach, as well as the phospholipids normally present in the diet.

The lipid emulsion enters the small intestine as fine lipid droplets with diameters of less than 500 nm. The combined action of bile and pancreatic juice markedly alters the chemical and physical form of the lipid emulsion in the upper part of the small intestine. Pancreatic lipase functions at the interface between oil and aqueous phases and hydrolyzes mainly the sn-1 and sn-3 positions of the triacylglycerol molecule to release monoacylglycerols and free fatty acids.[17–20] Further hydrolysis of monoacylglycerols by pancreatic lipase results in the formation of glycerol and free fatty acids. When fat digestion is observed by polarizing light microscopy *in vitro*, it is appreciated that at least three phases are present: an oil phase (mainly triglycerides, partial glycerides, and fatty acids), a calcium soap phase (Ca^{2+} ions and protonated long-chain fatty acids), and a viscous isotropic phase (monoacylglycerols and fatty acids).[21]

Pancreatic lipase is present in pancreatic juice. Its high concentration in pancreatic secretions taken together with its catalytic efficiency ensures the complete digestion of dietary fat. The very high capacity for fat digestion is underscored by the observation that severe pancreatic deficiency is required to produce fat malabsorption. Interestingly, purified pancreatic lipase is inefficient at hydrolyzing triglycerides in a model lipid mixture, even though it is highly efficient when present in pancreatic juice.[22,23] These observations led to the discovery of the colipase. Colipase is secreted by the pancreas as a procolipase.[24] After entering the small intestinal lumen, the procolipase is activated by the cleavage of a pentapeptide from the N-terminus. Whereas triglyceride lipid droplets covered with bile acids are not accessible to pancreatic lipase, the binding of the colipase to the triglyceride–aqueous interface allows the binding of the lipase molecule to the lipid–aqueous interface, greatly facilitating digestion of dietary fat.[25,26]

The digestion of phospholipids from bile and the diet also occurs in the lumen of the small intestine. In bile, phospholipids are solubilized primarily in mixed micelles together with bile acids and cholesterol. In the intestinal lumen, phospholipids are largely solubilized in mixed micelles but also participate in the emulsification of triglycerides. These phospholipids are hydrolyzed by pancreatic phospholipase A_2 at the sn-2 position to yield fatty acids and lysophosphatidylcholine molecules.

The enzyme involved in hydrolyzing cholesteryl esters is variably referred to as cholesterol esterase, carboxylic ester hydrolase, or sterol ester hydrolase. The human cholesterol esterase has a broad specificity, with the capacity to hydrolyze triglycerides, cholesteryl esters, and phospholipids.[27,28] Cholesterol esterase activity is greatly enhanced by the presence of bile acids, particularly the trihydroxy bile acid cholate.[29] As it enters the small intestine, dietary cholesterol is typically mixed in a lipid emulsion with triglycerides and phospholipids. The digestion of the phospholipids on the surface and triglycerides in the core of the lipid emulsion particles is required to liberate the dietary cholesterol.[30] This cholesterol is transferred to phospholipid vesicles and bile acid micelles for its transport to the brush border of enterocytes. Both cholesterol and lysophosphatidylcholine molecules are incorporated into disk-shaped micelles and liquid crystalline vesicles prior to their uptake by enterocytes.[31,32]

The detergent properties of bile acids are critical to intestinal lipid uptake because they coordinate micellar solubilization of intraluminal cholesterol.[33–35] Simple bile acid micelles (3 nm in diameter) are small, thermodynamically stable aggregates that can solubilize only minimal amounts of cholesterol. By contrast, phospholipids, monoacylglycerides, and free fatty acids are highly soluble in simple bile acid micelles. As a result, when combined together with ionized and nonionized fatty acids, monoacylglycerides, and lysophospholipids, bile acids form mixed micelles. Mixed micelles can solubilize much greater amounts of cholesterol compared with simple micelles. Mixed micelles are larger, thermodynamically stable aggregates and their sizes (4 to 8 nm in diameter) vary depending on the relative proportion of bile acids and phospholipids. Mixed micelles function as transport vehicles for cholesterol across the unstirred water layer toward the brush border, where they facilitate uptake of monomeric cholesterol by the enterocyte.[36–38]

Excess lipids that are not dissolved in mixed micelles reside in the intestinal lumen as a stable emulsion comprised mainly by bile acids, phospholipids, monoacylglycerides, and fatty acids in the intestinal lumen. During lipolysis, liquid crystals composed of multilamellar products of lipid digestion form at the surface of the emulsion droplets.[31,32] These liquid crystals give rise to vesicles, which are unilamellar spherical structures and contain phospholipids and cholesterol, with little, if any, bile acids. Vesicles (40 to 100 nm in diameter) are substantially larger than either simple or mixed micelles but much smaller than liquid crystals (500 nm in diameter), which are composed of multilamellar spherical structures. Both liquid crystals and vesicles provide an accessible source of cholesterol and other lipids for continuous formation and modification of mixed micelles in the presence of bile acids. Within the intestinal lumen, the presence of hydrophilic bile acids may reduce solubility of cholesterol by favoring the formation of liquid crystals and vesicles at the expense of mixed micelles.[39] Cholesterol molecules are poorly absorbed by enterocytes when incorporated into liquid crystals or vesicles. By contrast, hydrophobic bile acids markedly increase micellar cholesterol solubility and thereby augment cholesterol absorption.[39,40] This suggests that the hydrophobic bile acids are more effective at promoting cholesterol absorption than the hydrophilic bile acids. Luminal bile acids are derived from hepatic secretion and reabsorbed from the intestine (mainly the ileum) and returned to the liver via portal blood to complete the enterohepatic circulation.[8]

Intestinal Uptake of Sterols

Mixed micelles in the intestine promote cholesterol absorption by facilitating transport across the unstirred layer of water adjacent to the surface of the apical membrane of the enterocyte.[37] The particle itself does not penetrate the cell membrane. Rather, it facilitates passage across a diffusion barrier that is located at the intestinal lumen–membrane interface. Mucus coating the intestinal mucosa is also a diffusion-limiting barrier, especially because cholesterol molecules may be extensively bound to surface mucins prior to transfer into the enterocyte. Physiologic quantities of epithelial mucin encoded by the *MUC1* gene are necessary for normal intestinal uptake and absorption of cholesterol in mice, as evidenced by a reduction of cholesterol absorption efficiency by 50% in MUC1-knockout mice.[41]

Whereas it is clear that cholesterol incorporation into bile acid micelles is necessary for transport to the brush border membrane of enterocytes and for absorption, the mechanism by which the micellar cholesterol is taken up across the brush border membrane is unclear. One longstanding hypothesis suggests that cholesterol absorption occurs by an energy-independent, passive diffusion process in which micellar cholesterol is in equilibrium with monomolecular cholesterol in solution, and the monomeric cholesterol is in turn adsorbed to the brush border membrane down a concentration gradient.

A major advance in the effort to identify intestinal sterol transporters was the discovery that mutations in the genes encoding human ATP-binding cassette transporter G5 (ABCG5) and ABCG8 transporters constituted the molecular basis of sitosterolemia.[42,43] Patients with sitosterolemia absorb 20% to 30% of the dietary sitosterol, as opposed to the typically small amount (<5%) that is absorbed in normal individuals.[44–47] Interestingly, patients with sitosterolemia are hypercholesterolemic because they also absorb a greater fraction of dietary cholesterol and excrete less cholesterol into the bile compared with normal subjects. Studies in genetically engineered mice and *in vitro* have revealed that ABCG5 and ABCG8 are localized in the apical brush border membrane of enterocytes and in the canalicular membrane of hepatocytes.[48–50] They appear to function as an efficient efflux pump system for both cholesterol and plant sterols. In the small intestine, ABCG5 and ABCG8 transport sterols back into the intestinal lumen, whereas in the liver, they transport sterols into bile. Consistent with this hypothesis, there is a negative correlation between the efficiency of cholesterol absorption and the expression levels of ABCG5 and ABCG8 in the jejunum and ileum but not in the duodenum.[51] This suggests that under normal physiologic conditions, the jejunal and ileal ABCG5 and ABCG8 play major regulatory roles in modulating the amount of cholesterol that is absorbed from the intestine. Several polymorphisms in the *ABCG5* and *ABCG8* genes have been identified[52] that appear to exert moderate control over plasma sterol levels. The activity of these gene products may explain, in part, why cholesterol absorption occurs selectively and plant sterols and other noncholesterol sterols are absorbed poorly or not at all.

Not only are plant sterols poorly absorbed by the small intestine, but they also inhibit cholesterol absorption.[53–55] Plant sterols are more hydrophobic molecules than cholesterol and effectively displace cholesterol from mixed micelles.[56–59] This prevents cholesterol uptake by the enterocyte and presumably explains the more efficient uptake of cholesterol compared with β-sitosterol by the brush border membrane.

Studies in knockout mice have revealed that the liver X receptors (LXRs; LXR-α and LXR-β) are essential for diet-induced up-regulation of the *Abcg5* and *Abcg8* genes. Moreover, the stimulation of cholesterol excretion by a synthetic LXR agonist T0901317 requires intact *ABCG5* and *ABCG8* genes.[60] These studies suggest that the mRNA expression for ABCG5 and ABCG8 could be activated by dietary cholesterol via LXRs. It is currently unclear whether it is possible that plant sterols up-regulate expression levels of the *ABCG5* and *ABCG8* genes via the LXR pathway. If so, this could promote transport of plant sterols from enterocytes back into the intestinal lumen, serving a "gatekeeper" function to avoid increased plasma plant sterol concentrations.

The discovery of ezetimibe as a specific and potent inhibitor of intestinal cholesterol absorption has focused attention on a putative sterol influx transporter that might be a target for ezetimibe. Radiolabeled ezetimibe is localized to the brush border membrane of the enterocyte and appears to directly inhibit the uptake activity of the putative cholesterol transporter(s) at the intestinal brush border membrane.[61] Using a genomics–bioinformatics approach, the transcripts containing expression patterns and structural characteristics anticipated in cholesterol transporters (e.g., sterol-sensing and transmembrane domains, as well as extracellular signal peptides) were identified.[62,63] This led to discovery of the Niemann–Pick C1–like 1 (NPC1L1) protein and established it as a strong candidate for the ezetimibe-sensitive cholesterol transporter. Moreover, similarities in cholesterol absorption characteristics between ezetimibe-treated mice and NPC1L1–knockout mice supported the likelihood that NPC1L1 is the ezetimibe-inhibitable cholesterol transporter.[62] The NPC1L1 protein has 50% amino acid homology to NPC1, which functions in intracellular cholesterol trafficking and is defective in the cholesterol storage disease Niemann-Pick type C.[64] However, in contrast to broad expression pattern of *NPC1* in tissues, *Npc1l1* is expressed predominantly in the intestine in mice, with peak expression in the proximal jejunum,[62,63] paralleling the efficiency of cholesterol absorption along the gastrocolic axis. Subfractionation of the brush border membrane suggests that NPC1L1 is associated with the apical membrane fraction of enterocytes. A rat homologue of the human *NPC1L1* gene is unique in that it encodes a protein that contains an extracellular signal peptide, transmembrane sequences, N-linked glycosylation sites, and a sterol-sensing domain.[65] The binding affinities of ezetimibe and several key analogues to recombinant NPC1L1 were shown to be virtually identical to those observed for native enterocyte membranes, and ezetimibe did not bind to membranes from NPC1L1-knockout mice. These findings indicate that NPC1L1 is the direct molecular target of ezetimibe.[66,67] Nevertheless, attempts to reconstitute cholesterol transport activity in nonenterocyte cells by overexpression of NPC1L1 have so far been unsuccessful. This suggests that additional proteins could be required to reconstitute a fully functional cholesterol transporter. These could include caveolin-1, which forms a heterocomplex with annexin-2 (and cyclophilins) in zebrafish and mouse intestines.[68] A stable 55-kDa complex of annexin-2 and caveolin-1 appears to be involved in intracellular sterol trafficking. Incubation with ezetimibe led to a complete disruption of the caveolin-1–annexin-2 complex in the early state of zebrafish embryos. Pharmacologic treatment of mice with ezetimibe disrupts the complex only in mice rendered hypercholesterolemic by a high-cholesterol and high-fat diet or by LDL-receptor gene knockout,[68] suggesting that the caveolin-1 heterocomplex might represent an additional ezetimibe target that regulates intestinal cholesterol transport.

A number of important negative observations have also emerged from studies of ezetimibe. Inhibition of cholesterol absorption by ezetimibe is not mediated via changes in either the size or composition of the intestinal bile acid pool or the mRNA expression levels of *ABCG5*, *ABCG8*, *ABCA1*, or scavenger receptor class B type I (*SR-BI*).[69] Furthermore, ezetimibe neither inhibits pancreatic lipolytic enzyme activities in the intestinal lumen nor disrupts bile acid micelle solubilization of cholesterol.[70] Despite these collective advances, the exact molecular mechanism by which NPC1L1 regulates cholesterol absorption remains to be defined.

Over the past decade, the search for intestinal cholesterol transporters that are located at the apical brush border membrane of the enterocyte has led to additional protein candidates.[71–74] Using a photoreactive cholesterol derivative photocholesterol, that is, [3α-^{3}H]-6-azi-5α-cholestan-3β-ol, an 80-kDa and a 145-kDa integral membrane protein have been identified as putative components of the intestinal cholesterol transporters.[75] In addition, a photoreactive analogue of ezetimibe was found to bind to a distinct 145-kDa integral membrane protein. These proteins are different from the previously described candidate proteins for the intestinal cholesterol transporters (ABCA1, ABCG5, ABCG8, NPC1L1, and SR-BI). Recently, the 145-kDa ezetimibe-binding protein was purified by three different methods, and the protein sequencing revealed its identity to be the membrane-bound ectoenzyme aminopeptidase N (APN).[76,77] Because APN has a role in endocytotic processes, it was suggested that binding of ezetimibe to APN may block endocytosis of cholesterol-rich membrane microdomains, thereby inhibiting intestinal cholesterol absorption.[76,77] Nevertheless, the exact mechanism whereby APN influences intestinal cholesterol absorption remains to be defined.

The SR-BI protein is expressed in brush border membrane preparations and in Caco-2 cells. Preincubation with an anti–SR-BI antibody partially inhibited cholesterol and cholesteryl ester uptake by brush border membrane vesicles and Caco-2 cells compared with control incubations.[78] These *in vitro* experiments suggested that SR-BI might be a cholesterol transporter in the intestine and involved in the absorption of dietary cholesterol. The distribution of SR-BI along the gastrocolic axis and on the apical membrane of the enterocyte is also consistent with its participation in cholesterol absorption.[79] However, targeted disruption of the *Srb1* gene had little effect on intestinal cholesterol absorption in mice.[80–82] More importantly, the cholesterol absorption inhibitor ezetimibe, which has been shown to label SR-BI in the enterocyte, also inhibits cholesterol absorption in SR-BI–knockout mice,[80] indicating that SR-BI could not be the ezetimibe-sensitive target gene responsible for intestinal cholesterol absorption.

Initial observations showed that some retinoid X receptor (RXR) and LXR nuclear hormone receptor agonists, which up-regulate expression levels of ABCA1 in the intestine, resulted in a decrease in cholesterol absorption when these agents were administered to mice.[83] This led to the suggestion that the intestinal ABCA1 transporter may serve to efflux cholesterol from he enterocyte back into the intestinal lumen for excretion. However, studies in the ABCA1-knockout mouse revealed only marginal increases in cholesterol absorption in one study[84] and decreased cholesterol absorption in another.[85] Subsequent characterization of mice lacking ABCA1[86] and of the Wisconsin hypoalpha mutant (WHAM) chickens, which harbor a spontaneous mutation in the *ABCA1* gene,[87,88] revealed no impairment in percent cholesterol absorption, fecal neutral steroid excretion, or biliary cholesterol secretion. This was true even after challenge with a synthetic LXR agonist. The lack of a role for ABCA1 in cholesterol absorption is further evidenced by *in situ* hybridization studies in which ABCA1 was found predominately in cells present in the lamina propria in mice[60] and only occasionally in the enterocyte in the primate.[89] Instead, it has been hypothesized that ABCA1 may be involved in the transfer of cholesterol from enterocytes into lymph and/or to blood macrophages and may promote efficient cholesterol efflux from enterocytes to plasma high-density lipoprotein (HDL). Apart from ABCG5, ABCG8, and NPC1L1, other as yet unidentified sterol transporters in the intestine may play important roles in the regulation of intestinal absorption of cholesterol and plant sterols. The continued pursuit of these proteins should reveal the molecular and genetic mechanisms underlying the dominant rate-limiting step/factor in intestinal cholesterol absorption.

Intracellular Metabolism of Absorbed Lipids

Another potential step for sorting/regulation is the incompletely characterized intracellular pathway whereby the absorbed cholesterol molecule reaches the endoplasmic reticulum and is esterified to cholesteryl esters by the enzyme acyl-coenzyme A:cholesterol acyltransferase–2 (ACAT2).[90] Fatty acid binding protein (FABP) is present in the small intestine and may play an important role in the intracellular transport of the absorbed fatty acids.[91–93] This assertion is based on the higher concentration of FABP in villi compared with crypts, in jejunum compared with ileum, and in intestinal mucosa of animals fed a high-fat diet compared with those fed a low-fat diet.

Absorbed intestinal cholesterol enters a cholesterol pool within the enterocyte. This pool contains cholesterol from the diet, from nondietary sources (biliary cholesterol and cholesterol from cells shed from the intestinal mucosa), from newly synthesized cholesterol within the enterocyte, and from plasma lipoproteins. The enterocyte may treat these various sources of cholesterol differently. For example, in a fasting state, very little newly synthesized cholesterol is transported into lymph. By contrast, during active lipid absorption, significantly more of the newly synthesized cholesterol is transported into lymph following incorporation into chylomicrons. Cholesterol transported by the lymphatic system is almost exclusively esterified, and the rate of esterification of cholesterol may regulate lymphatic transport. In the small intestine, ACAT2 is highly specific for cholesterol and does not appreciably esterify plant sterols. Cholesteryl esters are incorporated into nascent chylomicrons. This process allows nascent chylomicrons to mature and exit the endoplasmic reticulum for eventual secretion as chylomicron particles into the lymph.[94]

During cholesterol absorption, there is little increase in the cholesterol content of the small intestinal wall, demonstrating that the absorbed cholesterol can be rapidly processed and exported from the enterocyte into the intestinal or thoracic duct lymph. Essentially all cholesterol molecules that move from the intestinal lumen into enterocytes are unesterified; however, cholesterol exported into intestinal lymph following a cholesterol-rich meal is largely esterified. This highlights the notion that the esterification may be an important step for bulk entry of cholesterol into the nascent chylomicrons and suggests that esterifying activity of the enterocyte is an important regulator of intestinal cholesterol absorption. Re-esterification of the absorbed cholesterol within the enterocyte would enhance the diffusion gradient from the lumen to the enterocyte, favoring cholesterol absorption. In this connection, it has been observed that pharmacologic inhibition of ACAT significantly reduces transmucosal transport of cholesterol in rats[95,96] and that deletion of the *Acat2* gene decreases intestinal cholesterol absorption in mice.[97] Moreover, the inhibition of intestinal 3-hydroxy-3-methylglutaryl-coenzyme A (HMG-CoA) reductase by pharmacologic treatment with statins also diminishes intestinal cholesterol absorption in laboratory animals[98,99] and in humans.[100]

Monoacylglycerols and fatty acids are largely reconstituted to form triacylglycerols, mainly via the consecutive actions of monoacylglycerol and diacylglycerol acyltransferases.[101,102] The locations of these enzymes on the cytoplasmic surface of the endoplasmic reticulum[103] suggest that triacylglycerols are formed in the cytoplasmic surface of the endoplasmic reticulum and gain entry into the cisternae of the endoplasmic reticulum. The second pathway present in intestinal mucosa for the formation of triacylglycerols is the α-glycerophosphate pathway that involves the stepwise acylation of glycerol-3-phosphate to form phosphatidic acid. In the presence of phosphatidate phosphohydrolase, phosphatidic acid is hydrolyzed to form diacylglycerols, which are then converted to triacylglycerols. The relative importance of these two pathways depends greatly on the supply of monoacylglycerols and fatty acids.[104] During normal lipid absorption, the monoacylglycerol pathway is the predominant route for the synthesis of triacylglycerols because monoacylglycerols and fatty acids are very efficiently converted to triacylglycerols. Monoacylglycerols also inhibit the α-glycerophosphate pathway. By contrast, when monoacylglycerols are insufficient, the α-glycerophosphate pathway becomes the major route for the formation of triacylglycerols.[104] Some of the absorbed lysophosphatidylcholines are reacylated to form phospholipids, and the others are hydrolyzed to form glycerol-3-phosphorylcholine, which may be transported to the liver via the portal vein. The liberated fatty acids are then used for triacylglycerol synthesis. Finally, some lysophosphatidylcholine molecules are combined to form one molecule of phospholipid and one molecule of glycerol-3-phosphorylcholine.

Assembly and Secretion of Intestinal Lipoproteins

The small intestine secretes predominantly chylomicrons. The assembly of chylomicrons (75 to 450 nm in diameter, $S_f \geq 60$, $d < 0.93$ g/mL) is a characteristic property of the enterocytes during the postprandial state. It is of interest that the small intestine also produces very-low-density lipoprotein (VLDL)–sized particles and HDLs to lesser degrees. The assembly of VLDL (30 to 80 nm in diameter, $S_f = 20$ to 60, $0.93 < d < 1.006$ g/mL) occurs constitutively and is the predominant lipoprotein secreted during the fasting state. VLDL may serve to transport lipids derived from the bile and sloughed enterocytes and fatty acids derived from the plasma. The assembly and secretion of HDL by the small intestine is beyond the scope of this chapter.

Chylomicrons are produced exclusively by the small intestine. These large, spherical particles are lipid rich: triglycerides (85% to 92%), phospholipids (6% to 12%), cholesterol (1% to 3%), and apolipoproteins (apos) (1% to 2%). The compositions indicate their primarily roles as triglyceride transport vehicles. The core of chylomicrons contains triglycerides and cholesteryl esters, whereas the surface of the particles comprises a monolayer of phospholipids, unesterified cholesterol, and apos.[105,106] The major apolipoproteins of chylomicrons are apoB-48, apoA-I, and apoA-IV. Traces of apoE and apoC detected in chylomicrons are added to the surface after interactions of chylomicrons with other plasma lipoproteins.

Chylomicron synthesis takes place within the enterocyte and requires apoB-48 expression that is translated from a common apoB mRNA following post-transcriptional editing in which enzymatic deamination of cytosine by the apoB-editing complex creates a uracil at nucleotide 6666. The nucleotide conversion results in truncation of apoB codon 2153, so that the mature protein is 48% as long as apoB-100 in units of amino acids.[107,108] Fatty acid compositions of triglycerides in intestinal lipoproteins reflect the dietary fatty acids.[109–112] By contrast, the fatty acid compositions of phospholipids (phosphatidylcholines, phosphatidylethanolamines, and sphingomyelins) and cholesteryl esters present in chylomicrons are not representative of the fatty acids present in the diet. Although the size and composition of the secreted chylomicrons are dependent on the rate of fat absorption and the type of fat absorbed, the molecular basis for the trafficking of different lipids for incorporation into chylomicrons by the enterocyte remains unclear.

It has been proposed that the assembly of chylomicrons involves three independent events.[113–117] First, the incorporation of preformed phospholipids and synthesis of smaller lipoproteins result in the formation of primordial lipoproteins. Second, triglyceride-rich lipid droplets of various sizes are synthesized during the postprandial state. Third, the fusion of primordial lipoproteins with triglyceride-rich lipid droplets results in the formation of various lipoproteins (VLDL-sized particles, small chylomicrons, and large chylomicrons), a process called *core expansion.* Core expansion appears to render lipid droplets "secretion competent." This notion is supported by the observation that the smooth endoplasmic reticulum contains lipid droplets without apoB-48 synthesis. In the absence of apoB-48, no droplets are found in the Golgi complex and the intercellular space.[118,119] However, after apoB-48 is synthesized, lipoprotein particles are detected in the Golgi complex and intercellular spaces. Moreover, triglycerides and apoB-48 are transported together from the endoplasmic reticulum to the Golgi complex. Therefore, core expansion may be a crucial step for the regulation of the assembly and secretion of large amounts of triglyceride-rich particles.

Intestinal microsomal triglyceride transfer protein (MTTP) transfers neutral lipids into newly formed chylomicrons in the endoplasmic reticulum.[120] *MTTP* mutations constitute the genetic basis for abetalipoproteinemia in humans, which is characterized by severe steatorrhea, neurologic symptoms, fatty liver, and very low plasma cholesterol levels.[121] Interestingly, targeted disruption of the *Cel* gene in mice induces a significant decrease in the number of chylomicron particles produced by the enterocyte after a lipid meal, with most of the intestinal lipoproteins produced by CEL-knockout mice being VLDL-sized particles.[9] Although the exact mechanism by which CEL participates in chylomicron assembly is unknown at this time, indirect evidence suggests that CEL may have an important effect on intracellular lipid trafficking. Intestinal apos A-I/C-III/A-IV have been proposed to play a role in the regulation of cholesterol absorption.[122] However, the regulatory effects of these proteins remain to be defined. Nevertheless, these collective observations concerning chylomicron assembly suggest that the later steps in the cholesterol absorption process are indeed critically important.

Following secretion into intestinal lymph, chylomicrons enter the blood through the thoracic duct. As they circulate, the triglycerides of chylomicrons undergo hydrolysis by lipoprotein lipase, an enzyme located on the surface of capillary endothelial cells of muscle and adipose tissues. This results in release of fatty acids and glycerol from the core of chylomicrons, as well as unesterified cholesterol from the surface coat of these particles. After lipolysis, chylomicron remnants are released back into the circulation and transform into remnant particles, which are cleared rapidly by the liver with the assistance of hepatic lipase.

FECAL EXCRETION OF INTESTINAL STEROLS

Cholesterol and bile acids that escape intestinal reabsorption are excreted as fecal neutral and acidic sterols, respectively. This constitutes the major route for sterol elimination from the body. Fecal sterol excretion in humans who are in the fasting state or consuming fat-free diets ranges from 0.7 to 1 g/day, but it must be emphasized that fecal sterols do not consist only of dietary residues. Likewise, fecal sterol excretion in patients with steatorrhea exceeds dietary intake, indicating that some of endogenous lipids entering the small intestinal lumen are excreted in feces.

GENETIC ANALYSIS OF INTESTINAL CHOLESTEROL ABSORPTION

There are significant interindividual differences and interstrain variations, respectively, in intestinal cholesterol absorption efficiency in humans[123–127] and in laboratory animals.[128–137] Because diet, the key environmental factor, was controlled in these studies, these observations strongly suggest that intestinal cholesterol absorption is regulated genetically. What is not clear is which cellular step(s) in the intestinal absorption of cholesterol could account for the genetic differences. Siblings of the higher-absorbing probands displayed significantly higher cholesterol absorption efficiency (49% ± 2%) than siblings of the lower-absorbing probands (37% ± 3%).[138] Likewise, there were significant differences in a systematic study of 12 inbred strains of mice in which 3 strains exhibited absorption efficiencies less than 25%, 5 strains from 25% to 30%, and 4 strains from 31% to 40%.[128] Importantly, differences among mouse strains have been shown to be independent of methods of measuring cholesterol absorption.[128,139]

Because a high cholesterol absorption rate is inherited as a dominant trait in certain genetic crosses between inbred mouse strains, quantitative trait locus (QTL) mapping techniques have been applied toward identifying the factors at the enterocyte level that are crucial for determining cholesterol absorption efficiency. Genetic loci that determine cholesterol absorption efficiency have been identified by genome-wide linkage studies in experimental crosses of inbred mouse strains.[134] As shown in Figure 3-3, a QTL that influences cholesterol absorption efficiency was detected on chromosome 2 (designated cholesterol absorption gene locus 1, *Chab1*), and a second suggestive QTL *(Chab2)* was found on chromosome 10. Additional loci were also found: *Chab3* on chromosome 6, *Chab4* on chromosome 15, *Chab5* on chromosome 19, *Chab6* on chromosome 1, and *Chab7* on chromosome 5.[134] Despite these numerous QTL identifications, positional cloning of the responsible genes remains to be accomplished.

FACTORS THAT INFLUENCE INTESTINAL CHOLESTEROL ABSORPTION EFFICIENCY

Because intestinal cholesterol absorption is a multistep process, any factor that can influence the transport of cholesterol from the intestinal lumen to the lymph may influence the efficiency of intestinal cholesterol absorption.[1] Table 3-1 lists dietary, pharmacologic, biliary, luminal, and cellular factors that could influence absorption. When dietary conditions are controlled, biliary factors may be shown to exert a major influence on the efficiency of cholesterol absorption. For example, hepatic output and pool size of biliary bile acids are markedly reduced in mice with homozygous disruption of the cholesterol 7α-hydroxylase *(Cyp7a1)* gene, which encodes the principal bile acid synthetic enzyme in the liver. Because of bile acid deficiency in bile, the mice absorb only trace amounts of cholesterol.[140] Similarly, disruption of the sterol 27-hydroxylase *(Cyp27)* gene, which encodes the main enzyme controlling the alternative pathway of bile acid synthesis, results in a significant reduction in bile acid synthesis. Consequently, intestinal cholesterol absorption decreases from 54% to 4%, and fecal excretion of sterols increases by 2.5-fold.[141] In both types of knockout mice, cholesterol absorption is reversed readily by feeding a bile acid–containing diet.[140,141] These findings confirm that biliary bile acids play a critical role in intestinal cholesterol absorption by regulating intraluminal micellar bile acid concentrations.

Changes in the detergency of biliary bile acids also influence cholesterol absorption. In mice with experimentally induced diabetes, percentages of cholesterol absorption are significantly increased. This is because the biosynthesis of a more detergent bile acid is augmented at the same time as the biosynthesis of a less detergent type of bile acid is reduced.[142] In addition, cholesterol absorption is reduced in a genetically engineered mouse model that does not secrete biliary phospholipids, which are necessary for intestinal cholesterol absorption.[143] Although disruption of the ileal bile acid transporter *(Ibat)* gene eliminates enterohepatic cycling of bile acids in mice, there is only a modest reduction in cholesterol absorption efficiency.[144] This can be explained by the fact that cholesterol absorption occurs predominantly in the proximal

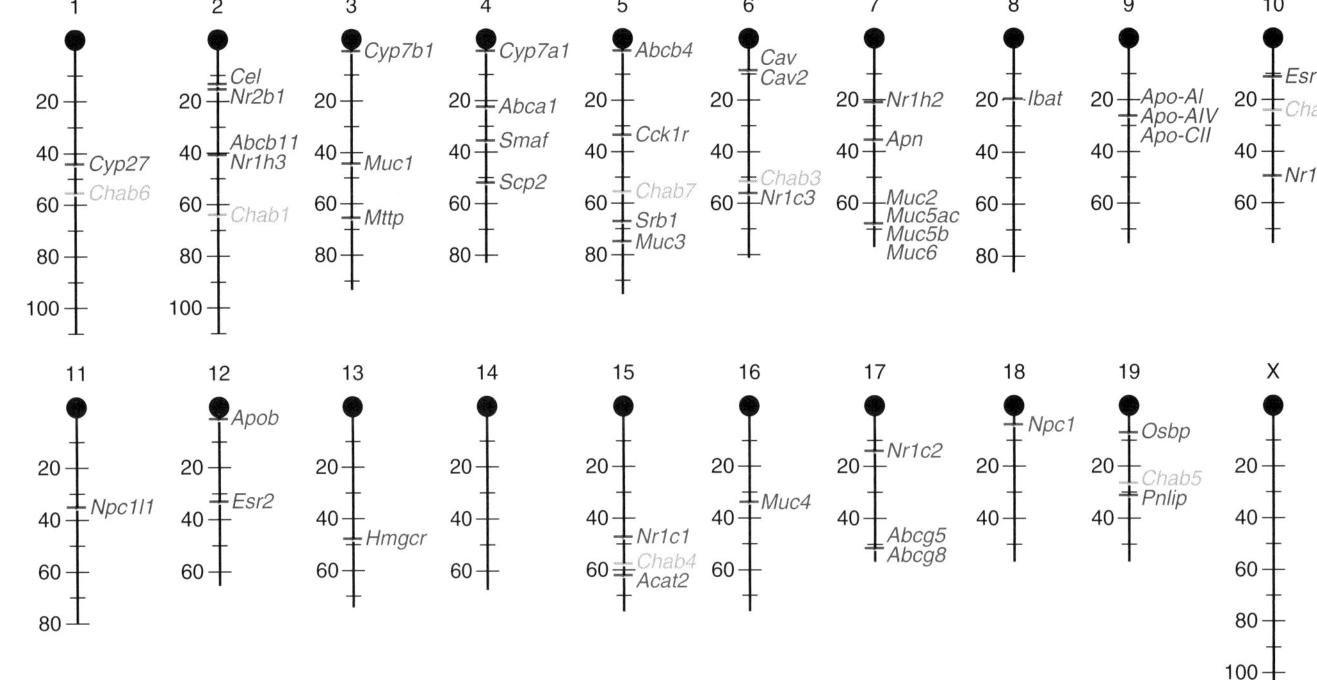

FIGURE 3-3 Composite map of the genes for intestinal sterol transporters and lipid metabolism; quantitative trait loci (QTLs) for cholesterol absorption *(Chab)* genes; and candidate genes for the regulation of cholesterol absorption on chromosomes, representing the entire mouse genome. A vertical line represents each chromosome, with the centromere at the top; genetic distances from the centromere *(horizontal black lines)* are indicated to the left of the chromosomes in centimorgans (cM). Chromosomes are drawn to scale, based on the estimated cM position of the most distally mapped locus taken from Mouse Genome Database (http://www.informatics.jax.org/). The locations of the genes for intestinal sterol transporters and lipid metabolism and candidate genes for the regulation of cholesterol absorption are represented by horizontal red lines; QTLs (*Chab* genes) are indicated by horizontal pink lines with the gene symbols to the right. Apn, Aminopeptidase N; Cav, Caveolin; Cck1r, cholecystokinin 1 receptor; Cel, carboxyl ester lipase; Cyp7a1, cholesterol 7α-hydroxylase; Cyp7b1, oxysterol 7α-hydroxylase; Cyp27, sterol 27α-hydroxylase; Esr1, estrogen receptor α; Esr2, estrogen receptor β; Npc1, Niemann-Pick C1 (protein); Pnlip, pancreatic triglyceride lipase; Smaf, sphingomyelinase (see also Table 3-1 for list of gene symbols and names). (Modified from Ref. 1, with permission.)

intestine, whereas intestinal uptake of bile acids occurs primarily in the distal intestine. In this connection, bile acid concentrations in the proximal intestine are not reduced in mice that are treated with inhibitors of intestinal bile acid reabsorption because of a compensatory increase in bile acid synthesis by the liver.

Small intestinal transit rate is an example of a luminal factor that can influence the efficiency of cholesterol absorption. Mice with deletion of the cholecystokinin-1 receptor *(Cck-1r)* gene absorb cholesterol at higher rates, which correlate with slower small intestinal transit rates.[145] By contrast, guinea pigs are resistant to the systemic effects of dietary cholesterol and display shorter small intestinal transit times than guinea pigs with hypercholesterolemia.[146] Furthermore, acceleration of small intestine transit induced by pharmacologic intervention is consistently associated with decreased cholesterol absorption in humans.[147] It was surprising to find that small intestinal transit times were similar among low, middle, and high cholesterol-absorbing inbred mouse strains.[128] This finding suggests that under normal physiologic conditions, luminal factors may not account for major differences in the efficiency of intestinal cholesterol absorption among diverse inbred strains of mice.

There are well-documented gender differences in the efficiency of cholesterol absorption in humans and in laboratory animals.[148–151] Estrogen increases biliary lipid secretion, which promotes cholesterol absorption.[148,152] In addition, estrogen appears to regulate expression of the sterol transporter genes in the intestine via the estrogen receptor pathway.[148]

Aging augments the efficiency of intestinal cholesterol absorption.[148–151] This is because aging significantly increases the secretion rate of biliary lipids and cholesterol content of bile, as well as size and hydrophobicity index of the bile acid pool. It would be instructive to explore whether aging per se enhances intestinal cholesterol absorption, perhaps via *Longevity* (aging) genes that could influence expression of the intestinal sterol transporter genes.

INHIBITORS OF INTESTINAL CHOLESTEROL ABSORPTION

Plasma cholesterol concentrations are sensitive to changes in the consumption of dietary cholesterol. This is evidenced by the observation that the maximal rise in plasma cholesterol concentrations in response to dietary cholesterol is reached at cholesterol intakes of 400 to 500 mg/day, corresponding to the typical cholesterol content of a Western diet. As a result, restriction of dietary calories, cholesterol, and saturated fat is a rational primary therapeutic intervention for the treatment of patients with dyslipidemia.

Despite significant restrictions in dietary intake, a reduction of dietary cholesterol frequently does not decrease circulating LDL cholesterol levels appreciably. This is due in part to the continued presence of

TABLE 3-1	Possible Factors Influencing Intestinal Cholesterol Absorption						
	Factors	**Effects on Percent Cholesterol Absorption and Type of Study**		**Mouse Chr***	**cM**	**Human Ortholog**	**References**
A. Dietary factors							
↑	Cholesterol	(-)	Animal feeding studies				51
	Fat						
↑	Monounsaturated	↓	African green monkey feeding studies				178
↑	ω-3 polyunsaturated	↓	African green monkey feeding studies				178
↑	Fish oils	↓	Rat lymphatic transport studies				179
↑	Sphingomyelin	↓	Animal feeding studies				180
↑	Fiber	↓	Human and animal feeding studies				181
↑	Plant sterols (phytosterols)	↓	Human and animal feeding studies				55, 59
B. Pharmacologic factors							
↑	Hydrophilic bile acids	↓	Human and animal feeding studies				39
↑	Hydrophobic bile acids	↑	Human and animal feeding studies				39, 182
↑	Ezetimibe	↓	Human and animal feeding studies				61, 158
↑	ACAT inhibitors	↓	Human and animal feeding studies				155, 183, 184
↑	Statins	↓	Human and animal feeding studies				185–187
↑	Bile acid sequestrants	↓	Human and animal feeding studies				188, 189
↑	Intestinal lipase inhibitors	↓	Human and animal feeding studies				153, 154
↑	Estrogen	↑	Animal feeding studies				148
C. Biliary factors							
↓	Biliary bile acid output	↓	Cholesterol 7α-hydroxylase (−/−) mice				140, 190
↓	Size of bile acid pool	↓	Cholesterol 7α-hydroxylase (−/−) mice				140, 190
↓	Biliary phospholipid output	↓	*Abcb4* (−/−) mice				143
↑	Biliary cholesterol output	↑	Animal studies				128, 139
↑	Cholesterol content of bile	↑	Animal studies				128, 139, 142
↑	HI of bile acid pool	↑	Animal studies				39, 142
D. Cellular factors							
↓	ACAT2	↓	ACAT2 inhibitors and *Acat2* (−/−) mice	15	61.7	12q13.13	155, 183, 184
↓	HMG-CoA reductase	↓	HMG-CoA reductase inhibitors in human and mouse studies	13	49.0	5q13.3–q14	185–187
↓	ABCA1	↓↑	*Abca1* (−/−) mice†	4	23.1	9q31.1	83–85
↓	ABCG5 and ABCG8	↑	*Abcg5/g8* (−/−) mice and *Abcg5/g8* transgenic mice; and sitosterolemia	17	54.5	2p21	42–50
↓	NPC1L1	↓	*Npc1l1* (−/−) mice and ezetimibe feeding studies	11	ND	7p13	61–63, 158
	Aminopeptidase N		To be identified	7	ND	15q25–q26	
↓	SR-BI	(-)↓	*Sr-b1* (−/−) mice and *Sr-b1* transgenic mice†	5	68.0	12q24.31	80–82
↓	IBAT	(-)	*Ibat* (−/−) mice	8	20	13q33	144
↓	Caveolin 1	(-)	Caveolin 1 (−/−) mice	6	A2‡	7q31.1	191
	Caveolin 2		To be identified	6	A2	7q31.1	
	MTTP		To be identified	3	66.2	4q24	
	SCP2		To be identified	4	52.0	1p32	

Continued

TABLE 3-1 Possible Factors Influencing Intestinal Cholesterol Absorption—cont'd

	Factors		Effects on Percent Cholesterol Absorption and Type of Study	Mouse Chr*	cM	Human Ortholog	References
	OSBP		To be identified	19	7.0	11q12–q13	
↓	ApoB-48	↓	*ApoB-48* (−/−) mice and "apoB-100-only" mice	12	2.0	2p24–p23	119, 192
	ApoA-I		To be identified	9	27.0	11q23–q24	
↓	ApoA-IV	(−)	*ApoA-IV* (−/−) mice and *ApoA-IV* transgenic mice	9	27.0	11q23	193, 194
	ApoC-III		To be identified	9	27.0	11q23.1–q23.2	
	Estrogen receptor-α		To be identified	10	12.0	6q25.1	
	Estrogen receptor-β		To be identified	12	33.0	14q23.2	
	NR1H4 (FXR)		To be identified	10	50.0	12q23.1	
	NR1H3 (LXR-α)		To be identified	2	40.4	11p11.2	
	NR1H2 (LXR-β)		To be identified	7	ND	19q13.3	
↑	NR2B1 (RXR-α)	↓	RXR agonist and mouse study	2	17.0	9q34.3	83
↑	NR1C1 (PPAR-α)	↓	PPAR-α agonist and PPAR-α (−/−) mice	15	48.8	22q13.31	195
↑	NR1C2 (PPAR-δ)	↓	PPAR-δ agonist and mouse study	17	13.5	6p21.2–p21.1	196
	NR1C3 (PPAR-γ)		To be identified	6	52.7	3p25	
E. Luminal factors							
↑	Small intestinal transit time	↑	Cck-1 receptor (−/−) mice				145
↑	Gastric emptying time	↑	Inbred strains of mice				197
↓	MUC1 mucin	↓	*Muc1* (−/−) mice	3	44.8	1q21	41
	MUC2 mucin		To be identified	7	69.0	11p15.5	
	MUC3 mucin		To be identified	5	75.0	7q22	
	MUC4 mucin		To be identified	16	ND	3q29	
	MUC5ac mucin		To be identified	7	69.0	11p15.5	
	MUC5b mucin		To be identified	7	69.0	11p15.5	
	MUC6 mucin		To be identified	7	69.0	11p15.5	
↓	Carboxyl ester lipase	(-)↓	Carboxyl ester lipase (−/−) mice	2	16.0	9q34.3	9, 10
↓	Pancreatic triglyceride lipase	↓	Pancreatic triglyceride lipase (−/−) mice	19	29.0	10q26.1	11
	Sphingomyelinase		To be identified	4	ND	8q12–q13	

↑, Increased; ↓, decreased; (−), no effect; ABC, ATP-binding cassette (transporter); ACAT, acyl-coenzyme A:cholesterol acyltransferase, apo, apolipoprotein; CCK, cholecystokinin; Chr, chromosome; cM, centimorgan; FXR, farnesoid X receptor; HI, hydrophobicity index; HMG, 3-hydroxy-3-methyglutaryl; IBAT, ileal bile acid transporter; LXR, liver X receptor; MTTP, microsomal triglyceride transfer protein; MUC, mucin gene; ND, not determined; NPC1L1, Niemann-Pick C1-like 1 (protein); NR, nuclear receptor; OSBP, oxysterol-binding protein; p, short arm of the Chr; q, long arm of the Chr; RXR, retinoid X receptor; PPAR, peroxisomal proliferator-activated receptor; SCP2, sterol carrier protein-2; SR-BI, scavenger receptor class B type I.

*Map position is based on conserved homology between mouse and human genomes and assigned indirectly from localization in other species. Information on homologous regions was retrieved from the mouse/human homology databases maintained at the Jackson Laboratory (http://www.informatics.jax.org/searches/marker_form.shtml) and the National Center for Biotechnology Information (http://www.ncbi.nlm.nih.gov/HomoloGene).

†Contradictory results were reported by different groups (see text for details).

‡As inferred from conserved map locations in mouse and human genomes, the mouse gene might be localized on proximal Chr 2 band A2.

Modified from Wang[1] with permission.

large amounts of biliary cholesterol in the intestine. Therefore, pharmacologic inhibition of cholesterol absorption is potentially an effective way of lowering plasma LDL cholesterol levels. Because intestinal cholesterol absorption is a complex process (see Fig. 3-2), there would be expected to be multiple potential therapeutic targets in the management of patients with hypercholesterolemia. For example, specific lipase inhibitors such as orlistat also suppress cholesterol absorption by blocking the digestive process within the gastrointestinal lumen,[153,154] resulting in decreased solubilization of cholesterol. The intestinal ACAT inhibitors have been considered and tested,[155] and the potential to alter ATP-binding cassette (ABC) transporter activity in the intestine is under investigation. Because they have been shown to lower plasma total and LDL cholesterol levels in humans, plant sterols and stanols (phytosterols), ezetimibe, and bile acids are the focus of the following sections.

Plant Sterols and Stanols (Phytosterols)

Over the past decade, plant sterols and stanols as ingredients in functional foods have been demonstrated to reduce plasma cholesterol concentrations.[53–55] The effective dosages are 1.5 to 3 g/day, leading to an 8% to 16% reduction in plasma LDL cholesterol concentrations. Although the dietary intake of cholesterol and plant sterols is almost equal, plant sterols are poorly absorbed. For example, the absorption efficiency of sitosterol and campesterol is 5% to 8% and 9% to 18%, respectively,[156] compared with 30% to 60% of intestinal cholesterol absorption in humans.[123–127] It is likely that most of the plant sterols that do enter the enterocyte are rapidly pumped back into the intestinal lumen for excretion by the actions of ABCG5 and ABCG8. In addition to poor net absorption, plant sterols are efficiently secreted into bile. These combined mechanisms maintain plasma plant sterol concentrations at less than 1 mg/dL in humans. Because plant sterols are insoluble, they must be esterified and incorporated into triglycerides in margarines in order to achieve high concentrations within the intestine.[157] The basic mechanism of inhibitory action of these compounds is that plant sterols can become efficiently incorporated into micelles in the intestinal lumen, displace the cholesterol, and lead to its precipitation with other, nonsolubilized plant sterols.[53–56] Furthermore, competition between cholesterol and plant sterols for incorporation into micelles and for transfer into the brush border membrane could partly explain the inhibitory effect of large amounts of plant sterols on cholesterol absorption. This reduces both hepatic cholesterol and triglyceride contents by reducing delivery of intestinal cholesterol to the liver via chylomicrons. LDL cholesterol is lowered by two different mechanisms: decreased availability of cholesterol for incorporation into VLDL particles and increased expression of the LDL receptor. Because cholesterol absorption from dietary and biliary sources is reduced in the presence of plant sterols, the unabsorbed cholesterol excreted in the feces is substantially increased.

Ezetimibe

Ezetimibe (SCH 58235), 1-(4-fluorophenyl)-(3*R*)-[3-(4-fluorophenyl)-(3*S*)-hydroxypropyl]-(4*S*)-(4-hydroxyphenyl)-2-azetidinone, and an analogue, SCH 48461, (3*R*)-(3-phenylpropyl)-1,(4*S*)-bis(4-methoxyphenyl)-2-azetidinone, are highly selective intestinal cholesterol absorption inhibitors that effectively and potently prevent the absorption of cholesterol by inhibiting the uptake of dietary and biliary cholesterol across the brush border membrane of the enterocyte. The high potency of these compounds is evidenced by a 50% inhibition at doses ranging from 0.0005 to 0.05 mg/kg in a series of different animal models.[61,158] Following oral administration, ezetimibe undergoes rapid glucuronidation in the enterocyte during its first pass.[158–160] Both ezetimibe and its glucuronide undergo enterohepatic cycling. As a result, there is repeated delivery back to the site of action in the intestine, resulting in multiple peaks of the drug and a long elimination half-life of approximately 22 hours.[161] This presumably explains why ezetimibe displays a longer duration of action and the effect of treatment persists for several days following its cessation. These kinetics provide the rationale for once-daily dosing to achieve a therapeutic effect. After oral administration of the glucuronide (SCH-60663), more than 95% of the compound remains in the intestine.[158] The observation that the glucuronide is more potent in inhibiting cholesterol absorption than the parent compound suggests that ezetimibe acts directly in the intestine as a glucuronide.[158] Because ezetimibe and its analogues are relatively small molecular structures and are effective at low concentrations, they do not appear to alter the physical chemistry of lipids within the intestinal lumen. Ezetimibe does not affect the enterohepatic circulation of bile acids and the absorption of fat-soluble vitamins. The wide variation in intestinal cholesterol absorption could explain the observation that the LDL cholesterol-lowering response to ezetimibe is also varied, with some nonresponders and some patients who have a greater-than-anticipated effect.

During ezetimibe treatment, there is a marked compensatory increase in cholesterol synthesis in the liver, but not in the peripheral organs, and an accelerated loss of cholesterol in the feces with little or no change in the rate of conversion of cholesterol to bile acids. Thus, the combination of ezetimibe with HMG-CoA reductase inhibitors has proved to be a potent therapeutic approach to reducing plasma LDL cholesterol levels.[162–168] It has also been used to lower plant sterol levels in patients with sitosterolemia.[169]

Bile Acids

Ursodeoxycholic acid (UDCA) has been used for more than 30 years to treat cholesterol gallstones.[170,171] Decreasing intestinal cholesterol absorption is one of its potential therapeutic actions.[172–175] The principal mechanism whereby hydrophilic bile acids inhibit cholesterol absorption appears to be via the uptake step of the enterocyte by curtailing micellar cholesterol solubilization intraluminally.[39,176] Decreased hydrophobicity of luminal bile acids reduces the bioavailability of cholesterol for absorption by enterocytes. Although previous reports examining cholesterol absorption after UDCA treatment have yielded conflicting results, most, but not all, studies showed that UDCA administration significantly reduced intestinal cholesterol absorption in humans. Nevertheless, in a recent randomized and carefully controlled study,[177] UDCA (15 mg/kg/day) did not decrease cholesterol absorption in adults consuming a controlled ("American Heart Association heart-healthy") diet, even though luminal bile was enriched with UDCA and intraluminal cholesterol solubilized in the aqueous phase was decreased in UDCA-treated subjects compared with controls.

CONCLUSIONS

Cholesterol absorption is a selective process, such that plant sterols are absorbed poorly. Recent research indicates that the activities of ABCG5 and ABCG8 provide an explanation for the selectivity against plant sterols and that NPC1L1-mediated uptake may play a critical role in the ezetimibe-sensitive cholesterol absorption. Accumulating genetic and biochemical evidence suggests the existence of a complex sterol transporter system that facilitates the movement and uptake of cholesterol into the enterocyte. The significant interindividual differences found in humans and the variations observed among inbred mouse strains provide evidence that multiple additional genes are involved in the regulation of intestinal cholesterol absorption. These differences also provide opportunities to apply state-of-the-art genetic techniques to identify the responsible genes. Improved understanding of the molecular mechanisms whereby cholesterol is absorbed in the intestine will no doubt lead to more molecular targets for the prevention and treatment of cardiovascular diseases.

Acknowledgments

This work was supported in part by research grants DK54012 DK73917 (to D.Q.-H.W.), DK56626, and DK48873 (to D.E.C.) from the National Institutes of Health (U.S. Public Health Service), and an Established Investigator Award from the American Heart Association to D.E.C.

REFERENCES

1. Wang DQ-H: Regulation of intestinal cholesterol absorption. *Annu Rev Physiol* 2007;69:221–248.
2. The National Cholesterol Education Program Expert Panel. Executive Summary of the Third Report of the National Cholesterol Education Program (NCEP) Expert Panel on Detection, Evaluation, and Treatment of High Blood Cholesterol in Adults (Adult Treatment Panel III). *JAMA* 2001;285:2486–2497.
3. Grundy SM, Cleeman JI, Merz CN, et al: Implications of recent clinical trials for the National Cholesterol Education Program Adult Treatment Panel III Guidelines. *J Am Coll Cardiol* 2004;44:720–732.
4. Smith SC Jr, Allen J, Blair SN, et al: AHA/ACC guidelines for secondary prevention for patients with coronary and other atherosclerotic vascular disease: 2006 update: endorsed by the National Heart, Lung, and Blood Institute. *Circulation* 2006;113: 2363–2372.
5. Grundy SM, Cleeman JI, Merz CN, et al: Implications of recent clinical trials for the National Cholesterol Education Program Adult Treatment Panel III guidelines. *Circulation* 2004;110: 227–239.
6. Hofmann AF: Bile acids. In Arias IM, Boyer JL, Fausto N, et al (eds): The Liver: Biology and Pathobiology, 3rd ed. *New York, Raven Press*, 1994, pp 677–718.
7. Heuman DM: Quantitative estimation of the hydrophilic-hydrophobic balance of mixed bile salt solutions. *J Lipid Res* 1989;30:719–730.
8. Carey MC, Duane WC: Enterohepatic circulation. In Arias IM, Boyer JL, Fausto N, et al (eds): The Liver: Biology and Pathobiology, 3rd ed. *New York, Raven Press*, 1994, pp 719–767.
9. Kirby RJ, Zheng S, Tso P, et al: Bile salt-stimulated carboxyl ester lipase influences lipoprotein assembly and secretion in intestine: a process mediated via ceramide hydrolysis. *J Biol Chem* 2002;277:4104–4109.
10. Weng W, Li L, van Bennekum AM, et al: Intestinal absorption of dietary cholesteryl ester is decreased but retinyl ester absorption is normal in carboxyl ester lipase knockout mice. *Biochemistry* 1999;38:4143–4149.
11. Huggins KW, Camarota LM, Howles PN, et al: Pancreatic triglyceride lipase deficiency minimally affects dietary fat absorption but dramatically decreases dietary cholesterol absorption in mice. *J Biol Chem* 2003;278:42899–42905.
12. Roberts IM, Montgomery RK, Carey MC: Rat lingual lipase: partial purification, hydrolytic properties, and comparison with pancreatic lipase. *Am J Physiol* 1984;247:G385–393.
13. Field RB, Scow RO: Purification and characterization of rat lingual lipase. *J Biol Chem* 1983;258:14563–14569.
14. Liao TH, Hamosh P, Hamosh M: Fat digestion by lingual lipase: mechanism of lipolysis in the stomach and upper small intestine. *Pediatr Res* 1984;18:402–409.
15. Regan PT, Malagelada JR, Dimagno EP, et al: Reduced intraluminal bile acid concentrations and fat maldigestion in pancreatic insufficiency: correction by treatment. *Gastroenterology* 1979;77:285–289.
16. Bouquet J, Sinaasappel M, Neijens HJ: Malabsorption in cystic fibrosis: mechanisms and treatment. *J Pediatr Gastroenterol Nutr* 1988;7 Suppl 1:S30–S35.
17. Borgstrom B: On the action of pancreatic lipase on triglycerides in vivo and in vitro. *Acta Physiol Scand* 1952;25:328–347.
18. Borgstrom B: On the mechanism of pancreatic lipolysis of glycerides. *Biochim Biophys Acta* 1954;13:491–504.
19. Mattson FH, Volpenhein RA: Hydrolysis of primary and secondary esters of glycerol by pancreatic juice. *J Lipid Res* 1968;9:79–84.
20. Mattson FH, Volpenhein RA: The digestion and absorption of triglycerides. *J Biol Chem* 1964;239:2772–2777.
21. Patton JS, Carey MC: Watching fat digestion. *Science* 1979;204: 145–148.
22. Borgstrom B, Erlanson C: Pancreatic juice co-lipase: physiological importance. *Biochim Biophys Acta* 1971;242:509–513.
23. Erlanson C, Borgstrom B: Purification and further characterization of co-lipase from porcine pancreas. *Biochim Biophys Acta* 1972;271:400–412.
24. Baskys B, Klein E, Lever WF: Lipases of blood and tissues. iii. Purification and properties of pancreatic lipase. *Arch Biochem Biophys* 1963;102:201–209.
25. Morgan RG, Barrowman J, Borgstrom B: The effect of sodium taurodesoxycholate and pH on the gel filtration behavior of rat pancreatic protein and lipases. *Biochim Biophys Acta* 1969;175:65–75.
26. Borgstrom B: On the interactions between pancreatic lipase and colipase and the substrate, and the importance of bile salts. *J Lipid Res* 1975;16:411–417.
27. Lombardo D, Fauvel J, Guy O: Studies on the substrate specificity of a carboxyl ester hydrolase from human pancreatic juice. I. Action on carboxyl esters, glycerides and phospholipids. *Biochim Biophys Acta* 1980;611:136–146.
28. Lombardo D, Guy O: Binding of human pancreatic carboxylic ester hydrolase to lipid interfaces. *Biochim Biophys Acta* 1981;659:401–410.
29. Blackberg L, Lombardo D, Hernell O, et al: Bile salt-stimulated lipase in human milk and carboxyl ester hydrolase in pancreatic juice: are they identical enzymes? *FEBS Lett* 1981;136:284–288.
30. Hofmann AF, Borgstrom B: Physico-chemical state of lipids in intestinal content during their digestion and absorption. *Fed Proc* 1962;21:43–50.
31. Staggers JE, Hernell O, Stafford RJ, et al: Physical-chemical behavior of dietary and biliary lipids during intestinal digestion and absorption. 1. Phase behavior and aggregation states of model lipid systems patterned after aqueous duodenal contents of healthy adult human beings. *Biochemistry* 1990;29:2028–2040.
32. Hernell O, Staggers JE, Carey MC: Physical-chemical behavior of dietary and biliary lipids during intestinal digestion and absorption. 2. Phase analysis and aggregation states of luminal lipids during duodenal fat digestion in healthy adult human beings. *Biochemistry* 1990;29:2041–2056.
33. Siperstein MD, Chaikoff IL, Reinhardt WO: C^{14}-Cholesterol. V. Obligatory function of bile in intestinal absorption of cholesterol. *J Biol Chem* 1952;198:111–114.
34. Hofmann AF, Small DM: Detergent properties of bile salts: correlation with physiological function. *Annu Rev Med* 1967;18: 333–376.

35. Simmonds WJ, Hofmann AF, Theodor E: Absorption of cholesterol from a micellar solution: intestinal perfusion studies in man. *J Clin Invest* 1967;46:874–890.
36. Borgstrom B: The micellar hypothesis of fat absorption: must it be revisited? *Scand J Gastroenterol* 1985;20:389–394.
37. Westergaard H, Dietschy JM: The mechanism whereby bile acid micelles increase the rate of fatty acid and cholesterol uptake into the intestinal mucosal cell. *J Clin Invest* 1976;58:97–108.
38. Wilson FA, Sallee VL, Dietschy JM: Unstirred water layers in intestine: rate determinant of fatty acid absorption from micellar solutions. *Science* 1971;174:1031–1033.
39. Wang DQ-H, Tazuma S, Cohen DE, et al: Feeding natural hydrophilic bile acids inhibits intestinal cholesterol absorption: studies in the gallstone-susceptible mouse. *Am J Physiol Gastrointest Liver Physiol* 2003;285:G494–G502.
40. Wang DQ-H, Lammert F, Cohen DE, et al: Cholic acid aids absorption, biliary secretion, and phase transitions of cholesterol in murine cholelithogenesis. *Am J Physiol* 1999;276: G751–G760.
41. Wang HH, Afdhal NH, Gendler SJ, et al: Lack of the intestinal Muc1 mucin impairs cholesterol uptake and absorption but not fatty acid uptake in Muc1$^{-/-}$ mice. *Am J Physiol Gastrointest Liver Physiol* 2004;287:G547–G554.
42. Berge KE, Tian H, Graf GA, et al: Accumulation of dietary cholesterol in sitosterolemia caused by mutations in adjacent ABC transporters. *Science* 2000;290:1771–1775.
43. Lee MH, Lu K, Hazard S, et al: Identification of a gene, ABCG5, important in the regulation of dietary cholesterol absorption. *Nat Genet* 2001;27:79–83.
44. Bhattacharyya AK, Connor WE: β-Sitosterolemia and xanthomatosis. A newly described lipid storage disease in two sisters. *J Clin Invest* 1974;53:1033–1043.
45. Miettinen TA: Phytosterolaemia, xanthomatosis and premature atherosclerotic arterial disease: a case with high plant sterol absorption, impaired sterol elimination and low cholesterol synthesis. *Eur J Clin Invest* 1980;10:27–35.
46. Salen G, Shore V, Tint GS, et al: Increased sitosterol absorption, decreased removal, and expanded body pools compensate for reduced cholesterol synthesis in sitosterolemia with xanthomatosis. *J Lipid Res* 1989;30:1319–1330.
47. Salen G, Tint GS, Shefer S, et al: Increased sitosterol absorption is offset by rapid elimination to prevent accumulation in heterozygotes with sitosterolemia. *Arterioscler Thromb* 1992;12: 563–568.
48. Yu L, Li-Hawkins J, Hammer RE, et al: Overexpression of ABCG5 and ABCG8 promotes biliary cholesterol secretion and reduces fractional absorption of dietary cholesterol. *J Clin Invest* 2002;110:671–680.
49. Yu L, Hammer RE, Li-Hawkins J, et al: Disruption of Abcg5 and Abcg8 in mice reveals their crucial role in biliary cholesterol secretion. *Proc Natl Acad Sci USA* 2002;99:16237–16242.
50. Wang HH, Patel SB, Carey MC, et al: Quantifying anomalous intestinal sterol uptake, lymphatic transport, and biliary secretion in Abcg8(-/-) mice. *Hepatology* 2007;45:998–1006.
51. Duan LP, Wang HH, Wang DQ-H: Cholesterol absorption is mainly regulated by the jejunal and ileal ATP-binding cassette sterol efflux transporters Abcg5 and Abcg8 in mice. *J Lipid Res* 2004;45:1312–1323.
52. Berge KE, von Bergmann K, Lutjohann D, et al: Heritability of plasma noncholesterol sterols and relationship to DNA sequence polymorphism in ABCG5 and ABCG8. *J Lipid Res* 2002;43:486–494.
53. Maki KC, Davidson MH, Umporowicz DM, et al: Lipid responses to plant-sterol-enriched reduced-fat spreads incorporated into a National Cholesterol Education Program Step I diet. *Am J Clin Nutr* 2001;74:33–43.
54. Miettinen TA, Puska P, Gylling H, et al: Reduction of serum cholesterol with sitostanol-ester margarine in a mildly hypercholesterolemic population. *N Engl J Med* 1995;333: 1308–1312.
55. Ostlund RE Jr, Racette SB, Okeke A, et al: Phytosterols that are naturally present in commercial corn oil significantly reduce cholesterol absorption in humans. *Am J Clin Nutr* 2002;75: 1000–1004.
56. Nissinen M, Gylling H, Vuoristo M, et al: Micellar distribution of cholesterol and phytosterols after duodenal plant stanol ester infusion. *Am J Physiol Gastrointest Liver Physiol* 2002;282: G1009–G1015.
57. Ikeda I, Tanabe Y, Sugano M: Effects of sitosterol and sitostanol on micellar solubility of cholesterol. *J Nutr Sci Vitaminol (Tokyo)* 1989;35:361–369.
58. Ikeda I, Tanaka K, Sugano M, et al: Discrimination between cholesterol and sitosterol for absorption in rats. *J Lipid Res* 1988;29:1583–1591.
59. Ikeda I, Tanaka K, Sugano M, et al: Inhibition of cholesterol absorption in rats by plant sterols. *J Lipid Res* 1988;29: 1573–1582.
60. Repa JJ, Berge KE, Pomajzl C, et al: Regulation of ATP-binding cassette sterol transporters ABCG5 and ABCG8 by the liver X receptors α and β. *J Biol Chem* 2002;277:18793–18800.
61. van Heek M, Farley C, Compton DS, et al: Comparison of the activity and disposition of the novel cholesterol absorption inhibitor, SCH58235, and its glucuronide, SCH60663. *Br J Pharmacol* 2000;129:1748–1754.
62. Altmann SW, Davis HR Jr, Zhu LJ, et al: Niemann-Pick C1 Like 1 protein is critical for intestinal cholesterol absorption. *Science* 2004;303:1201–1204.
63. Davis HR Jr, Zhu LJ, Hoos LM, et al: Niemann-Pick C1 Like 1 (NPC1L1) is the intestinal phytosterol and cholesterol transporter and a key modulator of whole-body cholesterol homeostasis. *J Biol Chem* 2004;279:33586–33592.
64. Carstea ED, Morris JA, Coleman KG, et al: Niemann-Pick C1 disease gene: homology to mediators of cholesterol homeostasis. *Science* 1997;277:228–231.
65. Davies JP, Levy B, Ioannou YA: Evidence for a Niemann-Pick C (NPC) gene family: identification and characterization of NPC1L1. *Genomics* 2000;65:137–145.
66. Iyer SP, Yao X, Crona JH, et al: Characterization of the putative native and recombinant rat sterol transporter Niemann-Pick C1 Like 1 (NPC1L1) protein. *Biochim Biophys Acta* 2005;1722:282–292.
67. Garcia-Calvo M, Lisnock J, Bull HG, et al: The target of ezetimibe is Niemann-Pick C1-Like 1 (NPC1L1). *Proc Natl Acad Sci USA* 2005;102:8132–8137.
68. Smart EJ, De Rose RA, Farber SA: Annexin 2-caveolin 1 complex is a target of ezetimibe and regulates intestinal cholesterol transport. *Proc Natl Acad Sci USA* 2004;101:3450–3455.
69. Repa JJ, Dietschy JM, Turley SD: Inhibition of cholesterol absorption by SCH 5805. in the mouse is not mediated via changes in the expression of mRNA for ABCA1, ABCG5, or ABCG8 in the enterocyte. *J Lipid Res* 2002;43:1864–1874.
70. van Heek M, Farley C, Compton DS, et al: Ezetimibe selectively inhibits intestinal cholesterol absorption in rodents in the presence and absence of exocrine pancreatic function. *Br J Pharmacol* 2001;134:409–417.
71. Sparrow CP, Patel S, Baffic J, et al: A fluorescent cholesterol analog traces cholesterol absorption in hamsters and is esterified in vivo and in vitro. *J Lipid Res* 1999;40:1747–1757.
72. Hernandez M, Montenegro J, Steiner M, et al: Intestinal absorption of cholesterol is mediated by a saturable, inhibitable transporter. *Biochim Biophys Acta* 2000;1486:232–242.
73. Detmers PA, Patel S, Hernandez M, et al: A target for cholesterol absorption inhibitors in the enterocyte brush border membrane. *Biochim Biophys Acta* 2000;1486:243–252.
74. Kramer W, Glombik H, Petry S, et al: Identification of binding proteins for cholesterol absorption inhibitors as components of the intestinal cholesterol transporter. *FEBS Lett* 2000;487: 293–297.
75. Kramer W, Girbig F, Corsiero D, et al: Intestinal cholesterol absorption: identification of different binding proteins for cholesterol and cholesterol absorption inhibitors in the enterocyte brush border membrane. *Biochim Biophys Acta* 2003;1633:13–26.
76. Kramer W, Girbig F, Corsiero D, et al: Aminopeptidase N (CD13) is a molecular target of the cholesterol absorption inhibitor ezetimibe in the enterocyte brush border membrane. *J Biol Chem* 2005;280:1306–1320.
77. Orso E, Werner T, Wolf Z, et al: Ezetimib influences the expression of raft-associated antigens in human monocytes. *Cytometry A* 2006;69:206–208.
78. Hauser H, Dyer JH, Nandy A, et al: Identification of a receptor mediating absorption of dietary cholesterol in the intestine. *Biochemistry* 1998;37:17843–17850.
79. Cai SF, Kirby RJ, Howles PN, et al: Differentiation-dependent expression and localization of the class B type I scavenger receptor in intestine. *J Lipid Res* 2001;42:902–909.

80. Altmann SW, Davis HR Jr, Yao X, et al: The identification of intestinal scavenger receptor class B, type I (SR-BI) by expression cloning and its role in cholesterol absorption. *Biochim Biophys Acta* 2002;1580:77–93.
81. Mardones P, Quinones V, Amigo L, et al: Hepatic cholesterol and bile acid metabolism and intestinal cholesterol absorption in scavenger receptor class B type I-deficient mice. *J Lipid Res* 2001;42:170–180.
82. Wang DQ-H, Carey MC: Susceptibility to murine cholesterol gallstone formation is not affected by partial disruption of the HDL receptor SR-BI. *Biochim Biophys Acta* 2002;1583:141–150.
83. Repa JJ, Turley SD, Lobaccaro JA, et al: Regulation of absorption and ABC1-mediated efflux of cholesterol by RXR heterodimers. *Science* 2000;289:1524–1529.
84. McNeish J, Aiello RJ, Guyot D, et al: High-density lipoprotein deficiency and foam cell accumulation in mice with targeted disruption of ATP-binding cassette transporter-1. *Proc Natl Acad Sci USA* 2000;97:4245–4250.
85. Drobnik W, Lindenthal B, Lieser B, et al: ATP-binding cassette transporter A1 (ABCA1) affects total body sterol metabolism. *Gastroenterology* 2001;120:1203–1211.
86. Plosch T, Kok T, Bloks VW, et al: Increased hepatobiliary and fecal cholesterol excretion upon activation of the liver X receptor is independent of ABCA1. *J Biol Chem* 2002;277: 33870–33877.
87. Attie AD, Hamon Y, Brooks-Wilson AR, et al: Identification and functional analysis of a naturally occurring E89K mutation in the ABCA1 gene of the WHAM chicken. *J Lipid Res* 2002;43:1610–1617.
88. Mulligan JD, Flowers MT, Tebon A, et al: ABCA1 is essential for efficient basolateral cholesterol efflux during the absorption of dietary cholesterol in chickens. *J Biol Chem* 2003;278: 13356–13366.
89. Lawn RM, Wade DP, Couse TL, et al: Localization of human ATP-binding cassette transporter 1 (ABC1) in normal and atherosclerotic tissues. *Arterioscler Thromb Vasc Biol* 2001;21: 378–385.
90. Lee RG, Willingham MC, Davis MA, et al: Differential expression of ACAT1 and ACAT2 among cells within liver, intestine, kidney, and adrenal of nonhuman primates. *J Lipid Res* 2000;41:1991–2001.
91. Abumrad N, Harmon C, Ibrahimi A: Membrane transport of long-chain fatty acids: evidence for a facilitated process. *J Lipid Res* 1998;39:2309–2318.
92. Stahl A, Hirsch DJ, Gimeno RE, et al: Identification of the major intestinal fatty acid transport protein. *Mol Cell* 1999;4:299–308.
93. Poirier H, Degrace P, Niot I, et al: Localization and regulation of the putative membrane fatty-acid transporter (FAT) in the small intestine. Comparison with fatty acid-binding proteins (FABP). *Eur J Biochem* 1996;238:368–373.
94. van Greevenbroek MM, Robertus-Teunissen MG, Erkelens DW, et al: Participation of the microsomal triglyceride transfer protein in lipoprotein assembly in Caco-2 cells: interaction with saturated and unsaturated dietary fatty acids. *J Lipid Res* 1998;39:173–185.
95. Heider JG, Pickens CE, Kelly LA: Role of acyl CoA:cholesterol acyltransferase in cholesterol absorption and its inhibition by 57-118 in the rabbit. *J Lipid Res* 1983;24:1127–1134.
96. Clark SB, Tercyak AM: Reduced cholesterol transmucosal transport in rats with inhibited mucosal acyl CoA:cholesterol acyltransferase and normal pancreatic function. *J Lipid Res* 1984;25:148–159.
97. Buhman KK, Accad M, Novak S, et al: Resistance to diet-induced hypercholesterolemia and gallstone formation in ACAT2-deficient mice. *Nat Med* 2000;6:1341–1347.
98. Hajri T, Ferezou J, Laruelle C, et al: Crilvastatin, a new 3-hydroxy-3-methylglutaryl-coenzyme A reductase inhibitor, inhibits cholesterol absorption in genetically hypercholesterolemic rats. *Eur J Pharmacol* 1995;286:131–136.
99. Nielsen LB, Stender S, Kjeldsen K: Effect of lovastatin on cholesterol absorption in cholesterol-fed rabbits. *Pharmacol Toxicol* 1993;72:148–151.
100. Vanhanen H, Kesaniemi YA, Miettinen TA: Pravastatin lowers serum cholesterol, cholesterol-precursor sterols, fecal steroids, and cholesterol absorption in man. *Metabolism* 1992;41: 588–595.
101. Manganaro F, Kuksis A: Purification and preliminary characterization of 2-monoacylglycerol acyltransferase from rat intestinal villus cells. *Can J Biochem Cell Biol* 1985;63: 341–347.
102. Rao GA, Johnston JM: Purification and properties of triglyceride synthetase from the intestinal mucosa. *Biochim Biophys Acta* 1966;125:465–473.
103. Bell RM, Ballas LM, Coleman RA: Lipid topogenesis. *J Lipid Res* 1981;22:391–403.
104. Polheim D, David JS, Schultz FM, et al: Regulation of triglyceride biosynthesis in adipose and intestinal tissue. *J Lipid Res* 1973;14:415–421.
105. Miller KW, Small DM: Surface-to-core and interparticle equilibrium distributions of triglyceride-rich lipoprotein lipids. *J Biol Chem* 1983;258:13772–13784.
106. Miller KW, Small DM: Triolein-cholesteryl oleate-cholesterol-lecithin emulsions: structural models of triglyceride-rich lipoproteins. *Biochemistry* 1983;22:443–451.
107. Chen SH, Habib G, Yang CY, et al: Apolipoprotein B-48 is the product of a messenger RNA with an organ-specific in-frame stop codon. *Science* 1987;238:363–366.
108. Powell LM, Wallis SC, Pease RJ, et al: A novel form of tissue-specific RNA processing produces apolipoprotein-B48 in intestine. *Cell* 1987;50:831–840.
109. Zilversmit DB: The composition and structure of lymph chylomicrons in dog, rat, and man. *J Clin Invest* 1965;44:1610–1622.
110. Redgrave TG, Dunne KB: Chylomicron formation and composition in unanaesthetised rabbits. *Atherosclerosis* 1975;22:389–400.
111. Karmen A, Whyte M, Goodman DS: Fatty acid esterification and chylomicron formation during fat absorption. 1. Triglycerides and cholesterol esters. *J Lipid Res* 1963;4:312–321.
112. Whyte M, Karmen A, Goodman DS: Fatty acid esterification and chylomicron formation during fat absorption. 2. Phospholipids. *J Lipid Res* 1963;4:322–329.
113. Hussain MM: A proposed model for the assembly of chylomicrons. *Atherosclerosis* 2000;148:1–15.
114. Dashti N: Synthesis and secretion of nascent lipoprotein particles. *Prog Lipid Res* 1991;30:219–230.
115. Levy E, Mehran M, Seidman E: Caco-2 cells as a model for intestinal lipoprotein synthesis and secretion. *FASEB J* 1995;9:626–635.
116. Field FJ, Mathur SN: Intestinal lipoprotein synthesis and secretion. *Prog Lipid Res* 1995;34:185–198.
117. Green PH, Glickman RM: Intestinal lipoprotein metabolism. *J Lipid Res* 1981;22:1153–1173.
118. Hamilton RL, Wong JS, Cham CM, et al: Chylomicron-sized lipid particles are formed in the setting of apolipoprotein B deficiency. *J Lipid Res* 1998;39:1543–1557.
119. Young SG, Cham CM, Pitas RE, et al: A genetic model for absent chylomicron formation: mice producing apolipoprotein B in the liver, but not in the intestine. *J Clin Invest* 1995;96: 2932–2946.
120. Gordon DA, Jamil H, Gregg RE, et al: Inhibition of the microsomal triglyceride transfer protein blocks the first step of apolipoprotein B lipoprotein assembly but not the addition of bulk core lipids in the second step. *J Biol Chem* 1996;271: 33047–33053.
121. Wetterau JR, Aggerbeck LP, Bouma ME, et al: Absence of microsomal triglyceride transfer protein in individuals with abetalipoproteinemia. *Science* 1992;258:999–1001.
122. Ordovas JM, Schaefer EJ: Genetic determinants of plasma lipid response to dietary intervention: the role of the APOA1/C3/A4 gene cluster and the APOE gene. *Br J Nutr* 2000;83 Suppl 1: S127–S136.
123. McNamara DJ, Kolb R, Parker TS, et al: Heterogeneity of cholesterol homeostasis in man. Response to changes in dietary fat quality and cholesterol quantity. *J Clin Invest* 1987;79:1729–1739.
124. Kesaniemi YA, Miettinen TA: Cholesterol absorption efficiency regulates plasma cholesterol level in the Finnish population. *Eur J Clin Invest* 1987;17:391–395.
125. Sehayek E, Nath C, Heinemann T, et al: U-shape relationship between change in dietary cholesterol absorption and plasma lipoprotein responsiveness and evidence for extreme interindividual variation in dietary cholesterol absorption in humans. *J Lipid Res* 1998;39:2415–2422.

126. Miettinen TA, Tilvis RS, Kesaniemi YA: Serum plant sterols and cholesterol precursors reflect cholesterol absorption and synthesis in volunteers of a randomly selected male population. *Am J Epidemiol* 1990;131:20–31.
127. Bosner MS, Lange LG, Stenson WF, et al: Percent cholesterol absorption in normal women and men quantified with dual stable isotopic tracers and negative ion mass spectrometry. *J Lipid Res* 1999;40:302–308.
128. Wang DQ-H, Paigen B, Carey MC: Genetic factors at the enterocyte level account for variations in intestinal cholesterol absorption efficiency among inbred strains of mice. *J Lipid Res* 2001;42:1820–1830.
129. Bhattacharyya AK, Eggen DA: Cholesterol absorption and turnover in rhesus monkeys as measured by two methods. *J Lipid Res* 1980;21:518–524.
130. Lofland HB, Jr., Clarkson TB, St Clair RW, et al: Studies on the regulation of plasma cholesterol levels in squirrel monkeys of two genotypes. *J Lipid Res* 1972;13:39–47.
131. Kirk EA, Moe GL, Caldwell MT, et al: Hyper- and hypo-responsiveness to dietary fat and cholesterol among inbred mice: searching for level and variability genes. *J Lipid Res* 1995;36:1522–1532.
132. Carter CP, Howles PN, Hui DY: Genetic variation in cholesterol absorption efficiency among inbred strains of mice. *J Nutr* 1997;127:1344–1348.
133. Jolley CD, Dietschy JM, Turley SD: Genetic differences in cholesterol absorption in 129/Sv and C57BL/6 mice: effect on cholesterol responsiveness. *Am J Physiol* 1999;276:G1117–G1124.
134. Schwarz M, Davis DL, Vick BR, et al: Genetic analysis of intestinal cholesterol absorption in inbred mice. *J Lipid Res* 2001;42:1801–1811.
135. Beynen AC, Meijer GW, Lemmens AG, et al: Sterol balance and cholesterol absorption in inbred strains of rabbits hypo- or hyperresponsive to dietary cholesterol. *Atherosclerosis* 1989;77: 151–157.
136. Van Zutphen LF, Fox RR: Strain differences in response to dietary cholesterol by JAX rabbits: correlation with esterase patterns. *Atherosclerosis* 1977;28:435–446.
137. Van Zutphen LF, Den Bieman MG: Cholesterol response in inbred strains of rats, Rattus norvegicus. *J Nutr* 1981;111: 1833–1838.
138. Gylling H, Miettinen TA: Inheritance of cholesterol metabolism of probands with high or low cholesterol absorption. *J Lipid Res* 2002;43:1472–1476.
139. Wang DQ-H, Carey MC: Measurement of intestinal cholesterol absorption by plasma and fecal dual-isotope ratio, mass balance, and lymph fistula methods in the mouse: an analysis of direct versus indirect methodologies. *J Lipid Res* 2003;44:1042–1059.
140. Schwarz M, Russell DW, Dietschy JM, et al: Alternate pathways of bile acid synthesis in the cholesterol 7a-hydroxylase knockout mouse are not upregulated by either cholesterol or cholestyramine feeding. *J Lipid Res* 2001;42:1594–1603.
141. Repa JJ, Lund EG, Horton JD, et al: Disruption of the sterol 27-hydroxylase gene in mice results in hepatomegaly and hypertriglyceridemia. Reversal by cholic acid feeding. *J Biol Chem* 2000;275:39685–39692.
142. Akiyoshi T, Uchida K, Takase H, et al: Cholesterol gallstones in alloxan-diabetic mice. *J Lipid Res* 1986;27:915–924.
143. Voshol PJ, Havinga R, Wolters H, et al: Reduced plasma cholesterol and increased fecal sterol loss in multidrug resistance gene 2 P-glycoprotein-deficient mice. *Gastroenterology* 1998;114:1024–1034.
144. Dawson PA, Haywood J, Craddock AL, et al: Targeted deletion of the ileal bile acid transporter eliminates enterohepatic cycling of bile acids in mice. *J Biol Chem* 2003;278: 33920–33927.
145. Wang DQ-H, Schmitz F, Kopin AS, et al: Targeted disruption of the murine cholecystokinin-1 receptor promotes intestinal cholesterol absorption and susceptibility to cholesterol cholelithiasis. *J Clin Invest* 2004;114:521–528.
146. Traber MG, Ostwald R: Cholesterol absorption and steroid excretion in cholesterol-fed guinea pigs. *J Lipid Res* 1978;19:448–456.
147. Ponz de Leon M, Iori R, Barbolini G, et al: Influence of small-bowel transit time on dietary cholesterol absorption in human beings. *N Engl J Med* 1982;307:102–103.
148. Duan LP, Wang HH, Ohashi A, et al: Role of intestinal sterol transporters Abcg5, Abcg8, and Npc1l1 in cholesterol absorption in mice: gender and age effects. *Am J Physiol Gastrointest Liver Physiol* 2006;290:G269–G276.
149. Turley SD, Schwarz M, Spady DK, et al: Gender-related differences in bile acid and sterol metabolism in outbred CD-1 mice fed low- and high-cholesterol diets. *Hepatology* 1998;28:1088–1094.
150. Hollander D, Morgan D: Increase in cholesterol intestinal absorption with aging in the rat. *Exp Gerontol* 1979;14:201–204.
151. Wang DQ-H: Aging per se is an independent risk factor for cholesterol gallstone formation in gallstone susceptible mice. *J Lipid Res* 2002;43:1950–1959.
152. Wang HH, Afdhal NH, Wang DQ-H: Estrogen receptor a, but not b, plays a major role in 17b-estradiol-induced murine cholesterol gallstones. *Gastroenterology* 2004;127:239–249.
153. Mittendorfer B, Ostlund RE Jr, Patterson BW, et al: Orlistat inhibits dietary cholesterol absorption. *Obes Res* 2001;9: 599–604.
154. Muls E, Kolanowski J, Scheen A, et al: The effects of orlistat on weight and on serum lipids in obese patients with hypercholesterolemia: a randomized, double-blind, placebo-controlled, multicentre study. *Int J Obes Relat Metab Disord* 2001;25: 1713–1721.
155. Insull W Jr, Koren M, Davignon J, et al: Efficacy and short-term safety of a new ACAT inhibitor, avasimibe, on lipids, lipoproteins, and apolipoproteins, in patients with combined hyperlipidemia. *Atherosclerosis* 2001;157:137–144.
156. Heinemann T, Axtmann G, von Bergmann K: Comparison of intestinal absorption of cholesterol with different plant sterols in man. *Eur J Clin Invest* 1993;23:827–831.
157. Hallikainen MA, Sarkkinen ES, Gylling H, et al: Comparison of the effects of plant sterol ester and plant stanol ester-enriched margarines in lowering serum cholesterol concentrations in hypercholesterolaemic subjects on a low-fat diet. *Eur J Clin Nutr* 2000;54:715–725.
158. Sudhop T, von Bergmann K: Cholesterol absorption inhibitors for the treatment of hypercholesterolaemia. *Drugs* 2002;62: 2333–2347.
159. Clader JW, Burnett DA, Caplen MA, et al: 2-Azetidinone cholesterol absorption inhibitors: structure-activity relationships on the heterocyclic nucleus. *J Med Chem* 1996;39:3684–3693.
160. Van Heek M, France CF, Compton DS, et al: In vivo metabolism-based discovery of a potent cholesterol absorption inhibitor, SCH58235, in the rat and rhesus monkey through the identification of the active metabolites of SCH48461. *J Pharmacol Exp Ther* 1997;283:157–163.
161. Ezzet F, Krishna G, Wexler DB, et al: A population pharmacokinetic model that describes multiple peaks due to enterohepatic recirculation of ezetimibe. *Clin Ther* 2001;23:871–885.
162. Melani L, Mills R, Hassman D, et al: Efficacy and safety of ezetimibe coadministered with pravastatin in patients with primary hypercholesterolemia: a prospective, randomized, double-blind trial. *Eur Heart J* 2003;24:717–728.
163. Feldman T, Koren M, Insull W Jr, et al: Treatment of high-risk patients with ezetimibe plus simvastatin co-administration versus simvastatin alone to attain National Cholesterol Education Program Adult Treatment Panel III low-density lipoprotein cholesterol goals. *Am J Cardiol* 2004;93:1481–1486.
164. Gagne C, Gaudet D, Bruckert E: Efficacy and safety of ezetimibe coadministered with atorvastatin or simvastatin in patients with homozygous familial hypercholesterolemia. *Circulation* 2002;105:2469–2475.
165. Knopp RH, Dujovne CA, Le Beaut A, et al: Evaluation of the efficacy, safety, and tolerability of ezetimibe in primary hypercholesterolaemia: a pooled analysis from two controlled phase III clinical studies. *Int J Clin Pract* 2003;57:363–368.
166. Dujovne CA, Bays H, Davidson MH, et al: Reduction of LDL cholesterol in patients with primary hypercholesterolemia by SCH 48461: results of a multicenter dose-ranging study. *J Clin Pharmacol* 2001;41:70–78.
167. Bays HE, Moore PB, Drehobl MA, et al: Effectiveness and tolerability of ezetimibe in patients with primary hypercholesterolemia: pooled analysis of two phase II studies. *Clin Ther* 2001;23:1209–1230.
168. Dujovne CA, Ettinger MP, McNeer JF, et al: Efficacy and safety of a potent new selective cholesterol absorption inhibitor,

ezetimibe, in patients with primary hypercholesterolemia. *Am J Cardiol* 2002;90:1092–1097.

169. Salen G, von Bergmann K, Lutjohann D, et al: Ezetimibe effectively reduces plasma plant sterols in patients with sitosterolemia. *Circulation* 2004;109:966–971.
170. Tokyo Cooperative Gallstone Study Group: Efficacy and indications of ursodeoxycholic acid treatment for dissolving gallstones. A multicenter double-blind trial. *Gastroenterology* 1980;78:542–548.
171. Makino I, Shinozaki K, Yoshino K, et al: Dissolution of cholesterol gallstones by long-term administration of ursodeoxycholic acid. *Jpn J Gastroenterol* 1975;72:690–702.
172. Ponz de Leon M, Carulli N, Loria P, et al: Cholesterol absorption during bile acid feeding. Effect of ursodeoxycholic acid (UDCA) administration. *Gastroenterology* 1980;78:214–219.
173. Lanzini A, Northfield TC: Effect of ursodeoxycholic acid on biliary lipid coupling and on cholesterol absorption during fasting and eating in subjects with cholesterol gallstones. *Gastroenterology* 1988;95:408–416.
174. Hardison WG, Grundy SM: Effect of ursodeoxycholate and its taurine conjugate on bile acid synthesis and cholesterol absorption. *Gastroenterology* 1984;87:130–135.
175. Leiss O, von Bergmann K, Streicher U, et al: Effect of three different dihydroxy bile acids on intestinal cholesterol absorption in normal volunteers. *Gastroenterology* 1984;87:144–149.
176. Watt SM, Simmonds WJ: Effects of four taurine-conjugated bile acids on mucosal uptake and lymphatic absorption of cholesterol in the rat. *J Lipid Res* 1984;25:448–455.
177. Woollett LA, Buckley DD, Yao L, et al: Effect of ursodeoxycholic acid on cholesterol absorption and metabolism in humans. *J Lipid Res* 2003;44:935–942.
178. Johnson FL, St Clair RW, Rudel LL. Effects of the degree of saturation of dietary fat on the hepatic production of lipoproteins in the African green monkey. *J Lipid Res* 1985;26:403–417.
179. Chen IS, Hotta SS, Ikeda I, et al: Digestion, absorption and effects on cholesterol absorption of menhaden oil, fish oil concentrate and corn oil by rats. *J Nutr* 1987;117:1676–1680.
180. Eckhardt ER, Wang DQ-H, Donovan JM, et al: Dietary sphingomyelin suppresses intestinal cholesterol absorption by decreasing thermodynamic activity of cholesterol monomers. *Gastroenterology* 2002;122:948–956.
181. Vahouny GV, Roy T, Gallo LL, et al: Dietary fiber and lymphatic absorption of cholesterol in the rat. *Am J Clin Nutr* 1978;31:S208–S210.
182. Huggins KW, Camarota LM, Howles PN, et al: Pancreatic triglyceride lipase deficiency minimally affects dietary fat absorption but dramatically decreases dietary cholesterol absorption in mice. *J Biol Chem* 2003;278:42899–42905.
183. Bennett Clark S, Tercyak AM: Reduced cholesterol transmucosal transport in rats with inhibited mucosal acyl CoA:cholesterol acyltransferase and normal pancreatic function. *J Lipid Res* 1984;25:148–159.
184. Heider JG, Pickens CE, Kelly LA: Role of acyl CoA:cholesterol acyltransferase in cholesterol absorption and its inhibition by 57-118 in the rabbit. *J Lipid Res* 1983;24:1127–1134.
185. Nielsen LB, Stender S, Kjeldsen K: Effect of lovastatin on cholesterol absorption in cholesterol-fed rabbits. *Pharmacol Toxicol* 1993;72:148–151.
186. Hajri T, Ferezou J, Laruelle C, et al: Crilvastatin, a new 3-hydroxy-3-methylglutaryl-coenzyme A reductase inhibitor, inhibits cholesterol absorption in genetically hypercholesterolemic rats. *Eur J Pharmacol* 1995;286:131–136.
187. Vanhanen H, Kesaniemi YA, Miettinen TA: Pravastatin lowers serum cholesterol, cholesterol-precursor sterols, fecal steroids, and cholesterol absorption in man. *Metabolism* 1992;41:588–595.
188. Davidson MH, Dillon MA, Gordon B, et al: Colesevelam hydrochloride holestagel: a new, potent bile acid sequestrant associated with a low incidence of gastrointestinal side effects. *Arch Intern Med* 1999;159:1893–1900.
189. Insull W Jr, Toth P, Mullican W, et al: Effectiveness of colesevelam hydrochloride in decreasing LDL cholesterol in patients with primary hypercholesterolemia: a 24-week randomized controlled trial. *Mayo Clin Proc* 2001;76:971–982.
190. Schwarz M, Russell DW, Dietschy JM, et al: Marked reduction in bile acid synthesis in cholesterol 7α-hydroxylase-deficient mice does not lead to diminished tissue cholesterol turnover or to hypercholesterolemia. *J Lipid Res* 1998;39:1833–1843.
191. Valasek MA, Weng J, Shaul PW, et al: Caveolin-1 is not required for murine intestinal cholesterol transport. *J Biol Chem* 2005;280:28103–28109.
192. Wang HH, Wang DQ-H. Reduced susceptibility to cholesterol gallstone formation in mice that do not produce apolipoprotein B48 in the intestine. *Hepatology* 2005;42:894–904.
193. Weinstock PH, Bisgaier CL, Hayek T, et al: Decreased HDL cholesterol levels but normal lipid absorption, growth, and feeding behavior in apolipoprotein A-IV knockout mice. *J Lipid Res* 1997;38:1782–1794.
194. Aalto-Setala K, Bisgaier CL, Ho A, et al: Intestinal expression of human apolipoprotein A-IV in transgenic mice fails to influence dietary lipid absorption or feeding behavior. *J Clin Invest* 1994;93:1776–1786.
195. Knight BL, Patel DD, Humphreys SM, et al: Inhibition of cholesterol absorption associated with a PPARα-dependent increase in ABC binding cassette transporter A1 in mice. *J Lipid Res* 2003;44:2049–2058.
196. van der Veen JN, Kruit JK, Havinga R, et al: Reduced cholesterol absorption upon PPARδ activation coincides with decreased intestinal expression of NPC1L1. *J Lipid Res* 2005;46:526–534.
197. Kirby RJ, Howles PN, Hui DY: Rate of gastric emptying influences dietary cholesterol absorption efficiency in selected inbred strains of mice. *J Lipid Res* 2004;45:89–98.

CHAPTER 4

High-Density Lipoprotein Metabolism

H. Bryan Brewer, Jr.

INTRODUCTION

Epidemiologic studies have firmly established that low-density lipoproteins (LDLs) and high-density lipoproteins (HDLs) are independent risk factors for the development of cardiovascular disease (CVD).[1,2] Over the past two decades, clinical trials in patients at both low and high risk have shown that a decrease in plasma LDL levels are associated with a 25% to 45% decrease in cardiac events.[3–8] Despite this reduction in risk there remains a significant residual risk for cardiovascular events in patients treated with statins.[9] Low HDL levels are often present in patients being treated for dyslipoproteinemia and are a current target for potential future therapy to decrease the residual risk of CVD.

Evidence from both experimental and clinical studies suggests that increasing HDL will be associated with a decrease in CVD risk. In addition to the epidemiologic evidence,[10] several animal models employing either HDL infusions in cholesterol-fed rabbits[11] or overexpression of apolipoprotein (apo) A-I in transgenic mice[12,13] and lecithin: cholesterol acyltransferase (LCAT) in transgenic rabbits[14] were associated with decreased atherosclerosis. Although limited in number, human clinical trials have supported the concept that increasing HDL may decrease clinical events. The follow-up of patients who received niacin in the Coronary Drug Project revealed a significant decrease in CVD events.[15] In the HDL Atherosclerosis Treatment Study (HATS), the combination of niacin plus statin was associated with decreased atherosclerosis by angiography as well as decreased clinical events.[16] In patients with acute coronary syndrome, in whom intravascular ultrasound was used to quantitate coronary atheroma, five weekly infusions of apoA-I_{Milano}/phospholipid complexes were associated with reduction of total atheroma volume.[17] In the Arterial Biology for the Investigation of the Treatment Effects of Reducing Cholesterol 3 (ARBITER 3), the addition of niacin to statin therapy resulted in regression of carotid intima–media thickness at both 12 and 24 months.[18] The combined results of the epidemiologic, animal, and clinical studies provide support for the concept that raising HDL will be an effective additional therapeutic target for CVD prevention.

HIGH-DENSITY LIPOPROTEINS

HDLs are composed of proteins, designated apolipoproteins, and lipids, including phospholipids, free cholesterol, and cholesteryl esters organized in a spherical micelle.[19] The two major apolipoproteins associated with HDL are apoA-I, a 243–amino acid protein,[20] which is the major structural apolipoprotein in HDL, and apoA-II, a homo-dimer of 154 amino acids.[21] In addition to apoA-I and apoA-II, HDL contains several minor apolipoproteins including apoE, apoC-I, apoC-II, apoC-III, apoA-IV, and apoA-V.[22] ApoE, apoC-I, apoC-II, and apoC-III are also associated with chylomicrons and very-low-density lipoproteins (VLDLs). ApoA-IV and apoA-V may be present in chylomicrons and VLDLs as well as the poorly lipidated very-high-density lipoprotein (VHDL) fraction. A structural characteristic of apoA-I and the other apolipoproteins is an amphipathic helical conformation with hydrophobic amino acids on one side of the helix that permit the binding of the apolipoprotein to lipid and a hydrophilic surface that is exposed to the aqueous plasma or lymph.[23,24] The apolipoproteins as well as the free cholesterol are intercalated between the polar head groups of the phospholipids. The neutral lipid, cholesteryl esters, fills the core of the HDL particle. The apolipoproteins are associated with the lipoprotein particle by protein–protein as well as protein–lipid interactions. Apolipoproteins function in lipoprotein metabolism as ligands for receptors and transporters, cofactors for enzymes, and structural proteins for lipoprotein particle biosynthesis. In addition to the apolipoproteins, HDL also contains 30 to 40 other minor proteins, based on analysis by mass spectrometry.[25] Further studies will be required to determine which of these proteins are clinically significant and play a role in lipoprotein function and metabolism.

CLASSIFICATION OF HIGH-DENSITY LIPOPROTEINS

HDLs are polydisperse and can be classified based on separation by hydrated density, size, charge, and apolipoprotein composition. HDLs can be separated by density gradient ultracentrifugation into HDL_2, HDL_3, and VHDL and by gradient gel electrophoresis into HDL_{2b}, $_{2a}$, $_{3a}$, $_{3b}$, and $_{3c}$.[26] Classification of individual HDL lipoprotein particles based on size can be achieved by nuclear magnetic resonance.[27] Moreover, 2-dimensional gel electrophoresis has been a very effective technique; it resolves HDL particles into lipid-poor pre-β_1 and pre-β_2 lipoproteins and the mature spherical cholesteryl ester containing α-HDL (α,–α_4) [28] (Fig. 4-1A). The classification of HDL into separate lipoprotein particles based on apolipoprotein composition has provided a major advance in our understanding of HDL function and metabolism. Lipoprotein (Lp) A-I and LpA-I:A-II are the two most abundant HDL particles, and LpE and LpE:A-I are important minor lipoprotein particles within HDL[29] (Fig. 4-1B).

SYNTHESIS OF HIGH-DENSITY LIPOPROTEIN APOLIPOPROTEIN A-I AND APOLIPOPROTEIN A-II

Four major pathways are involved in the synthesis of mature α-HDL. The major structural apolipoprotein of HDL, apoA-I is synthesized by the liver and intestine as a preproprotein and is secreted following cleavage of the prepeptide as lipid-poor proapoA-I into the circulation.[20,30] ProapoA-I is converted to mature apoA-I in the plasma during HDL metabolism.[30,31] ApoA-II is synthesized in the liver as a proprotein and secreted into plasma as the mature apoA-II.[31] Lipid-poor apoA-I and pre-β-HDL containing apoA-I are also formed by the intravascular metabolism and remodeling of both triglyceride-rich chylomicrons and hepatic VLDL (Fig. 4-2).

HIGH-DENSITY LIPOPROTEIN AND CHOLESTEROL EFFLUX

A schematic overview of the role of LDL and HDL in lipoprotein metabolism and the development of atherosclerosis is illustrated in Figure 4-3. Increased plasma levels of LDL result in the development of cholesterol-loaded macrophages in the vessel wall, leading to atherosclerosis. HDL has been proposed to function in removal of the excess cellular cholesterol by the process of “reverse cholesterol transport,” by which the cellular cholesterol is transported back to the liver where the excess cholesterol can be removed from the body.[32]

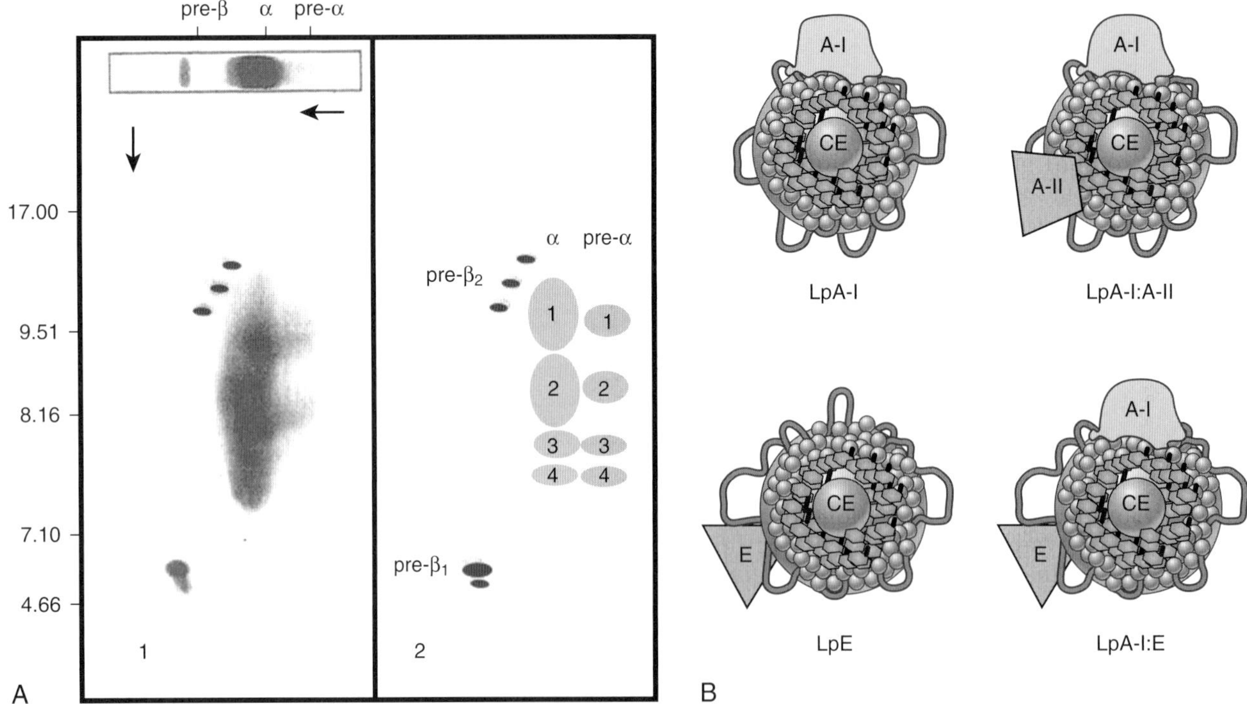

FIGURE 4-1 Plasma 2-D gel electrophoresis of plasma high-density lipoprotein (HDL) *(A)* and the major HDL particles classified based on apolipoprotein composition *(B)*.

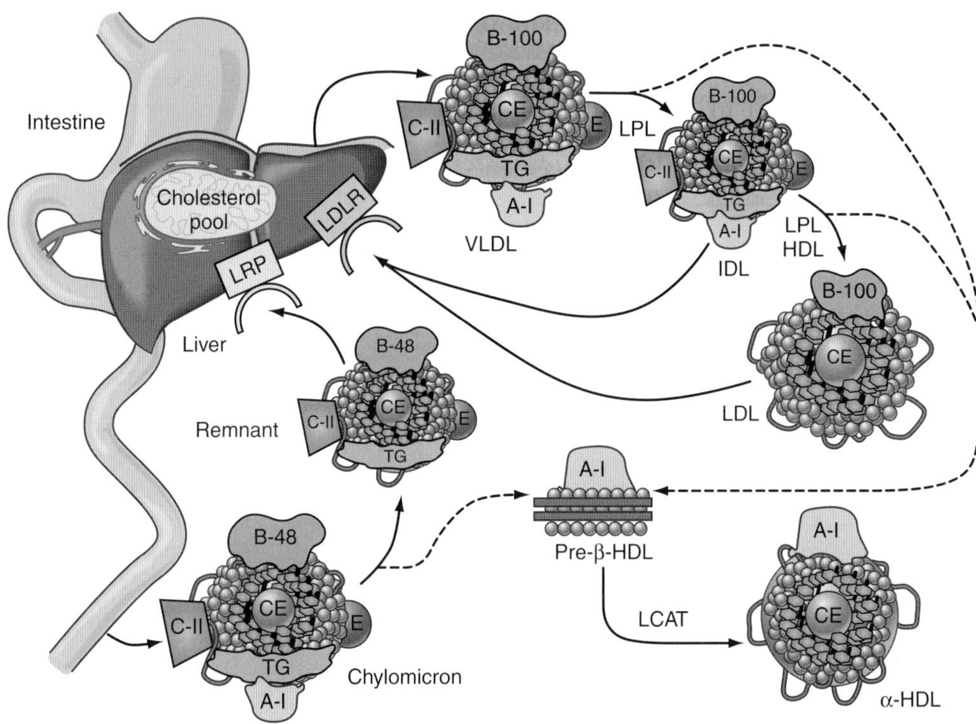

FIGURE 4-2 Lipid-poor apolipoprotein (apo) A-I is synthesized by the liver and intestine; apoA-II is synthesized by the liver. The lipids and apolipoproteins of high-density lipoprotein (HDL) are also derived from the remodeling of apoB-containing chylomicrons from the intestine and hepatically derived very-low-density lipoprotein (VLDL) by lipoprotein lipase (LPL) and hepatic lipase. CE, cholesteryl ester; IDL, intermediate-density lipoprotein; LCAT, lecithin:cholesterol acyltransferase; LDLR, low-density lipoprotein receptor; LRP, LDLR-related protein; TG, triglyceride.

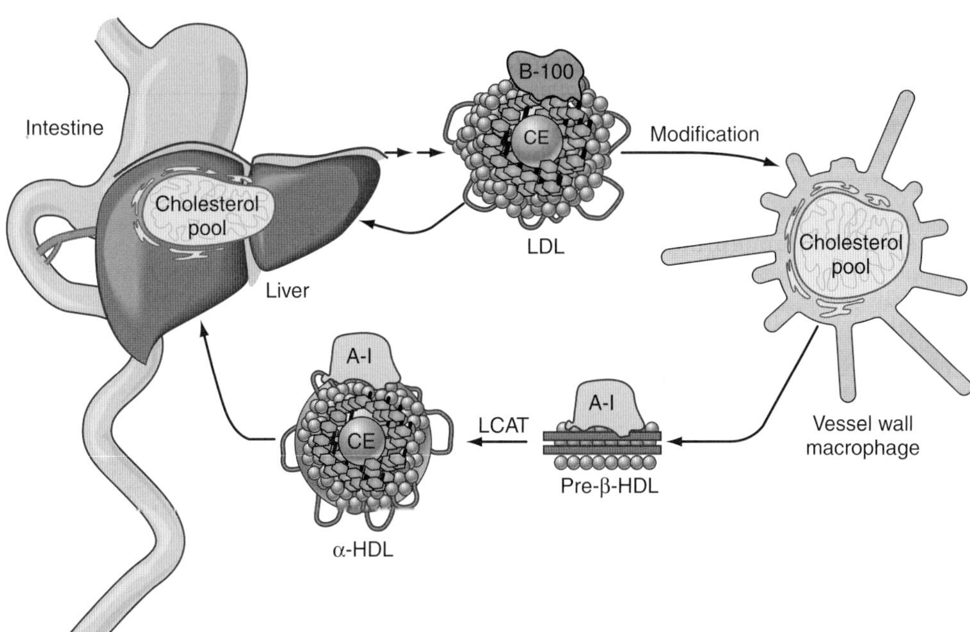

FIGURE 4-3 Schematic overview of low-density lipoprotein (LDL) and reverse cholesterol transport. LDL may either be taken up and degraded by the liver or become modified and catabolized by macrophages. Increased plasma levels of LDL are associated with the development of cholesterol-filled macrophages in the vessel wall. High-density lipoprotein (HDL) has been proposed to remove excess cholesterol from the macrophages and transport the cholesterol back to the liver for removal from the body in a process termed *reverse cholesterol transport*. A-I, apolipoprotein A-I; CE, cholesteryl ester; LCAT, lecithin:cholesterol acyltransferase.

A major breakthrough in our understanding of the molecular mechanism by which HDL selectively facilitates the removal of excess cellular cholesterol was the discovery of the genetic defect in patients with Tangier disease, which is characterized by orange tonsils, very low plasma levels of HDL, and increased risk of CVD.[33] HDL is unable to remove cholesterol from cholesterol-filled cells isolated from Tangier disease patients because of a genetic defect in the ATP-binding cassette A1 (ABCA 1) transporter, which binds to HDL and facilitates the removal of cellular cholesterol.[34–40] The ABCA1 transporter pathway provided a key insight into the mechanism for reverse cholesterol transport.

Following the discovery of the ABCA1 transporter, major advances were made in the elucidation of the mechanisms and regulation of the removal of excess cellular cholesterol. These studies led to the development of the concept of the dual pathway of cholesterol efflux from cholesterol-loaded cells and the mechanism for the regulation of the expression of the genes involved in cholesterol efflux. The concept of a dual pathway for cholesterol efflux from cholesterol-loaded cells is based on the two ligands involved in cholesterol efflux. The major ligand for the ABCA1 transporter, the key receptor pathway that regulates cellular cholesterol efflux to HDL, is lipid-poor apoA-I.[41] Cell culture studies have suggested that the ABCA1 transporter and apoA-I recycle from the cell membrane to the late endocytic compartment, which appears to be critical in the movement of the intracellular cholesterol to the cell surface for cholesterol efflux to lipid-poor apoA-I.[42,43] Following cholesterol efflux, lipid-poor apoA-I is converted to pre-β-HDL, which matures into the spherical α-HDL following the esterification of free cholesterol to cholesteryl esters by LCAT (Figs. 4-3, 4-4).

The second ligand in the dual pathway of cholesterol efflux is α-HDL, which is the ligand for both the scavenger receptor class B type I receptor (SR-BI)[44,45] and the ABCG1 transporter.[46–48] SR-BI has the capacity to transport cholesterol both out of and into cells depending on the increased or decreased intracellular cholesterol level, respectively[44,45] (see Fig. 4-4). The increased atherosclerosis observed following the exchange of bone marrow cells derived from SR-BI–knockout mice to control mice by bone marrow transplantation supports a physiologic role of SR-BI in the efflux of cellular cholesterol from vascular macrophages, thereby preventing the development of diet-induced atherosclerosis in the mice model.[49]

α-HDL facilitates cholesterol efflux through interaction with the ABCG1 transporter.[46–48] In addition to normal α-HDL, the large HDL isolated from patients with cholesteryl ester transfer protein (CETP) deficiency binds to the ABCG1 transporter and mediates cholesterol efflux.[48] An increased level of LCAT and apoE present on the large HDL particles that are isolated from patients with CETP deficiency have been reported to markedly increase the cholesterol efflux from cholesterol-loaded macrophages by the ABCG1 transporter. The effect on experimental atherosclerosis in control animals following bone marrow transplantation with cells derived from ABCG1 transporter–knockout mice is still controversial. In one report, the atherosclerosis was decreased,[50] whereas in a second report it was increased.[51]

In addition to the efflux mediated by interaction with SR-BI and ABCG1, α-HDL may efflux cholesterol by a nonspecific diffusion process (see Fig. 4-4).

The cellular levels of both the ABCA1 and ABCG1 transporters are major determinants regulating cholesterol efflux from cholesterol-loaded cells and thus play a key role in determining intracellular cholesterol levels. The expression of both the ABCA1 and ABCG1 transporter genes is modulated by the intracellular cholesterol concentration. Elevated levels of intracellular cholesterol result in increased levels of oxysterols, thereby stimulating the liver X receptor (LXR) transcription factor pathway. Increased intracellular levels of LXR coupled with retinoid X receptor (RXR) bind to the LXR response elements in the ABCA1 and ABCG1 promoters, resulting in increased *ABCA1* and *ABCG1* gene expression.[52–56] Enhanced expression of the ABCA1 and ABCG1 transporters increases intracellular cholesterol efflux to lipid-poor apoA-I to form pre-β-HDL and α-HDL, respectively. Thus, the overall effect is to decrease the cholesterol content of cholesterol-loaded cells by stimulation of the LXR/RXR

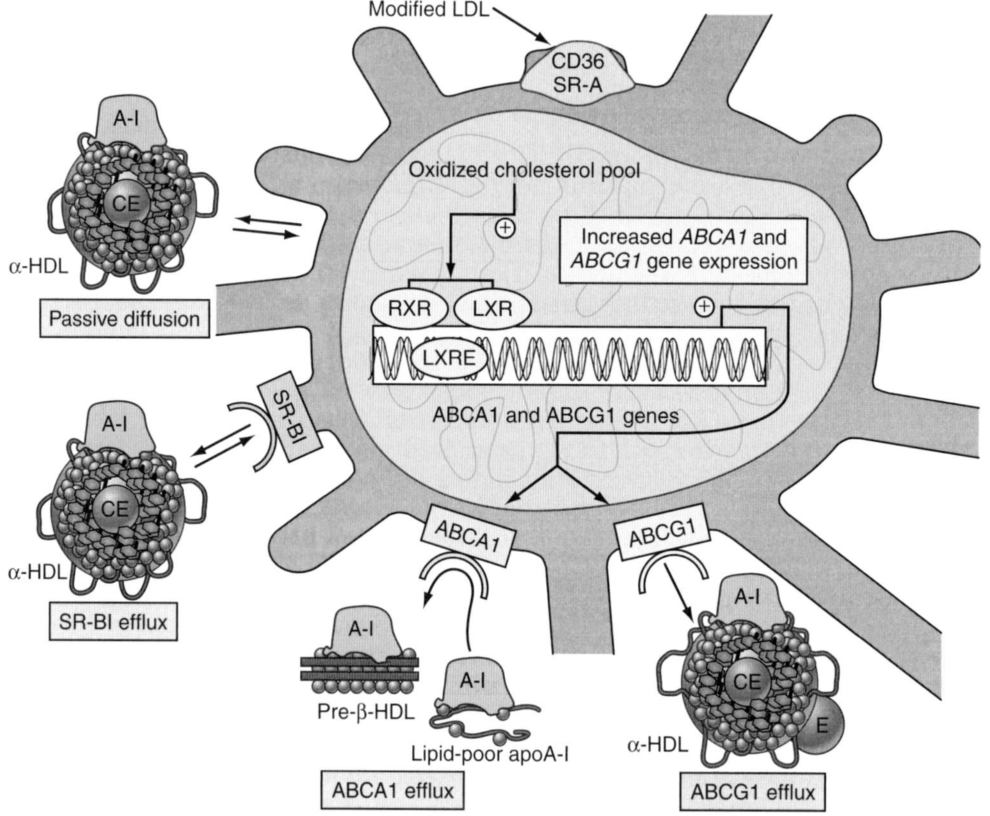

FIGURE 4-4 Illustration of the dual pathway for cholesterol efflux from cholesterol-filled macrophages. Two separate ligands, lipid-poor apolipoprotein (apo) A-I and α–high-density lipoprotein (HDL), interact with receptors and transporters to facilitate cholesterol efflux from the cholesterol-filled macrophage. Lipid-poor apo A-I interacts with the ATP-binding cassette A1 (ABCA1) transporter with the formation of cholesterol-filled pre-β-HDL, which is transformed into αHDL following the esterification of free cholesterol to cholesteryl esters (CE) by LCAT. α-HDL interacts with scavenger receptor class B type I receptor (SR-BI) and ABCG1 to increase cholesterol efflux. Cholesterol may also be removed by the low-affinity passive-diffusion process. The expression of both the ABCA1 and ABCG1 transporters are increased following the up-regulation of the liver X receptor/retinoid X receptor (LXR/RXR) pathway by an increased cellular level of oxysterols. At low levels of intracellular cholesterol, the ABCA1 and ABCG1 transporters are down-regulated and there will be minimal cellular cholesterol efflux.

pathway with increased cellular levels of both ABCA1 and ABCG1 transporters (see Fig. 4-4).

SCHEMATIC OVERVIEW OF HIGH-DENSITY LIPOPROTEIN METABOLISM AND REVERSE CHOLESTEROL METABOLISM

The metabolism of all of the major plasma lipoproteins is interrelated and involves the interplay of lipolytic enzymes, apolipoproteins, receptors, and transfer proteins. The major function of the triglyceride-rich chylomicrons secreted from the intestine is to transport dietary lipids to peripheral tissues and the liver. The triglycerides in chylomicrons undergo hydrolysis by lipoprotein lipase, and the particles are converted to remnants that are removed from the circulation by interaction with the hepatic LDL receptor–related protein (see Fig. 4-2). VLDL is secreted by the liver, and the triglycerides that are present in VLDL also undergo hydrolysis by lipoprotein lipase. With triglyceride hydrolysis, VLDL undergoes stepwise delipidation with the formation of particles with a hydrated density of intermediate-density lipoprotein (IDL) and finally LDL. VLDL remnants, IDL, and LDL are cleared from the plasma by interacting with the hepatic LDL receptor (LDLR) (see Fig. 4-2). The interaction of LDL with LDLR initiates receptor-mediated endocytosis and degradation of LDL in the liver and peripheral cells in the body.

HDL plays a pivotal role in lipoprotein and cholesterol metabolism by facilitating the efflux of excess cholesterol from the membranes of peripheral cells, including macrophages, by interaction with the ABCA1 transporter (Fig. 4-5). The ABCA1 transporter plays a central role in the regulation of intracellular cholesterol levels in the liver and intestine as well as the peripheral cells. An increase in intracellular cholesterol in both the liver and intestine results in increased expression of the ABCA1 transporter via the LXR/RXR pathway.[52–56] Lipid-poor apoA-I binds to the ABCA1 transporter generating pre-β-HDL, which is converted to α-HDL with esterification of the free cholesterol. Of particular clinical importance is the up-regulation of the ABCA1 transporter in cholesterol-filled macrophages in the coronary arteries. Lipid-poor apoA-I secreted by the liver and intestine is able to bind to the ABCA1 transporter in cholesterol-filled macrophages and decrease the cellular cholesterol content. The pre-β-HDL generated in this process contributes to the plasma α-HDL. The increased cholesterol present in the macrophages in the arterial wall may be also decreased by the interaction of α-HDL with the SR-BI receptor and the ABCG1 transporter. Thus, the combination of the dual pathway for cholesterol efflux with the lipid-poorapoA-I/ABCA1 transporter and the α-HDL/ABCG1 transporter–SR-BI receptor pathways effectively modulates cellular cholesterol metabolism.

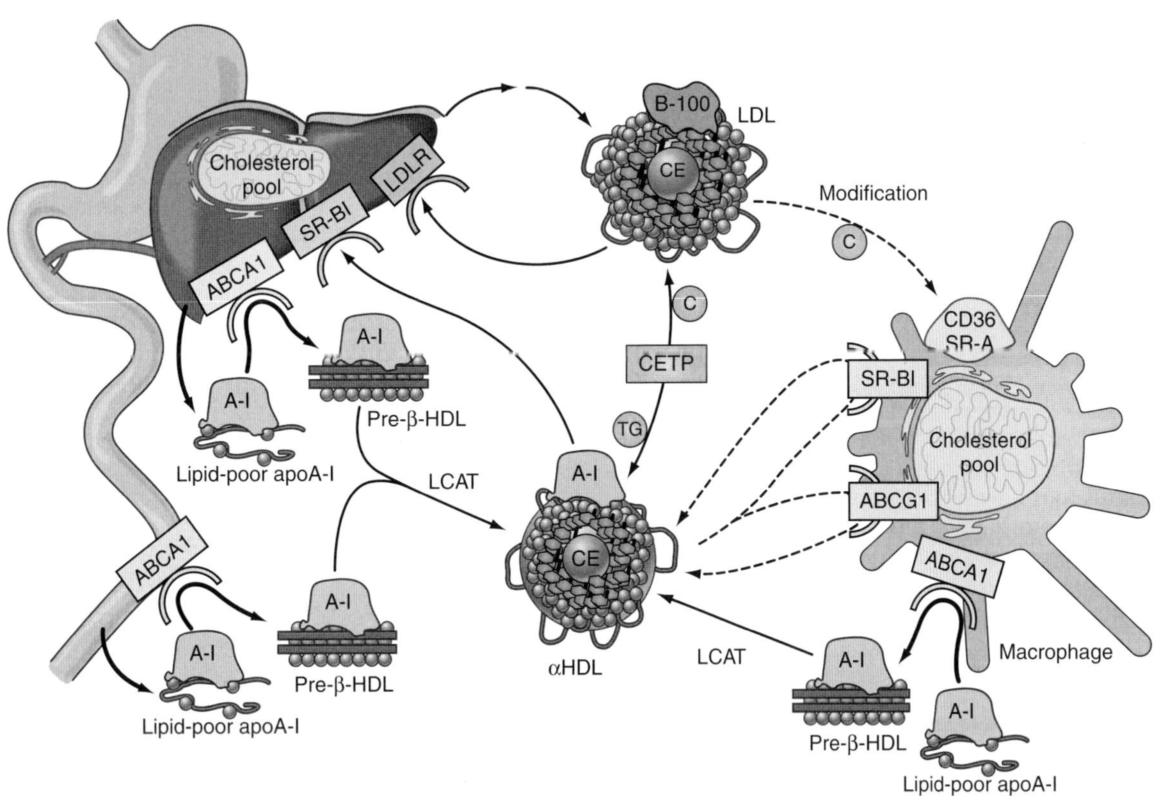

FIGURE 4-5 The cellular cholesterol level in the liver, intestine, and macrophage is modulated by high-density lipoprotein (HDL). An increased level of cellular cholesterol in the liver, intestine, or macrophage would up-regulate the level of expression of ATP-binding cassette A1 (ABCA1) and increase cholesterol-efflux to the lipid-poor apolipoprotein (apo) A-I with ultimate production of α-HDL following cholesterol esterification by lecithin:cholesterol acyltransferase (LCAT). Increased intracellular levels of cholesterol would also increase the ABCG1 transporter and, in conjunction with scavenger receptor class B type I receptor (SR-BI) would increase cholesterol efflux to α-HDL. Cholesterol is transported back to the liver either following transfer to apoB-containing lipoproteins by the cholesteryl ester transfer protein (CETP) or directly to the liver by selective update of HDL–free cholesterol by interaction of HDL with the hepatic SR-BI.

Plasma α-HDL transports cholesterol back to the liver by two separate pathways. In the first pathway, HDL cholesteryl esters are exchanged for triglycerides in the apoB-containing lipoproteins (chylomicrons, VLDL, IDL, and LDL) by CETP.[57] In humans, a significant fraction of cholesteryl esters present in HDL are transferred back to the liver by the LDL pathway.[58] The second pathway involves the direct delivery of cholesterol to the liver via SR-BI that functions to remove cholesterol selectively from lipoproteins without HDL particle uptake and degradation.[59,60] Following the transfer of cholesterol to the liver by SR-BI, HDL is remodeled by hepatic lipase, endothelial lipase, and the phospholipid transfer protein to generate lipid-poor apoA-I, pre-β-HDL, and poorly lipidated α-HDL. Thus, cholesterol may be transported back to the liver following exchange to chylomicrons, VLDL, IDL, and/or LDL or directly by HDL. It also has been proposed that a variable portion of tissue cholesterol may also be transported to the liver by HDL particles containing apoE (LpE), which may interact with both the hepatic LDLR related protein and LDLR. The major sites of catabolism of HDL are the liver and kidney. A major factor regulating HDL catabolism is HDL particle size, with small lipid-poor particles rapidly catabolized by the kidney.

REGULATION OF HEPATIC CHOLESTEROL

The intracellular level of hepatic cholesterol is regulated by modulation of 3-hydroxy-3-methylglutaryl–coenzyme A (HMG-COA) reductase, the rate-limiting enzyme in cholesterol biosynthesis, and by three separate integrated lipoprotein regulatory cycles (Fig. 4-6A–C). An increase in the hepatic level of cholesterol results in a decrease in cholesterol synthesis and a coordinate response in the three separate lipoprotein cycles. In the first cycle, the level of cholesterol can be reduced by increased secretion of cholesterol-enriched VLDL, which is converted to IDL and finally cholesterol-enriched LDL, and by a decrease in the level of LDLR expression reducing LDL uptake by the liver (see Fig. 4-6A). An increase in hepatic cholesterol results in an up-regulation of the LXR/RXR transcription factors, resulting in an increase in the level of the ABCA1 transporter; this would enhance hepatocyte cholesterol efflux to lipid-poor apoA-I with the formation of pre-β-HDL and conversion to α-HDL following cholesterol esterification by LCAT (see Fig. 4-6B). The up-regulation of the LXR pathway would also increase gene expression of ABCG5 and ABCG8,[61,62] which facilitates the secretion of cholesterol from the hepatocyte into the bile and would also increase the efflux of intracellular cholesterol in the enterocyte back into the lumen of the gastrointestinal tract, thereby decreasing the delivery of cholesterol back to the liver via the enterohepatic circulation[61,62] (see Fig. 4-6C).

A decrease in hepatic cholesterol would also involve regulation by the three circular cascades, and it would increase cholesterol synthesis as well as up-regulate the LDLR pathway with increased hepatic LDL uptake and cholesterol transport to the liver. A decrease in hepatic cholesterol also would result in a decreased level of LXR, resulting in a reduced expression of the ABCA1 transporter. The decreased level of the LXR system also would reduce hepatic biliary secretion of cholesterol and decrease cholesterol efflux from the enterocyte back into the gastrointestinal tract by down-regulation of ABCG5/ABCG8 in the enterocyte. The combined effects of reducing the LXR system would be to decrease biliary secretion of cholesterol, decrease the return of cholesterol to the gastrointestinal lumen, and increase cholesterol transport back to the liver by the enterohepatic circulation (see Fig. 4-6C).

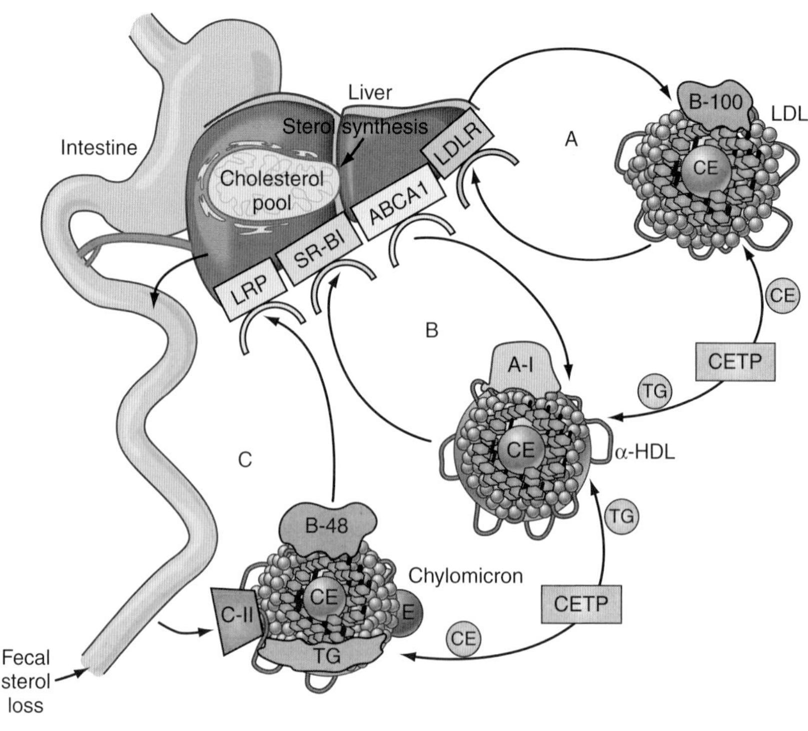

FIGURE 4-6 The intracellular hepatic cholesterol level is regulated by cholesterol synthesis by the rate-limiting enzyme 3-hydroxy-3-methylglutaryl-coenzyme A (HMG-CoA) reductase and three integrated lipoprotein cycles. An increase in hepatic cholesterol results in the coordinate down-regulation of HMG-CoA reductase and a decrease in the level of expression of the hepatic low-density lipoprotein receptor (LDLR), resulting in decreased uptake of plasma LDL. An increase in hepatic cholesterol would increase the liver X receptor (LXR) transcription factor, thereby increasing the level of expression of ATP-binding cassette transporter A1 ABC A1and ABCG5/ABCG8. The increase in the cellular level of these transporters will increase cholesterol efflux to lipid-poor apolipoprotein (apo)A-I/α-HDL and the HDL cycle (cycle B), and cholesterol transported into bile (cycle C), respectively. The increased delivery of cholesterol to the enterocyte via the Niemann–Pick C1–like (NPC1L1) receptor may increase enterocyte LXR/ABCG5/ABCG8, resulting in increased flux of cholesterol back to the intestinal lumen and decreased cholesterol returning to the liver by the enterohepatic circulation (cycle C). The three lipoprotein regulatory cycles are interconnected in the plasma by the exchange of triglycerides (TG) and cholesteryl esters (CE) by cholesteryl ester transfer protein (CETP). A decrease in hepatic cholesterol would be anticipated to have the reverse changes in the coordinated regulation of cholesterol synthesis and the cholesterol/lipoprotein pathways.

The three regulatory cycles, LDL, HDL, and the chylomicron enterohepatic circulation, are integrated in the plasma by the exchange of cholesteryl esters and triglycerides by CETP (see Fig. 4-6).

REGULATION OF THE PLASMA LEVEL OF HIGH-DENSITY LIPOPROTEIN

In the classic view of HDL metabolism (see Fig. 4-3), the plasma level of HDL was proposed to reflect HDL cholesterol removed from peripheral cells on the way back to the liver by the process of reverse cholesterol transport.[32] The marked increase in knowledge of the regulation of cholesterol efflux from the liver, intestine, and peripheral cells provided the unique opportunity to determine the tissue of origin of plasma HDL cholesterol. The ability to modulate the key genes involved in cholesterol metabolism in the mouse model system has been extremely useful in determining the major pathways that determine the plasma HDL levels. In the initial mouse studies, bone marrow transplantation of ABCA1-knockout macrophages resulted in increased atherosclerosis but no change in the plasma HDL levels.[63] Overexpression of the ABCA1 transporter in the liver[64,65] as well as the selective decrease in hepatic ABCA1 expression[66,67] resulted in increased and reduced plasma HDL cholesterol, respectively. Selective ABCA1 knockout in the intestine resulted in decreased plasma HDL levels.[68] The combined results from these studies in the mouse model suggested that ≈75% and ≈20% of HDL cholesterol was derived from the liver and intestine, respectively, and only a minor component (≈5%) of HDL cholesterol was derived from peripheral cells (Fig. 4-7). Thus, the level of plasma HDL cholesterol does not reflect reverse cholesterol transport and cannot be used to determine the efficiency of cholesterol efflux from peripheral cells, particularly cholesterol-filled macrophages in the coronary arteries.

HIGH-DENSITY LIPOPROTEIN METABOLISM

Changes in plasma HDL levels can be classified into those clinical conditions that are associated with changes in HDL synthesis or catabolism. The majority of studies in humans indicate that the rate of catabolism rather than synthesis is the major determinant of the plasma HDL level.

Genetic Dyslipoproteinemias Associated with Low Plasma High-Density Lipoprotein Levels

ApoA-I Variants

Subjects with a genetic variant of apoA-I, apoA-I_{Milano}, have a single amino acid substitution of a cysteine for an arginine at position 173.[69] Heterozygotes for the substitution have elevated triglycerides, low LDL, and low HDL; however, despite the low HDL levels there is no increased risk of CVD.[69–71] Kinetic studies using radiolabeled native apoA-I and apoA-I_{Milano} were

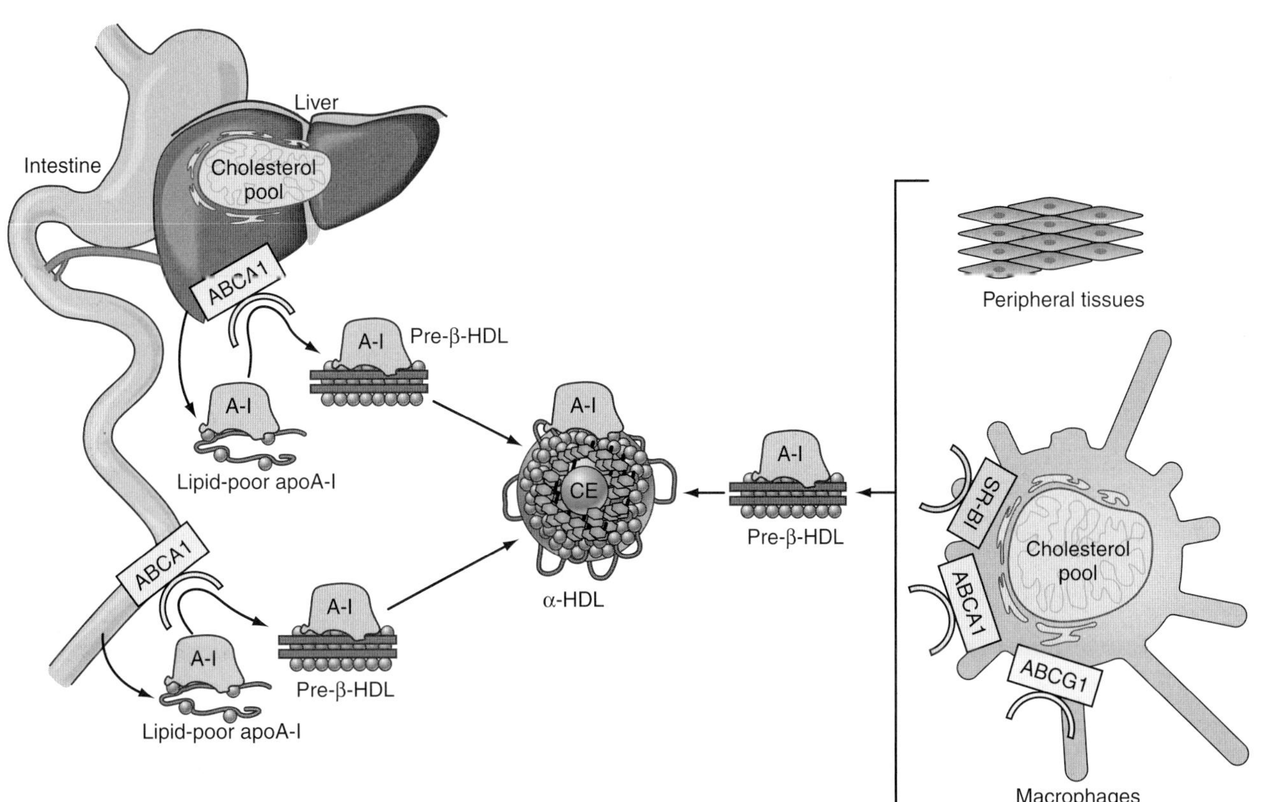

FIGURE 4-7 In the mouse model system, the plasma level of high-density lipoprotein (HDL) cholesterol is predominately determined by the cholesterol derived from the liver and intestine. A very small percentage of plasma HDL cholesterol (<5%) is derived from peripheral tissues including the macrophage.

performed in control subjects and heterozygotes for the apoA-I_{Milano} substitution.[72] In control subjects, apoA-I_{Milano} was catabolized at a faster rate than native apoA-I, consistent with the concept that the apoA-IMilano was abnormal with a faster catabolism in plasma. Kinetic studies in apoA-I_{Milano} heterozygotes revealed that both native and apoA-I_{Milano} were catabolized faster than native apoA-I in control subjects. The synthesis rate of apoA-I_{Milano} was normal. These studies established that apoA-I_{Milano} subjects have low HDL because of increased catabolism of an abnormal apoA-I variant but with no significant CVD. An intravascular ultrasound clinical trial using an infusion of apoA-I_{Milano}/phospholipid complex was shown to reduce coronary artery plaque in patients with acute coronary artery syndrome.[17] This imaging trial established that selectively increasing HDL without any major change in other lipoproteins could decrease CVD.

Individuals with another genetic variant of apoA-I, apoA-I_{Iowa}, have an amino acid substitution of an arginine for a glycine at position 26.[73] Patients with apoA-I_{Iowa} have a hereditary form of amyloidosis, and analysis of the amyloid protein established that the protein was a peptide fragment of apoA-I. Kinetic analysis of radiolabeled native and apoA-I_{Iowa} established that both native and apoA-I_{Iowa} had increased catabolism. In addition, the urinary excretion of radiolabeled amino acids derived from the catabolism of apoA-I_{Iowa} was approximately 50% less than native apoA-I in control subjects; this is consistent with retention of the abnormal apoA-I and the potential development of amyloidosis resulting from decreased clearance of the abnormal apoA-I_{Iowa} protein.[74]

In a kindred with familial hypoalphalipoproteinemia, the apoA-I gene was shown to contain a pancreatic secretory trypsin inhibitor (PSTI) restriction link polymorphism. Native apoA-I and apoA-I from the PSTI apoA-I kindred were radiolabeled, and kinetic studies were performed in control and PSTI apoA-I subjects.[75] Both native and PSTI apoA-I were catabolized at a faster rate, which is consistent with the hypoalphalipoproteinemia being due to increased catabolism rather than decreased synthesis.

In the apoA-I_{Milano}, apoA-I_{Iowa}, and PSTI apoA-I kinetic studies the increased catabolism of the native apoA-I in the patients with the apoA-I variants has been proposed to be due to the association of the native apolipoprotein with an HDL that is rapidly catabolized as a result of the presence of an abnormal apolipoprotein variant.

ABCA1

Patients with Tangier disease, as discussed earlier, have orange tonsils, low LDL, marked reductions in HDL, and increased risk of CVD. The structural mutation in the ABCA1 transporter prevents cholesterol efflux and the synthesis of normal αHDL. The failure of lipidation of apoA-I results in the formation of small, lipid-poor HDLs that are rapidly cleared through the kidney. Kinetic studies of HDL and apoA-I as well as apoA-II established that the low plasma HDL level was due to increased catabolism of a small, poorly lipidated HDL.[76,77]

Lecithin:Cholesterol Acyltransferase Deficiency

Classic LCAT deficiency as well as fish eye disease are due to mutations in the LCAT gene that result in complete or partial LCAT deficiency, respectively. The LCAT deficiency phenotype is characterized by cloudy corneas, low LDL, and very low HDL but no increased risk of CVD.[78] In this disease a deficiency of LCAT activity leads to increased levels of pre-β-HDL as a result of defective maturation of the pre-β-HDL to α-HDL. In kinetic studies, radiolabeled apoA-I and apoA-II were rapidly catabolized in classic LCAT deficiency as well as fish eye disease. The increased HDL catabolism leading to decreased HDL levels was due to rapid catabolism of the small, pre-β-HDL that failed to undergo maturation to α-HDL.[79]

Genetic Dyslipoproteinemias Associated with High Plasma High-Density Lipoprotein Levels

Cholesteryl Ester Transfer Protein Deficiency

The characteristic phenotype of patients with CETP deficiency includes markedly increased HDL levels, polydisperse LDL, and relatively normal triglycerides.[80] Controversy exists as to whether the homozygotes with CETP deficiency are at risk or protected against CVD. Kinetic analysis using both exogenous radiolabeled apolipoproteins and an endogenous primed constant infusion of $^{13}C_6$-phenylalaninne were performed in control subjects as well as homozygous patients with complete CETP deficiency. ApoA-I catabolism in CETP-deficient homozygotes was markedly slower when compared with control subjects.[81] Thus, the markedly increased plasma level of HDL is due to decreased catabolism of apoA-I and apoA-II. Decreased HDL catabolism was also reported in patients treated with torcetrapib, a CETP inhibitor.[82] Further studies will be required to definitively establish whether homozygotes with CETP deficiency do or do not have an increased risk of CVD.[83–85]

Hepatic Lipase Deficiency

Hepatic lipase plays a pivotal role in the remodeling of HDL to lipid-poor α-HDL and pre-β-HDL. Primed-constant infusion of D3-leucine was employed in kinetic studies of persons with complete and partial hepatic lipase deficiency and matched control subjects with increased triglycerides and normal triglycerides, respectively.[86] Those with complete hepatic lipase deficiency had increased levels of large HDL and decreased catabolism. In contrast, the subjects with partial hepatic lipase deficiency had normal HDL levels as well as normal HDL metabolism.

Familial Hyperalphalipoproteinemia

A single unique kindred has been identified with markedly increased HDL and apoA-I levels but normal apoA-II levels. The proband was healthy and the kindred was consistent with longevity; however, the number of kindred members was too small to make a definitive conclusion. Both radiolabeled apolipoproteins and primed constant infusion were used to determine HDL metabolism.[87] The apoA-I synthesis rate was markedly higher; however, the rate of catabolism was normal, indicating that there was no saturation of catabolism of apoA-I despite the markedly elevated apoA-I and HDL levels. In marked contrast, both the synthesis and catabolism of apoA-II was normal. The markedly increased HDL in this proband was due to a selective increase in synthesis of apoA-I with normal apoA-II production.

CONCLUSIONS

Residual CVD present in patients treated with statins represents a challenge to the cardiovascular field to develop additional therapeutic approaches to reduce these recurrent clinical events. The combined data from epidemiology, animal models, and initial clinical trials support the concept that raising HDL may be an effective new target to decrease CVD. Major advances have been made in our understanding of the mechanism by which HDL regulates plasma cholesterol metabolism and mediates cholesterol efflux from cholesterol-loaded cells. An improved understanding of HDL metabolism has led to a better understanding of the major role of the liver and intestine in determining the level of plasma HDL cholesterol and a revision of our concept that the level of HDL cholesterol reflects the efficiency of reverse cholesterol transport. However, despite the marked increase in our understanding of HDL metabolism, the question remains: What is the best method to increase HDL? Definitive clinical trials focusing on both safety and efficacy will be required to establish that increasing HDL will reduce clinical events and to determine the additional therapy necessary to further reduce CVD in patients at high risk.

REFERENCES

1. Castelli WP, Anderson K, Wilson PW, Levy D: Lipids and risk of coronary heart disease: the Framingham Study. *Ann Epidemiol* 1992;2:23–28.
2. Gordon DJ, Rifkind BM. High-density lipoprotein: the clinical implications of recent studies. *N Engl J Med* 1989;321:1311–1316.
3. Scandinavian Simvastatin Survival Study Group: Randomized trial of cholesterol lowering in 4444 patients with coronary heart disease: the Scandinavian Simvastatin Survival Study (4S). *Lancet* 1994;344:1383–1389.
4. Shepherd J, Cobbe SM, Ford I, et al: Prevention of coronary heart disease with pravastatin in men with hypercholesterolemia. *N Engl J Med* 1995;333:1350–1351.
5. Sacks FM, Pfeffer MA, Moye LA, et al: The effect of pravastatin on coronary events after myocardial infarction in patients with average cholesterol levels. *N Engl J Med* 1996;335:1001–1009.
6. Downs JR, Clearfield M, Weis S, et al: Primary prevention of acute coronary events with lovastatin in men and women with average cholesterol levels: results of AFCAPS/TexCAPS. Air Force/Texas Coronary Atherosclerosis Prevention Study. *JAMA* 1998;279:1615–1622.
7. Heart Protection Study Collaborative Group: MRC/BHF Heart Protection Study of cholesterol lowering with simvastatin in 20,536 high-risk individuals: a randomized placebo-controlled trial. *Lancet* 2002;360:7–22.
8. LaRosa JC, Grundy SM, Waters DD, et al: Intensive lipid lowering with atorvastatin in patients with stable coronary disease. *N Engl J Med* 2005;352:1425–1435.
9. Baigent C, Keech A, Kearney PM, et al: Efficacy and safety of cholesterol-lowering treatment: prospective meta-analysis of data from 90,056 participants in 14 randomised trials of statins. *Lancet* 2005;366:1267–1278.
10. Gordon T, Castelli WP, Hjortland MC, et al: High-density lipoprotein as a protective factor against coronary heart disease. The Framingham study. *Am J Med* 1977;62:707–714.
11. Badimon JJ, Badimon L, Fuster V, et al: Regression of atherosclerotic lesions by high-density lipoprotein plasma fraction in the cholesterol-fed rabbit. *J Clin Invest* 1990;85:1234–1241.
12. Rubin EM, Krauss RM, Spangler EA, et al: Inhibition of early atherogenesis in transgenic mice by human apolipoprotein AI. *Nature* 1991;353:265–267.
13. Plump AS, Scott CJ, Breslow JL, et al: Human apolipoprotein A-I gene expression increases high-density lipoprotein and suppresses atherosclerosis in the apolipoprotein E-deficient mouse. *Proc Natl Acad Sci USA* 1994;91:9607–9611.
14. Hoeg JM, Santamarina-Fojo S, Bérard AM, et al: Overexpression of lecithin:cholesterol acyltransferase in transgenic rabbits prevents diet-induced atherosclerosis. *Proc Natl Acad Sci USA* 1996;93:11448–11453.
15. Canner PL, Berge KG, Wenger NK, et al: Fifteen year mortality in Coronary Drug Project patients: long-term benefit with niacin. *J Am Coll Cardiol* 1986;8:1245–1255.
16. Brown BG, Zhao XQ, Chait A, et al: Simvastatin and niacin, antioxidant vitamins, or the combination for the prevention of coronary disease. *N Engl J Med* 2001;345:1583–1592.
17. Nissen SE, Tsunoda T, Tuzcu EM, et al: Effect of recombinant ApoA-I Milano on coronary atherosclerosis in patients with acute coronary syndromes: a randomized controlled trial. *JAMA* 2003;290:2292–2300.
18. Taylor A, Lee H, Sullenberger LE, et al: The effect of 24 months of combination statin and extended-release niacin on carotid intima-media thickness: ARBITER 3. *Curr Med Res Opin* 2006;22:2243–2250.
19. Assmann G, Sokoloski EA, Brewer HB Jr: ^{31}P nuclear magnetic resonance spectroscopy of native and recombined lipoproteins. *Proc Natl Acad Sci USA* 1974;71:549–553.
20. Brewer HBJ, Fairwell T, LaRue A, et al: The amino acid sequence of human ApoA-I, an apolipoprotein isolated from high-density lipoproteins. *Biochem Biophys Res Commun* 1978;80: 623–630.
21. Brewer HBJ, Lux SE, Ronan R, John KM: Amino acid sequence of human apoLp-Gln-II (apoA-II), an apolipoprotein isolated from the high-density lipoprotein complex. *Proc Natl Acad Sci USA* 1972;69:1304–1308.
22. Alaupovic P: Significance of apolipoproteins for structure, function, and classification of plasma lipoproteins. *Methods Enzymol* 1996;263:32–60.
23. Segrest JP, Jones MK, De Loof H, et al: The amphipathic helix in the exchangeable apolipoproteins: a review of secondary structure and function. *J Lipid Res* 1992;33:141–166.
24. Segrest JP, Garber DW, Brouillette CG, et al: The amphipathic alpha helix: a multifunctional structural motif in plasma apolipoproteins. *Adv Protein Chem* 1994;45:303–369.
25. Vaisar T, Pennathur S, Green PS, et al: Shotgun proteomics implicates protease inhibition and complement activation in the anti-inflammatory properties of HDL. *J Clin Invest* 2007;117: 746–756.
26. Blanche PJ, Gong EL, Forte TM, et al: Characterization of human high-density lipoproteins by gradient gel electrophoresis. *Biochim Biophys Acta* 1981;665:408–419.
27. Otvos JD: Measurement of lipoprotein subclass profiles by nuclear magnetic resonance spectroscopy. In Rifai N, Warnick GR, Dominiczak MH (eds): Handbook of Lipoprotein Testing. *Washington DC, AACC Press*, 2000, pp 609–623.
28. Asztalos BF, Schaefer EJ: High-density lipoprotein subpopulations in pathologic conditions. *Am J Cardiol* 2003;91:12E–17E.
29. Alaupovic P: The concept of apolipoprotein-defined lipoprotein families and its clinical significance. *Curr Atheroscler Rep* 2003;21:1459–1462.
30. Bojanovski D, Gregg RE, Ghiselli G, et al: Human apolipoprotein A-I isoprotein metabolism:proapoA-I conversion to mature ApoA-I. J. *Lipid Res* 1985;26:185–193.
31. Schaefer EJ, Zech LA, Jenkins LL, et al: Human apolipoprotein A-I and A-II metabolism. *J Lipid Res* 1982;23: 850–862.
32. Glomset JA: The plasma lecithin:cholesterol acyltransferase reaction. *J Lipid Res.* 1968;9:155–167.

33. Schaefer EJ, Zech LA, Schwartz DE, Brewer H Jr: Coronary heart disease prevalence and other clinical features in familial high-density lipoprotein deficiency (Tangier disease). *Ann Intern Med* 1980;93:261–266.
34. Brooks-Wilson A, Marcil M, Clee SM, et al: Mutations in ABC1 in Tangier disease and familial high-density lipoprotein deficiency. *Nat Genet* 1999;22:336–345.
35. Bodzioch M, Orso E, Klucken J, et al: The gene encoding ATP-binding cassette transporter 1 is mutated in Tangier disease. *Nat Genet* 1999;22:347–351.
36. Rust S, Rosier M, Funke H, et al: Tangier disease is caused by mutations in the ATP binding cassette transporter 1 (ABC1) gene. *Nat Genet* 1999;22:352–355.
37. Remaley AT, Rust S, Rosier M, et al: Human ATP-binding cassette transporter 1 (ABC1): genomic organization and identification of the genetic defect in the original Tangier disease kindred. *Proc Natl Acad Sci USA* 1999;96:12685–12690.
38. Brousseau ME, Schaefer EJ, Dupuis J, et al: Novel mutations in the gene encoding ATP-binding cassette 1 in four Tangier disease kindreds. *J Lipid Res* 2000;41:433–441.
39. Lawn RM, Wade DP, Garvin MR, et al: The Tangier disease gene product ABC1 controls the cellular apolipoprotein-mediated lipid removal pathway. *J Clin Invest* 1999;104:R25–R31.
40. Santamarina-Fojo S, Peterson K, Knapper C, et al: Complete genomic sequence of the human ABCA1 gene: analysis of the human and mouse ATP-binding cassette A promoter. *Proc Natl Acad Sci USA* 2000;97:7987–7992.
41. Oram JF, Vaughan AM: ABCA1-mediated transport of cellular cholesterol and phospholipids to HDL apolipoproteins. *Curr Opin Lipidol* 2000;11:253–260.
42. Neufeld EB, Remaley AT, Demosky SJ Jr, et al: Cellular localization and trafficking of the human ABCA1 transporter. *J Biol Chem 2001*;276:27584–27590.
43. Neufeld TB, Stonik JA, Demosky SJ Jr, et al: The ABCA1 transporter modulates late endocytic trafficking: insights from the correction of the genetic defect in Tangier disease. *J Biol Chem* 2004;279:15571–15578.
44. Williams DL, Connelly MA, Temel RE, et al: Scavenger receptor B1 and cholesterol trafficking. *Curr Opin Lipidol* 1999;10: 329–339.
45. Duong M, Collins HL, Jin W, et al: Relative contribution of ABCA1 and SR-BI to cholesterol efflux to serum from fibroblasts and macrophages. *Arterioscler Thromb Vasc Biol* 2006;26: 541–547.
46. Wang N, Lan D, Chen W, et al: ATP-binding cassette transporters G1 and G4 mediate cellular cholesterol efflux to high-density lipoproteins. *Proc Natl Acad Sci USA* 2004;31:9774–9779.
47. Kennedy MA, Barrera GC, Nakamura K, et al: ABCG1 has a critical role in mediating cholesterol efflux to HDL and preventing cellular lipid accumulation. *Cell Metab* 2005;1:121–131.
48. Matsuura F, Wang N, Chen W, et al: HDL from CETP-deficient subjects show enhanced ability to promote cholesterol efflux from macrophages in an apoE-and ABCG1-dependent pathway. *J Clin Invest* 2006;116:1435–1442.
49. Van Eck M, Bos ST, Hildebrand RB, et al: Dual role for scavenger receptor class B, type I on bone marrow-derived cells in atherosclerotic lesion development. *Am J Pathol* 2004;165:785–794.
50. Ranalletta M, Wang N, Han S, et al: Decreased atherosclerosis in low-density lipoprotein receptor knockout mice transplanted with Abcg1-/- bone marrow. *Arterioscler Thromb Vasc Biol* 2006;26:2308–2315.
51. Out R, Hoekstra M, Hildebrand RB, et al: Macrophage ABCG1 deletion disrupts lipid homeostasis in alveolar macrophages and moderately influences atherosclerotic lesion development in LDL receptor-deficient mice. *Arterioscler Thromb Vasc Biol* 2006;26:2295–2300.
52. Venkateswaran A, Laffitte BA, Joseph SB, et al: Control of cellular cholesterol efflux by the nuclear oxysterol receptor LXR alpha. *Proc Natl Acad Sci USA* 2000;97:12097–12102.
53. Schwartz K, Lawn RM, Wade DP: ABC1 gene expression and apoA-I-mediated cholesterol efflux are regulated by LXR. *Biochem Biophys Res Commun.* 2000;274:794–802.
54. Costet P, Luo Y, Wang N, Tall AR: Sterol-dependent transactivation of the ABC1 promoter by the liver X receptor/retinoid X receptor. *J Biol Chem 2000*;275:28240–28245.
55. Chawla A, Boisvert WA, Lee CH, et al: A PPAR gamma-LXR-ABCA1 pathway in macrophages is involved in cholesterol efflux and atherogenesis. *Mol Cell* 2001;7:161–171.
56. Wang N, Ranalletta M, Matsuura F, et al: LXR-induced redistribution of ABCG1 to plasma membrane in macrophages enhances cholesterol mass efflux to HDL. *Arterioscler Thromb Vasc Biol* 2006;26:1310–1316.
57. Tall AR: Metabolic and genetic control of HDL cholesterol levels. *J Intern Med* 1992;231:661–668.
58. Schwartz CC, Vlahcevic ZR, Halloran LG, Swell L: An in vivo evaluation in man of the transfer of esterified cholesterol between lipoproteins and into the liver and bile. *Biochim Biophys Acta* 1981;663:143–162.
59. Acton S, Rigotti A, Landschulz, KT et al: Identification of scavenger receptor SR-BI as a high-density lipoprotein receptor. *Science* 1996;271:518–520.
60. Trigatti BL, Krieger M, Rigotti A: Influence of the HDL receptor SR-BI on lipoprotein metabolism and atherosclerosis. *Arterioscler Thomb Vasc Biol* 2003;23:1732–1738.
61. Yu L, Gupta S, Xu F: Expression of ABCG5 and ABCG8 is required for regulation of biliary cholesterol secretion. *J Biol Chem* 2005;280:8742–8747.
62. Repa JJ, Berge KE, Pomajzl C, et al: Regulation of ATP-binding cassette sterol transporter ABCG5 and ABCG8 by the liver X receptors alpha and beta. *J Biol Chem* 2002;277:18793–18800.
63. Haghpassand M, Bourassa PA, Francone OL, et al.: Monocyte/macrophage expression of ABCA1 has minimal contribution to plasma HDL Levels. *J Clin Invest* 2001;108:1315–1320.
64. Vaisman BL, Lambert, G, Amar M, et al: ABCA1 overexpression leads to hyperalphalipoproteinemia. *J Clin Invest* 2001;108: 303–309.
65. Wellington CL, Brunham LR, Zhou S, et al: Alterations of plasma lipids in mice via adenoviral-mediated hepatic overexpression of human ABCA1. *J Lipid Res* 2003;44:1470–1480.
66. Timmins JM, Lee JY, Boudygiuuna E, et al: Targeted inactivation of hepatic Abca1 causes profound hypoalphalipoproteinemia and kidney hypercatabolism of apoA-I. *J Clin Invest* 2005;115: 1333–1342.
67. Ragozin S, Niemeier A, Laatsch A, et al: Knockdown of hepatic ABCA1 by RNA interference decreases plasma HDL cholesterol levels and influences postprandial lipemia in mice. *Arterioscler Thromb Vasc Biol* 2005;25:1433–1438.
68. Brunham LR, Kruit JK, Iqbal J, et al: Intestinal ABCA1 directly contributes to HDL biogenesis in vivo. *J Clin Invest* 2006;116: 1052–1062.
69. Weisgraber KH, Rall SC Jr, Bersot TP, et al: Apolipoprotein A-IMilano. Detection of normal apoA-I in affected subjects and evidence for a cysteine for arginine substitution in the variant A-I. *J Biol Chem* 1983;258:2508–2513.
70. Sirtori CR, Calabresi L, Franceschini G: Cardiovascular status of carriers of the apolipoprotein A-I(Milano) Mutant: the Limone sul Garda study. *Circulation* 2001;103:1949–1954.
71. Chiesa G, Sirtori CR: Apolipoprotein A-I(Milano): current perspectives. *Curr Opin Lipidol* 2003;14:159–163.
72. Roma P, Gregg RE, Meng MS, et al: In vivo metabolism of a mutant form of apolipoprotein A-I, apoA-I Milano, associated with familial hypoalphalipoproteinemia. *J Clin Invest* 1993;4:1445–1452.
73. Nichols WC, Gregg RE, Brewer HB Jr, Benson MD: A mutation in apolipoprotein A-I in the Iowa type of familial amyloidotic polyneuropathy. *Genomic* 1990;8:318–323.
74. Rader DJ, Gregg RE, Meng MS, et al: In vivo metabolism of a mutant apolipoprotein, apoA-I_{Iowa}, associated with hypoalphalipoproteinemia and hereditary systemic amyloidosis. *J Lipid Res* 1992;33:755–763.
75. Roma P, Gregg RE, Bishop C, et al: Apolipoprotein A-I metabolism in subjects with a PstI restriction fragment length polymorphism of the apoA-I gene and familial hypoalphalipoproteinemia. *J Lipid Res* 1990;10:1753–1760.
76. Schaefer EJ, Blum CB, Levy RI, et al: Metabolism of high-density lipoprotein apolipoproteins in Tangier disease. *N Engl J Med* 1978;299:905–910.
77. Bojanovski D, Gregg RE, Zech LA, et al: In vivo metabolism of proapolipoprotein A-I in Tangier disease *J Clin Invest* 1987;80: 1742–1747.
78. Assman G, von Eckardstein A, Brewer HB Jr: Familial Analphalipoproteinemia: Tangier disease. In Scriver CR, Beaudet AL, Sly WS, et al (eds): The Metabolic and Molecular Basis of Inherited Disease, 8th ed. *New York, McGraw Hill,* 2001, pp 2937–2980.
79. Rader DJ, Ikewaki K, Duverger N, et al: Markedly accelerated catabolism of apolipoprotein AII (ApoA-II) and high-density

lipoproteins containing apoA-II in classic lecithin:cholesterol acyltransferase deficiency and fish eye disease. *J Clin Invest* 1994;93:321–330.
80. Tall AR: Plasma cholesteryl ester transfer protein. *J Lipid Res* 1993;34:1255–1274.
81. Ikewaki K, Rader DJ, Sakamoto T, et al: Delayed catabolism of high-density lipoprotein apolipoproteins A-I and A-II in human cholesteryl ester transfer protein deficiency. *J Clin Invest* 1993;92:1650–1658.
82. Brousseau ME, Diffenderfer MR, Millar JS, et al: Effects of cholesteryl ester transfer protein inhibition on high-density lipoprotein subspecies, apolipoprotein A-I metabolism, and fecal sterol excretion. *Arterioscler Thromb Vasc Biol* 2005;25:1057–1064.
83. Hirano K, Yamashita S, Nakajima N, et al: Genetic cholesteryl ester transfer protein deficiency is extremely frequent in the Omagari area of Japan. Marked hyperalphalipoproteinemia caused by CETP gene mutations is not associated with longevity. *Arterioscler Thromb Vasc Biol* 1997;17:1053–1059.
84. Moriyama Y, Okamura T, Inazu A, et al: A low prevalence of coronary heart disease among subjects with increased high-density lipoprotein cholesterol levels including those with plasma cholesteryl ester transfer protein deficiency. *Prev Med* 1998;27:659–667.
85. Hirano K, Yamashita S, Matsuzawa Y: Pros and cons of inhibiting cholesteryl ester transfer protein. *Curr Opin Lipid* 2000;11:589–596.
86. Rue IL, Couture P, Cohn JS: Evidence that hepatic lipase deficiency in humans is not associated with proatherogenic changes in HDL composition and metabolism. *J Lipid Res* 2004:45:1528–1537.
87. Rader DJ, Schaefer JR, Lohse P, et al: Increased production of apolipoprotein A-I associated with elevated plasma levels of high-density lipoproteins, apolipoprotein A-I, and lipoprotein A-I in a patient with familial hyperalphalipoproteinemia. *Metabolism* 1993;42:1429–1434.

CHAPTER 5

Lipoproteins: Mechanisms for Atherogenesis and Progression of Atherothrombotic Disease

Peter Libby

INTRODUCTION

More than a century of laboratory and human findings link lipids with atherogenesis.[1] Fat-feeding studies in rabbits and subsequently in many other species demonstrated that diets enriched in cholesterol and saturated fat led to lesion formation.[2] Epidemiologic data secured the association of blood cholesterol levels and cardiovascular outcomes.[3–6] Pathoanatomic studies in humans supported a link between blood lipids and lesion formation.[7–10] Phylogenetic studies supported a link between cholesterol levels and the propensity to develop atherosclerosis. Low-density lipoprotein (LDL) levels in various species correlate fairly well with susceptibility to atherosclerosis.[11] Genetic studies detailed in subsequent chapters closed the loop of causality between cholesterol and atherosclerosis. The celebrated unraveling of the LDL receptor pathway showed that a single gene mutation that gave rise to hypercholesterolemia predisposed patients to the development of aggressive atherosclerosis.[12] More recent studies of the proprotein convertase subtilisin/kexin type 9 *(PCSK9)* gene in populations suggest that low cholesterol levels from birth confer protection from atherosclerotic disease.[13] This convincing constellation of data virtually fulfills Koch's postulates establishing a causal link between high LDL levels and atherosclerosis and its clinical consequences.

Despite the strength of these associations, even in the case of the relatively uncommon single gene mutations that predispose patients toward hypercholesterolemia and heightened atherogenesis, our understanding of the mechanisms that underlie these unassailable associations has lagged considerably. This chapter reviews the current state of our knowledge regarding this mechanistic link between lipoproteins and atherosclerosis.

INFLAMMATION: A FINAL COMMON PATH THAT LINKS MANY RISK FACTORS TO ATHEROGENESIS

Abundant data from the past several decades indicate that inflammation provides a common link between a number of atherogenic risk factors and altered arterial biology that promotes lesion formation and complication.[14] Subsequent sections dissect the inflammatory contributions to lesion initiation, progression, and complication. Popular schemes of the initiation of atherosclerosis posit a central role for modified lipoproteins and their constituents in instigating the inflammation that characterizes and drives atherosclerosis. In particular, the concept that oxidatively modified LDL or its constituents instigate inflammation and atherogenesis has gained considerable currency. However, the scientific basis for this popular viewpoint remains incomplete. Chapter 8 discusses in depth the oxidative modification of LDL. Much of the experimental literature about the effects of oxidized lipoproteins on vascular wall cells and inflammatory cells implicated in atherosclerosis has used transition metal–catalyzed oxidation as a tool. Fenton chemistry readily achieved in the laboratory may not apply so neatly to human atherosclerosis. Moreover, the "oxidized LDL" produced in the laboratory consists of an ill-defined and variable mixture of many mediators. Increasing chemical and biochemical rigor has identified specific structures that may activate inflammatory and immune responses that link dyslipidemia to atherogenesis mechanistically. Particular oxidized phospholipids with proinflammatory activity include palmitoyl oxovaleroyl phosphorylcholine (POVPC), 1-palmitoyl-2-glutaryl phosphatidylcholine (PGPC), and 1-palmitoyl-2-epoxyisoprostane-*sn*-glycero-3-phosphorylcholine (PEIPC) (Fig. 5-1). In addition to these specific oxidized phospholipids found in oxidized LDL, conformational epitopes of these phospholipids may elicit humoral and cellular immune responses that modulate inflammation during atherogenesis (see Chapter 8). Derivatization of the apolipoproteins (apos), for example, malondialdehyde-derivatized ε-amino groups of lysyl residues in apoB, may also engender immune responses that participate in atherogenesis.[15]

Molecular mechanisms by which the oxidized phospholipids can stimulate inflammation remain obscure for the most part. It appears reasonable that certain G-protein-coupled receptors on the surface of vascular or inflammatory cells may bind these oxidized phospholipids. In particular, heptahelical G-protein-coupled receptors can signal through class Ib phosphoinositide 3 kinase (PI3 kinase). Animals lacking the catalytic subunit of this class of PI3 kinases (p110γ) show attenuated atherosclerosis in response to hyperlipidemia.[16]

Beyond Fenton chemistry, modification of lipoproteins by reactive oxygen species may produce proinflammatory derivatives.[17] Notably, extracts of human atherosclerotic plaques bear the signatures of hypochlorous acid modification of amino acids such as chlorotyrosine. A subset of plaque macrophages contains myeloperoxidase, an enzyme that can generate hypochlorous acid and thus favor the derivatization of proteins and amino acids in the plaque.[18–20] In one well-studied example, chlorination of the specific tyrosine in apoA-I can interfere with the interaction of high-density lipoprotein (HDL) particles with the ATP-binding cassette A1 (ABCA1) transporter.[21,22] Thus, this "oxidative" modification of an apolipoprotein may indirectly promote inflammation by limiting the putative protective function of HDL particles during atherogenesis.

When activated by proinflammatory cytokines, arterial smooth muscle cells and mononuclear phagocytes increase the activity of oxidases that generate superoxide anion (O_2^-).[23,24] Activated phagocytes and smooth muscle cells may also generate high levels of nitric oxide (•NO). The capacity of human cells associated with atherosclerotic plaques to express the inducible isoform of nitric oxide synthase and, hence, produce excessive nitric oxide remains less well established than in rodents. Atherosclerotic plaques bear the signatures of nitration resulting from nitroxidation, including formation of the highly oxidant peroxynitrite radical by the combination of nitric oxide and superoxide.[25] This nitroxidation chemistry may also yield modification of lipoproteins implicated in atherogenesis.

In addition to oxidatively modified LDL and HDL, triglyceride-rich lipoproteins may promote inflammation (Fig. 5-2). Triglyceride-rich lipoproteins appear capable of stimulating inflammation by binding to the LDL receptor–related protein (LRP) through a pathway that involves p38 mitogen-activated protein (MAP) kinase and nuclear factor–κ B (NF-κB).[26] Triglyceride-rich lipoproteins abundant in apoC-III appear particularly proinflammatory. Recent evidence suggests that apoC-III can instigate inflammation through a pathway that involves protein kinase C (see Fig. 5-2).[27]

Thus, constituents of several classes of lipoproteins, LDL, HDL, and very-low-density lipoprotein (VLDL) and other triglyceride-rich lipoproteins can link to inflammatory pathways that operate during atherogenesis. These various mechanistic links have originated largely from laboratory studies and *in vitro* experiments correlated with *in situ* observations on retrieved atherosclerotic specimens. The following sections integrate these links between lipoproteins and inflammation with various temporal phases of lesion development, linking our current understanding of the cell and molecular biology of atherosclerosis and the clinical biology of its complications with lipoproteins. These sections aim to integrate lipoproteins and the pathogenesis of atherosclerosis.

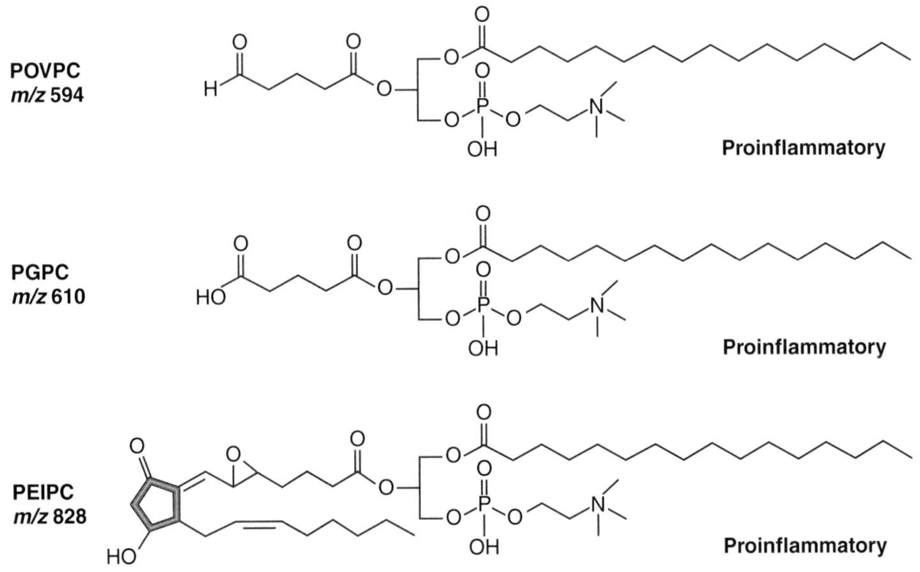

POVPC
***m/z* 594**
Proinflammatory

PGPC
***m/z* 610**
Proinflammatory

PEIPC
***m/z* 828**
Proinflammatory

FIGURE 5-1 Three proinflammatory oxidized phospholipids in minimally modified low-density lipoprotein (LDL). PEIPC, 1-palmitoyl-2-(5,6-epoxyisoprostane E_2)-*sn*-glycero-3-phosphorylcholine; PGPC, 1-palmitoyl-2-glutaryl-*sn*-glycero-3-phosphorylcholine; POVPC, 1-palmitoyl-2-oxovaleryl-*sn*-glycero-3-phosphorylcholine. *(Adapted from Ref. 38, with permission.)*

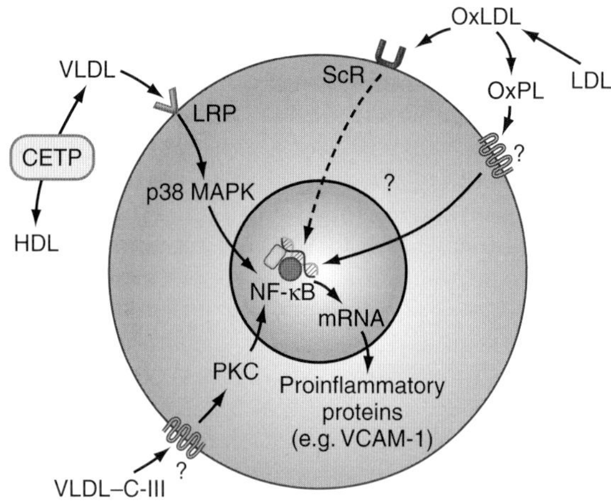

FIGURE 5-2 Atherogenic mechanisms of various lipoproteins. Low-density lipoprotein (LDL) modification generates forms of this lipoprotein that can undergo uptake by nonsuppressible scavenger receptors (ScR). This process advances the formation of foam cells of either macrophage or smooth muscle origin. Oxidation of LDL (OxLDL) provides bioactive lipids, including oxidized phospholipids (OxPL), which stimulate inflammation in vascular cells and leukocytes recruited to atherosclerotic lesions. These OxPL may interact with a cell surface receptor or trigger inflammatory pathways in target cells via other mechanisms. High-density lipoprotein (HDL) cholesterol and triglyceride levels fluctuate inversely partly because high levels of the triglyceride-rich lipoprotein very-low-density lipoprotein (VLDL) propel net transfer of cholesteryl ester from HDL particles to VLDL through cholesteryl ester transfer protein (CETP). HDL has anti-inflammatory properties as well as the capability to produce reverse cholesterol transport from foam cells. VLDL in turn putatively applies proinflammatory actions through binding and internalization via LDL receptor–related proteins (LRP) and downstream activation of p38 mitogen-activated protein (MAP) kinase and nuclear factor-κ B (NF-κB). Apolipoprotein C-III–containing lipoproteins, including VLDL (VLDL cholesterol-III), can trigger proinflammatory functions of endothelial cells, perhaps via a pertussis-sensitive, protein kinase C (PKC)–mediated pathway that can stimulate NF-κB. Vascular cell adhesion molecule–1 (VCAM-1), a sentinel proinflammatory gene regulated by NF-κB, plays a part in the recruitment of leukocytes to atheromata. Therefore, obesity- and diabetes mellitus–associated dyslipidemia, on the rise worldwide, can diminish endogenous anti-inflammatory pathways mediated by HDL and enhance proinflammatory actions of VLDL. *(Adapted from Ref. 1, with permission.)*

LIPOPROTEINS AND THE INITIATION OF ATHEROSCLEROSIS: RESPONSE TO LOW-DENSITY LIPOPROTEIN RETENTION AND BEYOND

In view of the strong evidence base supporting a causal role for LDL in atherogenesis, much attention to pathophysiologic mechanisms of this disease has centered on this family of lipoprotein particles. When in prolonged excess, LDL accumulates in the artery wall. Increased permeability of the endothelial monolayer may account for some of the LDL accumulation at sites prone to lesion formation. Classical observations have shown colocalization of sites predisposed to lesion formation and augmented accumulation of Evans blue, a dye that binds to albumin and the localization of which in the intima indicates permeability to proteins.[28] Quantitative studies using trapped ligand labels showed that increased retention of LDL in the intima contributed importantly to its accumulation.[29] Ultrastructural studies have shown entanglement of lipoprotein particles with extracellular matrix macromolecules in the arterial intima of animals that have consumed an atherogenic diet.[30]

Thus, morphologic observation provided a hint that increased dwelling of lipoprotein particles in the atherosclerotic intima might result from their retention by binding to extracellular matrix constituents (Fig. 5-3*A*). Considerable biochemical detail has emerged regarding the interaction of LDL particles with particular constituents of the arterial extracellular matrix (Fig. 5-4). A specific site in the apoB sequence influences the interaction of LDL particles with proteoglycan in a critical manner.[31] In particular, chondroitin sulfate–rich proteoglycan constituents of the arterial extracellular matrix appear to retard LDL.[32] In particular, biglycan and versican appear important in retaining apoB-containing particles in the arterial intima. In this regard, the excessive production of these chondroitin sulfate proteoglycans appears primordial in the pathogenesis of atherosclerosis. Human smooth muscle cells subjected to cyclic strain increase their production of proteoglycan molecules.[33] Thus, altered behavior of smooth muscle cells in response to biomechanical stimuli may promote the generation of an intimal extracellular matrix that provides a fertile field for the initiation of atherosclerosis.

The properties of different fractions of LDL appear to interact with extracellular matrix differentially. The small dense fraction of LDL appears to bind more readily to proteoglycan than does the larger "fluffier" fraction.[34,35] Small dense LDL particles tend to accumulate in individuals with high triglycerides and low levels of HDL, characteristics of the "metabolic syndrome" and diabetic dyslipidemia, as described in Chapter 37. The mechanistic link between heightened retention of small dense LDL and these metabolic conditions may provide part of the explanation for the propensity of these conditions to promote atherosclerosis. In particular, these qualitative aspects of LDL help us understand why diabetes often appears so intensely atherogenic in the face of average or near-average overall levels of LDL cholesterol.

In addition to defined biochemical interactions between LDL species and the intimal extracellular matrix, "accessory" enzymes may promote retention of LDL particles in the intima. In particular, lipoprotein lipase can bridge LDL particles to the extracellular matrix through a mechanism independent of its enzymatic activity.[32] Macrophages can synthesize lipoprotein lipase in the artery wall. Thus, whereas microvascular endothelial lipoprotein lipase appears to combat atherogenesis, local lipoprotein lipase in the intima may promote the retention of LDL and hence intensify atherogenesis. Secretory phospholipases overexpressed within atheromata may also process LDL particles in a way that increases their binding to intimal proteoglycan.[35] Likewise, processing by a secreted form of sphingomyelinase may augment the aggregation of lipoprotein particles in the artery wall, promoting their entrapment in this compartment. Sphingomyelinase action may also increase the binding of LDL particles to proteoglycan.[32] In sum, a variety of factors promote the accumulation of LDL in the intima at sites of early atherogenesis. In addition to locally increased permeability, retention resulting from electrostatic and sequence-specific interactions of LDL fractions with chondroitin sulfate–rich proteoglycan in the intima, augmented by the action of accessory enzymes, conspires to trap lipoproteins in the intima and increase their residence time.

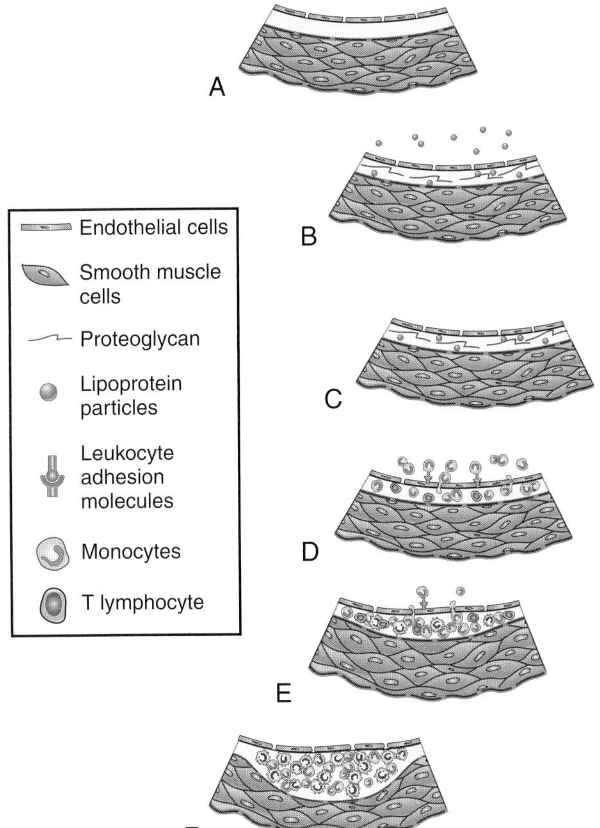

FIGURE 5-3 *A,* The normal artery. The normal artery consists of three layers: the intima, the media, and the adventitia. A monolayer of endothelial cells in contact with the blood lines the intima, which contains resident smooth muscle cells embedded in extracellular matrix. The internal elastic lamina comprises the border of the intima with the underlying tunica media. The middle layer, or tunica media, contains layers of smooth muscle cells invested with collagen- and elastin-rich extracellular matrix. Elastic arteries such as the aorta contain concentric lamellae of smooth muscle cells packed between dense bands of elastin. Muscular arteries have a looser organization of smooth muscle cells scattered within the matrix. The external elastic lamina serves as the border of the media with the adventitia, which contains nerves and some mast cells and is the origin of the vasa vasorum, which deliver blood to the outer two thirds of the tunica media. *B,* Accumulation of lipoprotein particles. Lipoprotein particles can amass in the intima of arteries, primarily because hypercholesterolemic states increase the ambient concentration. The lipoprotein particles often connect with constituents of the extracellular matrix, particularly proteoglycans, a key tenet of the "response to retention" concept. Sequestration within the intima separates lipoproteins from some plasma antioxidants and can advance oxidative modification. Such modified lipoprotein particles may produce a local inflammatory response responsible for signaling the ensuing steps of lesion formation, in part because of their content of specific lipid hydroperoxides shown in Figure 5-1. *C,* Adhesion of leukocytes. Adhesion of mononuclear leukocytes to the luminal endothelium takes place early in hypercholesterolemia. The increased expression of various adhesion molecules for leukocytes probably prompts this first step in the recruitment of white blood cells to a nascent arterial lesion. *D,* Penetration of leukocytes. Once adherent, some white blood cells migrate into the intima. The directed migration of leukocytes probably results from the action of chemoattractant factors, including modified lipoprotein particles and chemoattractant cytokines such as the chemokine monocyte chemoattractant protein–1 that vascular wall cells generate in response to modified lipoproteins. *E,* Accumulation of leukocytes. Leukocytes in the evolving fatty streak can divide and exhibit amplified expression of receptors for modified lipoproteins (scavenger receptors). These mononuclear phagocytes accumulate lipids and become foam cells, so called because of their lipid droplet–filled cytoplasm. *F,* Formation of the fibrous cap and lipid core. As the fatty streak develops into a more complex atherosclerotic lesion, smooth muscle cells amass within the expanding intima and the amount of extracellular matrix increases. The fibrous cap, which comprises extracellular matrix elaborated by the smooth muscle cells in the intima, characteristically covers a lipid core filled with macrophages. In addition to dividing, these cells in the lipid core can die, releasing their intracellular content and membrane-derived microparticles into the extracellular space. *(Adapted from Libby P: The pathogenesis of atherosclerosis. In: Harrison's Principles of Internal Medicine. New York, Blackwell Publishing, 2001, with permission.)*

The intima provides an environment sequestered from plasma antioxidants.[36] The increased dwelling time of LDL in atherosclerosis-prone regions of the intima may afford a greater opportunity for oxidative modification of the constituents of these particles in these regions relatively excluded from antioxidant protection. The various pro-oxidant mechanisms alluded to earlier have a greater opportunity to modify the lipoprotein particles residing for prolonged periods in the intima as a consequence of proteoglycan binding. Extravasation of erythrocytes from disrupted microvessels in more advanced lesions can lead to the deposition of heme in the extracellular space, a source of iron that may catalyze oxidation by Fenton chemistry. Myeloperoxidase and phospholipases have greater opportunity to modify lipoprotein particles with tardy transit caused by proteoglycan binding. As noted earlier, the oxidized phospholipids produced in this manner include biologically active species that can elicit an inflammatory response from surrounding intrinsic vascular wall cells and leukocytes as they accumulate. Thus, the "response to retention" provides a mechanistic link between accumulation of lipoprotein particles in the nascent atherosclerotic lesion and proinflammatory processes that amplify and sustain the atherogenic process.[32]

HIGH-DENSITY LIPOPROTEIN: THE ANTIATHEROGENIC LIPOPROTEIN

Abundant epidemiologic evidence establishes HDL as an inverse risk factor for atherosclerosis (see Chapters 4 and 10). Glomset first hypothesized a role for HDL in reverse cholesterol transport.[37] Recent evidence, reviewed in Chapter 4, has furnished a mechanistic understanding of the method by which HDL likely mediates egress of cholesterol from lipid-laden foam cells. ABCA1 mediates transfer of cholesterol to nascent HDL particles, whereas ABCG1 ferries cholesterol from cells to mature HDL particles. Scavenger receptor class B type I (SR-BI) appears to mediate uptake of cholesterol from HDL by steroidogenic organs and the liver. Human mutants (e.g., Tangier disease; see Chapter 4) verify a role for HDL in macrophage lipid accumulation. *In vitro* experiments verify the ability of HDL fractions to mediate lipid efflux from cholesterol-loaded cells. Thus, reverse cholesterol transport likely contributes to the cardiovascular benefit associated with increasing levels of plasma HDL.

Beyond the role of HDL in shuttling cholesterol, it may affect arterial biology as a carrier of anti-inflammatory and antioxidant proteins. Navab and colleagues have provided evidence that phospholipases associated with the HDL particle can catabolize some of the biologically active and proinflammatory oxidized phospholipids associated with modified LDL.[38] Proteins such as platelet-activating factor (PAF) acetylhydrolase and paraoxynase-1 (PON-1) exemplify such putative antioxidant proteins associated with HDL particles. Recent proteomic studies have further established the association of dozens of proteins with HDL particles, including a number that may favorably alter arterial biology. HDL particles associate with a number

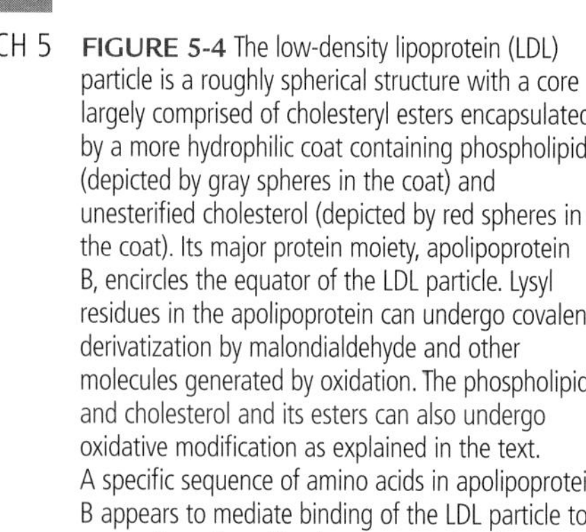

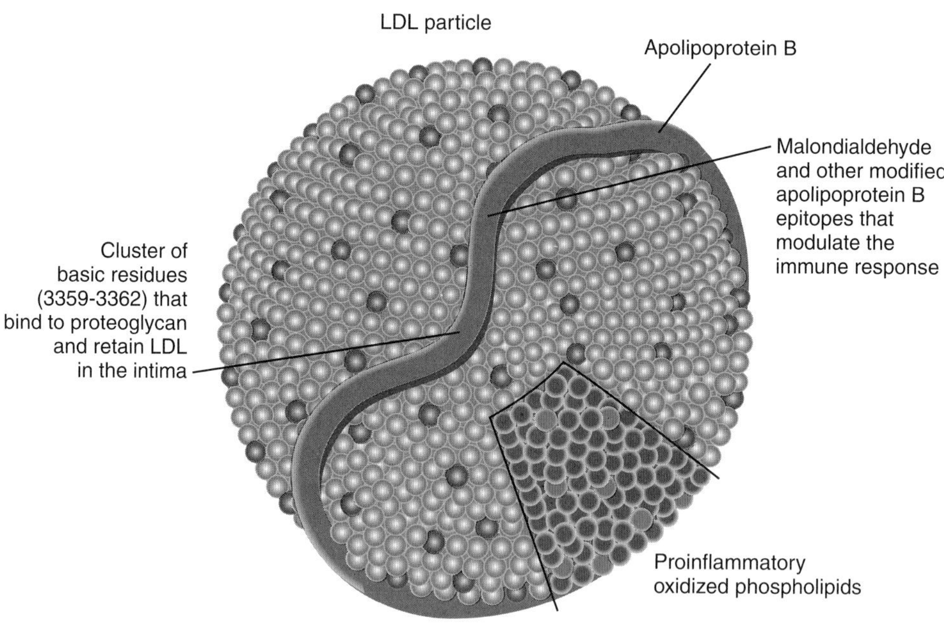

FIGURE 5-4 The low-density lipoprotein (LDL) particle is a roughly spherical structure with a core largely comprised of cholesteryl esters encapsulated by a more hydrophilic coat containing phospholipids (depicted by gray spheres in the coat) and unesterified cholesterol (depicted by red spheres in the coat). Its major protein moiety, apolipoprotein B, encircles the equator of the LDL particle. Lysyl residues in the apolipoprotein can undergo covalent derivatization by malondialdehyde and other molecules generated by oxidation. The phospholipids and cholesterol and its esters can also undergo oxidative modification as explained in the text. A specific sequence of amino acids in apolipoprotein B appears to mediate binding of the LDL particle to proteoglycan found in plaque, promoting the retention and oxidative modification of LDL in the arterial intima, an environment to which plasma antioxidants have limited accessibility.

of complement regulatory proteins and protease inhibitors (Fig. 5-5).[39] *In vivo* experiments in animals support an anti-inflammatory role of HDL.[40] For example, HDL infusions can limit expression of vascular cell adhesion molecule (VCAM) in injured arteries.[41]

However, not all HDL particles may exert anti-inflammatory actions. Some postulate the existence of proinflammatory HDL species. During systemic inflammatory states, levels of the acute-phase reactant serum amyloid A (SAA) mount. Levels of SAA, like those of C-reactive protein, can rise 10- to 100-fold during the acute-phase response to infection or tissue injury. The amphipathic acute-phase reactant SAA binds avidly to HDL and can displace certain other potentially atheroprotective proteins from these particles.[38] Thus, during acute inflammatory states, HDL may lose some of its anti-inflammatory properties. *In vitro* assays suggest that under some conditions HDL can actually promote inflammation.

Although the epidemiologic association between HDL and cardiovascular disease remains undisputed, whether manipulation of HDL can benefit atherosclerosis still remains hypothetical. Further investigations of the clinical consequences of manipulating HDL and its apolipoprotein species should clarify this clinically important area.

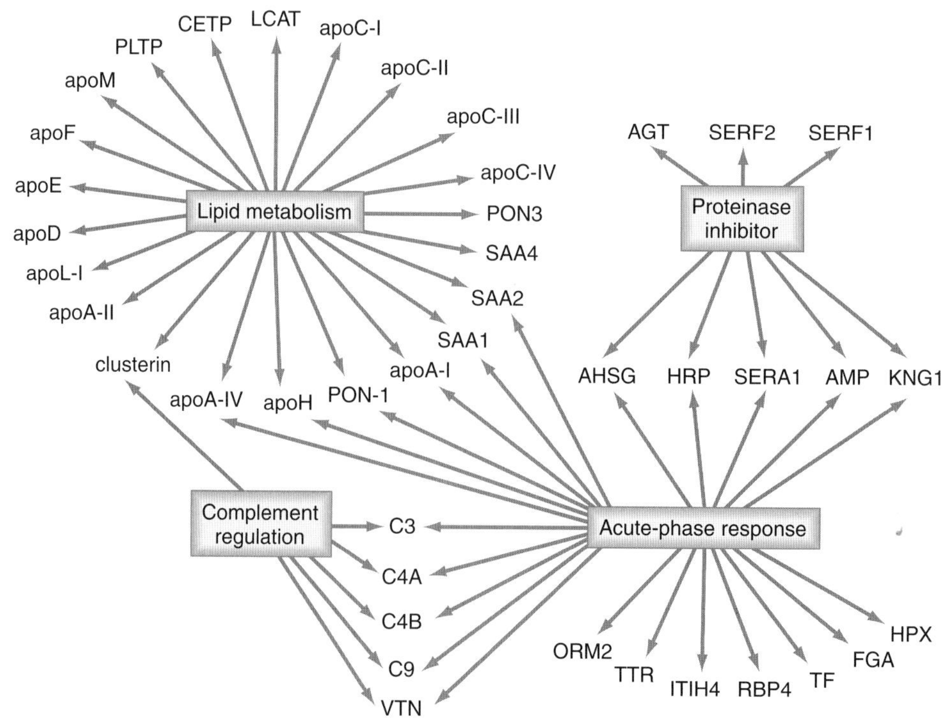

FIGURE 5-5 Global view of biologic processes and molecular functions of high-density lipoprotein (HDL) proteins. Proteins in total HDL and HDL_3 were identified through a proteomic analysis. This approach established significant over-representation of proteins involved in several categories, including lipid metabolism, the acute-phase response, protease inhibitor activity, and complement regulation. AGT, angiotensinogen; apo, apolipoprotein; AHSG, α-2-HS-glycoprotein; AMP, bikunin; apoH, β-2-glycoprotein I; CETP, cholesteryl ester transfer protein; FGA, fibrinogen; HPX, hemopexin; HRP, haptoglobin-related protein; ITIH4, inter-α-trypsin inhibitor heavy chain H4; KNG1, kininogen-1; LCAT, lecithin:cholesterol acyltransferase; ORM2, α-1-acid glycoprotein 2; PLTP, phospholipid transfer protein; PON-1, Paraoxynase-1; RBP4, retinol-binding protein; SAA, serum amyloid A; SERA1, α-1-antitrypsin; SERF1, serpin peptidase inhibitor (clade F, member 1); SERF2, α-2-antiplasmin; TF, transferrin; TTR, transthyretin; VTN, vitronectin. *(Adapted from Ref. 22, with permission.)*

FATTY STREAK FORMATION

The retardation and accumulation of LDL particles in the intima set the stage for the inflammatory processes that lead to lesion formation (see Fig. 5-3*B* and *C*). One of the first cellular consequences of hyperlipidemia, the recruitment of blood leukocytes, has undergone intensive scrutiny over the past few decades (see Fig. 5-3*D*).[42,43] The arterial endothelium usually resists prolonged contact with blood leukocytes. However, in response to constituents of oxidatively modified lipoproteins or protein mediators of inflammation such as cytokines, endothelial cells express structures on their luminal surface that promote leukocyte adhesion. The endothelial cell–leukocyte adhesion molecules implicated in atherogenesis fall into two major families: the selectins and the immunoglobulin G (IgG) superfamily members.[44] Of the selectins, considerable evidence supports the pathogenic involvement of P-selectin, found on platelets as well as endothelial cells, in the formation of experimental atherosclerotic lesions.[45] The selectins mediate the initial "rolling" or saltatory interaction of leukocytes with the endothelial monolayer. Members of the IgG superfamily appear responsible for the more prolonged adhesive interactions between arterial endothelium and the mononuclear leukocytes that accumulate at sites of atherosclerotic lesion formation.[46] Intercellular adhesion molecule–1 (ICAM-1) appears less important in this regard than VCAM-1.[47] Considerable experimental evidence in several species substantiates a causal role of VCAM-1 in early atherosclerotic lesion formation. Hypercholesterolemia prominently promotes VCAM-1 expression in a variety of species tested. Curiously, VCAM-1 does not consistently localize to the endothelium overlying early atherosclerotic lesions in humans. Rather, its expression prominently localizes to neovascular channels in more advanced lesions.[48] Nonetheless, the broad experimental literature strongly supports a link between hypercholesterolemia and elevated levels of adhesion molecule expression that promotes the adherence of blood leukocytes to endothelial cells at sites of lesion predilection.

The regionality of adhesion molecule expression and early leukocyte expression begs for explanation, given the homogeneity of the hypercholesterolemia that impinges on endothelial cells throughout the arterial tree. Strong evidence supports links between the local hydrodynamic environment and sites of early leukocyte recruitment.[42] Areas of low shear stress or disturbed flow appear particularly predisposed to lesion initiation. These local biomechanical conditions combat constitutive atheroprotective mechanisms characteristic of the normal endothelial monolayer. Laminar shear stress encountered in less atherosclerosis-prone regions of the circulation increases the expression of the endothelial isoform of nitric oxide synthase. This enzyme generates constitutive low levels of the endogenous vasodilator •NO, which may also inhibit the expression of VCAM-1 and thus limit leukocyte interaction with the normal endothelium. Laminar shear stress also augments the expression of superoxide dismutase, an endogenous antioxidant produced by endothelial cells. One of the orchestrators of a number of putative atheroprotective genes, Kruppel-like factor–2 (KLF2), also responds to shear stress.[49,50] When deprived of these usually atheroprotective functions of the endothelial cells at sites of disturbed flow, the adherence of leukocytes increases, providing a mechanistic explanation for the regional distributions of lesions in the presence of hypercholesterolemia.

Once bound to the endothelial cells, the leukocytes require a chemoattractant signal to penetrate into the intima (see Fig. 5-3*E*). A subclass of cytokines, protein mediators of inflammation and immunity, known as *chemokines,* promotes this process.[51,52] Abundant experimental studies and observations on human tissues support the involvement of a number of chemokines and chemokine receptors in leukocyte recruitment in early atherosclerotic plaques. These ligand–receptor pairs include monocyte chemoattractant protein–1 (MCP-1), interleukin-8 (IL-8), and fractalkine, *inter alii.* Loss-of-function studies in experimental atherosclerosis in mice support the pathogenic involvement of these chemokines in lesion formation.[53] Like the adhesion molecules, hyperlipidemia augments the expression of chemokines for mononuclear cells in arteries. Recent work has highlighted the importance of subpopulations of mononuclear cells in hyperlipemic conditions. In hypercholesterolemic mice, in particular, a subpopulation of proinflammatory monocytes identified by high levels of expression of Ly-6c prevails.[54,55] This proinflammatory population of monocytes preferentially enters the intima and contributes to clear cell accumulation in the nascent lesion. In addition to monocytes, T lymphocytes enter the arterial intima early during atherogenesis. Although less numerically abundant than the monocytes/macrophages, the T cells probably play important regulatory roles in the pathogenesis of atherosclerosis.[56,57] A separate set of adhesion molecules and the chemokine receptor CXCR-3 appear responsible for attracting the T cells to nascent atheromata. Notably, a trio of chemokines inducible by interferon-γ (IFN-γ) likely promotes T-cell accumulation in early lesions.[58]

Mast cells were first localized in atheromata in the 1950s; experimental evidence now supports a pathogenic role for these cells, at least in murine atherosclerosis. Products of mast cells may promote a number of proatherogenic processes. Mast cell products may also remodel lipoprotein particles in ways that increase their atherogenicity.[59,60] Recent pharmacologic gain-of-function and loss-of-function experiments and parallel experiments in genetically altered mice support a role for mast cells in atheroma formation.[61,62] However, mice may depend on mast cells for host defenses more than humans do, a fact that cautions against the facile extrapolation of the mouse results to the human situation.

Once resident in the arterial intima, blood monocytes mature into macrophages. In the atherosclerotic plaque, the characteristic tissue macrophage, that is, the foam cell, accumulates substantial intracellular cholesterol in droplets, yielding the characteristic foamy appearance of the cytoplasm on histologic study. Cells cannot accumulate excessive amounts of cholesterol via the classical apoB/apoE, or LDL, receptor. A number of exquisite regulatory mechanisms suppress the expression of this receptor as cells accumulate sufficient amounts of cholesterol for their cellular metabolism. A series of "scavenger" receptors can cause accumulation of cholesterol in the cytoplasm.[63] Scavenger receptors implicated in atherogenesis include the macrophage scavenger receptor class A (SR-A), CD36, and members of a lectin-like family. Scavenger receptors characteristically increase in expression in response to proinflammatory signals and do not exhibit suppression as intracellular cholesterol levels rise. Thus, inflammatory cells exposed to inflammatory mediators lead to formation of the hallmark of the early atherosclerotic lesion—the foam cell.

In sum, lipoproteins and their products appear essential in driving the formation of the initial lesion of atherosclerosis, the fatty streak, which is characterized by foam cell formation at sites of lesion predilection in arteries (see Fig. 5-3*F*). Increased adhesion leukocytes, their transmigration, and their maturation all link to aspects of hyperlipidemia, which appears permissive for all of these steps in early atherogenesis (see Fig. 5-3*A–F*).

LINKS BETWEEN LIPIDS AND LESION PROGRESSION

Fatty streaks, the initial lesion of atherosclerosis, seldom, if ever, cause clinical complications and may even regress. Atherosclerotic lesions progress by accumulating vascular smooth muscle cells and accumulating a complex extracellular matrix that consists not only of proteoglycans but also of collagens and elastin. The normal human arterial intima contains a scattering of smooth muscle cells.[64] In response to chemoattractant mediators and growth factors elaborated by activated inflammatory cells, as well as intrinsic vascular wall cells, smooth muscle cells normally found in the tunica intima can proliferate and augment their production of extracellular matrix constituents. Likewise, chemoattractants elaborated by the inflammatory cells in the intima can beckon normally quiescent smooth muscle cells from the tunica media to enter the intima. Mediators implicated in smooth muscle cell chemoattraction and proliferation include platelet-derived growth factor (PDGF) isoforms, forms of fibroblast growth factor, and heparin-binding epidermal growth factor. Extracellular matrix production by smooth muscle cells increases markedly when exposed to active forms of transforming growth factor–β (TGF-β). TGF-β may actually inhibit smooth muscle cell proliferation but strongly augments production of interstitial collagen, an important constituent of the evolving atherosclerotic plaque.

Curiously, as the volume of the intima increases because of accumulation of cells, and in particular, the complex extracellular matrix that they elaborate, the progressing atheroma seldom protrudes into the arterial lumen until it grows quite large. Rather, the artery wall expands in an abluminal, or outward, direction to accommodate lesion growth for much of the life history of the atherosclerotic plaque (Fig. 5-6*A* and *B*, Fig. 5-7, and Fig. 5-8). This geometric remodeling of the atherosclerotic plaque, known as *compensatory enlargement* or

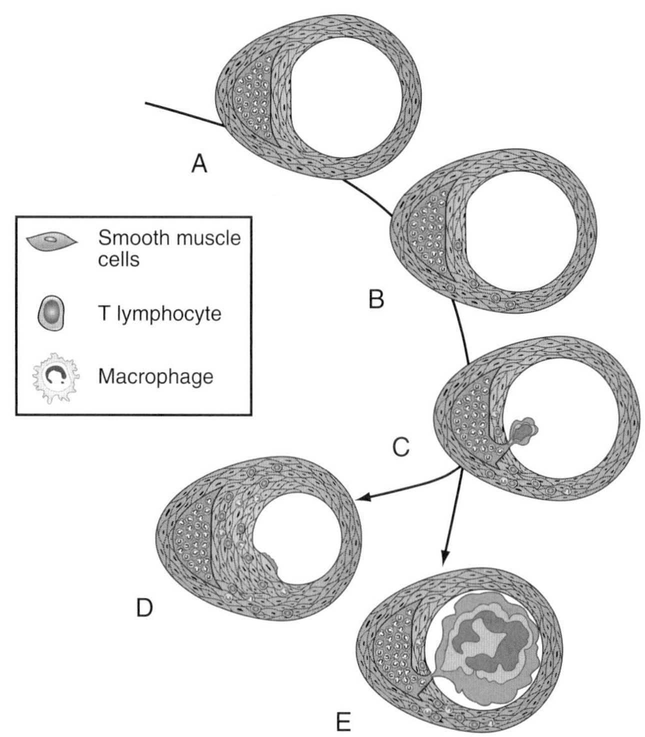

FIGURE 5-6 Plaque rupture, thrombosis, and healing. *A,* Arterial remodeling during atherogenesis. During the initial part of the existence of an atheroma, it often expands, conserving the caliber of lumen. This phenomenon, "compensatory enlargement," accounts in part for the tendency of coronary arteriography to underestimate the extent of atherosclerosis. *B,* Focal inflammation characterizes unstable atherosclerotic plaques. Foci of inflammation often arise in atheromata. Analyses of lesions that have ruptured and caused fatal myocardial infarction typically show prominent infiltration of macrophages and T lymphocytes. Both leukocytes and intrinsic vascular cells around sites of plaque rupture exhibit markers of inflammatory activation. *C,* Rupture of the plaque's fibrous cap causes thrombosis. Physical disruption of the atherosclerotic plaque generally causes arterial thrombosis by allowing blood coagulant factors to contact thrombogenic collagen in the arterial extracellular matrix and tissue factor generated by macrophage-derived foam cells in the lipid core of lesions. In this manner, sites of plaque rupture fashion the nidus for thrombi. The normal artery wall possesses several fibrinolytic or antithrombotic mechanisms that tend to withstand thrombosis and lyse clots that begin to form *in situ*. These antithrombotic or thrombolytic molecules include thrombomodulin, tissue and urokinase-type plasminogen activators, heparan sulfate proteoglycans, prostacyclin, and nitric oxide. When the clot overwhelms the endogenous fibrinolytic mechanisms, it may proliferate and lead to arterial occlusion *(E)*. In some cases, the thrombus may lyse or organize into a mural thrombus without obstructing the vessel. Such occurrences may remain clinically silent. The succeeding thrombin-induced fibrosis and healing causes a fibroproliferative reaction that can produce a more fibrous lesion, one that can generate an eccentric plaque that causes a hemodynamically significant stenosis *(D)*. *D,* Healing of a mural thrombus leads to lesion fibrosis and progression and luminal narrowing. Local thrombin activation can trigger smooth muscle production. Platelets release proteins, including platelet-derived growth factors and transforming growth factor–β that may also enhance collagen production by smooth muscle cells and modulate their growth. In this way, a nonocclusive mural thrombus, even if clinically silent or causing unstable angina rather than infarction, can prompt a healing response that can promote lesion fibrosis and luminal encroachment. Such a sequence of events may convert a "vulnerable" atheroma with a thin fibrous cap that is likely to rupture into a more "stable" fibrous plaque with a reinforced cap. Angioplasty of unstable coronary lesions may "stabilize" the lesions through a similar mechanism, causing a wound followed by healing. *E,* Plaque rupture with a propagated, occlusive thrombus can cause acute myocardial infarction. When a stable, occlusive thrombus forms in a coronary artery, the consequences hinge on the degree of existing collateral vessels. In a patient with chronic multivessel occlusive coronary artery disease, collateral channels have usually developed. Under such conditions, even a total arterial occlusion may not lead to myocardial infarction, or it may produce an unexpectedly modest or a non–ST elevation myocardial infarct because of collateral flow. In the patient with less advanced disease and without substantial stenotic lesions to provide a stimulus to collateral vessel formation, sudden plaque rupture and arterial occlusion generally beget ST-segment elevation myocardial infarction. These are the types of patients who may present with myocardial infarction or sudden death as a first sign of coronary atherosclerosis. *(Adapted from Libby P: The pathogenesis, prevention, and treatment, of atherosclerosis. In: Harrison's Principles of Internal Medicine. New York, Blackwell Publishing, 2008, with permission.)*

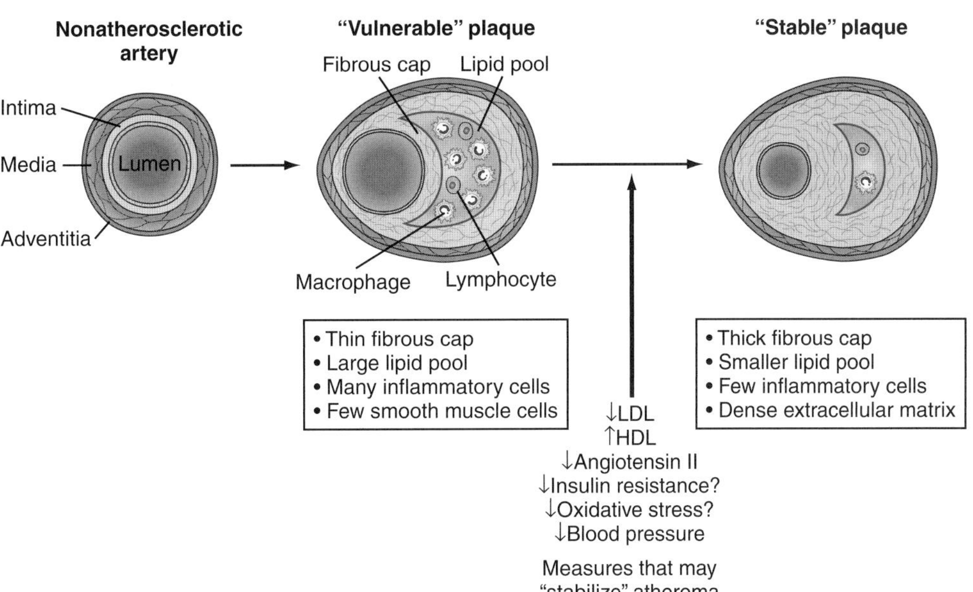

FIGURE 5-7 Evolution and stabilization of "vulnerable" atherosclerotic plaques. The nonatherosclerotic artery *(left)* has a trilaminar structure. During the early stage of atherosclerotic development, the atheroma often grows outward and maintains the caliber of the lumen *(middle)*. Pathologic studies have shown that the majority of atheromata that have ruptured and triggered an acute myocardial infarction contain a prominent lipid pool and numerous inflammatory cells, particularly macrophages. The activated inflammatory cells produce mediators that thin and weaken the fibrous cap that covers the lipid-rich core of the lesion by reducing synthesis and augmenting degradation of collagen. Smooth muscle cell apoptosis may also play a role in the depletion of collagen in the fibrous cap. Activated macrophages express tissue factor, a powerful activator of the coagulation cascade. Disruption of the thin fibrous cap of such vulnerable plaques leads to direct contact of blood coagulation factors with tissue factor and can initiate occlusive thrombus formation. Stabilization of lesions aims to lower the incidence of acute coronary events by influencing the nature of the vulnerable plaque qualitatively or functionally rather than by shrinking the lesion *(right)*. Lowering low-density lipoprotein (LDL) can diminish cholesterol delivery, and increased high-density lipoprotein (HDL) may enhance cholesterol efflux from the atheroma. Reducing LDL and inhibiting angiotensin II signaling may limit oxidative stress (e.g., reactive oxygen species production, lipid peroxidation, and oxidized LDL accumulation) in atheroma. Converting unstable plaques to stable plaques by modifying their biologic properties should prevent cardiovascular events such as myocardial infarction and stroke through a noninvasive strategy rather than helping in the conventional mechanical approach (bypass surgery, endarterectomy, or angioplasty). *(Adapted from Ref. 96, with permission.)*

positive remodeling, has been studied surprisingly little from a mechanistic perspective.[65–67] Clearly, extracellular matrix proteolysis must occur for smooth muscle cells to migrate through the dense arterial extracellular matrix. The elastic laminae must expand to accommodate lesion growth and also likely involve proteolysis. The positive remodeling characteristic of the progression phase of atherosclerosis conceals the disease beneath the clinical horizon by favoring lesion growth without luminal encroachment and consequent tissue ischemia that could produce clinical signs or symptoms.

As the early atherosclerotic lesion progresses, it acquires a characteristic distribution of constituents. A fibrous cap develops over a lipid-rich core in the typical eccentric atheroma.[68] The fibrous cap contains smooth muscle cells and a collagenous extracellular matrix. The lipid core accommodates the macrophage foam cells. Extracellular lipid accumulates, bound to the extracellular matrix in the fibrous cap and in the extracellular space, as well as intracellular deposits in the lipid core in particular. Cholesterol may accumulate either as cholesteryl ester or as cholesterol monohydrate, a chemical form that can develop crystals within plaques. Lipoprotein involvement in lesion progression probably results predominantly from perturbations that promote inflammation. Inflammatory mediators appear proximal in pathways that promote smooth muscle cell migration and proliferation as well as elaboration of extracellular matrix and of proteinases capable of remodeling the arterial extracellular matrix.

ATHEROTHROMBOSIS: THE COMPLICATIONS OF THE ATHEROSCLEROTIC PLAQUE

As atherosclerosis progresses, many changes occur in the plaque's lipid core. Macrophages not only proliferate but also die. Macrophage death in atherosclerotic plaques may occur by oncosis ("accidental" cell death) or by apoptosis (an energy-dependent and programmed process).[69–71] Oncosis, characterized by cell swelling, causes the lipid-laden macrophage to release its contents into the extracellular space. Deprived of the normal cellular antioxidant mechanisms and in contact with extracellular phospholipases and sphingomyelinase, as well as reactive oxygen species elaborated by activated cells, cholesteryl ester released by dying macrophages may have a particular propensity to undergo oxidative modification and perpetuate the proinflammatory state that prevails in the progressing atherosclerotic plaque.

As macrophages undergo programmed cell death (apoptosis), they can bud off membrane-bound microparticles known as *apoptotic bodies.* Lesional macrophages, in response to proinflammatory mediators such as CD154, also known as *CD40 ligand,* express the gene that encodes tissue factor, a potent procoagulant.[72] The apoptotic bodies bear this intrinsic membrane protein on their surface, thus providing a ready store of triggers for thrombus formation in the heart of the lesion.

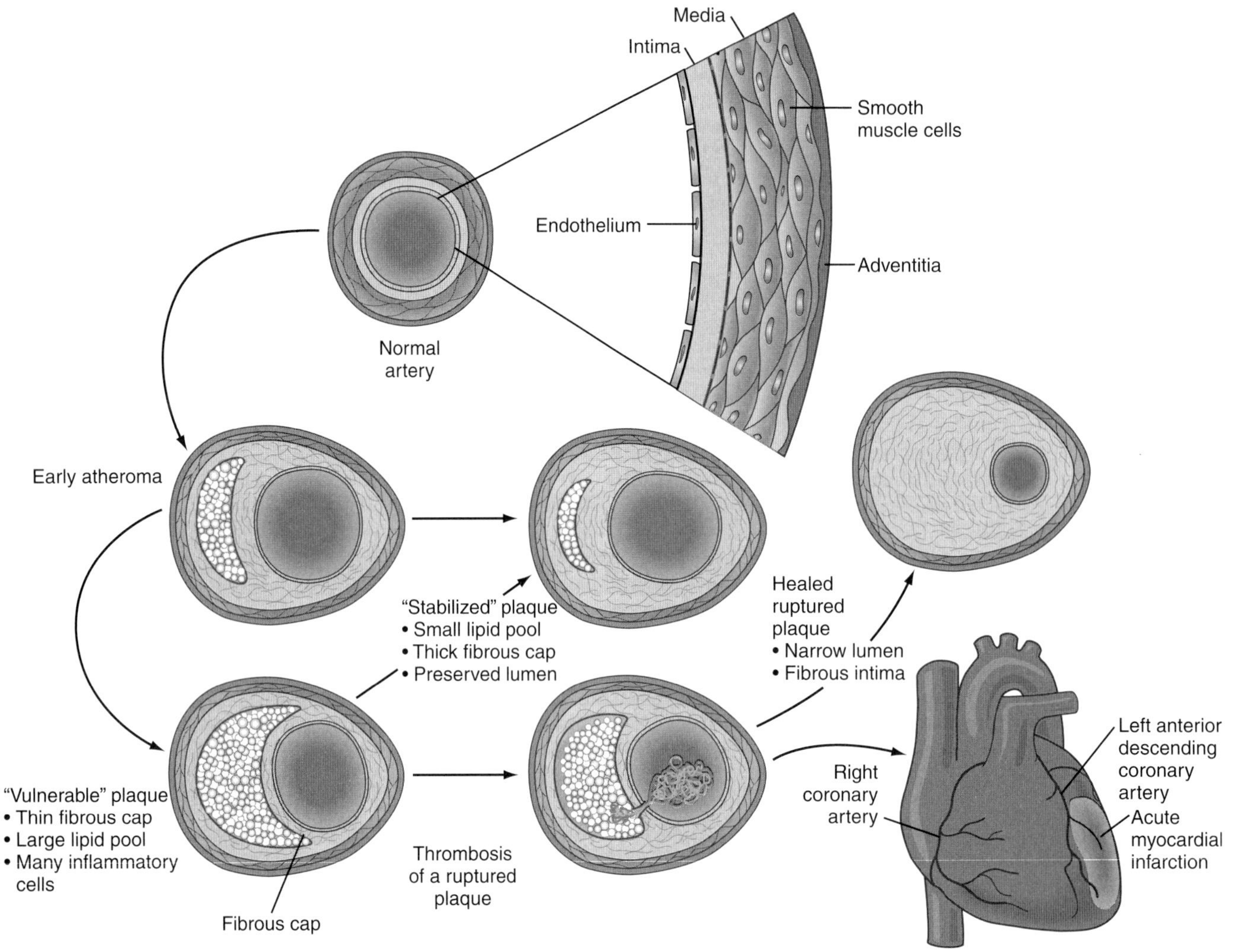

FIGURE 5-8 Schematic of the life history of an atheroma. The normal human coronary artery has a typical trilaminar structure. The intimal layer in adult humans typically contains a smattering of smooth muscle cells scattered in the extracellular matrix. The media comprises several layers of smooth muscle cells, much more tightly packed than in the diffusely thickened intima, and embedded in a matrix rich in elastin and collagen. In early atherogenesis, inflammatory cell recruitment and lipid buildup form a lipid-rich core, as the artery enlarges in an outward, abluminal direction to accommodate the growth of the intima. If inflammatory conditions exist and risk factors such as dyslipidemia continue, the lipid core can grow; in addition, activated leukocytes secrete proteinases that can degrade the extracellular matrix, while proinflammatory cytokines such as interferon-γ (IFN-γ) can restrict the production of new collagen. These changes can weaken the fibrous cap, rendering it friable and vulnerable to rupture. Upon rupture of the plaque, blood coming in contact with the tissue factor in the plaque coagulates. Platelets activated by thrombin produced by the coagulation cascade and by contact with the intimal compartment prompt thrombus formation. Persistent occlusion of the vessel by the thrombus can result in an acute myocardial infarction (the shadowy area in the anterior wall of the left ventricle, *lower right*). The thrombus may eventually resorb as a result of endogenous or therapeutic thrombolysis. However, a wound-healing response triggered by thrombin generated during blood coagulation can trigger smooth muscle production. Activated platelets release platelet-derived growth factor, which prompts smooth muscle cell migration. Transforming growth factor–β (TGF–β), also released from activated platelets, induces interstitial collagen production. This increased migration, proliferation, and extracellular matrix synthesis by smooth muscle cells thickens the fibrous cap and causes further expansion of the intima, often now in an inward direction, constricting the lumen. Stenotic lesions generated by the luminal advance of the fibrosed plaque may diminish flow, particularly under conditions of increased cardiac demand; this leads to ischemia, which commonly triggers symptoms such as angina pectoris. Advanced stenotic plaques, being more fibrous, may prove less prone to rupture and renewed thrombosis. Lipid-lowering therapy can reduce lipid content and calm the intimal inflammatory response, producing a more "stable" plaque with a thick fibrous cap and a preserved lumen *(center)*. *(Adapted from Ref. 53, with permission.)*

Meanwhile, the biology of the plaque's fibrous cap evolves. The smooth muscle cells that populate the fibrous cap do not escape apoptotic cell death. Smooth muscle cells in the intima express FAS, a receptor for the death signal Fas ligand, expressed by activated leukocytes in lesions.[73] A milieu rich in proinflammatory cytokines primes smooth muscle cells for apoptotic cell death. Smooth muscle cells furnish most of the collagen and elastin that lend strength to the plaque's fibrous cap. The loss of smooth muscle cells in the fibrous cap as a result of cell death impairs the ability of this cell population to repair and maintain the extracellular matrix that provides biomechanical integrity to this crucial structure that lies between the blood compartment and the prothrombotic material in the lipid core.[74,75]

In the base of the plaque, underlying the lipid core, plexi of newly formed microvessels arise generally from vasa vasorum that penetrate the plaque from the outermost layer of the arterial wall, the adventitia. These plexi of microvessels provide a relatively large surface area for recruitment of leukocytes that may amplify the inflammatory environment within the lesion. As noted earlier, these plaque microvessels display considerable VCAM-1 expression and hence appear poised for mononuclear cell recruitment. These microvessels provide a source of nutrition to the growing atherosclerotic plaque analogous to the neovessels that foster tumor growth. Like newly formed vessels in the retina and elsewhere, the plaque's neovasculature may prove particularly permeable and promote erythrocyte extravasation with attendant heme and iron deposition in the extracellular space, catalyzing oxidant chemistry as noted earlier.[76] Membrane lipids from extravasated erythrocytes may also contribute to lipid accumulation within lesions.[77]

Thrombosis *in situ* resulting from microvascular hemorrhage can lead to thrombin formation. Thrombin potently promotes smooth muscle cell migration and proliferation. Thus, episodes of intraplaque hemorrhage well below the clinical threshold may predispose patients to plaque complications by initiating a round of smooth muscle cell migration and proliferation. Platelets, when activated at these sites of intraplaque hemorrhage, can elaborate chemokines and growth factors that enhance leukocyte recruitment as well as smooth muscle cell activation.[78] TGF-β derived from activated platelets probably promotes collagen deposition in the complicating plaque. The fibrotic response that ensues after episodes of intraplaque hemorrhage may promote constrictive remodeling that causes the plaque to protrude into the lumen and provoke stenosis (see Fig. 5-6*C–E*). Lesions that thus embarrass arterial flow can cause ischemia and its well-known clinical consequences, including chronic stable angina, when it affects the coronary arteries.

A great deal of clinical and morphologic data indicate that thrombosis-complicating atherosclerotic lesions provoke most acute coronary syndromes, such as episodes of unstable angina pectoris or acute myocardial infarction (see Fig. 5-6*D*). Interestingly, many plaques that promote sudden arterial occlusion that cause a fatal myocardial infarction do not arise at sites of severe stenosis. Many morphologic studies point to a physical disruption of the atherosclerotic plaque as the most common precipitant of fatal coronary thrombi and presumably many acute myocardial infarctions.

Of the forms of physical disruption that precipitate acute coronary syndromes, a rupture of the plaque's fibrous cap appears most prominent (see Fig. 5-6*C*).[79] Plaques that have ruptured and precipitated death from myocardial infarction typically have large lipid pools, abundant inflammatory cells, and a characteristically thin fibrous cap. Mechanisms described earlier probably predispose patients to plaque disruption by promoting friability of the plaque's cap. Smooth muscle cell death depletes the plaque of the major cellular source of collagen and elastin that lend strength to the plaque's cap. Inflammatory mediators promote overproduction of proteinases that can catabolize collagen and weaken the plaque's protective cap. Plaques prominently overexpress a number of proteases capable of degrading extracellular matrix macromolecules.[80] Members of the matrix metalloproteinase (MMP) family include the interstitial collagenases, which are rate-limiting enzymes in the catabolic pathway of forms of collagen that strengthen the plaque's fibrous cap. MMP gelatinases continue collagen catabolism. Prominent elastases overexpressed in plaque include not only MMP-9, which possesses both elastinolytic and gelatinolytic activity, but also members of the papain-like cysteinyl proteinases.[81] Cathepsins S, K, and L have substantial elastolytic activity and contribute to arterial remodeling during atherogenesis and disruption of the elastic laminae characteristic of inflamed atherosclerotic plaques. Considerable experimental evidence supports the causal involvement of these matrix-degrading proteinases in collagenolysis and elastolysis in atherosclerotic plaques. Mice with a form of interstitial collagen that resists the action of MMP collagenases accumulate excessive collagen in their atheromata.[82] Animals deficient in a major murine interstitial collagenase, MMP-13, likewise accumulate collagen in their plaques.[83] Mice with bone marrow–derived cells deficient in membrane type 1 MMP, or MMP-14, also accumulate plaque collagen.[84] MMP-14 may act directly as an interstitial collagenase and activate other enzymes involved in collagen degradation. Serine proteinases derived from mast cells, such as tryptase and chymase, can activate latent zymogen forms of the MMP.[85] In addition, plasmin produced by endogenous plasminogen activators can also activate matrix metalloproteinases.[86] Not only do inflammatory mediators prompt overexpression of MMP by cells involved in atherosclerosis, but also lipid-laden macrophages in lesions prominently overexpress these enzymes.[87] Experimental studies in rabbits documented overexpression of MMPs, including interstitial collagenase, in hypercholesterolemia-induced foam cells.[88] These observations furnish an important link between hyperlipidemia, inflammation, and impaired integrity of the plaque's protective fibrous cap.

The disrupted plaque triggers thrombosis by exposing platelets to collagen, thereby promoting their aggregation and degranulation. After rupture, tissue factor, produced by lipid-laden macrophages in response to the proinflammatory mediator CD154, can contact factors VII and X in the blood compartment and cause coagulation that culminates in thrombin formation with the downstream consequences. Local generation of thrombin from prothrombin not only favors formation of fibrin clots but also promotes smooth muscle cell migration and proliferation. TGF-β and chemokines released from the platelets as they degranulate further prompt fibrosis and perpetuate inflammation at sites of plaque disruption (see Fig. 5-6*E*).

Neutrophils entrapped in thrombi, formed as a consequence of plaque disruption, can elaborate high levels of reactive oxygen species, including superoxide anion and hypochlorous acid derived from myeloperoxidase.[89] These reactive oxygen species can mediate further modification of lipoproteins and other adverse consequences of oxidative stress in the atheroma. Degranulating platelets and neutrophils can release myeloid-related protein–8/14, a marker and putative mediator of acute cardiovascular events.[90,91] The tissue factor–rich microparticles derived from the apoptotic bodies of lesional macrophages and smooth muscle cells can enter the bloodstream after plaque disruption.[92–94] These microparticles may provoke downstream thrombosis in microvessels distal to the disrupted plaque, propagating the ischemia and impairing reflow after mechanical intervention or therapeutic or endogenous fibrinolysis of the culprit arterial thrombus. Thus, the lipid-laden foam cell plays a prominent role in several aspects of atherothrombosis and acute plaque complication.

Most plaque disruptions occur well below the threshold for clinical manifestation. Many limited mural thrombi evade clinical detection, because they do not lead to a persistent total arterial occlusion (see Fig. 5-6*C*). However, the resorbing thrombus, with its local generation of thrombin and release of chemoattractants, growth factors, and fibrogenic mediators from platelets, can provoke a local fibrotic response akin to wound healing (see Fig. 5-6*E*). The provisional matrix of the thrombus provides a scaffold for collagen and elastin elaborated by smooth muscle cells, recruited by and responding to PDGF, TGF-β, and other mediators. As the healing response matures, the artery may undergo constrictive remodeling. In this manner, plaque disruption, with consequent thrombosis and ultimate healing, can lead to the transition from a lipid-rich fibrofatty plaque into a paucicellular matrix-rich inwardly remodeled plaque that can create a stenosis (see Fig. 5-7). Calcification often complicates such maturing plaques. Despite the lack of rigorous evidence, the scenario that the lipid-rich, highly inflamed plaque serves as the precursor to the stenotic, calcified, and fibrotic plaque by the scenario described previously certainly fits much of the evidence currently at hand.[95]

EFFECTS OF LIPID LOWERING ON THE ATHEROSCLEROTIC PLAQUE

In the current era, the success of lipid-lowering therapy renders highly relevant the concept of plaque regression. Indeed, considerable current evidence suggests that plaque evolution can occur not only in ways that aggravate atherosclerosis but also in ways that can favorably alter plaque biology. Our current understanding of the vascular biology of atherosclerosis provides a subtler framework than in previous eras for understanding potentially beneficial changes in plaques (see Fig. 5-7).[96] Classical studies published in the 1970s by Mark Armstrong and colleagues showed that cessation of atherogenic diets in nonhuman primates could result in lesional changes.[97] These early morphologic observations showed a lowering of lipid content of plaques with a relative increase in the amount of fibrous tissue in the intima. More contemporary studies of lipid lowering have extended these pioneering observations on the effects of lipid lowering on atherosclerotic plaques. Our studies in rabbits have shown that lipid lowering, either by dietary intervention or by statin treatment, can reduce inflammation as gauged by macrophage accumulation and the expression of inflammatory mediators and effectors such as MCP-1 and VCAM-1.[98] In particular, we found that lowering lipid content reduces levels of interstitial collagenases and other MMPs associated with plaque complication (see Fig. 5-7).[99] Lipid-lowering therapy can also reduce reactive oxygen species production and improve endothelial vasodilator function in experimental animals and human subjects.[100,101]

Interestingly, such beneficial changes in plaque biology do not necessarily correspond to substantial improvements in the caliber of fixed stenoses. Quantitative coronary arteriographic studies have shown very modest improvement in the mean luminal caliber at sites of fixed stenoses of arteries.[102] Recent studies using magnetic resonance imaging of arteries have shown that the volume of plaque can decrease without substantial improvement in luminal caliber.[103] Indeed, the compensatory enlargement, or positive remodeling, that accompanies plaque growth appears to operate in reverse in response to lipid lowering. The compensatory enlargement phenomenon described by Clarkson and colleagues in nonhuman primates[68] and by Glagov[11] in human specimens appears bidirectional.

These various findings suggest that lipid-lowering therapy may not yield regression of plaques in the sense of shrinking stenoses. The new understanding of the role of plaque disruption in triggering thrombotic complications of atherosclerosis, and the primordial importance of the extracellular matrix in protecting plaques from disruption, should lead us to recast our emphasis from "regression" per se to a subtler therapeutic goal of lesion "stabilization." The term *stabilization* signifies alterations in plaque morphology from those associated with plaques that have caused thromboses, such as thin fibrous caps, large lipid pools, and abundant macrophages, toward plaques with a thicker fibrous cap and smaller lipid pool (see Fig. 5-7).[104] In addition to these morphologic changes, functional alterations, such as reductions in tissue factor and tissue factor activity, accompany the reduced expression of proinflammatory mediators, including CD154, and reduced numbers of macrophages in plaques of animals subjected to lipid-lowering or statin treatment.[96]

Although lifestyle interventions remain the cornerstone of antiatherosclerotic therapy, the success of statins in reducing clinical events has led to their widespread adoption in clinical practice. The lipid-lowering effect alone appears to confer some of the biologic benefits described earlier. Indeed, lipid lowering, per se, in the dietary lipid experiments described previously can reduce manifestations of inflammation.[98,99,105] However, beyond their lipid-lowering effects, statins appear capable of direct anti-inflammatory actions that may explain some of their clinical benefit. In experimental animals, statin administration can decrease signs of inflammation, even under conditions that alter LDL levels much more modestly than the exaggerated fluctuations in cholesterolemia in response to dietary manipulation.[106] In human studies, statins consistently lower levels of inflammatory markers such as C-reactive protein, an acute-phase reactant that correlates with clinical cardiovascular events.[107] This finding in itself theoretically could reflect an anti-inflammatory benefit resulting from reduction in LDL levels. Yet, many clinical studies have shown independently a lack of correlation between statin-induced reductions in LDL and the reduction in C-reactive protein in individuals. This finding suggests that statins have anti-inflammatory actions independent of their LDL-lowering effects.

Declines in C-reactive protein do not correlate well with statin-induced increases in HDL levels, a further indication for a non-lipoprotein-mediated anti-inflammatory effect of statins. Many preclinical studies support the concept of so-called pleiotropic effects of statins attributed to altered prenylation of G proteins implicated in regulation of cell functions.[108] Clinical studies have begun to provide support for the proposition that statin therapy can confer an anti-inflammatory benefit beyond LDL lowering. A prespecified analysis of the Pravastation or Atorvastatin Evaluation and Infection Therapy–Thrombolysis in Myocardial Infarction (PROVE IT-TIMI 22) indicated that a substantial portion of the reduction in recurrent coronary events arose from an anti-inflammatory effect of the statins reflected in C-reactive protein lowering (see Chapters 33 and 39).[109] A post hoc analysis of another study of the effects of statins on survivors of acute coronary syndromes (The -A to -Z Study) provided independent support for the prespecified analysis performed in PROVE IT.[110] Thus, although LDL lowering itself undoubtedly can confer changes on plaques associated with their "stability," direct anti-inflammatory actions may act in concert with LDL lowering to provide clinical benefit.

PERSPECTIVES ON LINKS BETWEEN LIPOPROTEINS AND MECHANISMS OF ATHEROSCLEROSIS

The advent of genetically modified mice and the ready testing of mechanistic hypotheses in these animals have profoundly influenced our thinking about the links between lipoproteins and atherosclerosis. The use of genetically modified mice has permitted researchers to close the loop of causality and test many hypotheses regarding the roles of specific mediators in aspects of atherogenesis. Still, we must bear in mind the profound differences between atherosclerosis in our experimental preparations, including mice, and the human disease. The levels and types of dyslipidemia achieved in commonly used atherosclerosis-prone mice differ considerably from clinical circumstances. The LDL levels in many patients with acute myocardial infarction do not exceed the average for the population and are certainly well beneath the levels produced by genetic modifications to confer atherosclerosis susceptibility in mice.

Our experimental atherosclerosis preparations permit us to perform experiments in a timescale of months, whereas the human disease requires years and in many cases several decades. Most of the acute clinical complications of atherosclerosis in humans result from plaque disruption and thrombosis. Only exaggerated experimental circumstances reliably give rise to thrombotic complications in mice. Thus, we should have considerable humility regarding the direct applicability of our animal experiments to clinical atherosclerosis. These cautionary considerations by no means vitiate the profound importance of mechanistic insights gained from the use of experimental preparations. However, these caveats should cause us to pause before glib extrapolations of our experimental results to human atherosclerosis.

We should also bear in mind that in part because of secular trends in diet and the adoption of statin therapy, we are witnessing a shift in the pattern of lipoprotein abnormalities associated with clinical complications of atherosclerosis. LDL levels are waning in Western societies at a time when we face an obesity epidemic and the associated increase in dyslipidemia (see Chapters 19, 21, and 37). Increased triglyceride-rich lipoproteins and decreased HDL thus loom large as lipoprotein-related risk factors in the future. As we gain increasing mastery over LDL levels, the convincing and consistent links between LDL levels and cardiovascular events may not apply so readily to other lipoprotein fractions. In particular, HDL metabolism appears more perplexing and challenging to manipulate than LDL metabolism (see Chapters 4, 10, and 45). Although we have increasing sophistication in our understanding of the roles of HDL in reverse cholesterol transport, and perhaps as a carrier of antioxidant and anti-inflammatory proteins, we have much to learn about manipulation of various HDL fractions and their biologic consequences on atherogenesis. Only a few decades ago, respected authorities challenged the cholesterol hypothesis.[111] The progression of basic and clinical science has silenced most of this skepticism.[112,113] Continued quests to probe the underlying vascular biology of atherosclerosis and rigorously investigate the links between lipoproteins beyond LDL should lead us toward a deeper and more rigorous understanding of these remaining gaps in our knowledge in the future.

Acknowledgments

Dr. Libby's research has been supported by the Donald W. Reynolds Foundation, the Fondation Leducq, the American Heart Association, and the National Heart, Lung, and Blood Institute (HL080472 and HL34636).

REFERENCES

1. Libby P, Aikawa M, Schonbeck U: Cholesterol and atherosclerosis. *Biochim Biophys Acta* 2000;1529:299–309.
2. Anitschkow N, Chalatow S: On experimental cholesterin steatosis and its significance in the origin of some pathological processes (1913). *Reprinted in Arteriosclerosis* 1983;3:178–182.
3. Assmann G, Cullen P, Schulte H: The Munster Heart Study (PROCAM). Results of follow-up at 8 years. *Eur Heart J* 1998;19(Suppl A):A2–11.
4. Kannel WB, Dawber TR, Kagan A: Factors of risk in the development of coronary heart disease—six year follow-up experience: The Framingham Study. *Ann Intern Med* 1961;44:33–50.
5. Keys A: Seven Countries. A Multivariate Analysis of Death and Coronary Heart Disease. Cambridge, Harvard University Press, 1980.
6. Ridker PM, Libby P: Risk factors for atherothrombotic disease. In Libby P, Bonow RO, Mann DL, et al (eds): Braunwald's Heart Disease: A Textbook of Cardiovascular Medicine, vol 1, 8th ed. Philadelphia, Elsevier Saunders, 2007.
7. Li S, Chen W, Srinivasan SR, et al: Childhood cardiovascular risk factors and carotid vascular changes in adulthood: the Bogalusa Heart Study. *JAMA* 2003;290:2271–2276.
8. McGill HC Jr, McMahan CA, Herderick EE, et al: Effects of coronary heart disease risk factors on atherosclerosis of selected regions of the aorta and right coronary artery. PDAY Research Group. Pathobiological Determinants of Atherosclerosis in Youth. *Arterioscler Thromb Vasc Biol* 2000;20:836–845.

9. Strong JP, Malcom GT, McMahan CA, et al: Prevalence and extent of atherosclerosis in adolescents and young adults: Implications for prevention from the Pathobiological Determinants of Atherosclerosis in Youth Study. *JAMA* 1999;281:727–735.
10. Strong JP, Malcom GT, Oalmann MC, et al: The PDAY Study: Natural history, risk factors, and pathobiology. Pathobiological Determinants of Atherosclerosis in Youth. *Ann N Y Acad Sci* 1997;811:226–235.
11. Libby P: The forgotten majority: unfinished business in cardiovascular risk reduction. *J Am Coll Cardiol* 2005;46:1225–1228.
12. Brown MS, Goldstein JL: A receptor-mediated pathway for cholesterol homeostasis. *Science* 1986;232:232–247.
13. Cohen JC, Boerwinkle E, Mosley TH Jr, et al: Sequence variations in PCSK9, low LDL, and protection against coronary heart disease. *N Engl J Med* 2006;354:1264–1272.
14. Libby P, Ridker PM: Inflammation and atherothrombosis: from population biology and bench research to clinical practice. *J Am Coll Cardiol* 2006;48:A33–46.
15. Binder CJ, Chang MK, Shaw PX, et al: Innate and acquired immunity in atherogenesis. *Nat Med* 2002;8:1218–1226.
16. Chang JD, Sukhova GK, Libby P, et al: Deletion of the phosphoinositide 3-kinase p110gamma gene attenuates murine atherosclerosis. *Proc Natl Acad Sci U S A* 12007;04:8077–8082.
17. Heinecke JW: Is lipid peroxidation relevant to atherogenesis? *J Clin Invest* 1999;104:135–136.
18. Daugherty A, Dunn JL, Rateri DL, et al: Myeloperoxidase, a catalyst for lipoprotein oxidation, is expressed in human atherosclerotic lesions. *J Clin Invest* 1994;94:437–444.
19. Hazen SL: Myeloperoxidase and plaque vulnerability. *Arterioscler Thromb Vasc Biol* 2004;24:1143–1146.
20. Sugiyama S, Okada Y, Sukhova GK, et al: Macrophage myeloperoxidase regulation by granulocyte macrophage colony-stimulating factor in human atherosclerosis and implications in acute coronary syndromes. *Am J Pathol* 2001;158:879–891.
21. Nicholls SJ, Zheng L, Hazen SL: Formation of dysfunctional high-density lipoprotein by myeloperoxidase. *Trends Cardiovasc Med* 2005;15:212–219.
22. Vaisar T, Pennathur S, Green PS, et al: Shotgun proteomics implicates protease inhibition and complement activation in the antiinflammatory properties of HDL. *J Clin Invest* 2007;117:746–756.
23. Griendling KK, Harrison DG: Out, damned dot: studies of the NADPH oxidase in atherosclerosis. *J Clin Invest* 2001;108:1423–1424.
24. Landmesser U, Harrison DG, Drexler H: Oxidant stress—a major cause of reduced endothelial nitric oxide availability in cardiovascular disease. *Eur J Clin Pharmacol* 2006;62(Suppl 1):13–19.
25. Beckman JS: Protein tyrosine nitration and peroxynitrite. *Faseb J* 2002;16:1144.
26. Ting HJ, Stice JP, Schaff UY, et al: Triglyceride-rich lipoproteins prime aortic endothelium for an enhanced inflammatory response to tumor necrosis factor-alpha. *Circ Res* 2007;100:381–390.
27. Kawakami A, Aikawa M, Alcaide P, et al: Apolipoprotein CIII induces expression of vascular cell adhesion molecule-1 in vascular endothelial cells and increases adhesion of monocytic cells. *Circulation* 2006;114:681–687.
28. Gerrity RG, Naito HK, Richardson M, et al: Dietary induced atherogenesis in swine: morphology of the intima in prelesion stages. *Am J Pathol* 1979;95:775–786.
29. Schwenke DC, Carew TE: Initiation of atherosclerotic lesions in cholesterol-fed rabbits. II. Selective retention of LDL vs. selective increases in LDL permeability in susceptible sites of arteries. *Arteriosclerosis* 1989;9:908–918.
30. Nievelstein PF, Fogelman AM, Mottino G, et al: Lipid accumulation in rabbit aortic intima 2 hours after bolus infusion of low-density lipoprotein. A deep-etch and immunolocalization study of ultrarapidly frozen tissue. *Arterioscler Thromb* 1991;11:1795–1805.
31. Boren J, Olin K, Lee I, et al: Identification of the principal proteoglycan-binding site in LDL. A single-point mutation in apo-B100 severely affects proteoglycan interaction without affecting LDL receptor binding. *J Clin Invest* 1998;101:2658–2664.
32. Tabas I, Williams KJ, Boren J: Subendothelial lipoprotein retention as the initiating process in atherosclerosis: update and therapeutic implications. *Circulation* 2007;116:1832–1844.
33. Lee RT, Yamamoto C, Feng Y, et al: Mechanical strain induces specific changes in the synthesis and organization of proteoglycans by vascular smooth muscle cells. *J Biol Chem* 2001;276:13847–13851.
34. Berneis KK, Krauss RM: Metabolic origins and clinical significance of LDL heterogeneity. *J Lipid Res* 2002;43:1363–1379.
35. Sartipy P, Camejo G, Svensson L, et al: Phospholipase A2 modification of lipoproteins: Potential effects on atherogenesis. *Adv Exp Med Biol* 2002;507:3–7.
36. Steinberg D: Atherogenesis in perspective: hypercholesterolemia and inflammation as partners in crime. *Nat Med* 2002;8:1211–1217.
37. Glomset JA: The plasma lecithins cholesterol acyltransferase reaction. *J Lipid Res* 1968;9:155–167.
38. Navab M, Ananthramaiah GM, Reddy ST, et al: The oxidation hypothesis of atherogenesis: the role of oxidized phospholipids and HDL. *J Lipid Res* 2004;45:993–1007.
39. Vaisar T, Shao B, Green PS, et al: Myeloperoxidase and inflammatory proteins: pathways for generating dysfunctional high-density lipoprotein in humans. *Curr Atheroscler Rep* 2007;9:417–424.
40. Barter PJ, Nicholls S, Rye KA, et al: Antiinflammatory properties of HDL. *Circ Res* 2004;95:764–772.
41. Ashby DT, Rye KA, Clay MA, et al: Factors influencing the ability of HDL to inhibit expression of vascular cell adhesion molecule-1 in endothelial cells. *Arterioscler Thromb Vasc Biol* 1998;18:1450–1455.
42. Gimbrone MA Jr, Topper JN, Nagel T, et al: Endothelial dysfunction, hemodynamic forces, and atherogenesis. *Ann N Y Acad Sci* 2000;902:230–239; discussion 239–240.
43. Ley K, Reutershan J: Leucocyte-endothelial interactions in health and disease. *Handb Exp Pharmacol* 2006;97–133.
44. Ley K: The role of selectins in inflammation and disease. Trends Mol Med 2003;9:263–268.
45. Burger PC, Wagner DD: Platelet P-selectin facilitates atherosclerotic lesion development. *Blood* 2003;101:2661–2666.
46. Cybulsky MI, Won D, Haidari M: Leukocyte recruitment to atherosclerotic lesions. *Can J Cardiol* 2004;20(Suppl B):24B–28B.
47. Cybulsky MI, Iiyama K, Li H, et al: A major role for VCAM-1, but not ICAM-1, in early atherosclerosis. *J Clin Invest* 2001;107:1255–1262.
48. O'Brien K, Allen M, McDonald T, et al: Vascular cell adhesion molecule-1 is expressed in human coronary atherosclerotic plaques: implications for the mode of progression of advanced coronary atherosclerosis. *J Clin Invest* 1993;92:945–951.
49. Libby P, Aikawa M, Jain MK: Vascular endothelium and atherosclerosis. *Handb Exp Pharmacol* 2006;285–306.
50. Parmar KM, Larman HB, Dai G, et al: Integration of flow-dependent endothelial phenotypes by Kruppel-like factor 2. *J Clin Invest* 2006;116:49–58.
51. Charo IF, Ransohoff RM: The many roles of chemokines and chemokine receptors in inflammation. *N Engl J Med* 2006;354:610–621.
52. Gerszten RE, Mach F, Sauty A, et al: Chemokines, leukocytes, and atherosclerosis. *J Lab Clin Med* 2000;136:87–92.
53. Libby P: Inflammation in atherosclerosis. *Nature* 2002;420:868–874.
54. Swirski FK, Libby P, Aikawa E, et al: Ly-6C monocytes dominate hypercholesterolemia-associated monocytosis and give rise to macrophages in atheromata. *J Clin Invest* 2007;117:195–205.
55. Tacke F, Alvarez D, Kaplan TJ, et al: Monocyte subsets differentially employ CCR2, CCR5, and CX3CR1 to accumulate within atherosclerotic plaques. *J Clin Invest* 2007;117:185–194.
56. Hansson GK: Inflammation, atherosclerosis, and coronary artery disease. *N Engl J Med* 2005;352:1685–1695.
57. Hansson GK, Libby P: The immune response in atherosclerosis: a double-edged sword. *Nat Rev Immunol* 2006;6:508–519.
58. Mach F, Sauty A, Iarossi AS, et al: Differential expression of three T lymphocyte-activating CXC chemokines by human atheroma-associated cells. *J Clin Invest* 1999;104:1041–1050.
59. Forrester JS, Libby P: The inflammation hypothesis and its potential relevance to statin therapy. *Am J Cardiol* 2007;99:732–738.
60. Kovanen PT: Role of mast cells in atherosclerosis [review]. *Chem Immunol* 1995;62:132–170.
61. Bot I, de Jager SC, Zernecke A, et al: Perivascular mast cells promote atherogenesis and induce plaque destabilization in apolipoprotein E-deficient mice. *Circulation* 2007;115:2516–2525.
62. Sun J, Sukhova GK, Wolters PJ, et al: Mast cells promote atherosclerosis by releasing proinflammatory cytokines. *Nat Med* 2007;13:719–724.

63. van Berkel TJ, Out R, Hoekstra M, et al: Scavenger receptors: friend or foe in atherosclerosis? *Curr Opin Lipidol* 2005;16: 525–535.
64. Schwartz SM: The intima: a new soil [editorial; comment]. *Circ Res* 1999;85:877–879.
65. Armstrong ML, Megan MB, Heistad DD (eds): Adaptive Responses of the Artery Wall as Human Atherosclerosis Develops (Pathobiology of the Human Atherosclerotic Plaque). *New York, Springer-Verlag*, 1989.
66. Clarkson TB, Prichard RW, Morgan TM, et al: Remodeling of coronary arteries in human and nonhuman primates. *JAMA* 1994;271:289–294.
67. Glagov S, Weisenberg E, Zarins C, et al: Compensatory enlargement of human atherosclerotic coronary arteries. *N Engl J Med* 1987;316:371–375.
68. Libby P: The vascular biology of atherosclerosis. In Libby P, Bonow RO, Mann DL, et al (eds): Braunwald's Heart Disease: a Textbook of Cardiovascular Medicine, vol 1, 8th ed. Philadelphia, Elsevier Saunders, 2007.
69. Geng Y-J, Libby P: Evidence for apoptosis in advanced human atheroma. Co-localization with interleukin-1 b-converting enzyme. *Am J Pathol* 1995;147:251–266.
70. Han D, Haudenschild C, Hong M, et al: Evidence for apoptosis in human atherogenesis and in a rat vascular injury model. *Am J Pathol* 1995;147:267–277.
71. Littlewood TD, Bennett MR: Apoptotic cell death in atherosclerosis. *Curr Opin Lipidol* 2003;14:469–475.
72. Mach F, Schoenbeck U, Bonnefoy J-Y, et al: Activation of monocyte/macrophage functions related to acute atheroma complication by ligation of CD40. Induction of collagenase, stromelysin, and tissue factor. *Circulation* 1997;96:396–399.
73. Geng Y-J, Henderson L, Levesque E, et al: Fas is expressed in human atherosclerotic intima and promotes apoptosis of cytokine-primed human vascular smooth muscle cells. *Arterioscler Thromb Vasc Biol* 1997;17:2200–2208.
74. Clarke MC, Figg N, Maguire JJ, et al: Apoptosis of vascular smooth muscle cells induces features of plaque vulnerability in atherosclerosis. *Nat Med* 2006;12:1075–1080.
75. Libby P: The molecular bases of the acute coronary syndromes. *Circulation* 1995;91:2844–2850.
76. Brogi E, Winkles J, Underwood R, et al: Distinct patterns of expression of fibroblast growth factors and their receptors in human atheroma and non-atherosclerotic arteries: association of acidic FGF with plaque microvessels and macrophages. *J Clin Invest* 1993;92:2408–2418.
77. Kolodgie FD, Gold HK, Burke AP, et al: Intraplaque hemorrhage and progression of coronary atheroma. *N Engl J Med* 2003;349:2316–2325.
78. Croce K, Libby P: Intertwining of thrombosis and inflammation in atherosclerosis. *Curr Opin Hematol* 2007;14:55–61.
79. Libby P, Theroux P: Pathophysiology of coronary artery disease. *Circulation* 2005;111:3481–3488.
80. Dollery CM, Libby P: Atherosclerosis and proteinase activation. *Cardiovasc Res* 2006;69:625–635.
81. Liu J, Sukhova GK, Sun JS, et al: Lysosomal cysteine proteases in atherosclerosis. *Arterioscler Thromb Vasc Biol* 2004;24:1359–1366.
82. Fukumoto Y, Deguchi JO, Libby P, et al: Genetically determined resistance to collagenase action augments interstitial collagen accumulation in atherosclerotic plaques. *Circulation* 2004;110:1953–1959.
83. Deguchi JO, Aikawa E, Libby P, et al: Matrix metalloproteinase-13/collagenase-3 deletion promotes collagen accumulation and organization in mouse atherosclerotic plaques. *Circulation* 2005;112:2708–2715.
84. Schneider F, Sukhova GK, Aikawa M, et al: Matrix metalloproteinase-14 deficiency in bone marrow-derived cells promotes collagen accumulation in mouse atherosclerotic plaques. *Circulation* 2008; 117: 931–939.
85. Kovanen PT, Kaartinen M, Paavonen T: Infiltrates of activated mast cells at the site of coronary atheromatous erosion or rupture in myocardial infarction [see comments]. *Circulation* 1995;92:1084–1088.
86. Carmeliet P, Moons L, Lijnen R, et al: Urokinase-generated plasmin activates matrix metalloproteinases during aneurysm formation. *Nat Genet* 1997;17:439–444.
87. Sukhova GK, Schonbeck U, Rabkin E, et al: Evidence for increased collagenolysis by interstitial collagenases-1 and -3 in vulnerable human atheromatous plaques. *Circulation* 1999;99: 2503–2509.
88. Galis Z, Sukhova G, Kranzhöfer R, et al: Macrophage foam cells from experimental atheroma constitutively produce matrix-degrading proteinases. *Proc Natl Acad Sci U S A* 1995;92: 402–406.
89. Naruko T, Ueda M, Haze K, et al: Neutrophil infiltration of culprit lesions in acute coronary syndromes. *Circulation* 2002;106:2894–2900.
90. Healy AM, Pickard MD, Pradhan AD, et al: Platelet expression profiling and clinical validation of myeloid-related protein-14 as a novel determinant of cardiovascular events. *Circulation* 2006;113:2278–2284.
91. Morrow DA, Wang Y, Croce K, et al: Myeloid-related protein 8/14 and the risk of cardiovascular death or myocardial infarction after an acute coronary syndrome in the Pravastatin or Atorvastatin Evaluation and Infection Therapy: Thrombolysis in Myocardial Infarction (PROVE IT-TIMI 22) trial. *Am Heart J* 2008;155:49–55.
92. Rauch U, Nemerson Y: Circulating tissue factor and thrombosis. *Curr Opin Hematol* 2000;7:273–277.
93. Schecter AD, Spirn B, Rossikhina M, et al: Release of active tissue factor by human arterial smooth muscle cells. *Circ Res* 2000;87:126–132.
94. Schonbeck U, Mach F, Sukhova GK, et al: CD40 ligation induces tissue factor expression in human vascular smooth muscle cells. *Am J Pathol* 2000;156:7–14.
95. Burke AP, Kolodgie FD, Farb A, et al: Healed plaque ruptures and sudden coronary death: evidence that subclinical rupture has a role in plaque progression. *Circulation* 2001;103:934–940.
96. Libby P, Aikawa M: Stabilization of atherosclerotic plaques: New mechanisms and clinical targets. *Nat Med* 2002;8:1257–1262.
97. Armstrong ML, Megan MB: Lipid depletion in atheromatous coronary arteries in rhesus monkeys after regression diets. *Circ Res* 1972;30:675–680.
98. Aikawa M, Sugiyama S, Hill C, et al: Lipid lowering reduces oxidative stress and endothelial cell activation in rabbit atheroma. *Circulation* 2002;106:1390–1396.
99. Aikawa M, Rabkin E, Okada Y, et al: Lipid lowering by diet reduces matrix metalloproteinase activity and increases collagen content of rabbit atheroma: a potential mechanism of lesion stabilization. *Circulation* 1998;97:2433–2444.
100. Anderson T, Meredith I, Yeung A, et al: The effect of cholesterol lowering and antioxidant therapy on endothelium-dependent coronary vasomotion. *N Engl J Med* 1995;332:488–493.
101. Benzuly KH, Padgett RC, Kaul S, et al: Functional improvement precedes structural regression of atherosclerosis. *Circulation* 1994;89:1810–1818.
102. Brown BG, Zhao XQ, Sacco DE, et al: Lipid lowering and plaque regression. New insights into prevention of plaque disruption and clinical events in coronary disease [review]. *Circulation* 1993;87:1781–1791.
103. Corti R, Fuster V, Fayad ZA, et al: Effects of aggressive versus conventional lipid-lowering therapy by simvastatin on human atherosclerotic lesions: a prospective, randomized, double-blind trial with high-resolution magnetic resonance imaging. *J Am Coll Cardiol* 2005;46:106–112.
104. Davies MJ: Stability and instability: the two faces of coronary atherosclerosis. The Paul Dudley White Lecture, 1995. *Circulation* 1996;94:2013–2020.
105. Aikawa M, Rabkin E, Voglic SJ, et al: Lipid lowering promotes accumulation of mature smooth muscle cells expressing smooth muscle myosin heavy chain isoforms in rabbit atheroma. *Circ Res* 1998;83:1015–1026.
106. Aikawa M, Rabkin E, Sugiyama S, et al: An HMG-CoA reductase inhibitor, cerivastatin, suppresses growth of macrophages expressing matrix metalloproteinases and tissue factor *in vivo* and *in vitro*. *Circulation* 2001;103:276–283.
107. Ridker PM, Rifai N, Pfeffer MA, et al: Long-term effects of pravastatin on plasma concentration of C-reactive protein. The Cholesterol and Recurrent Events (CARE) Investigators. *Circulation* 1999;100:230–235.

108. Jain MK, Ridker PM: Anti-inflammatory effects of statins: clinical evidence and basic mechanisms. *Nat Rev Drug Discov* 2005;4:977–987.
109. Ridker PM, Cannon CP, Morrow D, et al: C-reactive protein levels and outcomes after statin therapy. *N Engl J Med* 2005;352:20–28.
110. Morrow DA, de Lemos JA, Sabatine MS, et al: Clinical relevance of C-reactive protein during follow-up of patients with acute coronary syndromes in the Aggrastat-to-Zocor Trial. *Circulation* 2006;114:281–288.
111. Oliver MF: Serum cholesterol—the knave of hearts and the joker. *Lancet* 1981;2:1090–1095.
112. Steinberg D: Thematic review series: the pathogenesis of atherosclerosis. An interpretive history of the cholesterol controversy, part II: the early evidence linking hypercholesterolemia to coronary disease in humans. *J Lipid Res* 2005;46:179–190.
113. Steinberg D: Thematic review series: the pathogenesis of atherosclerosis. An interpretive history of the cholesterol controversy: part I. *J Lipid Res* 2004;45:1583–1593.

CHAPTER 6

Genetic Dyslipidemia

John D. Brunzell

INTRODUCTION

General Comments

Disorders of lipoprotein metabolism, together with the prevalence of high-fat diets, obesity, and physical inactivity, have resulted in an epidemic of atherosclerotic disease in the United States and other developed countries. The interaction of common genetic and acquired disorders of lipoproteins with these adverse environmental factors predisposes to premature atherosclerosis. In the United States, mortality from coronary artery disease (CAD), particularly in middle-aged persons, has been declining since 1970; however, atherosclerotic cardiovascular disease remains the most common cause of death among both men and women.

Hyperlipidemia has been defined as an elevation of a lipoprotein level. The recognition that low levels of high-density lipoprotein (HDL) and the presence of small-dense low-density lipoprotein (LDL) particles are clinically important in the development of CAD has led to the use of the term *dyslipidemia* to describe a range of disorders that include both abnormally high and low lipoprotein levels as well as abnormalities in the composition of these particles. Dyslipidemias are clinically important principally because of their contribution to atherogenesis; however, pancreatitis and fatty liver disease are other clinically significant manifestations of lipid disorders.

Lipoprotein Metabolism

After a meal, the intestinal absorptive cells process monoglyceride, fatty acids, and cholesterol into triglyceride and cholesteryl ester and incorporate them into the core of chylomicrons containing apolipoprotein (apo) B-48.[1] Triglyceride greatly exceeds cholesteryl ester in the chylomicron core. Chylomicrons are secreted into the lymphatics, then into plasma, where apoC-II on the chylomicron surface activates endothelial-bound lipoprotein lipase (LPL). LPL in turn hydrolyzes the core triglyceride of the chylomicron and releases free fatty acids (FFA). These fatty acids are taken up by adipose tissue for storage and by muscle for energy. During lipolysis, the chylomicron decreases in size, and the phospholipid and cholesterol surface components are transferred to HDL via phospholipid transfer protein; the remaining lipoprotein is the chylomicron remnant particle. This chylomicron remnant next acquires apoE from HDL and, after binding to sites that recognize apoE, is subsequently taken up by the liver, where it is then degraded. This process delivers dietary cholesterol to the liver.

The liver also synthesizes triglyceride and secretes the triglyceride-rich, apoB-100–containing very-low-density lipoproteins (VLDLs) into plasma.[1] VLDL also acquires apoC-II from HDL and interacts with LPL on the capillary endothelium, where the core triglyceride is hydrolyzed to provide fatty acids to adipose and muscle tissues. About half of the catabolized VLDL remnants (intermediate density lipoproteins [IDLs]) are taken up by hepatic receptors that bind to apoE for degradation; the other half, depleted of triglyceride relative to cholesteryl ester, is converted by the liver to apoB-100–containing cholesteryl ester–rich LDL. As IDL is converted to LDL, apoE is transferred back to HDL, leaving only one apolipoprotein, apoB-100.

In the metabolism of both chylomicrons and VLDL, apoC-II promotes the hydrolysis of triglyceride by LPL, and apoE enhances hepatic uptake of remnants. A major difference is that chylomicrons contain a truncated form of apoB (i.e., apoB-48), whereas VLDL contains the complete form (i.e., apoB-100). Another difference is that chylomicron remnants are degraded after they have been absorbed by the liver, whereas many of the VLDL remnants are most likely processed in the hepatic sinusoids or hepatocytes to become LDL.

Regulation of Apolipoprotein B-100 Lipoprotein Assembly and Catabolism

Four major clinically significant physiologic steps take place in the lipoprotein cascade from VLDL to LDL: one is a VLDL assembly anabolic disorder, and three are catabolic disorders of hydrolysis by LPL, remnant catabolism, and LDL catabolism (Fig. 6-1).[1,2] Defects at each step in the cascade can lead to dyslipidemia. These defects can be genetic or acquired (i.e., secondary to other disease or the effects of certain drugs) or the result of an interaction of genetic and acquired factors. The genetic dyslipidemias can be classified into anabolic or catabolic disorders. Although the mechanism of every disorder is not well understood, it is convenient to classify each in order to understand the known differences between them.

Lipoprotein Assembly

ApoB-100 is synthesized constitutively in the endoplasmic reticulum of the hepatocyte, and much of it is degraded in the proteosome. Triglyceride is added to the surviving apoB and transported to the Golgi complex for additional core lipid, forming the nascent VLDL particle. This particle is secreted into plasma, where it acquires other apolipoproteins (e.g., apoC-II and apoE) from HDL.[1]

An abnormality in VLDL secretion occurs in two genetic forms of hyperlipidemia: familial hypertriglyceridemia (FHTG) and familial combined hyperlipidemia (FCHL). FHTG is characterized by the overproduction of triglyceride secreted within a normal number of VLDL particles; this results in each particle having a high triglyceride-to-apoB ratio. In FCHL, an increased amount of apoB-100 is secreted into plasma as VLDL or LDL particles; these particles tend to be smaller than normal.[3]

The metabolic syndrome, a common condition in the general population, is a component of most cases of FCHL and also contributes to the residual dyslipidemia seen in patients with type 2 diabetes mellitus who have been treated chronically with insulin or insulin secretagogues. The potential molecular basis of the hepatic triglyceride or apoB oversecretion in these disorders is discussed later.

Decreased hepatic secretion of lipoproteins containing apoB also can occur. Abetalipoproteinemia may occur because of a molecular defect in both apoB genes that prevents the production of apoB. It also may occur in individuals who are homozygous for mutations in the microsomal triglyceride transport protein, a protein critical for apoB transport in the endoplasmic reticulum. Homozygous hypobetalipoproteinemia and abetalipoproteinemia lead to deficiencies in fat-soluble vitamins because each of these conditions results in the absence of apoB-containing lipoproteins needed to transport fat-soluble vitamins. Hypobetalipoproteinemia can be caused by a defect in a single apoB gene and is characterized by apoB levels that are 50% of normal.[4]

Lipoprotein(a). Lipoprotein(a) (Lp[a]) is a separate class of lipoprotein particles similar to LDL that are synthesized in the liver. Lp(a) differs from LDL by the addition of apo(a), a protein with a structure that is homologous to plasminogen.[5] The apo(a) protein is bound by a disulfide linkage to apoB-100 to form the Lp(a) particle. High levels of Lp(a) are both prothrombotic and proatherogenic. Levels of Lp(a) in plasma are almost completely determined by genetic variation in the two Lp(a) alleles.

Lipoprotein Catabolism

Lipoprotein Lipase–Mediated Triglyceride Removal. LPL is synthesized in adipose tissue and muscle and then transported to the luminal surface of the endothelial lining of the adjacent capillary, where it hydrolyses triglyceride in triglyceride-rich lipoproteins. The fatty acids released during the processing of triglyceride-rich particles (i.e., chylomicrons and VLDL) can be used for energy by muscle or they can be re-esterified into triglyceride and stored in adipocytes for later use.[6] ApoC-II, the LPL activator, is carried on the triglyceride-rich lipoproteins chylomicrons and VLDL. ApoAV carried on the lipoprotein also contributes to LPL-mediated triglyceride hydrolysis.

Autosomal recessive genetic defects that result in impaired lipoprotein lipase synthesis or function are rare causes of hyperlipidemia that usually present in neonates or infants as severe hypertriglyceridemia. Obligate heterozygote parents of these children often have mild hypertriglyceridemia. Acquired defects of LPL such as untreated diabetes, hypothyroidism, or uremia are more common causes of hyperlipidemia. When an acquired defect of LPL occurs with a genetic disorder characterized by excessive input of VLDL, marked hypertriglyceridemia can ensue. The coexistence of two or more disorders that each increase the level of triglycerides in plasma (e.g., FHTG or FCHL coexistent with

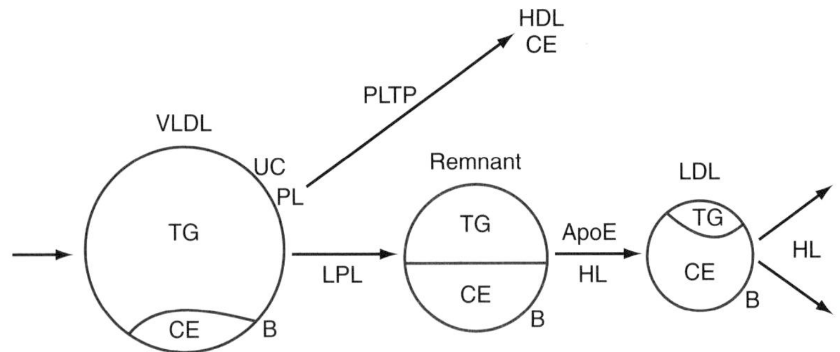

FIGURE 6-1 The apolipoprotein B-100 (apoB-100) cascade. Very-low-density lipoprotein (VLDL) particles are secreted from the liver with one apoB on the surface and triglyceride (TG) and cholesteryl ester (CE) in the core. Core triglyceride is hydrolyzed by lipoprotein lipase (LPL) to become a remnant lipoprotein recognized by the liver by apoE. The remnant lipoprotein is further processed to form low-density lipoprotein (LDL) particles, which have a cholesteryl ester–rich core and one molecule of apoB-100. The LDL particles apoB is the ligand for the peripheral or hepatic LDL receptors. As the VLDL core is hydrolyzed, the unesterified cholesterol (UC) and phospholipid (PL) are transferred to high-density lipoprotein (HDL) by phospholipid transfer protein (PLTP). HL, hepatic lipase. Modified from Ref. 2.

untreated diabetes) can lead to marked hypertriglyceridemia.[6] (See Chylomicronemia Syndrome, later.)

Remnant Catabolism. Both chylomicron and VLDL remnant particles acquire apoE from HDL before they can bind to hepatic receptors for either uptake and degradation or further processing to LDL. Three common alleles of the *APOE* gene (i.e., *APOE*E$_2$*, *APOE*E3*, and *APOE*E4*) result in six possible combinations. The *APOE*E4* allele product has the greatest affinity for hepatic receptors, followed by the *APOE*E3* allele product, whereas the *APOE*E$_2$* allele product has markedly reduced receptor affinity.

Individuals who are homozygous for the *APOE*E$_2$* allele (E_2/E_2), about 1% of white populations, have marked impairment of hepatic remnant lipoprotein uptake. This results in the accumulation of these remnants in the plasma associated with very low levels—or absence—of LDL particles. Interestingly, most individuals with E_2/E_2 have either normal or low cholesterol levels because of the Paucity of LDL particles characteristic of this disorder.[7] However, if an individual who is homozygous for the *APOE*E$_2$* allele (E_2/E_2) has either an inherited or acquired defect that causes excessive input of VLDL from the liver, an accumulation of VLDL remnants with hyperlipidemia results; this is termed *remnant removal disease.* Because chylomicron and VLDL remnants contain approximately equal amounts of triglyceride and cholesterol, the hyperlipidemia of remnant removal disease is characterized by both hypercholesterolemia and hypertriglyceridemia.[7] $ApoE_3$ or $ApoE_4$ alone or in combination with $ApoE_2$ modulates the level of LDL cholesterol but not IDL levels.[8]

LDL Catabolism. The final step in the apoB cascade at which a defect in lipoprotein metabolism can occur is in LDL catabolism. ApoB-100 on the surface of LDL binds to its receptor on the cell surface; LDL is then taken into the cell, where it is catabolized (Fig. 6-2). After hydrolysis of the core lipids, unesterified cholesterol is used by cells for synthesis of membranes, bile acids, and steroid hormones and for various regulatory actions to limit the accumulation of cholesterol within the cell. The vast majority of LDL particles in plasma are taken up by the liver via the LDL receptor.

Mutations of the LDL receptor (as found in familial hypercholesterolemia [FH]) or, less commonly, mutations in the apoB-100 molecule (as found in familial defective apoB-100) lead to an impairment in the interaction of LDL with its receptor and elevated LDL levels.[9] A variant in a serine protease (PCSK9) affects the LDL receptor and is associated with low LDL cholesterol levels.[10] LDL levels also can be influenced by dietary factors by several pathways. For example, dietary cholesterol delivered to the liver by chylomicron remnants can suppress hepatic LDL receptors, leading to decreased LDL removal from plasma. Dietary saturated fats also reduce LDL receptor activity and increase LDL production. Hypothyroidism also is associated with defective LDL receptor–mediated cholesterol removal.[9]

Function and Regulation of High-Density Lipoprotein

The major HDL apolipoproteins are apoA-I and apoA-II, which are formed in the liver and in the small intestine and secreted into plasma as an AI–phospholipid disk.[11] Most of the apolipoproteins and phospholipid destined to become nascent HDL are initially secreted on the surface of chylomicrons and VLDL. After LPL hydrolyzes triglyceride in chylomicrons and VLDL, the core lipid content in these lipoprotein particles becomes smaller, and excess surface unesterified cholesterol and phospholipid are transferred to HDL by phospholipid transfer protein. In addition, nascent HDL particles pick up excess unesterified cholesterol and phospholipid from peripheral tissues including macrophages via ATP-binding cassette transporter A1 (ABCA1). This unesterified cholesterol in HDL then undergoes esterification by the plasma enzyme lecithin: cholesterol acyltransferase (LCAT). This enzyme is activated by apoA-I on the HDL surface to esterify free cholesterol into cholesteryl ester, causing it to transfer into the core. Through this process, the HDL particle becomes the larger, more buoyant HDL_3 particle and progresses to the even larger HDL_2 particle.[11,12] At some point, apoA-II is added to the HDL particle. The function of apoA I in humans is not clear. Cholesteryl ester

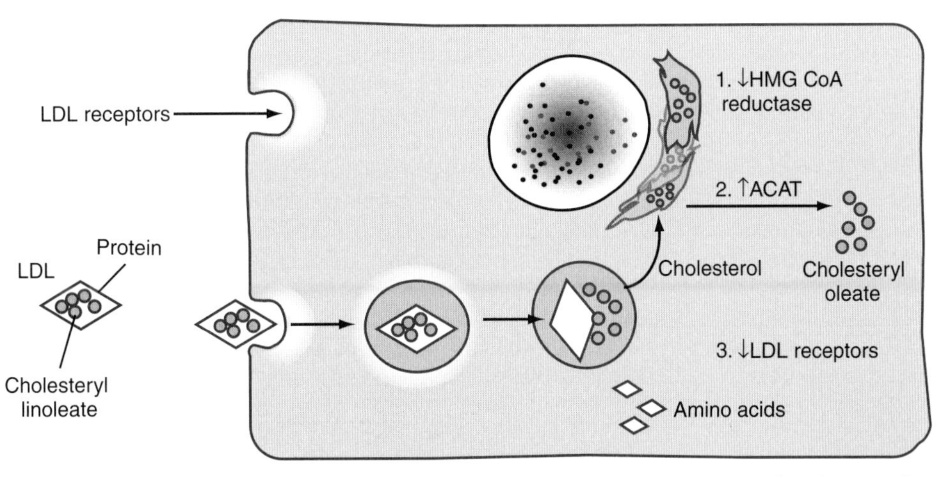

FIGURE 6-2 The LDL Receptor pathway in mammalion cells. Low-density lipoprotein (LDL) is endocytosed by cells via the LDL receptor recognition of apolipoprotein (apo) B. Once internalized, the lipoprotein is catabolized, releasing free cholesterol, cholesteryl ester, and amino acids. The free cholesterol is converted to cholesteryl oleate by the enzyme acyl–coenzyme A:cholesterol acyltransferase (ACAT). The LDL receptor subsequently is recycled back to the cell surface. HMG- CoA, 3-hydroxy-3-methylglutaryl–coenzyme A. From reference 9. Used with permission.

transfer protein (CETP) directs cholesteryl ester to the liver via apoB-containing lipoproteins. Hepatic lipase activity on the hepatocyte surface hydrolyzes the phospholipid and triglyceride in the HDL_2 particle, promoting a decrease in size and density to HDL_3 and then to even smaller HDL particles.[12] Recycling of some of the apoA-I causes the process to repeat itself (Fig. 6-3). These HDL particles interact with scavenger receptor B1 in the liver to remove intact HDL particles or specifically cholesteryl ester.

Genetic defects leading to abnormally high or low levels of HDL cholesterol are rare (see Chapter 7).[13–16] Elevations in the HDL cholesterol level may result from genetic CETP deficiency. Markedly reduced HDL cholesterol levels may be caused by (1) an apoA-I structural mutation; (2) homozygosity for mutations in ABCA1,[13] leading to Tangier disease; or (3) homozygosity for mutations in the enzyme LCAT, leading to LCAT deficiency and fish eye disease. Factors associated with an increase in HDL levels include female sex, aerobic exercise, weight reduction, high-fat diets, and certain drugs (e.g., alcohol, estrogens, fibrates, and nicotinic acid). Factors associated with a decrease in HDL levels include male sex, central obesity, cigarette smoking, low-fat diets, hypertriglyceridemia, uremia, being heterozygous for Tangier disease, and certain drugs (e.g., androgens, progestins, and some antihypertensive agents). Low HDL particle number is commonly associated with increased triglyceride levels, as seen in the metabolic syndrome, and in familial hypoalphalipoproteinemia (FHA).

Hepatic lipase is synthesized in the hepatocyte and binds to endothelial surfaces in the liver sinusoids to interact with lipoproteins.[12] After triglyceride-rich VLDL particles exchange triglyceride for the cholesteryl ester in LDL and HDL, hepatic lipase hydrolyzes the phospholipid and triglyceride in LDL and HDL (Fig. 6-4), leading to the formation of smaller, denser LDL and HDL particles. This process may be driven by the presence of particularly triglyceride-rich VLDL in the presence of normal hepatic lipase activity or by increases in the level of hepatic lipase. Factors such as male sex and the accumulation of intra-abdominal fat predispose to increased hepatic lipase levels and are associated with an increase in small dense LDL levels and a decrease in HDL_2 levels. An increase in hepatic lipase levels is an important factor in the dyslipidemia of the metabolic syndrome.[12,17] Hepatic lipase also facilitates hepatic recognition and uptake of chylomicron and VLDL remnant lipoproteins.

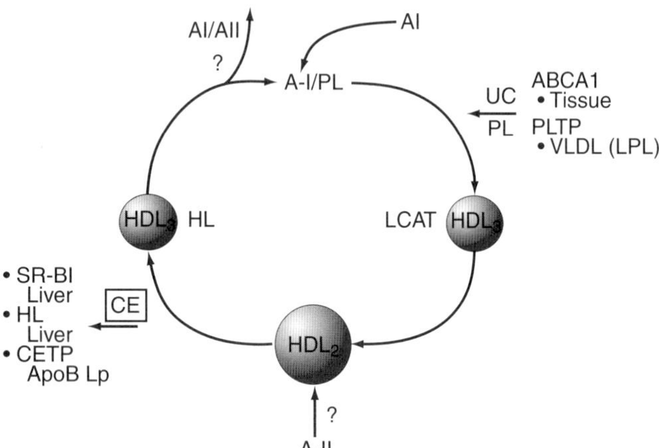

FIGURE 6-3 The circular pathway of high-density lipoprotein (HDL) formation and catabolism. HDL begins as an apolipoprotein (apo) A-I–phospholipid (PL) complex. Unesterified cholesterol (UC) and phospholipid are added to the nascent HDL via ATP-binding cassette transporter A1 (ABCA1) transporter from tissues, and via phospholipid transfer protein (PLTP) from apoB–lipoprotein surfaces to begin the formation of the smaller HDL_3 particle. Lecithin: cholesterol acyltransferase (LCAT) acid hydrolyses phospholipid to a free fatty acid and a lysophospholipid and esterifies the cholesterol, which moves to the HDL core. In this process, the HDL particle becomes the larger, more buoyant HDL_3 particle. As this process progresses, the even larger HDL_2 particle is formed. Cholesteryl ester transfer protein (CETP) transfers cholesteryl ester (CE) from HDL_2 to the liver and various apoB-containing lipoproteins. With loss of cholesteryl ester, the HDL particle shrinks in size. Hepatic lipase (HL) hydrolyzes the phospholipid and triglyceride in the HDL_2 particle, furthering the decrease in size and density to HDL_3 and then to even smaller HDL particles. Recycling of some of the apoA-I causes the process to repeat itself. The role of apoA-II in this process in humans is not clear. LPL, lipoprotein lipase; SR-BI, scavenger receptor class B type 1. Modified from Ref. 12.

Approach to the Patient with Abnormal Lipid Levels

Patients with Isolated Elevation of Low-Density Lipoprotein Cholesterol Levels (type IIA Hyperlipidemia Adult Treatment Panel III)

The National Cholesterol Education Program (NCEP) defines a patient's LDL cholesterol level as "borderline high" in an individual with low atherosclerotic risk if the LDL cholesterol level exceeds 130 mg/dL. High LDL levels are those above 160 mg/dL with isolated high LDL cholesterol level. The patient's triglyceride level is by definition normal,[18] and the HDL cholesterol level is variable but often normal. The dyslipidemia in these patients is often discovered through routine cholesterol screening. Although some observers question the cost-effectiveness of screening all men and women older than age 20 years, the high prevalence of elevated LDL cholesterol in the United States warrants population screening, as recommended by the NCEP ATPIII and other authorities. Severely elevated cholesterol levels suggest FH. The ability to diagnose FH is valuable

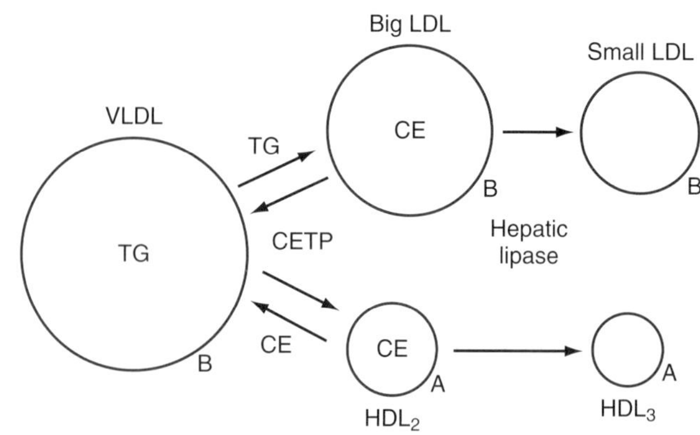

FIGURE 6-4 Dyslipidemia in the hypertriglyceridemic syndromes. Triglyceride-rich very-low-density lipoprotein (VLDL) exchanges triglyceride (TG) for the cholesteryl ester (CE) in low-density lipoprotein (LDL) and high-density lipoprotein (HDL) particles. This change in lipoprotein composition is initiated by cholesteryl ester transfer protein (CETP). Hepatic lipase hydrolyzes the triglyceride and phospholipid in large LDL and HDL particles, decreasing the size of each particle. Modified from Ref. 17.

because affected individuals will require initiation of drug therapy during late adolescence.

Isolated hypercholesterolemia may be present intermittently in patients with FCHL. A family history that is strongly positive for premature cardiovascular disease will provide clues to the diagnosis of this disorder. Not all cases of isolated hypercholesterolemia are indicative of FH or FCHL; some cases may result from interactions of acquired and environmental factors, particularly dietary factors, with unknown genetic factors that confer susceptibility to hypercholesterolemia.

Patients with Isolated Elevation of Triglyceride Levels (Type IV and Mild Type V, Hyperlipidemia)

An isolated elevation in triglyceride levels may be caused by a primary disorder of lipid metabolism (e.g., FHTG or FCHL); it may arise secondary to the use of therapeutic drugs; or it may be a component of untreated diabetes mellitus, human immunodeficiency virus/acquired immunodeficiency syndrome, or chronic kidney disease. Unlike with cholesterol levels, it has been difficult to determine the level of triglyceride associated with risk of CAD. It is valuable to determine the cause of the hypertriglyceridemia because the therapeutic approaches may differ.

For example, it is important to distinguish FHTG, which confers no risk of premature CAD, from FCHL, which is associated with a high incidence of premature CAD.[19] It is often difficult to distinguish these disorders when FCHL is associated with hypertriglyceridemia. A positive personal or family history of premature atherosclerosis with hypertriglyceridemia suggests FCHL. In addition, patients with FCHL frequently have nonlipid cardiovascular risk factors (i.e., central obesity, hypertension, insulin resistance, and impaired glucose tolerance). The presence of hypertriglyceridemia in FCHL indicates increased numbers of small dense LDL particles, even though the LDL cholesterol level may be normal, and confers an increased risk of premature cardiovascular disease.[17] Similarly, hypertriglyceridemia associated with treated type 2 diabetes mellitus with the metabolic syndrome is an important marker for cardiovascular risk. Other cardiovascular risk factors are usually present in patients with type 2 diabetes mellitus or FCHL. Therefore, the therapeutic strategy must consider treating factors beyond the lipid disorder.

Patients with FHTG do not appear to be at significantly increased risk for the premature development of CAD.[19] However, they are at increased risk for the development of the chylomicronemia syndrome when secondary forms of hypertriglyceridemia are present, such as untreated diabetes or the hypertriglyceridemia caused by the use of triglyceride-raising drugs. The chylomicronemia syndrome occurs in FCHL in combination with other causes of hypertriglyceridemia as well. In patients with pancreatitis caused by hypertriglyceridemia, triglyceride levels exceed 2000 mg/dL and can be much higher. It is recommended that plasma triglyceride levels always be maintained below 2000 mg/dL to prevent recurrent acute pancreatitis. A safe goal would be a level of less than 1000 mg/dL.[6] In patients with severe hypertriglyceridemia, the increase in total plasma cholesterol is a result of the cholesterol in VLDL and chylomicrons. Fibrates are often the drug of choice. However, it is very important to determine the etiology of the severe hypertriglyceridemia and remove any offending drug or treat any secondary cause of hypertriglyceridemia.[6]

Patients with Elevations in Cholesterol and Triglyceride Levels (Type IIb and Type III Hyperlipidemia)

Patients with elevations in the levels of both total plasma cholesterol and triglyceride can be divided into three categories. In the first category, VLDL and LDL are elevated, as in FCHL. In the second category VLDL and chylomicron remnants are elevated, as in remnant removal disease. The third category consists of patients with very high triglyceride levels in whom the increase in plasma cholesterol is a result of the cholesterol in VLDL and chylomicrons.

In patients with FCHL, an increase in triglycerides and in LDL cholesterol is often found. These patients always have elevated apoB levels and small dense LDL particles. Therapy for these individuals often requires several drugs, one aimed at lowering the cholesterol level and one aimed at reducing the amount of small dense LDL and HDL particles.

In patients with remnant removal disease, the levels of plasma cholesterol and triglyceride are often equal. It is important to consider remnant removal disease when both cholesterol and triglyceride are elevated. Therapy should be directed at decreasing hepatic lipoprotein secretion with statins, fibrates, or niacin.

Patients with Low High-Density Lipoprotein Cholesterol Levels

Many, if not most, patients with hypertriglyceridemia have a concomitant reduction in HDL cholesterol levels. Therefore, the management of low HDL cholesterol levels should be considered in the context of the management of the underlying disorder (e.g., FCHL or treated type 2 diabetes mellitus). Isolated low HDL cholesterol levels of 20 to 30 mg/dL without concomitant hypertriglyceridemia or other changes in lipid and lipoprotein levels are rare, but such low levels are a risk factor for cardiovascular disease.[11] In the past, reductions in HDL levels were often missed; the screening strategies used were based on the assessment of total cholesterol levels, and total cholesterol levels often are not elevated in patients with isolated reductions in HDL. Specific measurement of HDL cholesterol is required to identify these patients. The treatment of those rare patients with isolated low levels of HDL cholesterol remains somewhat controversial. There are no currently available drugs that effectively increase HDL cholesterol levels only (see Chapter 45).

COMMON GENETIC DISORDERS OF LIPOPROTEIN METABOLISM

Primary disorders of lipoprotein metabolism are those that arise from genetic defects in the metabolic pathways of lipoproteins (i.e., familial disorders caused by increased hepatic secretion of lipoproteins or by catabolic defects in lipoproteins). The disorders that cause increased lipoprotein secretion are the metabolic syndrome, FCHL type 2 diabetes mellitus, and FHTG; elevations of Lp(a) also can be due to increased lipoprotein secretion. Genetic disorders of the LPL-related triglyceride removal system are rare. Remnant removal disease is a defect in remnant catabolism. Disorders of LDL receptor–mediated catabolism of LDL are FH and familial defective apoB-100.

Metabolic Syndrome

The metabolic syndrome consists of a central distribution of adiposity or visceral obesity, insulin resistance, elevations in plasma FFA levels, impaired glucose tolerance, hypertension, dyslipidemia, and an abnormal procoagulant and proinflammatory state. Many individual components of this syndrome are known to predispose men and women to premature CAD.[17]

Etiology and Risk Factors

A selective accumulation of visceral rather than subcutaneous fat has been observed in individuals with the central body fat distribution characteristic of the metabolic syndrome. Men have more visceral fat than premenopausal women, even when matched for body mass index. It has been suggested that these differences in visceral fat and insulin resistance and the associated changes in lipoproteins and blood pressure could account, in part, for the difference between men and premenopausal women for risk of premature CAD.[20,21] Increased visceral fat is associated with insulin resistance and hyperinsulinemia, low plasma adiponectin levels, and elevations in plasma FFA levels.[22] It has been suggested that the accumulation of visceral fat precedes and causes insulin resistance and the resultant hyperinsulinemia because insulin sensitivity increases and FFA levels fall when visceral fat is decreased after caloric restriction.[23]

The levels of insulin, glucose, triglyceride, blood pressure, and plasminogen activator inhibitor type–1 (PAI-1) are increased above the mean normal in patients with the metabolic syndrome. Although these variables are often shifted to quite high levels, some of these variables are usually in the high-normal range in affected individuals. HDL levels tend to be lower than mean normal for men and women. Genetic and environmental factors appear to affect the distribution of these variables in both normal individuals and those with the metabolic syndrome. Because the metabolic syndrome is associated with multiple risk factors for premature CAD, individuals with the metabolic syndrome are at increased risk for atherosclerosis. Whether all individuals who meet the NCEP guidelines for the metabolic syndrome[24] are at increased risk for premature CAD is unknown. However, treated type 2 diabetes mellitus and FCHL are specific disorders of which the metabolic syndrome is a component.[17] These two disorders account for at least 40% to 50% of cases of premature CAD and must be considered in the context of the metabolic syndrome.

The risk of abdominal fat accumulation, insulin resistance, dyslipidemia, impaired glucose metabolism, and hypertension—the sentinel symptoms of the metabolic syndrome—increases with age.[25] Central obesity associated with the metabolic syndrome may occur in young adults; however, central obesity and insulin resistance more typically manifest in midlife. Whereas elevations in LDL cholesterol levels may not predict the onset of atherosclerosis in the elderly, central obesity, hypertension, and insulin resistance are risk factors for atherosclerosis and their prevalence increases with age, possibly because of the metabolic syndrome.[25–29]

Pathophysiology

Although the association of central obesity and insulin resistance with dyslipidemia is well established, the underlying mechanisms remain unclear. One abnormality that may explain the association of central obesity and insulin resistance with dyslipidemia is an increase in the level of portal vein long-chain FFAs. Such an increase would inhibit hepatic apoB from undergoing degradation in the hepatic proteosome and would increase the likelihood of apoB undergoing hepatic secretion in triglyceride-containing lipoproteins. This would account for the increased levels of triglyceride and the increased number of VLDL and LDL particles seen in patients with insulin resistance.[30] Another effect of long-chain FFAs is to increase hepatic lipase on the surface of hepatocytes. Hepatic lipase hydrolyzes triglyceride and phospholipid in LDL and HDL particles, decreasing the size of each particle (see Fig. 6-4).[17] CETP also contributes to this lipoprotein remodeling process; whether hepatic lipase or CETP has the predominate effect on the size and density of LDL and HDL particles depends on the triglyceride content of VLDL and the hepatic secretion rate of VLDL. The differences in LDL particle size and HDL_2 levels between men and premenopausal women can largely be explained by the excess of visceral fat in men.

Diagnosis

The NCEP ATP III has suggested five clinical variables as diagnostic criteria for the metabolic syndrome: (1) increased waist circumference, (2) increased triglyceride level, (3) decreased HDL cholesterol level, (4) increased blood pressure, and (5) elevated level of fasting plasma glucose.[18] A diagnosis of the metabolic syndrome is made when three or more of these clinical variables are present. When these five variables were assessed in a survey of 8814 adult men and women, approximately 24% of those surveyed met the criteria for diagnosis of the metabolic syndrome.[31,32] The World Health Organization and the International Diabetes Federation also established criteria for the metabolic syndrome. The recognition of the syndrome and its components is more important than determining the factors included in attempts to categorize patients. These components occur more commonly than would be expected by chance alone.

Visceral obesity and the resultant insulin resistance are major contributors to the dyslipidemia associated with the metabolic syndrome. The following lipid abnormalities are associated with the metabolic syndrome: increased levels of triglyceride, increased numbers of small dense LDL particles, increased apoB levels, and decreased levels of HDL_2 cholesterol. However, in normal, randomly selected populations, isolated visceral obesity and insulin resistance have been found to be associated with only a slight increase in triglyceride levels and only a slight decrease in HDL cholesterol levels.[22] In contrast, visceral obesity and insulin resistance can contribute to a more severe dyslipidemia when combined with an additional genetic dyslipidemia such as that associated with treated type 2 diabetes mellitus and FCHL.[17] The dyslipidemia of the metabolic syndrome can be diagnosed by demonstrating mild to moderate increases in plasma triglyceride and apoB levels above population means and decreased levels of HDL cholesterol in the presence of normal levels of LDL cholesterol. Although the LDL cholesterol level is normal in patients with this disorder, the number of LDL particles is generally increased because of increased small dense LDL particle number. These particles are cholesterol poor relative to large buoyant LDL particles. The presence of small dense LDL particles can be determined by direct measurement of LDL size or density or estimated by measurement of plasma apoB levels in clinical practice. It is not necessary to measure LDL size or density for the diagnosis of this disorder; however, measurement of plasma apoB levels can indicate the presence of increased numbers of small dense LDL particles. Similarly, total HDL levels reflect changes in the HDL_2 values, indicating that measurement of HDL subfractions is not required.[33]

It is possible that patients with the metabolic syndrome but without FCHL or type 2 diabetes may not be at risk for premature CAD. This study has not been undertaken and the answer remains unknown.

Familial Combined Hyperlipidemia

FCHL was first defined in the early 1970s. Goldstein and colleagues studied survivors of myocardial infarction and their families and reported different combinations of hyperlipidemia to be present in single families—elevated triglyceride, elevated cholesterol, or both.[34–36] Nikkilä and Aro reported multiple lipoprotein phenotypes occurring in Finnish families at about the same time.[37] Subsequently, families with FCHL have been described in Holland,[38,39] United Kingdom,[40] Canada,[41] Germany and China,[42] and Mexico.[43]

Premature Coronary Artery Disease

Goldstein and coworkers estimated the prevalence of FCHL in the population to be 1% to 2% and of CAD to be at least 10%.[35] FCHL also was found in families of middle-aged adult probands with hypertriglyceridemia in the absence of CAD.[44] In these studies, the prevalence of CAD in the families with FCHL was double that of the families with monogenic FHTG or the spouses of both families. Death attributable to CAD was found to be increased in both FCHL and FHTG in both of the Seattle-based families at 20-year follow-up.[19] However, premature CAD occurred only in the individuals with FCHL, with no premature CAD in FHTG families (Fig. 6-5). A further estimate of the prevalence of FCHL in premature CAD can be made from the Familial Atherosclerosis Treatment Study (FATS) of Brown and colleagues.[45] They screened 1300 men with premature CAD under the age of 62 years in two community-based hospitals in Seattle. One third of these men with premature CAD had an elevated apoB level. When family studies were performed on the men with elevated apoB levels who ultimately enrolled in FATS, 23% had familial hypercholesterolemia, 54% had FCHL, and the rest (23%) had an isolated, elevated Lp(a) level.[46] This one third of 54% with FCHL would be a coronary population estimate of 15% to 20%, not too dissimilar from the minimal estimate of Goldstein and coworkers.[35]

Phenotype

The variable lipid phenotype in FCHL has been confusing. In most affected individuals the lipoprotein phenotype can vary from isolated hypertriglyceridemia to isolated hypercholesterolemia within families and in single individuals.[3] This suggests that the variation in the lipid phenotype is often due to environmental changes. However, in some individuals the lipoprotein phenotype seems to be fixed; one such subset of individuals might be those with one half the normal levels of postheparin plasma LPL activity.[47] These individuals are more hypertriglyceridemic and less hypercholesterolemic. It has been suggested that an elevation in apoB levels is a consistent finding in FCHL[3,48,49] because of increased hepatic apoB secretion.[50–53] Indeed, if one measures lipoprotein phenotype, apoB levels, and size or density of LDL particles,[54–56] an increase in apoB levels in the presence of dense LDL particles is noted and is present in all subjects whether they have hypertriglyceridemia, hypercholesterolemia, or both.[57] In a society that has focused on LDL cholesterol levels, and recently HDL cholesterol levels, as risk factors for premature CAD, the dyslipidemia of FCHL has been deemphasized.[18] An attempt to account for this dyslipidemia was incorporated into NCEP ATP III by defining

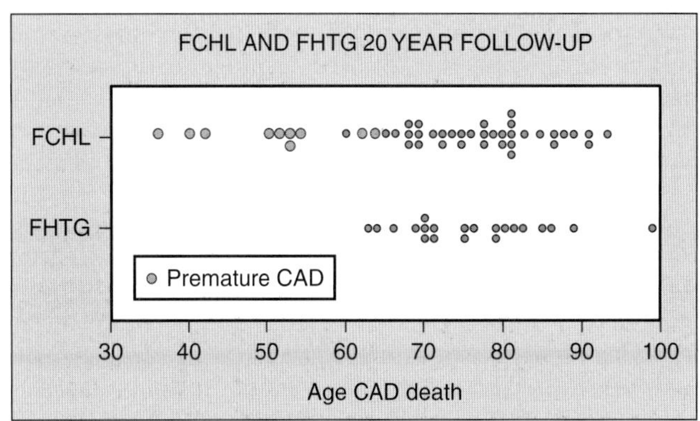

FIGURE 6-5 Age of death attributable to coronary artery disease (CAD) in familial combined hyperlipidemia (FCHL) and familial hypertriglyceridemia (FHTG). Patients and their families from the Seattle MI Study[35] and the Seattle Hypertriglyceridemia Study[110] were followed for 20 years. Death from CAD was documented by death certificate.[19] The age of CAD death occurred over a wide range in FCHL; there was no premature CAD death in the families with FHTG. Modified from reference 101.

the metabolic syndrome as a risk factor for CAD and including elevated triglyceride, decreased HDL cholesterol, and waist circumference in the definition.[18] Two entities enriched in the metabolic syndrome are FCHL and type 2 diabetes.[16] It may be that measurement of apoB levels, in addition to assessment of LDL and HDL cholesterol levels, will suffice to identify these individuals at risk for premature CAD with FCHL.[48,58–60]

Goldstein and colleagues initially described FCHL to be a monogenic disorder resulting from the apparently vertical transmission in families with the appropriate prevalence in adult offspring.[35] Nikkilä and Aro felt that FCHL was due to several genetic "hits."[37] Perhaps FCHL does have a major gene transmitted as a less common monogenic trait, interacting with common population traits. Jarvik and coworkers, using complex segregation analyses in the Seattle FCHL families, suggested that the putative locus for apoB levels segregated independently from the putative locus for LDL size.[61] This was consistent with the notion that apoB levels were bimodally distributed in individuals with FCHL who had small LDL particles.[62] Clinical studies support this "two-hit" hypothesis. Central obesity and insulin resistance have been reported to be very common in patients with FCHL.[63] However, central obesity and insulin resistance could not account for the elevated apoB levels seen in FCHL.[64] One hypothesis for FCHL is that a locus for apoB is transmitted as a monogenic trait[61] that interacts with a common population trait such as the metabolic syndrome[18] or the less common defect of decreased LPL activity.[48] In the initial Finnish FCHL family studies, the variant on chromosome 1q23, found to be in *USF1*, was associated with lipid values but not with apoB levels[65] compatible with a "two-hit" oligogenic disorder. Some investigators suggest that this heterogenous dyslipidemia is due to the interaction of many genes.[66]

In contrast, others believe that FCHL can be explained on the basis of a single defect,[67] perhaps in adipose tissue.[68] In this scenario, an abnormality in adipose tissue can lead to accumulation of adipose tissue triglyceride stores and to increased FFA mobilization with increased presentation of FFA to the liver. This increase in FFA flux may lead to increased hepatic triglyceride synthesis or, more likely, to decreased hepatic apoB degradation with resultant elevated hepatic apoB lipoprotein secretion.

A candidate protein for this abnormality has been suggested to be acylation-stimulating protein (ASP).[69] This is a 76-amino-acid fragment of the third component of complement (C3) that is generated by the interaction of adipsin and factor B with C3. The ASP pathway is a newly described biologic pathway that appears to play an important role in regulating adipose tissue triglyceride synthesis. Impaired function of this pathway may be the reason for the increased fatty acid traffic in the adipocyte–hepatocyte axis leading to the hyperapoB version of FCHL.[70] HyperapoB is the atherogenic dyslipoproteinemia characterized by increased numbers of LDL particles in plasma resulting from increased secretion of B1-00–containing lipoprotein particles by the liver. The lipid phenotype in affected patients is variable, but an increased plasma apoB points to the increased LDL particle number. For these reasons, ASP is also considered a candidate protein for FCHL[37]; however, in contrast to upstream transcription factor–1, the evidence for ASP as a candidate for FCHL rests primarily on biologic plausibility.[71]

Genetic Influences on Familial Combined Hyperlipidemia

Although numerous studies have demonstrated evidence for genetic linkage with various FCHL phenotypes,[72–78] attempts to fully understand the genetic basis for FCHL have been hampered by genetic heterogeneity, an unknown mode of inheritance, lack of standardized diagnostic criteria for FCHL, and a complex phenotype that likely includes pleiotropic effects.[79] In addition, small dense LDL particles, a component of FCHL, have been shown to be in association with many gene variants.[80,81] In spite of these challenges, several groups have reported linkage of a variety of FCHL lipid and lipoprotein phenotypes to regions on many chromosomes.[66,82–84] Until recently, evidence for effects of specific candidate genes in these regions had not been reported. An FCHL locus on chromosome 1q21-23 was the first to be identified and was based on an initial report of linkage to FCHL-related phenotypes in a sample of Finnish families,[72] subsequently confirmed in the National Heart, Lung, and Blood Institute (NHLBI) Family Heart Study,[85] German and Chinese FCHL families,[75] in British families,[86] and more recently in extended Mexican families.[82] The association of the A-I/C-III/A-IV locus on chromosome 11q13-pter with FCHL has been confirmed in almost all studies.[72,76,87–90] This locus seems a feasible candidate for the hypertriglyceridemia and hypercholesterolemia of FCHL, but no gene defect has been recognized. Finally, the hepatic lipase gene has been implicated in FCHL[91] and in the determination of LDL particle size and density.[92] It also has been linked to lipids in the NHLBI Family Heart Study.[93] An aggressive approach to modify reversible cardiovascular risk factors should be undertaken in individuals affected by this disorder. Diet therapy and therapeutic lifestyle modification that includes physical activity should be undertaken, together with lipid-lowering drug therapy and management of other cardiovascular risk factors.

Type 2 Diabetes Mellitus

Patients with untreated type 2 diabetes and insulin deficiency often have hypertriglyceridemia either because of a decrease in adipose tissue LPL-related plasma triglyceride removal or increased hepatic VLDL triglyceride secretion. These defects are corrected after treatment of the hyperglycemia for several months.[94–96] Patients undergoing chronic treatment of type 2 diabetes mellitus characteristically have a milder dyslipidemia, visceral obesity, and insulin resistance. First-degree relatives of individuals with type 2 diabetes mellitus may be centrally obese and have insulin resistance, or they may have decreased insulin secretion in response to glucose; first-degree relatives who both are centrally obese and have a defect in insulin secretion invariably develop type 2 diabetes mellitus. Type 2 diabetes mellitus is a classic example of an oligogenic disorder. The genes contributing to central obesity, insulin resistance, and defective insulin secretion have been extensively characterized in the past several years. In 2007, multiple centers reported and confirmed up to 10 common single nucleotide polymorphisms, found in multiple populations, that are associated with type 2 diabetes, obesity, and dyslipidemia.[97–100] Learning how these genes interact to cause diabetes will be of great interest.

The dyslipidemia of treated type 2 diabetes mellitus is probably genetic and is similar to that of the metabolic syndrome and FCHL; it is characterized by a mild increase in triglyceride levels, decreased HDL_2 cholesterol levels, and increased numbers of small dense LDL particles. Treatment entails diet therapy, increased physical activity, and lipid-lowering drug therapy.

Familial Hypertriglyceridemia

FHTG is a common inherited disorder, thought to be autosomal dominant, which affects about 1% of the population. FHTG is characterized by an increase in triglyceride synthesis that results in VLDL particles that are being enriched with triglyceride secreted in normal quantities. Affected people have elevated VLDL levels but low levels of LDL and HDL and are generally asymptomatic unless severe hypertriglyceridemia (i.e., chylomicronemia syndrome) develops. Plasma VLDL in FHTG are particles larger than normal or those seen in FCHL and are associated with very triglyceride-rich HDL particles,[3,101] presumably excluding some core cholesteryl ester leading to low HDL cholesterol but normal apoA-I levels.[101] FHTG does not appear to be associated with an increased risk of premature CAD.[19,44]

A defect in bile acid metabolism has been suggested to account for FHTG. Elevated hepatic cholic acid and chenocholic acid synthesis are present in FHTG compared with FCHL and with normal.[102,103] Preliminary studies demonstrated a defect in bile acid absorption in a small number of subjects with FHTG. Only one of 20 probands collected at three sites was found to have a mutation in the sodium-sensitive intestinal bile acid transporter gene.[104] Other defects in bile acid metabolism should be sought. The dyslipidemia of FHTG is much like that seen with bile acid–binding resin therapy.

A diagnosis is made by family history and examination of fasting lipoprotein profiles of the patient and relatives. The triglyceride level ranges from about 250 to 1000 mg/dL in approximately one half of first-degree relatives; a strong family history of premature CAD usually is lacking, and elevated LDL cholesterol levels should not be present.

Patients with FHTG should lose weight with regular exercise and reduce their intake of saturated fatty acids and cholesterol. Alcohol, exogenous estrogens, and other drugs that increase VLDL levels may need to be restricted. Diabetes, if present, should be well controlled. Hypertriglyceridemia in patients with FHTG often responds to these measures. If triglyceride levels exceed 500 mg/dL after 6 months of nonpharmacologic therapy, drug therapy with a fibrate might be considered[18]; at levels above 1000 mg/dL, drug therapy should be instituted.[105]

Familial Hypoalphalipoproteinemia with High Triglyceride

In 1992, Genest and colleagues proposed that FHA, a disorder with elevated triglyceride and low HDL cholesterol, was a common genetic dyslipidemia associated with premature CAD.[106,107] The HDL Atherosclerosis Treatment Study (HATS) selected middle-aged men and women with premature CAD for an intervention study.[108] In HATS, 87 men with low HDL selected to not have diabetes or elevated apoB levels were proposed to have FHA.[101] These men had normal levels of apoB compared with FCHL.[101] In contrast to FHTG, men with FHA had lower plasma apoA-I levels and did not have triglyceride-rich HDL particles as seen in FHTG. Furthermore, the FHA patients had a selective decrease in the HDL_2 apoA-I (without apoA-II) particle.[109]

It is not known whether FHA is a discrete genetic disorder. Low HDL cholesterol is commonly seen with premature CAD and has been proposed to be related, in part, to mutations in proteins of HDL metabolism (see Chapter 7). However, mutations in these candidate genes are rare and account for little FHA.

FHA is often confused with FHTG. In the Seattle Myocardial Infarction Study,[35] the patients classified as having FHTG may have had FHA. The Seattle Hypertriglyceridemia Study conducted at the same time with hypertriglyceridemic probands, who did not have clinical atherosclerosis, found no evidence for premature CAD in the FHTG families.[110] This was confirmed by a 20-year follow-up study.[19] It also is possible that the families termed FHTG in the NHLBI Family Heart Study[111] actually had FHA. More studies are needed to understand FHA. It is important to hypothesize that such a disorder exists for research purposes when performing pathophysiologic or genetic studies.

Chylomicronemia Syndrome

Pancreatitis is associated with chylomicronemia, usually associated with elevated levels of VLDL. The mechanism by which chylomicronemia causes pancreatitis is unclear. Pancreatitis may result from the release of more FFAs and lysolecithin from chylomicrons than can be bound by albumin in the pancreatic capillaries.

The chylomicronemia syndrome occasionally occurs when LPL is defective as a result of genetic variation in the enzyme or its cofactors, apoC-II and apoA-V. Much more commonly, chylomicronemia is caused by the coexistence of a genetic form of hypertriglyceridemia combined with an acquired disorder of plasma triglyceride metabolism, the most common being untreated diabetes.[6] Other conditions that may be implicated are the use of drugs that raise triglyceride levels.

The chylomicronemia syndrome is associated with abdominal pain, eruptive xanthomas, and transient memory loss. Eruptive xanthomas occur most frequently on the buttocks and the extensor surfaces of the upper limb. A reversible loss of memory, particularly for recent events, and peripheral neuropathy, which sometimes mimics the carpal tunnel syndrome, also may occur. The retinal vessels occasionally demonstrate lipemia retinalis. If the chylomicronemia syndrome is not corrected, it may lead to acute, recurrent pancreatitis. Acute pancreatitis often recurs until low triglyceride levels are maintained and can be fatal. The risk of pancreatitis caused by severe hypertriglyceridemia markedly increases with triglyceride levels greater than 2000 mg/dL.[6]

Familial Hypercholesterolemia

FH is an autosomal dominant disorder caused by a mutation in the gene encoding the LDL receptor. The extremely rare homozygote with FH has two mutant alleles at the LDL receptor locus, leaving the person with an absolute or nearly absolute inability to clear LDL from the circulation by the LDL receptor.[9] Heterozygotes with FH possess one normal allele, giving them approximately one half the normal receptor activity. Because the LDL receptor also contributes to VLDL remnant clearance from the plasma, a deficiency of LDL receptors may lead to some accumulation of remnant lipoproteins as well. High concentrations of LDL result in uptake of LDL by the extracellular matrix, including that of the arterial wall, leading to the formation of xanthomas and atherosclerosis. The heterozygous form of this disorder has a prevalence of about one in 500 people, making it a common genetic disease.[9]

Diagnosis

FH can be detected at birth in umbilical cord blood. Tendon xanthomas are a highly specific sign of FH; they begin to appear by age 20 years and may be present in up to 70% of older patients. Because xanthomas are subtle, careful examination of the dorsal hand tendons and Achilles tendon is required for their detection. Xanthelasma (cutaneous xanthomas on the palpebra) and corneal arcus are common in patients with FH after age 30 years; however, they are not specific for FH. Early corneal arcus is seen superiorly and inferiorly at the edge of the cornea and later becomes totally circumferential.

CAD develops early, with symptoms often manifesting in men in the fourth or fifth decade and in women about 10 years later. Approximately 5% of all cases of premature myocardial infarction occur in patients with heterozygous FH.[9,54] Before the development of statin therapy, at least 50% of patients for men with heterozygous FH experienced myocardial infarction by age 60 years, and about 10 years later for women. The LDL cholesterol level in heterozygous patients generally ranges from 200 to 400 mg/dL and increases with age. The triglyceride level may be mildly elevated, and the HDL cholesterol level occasionally is reduced.

Heterozygous FH should be suspected when severe hypercholesterolemia from elevated LDL is present. If tendon xanthomas are present, the diagnosis is virtually certain; if tendon xanthomas are absent, secondary causes of hypercholesterolemia should be sought, but the diagnosis of familial hypercholesterolemia is not excluded. A comprehensive family history should reveal a strong history of premature CAD and hypercholesterolemia with tendon xanthomas but without hypertriglyceridemia; the disorder affects approximately one half of first-degree relatives. The presence of hypercholesterolemia and tendon xanthomas in a parent or sibling is virtually diagnostic, as is hypercholesterolemia in a child in the family because other forms of elevated LDL cholesterol are rare in children. Careful screening of family members is mandatory because 50% of first-degree relatives will be affected and will require aggressive lipid-lowering therapy.[112] Management of FH requires both dietary intervention and drug therapy. The goal of therapy is to lower the LDL cholesterol level to less than 130 mg/dL, or even lower if the patient exhibits CAD. Aggressive reduction of LDL cholesterol in men and women who have heterozygous FH may cause a regression of coronary atherosclerosis.[101]

Familial Defective Apolipoprotein B-100

A mutation in apoB-100 that inhibits its binding to the LDL receptor is another genetic cause of elevations in LDL cholesterol. The prevalence of this disorder is unknown but is estimated to be 5% to 10% that seen in FH. The LDL receptor is normal. A full-length apoB-100 molecule is produced with a single amino acid substitution at residue 3500; this results in apoB that binds poorly to the LDL receptor, leading to LDL accumulation in the plasma. Affected individuals are clinically indistinguishable from patients with heterozygous FH: they may present with severe hypercholesterolemia, tendon xanthomas, and premature atherosclerosis. Treatment is similar to that for patients with LDL receptor mutations.

Increased Levels of Lipoprotein(a)

Lp(a) is a specific lipoprotein particle synthesized in the liver.[5] An important component of Lp(a) is apo(a), which has a structure homologous with plasminogen, a key protein in the fibrinolytic pathway. Plasma concentrations of Lp(a) vary markedly among individuals, ranging from undetectable to greater than 200 mg/dL. Lp(a) plasma concentration is strongly controlled by inheritance.

Most epidemiologic studies indicate that Lp(a) is a risk factor for CAD and stroke. Lp(a) may be atherogenic because of its LDL-like properties: Lp(a) has been shown to undergo endothelial uptake and oxidative modification and to promote foam cell formation. Because Lp(a) has a high degree of homology with plasminogen, it may play a role in thrombosis by interfering with the binding of plasminogen to fibrin. Elevated Lp(a) levels appear to complement the atherogenicity of other cardiovascular risk factors, with earlier onset of cardiovascular events.

Reduction of LDL cholesterol levels in patients with high levels of Lp(a) may be an effective strategy to slow the progression of atherosclerosis and to prevent coronary events.[10] The Lp(a) level itself can be reduced with high-dose niacin or estrogen. No data exist regarding the efficacy of lowering the Lp(a) level per se to inhibit atherosclerosis or to prevent coronary events.[5]

Remnant Removal Disease

Remnant removal disease, also called type III hyperlipoproteinemia, dysbetalipoproteinemia, or broad-beta disease, is defined as the presence of VLDL particles that migrate in the beta position on electrophoresis (normal VLDL particles migrate in the pre-beta location) as chylomicron and VLDL remnants.

Remnant removal disease is caused in part by a mutation in the *APOE* gene[7] that leads to an impairment in the hepatic uptake of apoE-containing lipoproteins and stops the conversion of VLDL and IDL to LDL particles. In the absence of additional genetic, hormonal, or environmental factors, remnants do not accumulate to a degree sufficient to cause hyperlipidemia because they are cleared by hepatic receptors that also bind, with less avidity, to apoB-48 and apoB-100. Remnant removal disease results when an apoE defect (almost always the E_2/E_2 genotype) occurs in conjunction with a second genetic or acquired defect that causes either overproduction of VLDL (such as FCHL) or a reduction in LDL receptor activity (such as occurs in heterozygous FH or hypothyroidism). The E_2/E_2 genotype is found in 1% of the white population and in virtually all persons with remnant removal disease, about 1 per 1000 individuals.

Diagnosis

Persons with remnant removal disease have elevations in both cholesterol and triglyceride levels, are likely to develop premature CAD, and are at particularly increased risk for peripheral vascular disease. Clinical dyslipidemia usually does not develop before adulthood. Palmar xanthomas (xanthoma striata palmaris), orange lipid deposits in the palmar creases, are pathognomonic for genetic remnant removal disease but are not always present. Palmar xanthomas may be difficult to see and should be sought using good lighting. Tuberoeruptive xanthomas are occasionally found at pressure sites on the elbows, buttocks, and knees.

The presence of remnant removal disease should be suspected in a person with elevated total cholesterol and triglyceride levels, elevated VLDL and IDL cholesterol levels, and reduced LDL and HDL cholesterol levels. Cholesterol and triglyceride levels range from 300 to 1000 mg/dL and are roughly equal, except during an acute exacerbation of the hypertriglyceridemia. Beta-migrating VLDLs are seen on agarose gel electrophoresis, although this test is no longer commonly used. Ultracentrifugation demonstrates that the ratio of VLDL cholesterol to total plasma triglyceride is greater than 0.3. Definitive diagnosis is made by detecting the E_2/E_2 phenotype by isoelectric focusing of plasma lipoproteins or the genotype by genetic analysis. Generally, therapy for remnant removal disease is the same as that for other forms of hypertriglyceridemia. Drugs that increase triglyceride levels, such as bile acid-binding resins, must be avoided.

Rare Disorders

Severe hypertriglyceridemia can present in childhood as a result of LPL deficiency or, extremely rarely, as apoC-II or apoA-V deficiency. These patients are at risk for acute, recurrent pancreatitis with severe hypertriglyceridemia and must be treated with moderate to severe dietary fat restriction until plasma triglyceride levels are below 1000 to 2000 mg/dL.

Homozygous FH is extremely rare and leads to severe hypercholesterolemia, unusual xanthomas, atherosclerosis, and death, often in the first two decades of life. Patients with homozygous FH may benefit from LDL apheresis. At the other extreme, the absence of apoB-containing lipoproteins can result from defects in the synthesis of apoB (e.g., homozygous hypobetalipoproteinemia) or from homozygous defects in the transport of apoB into the hepatic endoplasmic reticulum by the microsomal triglyceride transfer protein. Individuals with very low apoB levels are not at risk for atherosclerosis.

Miscellaneous Common Dyslipidemias

Polygenic hypercholesterolemia was once thought to be very common. The term *polygenic hypercholesterolemia* has been used to refer to the occurrence of mild elevations in LDL cholesterol in the apparent absence of a familial form of dyslipidemia or of dyslipidemia of secondary cause. This category of dyslipidemia continues to diminish as LDL variants such as Lp(a) and small dense LDL particles are discovered.

Mild to moderate hypertriglyceridemia may occur in the presence of modest defects in LPL in conjunction with a decrease in HDL cholesterol levels. It is seen in the obligate heterozygote parents of children with LPL deficiency. This defect may predispose to premature atherosclerosis.

SUMMARY AND CONCLUSIONS

Many genetic disorders of lipoproteins are associated with premature CAD. As the understanding of human lipoprotein has developed, it has been recognized that defects occur at many different sites, some very common. In the past 20 years, drugs have been developed that allow the delay of the onset of premature CAD for years, particularly when used in combination and with modification of lifestyle. One can treat all patients at risk with statins and follow the course of therapy with LDL cholesterol levels. Alternatively, we can develop specific courses of combination drug therapy based on the genetic basis of the lipoprotein disorder.[105] As we better understand the genetic lipoprotein disorders, newer and more specific drugs will be developed.

Acknowledgment

The work was supported by National Institutes of Health grant HL30086.

REFERENCES

1. Havel R, Kane J: Introduction: structure and metabolism of plasma lipoproteins. In Scriver CR, Beaudet AL, Sly WS, et al (eds): The Metabolic and Molecular Bases of Inherited Disease, 8th edition. *New York, McGraw-Hill,* 2001, pp 2705–2716.
2. Brunzell JD, Chait A, Bierman EL: Pathophysiology of lipoprotein transport. *Metabolism* 1978;27:1109–1127.
3. Brunzell JD, Albers JJ, Chait A, et al: Plasma lipoproteins in familial combined hyperlipidemia and monogenic familial hypertriglyceridemia. *J Lipid Res* 1983;24:147–155.
4. Kane JP, Havel RJ: Disorders of the biogenesis and secretion of lipoproteins containing the B apolipoproteins. In Scriver CR, Beaudet AL, Sly WS, et al (eds): The Metabolic and Molecular Bases of Inherited Disease, 8th edition. *New York, McGraw-Hill,* 2001, pp 2717–2752.
5. Utermann G: Lipoprotein(a). In Scriver CR, Beaudet AL, Sly WS, et al (eds): The Metabolic and Molecular Bases of Inherited Disease, 8th edition. *New York, McGraw-Hill,* 2001, pp 2753–2787.
6. Brunzell J, Deeb S: Familial lipoprotein lipase deficiency, apoCII deficiency, and hepatic lipase deficiency. In Scriver CR, Beaudet AL, Sly WS, et al (eds): The Metabolic and Molecular Bases of Inherited Disease, 8th edition. *New York, McGraw-Hill,* 2001, pp 2789–2816.
7. Mahley R, Rall S: Type III hyperlipoproteinemia (dysbetalipoproteinemia): the role of apolipoprotein E in normal and abnormal lipoprotein metabolism. In Scriver CR, Beaudet AL, Sly WS, et al (eds): The Metabolic and Molecular Bases of Inherited Disease, 8th edition. *New York, McGraw-Hill,* 2001, pp 2835–2862.
8. Murdoch SJ, Boright AP, Paterson, AD, et al: LDL composition in E_2/2 subjects and LDL distribution by Apo E genotype in type 1 diabetes. *Atherosclerosis* 2007;192:138–147.
9. Goldstein JL, Hobbs HH, Brown MS: Familial hypercholesterolemia. In Scriver CR, Beaudet AL, Sly WS, et al (eds): The Metabolic and Molecular Bases of Inherited Disease, 8th edition. *New York, McGraw-Hill,* 2001, pp 2863–2913.
10. Cohen JC, Boerwinkle E, Mosley TH Jr, et al: Sequence variations in PCSK9, low LDL, and protection against coronary heart disease. *N Engl J Med* 2006;354:1264–12.
11. Tall A, Breslow J, Rubin E: Genetic disorders affecting plasma high-density lipoproteins. In Scriver CR, Beaudet AL, Sly WS, et al (eds): The Metabolic and Molecular Bases of Inherited Disease, 8th edition. *New York, McGraw-Hill,* 2001, pp 2915–2936.
12. Deeb SS, Zambon A, Carr MC, et al: Hepatic lipase and dyslipidemia: interactions among genetic variants, obesity, gender, and diet. *J Lipid Res* 2003;44:1279–1286.
13. Frikke-Schmidt R, Nordestgaard BG, Jensen GB, et al: Genetic variation in ABC transporter A1 contributes to HDL cholesterol in the general population. *J Clin Invest* 2004;114:1343–1353.
14. Cohen JC, Kiss RS, Pertsemlidis A, et al: Multiple rare alleles contribute to low plasma levels of HDL cholesterol. *Science* 2004;305:869–872.
15. Boekholdt SM, Souverein OW, Tanck MW, et al: Common variants of multiple genes that control reverse cholesterol transport together explain only a minor part of the variation of HDL cholesterol levels. *Clin Genet* 2006;69:263–270.
16. Kiss RS, Kavaslar N, Okuhira K, et al: Genetic etiology of isolated low HDL syndrome: incidence and heterogeneity of efflux defects. *Arterioscler Thromb Vasc Biol* 2007;27:1139–1145.
17. Carr MC, Brunzell JD: Abdominal obesity and dyslipidemia in the metabolic syndrome: importance of type 2 diabetes and familial combined hyperlipidemia in coronary artery disease risk. *J Clin Endocrinol Metab* 2004;89:2601.
18. Executive summary of the third report of the National Cholesterol Education Program (NCEP) expert panel on detection, evaluation, and treatment of high blood cholesterol in adults (adult treatment panel III). Expert Panel on Detection, Evaluation, and Treatment of High Blood Cholesterol in Adults. *JAMA* 2001;285:2486–2497. Available at www.nhlbi.nih.gov/guidelines/cholesterol/atp_iii.htm.
19. Austin MA, McKnight B, Edwards KL, et al: Cardiovascular disease mortality in familial forms of hypertriglyceridemia: a 20-year prospective study. *Circulation* 2000;101:2777.
20. Carr MC: The emergence of the metabolic syndrome with menopause. *J Clin Endocrinol Metab* 2003;88:2404–2411.
21. Lemieux S, Despres JP, Moorjani S, et al: Are gender differences in cardiovascular disease risk factors explained by the level of visceral adipose tissue? *Diabetologia* 1994;37:757–764.
22. Nieves D, Cnop M, Retzlaff B, et al: The atherogenic lipoprotein profile associated with obesity and insulin resistance is largely attributable to intra-abdominal fat. *Diabetes* 2003;52:172–179.
23. Purnell JQ, Kahn SE, Albers JJ, et al: Effect of weight loss with reduction of intra-abdominal fat on lipid metabolism in older men. *J Clin Endocrinol Metab* 2000;85:977.
24. Grundy SM: Approach to lipoprotein management in 2001 National Cholesterol Guidelines. *Am J Cardiol* 2002;90:11i–22i.
25. Cefalu WT, Wang ZQ, Werbel S, et al: Contribution of visceral fat mass to the insulin resistance of aging. *Metabolism* 1995;44:954–959.
26. Bermudez OI, Tucker KL: Total and central obesity among elderly Hispanics and the association with type 2 diabetes. *Obes Res* 2001;9:443–451.
27. Lempiainen P, Mykkanen L, Pyorala K, et al: Insulin resistance syndrome predicts coronary heart disease events in elderly nondiabetic men. *Circulation* 1999;100:123–128.
28. Mykkanen L, Kuusisto J, Haffner SM, et al: Hyperinsulinemia predicts multiple atherogenic changes in lipoproteins in elderly subjects. *Arterioscler Thromb* 1994;14:518–526.
29. Cefalu WT, Werbel S, Bell-Farrow AD, et al: Insulin resistance and fat patterning with aging: relationship to metabolic risk factors for cardiovascular disease. *Metabolism* 1998;47:401–408.
30. Ginsberg HN: Insulin resistance and cardiovascular disease. *J Clin Invest* 2000;106:453–458.
31. Ford E, Giles W, Dietz W: Prevalence of the metabolic syndrome among US adults: findings from the third National Health and Nutrition Examination Survey. *JAMA* 2002;287:356–359.
32. Alexander CM, Landsman PB, Teutsch SM, et al: NCEP-defined metabolic syndrome, diabetes, and prevalence of coronary heart disease among NHANES III participants age 50 years and older. *Diabetes* 2003;52:1210–1214.
33. Lamarche B, Moorjani S, Cantin B, et al: Associations of HDL_2 and HDL3 subfractions with ischemic heart disease in men. *Arterioscler Thromb Vasc Biol* 1997;17:1098–1105.
34. Goldstein JL, Hazzard WR, Schrott HG, et al: Hyperlipidemia in coronary heart disease. I. Lipid levels in 500 survivors of myocardial infarction. *J Clin Invest* 1973;52:1533–1543.
35. Goldstein JL, Schrott HG, Hazzard WR, et al: Hyperlipidemia in coronary heart disease. II. Genetic analysis of lipid levels in 176 families and delineation of a new inherited disorder, combined hyperlipidemia. *J Clin Invest* 1973;52:1544–1568.
36. Hazzard WR, Goldstein JL, Schrott MG, et al: Hyperlipidemia in coronary heart disease. III. Evaluation of lipoprotein phenotypes of 156 genetically defined survivors of myocardial infarction. *J Clin Invest* 1973;52:1569–1577.
37. Nikkilä EA, Aro A: Family study of serum lipids and lipoproteins in coronary heart disease. *Lancet* 1973;1:954–9.
38. Aouizerat BE, Allayee H, Cantor RM, et al: A genome scan for familial combined hyperlipidemia reveals evidence of linkage with a locus on chromosome 11. *Am J Hum Genet* 1999;65:397–412.
39. de Graaf J, Stalenhoef AF: Defects of lipoprotein metabolism in familial combined hyperlipidaemia. *Curr Opin Lipidol* 1998;9:189–196.
40. Wojciechowski AP, Farrall M, Cullen P, et al: Familial combined hyperlipidaemia linked to the apolipoprotein AI-CII-AIV gene cluster on chromosome 11q23-q24. *Nature* 1991;349:161–164.
41. Gagne E, Genest J Jr, Zhang H, et al: Analysis of DNA changes in the LPL gene in patients with familial combined hyperlipidemia. *Arterioscler Thromb* 1994;14:1250–7.
42. Pei W, Baron H, Muller-Myhsok B, et al: Support for linkage of familial combined hyperlipidemia to chromosome 1q21-q23 in Chinese and German families. *Clin Genet.* 2000;57:29–34.
43. Huertas-Vázquez A, del Rincón JP, Canizales-Quinteros S, et al: Contribution of chromosome 1q21-q23 to familial combined hyperlipidemia in Mexican families. *Ann Hum Genet* 2004;68:419–427.
44. Brunzell JD, Schrott HG, Motulsky AG, Bierman EL: Myocardial infarction in the familial forms of hypertriglyceridemia. *Metabolism* 1976;25:313–320.
45. Brown G, Albers JJ, Fisher LD, et al: Regression of coronary artery disease as a result of intensive lipid-lowering therapy in men with high levels of apolipoprotein B. *N Engl J Med* 1976;323:1289–1290.

46. Zambon A, Brown BG, Hokanson JE, et al: Genetically determined apoB levels and peak LDL density predict angiographic response to intensive lipid-lowering therapy. *J Intern Med* 2006;259:401–409.
47. Babirak SP, Brown BG, Brunzell JD, et al: Familial combined hyperlipidemia and abnormal lipoprotein lipase. *Arterioscler Thromb* 1992;12:1176.
48. Sniderman A, Shapiro S, Marpole D, et al: Association of coronary atherosclerosis with hyperapobetalipoproteinemia [increased protein but normal cholesterol levels in human plasma low-density (beta) lipoproteins]. *Proc Natl Acad Sci USA.* 1980;77:604–608.
49. Castro Cabezas M, Erkelens DW, Kock LA, De Bruin TW: Postprandial apolipoprotein B100 and B48 metabolism in familial combined hyperlipidaemia before and after reduction of fasting plasma triglycerides. *Eur J Clin Invest.* 1994;24:669–678.
50. Chait A, Albers JJ, Brunzell JD: Very low-density lipoprotein overproduction in genetic forms of hypertriglyceridemia. *Eur J Clin Invest* 1980;10:17–22.
51. Janus ED, Nicoll AM, Turner PR, et al: Kinetic bases of the primary hyperlipidaemias: studies of apolipoprotein B turnover in genetically defined subjects. *Eur J Clin Invest* 1980;10: 161–172.
52. Kissebah AH, Alfarsi S, Adams PW: Integrated regulation of very low-density lipoprotein triglyceride and apolipoprotein-B kinetics in man: normolipemic subjects, familial hypertriglyceridemia and familial combined hyperlipidemia. *Metabolism.* 1981;30:856–868.
53. Venkatesan S, Cullen P, Pacy P, et al: Stable isotopes show a direct relation between VLDL apoB overproduction and serum triglyceride levels and indicate a metabolically and biochemically coherent basis for familial combined hyperlipidemia. *Arterioscler Thromb* 1993;13:1110–1118.
54. Bredie SJ, Kiemeney LA, de Haan AF, et al: Inherited susceptibility determines the distribution of dense low-density lipoprotein subfraction profiles in familial combined hyperlipidemia. *Am J Hum Genet* 1996;58:812–822.
55. Hokanson JE, Krauss RM, Albers JJ, et al: Low-density lipoprotein physical and chemical properties in familial combined hyperlipidemia. *Arterioscler Thromb Vasc Biol* 1995;15: 452–459.
56. Sniderman AD, Castro Cabezas M, Ribalta J, et al: A proposal to redefine familial combined hyperlipidaemia—third workshop on FCHL held in Barcelona from 3 to 5 May 2001, during the scientific sessions of the European Society for Clinical Investigation. *Eur J Clin Invest* 2002;32:71–73.
57. Ayyobi AF, McGladdery SH, McNeely MJ, et al: Small dense LDL and elevated apolipoprotein B are the common characteristics for the three major lipid phenotypes of familial combined hyperlipidemia. *Arterioscler Thromb Vasc Biol* 2003;23: 1289–1294.
58. Yusuf S, Hawken S, Ounpuu S, et al: Effect of potentially modifiable risk factors associated with myocardial infarction in 52 countries (the INTERHEART study): case–control study. *Lancet* 2004;364:937–952.
59. Lamarche B, Tchernof A, Moorjani S, et al: Small, dense low-density lipoprotein particles as a predictor of the risk of ischemic heart disease in men. Prospective results from the Quebec Cardiovascular Study. *Circulation* 1997;95:69–75.
60. Jungner I, Sniderman AD, Furberg C, et al: Does low-density lipoprotein size add to atherogenic particle number in predicting the risk of fatal myocardial infarction? *Am J Cardiol* 2006;97:943–946.
61. Jarvik GP, Brunzell JD, Austin MA, et al: Genetic predictors of FCHL in four large pedigrees: influence of ApoB level major locus predicted genotype and LDL subclass phenotype. *Arterioscler Thromb* 1994;14:1687.
62. Steinberg D, Pearson TA, Kuller LH: Alcohol and atherosclerosis. *Ann Intern Med* 1991;114:967–976.
63. Aitman TJ, Godsland IF, Farren B, et al: Defects of insulin action on fatty acid and carbohydrate metabolism in familial combined hyperlipidemia. *Arterioscler Thromb Vasc Biol* 1997;17: 748–754.
64. Purnell JQ, Kahn SE, Schwartz RS, Brunzell JD: Relationship of insulin sensitivity and apoB levels to intra-abdominal fat in subjects with familial combined hyperlipidemia. *Arterioscler Thromb Vasc Biol* 2001;21:567–572.
65. Lee JC, Weissglas-Volkov D, Kyttala M, et al: USF1 contributes to high serum lipid levels in Dutch FCHL families and U.S. whites with coronary artery disease. *Arterioscler Thromb Vasc Biol* 2007;27:2222–2227.
66. Lee JC, Lusis AJ, Pajukanta P: Familial combined hyperlipidemia: upstream transcription factor 1 and beyond. *Curr Opin Lipidol* 2006;17:101–109.
67. Juo SH, Bredie SJ, Kiemeney LA, et al: A common genetic mechanism determines plasma apolipoprotein B levels and dense LDL subfraction distribution in familial combined hyperlipidemia. *Am J Hum Genet* 1998;63:586–594.
68. de Graaf J, Veerkamp MJ, Stalenhoef AF: Metabolic pathogenesis of familial combined hyperlipidaemia with emphasis on insulin resistance, adipose tissue metabolism and free fatty acids. *J R Soc Med* 2002;95(Suppl 42):46–53.
69. Cianflone KM, Maslowska MH, Sniderman AD: Impaired response of fibroblasts from patients with hyperapobetalipoproteinemia to acylation-stimulating protein. *J Clin Invest* 1990;85: 722–730.
70. Brunzell JD, Sniderman AD, Albers JJ, Kwiterovich PO: Apoproteins B and AI and coronary artery disease in humans. *Arteriosclerosis* 1984;4:79–83.
71. Cianflone K, Maslowska M, Sniderman A: The acylation stimulating protein-adipsin system. *Int J Obes Relat Metab Disord* 1995;19(Suppl 1):S34–S38.
72. Pajukanta P, Nuotio I, Terwilliger JD, et al: Linkage of familial combined hyperlipidaemia to chromosome 1q21-q23. *Nature Gen* 1998;18:369–373.
73. Pajukanta P, Terwilliger JD, Perola M, et al: Genomewide scan for familial combined hyperlipidemia genes in Finnish families, suggesting multiple susceptibility loci influencing triglyceride, cholesterol, and apolipoprotein B levels. *Am J Hum Genet* 1999;64:1453–1463.
74. Aouizerat BE, Allayee H, Cantor RM, et al: A genome scan for familial combined hyperlipidemia reveals evidence of linkage with a locus on chromosome 11. *Am J Hum Genet* 1999;65: 397–412.
75. Pei W, Baron H, Müller-Myhsok B, et al: Support for linkage of familial combined hyperlipidemia to chromosome 1q21-q23 in Chinese and German families. *Clin Genet* 2000;57:29–34.
76. Coon H, Myers RH, Borecki IB, et al: Replication of linkage of familial combined hyperlipidemia to chromosome 1q with additional heterogeneous effect of apolipoprotein A-I/C-III/A-IV locus. The NHLBI Family Heart Study. *Arterioscler Thromb Vasc Biol* 2000;20:2275–2280.
77. van der Kallen CJ, Cantor RM, van Greevenbroek MM, et al: Genome scan for adiposity in Dutch dyslipidemic families reveals novel quantitative trait loci for leptin, body mass index and soluble tumor necrosis factor receptor superfamily 1A. *Int J Obes Relat Metab Disord* 2000;24:1381–1391.
78. Allayee H, de Bruin TW, Michelle Dominguez K, et al: Genome scan for blood pressure in Dutch dyslipidemic families reveals linkage to a locus on chromosome 4p. *Hypertension* 2001;38: 773–778.
79. Edwards KL, Mahaney MC, Motulsky AG, Austin MA: Pleiotropic genetic effects on LDL size, plasma triglyceride, and HDL cholesterol in families. *Arterioscler Thromb Vasc Biol* 1999;19: 2456–2464.
80. Bossé Y, Pérusee L, Vohl MC: Genetics of LDL particle heterogeneity: from genetic epidemiology to DNA-based variations. *J Lipid Res* 2004;45:1008–1026.
81. Badzioch MD, Igo RP, Gagnon F, et al: LDL particle size loci in familial combined hyperlipidemia: evidence for multiple loci from a genome scan. *Arterioscler Thromb Vasc Biol* 2004;24: 1942–1950.
82. Huertas-Vazquez A, Aguilar-Salinas C, Lusis AJ, et al: Familial combined hyperlipidemia in Mexicans: association with upstream transcription factor 1 and linkage on chromosome 16q24.1. *Arterioscler Thromb Vasc Biol* 2005;25:1985–1991.
83. Naukkarinen J, Ehnholm C, Peltonen L: Genetics of familial combined hyperlipidemia. *Curr Opin Lipidol* 2006;17:285–290.
84. Suviolahti E, Lilja HE, Pajukanta P: Unraveling the complex genetics of familial combined hyperlipidemia. *Ann Med* 2006;38:337–351.
85. Coon H, Myers RH, Borecki IB, et al: Replication of linkage of familial combined hyperlipidemia to chromosome 1q with additional heterogeneous effect of apolipoprotein A-I/C-III/A-IV

locus. The NHLBI Family Heart Study. *Arterioscler Thromb Vasc Biol* 2000;20:2275–2280.

86. Shoulders CC, Naoumova RP: USF1 implicated in the aetiology of familial combined hyperlipidaemia and the metabolic syndrome. *Trends Mol Med* 2004;10:362–365.
87. Wojciechowski AP, Farrall M, Cullen P, et al: Familial combined hyperlipidaemia linked to the apolipoprotein AI-CII-AIV gene cluster on chromosome 11q23-q24. *Nature* 1991;349:161–164.
88. Gagnon F, Jarvik GP, Motulsky AG, et al: Evidence of linkage of HDL level variation to APOC3 in two samples with different ascertainment. *Hum Genet* 2003;113:522–533.
89. Eichenbaum-Voline S, Olivier M, Jones EL, et al: Linkage and association between distinct variants of the APOA1/C3/A4/A5 gene cluster and familial combined hyperlipidemia. *Arterioscler Thromb Vasc Biol* 2004;24:167–174.
90. Aouizerat BE, Allayee H, Cantor RM, et al: Linkage of a candidate gene locus to familial combined hyperlipidemia: lecithin: cholesterol acyltransferase on 16q. *Arterioscler Thromb Vasc Biol* 1999;19:2730–2736.
91. Allayee H, Dominguez KM, Aouizerat BE, et al: Contribution of the hepatic lipase gene to the atherogenic lipoprotein phenotype in familial combined hyperlipidemia. *J Lipid Res* 2000;41:245–252.
92. Zambon A, Hokanson JE, Brown BG, et al: Evidence for a new pathophysiological mechanism for coronary artery disease regression: hepatic lipase-mediated changes in LDL density. *Circulation* 1999;99:1959.
93. Feitosa MF, Province MA, Heiss G, et al: Evidence of QTL on 15q21 for high-density lipoprotein cholesterol: the National Heart, Lung, and Blood Institute Family Heart Study (NHLBI FHS). *Atherosclerosis* 2007;190:232–237.
94. Pykälistö OJ, Smith PH, Brunzell JD: Determinants of human adipose tissue lipoprotein lipase: effects of diabetes and obesity on basal and diet induced activity. *J Clin Invest* 1975;56:1108–1117.
95. Brunzell JD, Porte D Jr., Bierman EL: Abnormal lipoprotein lipase mediated plasma triglyceride removal in untreated diabetes mellitus associated with hypertriglyceridemia. *Metabolism* 1979;28:897–903.
96. Tavangar K, Murata Y, Pedersen ME, et al: Regulation of lipoprotein lipase in the diabetic rat. *J Clin Invest* 1992;90:1672–1678.
97. Sladek R, Rocheleau G, Rung J, et al: A genome-wide association study identifies novel risk loci for type 2 diabetes. *Nature* 2007;445:881–885.
98. Diabetes Genetics Initiative of Broad Institute of Harvard and MIT, Lund University, Novartis Institutes of Biomedical Research, et al: Genome-wide association analysis identifies loci for type 2 diabetes and triglyceride levels. *Science* 2007;316:1331–1336.
99. Zeggini E, Weedon MN, Lindgren CM, et al: Replication of genome-wide association signals in UK samples reveals risk loci for type 2 diabetes. *Science* 2007;316:1336–1341.
100. Scott LJ, Mohike KL, Bonnycastle LL, et al: A genome-wide association study of type 2 diabetes in Finns detects multiple susceptibility variants. *Science* 2007;316:1341–1345.
101. Zambon A, Brown BG, Deeb S, Brunzell JD: Genetics of apolipoprotein B and apolipoprotein A1 and premature cardiovascular disease. *J Intern Med* 2006;259:473–480.
102. Angelin B, Hershon KS, Brunzell JD: Bile acid metabolism in hereditary forms of hypertriglyceridemia: evidence for an increased synthesis rate in monogenic familial hypertriglyceridemia. *Proc Natl Acad Sci USA* 1987;84:5434–5438.
103. Duane WC: Abnormal bile acid absorption in familial hypertriglyceridemia. *J Lipid Res* 1995;36:96–107.
104. Love MW, Craddock AL, Angelin B, et al: Analysis of the ileal bile acid transporter gene, SLC10A2, in subjects with familial hypertriglyceridemia. *Arterioscler Thromb Vasc Biol* 2001;21:2039–2045.
105. Brunzell JD: Clinical practice: hypertriglyceridemia. *New Engl J Med* 2007;357:1009–1017.
106. Genest JJ Jr, Martin-Munley SS, McNamara JR, et al: Familial lipoprotein disorders in patients with premature coronary artery disease. *Circulation* 1992;85:2025–2033.
107. Genest J Jr, Bard JM, Fruchart JC, et al: Familial hypoalphalipoproteinemia in premature coronary artery disease. *Arterioscler Thromb* 1993;13:1728–1737.
108. Brown BG, Zhao XQ, Chait A, et al: Simvastatin and niacin, antioxidant vitamins, or the combination for the prevention of coronary disease. *N Engl J Med* 2001;345:1583–1592.
109. Cheung MC, Wolfbauer G, Brown BG, Albers JJ: Relationship between plasma phospholipid transfer protein activity and HDL subclasses among patients with low HDL and cardiovascular disease. *Atherosclerosis* 1999;142:201–205.
110. Williams RR, Hopkins PN, Hunt SC, et al: Population-based frequency of dyslipidemia syndromes in coronary-prone families in Utah. *Arch Intern Med* 1990;150:582.
111. Marks D, Thorogood M, Neil HA, et al: A review on the diagnosis, natural history, and treatment of familial hypercholesterolaemia. *Atherosclerosis* 2003;168:1.
112. Maher VM, Brown BG, Marcovina SM, et al: Effects of lowering elevated LDL cholesterol on the cardiovascular risk of lipoprotein(a). *JAMA* 1995;274:1771–1774.

CHAPTER 7

High-Density Lipoprotein Mutations

Gerd Assmann and Udo Seedorf

HIGH-DENSITY LIPOPROTEIN CHOLESTEROL LEVELS IN POPULATIONS

In most populations, high-density lipoprotein (HDL) cholesterol levels show a broad distribution ranging from less than 20 to greater than 80 mg/dL. Figure 7-1 shows the distribution of HDL cholesterol concentrations according to myocardial infarction status in the male population of the Prospective Cardiovascular Münster (PROCAM) Study, a large prospective epidemiologic study on the risk factors for myocardial infarction, stroke, and other diseases performed in the northwestern part of Germany. Whereas the highest frequency of the HDL cholesterol distribution occurred at 44 mg/dL in men who did not have a major coronary event within 10 years of follow-up, the corresponding HDL cholesterol level in men who had an event occurred at 34 mg/dL, a value 10 mg/dL lower. Similar results have been obtained in the United States, notably by the Framingham Heart Study.[1]

The variation of HDL cholesterol observed in the general population relates to complex multifactorial causes, notably dietary and lifestyle habits, age, gender, hormones, drugs, and infectious diseases, as well as socioeconomic status in some populations. Moreover, ethnic differences play a role. In Turkish adults, for instance, HDL cholesterol levels are 10 to 15 mg/dL lower than those of adults in Western Europe and the United States. It has been shown that HDL cholesterol levels in Turks are low from birth to adulthood and depend significantly on the socioeconomic status in children but not in adults.[2] Mean levels of HDL cholesterol that deviate from those of whites have also been reported for many populations from developing countries. These differences are presumably a function of the frequency of specific genotypes and interaction with environmental factors such as lower or higher fat intake, alcohol consumption, or a higher level of physical activity that is normally associated with a rural lifestyle.[3] Although HDL cholesterol levels are influenced considerably by environmental and lifestyle factors, it is well established that genetic factors also play a very prominent role; they account for 40% to 60% of the HDL cholesterol variation in the population.[4] The known monogenic disorders affecting HDL cholesterol levels play a role in both extremes of the cholesterol distribution (at levels <20 mg/dL or >70 mg/dL; see Fig. 7-1), but these disorders likely do not account for the relationship existing between HDL cholesterol and coronary heart disease risk in the general population.

An important condition related to low HDL cholesterol levels in the population is the metabolic syndrome, which has a high prevalence in many countries of the world.[5] The metabolic syndrome is characterized by the simultaneous presence of multiple metabolic abnormalities that likely result from complex interactions between lifestyle habits and genetic factors.[6] Of special importance is the presence of central obesity, which often is accompanied by dyslipidemia (high triglycerides, low HDL cholesterol, and the presence of small dense, low-density lipoproteins [LDLs]) combined with elevated blood pressure and/or insulin resistance or glucose intolerance. Additional frequently observed anomalies include a prothrombotic state (i.e., high fibrinogen or plasminogen activator inhibitor–1 in the blood) and/or a proinflammatory state (i.e., elevated C-reactive protein in the blood).

Two widely used clinical definitions of the metabolic syndrome have been proposed that both incorporate low HDL cholesterol as a diagnostic criterion. The latest version of the definition developed by the National Cholesterol Education Program Adult Treatment Program III (NCEP ATP III) panel[7] relies on the presence of at least three of the following five criteria: (1) increased waist circumference with population-specific cut-off values, (2) increased levels of fasting triglycerides or treatment for hypertriglyceridemia, (3) low HDL

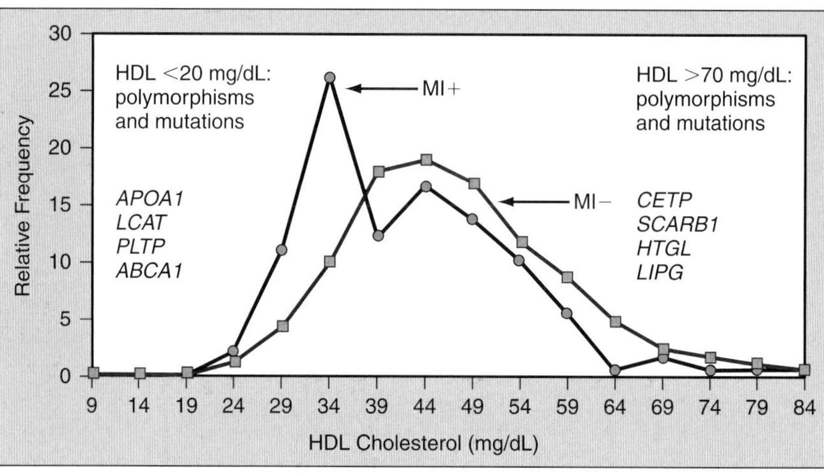

FIGURE 7-1 Relative frequency of high-density lipoprotein (HDL) cholesterol levels in male participants of the Prospective Cardiovascular Münster (PROCAM) Study who experienced a major coronary event (MI+) in comparison with those who remained event-free (MI–) within 10 years of follow-up. ABCA1, ATP-binding cassette transporter A1; APOA1, apoliprotein A-I; CETP, cholesteryl ester transfer protein; HTGL, hepatic triglyceride lipase; LCAT, lecithin:cholesterol acyltransferase; LIPG, endothelial lipase gene; MI, myocardial infarction; PLTP, phospholipid transfer protein; SR-BI, scavenger receptor class B type I.

cholesterol levels or treatment for this condition, (4) elevated blood pressure or antihypertensive treatment, and (5) elevated blood glucose or treatment with a hypoglycemic agent. The definition by the International Diabetes Federation (IDF) requires presence of central obesity with population-specific waist circumference cut-off values that are lower than in the NCEP-ATP III definition plus any two of the following four criteria: (1) elevated fasting triglycerides, (2) reduced HDL cholesterol, (3) hypertension, and (4) raised plasma glucose or previous diagnosis of type 2 diabetes.[8]

In both male and female participants of the PROCAM study, the metabolic syndrome is highly prevalent. Of all men aged 35 to 65 years, 26.8% fulfill the definition of the NCEP ATP III and 23.9% fulfill the IDF criteria. In women aged 45 to 65 years, the respective prevalence values are somewhat lower, but still 15.5% fulfill the criteria according to NCEP ATP III and 17.7% according to the IDF definition. As shown in Table 7-1, for male participants of the PROCAM study the HDL cholesterol cut-off value is included in three of the five most common combinations of the individual components of the metabolic syndrome based on the NCEP ATP III definition and two of the five most common combinations based on the IDF definition. Thus, it may be assumed that the high prevalence of low HDL cholesterol levels in individuals with the metabolic syndrome is a major determinant of low HDL cholesterol levels in the population.

There is evidence that HDL cholesterol is causally related to protection against coronary heart disease by virtue of its role in reverse cholesterol transport and other atheroprotective effects that are associated with this lipoprotein class.[9] Although some clinical trials suggest a benefit from raising HDL cholesterol to reduce risk, a recently published important trial on the cholesteryl ester transfer protein (CETP) inhibitor torcetrapib showed no beneficial effect on coronary atherosclerosis despite the fact that the drug was associated with a substantial increase in HDL cholesterol and decrease in LDL cholesterol.[10] It should be noted, however, that this negative result may have been due to the specific mechanism of torcetrapib, which blocks the activity of CETP, representing an important component of the reverse cholesterol transport pathway. Moreover, the drug was associated with increased blood pressure in the study by Nissen and colleagues.[10] Thus, it cannot be excluded that future attempts to raise HDL cholesterol by other means will be effective to reduce coronary atherosclerosis. Nevertheless, HDL cholesterol is currently not considered a primary target of therapy in the NCEP ATP III guidelines; however, HDL cholesterol is part of a patient's overall profile of established risk factors in determining the risk for myocardial infarction and deciding on treatment strategies.

IMPACT OF GENES ON HIGH-DENSITY LIPOPROTEIN CHOLESTEROL

The search for specific genes and gene variants that account for the genetic impact on HDL cholesterol levels has been a matter of intense research over the past

TABLE 7-1 Prevalence of the Five Most Frequent Combinations of Abnormalities in Male Participants of the PROCAM Study with Metabolic Syndrome According to the NCEP ATP III and the IDF Definitions

NCEP ATP III Definition of Metabolic Syndrome		IDF Definition of Metabolic Syndrome	
	Prevalence (%)		*Prevalence (%)*
TG+BP+Gluc	16.6	WC+BP+Gluc	21.8
TG+HDL+BP+Gluc	13.9	WC+TG+HDL+BP+Gluc	16.9
TG+HDL+BP	13.4	WC+TG+BP+Gluc	14.4
WC+TG+HDL+BP+Gluc	8.3	WC+TG+HDL+BP	10.8
WC+BP+Gluc	7.7	WC+TG+BP	9.0

TG, triglycerides; BP, systolic blood pressure; Gluc, glucose; WC, waist circumference; HDL, high-density lipoprotein cut-off values according to the indicated definitions; IDF, International Diabetes Federation; NCEP ATP III, National Cholesterol Education Program Adult Treatment Program III; PROCAM III, Prospective Cardiovascular Münster Study.

20 years. Early studies used the candidate gene approach; however, the outcome was rather disappointing.[11] In many cases, initially observed significant associations between specific genetic markers and plasma lipid levels could not be replicated if investigated in other populations or larger sample sizes. Those initial studies were frequently statistically underpowered, and the effect sizes of the marked loci were rather small. Even for genes showing consistent and significant association between genotypes and phenotypes such as apolipoprotein (apo)E, hepatic lipase or CETP, each locus explained less than 5% of the HDL cholesterol variability in the general population. More recently performed studies showed moderate effects on HDL cholesterol levels for several common polymorphisms in ATP-binding cassette transporter A1 (ABCA1),[12] and a range of rare ABCA1 alleles were identified in subjects with low HDL cholesterol levels.[13] Studies in mouse models have shown that hypoalphalipoproteinemia and postprandial lipemia observed in patients with Tangier disease relate to absence of ABCA1 from the liver rather than from macrophages.[14] Thus, variation of ABCA1 may be a determinant of plasma HDL cholesterol levels and possibly atherosclerosis risk in the general population.

In addition to candidate gene association studies, quantitative trait locus (QTL) analysis has been used successfully to identify chromosomal regions that contain genes regulating HDL cholesterol levels. These studies have led to more than 30 human QTLs for plasma HDL cholesterol levels; many are located in regions homologous to corresponding mouse QTLs.[15] Some of these QTLs coincide with well-established candidate genes for the low HDL cholesterol trait (Figure 7-2). Of particular current interest is a region on chromosome 9p that was shown to be linked to HDL cholesterol levels in Mexican Americans.[16] The region was located approximately 25 cM centromeric to a region between markers D9S288 and D9S925 that had previously been shown to be linked to type 2 diabetes (LOD score = 2.4) and age of diabetes onset (LOD score = 2.1) in the same population.[17] The specific location of both regions between markers D9S288 and D9S925 and between D9S925 and D9S741 suggested a considerable degree of overlap for both traits. Interestingly, several single nucleotide polymorphisms that were highly significantly associated with coronary heart disease in several recently performed high-density whole genome association scans were identified in the same region of chromosome 9p.[18–21] The approximately 100-kb region of interest contains the coding sequences of two cyclin-dependent kinase inhibitors, CDKN2A and CDKN2B.

INBORN ERRORS OF HIGH-DENSITY LIPOPROTEIN METABOLISM

The search for genes and mutations that cause less common forms of HDL cholesterol deficiency (also called hypoalphalipoproteinemia) or elevated HDL cholesterol (also called hyperalphalipoproteinemia) has been very successful over the past 20 years. It could be shown that altered levels of HDL cholesterol can result from mutations in a number of genes that regulate HDL production, maturation, or catabolism (Table 7-2). ApoA-I is the main structural protein of HDL, and *APOA1* mutations can lead to severe HDL deficiency.[22,23] Mutations in lecithin: cholesterol acyltransferase (LCAT), which promotes the maturation of HDL particles by catalyzing the esterification of cholesterol in HDL particles, cause two autosomal recessive forms of low HDL cholesterol: familial LCAT deficiency and fish eye disease.[24–26] Phospholipid transfer protein (PLTP) is involved in HDL remodeling, and low HDL cholesterol results from PLTP deficiency in mice.[27,28] PLTP missense mutations have been identified in humans with low HDL cholesterol levels; one of these mutations was associated with decreased lipid transfer *in vitro*.[29] Conversely, mutations in CETP are associated with increases of HDL cholesterol levels.[30] CETP catalyzes the transfer of cholesteryl esters and triglycerides among HDL, LDL, intermediate-density lipoprotein (IDL), and very-low-density lipoprotein (VLDL) particles.[31]

Tangier disease is a rare autosomal recessive disorder associated with almost complete HDL deficiency.[32] The disease is characterized by defective cellular lipid efflux to apoA-I, resulting from homozygosity or compound heterozygosity for mutations in the *ABCA1* gene.[33–39] Defective lipid efflux is also a significant factor in familial HDL deficiency, a more common and clinically milder form of HDL deficiency than Tangier disease.[40] It could be shown that some of the affected subjects are heterozygous carriers of *ABCA1* mutations.[37,41,42] In addition, rare ABCA1 alleles have also been identified in subjects with low HDL cholesterol levels who do not have Tangier disease or familial HDL deficiency.[12] Studies in mouse models showed that hypoalphalipoproteinemia and postprandial lipemia associated with Tangier disease relate primarily to absence of ABCA1 from the liver.[14]

Low HDL cholesterol is also associated with several monogenic disorders that are due to mutations in genes that are not directly involved HDL cholesterol metabolism (see Table 7-2). Fabry disease, a lysosomal storage disease resulting from deficient α-galactosidase A activity, is associated with elevated levels of HDL cholesterol.[43] Conversely, Gaucher disease, the most common lysosomal storage disorder caused by deficiency of glucocerebrosidase, is associated with decreased levels of HDL cholesterol.[44] Based on the high frequency of glucocerebrosidase mutations in various populations, it was estimated that the glucocerebrosidase locus might be responsible for familial hypoalphalipoproteinemia in up to 2% of the general population, suggesting that these mutations may represent one of the most common monogenic causes of low HDL cholesterol in some populations. Another autosomal recessive disorder that is consistently associated with low HDL cholesterol levels is cholesteryl ester storage disease.[45] It was shown recently that mutations in the gene for lysosomal acid lipase that cause cholesteryl ester storage disease have a relatively high frequency in some populations.[46]

An important topic of current research in the field of monogenic disorders affecting HDL cholesterol relates to the question of whether these disorders are associated with altered risk for cardiovascular disease. In a recent study, Hovingh and colleagues compared carotid intima–media thickness of a substantial number of individuals with rare mutations in HDL cholesterol–modulating genes, including *APOA*1, *ABCA*1, *LCAT*, and *CETP*.[47]

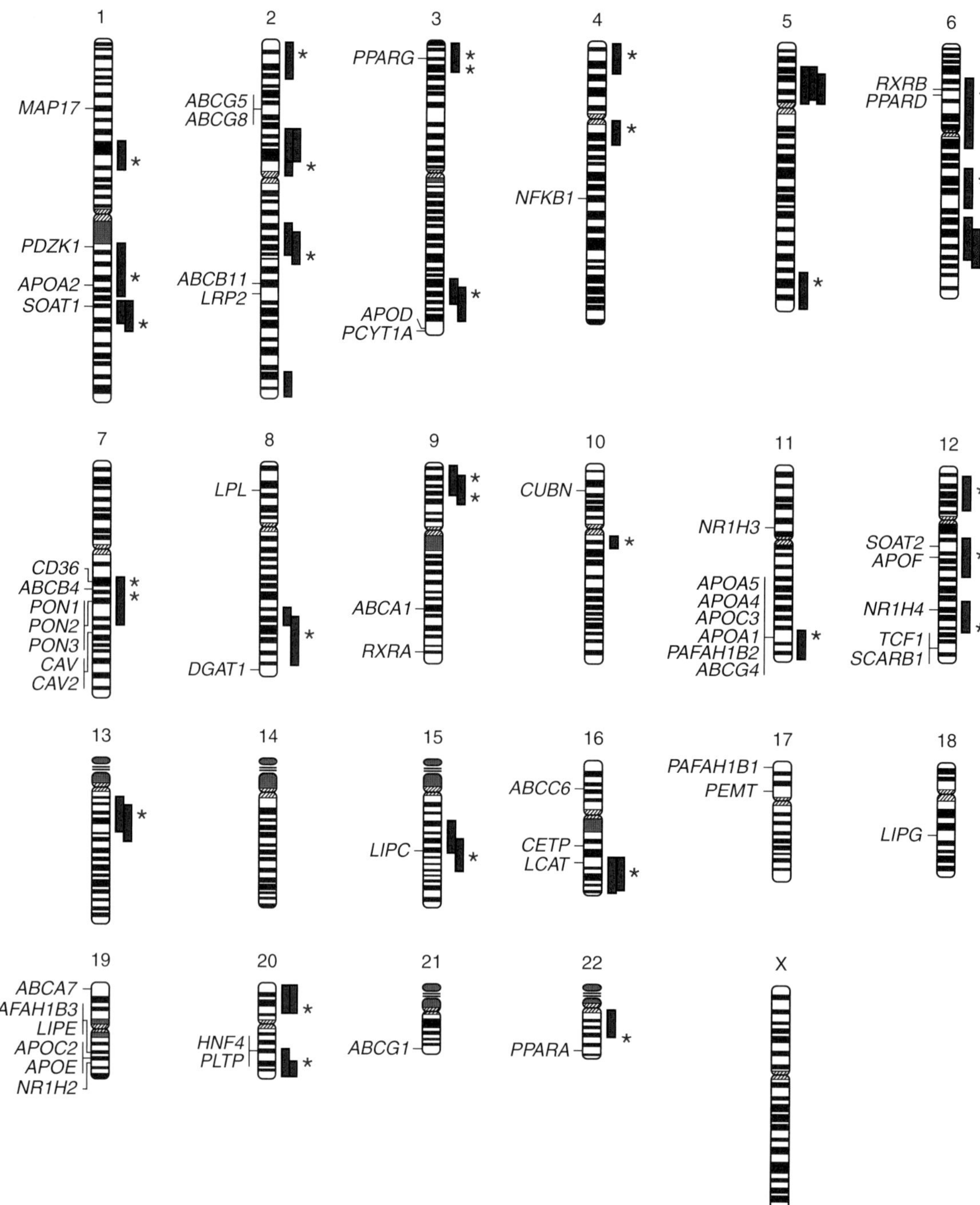

FIGURE 7–2 Chromosome map of human quantitative trait loci (QLTs) for plasma high-density lipoprotein (HDL) Cholesterol levels. Candidate genes are indicated to the left of the chromosomes. Human HDL cholesterol QTLs that overlap with homologous regions of mouse HDL cholesterol QTLs are represented by asterisks. *(From Ref. 15, with permission.)*

ABC, ATP-binding cassette transporter; APO, apolipoprotein; CAV, caveolin; CD, cluster of differentiation; CETP, cholesteryl ester transfer protein; CUBN, cubilin; DGAT, diacylglycerol acyltransferase; HDL, high-density lipoprotein; HNF, hepatocyte nuclear factor; LCAT, lecithin:cholesterol acyltransferase; LIPC, hepatic lipase; LIPE, hormone-sensitive lipase; LIPG, endothelial lipase; LPL, lipoprotein lipase; LRP, low-density lipoprotein receptor–related protein; MAP, membrane-associated proteni; NFKB, nuclear-factor–κB; NR1H, nuclear-receptor–1H; PAFAH1B, platelet-activating factor acetylhydrolase–1b; PEMT, phosphatidylethanolamine methyltransferase; PDZK1, postsynaptic density–95/disc-large/zona occludens domain–containing 1; PLTP, phospholipid transfer protein; PPARA, peroxisome proliferator–activated receptor; PON, paraoxonase; PCYT1A, phosphate cytidylyltransferase–1; QTL, quantitative trait locus; RXR, retinoid X receptor; SCARB1, scavenger receptor class B type 1; SOAT, sterol O-acyltransferase; TCF, transcription factor.

Their data showed that carriers of an *APOA1* mutation exhibited the most pronounced accelerated increase of intima media thickness compared with those carrying mutations in *ABCA1* or *LCAT*. Conversely, heterozygosity for a nonsense *CETP* mutation associated with elevated HDL cholesterol levels did not significantly affect intima–media thickness progression. Studies on patients with Fabry disease, who have elevated HDL cholesterol plasma levels, have shown that these patients are at increased risk to develop vascular disease, including stroke and coronary heart disease.[48]

The following section summarizes clinical features of the most important monogenic disorders affecting human HDL metabolism. It should be noted, however, that a recently published survey of mutations in more than 100 cases of sporadic HDL cholesterol deficiency

TABLE 7-2 Genetic Variation and Monogenic Disorders Associated with HDL Cholesterol Levels in the Human

Gene Symbol	Gene Product	Phenotype
ABCA1	ABC transporter A-I	Tangier disease; Familial HDL deficiency; Association with low HDL cholesterol levels
APOA1	Apolipoprotein A-I	HDL deficiency; HDL deficiency with periorbital xanthelasmas; HDL deficiency with amyloidosis; Association with high HDL cholesterol levels
LCAT	Lecithin:cholesterol acyltransferase	Familial LCAT deficiency; fish eye disease; association with low HDL cholesterol levels
CETP	Cholesteryl ester transfer protein	Hyperalphalipoproteinemia; association with high HDL cholesterol levels
APOD	Apolipoprotein D	Association with low HDL_3-C and apoA-I levels in females
APOC3	Apolipoprotein C-III	Association with elevated HDL cholesterol levels
APOA5	Apolipoprotein A-V	Association with low HDL cholesterol levels
GHR	Growth hormone receptor	Association of the *GHR* Leu *allele with low* HDL cholesterol levels in hypercholesterolemia
LIPC	Hepatic lipase	Association with elevated HDL cholesterol levels
LIPI	LPD lipase	Association with low plasma HDL cholesterol levels
LPL	Lipoprotein lipase	Association with low HDL cholesterol levels
ESR1	Estrogen receptor-1	Association with high HDL cholesterol after hormone replacement therapy
LIPG	Endothelial lipase	Association with elevated HDL cholesterol levels
PLTP	Phospholipid transfer protein	Association with low HDL cholesterol levels except for -34C, which is associated with elevated HDL cholesterol levels
PTGDS	Prostaglandin D2 synthase 21kDa (brain)	Association with low HDL cholesterol levels
SCARB1	Scavenger receptor class B type 1	Association with high HDL cholesterol levels
LIPA	Lysosomal acid lipase	Cholesteryl ester storage disease associated with low HDL cholesterol
GLA	α-galactosidase A	Fabry disease associated with high HDL cholesterol
GBA	Glucocerebrosidase	Gaucher disease associated with low HDL cholesterol
PPARD	Peroxisome proliferator-activated receptor-δ	Association with low HDL cholesterol levels
SMPD1	Sphingomyelin phosphodiesterase-1	Niemann-Pick disease type B associated with low HDL cholesterol levels
NPC1	Niemann-Pick disease type C1	Niemann-Pick disease type C associated with low HDL cholesterol levels

HDL, high-density lipoprotein.

implied that only a little more than 10% could be attributed to mutations in known candidate genes of HDL metabolism, whereas almost 90% were left without a genetic diagnosis.[49] Thus, there still may be a considerable number of genes that may be mutated in these cases but have not yet been discovered.

Apolipoprotein A-I

Apo A-I serves as ligand for binding of HDL particles to cellular receptors, such as scavenger receptor class B type I (SR-BI) and ABCA1.[50,51] To date, 46 mutations, most of them missense or nonsense mutations, have been identified in *APOA1*. In addition, three complex gene rearrangements were found, all of them exceedingly rare.[52–54] A DNA inversion involving *APOA1* and *APOC3* as well as a gross deletion involving *APOA1*, *APOC3*, and *APOA4* were associated with complete apoA-I deficiency and severe premature coronary heart disease.[52,54] Moreover, a deletion/insertion mutation affecting exon 4 of *APOA1* was associated with a unique non-neuropathic form of hereditary amyloidosis characterized by pronounced hepatic involvement.[53] Various forms of amyloidosis have also been observed in the presence of 9 different *APOA1* missense mutations, suggesting that amyloidosis is relatively commonly associated with *APOA1* mutations.

Several *APOA1* mutations were identified in homozygotes affected by severe premature coronary heart disease. Support for an antiatherogenic role of apoA-I was also obtained from studying mouse models, that lack *Apoa1* and develop more severe atherosclerosis compared with respective controls.[55] Moreover, overexpression of human apoa-I in mouse models resulted in decreased aortic lesion development.[56] Conversely, two apoA-I variants known as apoA-I_{Paris} and apoA-I_{Milano} were found to be associated with low HDL cholesterol levels but apparently lower rates of coronary heart disease. The apoA-I_{Milano} variant is due to an amino acid substitution of cysteine for arginine (R173C). apoA-I_{Milano} homodimers induce enhanced RCT[57] and, when complexed with phospholipids, inhibit platelet aggregation.[58] *apoA-I*$_{Paris}$ lacks the LCAT-cofactor activity, whereas its lipid-binding and cholesterol efflux–promoting activities were essentially normal.[59]

In addition to low HDL cholesterol, elevated HDL cholesterol levels may be due to genetic variation in *APOA1*. High HDL cholesterol levels were found to be associated with a G-to-A transition at position −75 relative to the transcriptional start site and with two polymorphisms located at positions +83 and +84 of the *APOA1* gene.[60,61] All three sites are in considerable linkage disequilibrium, and it was calculated that these polymorphisms account for up to 6.5% of the variance in circulating HDL cholesterol levels when age and gender were controlled as covariates.[61] Whether or not these substitutions are associated with protection against coronary heart disease is currently unknown.

Familial Lecithin:Cholesterol Acyltransferase Deficiency and Fish Eye Disease

LCAT plays an important role in reverse cholesterol transport by catalyzing the conversion of cholesterol and phosphatidylcholine to cholesteryl esters and lysophosphatidylcholine on the surface of lipoproteins. More than 45 mutations have been identified that cause either familial LCAT deficiency (also called Norum disease) or fish eye disease. In fish eye disease, there is a selective inability of LCAT to esterify cholesterol in HDL, a deficiency of α-LCAT function, whereas Norum disease results from impairment of α- and β-LCAT function, leading to a generalized deficiency of cholesterol esterification in HDL, LDL, IDL, and VLDL.[62] Both recessive disorders result in pronounced decreases of HDL cholesterol levels in homozygous and compound heterozygous patients. Typical clinical features of Norum disease consist of diffuse corneal opacities, hemolytic anemia, and proteinuria with renal failure. In contrast, fish eye disease represents the clinically milder form of LCAT deficiency, and visual impairment is essentially the only clinical problem associated with the disease. The term "fish eye disease" relates to the striking corneal opacities that give the patient's eyes the appearance of those of boiled fish. According to Norum and coworkers, neither fish eye disease nor Norum disease is apparently associated with increased risk of premature atherosclerotic cardiovascular disease.[63] This is remarkable in light of the important role of LCAT in reverse cholesterol transport and the markedly low levels of HDL cholesterol, apoA-I, and apoA-II in both disorders.

Cholesteryl Ester Transfer Protein Deficiency

CETP catalyzes the transfer of cholesteryl esters and triglycerides among lipoprotein particles. To date, 17 mutations have been identified in homozygous or compound heterozygous carriers who had pronounced increases of HDL cholesterol levels. Four nucleotide substitutions, all of which were located upstream of the *CETP* gene, were implicated in association with elevated HDL cholesterol levels.[64–67]

CETP deficiency is the most common cause of hyperalphalipoproteinemia in Japan. Based on a study of 3469 men of Japanese ancestry in the Honolulu Heart Study, a high prevalence of two different *CETP* gene mutations, D442G (prevalence 5.1%) and a G-to-A substitution in the intron 14 splice donor site (prevalence 0.5%), were observed.[68] Both mutations were associated with decreased CETP activity and an approximate increase of 10% in HDL cholesterol levels. Remarkably, the overall prevalence of coronary heart disease was somewhat higher in men with the CETP mutations (21%) compared with men without mutations (16%).

ATP-Binding Cassette Transporter A1 Deficiency: Tangier Disease and Familial High-Density Lipoprotein Deficiency

Tangier disease is a rare autosomal recessive disorder characterized by extremely low levels of plasma HDL cholesterol, abnormal deposition of cholesteryl esters in the reticuloendothelial system, and impairment of cellular cholesterol efflux.[32] The most prominent features are very large, orange tonsils; enlarged spleen and lymph nodes; hypocholesterolemia; abnormal chylomicron remnants; and markedly reduced HDL cholesterol levels in the plasma. The main neurologic manifestations consist of relapsing asymmetric mono- or polyneuropathy or slowly progressive symmetrical polyneuropathy, which are more frequent than the most severe form of a syringomyelia-like syndrome. The disease is caused by mutations in the *ABCA1* gene,[33–35] and more than 70 mutations have been described. Many mutations cluster in the first large extracellular loop and the two nucleotide-binding folds that are essential for the function of ABCA1 in the apoA-1–mediated lipid-removal pathway from cells.[69] Mutations in *ABCA1* have also been found in patients with familial HDL deficiency,[37] a more common disorder with a more benign course than Tangier disease. In addition, common polymorphisms in *ABCA1* are associated with changes in plasma lipoprotein levels and atherosclerosis risk, and a range of rare ABCA1 alleles has been identified in subjects with low HDL cholesterol levels.[13]

In several well-documented cases of Tangier disease patients had very low HDL cholesterol levels but no signs of premature atherosclerosis, whereas others had premature atherosclerosis and developed coronary artery disease well before age 50 years. Moreover, the time of onset and extent of peripheral neuropathy is known to vary extensively between different Tangier disease families.[32] In general, ABCA1 null alleles are associated with a clinically more severe course of the disease than alleles that determine residual cholesterol efflux activity. This supports the hypothesis that the clinical variability of the disease may be related to some extent to the level of residual cholesterol efflux activity that is determined by the underlying *ABCA1* mutations.

REFERENCES

1. Castelli WP, Garrison RJ, Wilson PW, et al: Incidence of coronary heart disease and lipoprotein cholesterol levels. The Framingham Study. *JAMA* 1986;256:2835–2838.
2. Mahley RW, Arslan P, Pekcan G, et al: Plasma lipids in Turkish children: impact of puberty, socioeconomic status, and nutrition on plasma cholesterol and HDL. *J Lipid Res* 2001;42:1996–2006.
3. Kuller LH: Ethnic differences in atherosclerosis, cardiovascular disease and lipid metabolism. *Curr Opin Lipidol* 2004;15: 109–113.
4. Heller DA, de Faire U, Pedersen NL, et al: Genetic and environmental influences on serum lipid levels in twins. *N Engl J Med* 1993;328:1150–1156.
5. Bonow RO, Smaha LA, Smith SC Jr, et al: World Heart Day 2002. the international burden of cardiovascular disease: responding to the emerging global epidemic. *Circulation* 2002;106:1602–1605.
6. Eckel RH, Grundy SM, Zimmet PZ: The metabolic syndrome. *Lancet* 2005;365:1415–1428.
7. Grundy SM, Cleeman JI, Daniels SR, et al: Diagnosis and management of the metabolic syndrome: an American Heart Association/National Heart, Lung, and Blood Institute Scientific Statement. *Circulation* 2005;112:2735–2752.
8. Alberti KG, Zimmet P, Shaw J: The metabolic syndrome — a new worldwide definition. *Lancet* 2005;366:1059–1062.
9. Assmann G, Nofer JR: Atheroprotective effects of high-density lipoproteins. *Annu Rev Med* 2003;54:321–341.
10. Nissen SE, Tardif JC, Nicholls SJ, et al: ILLUSTRATE Investigators: Effect of Torcetrapib on the Progression of Coronary Atherosclerosis. *N Engl J Med* 2007;356:1304–1316.
11. Ordovas JM: HDL genetics: candidate genes, genome wide scans and gene-environment interactions. *Cardiovasc Drugs Ther* 2002;16:273–281.
12. Clee SM, Zwinderman AH, Engert JC, et al: Common genetic variation in ABCA1 is associated with altered lipoprotein levels and a modified risk for coronary artery disease. *Circulation* 2001;103:1198–1205.
13. Cohen JC, Kiss RS, Pertsemlidis A, et al: Multiple rare alleles contribute to low plasma levels of HDL cholesterol. *Science* 2004;305:869–872.
14. Timmins JM, Lee JY, Boudyguina E, et al: Targeted inactivation of hepatic ABCA1 causes profound hypoalphalipoproteinemia and kidney hypercatabolism of apoA-I. *J Clin Invest* 2005;115: 1333–1342.
15. Wang X, Paigen B: Genetics of variation in HDL cholesterol in humans and mice. *Circ Res* 2005;96:27–42.
16. Arya R, Duggirala R, Almasy L, et al: Linkage of high-density lipoprotein-cholesterol concentrations to a locus on chromosome 9p in Mexican Americans. *Nat Genet* 2002;30:102–105.
17. Duggirala, R, Blangero J, Almasy L, et al: Linkage of type 2 diabetes mellitus and of age of onset to a genetic location of chromosome 10q in Mexican Americans. *Am J Hum Genet* 1999;64: 1127–1140.
18. The Wellcome Trust Case–Control Consortium: Genome-wide association study of 14,000 cases of seven common diseases and 3,000 shared controls. *Nature* 2007;447:661–683.
19. Helgadottir A, Thorleifsson G, Manolescu A, et al: A common variant on chromosome 9p21 affects the risk of myocardial infarction. *Science* 2007;316:1491–1493.
20. Scott LJ, Mohlke KL, Bonnycastle LL, et al: A genome-wide association study of type 2 diabetes in Finns detects multiple susceptibility variants. *Science* 2007;316:1341–1345.
21. McPherson R, Pertsemlidis A, Kavaslar N, et al: A common allele on chromosome 9 associated with coronary heart disease. *Science* 2007;316:1488–1491.
22. Miccoli R, Zhu YH, Daum U, et al: A natural apolipoprotein A-I variant, apoA-I(L141R)Pisa, interferes with the formation of α-high-density lipoproteins (HDL) but not with the formation of preβ1-HDL and influences efflux of cholesterol into plasma. *J Lipid Res* 1997;38:1242–1253.
23. Daum U, Leren TP, Langer C, et al: Multiple dysfunctions of two apolipoprotein A-I variants, apoA-I (R160L)Oslo and apoA-I(P165R), that are associated with hypoalphalipoproteinemia in heterozygous carriers. *J Lipid Res* 1999;40:486–494.
24. Funke H, von Eckardstein A, Pritchard PH, et al: A molecular defect causing fish eye disease: an amino acid exchange in lecithin:cholesterol acyltransferase (LCAT) leads to the selective loss of alpha-LCAT activity. *Proc Natl Acad Sci USA* 1991;88:4855–4859.
25. Miettinen HE, Gylling H, Tenhunen J, et al: Molecular genetic study of Finns with hypoalphalipoproteinemia and hyperalphalipoproteinemia—a novel Gly230Arg mutation (LCATFin) of lecithin:cholesterol acyltransferase (LCAT) accounts for 5% of cases with very low serum HDL cholesterol levels. *Arterioscler Thromb Vasc Biol* 1998;18:591–598.
26. Lambert G, Sakai N, Vaisman BL, et al: Analysis of glomerulosclerosis and atherosclerosis in lecithin: cholesterol acyltransferase-deficient mice. *J Biol Chem* 2001;276:15090–15098.
27. Jiang XC, Bruce C, Mar J, et al: Targeted mutation of plasma phospholipid transfer protein gene markedly reduces high-density lipoprotein levels. *J Clin Invest* 1999;103:907–914.
28. Qin SC, Kawano K, Bruce C, et al: Phospholipid transfer protein gene knock-out mice have low high-density lipoprotein levels, due to hypercatabolism, and accumulate apoA-IV-rich lamellar lipoproteins. *J Lipid Res* 2000;41:269–276.
29. Aouizerat BE, Engler MB, Natanzon Y, et al:. Genetic variation of PLTP modulates lipoprotein profiles in hypoalphalipoproteinemia. *J Lipid Res* 2006;47:787–793.
30. Assmann G, von Eckardstein A, Funke H: High-density lipoproteins, reverse transport of cholesterol, and coronary artery disease. Insights from mutations. *Circulation* 1993;87(4 Suppl): III28–34.
31. Inazu A, Brown ML, Hesler CB, et al: Increased high-density lipoprotein levels caused by a common cholesteryl-ester transfer protein gene mutation. *N Engl J Med* 1990;323:1234–1238.
32. Assmann G, von Eckardstein A, Brewer HB: Familial high density lipoprotein deficiency: Tangier disease. In Scriver CR, Beaudet AL, Sly WS, Valle D (eds): The Metabolic and Molecular Basis of Inherited Disease, 7th ed. *New York, McGraw-Hill,* 1995, pp 2053–2072.
33. Brooks-Wilson A, Marcil M, Clee SM, et al: Mutations in ABC1 in Tangier disease and familial high-density lipoprotein deficiency. *Nat Genet* 1999;22:336–345.
34. Bodzioch M, Orsó E, Klucken T, et al: The gene encoding ATP-binding cassette transporter 1 is mutated in Tangier disease. *Nat Genet* 1999;22:347–351.
35. Rust S, Rosier M, Funke H, et al: Tangier disease is caused by mutations in the gene encoding ATP-binding cassette transporter 1. *Nat Genet* 1999;22:352–355.
36. Remaley AT, Rust S, Rosier M, et al: Human ATP-binding cassette transporter 1 (ABC1): genomic organization and identification of the genetic defect in the original Tangier disease kindred. *Proc Natl Acad Sci USA* 1999;96:12685–12690.
37. Marcil M, Brooks-Wilson A, Clee SM, et al: Mutations in the ABC1 gene in familial HDL deficiency with defective cholesterol efflux. *Lancet* 1999;354:1341–1346.
38. Walter M, Gerdes U, Seedorf U, Assmann G: The high-density lipoprotein- and apolipoprotein A-I-induced mobilization of cellular cholesterol is impaired in fibroblasts from Tangier disease subjects. *Biochem Biophys Res Commun* 1994;205: 850–856.
39. Marcil M, Yu L, Krimbou L, et al: Cellular cholesterol transport and efflux in fibroblasts are abnormal in subjects with familial HDL deficiency. *Arterioscler Thromb Vasc Biol* 1999;19: 159–169.
40. Mott S, Yu L, Marcil M, et al: Decreased cellular cholesterol efflux is a common cause of familial hypoalphalipoproteinemia: role of the ABCA1 gene mutations. *Atherosclerosis* 2000;152: 457–468.
41. Eberhart GP, Mendez AJ, Freeman MW: Decreased cholesterol efflux from fibroblasts of a patient without Tangier disease, but with markedly reduced high-density lipoprotein cholesterol levels. *J Clin Endocrinol Metab* 1998;83:836–846.
42. Batal R, Tremblay M, Krimbou L, et al: Familial HDL deficiency characterized by hypercatabolism of mature apoA-I but not proapoA-I. *Arterioscler Thromb Vasc Biol* 1998;18:655–664.
43. Cartwright DJ, Cole AL, Cousins AJ, Lee PJ: Raised HDL cholesterol in Fabry disease: response to enzyme replacement therapy. *J Inherit Metab Dis* 2004;27:791–793.
44. Pocovi M, Cenarro A, Civeira F, et al: Beta-glucocerebrosidase gene locus as a link for Gaucher's disease and familial hypo-alpha-lipoproteinaemia. *Lancet* 1998;351:1919–1923.
45. Assmann G, Seedorf U: Acid lipase deficiency: Wolman disease and cholesteryl ester storage disease. In Scriver CR,

Beaudet AL, Sly WS, Valle D (eds): The Metabolic and Molecular Basis of Inherited Disease, 7th ed. New York, McGraw-Hill, 1995, pp 2563–2587.

46. Muntoni S, Wiebusch H, Jansen-Rust M, et al: Prevalence of Cholesteryl Ester Storage Disease. *Arterioscler Thromb Vasc Biol* 2007;27:1866–1868.
47. Hovingh GK, de Groot E, van der Steeg W, et al: Inherited disorders of HDL metabolism and atherosclerosis. *Curr Opin Lipidol* 2005;16:139–145.
48. Schiffmann R, Ries M: Fabry's disease—an important risk factor for stroke. *Lancet* 2005;366:1754–1756.
49. Kiss RS, Kavaslar N, Okuhira K, et al: Genetic etiology of isolated low HDL syndrome: incidence and heterogeneity of efflux defects. *Arterioscler Thromb Vasc Biol* 2007;27:1139–1145.
50. Rigotti A, Trigatti B, Babitt J, et al: Scavenger receptor BI—a cell surface receptor for high-density lipoprotein. *Curr Opin Lipidol* 1997;8:181–188.
51. Remaley AT, Stonik JA, Demosky SJ, et al: Apolipoprotein specificity for lipid efflux by the human ABCAI transporter. *Biochem Biophys Res Commun* 2001;280:818–823.
52. Karathanasis SK, Ferris E, Haddad IA: DNA inversion within the apolipoproteins AI/CIII/AIV-encoding gene cluster of certain patients with premature atherosclerosis. *Proc Natl Acad Sci USA* 1987;84:7198–7202.
53. Booth DR, Tan SY, Booth SE, et al: Hereditary hepatic and systemic amyloidosis caused by a new deletion/insertion mutation in the apolipoprotein AI gene. *J Clin Invest* 1996;97:2714–2721.
54. Ordovas JM, Cassidy DK, Civeira F, et al: Familial apolipoprotein A-I, C-III, and A-IV deficiency and premature atherosclerosis due to deletion of a gene complex on chromosome 11. *J Biol Chem* 1989;264:16339–16342.
55. Ikewaki K, Matsunaga A, Han H, et al: A novel two nucleotide deletion in the apolipoprotein A-I gene, apoA-I Shinbashi, associated with high-density lipoprotein deficiency, corneal opacities, planar xanthomas, and premature coronary artery disease. *Atherosclerosis* 2004;172:39–45.
56. Belalcazar LM, Merched A, Carr B, et al: Long-term stable expression of human apolipoprotein A-I mediated by helper-dependent adenovirus gene transfer inhibits atherosclerosis progression and remodels atherosclerotic plaques in a mouse model of familial hypercholesterolemia. *Circulation* 2003;107: 26–32.
57. Franceschini G, Calabresi L, Chiesa G, et al: Increased cholesterol efflux potential of sera from ApoA-I Milano carriers and transgenic mice. *Arterioscler Thromb Vasc Biol* 1999;19:1257–1262.
58. Li D, Weng S, Yang B, et al: Inhibition of arterial thrombus formation by ApoA1 Milano. *Arterioscler Thromb Vasc Biol* 1999;19:378–383.
59. Daum U, Langer C, Duverger N, et al: Apolipoprotein A-I (R151C)Paris is defective in activation of lecithin: cholesterol acyltransferase but not in initial lipid binding, formation of reconstituted lipoproteins, or promotion of cholesterol efflux. *J Mol Med* 1999;77:614–622.
60. Jeenah M, Kessling A, Miller N, Humphries S: G to A substitution in the promoter region of the apolipoprotein AI gene is associated with elevated serum apolipoprotein AI and high-density lipoprotein cholesterol concentrations. *Mol Biol Med* 1990;7:233–241.
61. Wang XL, Badenhop R, Humphrey KE, Wilcken DE: New MspI polymorphism at +83 bp of the human apolipoprotein AI gene: association with increased circulating high-density lipoprotein cholesterol levels. *Genet Epidemiol* 1996;13:1–10.
62. Carlson LA, Holmquist L: Paradoxical esterification of plasma cholesterol in fish eye disease. *Acta Med Scand* 1985;217: 491–499.
63. Norum KR, Gjone E, Glomset JA: Familial lecithin:cholesterol acyltransferase deficiency including fish eye disease. In Scriver CR, Beaudet AL, Sly WS, Valle D (eds): The Metabolic and Molecular Basis of Inherited Disease, 7th ed. New York, McGraw-Hill, 1995, pp 1181–1194.
64. Klerkx AH, Tanck MW, Kastelein JJ, et al: Haplotype analysis of the CETP gene: not TaqIB, but the closely linked -629C→A polymorphism and a novel promoter variant are independently associated with CETP concentration. *Hum Mol Genet* 2003;12:111–123.
65. Dachet C, Poirier O, Cambien F, et al: New functional promoter polymorphism, CETP/-629, in cholesteryl ester transfer protein (CETP) gene related to CETP mass and high-density lipoprotein cholesterol levels: role of Sp1/Sp3 in transcriptional regulation. *Arterioscler Thromb Vasc Biol* 2000;20:507–515.
66. Nagano M, Yamashita S, Hirano K, et al: Point mutation (-69 G→A) in the promoter region of cholesteryl ester transfer protein gene in Japanese hyperalphalipoproteinemic subjects. *Arterioscler Thromb Vasc Biol* 2001;21:985–990.
67. Thompson JF, Lloyd DB, Lira ME, Milos PM: Cholesteryl ester transfer protein promoter single-nucleotide polymorphisms in Sp1-binding sites affect transcription and are associated with high-density lipoprotein cholesterol. *Clin Genet* 2004;66: 223–228.
68. Zhong S, Sharp DS, Grove JS, et al: Increased coronary heart disease in Japanese-American men with mutation in the cholesteryl ester transfer protein gene despite increased HDL levels. *J Clin Invest* 1996;97:2917–2923.
69. Lawn RM, Wade DP, Garvin MR, et al:. The Tangier disease gene product ABC1 controls the cellular apolipoprotein-mediated lipid removal pathway. *J Clin Invest* 1999;104:R25–R31.

CHAPTER 8

Lipoprotein Oxidation and Modification

Yury I. Miller and Sotirios Tsimikas

INTRODUCTION

The oxidation hypothesis of atherosclerosis, summarized by Steinberg and colleagues in 1989 in their classic article, "Beyond cholesterol: modifications of low-density lipoprotein that increase its atherogenicity,"[1] suggests that oxidative modifications of low-density lipoprotein (LDL) promote LDL atherogenicity. In this chapter, we will describe the concept of oxidized LDL (OxLDL), describe its cellular, immunologic, and proinflammatory effects, demonstrate its relevance to the development of experimental atherosclerotic lesions, discuss the results of clinical trials, and review the emerging data on OxLDL biomarkers for clinical risk prediction.

The Low-Density Lipoprotein Paradox and Oxidatively Modified Low-Density Lipoprotein

After much debate in the 1970s and 1980s, it has now become widely accepted that an elevated plasma level of LDL cholesterol is a foremost pathogenic factor in the development of atherogenesis. Primary evidence for this is reflected by the reduction in the incidence of all-cause mortality and recurrent cardiovascular events with statin therapy.[2] Furthermore, the homozygous form of familial hypercholesterolemia (HFH), a monogenetic disorder, results in LDL cholesterol levels of approximately 600 to 800 mg/dL, and patients with HFH often develop myocardial infarction (MI) in the first two decades of life.[3] The landmark studies of Brown and Goldstein established that the affected gene in these patients encoded the LDL receptor, a membrane protein to which LDL binds with high affinity, leading to its internalization and degradation within the cell.[4] However, patients with HFH have very few or no LDL receptors, yet they accumulate cholesterol in subcutaneous and tendon xanthomas and in arterial lesions despite having LDL that is structurally and metabolically similar to LDL from normal subjects. Therefore, cholesterol accumulation must be occurring by a pathway other than the LDL receptor. Furthermore, incubation of monocyte/macrophages with native LDL *in vitro* does not lead to significant accumulation of cellular cholesterol.[5]

This apparent paradox was explained by demonstrating the presence of oxidized or modified LDL as well as complementary scavenger receptors that mediate the unregulated uptake of OxLDL (Fig. 8-1). Goldstein and coworkers[5] initially described the *acetyl LDL receptor,* which binds LDL modified *in vitro* with acetic anhydride. Unlike the LDL receptor, which down-regulates as the cell cholesterol content increases, the acetyl-LDL receptor was not down-regulated but continued to be fully active even as the cell cholesterol content increased markedly. Subsequently Kodama et al.[6] cloned and sequenced the acetyl-LDL receptor, which was redesignated *scavenger receptor, type A,* or SR-A. Acetoacetylation or conjugation with malondialdehyde (MDA) also generated modified LDL recognized by the acetyl-LDL receptor or SR-A.[7,8] However, all these studies were performed *in vitro,* and the biological significance was uncertain until Henriksen and colleagues[9] reported in 1981 that in cell culture experiments, all cells in the vessel wall could modify LDL in a way to make it a ligand for scavenger receptors on macrophages. Interestingly, the binding and uptake of the modified LDL was competitively inhibited by unlabeled acetyl-LDL by only 60%, implying the presence of additional receptors, which were later described and labeled as SR-B and CD36. Later studies by Steinbrecher et al.[10] showed that all these cell-induced changes are blocked by a number of antioxidants, such as vitamin E, or by addition of 5% to 10% serum to the media, and that all these

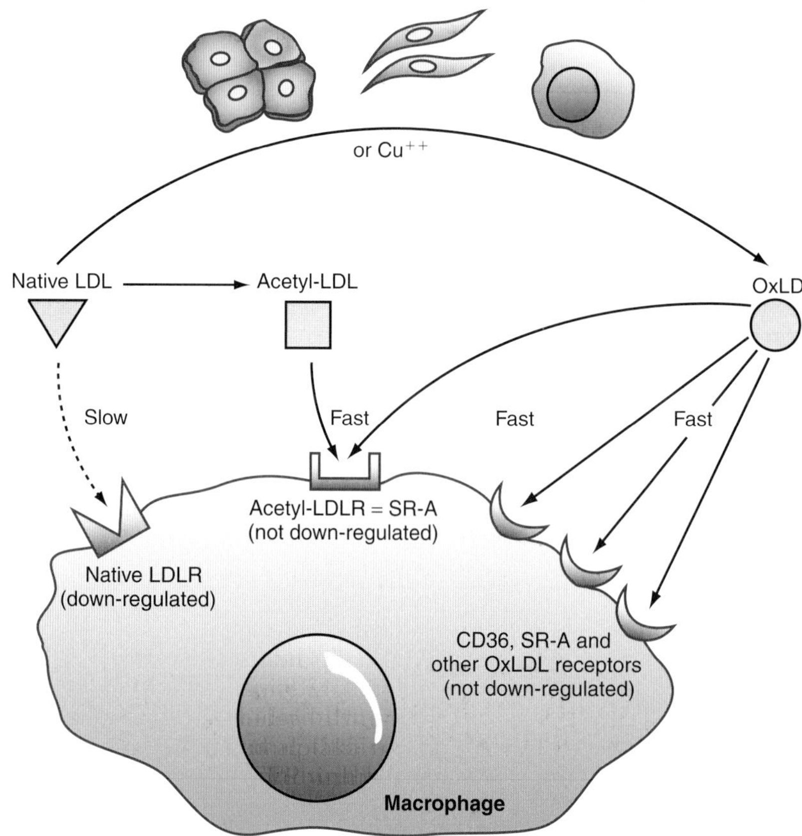

FIGURE 8-1 Mechanisms of oxidized low-density lipoprotein (OxLDL) uptake by macrophages. Native LDL cannot induce foam-cell formation because uptake is slow and because the LDL receptor is down-regulated. Either acetyl-LDL or OxLDL can induce cholesterol accumulation in macrophages resulting in foam-cell formation because uptake is rapid and the scavenger receptors are not down-regulated in response to an increase in cellular cholesterol. *(From Ref. 105, with permission.)* LDLR, low-density lipoprotein receptor; SR-A, scavenger receptor class A.

changes could be reproduced by simply incubating the LDL with copper to catalyze nonenzymatic oxidation. Thus, oxidative modification of LDL seemed to be a biologically plausible mechanism in that it explained foam cell formation.

Although this chapter deals primarily with oxidation of LDL, it is important to recognize the significance of high-density lipoprotein (HDL) modification resulting in the formation of dysfunctional HDL, as well as a number of alternative mechanisms by which foam cells might be generated. These include but are not limited to macrophage uptake of aggregated and extracellular matrix–trapped LDL and immunoglobulin G (IgG) immune complexes with aggregated or modified LDL.[11–15]

MECHANISMS OF LOW-DENSITY LIPOPROTEIN OXIDATION

Nonenzymatic Oxidation of Low-Density Lipoprotein

The LDL particle is exquisitely sensitive to oxidative damage because of its complex lipid–protein composition. Each LDL particle contains about 700 molecules of phospholipids, 600 of free cholesterol, 1600 of cholesteryl esters, 185 of triglycerides, and 1 molecule of apolipoprotein (apo) B, which in turn is made of 4536 amino acid residues. LDL in plasma is reasonably stable, but once it has been purified it begins to deteriorate rapidly. Both the protein and the lipid moieties undergo oxidative damage, and the overall process is enormously complex.

Low-density Lipoprotein Oxidation by Copper

Overnight exposure of LDL to copper sulfate (Cu^{2+}) leads to profound oxidative degradation.[10] This type of Cu^{2+}-catalyzed oxidative attack on the polyunsaturated fatty acids (PUFAs) in the *sn*-2 position of phospholipids may lead to degradation of 40% of the phosphatidylcholine and 50% to 75% of the PUFA.[16,17] The hydrated density of the LDL particle increases markedly, in some cases even to a density as high as that of HDL. Finally, the apoB also undergoes drastic alterations, partly as a result of direct oxidative attack and partly as a result of conjugation of lipid fragments with the protein. The recognition of OxLDL by scavenger receptors probably depends in part on the generation of neoepitopes created by the masking of ε-amino groups of lysine residues by aldehyde fragments generated from the PUFAs. Nonenzymatic oxidation catalyzed by Cu^{2+} is believed to depend on the presence of lipid hydroperoxides in the starting material.[18] These hydroperoxides are degraded to peroxy radicals and alkoxy radicals by Cu^{2+}, and those radicals in turn can initiate a chain reaction that can generate many more hydroperoxides. The fatty acid side chains of cholesterol esters are susceptible to oxidative damage, and the polycyclic sterol ring structure of cholesterol is also subject to oxidative attack. Incubation of LDL with Cu^{2+} for even a few hours, or with 15-lipoxygenase, is sufficient to oxidize it to the point that it develops important new biological properties.[19,20] This form of LDL, designated *mildly oxidized*, or *minimally modified*, LDL (mmLDL), is still recognized by the LDL receptor and it is not, at this stage of oxidation, a ligand for the scavenger receptors.[19,21] *In vitro* experiments have indicated a large number of biological properties that could in principle make it proatherogenic.[22]

Low-Density Lipoprotein Oxidation by Heme

Divalent iron cations ($FeCl_2$) can also induce LDL oxidation but to a lesser degree than the Cu^{2+}. However, heme, an iron complex with protoporphyrin IX, is a very strong LDL-oxidizing agent, especially when activated by low concentrations of peroxides. Heme is the oxygen-binding prosthetic group of hemoglobin. LDL oxidation by hemoglobin (Hb) results in apoB–apoB crosslinking and in Hb–apoB crosslinking in blood, as well as robust lipid peroxidation.[23] Small amounts of Hb are constantly leaking from damaged erythrocytes, particularly in the vascular regions with turbulent flow, such as vessel bifurcations and aortic curvatures. These processes are exacerbated in hemodialysis patients with high rates of hemolysis. Hb-induced LDL oxidation has been suggested to significantly contribute to the increased levels of OxLDL found in the plasma of the patients on hemodialysis.[24–26]

In plasma, the oxidative damage by free Hb is prevented by Hb binding to haptoglobin (Hp).[27] Hp is a dimer, and its two allelic variants, Hp1 and Hp2, are known. The Hp2 variant is less effective than Hp1 in preventing Hb-induced oxidation, and the antioxidative efficiency of Hp2 is further reduced when it is complexed with glycated HbA1c, present in patients with diabetes.[28] Remarkably, subjects with the Hp2/2 phenotype, present in up to 37% of whites, have a higher risk of cardiovascular events than the Hp1/1 and Hp2/1 populations.[29] The odds ratio of having cardiovascular disease (CVD) in patients with diabetes who have the Hp2/2 phenotype is five times greater than in the patients with the Hp1/1 phenotype. An intermediate risk of CVD is associated with the Hp2/1 phenotype.[30–32] Furthermore, transgenic Hp2/2 mice on an apoE−/− background have more iron deposits and lipid peroxidation products as well as macrophage accumulation in atherosclerotic lesions compared with apoE−/− controls that have wild-type mouse Hp1/1 genotype.[33]

Even intact erythrocytes can be a source of catalytically active heme. Hemoglobin catabolism yields low levels of free hemin (Fe^{3+}), which accumulates in the membrane of erythrocytes. Under normal circumstances, hemopexin and albumin clear hemin from the erythrocyte membrane. However, an *in vitro* study of the kinetics of hemin clearance demonstrates that under conditions of hyperlipidemia and inflammation, LDL and HDL can transiently bind hemin in whole blood and thus become mildly oxidized.[34]

Enzymatic and Cell-Mediated Oxidation of Low-Density Lipoprotein

Incubation of LDL with several cell types *in vitro* accelerates its oxidative modification. Included among these are endothelial cells, smooth muscle cells, and monocyte/macrophages (i.e., all the cell types that are found in an atherosclerotic lesion). However, a number of other cell types can also oxidize LDL *in vitro*, including neutrophils and fibroblasts. LDL is oxidized not only within the artery wall but also at peripheral sites of inflammation.[35]

Many mechanisms have been postulated by which LDL could become oxidized within the artery wall. A number of different enzyme systems such as lipoxygenases,[36–40] myeloperoxidase,[41] nicotinamide adenine dinvcleotide phosphate (NADPH) oxidase,[42] and other peroxidases[43] have been shown to have the potential to contribute to the oxidation of LDL. Macrophages and/or other phagocytes express these enzymes and, in particular, use myeloperoxidase (MPO), inducible nitric oxide synthase, and NADPH oxidase as mechanisms for generating antimicrobial reactive oxygen species essential for native immunity.[44] Although macrophages may not be required to initiate LDL oxidation, they are likely to amplify oxidative reactions in macrophage-rich areas of atherosclerotic lesions.

For example, the enzyme 12/15-lipoxygenase (LO) initiates the "seeding" of LDL in the tissue fluids with hydroperoxides, leading to the subsequent initiation of lipid peroxidation and the changes that render the OxLDL proinflammatory. Treatment of hypercholesterolemic rabbits with specific inhibitors of 15-LO reduces the progression of atherosclerosis,[45,46] and studies in transgenic mice in which 12/15-LO was deleted demonstrated reduced lesion formation.[47,48] However, paradoxically, overexpression of 15-LO in the rabbit reduced atherosclerosis.[49] Similarly, conflicting results have been observed for the contributions of endothelial and inducible nitric oxide synthases to the development of atherosclerosis in mouse models.[50–52] It is possible that mechanisms responsible for LDL oxidation differ between humans and animal models. For example, MPO is a heme enzyme secreted by neutrophils and monocytes that generates a number of oxidants, including hypochlorous acid and peroxynitrite, which can initiate lipid and protein oxidation. MPO has been identified in human atherosclerotic lesions and is of particular interest because modifications found in human atherosclerosis bear similarities to hypochlorous acid–mediated derivation of lipoprotein components *in vitro*.[53] MPO was recently shown to specifically bind to HDL within human atherosclerotic lesions, with selective targeting of apoA-I for site-specific chlorination and nitration by MPO-generated reactive oxidants *in vivo*. One apparent consequence of MPO-catalyzed apoA-I oxidation is the functional impairment of the ability of HDL to promote cellular cholesterol efflux, thereby generating dysfunctional HDL.[54,55] However, in bone marrow transplantation experiments in which LDL receptor (LDLR)−/− mice received MPO-deficient bone marrow progenitor cells, larger lesions were observed than in LDLR−/− mice transplanted with wild-type progenitor cells. Similar results were seen when MPO-deficient mice were crossed into LDLR−/− mice. However, there was no evidence for the presence of MPO in murine lesions, and the types of MPO-dependent oxidation products found in human lesions were not present in murine lesions,[56] suggesting that MPO could not be directly related to lesion formation in mice.

Evidence that Oxidation of Low-Density Lipoprotein Takes Place *in vivo*

Many lines of evidence now indicate that oxidation of lipoproteins does occur *in vivo* and that this process is quantitatively important. This evidence has been extensively reviewed elsewhere[57,58] and is summarized in Table 8-1.

PROPERTIES OF OXIDIZED LOW-DENSITY LIPOPROTEIN THAT MAKE IT ATHEROGENIC

It is well documented that biological properties of OxLDL make it more atherogenic than native LDL (see summary in Table 8-2). Several of these features are now discussed in detail.

Recruitment of Monocytes from the Circulation into the Artery Wall

OxLDL present in the vessel wall acts as a chemoattractant for monocytes[59] and for T lymphocytes[60] but not for B lymphocytes. Furthermore, OxLDL inhibits the motility of tissue macrophages and might therefore suppress any tendency for macrophages to exit from an atherosclerotic lesion.[61] mmLDL can indirectly participate in the recruitment of monocytes by stimulating the release from endothelial cells of chemokines interleukin-8 (IL-8) and monocyte chemotactic protein–1 (MCP-1).[62] Recent studies suggest that some of the biological effects of mmLDL and OxLDL are in large part attributable to oxidized phospholipids (OxPLs), in which the fatty acids in the *sn*-2 position have been oxidized.[62,63] The endothelial cell receptors that mediate OxPL-induced IL-8 release may include toll-like receptor–4 (TLR-4) and EP2, a prostaglandin E_2 receptor.[64,65] OxPL-induced monocyte adhesion depends on the activation of protein kinases A and C, mitogen-activated protein (MAP) kinases, and cytosolic phospholipase A_2 in endothelial cells.[63,66] This phospholipase releases arachidonic acid, which is then oxygenated by 12/15-LO, and the oxidized arachidonic acid products play an important role in priming endothelial cells for monocyte adhesion.[66,67]

TABLE 8-1	Evidence that Low-Density Lipoprotein Undergoes Oxidation *In Vivo*
LDL gently extracted from the atherosclerotic tissue of rabbits and humans has all the physical, biological, and immunological properties observed with LDL oxidized *in vitro*	
A small fraction of circulating LDL particles display a number of chemical indices consistent with early stages of LDL oxidation	
Subtle modifications of LDL renders autologous LDL immunogenic	
“Oxidation-specific” epitopes are present in atherosclerotic lesions	
Autoantibodies to a variety of epitopes of OxLDL can be found in plasma of experimental animals with atherosclerosis	
“Oxidation-specific” antibodies avidly bind to atherosclerotic lesions	
The presence of OxLDL in the vessel wall can be imaged *in vivo* using radiolabeled oxidation-specific antibodies	

LDL, low-density lipoprotein; OxLDL, oxidized LDL.

Macrophage Foam Cell Formation

Macrophage Scavenger Receptors

Macrophages express scavenger receptors that mediate binding and uptake of OxLDL, including SR-A, CD36, SR-BI, CD68, lectin-like OxLDL receptor-1 (LOX-1) and scavenger receptor for phosphatidylserine and oxidized lipoprotein (SR-PSOX)[68–71] (Fig. 8-2). It is unlikely that scavenger receptors evolved as a mechanism for clearing OxLDL because atherosclerosis is a disease essentially limited to humans, whereas these receptors are found in lower mammals and even Drosophila.[72] These proteins comprise a class of pattern recognition receptors (PRRs), which are capable of recognizing pathogen-associated molecular patterns (PAMPs) rather than individual molecules. PRRs have been proposed to play physiologic roles in the recognition and clearance of pathogens and apoptotic cells. It appears that OxLDL has chemical moieties exposed on its surface that precisely match or resemble PAMPs and, accordingly, are recognized by PRRs.

In contrast to the native LDLR, scavenger receptors are not down-regulated as the cholesterol content of the cell increases and can therefore mediate massive cholesterol accumulation in the macrophage. Indeed, *in vitro* experiments demonstrate that macrophages from mice with combined SR-A and CD36 deficiency show a 75% decrease in uptake of OxLDL.[73] A comparison of monocyte/macrophages from patients with a total deficiency of CD36 with normal monocyte/macrophages suggests that about 50% of the uptake of OxLDL is attributable to this receptor under the conditions studied.[74] However, no human data correlating CD36 deficiency with atherosclerosis are yet available, and mouse model studies have produced mixed results. Gene deletion and bone marrow transplantation experiments suggest that SR-A and CD36 play quantitatively important roles in mediating uptake of OxLDL and promoting the development of atherosclerosis in apoE−/− mice.[75–77] In contrast, a recent study by a different group demonstrated that SR-A/apoE– and CD36/apoE– double knockout mice, although having significant reductions in peritoneal macrophage lipid accumulation *in vivo*, had increased atherosclerosis.[78] This discrepancy underscores the complexity of the mechanisms of macrophage lipid accumulation and atherosclerosis.[79]

Genetic studies of SR-BI indicate that it plays an antiatherogenic role,[80,81] presumably because of its function in mediating reverse cholesterol transport by HDL. The overall actions of SR-BI in the arterial wall appear to be protective, although it may depend on the cell type expressing SR-BI and on the stage in the development of atherosclerosis.[80,82] ApoE knockout mice with total or hepatic deficiency of SR-BI exhibit severe atherosclerosis with evidence of plaque rupture and acute MI, complications that are rare in other murine models of atherosclerosis.[80,83]

TABLE 8-2 Potential Mechanisms by Which Oxidized Low-Density Lipoprotein May Influence Atherogenesis
OxLDL has enhanced uptake by macrophages leading to foam cell formation
Products of OxLDL are chemotactic for monocytes and T cells and inhibit the motility of tissue macrophages
Products of OxLDL are cytotoxic, in part because of oxidized sterols, and can induce apoptosis
OxLDL or products are mitogenic for smooth muscle cells and macrophages
OxLDL or products can alter gene expression in vascular cells, e.g., induction of MCP-1, colony-stimulating factors, IL-1 and expression of adhesion molecules
OxLDL or products can increase expression of macrophage scavenger receptors, thereby enhancing its own uptake
OxLDL can induce expression and activate PPARγ, thereby influencing many gene functions
OxLDL is immunogenic and elicits autoantibody formation and activated T cells
Oxidation renders LDL more susceptible to aggregation, which independently leads to enhanced uptake. Similarly, OxLDL is a better substrate for sphingomyelinase, which also aggregates LDL
OxLDL may enhance procoagulant pathways, e.g., by induction of tissue factor and platelet aggregation
Products of OxLDL can adversely affect arterial vasomotor properties
OxLDL is involved in acute coronary syndromes and may potentially lead to plaque disruption

(Modified from Ref. 139, with permission.)

IL, interleukin; LDL, low-density lipoprotein; MCP, monocyte chemotactic protein; OxLDL, oxidized LDL; PPAR, peroxisome proliferator-activated receptor.

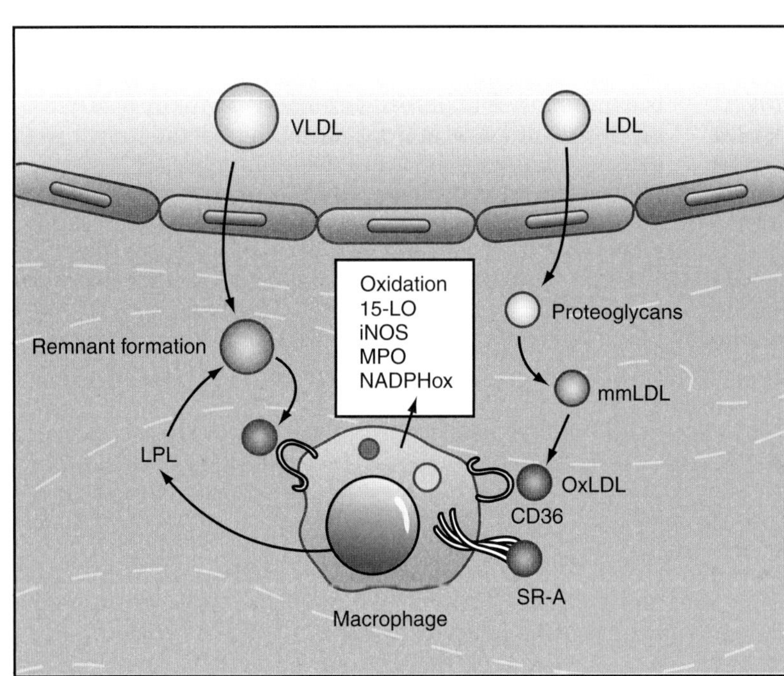

FIGURE 8-2 Mechanisms contributing to foam cell formation. Low-density lipoprotein (LDL) penetrates into the artery wall, where it is trapped after adhering to proteoglycans. It is then highly susceptible to oxidation by enzymes such as lipoxygenases (LOs), myeloperoxidase (MPO), and iNOS. Very-low-density lipoprotein (VLDL) particles are subject to modification by lipoprotein lipase (LPL). The resulting remnant particles are also subject to trapping by proteoglycans, oxidative modification, and uptake by macrophages. *(From Ref. 71, with permission.)* LO, lipoxygenase; *mmLDL, minimally modified LDL; NADPHox, nicotin amide adenine dinucleotide phosphate oxidase; OxLDL, oxidized LDL;SR-A, scavenger receptor class A.*

The relative contributions of additional scavenger receptors to foam cell formation have not yet been addressed through genetic loss-of-function experiments. Although inhibition of macrophage scavenger receptor activity could potentially provide the basis of an antiatherogenic therapy, it may be the case that several classes of proteins will have to be targeted simultaneously. Since these receptors are also involved in clearing microorganisms, enhanced susceptibility to specific infectious pathogens may also occur. Finally, it is also possible that inhibition of scavenger receptor function could have deleterious effects if scavenger receptors play an important role in the clearance of apoptotic cells.

Cholesterol Homeostasis and Foam Cell Formation

Macrophages possess robust feed-forward mechanisms for preserving cholesterol homeostasis that involve its export to extracellular acceptors and conversion to cholesteryl esters. However, these pathways appear to be overwhelmed in the setting of atherosclerosis through scavenger receptor–mediated uptake of modified lipoproteins. When cholesterol uptake exceeds the capacity of cholesterol efflux pathways, cholesterol esterification results in the formation of lipid droplets that are characteristic of macrophage foam cells. A detailed analysis of cholesterol homeostasis in macrophages was recently reviewed.[84]

Roles of Peroxisome Proliferator-Activated Receptors and Liver X Receptors in Regulating Scavenger Receptor Activity and Cholesterol Homeostasis

Peroxisome proliferator–activated receptors are members of the nuclear receptor superfamily of ligand activated transcription factors. The PPAR subfamily consists of PPAR-α, PPAR-γ, and PPAR-δ (also known as PPAR-β).[85] The endogenous ligands that regulate PPAR activity remain poorly characterized but are presumed to include fatty acids and their metabolites. Recent studies indicate that PPAR-α and PPAR-δ are regulated by fatty acids liberated from triglyceride-rich lipoproteins by lipoprotein lipase.[86,87] The prostaglandin 15-deoxy-Δ-prostaglandin J_2[12,14] and lipoxygenase products including 12-HETE and 13-HODE present in OxLDL have been suggested to be endogenous ligands for PPAR-γ in macrophages,[88–91] and cholesteryl ester hydroperoxides, also the components of OxLDL, may activate PPAR-α.[92] Several lines of evidence suggest that PPAR-γ agonists can exert both atherogenic and antiatherogenic effects on patterns of gene expression.[91,93–95] PPAR-γ stimulates expression of the scavenger receptor CD36.[95] PPAR-γ agonists also inhibit the program of macrophage activation in response to inflammatory mediators such as interferon-γ (IFN-γ) and lipopolysaccharide (LPS).[94,96,97]

Liver X receptors (LXRs) –α and –β compose a second subfamily of nuclear receptors that have more recently emerged as transcription factors that function in concert with sterol regulatory element–binding proteins (SREBPs) to regulate cholesterol homeostasis.[98] At least three important classes of LXR target genes have been identified that influence cholesterol homeostasis and foam cell formation in macrophages. First, LXRs induce the expression of ATP-binding cassette (ABC) transporters that have been linked to cholesterol efflux.[99] Second, LXRs induce the expression of apoE, which can potentially serve as an acceptor of cholesterol transported by ABCA1-dependent processes.[100] Third, LXR-α appears to induce synthesis of fatty acids that are preferential substrates of acyl-coenzymeA: cholesterol acyltransferase (ACAT) in cholesterol esterification reactions.[98] Thus, these genes act in concert to reduce free cholesterol levels and protect macrophages from its cytotoxic effects. LXRs are activated by specific intracellular oxysterols,[98] and it is yet a matter of controversy whether exogenous oxysterols delivered by OxLDL activate or suppress LXRs.[101–103]

Cellular Proinflammatory Responses to Oxidized Low-Density Lipoprotein

The appreciation that inflammation is a fundamentally important component of atherosclerotic lesion initiation and progression has fundamentally altered our view of the pathogenesis of atherosclerosis.[104,105] With the exception of the absence of neutrophils, the chronic atherosclerotic lesion has all the pathologic components of a typical inflammatory response, including the presence of monocyte/macrophages, dendritic cells, T cells, proinflammatory and anti-inflammatory cytokines, antibodies (many of which bind oxidation-specific epitopes), activated complement, and even mast cells (Fig. 8-3).

The recent discovery of TLRs provided an answer to long unresolved question in innate immunity: what receptors initiate proinflammatory intracellular signaling and sustain the inflammatory response? The signaling cascade initiated by TLRs is now relatively well understood, and bacterial and viral pathogens

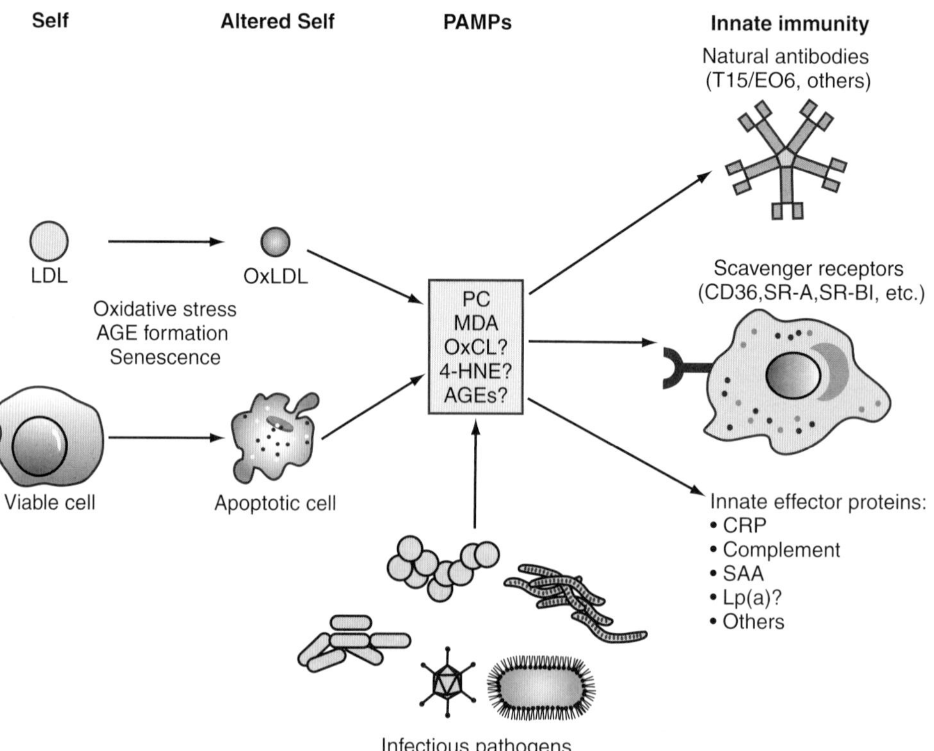

FIGURE 8-3 Oxidation-specific epitopes are a class of pathogen-associated molecular patterns (PAMPs) that are recognized by natural antibodies and other innate immune receptors. Physiologic and pathologic stress can lead to the generation of oxidation-specific epitopes (altered self) on membranes of lipoproteins as well as cells (self), which are subsequently recognized by natural antibodies, scavenger receptors, and other innate effector proteins via these motifs. In many, if not all, cases, molecular mimicry exists between oxidation-specific epitopes of self-antigens and epitopes of infectious pathogens. *(From Ref. 135, with permission.)* AGE, advanced glycation endproduct; CRP, C-reactive protein; 4-HNE, 4-hydroxynonenal; LDL, low-density lipoprotein; Lp(a), lipoprotein(a); MDA, malondialdehyde; OxCL, oxidized cardiolipin; OxLDL, oxidized LDL PC, phosphoycholine; SAA, serum amyloid A; SR, scavenger receptor.

are identified that activate specific TLRs, 12 of which are known so far.[106] TLRs are signaling receptors and, like scavenger receptors, are also PRRs capable of recognizing a variety of PAMPs. In many cases, efficient proinflammatory response requires association of binding and signaling receptors. As such, a complex of the binding receptor CD36 with signaling receptors TLR-2 and TLR-6 provides the sensing and the signaling components to the response to bacterial diacylated lipopeptides.[107]

The role of TLRs in atherogenesis is supported by studies with MyD88/apoE–double knockout mice. MyD88 is a signaling molecule downstream from many TLRs and is essential for the majority of TLR proinflammatory effects. Targeted deletion of MyD88 in apoE−/− mice resulted in a reduction in lesion size, a reduction in the number of lesional macrophages, and lower circulating MCP-1 levels.[108,109] TLR4 deficiency in apoE−/− mice also reduced the lesion size.[109] Similarly, TLR-2 deficiency in LDLR−/− mice significantly reduced atherosclerosis.[110] Human epidemiologic studies provide less definitive answers than the experimental animal models. The Asp299Gly polymorphism in the *TLR4* gene, which is associated with muted TLR-4 responses, has been associated with both decreased risk for atherosclerosis and acute coronary events.[111,112] Other studies, however, did not find a connection between the same TLR-4 polymorphism and carotid atherosclerosis and stroke.[113,114]

It has been proposed that mmLDL generated by 15-lipoxygenase–expressing cells is an agonist for the TLR-4 signaling. MmLDL triggers cytoskeletal rearrangements in macrophages via CD14/TLR-4/MD2, induces TLR-4– and MyD88-dependent macrophage inflammatory protein–2 (MIP-2) (a mouse analogue of human chemokine IL-8) secretion by macrophages,[115,116] and enhances MyD88-dependent monocyte adhesion to endothelial cells.[109] In addition, oxidized phosphatidylcholine has been suggested to increase IL-8 expression in endothelial cells via TLR-4.[64] However, evidence that OxLDL activates TLR-2 signaling is not yet available, and the precise chemical moieties of modified LDL that activate TLRs are yet to be identified.

Oxidized Low-Density Lipoprotein-Induced Apoptosis and Apoptotic Cell Clearance

In addition to the important roles of living macrophages in lesion development and progression, macrophage apoptosis also occurs throughout all stages of atherosclerosis. Recent *in vivo* studies suggest that macrophage death in early lesions, which appears to be accompanied by rapid phagocytic clearance of the apoptotic cells, decreases macrophage burden and slows lesion progression.[117–119] In late lesions, however, macrophage death causes necrotic core formation, which is thought to promote plaque rupture.[119] Postapoptotic necrosis of macrophages likely is due to inefficient phagocytosis of apoptotic macrophages in advanced atherosclerotic lesions.[119,120] Thus, the balance between macrophage survival and death throughout atherosclerosis is an important determinant of lesion development and progression.

In this context, OxLDL accumulation induces apoptosis of cultured macrophages *in vitro*, and there is circumstantial evidence that OxLDL may be important in macrophage death in atherosclerotic lesions.[119,121–124] Interestingly, unlike OxLDL, mmLDL promotes cell survival via a phosphoinositide-3–kinase (PI3K)/Akt mechanism, and phosphorylated (activated) Akt has been demonstrated in atherosclerotic lesions.[125] However, given that mmLDL may contribute to decreased phagocytosis of apoptotic cells through initiating adverse cytoskeletal rearrangements in macrophages,[115] mmLDL may promote necrotic core formation even as it lessens macrophage apoptosis. It is still unclear which in OxLDL and in mmLDL determine their opposite effects on cell survival.

OXIDIZED LOW-DENSITY LIPOPROTEIN AND THE HUMORAL IMMUNE RESPONSES IN ATHEROGENESIS

Immune activation that occurs in the atherosclerotic lesion must be viewed in the context of a coordinated response to perceived pathogens. A variety of candidate pathogens, including microbial and viral agents, aberrant expression of endogenous proteins such as heat shock proteins, and other modifications of proteins such as the generation of nonenzymatic glycation and advanced glycation endproducts, occur secondary to hyperglycemia. Chief among the potential pathogens are various forms of mmLDL and heavily OxLDL. The generation of a wide spectrum of oxidized moieties that occur when LDL is oxidized produces not only bioactive molecules with diverse proinflammatory effects but also enhanced immunogenicity to oxidation-specific epitopes, resulting in a profound cellular and humoral immune response.[126]

A wide variety of both adaptive and innate immune responses have been shown to be capable of modulating lesion formation in animal models of atherosclerosis. For example, both apoE−/− and LDLR−/− models have been crossed into recombination-activating gene (RAG)–deficient mice, which lack both T and B cells. When such mice are fed an atherogenic diet, achieving very high cholesterol levels, the extent of lesion formation is not altered. However, when these same mice are examined at very early time points or even over more extended periods of time, but in the presence of more modest elevations of plasma cholesterol, immune deficiency results in a 40% to 80% decrease in lesion formation.[127] These data indicate that immune cells are not obligatory for lesion formation in the presence of the extreme atherogenic pressure generated by marked hypercholesterolemia. However, in the presence of a lesser atherogenic pressure, these immune responses are capable of modulating atherogenesis. Although these studies indicate a net proatherogenic effect of adaptive immunity, many examples exist in which specific components of adaptive immunity can be protective as well. For instance, immunization of mice with OxLDL has been shown to reduce the extent of lesion formation despite very high plasma cholesterol levels.[128]

Adaptive immunity represents a somewhat delayed but precise response of the immune system to newly exposed antigens. Adaptive immunity is mediated by somatic mutations of antigen receptors, such as T-cell receptors and B-cell receptors, which give rise to specific and high-affinity cellular and humoral immunity. In contrast, innate immunity is mediated by highly conserved and phylogenetically ancient PRRs that provide a rapid if less precise response to PAMPs. Natural antibodies, which are usually IgM or IgA subtypes, are so-called germ-line–encoded antibodies that arise without known antigenic stimulation and contain evolutionarily conserved antigen-binding sites that are thought to provide rapid recognition of PAMPs on pathogens.

Recent studies have uncovered an example of a common PAMP that is found on OxLDL, apoptotic cells, and the cell wall of many common pathogens. The natural IgM autoantibody EO6 was cloned from apoE-deficient mice for its ability to bind to OxLDL.[129] Subsequently it was shown to bind to the phosphocholine (PC) moiety of the oxidized phospholipids but not native, unoxidized phospholipids, even though they contain the same PC motif.[130] Thus, oxidation of phospholipids appears to generate specific and quite subtle conformational changes that "expose" the PC headgroup leading to recognition by EO6.[131] Subsequently, it was shown that cells undergoing apoptosis, which are also subjected to enhanced oxidative stress, also "expose" the PC moiety of their oxidized phospholipids and enable binding of EO6. EO6 does not bind to viable cells.[132] It was also shown that EO6 could inhibit the binding and uptake of OxLDL and apoptotic cells by macrophages, and specifically by CD36-transfected cells.[68] Thus, the oxidized phospholipid containing the PC moiety is a ligand on OxLDL and apoptotic cells mediating binding and uptake by macrophage scavenger receptors; for example, PC is a PAMP on OxLDL and apoptotic cells recognized by the PRR CD36. Cloning and sequencing studies of the antigen-binding domains of EO6 revealed that this antibody was identical to an antibody named T15 that was studied more than 30 years ago.[133] T15 is an anti-PC antibody that binds to the PC moiety that is covalently linked to the cell wall polysaccharide of common pathogens such as *Streptococcus pneumoniae,* and this single antibody class provides the optimal protection to mice against lethal infection with this pathogen. Interestingly, pneumococcal vaccination of $LDLR^{-/-}$ mice increased the EO6/T15 titers and, most strikingly, reduced the progression of atherosclerosis.[134] Thus, there is molecular mimicry between the exposed PC of OxLDL and apoptotic cells and the PC of many pathogens; this is an important modulator of atherogenic precesses.[135] A number of natural antibodies against epitopes of oxidatively modified LDL other than EO6 have been cloned from humans and nonimmunized atherosclerotic mice.[136,137] Interestingly, immunization with MDA-LDL, which does not contain OxPL, induces a preferential expansion of MDA-LDL-specific Th2 cells that prominently secrete IL-5 and also lead to the expansion of T15/EO6 antibodies through noncognate stimulation to innate B-1 cells.[138] These observations exemplify the intimate relationships between the adaptive immune system and the innate immune system, leading to a coordinated response to pathogenic stimuli.

LOW-DENSITY LIPOPROTEIN OXIDATION AND ATHEROGENESIS

Animal Models

If oxidation of LDL promotes atherogenesis, the most convincing evidence would be the direct demonstration that inhibition of oxidation leads to inhibition of the progression of atherosclerosis and that this occurs independently of any effects on plasma lipoprotein levels. Many studies in a variety of animal models have been published demonstrating that chemically different antioxidants retard the progression of atherosclerosis (for detailed discussion see references 58 and 139). For example, most antioxidant studies in both cholesterol-fed New Zealand white and LDLR−/− rabbits (Watanabe heritable hyperlipidemic rabbits), such as with probucol, probucol analogues, diphenylphenylediamine (DPPD), carvedilol, and butylated hydroxytoluene (BHT) but not vitamin E, have shown protection against progression of atherosclerosis. In fact in several different rabbit studies, probucol inhibited atherosclerosis by 40% to 80%, despite the fact that it lowered HDL levels. In rodents, the data are less consistent, perhaps because of the fact that rodents carry most of their cholesterol on HDL rather than LDL and thus may have different responses. AGI-1067, a probucol analogue, has shown significant reductions in atherosclerosis in both LDLR−/− and apoE−/− mice, which were also associated with reduced expression of inflammatory genes such as vascular cell adhesion molecule–1 (VCAM-1) and MCP-1.[140] However, the underlying mechanisms by which these compounds inhibit atherosclerosis has not been fully determined.

Additional studies in 12/15-LO−/−/apoE−/− mice and 12/15-LO−/−/LDLR−/− mice demonstrated significant reductions in the extent of early lesion formation.[47,141–143] Urinary and plasma levels of F_2-isoprostanes, nonenzymatic breakdown products resulting from lipid peroxidation of arachidonic acid, and OxLDL autoantibodies were also reduced and were highly correlated both with plaque burden and with each other. Although it is possible that 12/15-LO affected atherogenesis by other mechanisms, these studies lend strong support to the concept that a major mechanism by which LO deficiency decreased atherosclerosis was that of decreasing the extent of lipid peroxidation and specifically the generation of OxLDL. Conversely, overexpression of 15-LO in endothelial cells led to an enhancement of atherosclerosis in LDLR−/− mice.[48] In contrast, macrophage-specific overexpression of 15-LO led to protection against atherosclerosis in cholesterol-fed rabbits. The 12/15-LO deletion was global, whereas the studies with 15-LO overexpression were tissue specific. Whether this explains the difference in the latter two studies is unclear. It is likely that there are many mechanisms in addition to 12/15-LO by which LDL is oxidized within the artery wall.[144] Additional studies have shown that combined paraoxonase/apoE–double knockout mice have enhanced LDL oxidation, detected by enhanced clearance of intravenously injected LDL and faster generation of plasma levels of circulating OxLDL and immune complexes, and attendant enhanced atherosclerosis.[145]

In experimental studies of atherosclerosis regression, evidence has accumulated that in conjunction with dietary lipid lowering, reduced OxLDL content in the vessel wall has been strongly associated with plaque regression and possibly plaque stabilization, as measured by direct immunostaining and with imaging with radiolabeled oxidation-specific antibodies.[146,147] Remarkably, the vessel wall OxLDL content was strongly correlated with OxLDL autoantibody titers, which also correlated with extent of atherosclerosis progression and regression.[47,147–149] Reduction in OxLDL markers was also associated with features of plaque stabilization, such as reduction in expression of VCAM-1 and MCP-1 and improvement in eNOS expression.

Epidemiologic Data and Clinical Trials

Epidemiologic Correlations between Antioxidant Vitamin Intake and Cardiovascular Disease Risk

Many epidemiologic studies demonstrate an inverse relationship between dietary intake and/or serum levels of antioxidants and CVD (for detailed review see reference 139). However, epidemiologic studies only generate hypotheses and do not substitute for prospective interventional trials.

Randomized Trials Assessing Plaque Morphology and Restenosis

Table 8-3 lists the major randomized placebo-controlled trials that examined plaque progression/regression with antioxidants. (A detailed description of these studies can be found in reference 139.) In general probucol or the probucol analogue AGI-1067 and the combination of vitamin E and vitamin C have been modestly successful in reducing plaque progression.

Similar to the studies on plaque morphology, probucol or probucol analogues appear to prevent restenosis (Table 8-4).

Randomized Clinical Trials Assessing Cardiovascular Events

A workshop to review the available data on antioxidants by leading experts was convened by the National Heart, Lung, and Blood Institute (NHLBI) in 1991 and suggested that clinical trials were justified, primarily based on a large body of epidemiologic data and animal data, mostly with probucol.[150] The NHLBI recommended that the first trials be performed with naturally occurring antioxidants on the premise that they would be safe. Unfortunately, the mechanisms underlying any potential reduction in atherosclerosis or clinical events were inferred, and not proved, as would be required for any other drug undergoing evaluation. In addition, dietary antioxidants were assumed to share similar biological properties and could be used interchangeably. This has proved to be a false assumption. For example, beta-carotene is a potent trap for singlet oxygen but much less effective in terminating free radical chain reactions. Vitamin E, on the other hand, is an excellent terminator of chain

TABLE 8-3 Effects of Antioxidant Supplementation on Plaque Progression/Regression

Study/Year	N	Imaging Modality	Antioxidant	Duration	Effect on CVD
PQRST 1994[190]	303	Femoral QCA	Probucol 500 mg twice daily	3 years	No benefit
SECURE 2001[191]	732	B-mode US Carotid IMT	Vit E (N) 400 IU+	4–6 years	No benefit
HATS 2001[192]	160	Coronary QCA	Vit E (N) 800 IU+ Vit C 1000 mg+ BetaC 25 mg+ Selenium 100 μg	3 years	No benefit
FAST 2002[193]	246	B-mode US carotid IMT	Probucol 500 mg/day or Pravastatin 10 mg/day	2 years	14% reduction in IMT with either probucol or pravastatin Probucol reduced cardiac events
Transplant-Associated Atherosclerosis 2002[194]	40	Coronary IVUS	Vit E (N) 400 IU+ Vit C 500 mg	1 year	Reduced intimal index 0.8% vs 8% with placebo, $P = 0.008$
VEAPS 2002[195]	332	B-mode US carotid IMT	Vit E (S) 400 IU	3 years	No benefit
CART-1 2003[196]	305	Coronary IVUS	AGI-1067 280 mg daily	6 months	AGI-1067 induced regression of reference segments
ASAP 2003[197]	440	B-mode US carotid IMT	Vit E (N) 136 IU+ Vit C 250 mg Both twice daily	6 years	−26%, $P = 0.014$
MAVET 2006[198]	409	B-mode US carotid IMT	Vit E 500 IU in smokers	4 years	No benefit

BetaC, betacarotene; CVD, cardiovascular disease; IMT, intima-media thickness; IVUS, intravascular ultrasound; QCA, quantitative coronary angiography; US, ultrasound; Vit C, vitamin C; Vit E (S), synthetic vitamin E; Vit E (N), natural vitamin E. Intimal index defined as plaque area divided by vessel area.

TABLE 8-4 Effects of Antioxidant Supplementation on Angiographic Coronary Restenosis

Study/Year	N	Imaging Modality	Antioxidant	Duration	Effect on CVD
MVP 1997[199] Balloon angioplasty	317	Coronary QCA	Vit E (N) 700 IU+ Vit C 500 mg+ BetaC 30,000 IU Probucol 500 mg All twice daily	6 months	Restenosis reduced with (probucol 20.7% vs 38.9% with placebo, $P = 0.003$; 40.3% with multivitamin)
PART 1997[200] Balloon angioplasty	101	Coronary QCA	Probucol 1000 mg daily	6 months	Restenosis reduced with probucol (23% vs 58% with no lipid lowering, $P = 0.001$)
EUROCARE 2000[201] Atherectomy	292	Coronary QCA	Carvedilol 25 mg twice daily	6 months	No reduction in restenosis
CART-1 2003[196] Stent	305	Coronary QCA IVUS	AGI-1067 280 mg daily or Probucol 500 mg twice daily	6 months	AGI-1067 and probucol reduced restenosis

BetaC, beta-carotene; CVD, cardiovascular disease; QCA, quantitative coronary angiography; Vit C, vitamin C; Vit E (N), natural vitamin E.

reactions. Beta-carotene does not significantly protect LDL against *ex vivo* oxidation,[151] but vitamin E is moderately effective.[152] However, this reduction in plasma LDL oxidation is orders of magnitude lower than the rate of reaction of superoxide radicals in initiating oxidation.[153] Presumably inhibiting oxidation in the vessel wall is much more important than inhibiting oxidation in plasma, which is enriched in antioxidants. In addition, because it has not been established where and how LDL gets oxidized *in vivo*, it is not possible to make meaningful comparisons of these various antioxidants. There are also large differences in the pharmacokinetics of the several nutrient antioxidants. For example, vitamin C is distributed exclusively in the aqueous phase, whereas vitamin E is lipophilic and is transported in lipoproteins.

Table 8-5 presents the major trials of antioxidants that examined clinical events. In general, it can be summarized that no trials showed a benefit of antioxidant vitamins with the exception of the Cambridge Heart Antioxidant Study (CHAOS) and the Secondary Prevention with Antioxidants of Cardiovascular Disease in End-Stage Renal Disease (SPACE) trial. Taking these trials as a whole, one would, conclude that in unselected patients with established, well-advanced CVD, vitamin E at doses up to 800 IU/day does not have any measurable benefit in preventing cardiovascular events over 5 years of treatment.

The latest randomized clinical trial was the Aggressive Reduction of Inflammation Stops Events (ARISE) trial, which tested the hypothesis that succinobucol (AGI-1067) would reduce the length of time to the first occurrence of cardiovascular mortality, resuscitated cardiac arrest, nonfatal MI, nonfatal stroke, hospitalization for angina pectoris, or use of coronary revascularization in patients with preexisting CVD.[153] The study showed that succinobucol was not better than placebo for the primary endpoint.

TABLE 8-5 Effects of Antioxidant Supplements on Cardiovasculor Disease Endpoints

Study/Year	N	Prevention	Antioxidant	Duration	Effect on CVD
ATBC 1994[202]	29,133	Primary	Vit E (S) 50 mg+ BetaC 20 mg	5–8 years	No benefit
CHAOS 1996[203]	2,002	Secondary	Vit E (N) 400/800 IU	510 days	-47% ($P = 0.005$)
GISSI 1999[204]	11,324	Secondary	Vit E (S) 300 mg	3.5 years	No benefit
HOPE 2000[205]	9,541	Secondary	Vit E (N) 400 IU	4–6 years	No benefit
SPACE 2000[206]	196	Secondary	Vit E (N) 400 IU	519 days	-46% ($P = 0.014$)
PPP 2001[207]	4,495	Primary	Vit E (S) 300 mg	3.6 years	No benefit
HPS 2002[208]	20,536	Secondary	Vit E (N) 400 IU+ 250 mg Vit C+ 20 mg BetaC	5 years	No benefit
ARISE 2007[153a]	6,144	Secondary	Succinobucol (AGI-1067)	5 years	No benefit for primary endpoint but a 19% decrease in secondary endpoint (cardiovascular death, cardiac arrest, MI, and stroke)

BetaC, beta carotene; MI, myocardial infarction; Vit E (N), natural vitamin E; Vit E (S), synthetic vitamin E.

However, a significant 19% reduction in cardiovascular death, cardiac arrest, MI, and stroke, a prespecified secondary endpoint, was noted, as was a significant reduction in new-onset diabetes. It remains to be seen whether this drug will be tested in further clinical studies that are better designed to address the issue of whether a benefit may be seen in specific patient subsets.

Why Have the Vitamin E Clinical Endpoint Trials Been Largely Negative?

It is unlikely that the pathogenesis of atherosclerosis in humans is fundamentally different from that in mice, rabbits, or primates. The reasons for the negative results have been previously discussed in detail, summarized as follows[58,154]:

1. Although more data are emerging with regard to mechanisms of oxidation (e.g., 12/15 LO, MPO), the underlying mechanisms and location of oxidation are still not well understood.
2. It has not been possible to measure oxidative stress in humans with quantitative methods to enroll patients with the highest risk. Therefore, this limits the effectiveness of therapy because many patients would be unlikely to benefit. This is analogous to treating patients with statins without knowing their baseline LDL cholesterol levels and having no way to measure effectiveness.
3. The antioxidants evaluated clinically have been mainly natural vitamins, which are relatively weak in antioxidant efficacy and may also have pro-oxidant effects. The rates of oxidation *in vivo* are generally orders of magnitude higher than can be prevented with antioxidant vitamins.
4. In humans, the rate of generation of reactive free radical oxygen species is much lower per unit of body weight than in small mammals. The role of oxidation in atherogenesis may be less robust, and thus it may take longer to demonstrate the effectiveness of antioxidant intervention.
5. Data on the pharmacokinetics of the antioxidants and independent measures of the effectiveness of these compounds *in vivo* have been lacking.
6. Treatment may need to be started earlier and continued longer. Most of the animal model studies evaluated early lesions. Oxidation may have less of an effect on the later, advanced lesions.
7. The effectiveness of agents such as statins that reduce CVD events suggests that effectively reducing substrate for oxidation is an important pathway to reduce CVD risk. However, the risk reduction of statins is only in the order of approximately 20% to 30%; therefore, additional therapeutic measures are needed to further improve clinical outcomes.

OXIDIZED LOW-DENSITY LIPOPROTEIN PLASMA BIOMARKERS

The generation of monoclonal antibodies recognizing distinct oxidation-specific epitopes has allowed the development of sensitive and specific assays to measure circulating OxLDL in plasma. Previous assays were limited by the nonspecific nature of *in vitro* measures such as thiobarbiturate reactive substances (TBARS) and MDA measures because these can be generated by cell membranes, platelet, and DNA, poor reflection of *in vitro* LDL susceptibility measures to *in vivo* oxidation, poor precision, and inability to adapt to large-scale studies.[155]

The development of monoclonal antibodies binding oxidation-specific epitopes has allowed the development of sensitive and specific assays to measure circulating OxLDL.[156–158] Fig. 8-4 displays the methodology for three well-described OxLDL assays from which the majority of published clinical data exists. These assays are not necessarily comparable because they either use antibodies detecting different epitopes or are

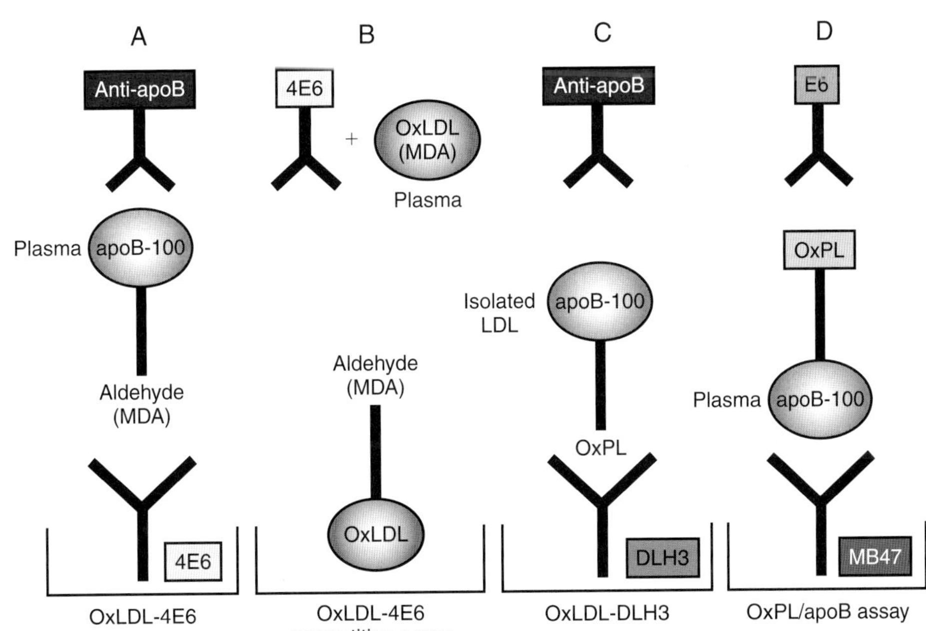

FIGURE 8-4 Schematic representation of plasma oxidized low-density lipoprotein (OxLDL) assays. *A,* Standard OxLDL-4E6 assay; *B,* competition OxLDL-4E6 assay; *C,* OxLDL-DLH3 assay; *D,* OxPL/apoB assay. *(From Ref. 159, with permission.)* apo, apolipoprotein; MDA, malondialdehyde. *From Ref. 159, with permission.*

set up in different formats and units of measurement (for a detailed description of these assays, see reference 159). The characteristics of these assays are shown in Table 8-6. All these assays have some advantages and disadvantages, and comparative data are awaited to assess if any one provides enhanced clinical utility compared with the others. None of these assays are currently approved for routine clinical use.

Circulating Oxidized Low-Density Lipoprotein As a Marker of Preclinical Cardiovascular Disease

In vitro and *in vivo* studies have shown that OxLDL promotes endothelial cell toxicity and vasoconstriction. Circulating OxLDL levels correlate with impaired endothelial function, and reduction in circulating OxLDL correlates with improvement following lipid-lowering therapy with apheresis or statins (reviewed in reference 62). Plasma levels of OxLDL measured by antibody DLH3 were recently shown to be an independent determinant of coronary macrovasomotor and microvasomotor responses to bradykinin in humans.[160] The value of OxLDL in screening selected high-risk subjects is more controversial at this point, because some studies[161,162] have shown a correlation with increased carotid intima–media thickness (IMT), whereas others[163,164] have not. Because IMT is strongly correlated with hypertension and also represents a very small atherosclerotic burden at best, it is not surprising that a stronger association with OxLDL has not been found.

Circulating Oxidized Low-Density Lipoprotein and Coronary Artery Disease

There are now several studies that show a strong association of circulating OxLDL with stable coronary artery disease (CAD).[165–168] For example, OxPL/apoB levels measured with antibody EO6 were strongly correlated with both the presence and extent of angiographically determined CAD.[169] Interestingly, in that study lipoprotein(a) [Lp(a)] had a strikingly similar association with CAD and strongly correlated ($R = 0.83$, $P < 0.001$) with OxPL/apoB. This association has been confirmed in all studies performed to date, with a consistent correlation coefficient of $R = 0.80$ to 90.[169–173] Additional studies have shown that OxPL accumulate preferentially on Lp(a) particles as opposed to other non-Lp(a) apoB-containing particles.[171,174] This has led to the hypothesis that Lp(a) may act as a potent binder and transporter of OxPL, and its contribution to atherothrombosis may be additionally mediated by its association with proinflammatory OxPL.

Association of Oxidized Low-Density Lipoprotein with Acute Coronary Syndromes, Percutaneous Coronary Intervention, and Vulnerable Plaques

The association of OxLDL with acute coronary syndromes (ACSs) makes a strong argument that OxLDL may be integrally involved in plaque destabilization.[170,175–178] Monocytes derived from patients with unstable angina induced a significant amount of nuclear factor–κB (NF-κB) when exposed to patients' serum with elevated OxLDL levels.[179] Furthermore, correlations have been noted between circulating plasma levels of OxLDL and coronary plaque wall content of OxLDL derived with atherectomy techniques and measured immunohistochemically. Additionally, "vulnerable" carotid plaques are highly enriched in macrophages and OxLDL (with ≈100-fold greater levels in lesions than plasma) compared with stable carotid plaques.[180] It has also been shown that pravastatin treatment prior to carotid endarterectomy significantly reduces OxLDL content in carotid plaques.[181] Additionally, percutaneous coronary

TABLE 8-6 Characteristics of the Three Well-Described Oxidized Low-Density Lipoprotein Assays

	OxLDL-4E6	OxLDL-DLH3	OxPL/apoB
Year described	1995	1995	1996
Monoclonal antibody	4E6	DLH3/FOH1a	EO6
Epitope	Aldehyde-lysine on apoB	OxPL	PC-OxPL
Source material	Plasma	Isolated LDL	Plasma
Detection method	Absorbance 450	Absorbance 405	Chemiluminescence
Units	U/L	ng/μg LDL protein	RLU
Standardized to reference	No	No	No
Calibration	"Standard" OxLDL	"Standard" OxLDL	RLU
Coefficient of variation	4.0%–8.3%	4.7%–7.7%	6%–10%
Stability of frozen samples	6 months	No	>5 years
High throughput	Yes	No	Yes
Commercially available for research use	Yes (Mercodia)	Yes (Kyowa Medex MX kit)	No
Correlates with LDL cholesterol	Yes	No	No
Correlates with Lp(a)	?	Yes	Yes

LDL, low-density lipoprotein; OxLDL, oxidized LDL; PC-OxPL, phosphocholine-containing oxidized phospholipids; RLU, relative light units.
(Modified from Ref. 139, with permission.)

intervention induces a strikingly acute increase in OxPL immediately following the procedure, suggesting release from the iatrogenically disrupted atherosclerotic plaque.[171] However, circulating OxLDL seems not to predict restenosis.[182–184]

Association of Oxidized Low-Density Lipoprotein with Progression of Cardiovascular Disease and Prognosis of New Cardiovascular Events

Elevated baseline OxPL/apoB levels were recently shown to predict the presence, extent, and interim development of carotid and femoral atherosclerosis over the 5-year period in the Bruneck study, a community-based, prospectively followed cohort of 40- to 79-year-old men and women.[173] Furthermore, during the follow-up period of 10 years, 82 subjects developed CVD. In multivariable analysis, which included traditional risk factors, high sensitivity C-reactive protein (hsCRP) and lipoprotein-associated phospholipase A_2 (Lp-PLA_2) activity, subjects in the highest tertile of OxPL/apoB had a significantly higher risk of cardiovascular events than those in the lowest tertile (hazard ratio 2.4 [95% confidence interval (CI) 1.3 to 4.3], $P = 0.004$). The strength of the association between OxPL/apoB and CVD risk was amplified with increasing Lp-PLA_2 activity ($P = 0.018$ for interaction). Moreover, OxPL/apoB levels predicted future cardiovascular events beyond the information provided by the Framingham Risk Score (Fig. 8-5).[185]

Additionally, a small number of recent studies with other OxLDL assays have shown that circulating OxLDL predicts secondary cardiovascular events, with odds ratios of 2 to 3.[186–188] Additional studies are required in large, diverse populations taking into account both traditional and emerging cardiovascular risk factors. In the future, the role of different oxidative biomarkers will need to be evaluated in the same data sets to evaluate whether they provide complementary or similar information and to assess how to apply these in clinical settings.[189]

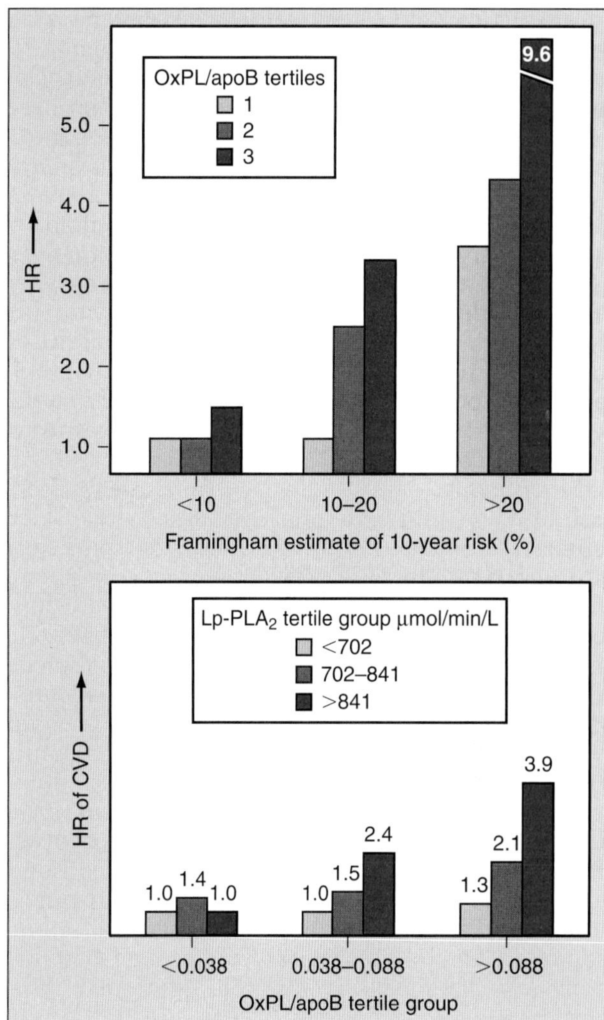

FIGURE 8-5 *Upper panel,* Relationship between tertile groups of OxPL/apoB (<0.0379, 0.0379 to 0.0878, >0.0878) and cardiovasular disease (CVD) risk within each Framingham Risk Score group in the Bruneck Study. Framingham Risk Score was calculated as low risk (<10% risk of events over 10 years), moderate risk (10% to 20%), and high risk (>20%). *Lower panel,* Relationship between OxPL/apoB tertile groups and CVD risk according to tertiles of Lipoprotein-associated phospholipase A_2 ($LpPLA_2$) activity ($P = 0.018$ for interaction). *(From Ref. 185, with permission.)* apo, apoliprotein; HR, hazard ratio; OxPL, oxidized phospholipid.

SUMMARY

The field of oxidation of LDL is now entering its fourth decade. Initial studies focused on how LDL enters monocyte/macrophages and understanding how oxidation occurs *in vitro*; which reactive oxygen species, enzymes, cells, and microdomains mediate oxidation; and how natural antioxidant vitamins reduce oxidation. The field then transitioned to studying macrophage scavenger receptors and assessing the role of antioxidant vitamins on atherosclerosis in animal models. Knockout mouse models provided a robust scientific basis for fully understanding the role of scavenger receptors and oxidant enzymes. Concurrent with this, and before a robust clinical database was accumulated, antioxidant vitamins were tested in large-scale human studies and generally failed to provide clinical protection except in specific high-risk groups such as patients with renal failure. While these studies were ongoing, a strong consensus emerged and became dominant in showing that chronic inflammation was a dominant mechanism through which atherosclerosis was initiated and progressed. Oxidation and inflammation have become intimately associated in the pathophysiology of atherogenesis.[104,105]

The new paradigms that are now emerging are not only going "beyond cholesterol" but are also going beyond simple approaches to reduce cardiovascular risk. A strong understanding has emerged that the immune system is significantly involved in modifying responses to the presence of oxidized species, and the immunologic aspects of oxidation are now emerging as dominant areas to examine the role in human disease. In addition, oxidative biomarkers are now showing strong associations with both progression of CAD and predicting future events, suggesting that they may be used as surrogates and may complement diagnostic investigations in future studies.

Immunomodulation involving oxidized species may become a dominant theory in the coming decade in treating atherosclerosis. Thus, it is likely that the field will come full circle, with much scientific data showing that oxidation is intimately involved in atherogenesis, but now with a greater understanding of the role of both innate and adaptive immunity and the ability to quantitate oxidized species to rationally test new therapies. Targeting only one aspect of this complex disease is not likely to be as fruitful as targeting all aspects, particularly upstream targets such as the substrate for inflammation and oxidation. As we search for new insights into the pathogenesis of atherogenesis and try to develop new therapies, it will be important to better understand the fundamental interactions among hypercholesterolemia, inflammation, and oxidation.

REFERENCES

1. Steinberg D, Parthasarathy S, Carew TE, et al: Beyond cholesterol: modifications of low-density lipoprotein that increase its atherogenicity. *New Engl J Med* 1989;320:915–924.
2. Steinberg D: Thematic review series: the pathogenesis of atherosclerosis. An interpretive history of the cholesterol controversy, part V: The discovery of the statins and the end of the controversy. *J Lipid Res* 2006;47:1339–1351.
3. Goldstein JL, Kita T, Brown MS: Defective lipoprotein receptors and atherosclerosis. Lessons from an animal counterpart of familial hypercholesterolemia. *N Engl J Med* 1983;309:288–296.
4. Brown MS, Goldstein JL: A receptor-mediated pathway for cholesterol homeostasis. *Science* 1986;232:34–47.
5. Goldstein JL, Ho YK, Basu SK, et al: Binding site on macrophages that mediates uptake and degradation of acetylated low-density lipoprotein, producing massive cholesterol deposition. *Proc Natl Acad Sci USA* 1979;76:333–337.
6. Kodama T, Freeman M, Rohrer L, et al: Type I macrophage scavenger receptor contains alpha-helical and collagen-like coiled coils. *Nature* 1990;343:531–535.
7. Fogelman AM, Shechter I, Seager J, et al: Malondialdehyde alteration of low-density lipoproteins leads to cholesteryl ester accumulation in human monocyte-macrophages. *Proc Natl Acad Sci USA* 1980;77:2214–2218.
8. Mahley RW, Innerarity TL, Weisgraber KB, et al: Altered metabolism (*in vivo* and *in vitro*) of plasma lipoproteins after selective chemical modification of lysine residues of the apoproteins. *J Clin Invest* 1979;64:743–750.
9. Henriksen T, Mahoney EM, Steinberg D: Enhanced macrophage degradation of low-density lipoprotein previously incubated with cultured endothelial cells: recognition by receptors for acetylated low-density lipoproteins. *Proc Natl Acad Sci USA* 1981;78:6499–6503.
10. Steinbrecher UP, Parthasarathy S, Leake DS, et al: Modification of low-density lipoprotein by endothelial cells involves lipid peroxidation and degradation of low-density lipoprotein phospholipids. *Proc Natl Acad Sci USA* 1984;81:3883–3887.
11. Khoo JC, Miller E, McLoughlin P, et al: Enhanced macrophage uptake of low-density lipoprotein after self-aggregation. *Arteriosclerosis* 1988;8:348–358.
12. Camejo G: The interaction of lipids and lipoproteins with the intercellular matrix of arterial tissue: its possible role in atherogenesis. *Adv Lipid Res* 1982;19:1–53.
13. Kaplan M, Aviram M: Retention of oxidized LDL by extracellular matrix proteoglycans leads to its uptake by macrophages: an alternative approach to study lipoproteins cellular uptake. *Arterioscler Thromb Vasc Biol* 2001;21:386–393.
14. Khoo JC, Miller E, Pio F, et al: Monoclonal antibodies against LDL further enhance macrophage uptake of LDL aggregates. *Arterioscler Thromb* 1992;12:1258–1266.
15. Lopes-Virella MF, Griffith RL, Shunk KA, et al: Enhanced uptake and impaired intracellular metabolism of low-density lipoprotein complexed with anti-low-density lipoprotein antibodies. *Arterioscler Thromb* 1991;11:1356–1367.
16. Esterbauer H, Jurgens G, Quehenberger O, et al: Autoxidation of human low-density lipoprotein: loss of polyunsaturated fatty acids and vitamin E and generation of aldehydes. *J Lipid Res* 1987;28:495–509.
17. Reaven P, Parthasarathy S, Grasse BJ, et al: Effects of oleate-rich and linoleate-rich diets on the susceptibility of low-density lipoprotein to oxidative modification in mildly hypercholesterolemic subjects. *J Clin Invest* 1993;91:668–676.
18. Esterbauer H, Gebicki J, Puhl H, et al: The role of lipid peroxidation and antioxidants in oxidative modification of LDL. *Free Radic Biol Med* 1992;13:341–390.
19. Berliner JA, Territo MC, Sevanian A, et al: Minimally modified low-density lipoprotein stimulates monocyte endothelial interactions. *J Clin Invest* 1990;85:1260–1266.
20. Sigari F, Lee C, Hörkkö S, et al: Fibroblasts that overexpress 15-lipoxygenase generate bioactive and minimally modified low-density lipoprotein. *Arterioscler Thromb Vasc Biol* 1997 (in press);17:3639–3645.
21. Navab M, Berliner JA, Watson AD, et al: The Yin and Yang of oxidation in the development of the fatty streak. *Arterioscler Thromb Vasc Biol* 1996;16:831–842.
22. Berliner JA, Subbanagounder G, Leitinger N, et al: Evidence for a role of phospholipid oxidation products in atherogenesis. *Trends Cardiovasc Med* 2001;11:142–147.
23. Ziouzenkova O, Asatryan L, Akmal M, et al: Oxidative cross-linking of ApoB100 and hemoglobin results in low-density lipoprotein modification in blood. Relevance to atherogenesis caused by hemodialysis. *J Biol Chem* 1999;274:18916–18924.
24. Ziouzenkova O, Asatryan L, Sevanian A: Oxidative stress resulting from hemolysis and formation of catalytically active hemoglobin: protective strategies. *Int J Clin Pharmacol Ther* 1999;37:125–132.
25. Ziouzenkova O, Asatryan L, Tetta, C et al: Oxidative stress during ex vivo hemodialysis of blood is decreased by a novel hemolipodialysis procedure utilizing antioxidants. *Free Radic Biol Med* 2002;33:248–258.
26. Sevanian A, Asatryan L: LDL modification during hemodialysis. Markers for oxidative stress. *Contrib Nephrol* 2002; 386–395.
27. Miller YI, Altamentova SM, Shaklai N: Oxidation of low-density lipoprotein by hemoglobin stems from a heme-initiated globin radical: antioxidant role of haptoglobin 248. *Biochemistry* 1997;36:12189–12198.
28. Asleh R, Marsh S, Shilkrut M, et al: Genetically determined heterogeneity in hemoglobin scavenging and susceptibility to diabetic cardiovascular disease. *Circ Res* 2003;92:1193–1200.
29. Asleh R, Guetta J, Kalet-Litman S, et al: Haptoglobin genotype- and diabetes-dependent differences in iron-mediated oxidative stress *in vitro* and *in vivo*. *Circ Res* 2005;96:435–441.
30. Burbea Z, Nakhoul F, Zoabi R, et al: Haptoglobin phenotype as a predictive factor of mortality in diabetic haemodialysis patients. *Ann Clin Biochem* 2004;41:469–473.
31. Levy AP, Hochberg I, Jablonski K, et al: Haptoglobin phenotype is an independent risk factor for cardiovascular disease in individuals with diabetes: the strong heart study. *J Am Coll Cardiol* 2002;40:1984–1990.
32. Roguin A, Koch W, Kastrati A, et al: Haptoglobin genotype is predictive of major adverse cardiac events in the 1-year period after percutaneous transluminal coronary angioplasty in individuals with diabetes. *Diabetes Care* 2003;26:2628–2631.
33. Levy AP, Levy JE, Kalet-Litman S, et al: Haptoglobin genotype is a determinant of iron, lipid peroxidation, and macrophage accumulation in the atherosclerotic plaque. *Arterioscler Thromb Vasc Biol* 2007;27:134–140.
34. Miller YI, Shaklai N: Kinetics of hemin distribution in plasma reveals its role in lipoprotein oxidation 246. *Biochim Biophys Acta* 1999;1454:153–164.
35. Liao F, Andalibi A, Qiao JH, et al: Genetic evidence for a common pathway mediating oxidative stress, inflammatory gene induction, and aortic fatty streak formation in mice. *J Clin Invest* 1994;94:877–884.
36. Sparrow CP, Parthasarathy S, Steinberg D: Enzymatic modification of low-density lipoprotein by purified lipoxygenase plus phospholipase A2 mimics cell-mediated oxidative modification. *J Lipid Res* 1988;29:745–753.
37. Benz DJ, Mol M, Ezaki M, et al: Enhanced levels of lipoperoxides in low-density lipoprotein incubated with murine fibroblast expressing high levels of human 15-lipoxygenase. *J Biol Chem* 1995;270:5191–5197.
38. Parthasarathy S, Wieland E, Steinberg D: A role for endothelial cell lipoxygenase in the oxidative modification of low-density lipoprotein. *Proc Natl Acad Sci USA* 1989;86:1046–1050.
39. Cathcart MK, McNally AK, Chisolm GM: Lipoxygenase-mediated transformation of human low-density lipoprotein to an oxidized and cytotoxic complex. *J Lipid Res* 1991;32: 63–70.

40. Rankin SM, Parthasarathy S, Steinberg D: Evidence for a dominant role of lipoxygenase(s) in the oxidation of LDL by mouse peritoneal macrophages. *J Lipid Res* 1991;32:449–456.
41. Savenkova ML, Mueller DM, Heinecke JW: Tyrosyl radical generated by myeloperoxidase is a physiological catalyst for the initiation of lipid peroxidation in low-density lipoprotein. *J Biol Chem* 1994;269:20394–20400.
42. McNally AK, Chisolm GM III, Morel DW, et al: Activated human monocytes oxidize low-density lipoprotein by a lipoxygenase-dependent pathway. *J Immunol* 1990;145:254–259.
43. Wieland E, Parthasarathy S, Steinberg D: Peroxidase-dependent metal-independent oxidation of low-density lipoprotein *in vitro*: a model for *in vivo* oxidation? *Proc Natl Acad Sci USA* 1993;90:5929–5933.
44. Babior BM: Phagocytes and oxidative stress. *Am J Med* 2000;109:33–44.
45. Sendobry SM, Cornicelli JA, Welch K, et al: Attenuation of diet-induced atherosclerosis in rabbits with a highly selective 15-lipoxygenase inhibitor lacking significant antioxidant properties. *Br J Pharmacol* 1997;120:1199–1206.
46. Bocan TM, Rosebury WS, Mueller SB, et al: A specific 15-lipoxygenase inhibitor limits the progression and monocyte-macrophage enrichment of hypercholesterolemia-induced atherosclerosis in the rabbit. *Atherosclerosis* 1998;136:203–216.
47. Cyrus T, Witztum JL, Rader DJ, et al: Disruption of the 12/15-lipoxygenase gene diminishes atherosclerosis in apoE-deficient mice. *J Clin Invest* 1999;103:1597–1604.
48. Harats D, Shaish A, George J, et al: Overexpression of 15-lipoxygenase in vascular endothelium accelerates early atherosclerosis in LDL receptor-deficient mice. *Arterioscler Thromb Vasc Biol* 2000;20:2100–2105.
49. Shen J, Herderick E, Cornhill JF, et al: Macrophage-mediated 15-lipoxygenase expression protects against atherosclerosis development. *J Clin Invest* 1996;98:2201–2208.
50. Detmers PA, Hernandez M, Mudgett J, et al: Deficiency in inducible nitric oxide synthase results in reduced atherosclerosis in apolipoprotein E-deficient mice. *J Immunol* 2000;165:3430–3435.
51. Ihrig M, Dangler CA, Fox JG: Mice lacking inducible nitric oxide synthase develop spontaneous hypercholesterolaemia and aortic atheromas. *Atherosclerosis* 2001;156:103–107.
52. Shi W, Wang X, Shih DM, et al: Paradoxical reduction of fatty streak formation in mice lacking endothelial nitric oxide synthase. *Circulation* 2002;105:2078–2082.
53. Daugherty A, Dunn JL, Rateri DL, et al: Myeloperoxidase, a catalyst for lipoprotein oxidation, is expressed in human atherosclerotic lesions. *J Clin Invest* 1994;94:437–444.
54. Nicholls SJ, Zheng L, Hazen SL: Formation of dysfunctional high-density lipoprotein by myeloperoxidase. *Trends Cardiovasc Med* 2005;15:212–219.
55. Shao B, Oda MN, Bergt C, et al: myeloperoxidase impairs ABCA1-dependent cholesterol efflux through methionine oxidation and site-specific tyrosine chlorination of apolipoprotein A-I. *J Biol Chem* 2006;281:9001–9004.
56. Brennan ML, Anderson MM, Shih DM, et al: Increased atherosclerosis in myeloperoxidase-deficient mice. *J Clin Invest* 2001;107:419–430.
57. Tsimikas S, Witztum JL: The oxidative modification hypothesis of atherosclerosis. In Keaney JF (ed): Oxidative Stress and Vascular Disease. Boston, Kluwer Academic Publishers, 2000, pp 49–74.
58. Witztum JL, Steinberg D: The oxidative modification hypothesis of atherosclerosis: does it hold for humans? *Trends Cardiovasc Med* 2001;11:93–102.
59. Quinn MT, Parthasarathy S, Fong LG, et al: Oxidatively modified low-density lipoproteins: a potential role in recruitment and retention of monocyte/macrophages during atherogenesis. *Proc Natl Acad Sci USA* 1987;84:2995–2998.
60. McMurray HF, Parthasarathy S, Steinberg D: Oxidatively modified low-density lipoprotein is a chemoattractant for human T lymphocytes. *J Clin Invest* 1993;92:1004–1008.
61. Quinn MT, Parthasarathy S, Steinberg D: Endothelial cell-derived chemotactic activity for mouse peritoneal macrophages and the effects of modified forms of low-density lipoprotein. *Proc Natl Acad Sci USA* 1985;82:5949–5953.
62. Navab M, Ananthramaiah GM, Reddy ST, et al: Thematic review series: The pathogenesis of atherosclerosis: The oxidation hypothesis of atherogenesis: the role of oxidized phospholipids and HDL. *J Lipid Res* 2004;45:993–1007.
63. Leitinger N: Oxidized phospholipids as modulators of inflammation in atherosclerosis. *Curr Opin Lipidol* 2003;14:421–430.
64. Walton KA, Hsieh X, Gharavi N, et al: Receptors involved in the oxidized 1-palmitoyl-2-arachidonoyl-*sn*-glycero-3-phosphorylcholine-mediated synthesis of interleukin-8: a role for toll-like receptor 4 and a glycosylphosphatidylinositol-anchored protein. *J Biol Chem* 2003;278:29661–29666.
65. Li R, Mouillesseaux KP, Montoya D, et al: Identification of prostaglandin E_2 receptor subtype 2 as a receptor activated by Ox-PAPC. *Circ Res* 2006;98:642–650.
66. Huber J, Furnkranz A, Bochkov VN, et al: Specific monocyte adhesion to endothelial cells induced by oxidized phospholipids involves activation of cPLA2 and lipoxygenase. *J Lipid Res* 2006;47:1054–1062.
67. Bolick DT, Srinivasan S, Whetzel A, et al: 12/15 Lipoxygenase mediates monocyte adhesion to aortic endothelium in apolipoprotein E-deficient mice through activation of RhoA and NF-κB. *Arterioscler Thromb Vasc Biol* 2006;26:1260–1266.
68. Boullier A, Gillotte KL, Hörkkö S, et al: The binding of oxidized low-density lipoprotein to mouse CD36 is mediated in part by oxidized phospholipids that are associated with both the lipid and protein moieties of the lipoprotein. *J Biol Chem* 2000;275:9163–9169.
69. Febbraio M, Hajjar DP, Silverstein RL: CD36: a class B scavenger receptor involved in angiogenesis, atherosclerosis, inflammation, and lipid metabolism. *J Clin Invest* 2001;108:785–791.
70. Linton MF, Fazio S: Class A scavenger receptors, macrophages, and atherosclerosis. *Curr Opin Lipidol* 2001;12:489–495.
71. Li AC, Glass CK: The macrophage foam cell as a target for therapeutic intervention. *Nat Med* 2002;8:1235–1242.
72. Krieger M, Herz J: Structures and functions of multiligand lipoprotein receptors: macrophage scavenger receptors and LDL receptor-related protein (LRP). *Annu Rev Biochem* 1994;63:601–637.
73. Kunjathoor VV, Febbraio M, Podrez EA, et al: Scavenger receptors class A-I/II and CD36 are the principal receptors responsible for the uptake of modified low-density lipoprotein leading to lipid loading in macrophages. *J Biol Chem* 2002;277:49982–49988.
74. Nozaki S, Kashiwagi H, Yamashita S, et al: Reduced uptake of oxidized low-density lipoproteins in monocyte-derived macrophages from CD36-deficient subjects. *J Clin Invest* 1995;96:1859–1865.
75. Febbraio M, Podrez EA, Smith JD, et al: Targeted disruption of the class B scavenger receptor CD36 protects against atherosclerotic lesion development in mice. *J Clin Invest* 2000;105:1049–1056.
76. Suzuki H, Kurihara Y, Takeya M, et al: A role for macrophage scavenger receptors in atherosclerosis and susceptibility to infection. *Nature* 1997;386:292–296.
77. Sakaguchi H, Takeya M, Suzuki H, et al: Role of macrophage scavenger receptors in diet-induced atherosclerosis in mice. *Lab Invest* 1998;78:423–434.
78. Moore KJ, Kunjathoor VV, Koehn SL, et al: Loss of receptor mediated lipid uptake via scavenger receptor A or CD36 pathways does not ameliorate atherosclerosis in hyperlipidemic mice. *J Clin Invest* 2005;115:2192–2201.
79. Witztum JL: You are right too! *J Clin Invest* 2005;115:2072–2075.
80. Braun A, Trigatti BL, Post MJ, et al: Loss of SR-BI expression leads to the early onset of occlusive atherosclerotic coronary artery disease, spontaneous myocardial infarctions, severe cardiac dysfunction, and premature death in apolipoprotein E-deficient mice. *Circ Res* 2002;90:270–276.
81. Huszar D, Varban ML, Rinninger F, et al: Increased LDL cholesterol and atherosclerosis in LDL receptor-deficient mice with attenuated expression of scavenger receptor B1. *Arterioscler Thromb Vasc Biol* 2000;20:1068–1073.
82. Van Eck M, Bos IS, Hildebrand RB, et al: Dual role for scavenger receptor class B, type I on bone marrow-derived cells in atherosclerotic lesion development. *Am J Pathol*2004;165:785–794.
83. Huby T, Doucet C, Dachet C, et al: Knockdown expression and hepatic deficiency reveal an atheroprotective role for SR-BI in liver and peripheral tissues. *J Clin Invest* 2006;116:2767–2776.
84. Pennings M, Meurs I, Ye D, et al: Regulation of cholesterol homeostasis in macrophages and consequences for atherosclerotic lesion development. *FEBS Lett* 2006;580:5588–5596.

85. Willson TM, Brown PJ, Sternbach DD, et al: The PPARs: from orphan receptors to drug discovery. *J Med Chem* 2000;43: 527–550.
86. Chawla A, Lee CH, Barak Y, et al: PPAR delta is a very low-density lipoprotein sensor in macrophages. *Proc Natl Acad Sci USA* 2003;100:1268–1273.
87. Ziouzenkova O, Perrey S, Asatryan L, et al: Lipolysis of triglyceride-rich lipoproteins generates PPAR ligands: Evidence for an antiinflammatory role for lipoprotein lipase. *Proc Natl Acad Sci USA* 2003;100:2730–2735.
88. Forman BM, Tontonoz P, Chen J, et al: 15-Deoxy-delta 12, 14-prostaglandin J2 is a ligand for the adipocyte determination factor PPAR gamma. *Cell* 1995;83:803–812.
89. Kliewer SA, Lenhard JM, Willson TM, et al: A prostaglandin J2 metabolite binds peroxisome proliferator-activated receptor gamma and promotes adipocyte differentiation. *Cell* 1995;83: 813–819.
90. Huang JT, Welch JS, Ricote M, et al: Interleukin-4-dependent production of PPAR-gamma ligands in macrophages by 12/15-lipoxygenase. *Nature* 1999;400:378–382.
91. Nagy L, Tontonoz P, Alvarez JG, et al: Oxidized LDL regulates macrophage gene expression through ligand activation of PPARgamma. *Cell* 1998;93:229–240.
92. Jedidi I, Couturier M, Therond P, et al: Cholesteryl ester hydroperoxides increase macrophage CD36 gene expression via PPAR[alpha]. *Biochem Biophys Res Commun* 2006;351: 733–738.
93. Ricote M, Huang J, Fajas L, et al: Expression of the peroxisome proliferator-activated receptor gamma (PPARgamma) in human atherosclerosis and regulation in macrophages by colony stimulating factors and oxidized low-density lipoprotein. *Proc Natl Acad Sci USA* 1998;95:7614–7619.
94. Ricote M, Li AC, Willson TM, et al: The peroxisome proliferator-activated receptor-gamma is a negative regulator of macrophage activation. *Nature* 1998;391:79–82.
95. Tontonoz P, Nagy L, Alvarez JG, et al: PPARgamma promotes monocyte/macrophage differentiation and uptake of oxidized LDL. *Cell* 1998;93:241–252.
96. Jiang C, Ting AT, Seed B: PPAR-gamma agonists inhibit production of monocyte inflammatory cytokines. *Nature* 1998;391:82–86.
97. Marx N, Schonbeck U, Lazar MA, et al: Peroxisome proliferator-activated receptor gamma activators inhibit gene expression and migration in human vascular smooth muscle cells. *Circ Res* 1998;83:1097–1103.
98. Repa JJ, Liang G, Ou J, et al: Regulation of mouse sterol regulatory element-binding protein-1c gene (SREBP-1c) by oxysterol receptors, LXRalpha and LXRbeta. *Genes Dev* 2000;14: 2819–2830.
99. Chawla A, Repa JJ, Evans RM, et al: Nuclear receptors and lipid physiology: opening the X-files. *Science* 2001;294: 1866–1870.
100. Laffitte BA, Repa JJ, Joseph SB, et al: LXRs control lipid-inducible expression of the apolipoprotein E gene in macrophages and adipocytes. *Proc Natl Acad Sci USA* 2001;98:507–512.
101. Zhu Y, Liao H, Xie X, et al: Oxidized LDL downregulates ATP-binding cassette transporter-1 in human vascular endothelial cells via inhibiting liver X receptor (LXR). *Cardiovasc Res* 2005;68:425–432.
102. Kim OS, Lee CS, Joe EH, et al: Oxidized low-density lipoprotein suppresses lipopolysaccharide-induced inflammatory responses in microglia: Oxidative stress acts through control of inflammation. *Biochem Biophys Res Commun* 2006; 342:9–18.
103. Chawla A, Boisvert WA, Lee CH, et al: A PPAR[gamma]-LXR-ABCA1 pathway in macrophages is involved in cholesterol efflux and atherogenesis. *Mol Cell* 2001;7:161–171.
104. Libby P: Inflammation in atherosclerosis. *Nature* 2002;420: 868–874.
105. Steinberg D: Atherogenesis in perspective: hypercholesterolemia and inflammation as partners in crime. *Nat Med* 2002;8:1211–1217.
106. Kawai T, Akira S: TLR signaling. *Cell Death Differ* 2006;13: 816–825.
107. Hoebe K, Georgel P, Rutschmann S, et al: CD36 is a sensor of diacylglycerides. *Nature* 2005;433:523–527.
108. Bjorkbacka H, Kunjathoor VV, Moore KJ, et al: Reduced atherosclerosis in MyD88-null mice links elevated serum cholesterol levels to activation of innate immunity signaling pathways. *Nat Med* 2004;10:416–421.
109. Michelsen KS, Wong MH, Shah PK, et al: Lack of Toll-like receptor 4 or myeloid differentiation factor 88 reduces atherosclerosis and alters plaque phenotype in mice deficient in apolipoprotein E. *Proc Nat Acad Sci USA* 2004;101:10679–10684.
110. Mullick AE, Tobias PS, Curtiss LK: Modulation of atherosclerosis in mice by Toll-like receptor 2. *J Clin Invest* 2005;115: 3149–3156.
111. Kiechl S, Lorenz E, Reindl M, et al: Toll-like receptor 4 polymorphisms and atherogenesis. *N Engl J Med* 2002;347: 185–192.
112. Ameziane N, Beillat T, Verpillat P, et al: Association of the Toll-like receptor 4 gene Asp299Gly polymorphism with acute coronary events. *Arterioscler Thromb Vasc Biol* 2003;23: 61e–664.
113. Norata GD, Garlaschelli K, Ongari M, et al: Effect of the Toll-like receptor 4 (TLR-4) variants on intima–media thickness and monocyte-derived macrophage response to LPS. *J Intern Med* 2005;258:21–27.
114. Zee RYL, Hegener HH, Gould J, et al: Toll-like receptor 4 Asp-299Gly gene polymorphism and risk of atherothrombosis. *Stroke* 2005;36:154–157.
115. Miller YI, Viriyakosol S, Binder CJ, et al: Minimally modified LDL binds to CD14, induces macrophage spreading via TLR4/ MD-2, and inhibits phagocytosis of apoptotic cells. *J Biol Chem* 2003;278:1561–1568.
116. Miller YI, Viriyakosol S, Worrall DS, et al: Toll-like receptor 4-dependent and -independent cytokine secretion induced by minimally oxidized low-density lipoprotein in macrophages. *Arterioscler Thromb Vasc Biol* 2005;25:1213–1219.
117. Liu J, Thewke DP, Su YR, et al: Reduced macrophage apoptosis is associated with accelerated atherosclerosis in low-density lipoprotein receptor-null mice. *Arterioscler Thromb Vasc Biol* 2005;25:174–179.
118. Arai S, Shelton JM, Chen M, et al: A role for the apoptosis inhibitory factor AIM/Spalpha/Api6 in atherosclerosis development. *Cell Metab* 2005;1:201–213.
119. Tabas I. Consequences and therapeutic implications of macrophage apoptosis in atherosclerosis. The importance of lesion stage and phagocytic efficiency. *Arterioscler Thromb Vasc Biol* 2005;25:2255–2264.
120. Schrijvers DM, De Meyer GRY, Kockx MM, et al: Phagocytosis of apoptotic cells by macrophages is impaired in atherosclerosis. *Arterioscler Thromb Vasc Biol* 2005;25:1256–1261.
121. Yuan XM, Li W, Brunk UT, et al: Lysosomal destabilization during macrophage damage induced by cholesterol oxidation products. *Free Rad Biol Med* 2000;28:208–218.
122. Napoli C, Quehenberger O, de Nigris F, et al: Mildly oxidized low-density lipoprotein activates multiple apoptotic signaling pathways in human coronary cells. *FASEB J* 2000;14:1996–2007.
123. Colles SM, Maxson JM, Carlson SG, Chisoim 6M: Oxidized LDL-induced injury and apoptosis in atherosclerosis. Potential roles for oxysterols. *Trends Cardiovasc Med* 2001;11:131–138.
124. Salvayre R, Auge N, Benoist H, et al: Oxidized low-density lipoprotein-induced apoptosis. *Biochim Biophys Acta* 2002;1585: 213–221.
125. Boullier A, Li Y, Quehenberger O, et al: Minimally oxidized LDL offsets the apoptotic effects of extensively oxidized LDL and free cholesterol in macrophages. *Arterioscler Thromb Vasc Biol* 2006;26:1169–1176.
126. Witztum JL: The oxidation hypothesis of atherosclerosis. *Lancet* 1994;344:793–795.
127. Song L, Leung C, Schindler C: Lymphocytes are important in early atherosclerosis. *J Clin Invest* 2001;108:251–259.
128. Binder CJ, Chang MK, Shaw PX, et al: Innate and acquired immunity in atherogenesis. *Nat Med* 2002;8:1218–1226.
129. Palinski W, Hörkkö S, Miller E, et al: Cloning of monoclonal autoantibodies to epitopes of oxidized lipoproteins from apolipoprotein E-deficient mice. Demonstration of epitopes of oxidized low-density lipoprotein in human plasma. *J Clin Invest* 1996;98:800–814.
130. Hörkkö S, Bird DA, Miller E, et al: Monoclonal autoantibodies specific for oxidized phospholipids or oxidized phospholipid-protein adducts inhibit macrophage uptake of oxidized low-density lipoproteins. *J Clin Invest* 1999;103:117–128.

131. Friedman P, Hörkkö S, Steinberg D, et al: Correlation of antiphospholipid antibody recognition with the structure of synthetic oxidized phospholipids: importance of Schiff base formation and Aldol condensation. *J Biol Chem* 2001;277:7010–7020.
132. Chang MK, Bergmark C, Laurila A, et al: Monoclonal antibodies against oxidized low-density lipoprotein bind to apoptotic cells and inhibit their phagocytosis by elicited macrophages: evidence that oxidation-specific epitopes mediate macrophage recognition. *Proc Natl Acad Sci USA.* 1999;96:6353–6358.
133. Shaw PX, Hörkkö S, Chang MK, et al: Natural antibodies with the T15 idiotype may act in atherosclerosis, apoptotic clearance, and protective immunity. *J Clin Invest* 2000;105:1731–1740.
134. Binder CJ, Hörkkö S, Dewan A, et al: Pneumococcal vaccination decreases atherosclerotic lesion formation: molecular mimicry between Streptococcus pneumoniae and oxidized LDL. *Nat Med* 2003;9:736–743.
135. Binder CJ, Shaw PX, Chang MK, et al: Thematic review series: the immune system and atherogenesis. The role of natural antibodies in atherogenesis. *J Lipid Res*2005;46:1353–1363.
136. Shaw PX, Hörkkö S, Tsimikas S, et al: Human-derived anti-oxidized LDL autoantibody blocks uptake of oxidized LDL by macrophages and localizes to atherosclerotic lesions *in vivo*. *Arterioscler Thromb Vasc Biol* 2001;21:1333–1339.
137. Tuominen A, Miller YI, Hansen LF, et al: A natural antibody to oxidized cardiolipin binds to oxidized low-density lipoprotein, apoptotic cells, and atherosclerotic lesions. *Arterioscler Thromb Vasc Biol* 2006;26:2096–2102.
138. Binder CJ, Hartvigsen K, Chang MK, et al: IL-5 links adaptive and natural immunity specific for epitopes of oxidized LDL and protects from atherosclerosis. *J Clin Invest* 2004;114: 427–437.
139. Tsimikas S, Glass C, Steinberg D, et al: Lipoproteins, lipoprotein oxidation and atherogenesis. In Chien KR (ed): Molecular Basis of Cardiovascular Disease. A Companion to Braunwald's Heart Disease. Philadelphia, W.B Saunders, 2004, pp 385–413.
140. Sundell CL, Somers PK, Meng CQ, et al: AGI-1067: A multifunctional phenolic antioxidant, lipid modulator, anti-inflammatory and anti-atherosclerotic agent. *J Pharmacol Exp Ther* 2003.
141. Cyrus T, Praticó D, Zhao L, et al: Absence of 12/15-lipoxygenase expression decreases lipid peroxidation and atherogenesis in apolipoprotein E-deficient mice. *Circulation* 2001;103: 2277–2282.
142. Steinberg D: At last, direct evidence that lipoxygenases play a role in atherogenesis. *J Clin Invest* 1999;103:1487–1488.
143. George J, Afek A, Shaish, A et al: 12/15-Lipoxygenase gene disruption attenuates atherogenesis in LDL receptor-deficient mice. *Circulation* 2001;104:1646–1650.
144. Heinecke JW: Is lipid peroxidation relevant to atherogenesis? *J Clin Invest* 1999;104:135–136.
145. Shih DM, Xia YR, Wang XP, et al: Combined serum paraoxonase knockout/apolipoprotein E knockout mice exhibit increased lipoprotein oxidation and atherosclerosis. *J Biol Chem* 2000;275:17527–17535.
146. Tsimikas S, Palinski W, Halpern SE, et al: Radiolabeled MDA2, an oxidation-specific, monoclonal antibody, identifies native atherosclerotic lesions *in vivo*. *J Nucl Cardiol* 1999;6: 41–53.
147. Aikawa M, Sugiyama S, Hill CC, et al: Lipid lowering reduces oxidative stress and endothelial cell activation in rabbit atheroma. *Circulation* 2002;106:1390–1396.
148. Tsimikas S, Palinski W, Witztum JL: Circulating autoantibodies to oxidized LDL correlate with arterial accumulation and depletion of oxidized LDL in LDL receptor-deficient mice. *Arterioscler Thromb Vasc Biol* 2001;21:95–100.
149. Tsimikas S, Aikawa M, Miller FJ Jr, et al: Increased plasma oxidized phospholipid:apolipoprotein b-100 ratio with concomitant depletion of oxidized phospholipids from atherosclerotic lesions after dietary lipid-lowering: a potential biomarker of early atherosclerosis regression. *Arterioscler Thromb Vasc Biol* 2007;27:175–181.
150. Steinberg D: Antioxidants in the prevention of human atherosclerosis. Summary of the proceedings of a National Heart, Lung, and Blood Institute Workshop: September 5–6, 1991, Bethesda, Maryland. *Circulation* 1992;85:2337–2344.
151. Reaven PD, Khouw A, Beltz WF, et al: Effect of dietary antioxidant combinations in humans. Protection of LDL by vitamin E but not by beta-carotene. *Arterioscler Thromb* 1993;13: 590–600.
152. Reaven PD, Witztum JL: Comparison of supplementation of RRR-alpha-tocopherol and racemic alpha-tocopherol in humans. Effects on lipid levels and lipoprotein susceptibility to oxidation. *Arterioscler Thromb* 1993;13:601–608.
153. Landmesser U, Harrison DG: Oxidant stress as a marker for cardiovascular events: Ox marks the spot. *Circulation* 2001;104: 2638–2640.
153a. Tardif J-C, McMurray JJ, Klug E, et al: Effects of succinobucol (ABI-1067) after an acute coronary syndrome: a randomized, double-blind, placebo-controlled trial. *Lancet* 2008;371: 1761–1768.
154. Steinberg D, Witztum JL: Is the oxidative modification hypothesis relevant to human atherosclerosis? Do the antioxidant trials conducted to date refute the hypothesis? *Circulation* 2002;105:2107–2111.
155. Shoenfeld Y, Wu R, Dearing LD, et al: Are anti-oxidized low-density lipoprotein antibodies pathogenic or protective? *Circulation* 2004;110:2552–2558.
156. Holvoet P, Perez G, Zhao Z, et al: Malondialdehyde-modified low-density lipoproteins in patients with atherosclerotic disease. *J Clin Invest* 1995;95:2611–2619.
157. Hörkkö S, Bird DA, Miller E, et al: Monoclonal autoantibodies specific for oxidized phospholipids or oxidized phospholipid-protein adducts inhibit macrophage uptake of oxidized low-density lipoproteins. *J Clin Invest* 1999;103:117–128.
158. Itabe H, Yamamoto H, Imanaka T, et al: Sensitive detection of oxidatively modified low-density lipoprotein using a monoclonal antibody. *J Lipid Res* 1996;37:45–53.
159. Tsimikas S: Measures of oxidative stress. *Clin Lab Med* 2006;26:571–590.
160. Matsumoto T, Takashima H, Ohira N, et al: Plasma level of oxidized low-density lipoprotein is an independent determinant of coronary macrovasomotor and microvasomotor responses induced by bradykinin. *J Am Coll Cardiol* 2004;44:451–457.
161. Liu ML, Ylitalo K, Salonen R, et al: Circulating oxidized low-density lipoprotein and its association with carotid intima–media thickness in asymptomatic members of familial combined hyperlipidemia families. *Arterioscler Thromb Vasc Biol* 2004;24:1492–1497.
162. Hulthe J, Fagerberg B: Circulating oxidized LDL is associated with subclinical atherosclerosis development and inflammatory cytokines (AIR Study). *Arterioscler Thromb Vasc Biol* 2002;22:1162–1167.
163. van Tits LJH, van Himbergen TM, Lemmers HLM, et al: Proportion of oxidized LDL relative to plasma apolipoprotein B does not change during statin therapy in patients with heterozygous familial hypercholesterolemia. *Atherosclerosis* 2006;185: 307–312.
164. Rodenburg J, Vissers MN, Wiegman A, et al: Oxidized low-density lipoprotein in children with familial hypercholesterolemia and unaffected siblings: effect of pravastatin. *J Am Coll Cardiol* 2006;47:1803–1810.
165. Holvoet P, Mertens A, Verhamme P, et al: Circulating oxidized LDL is a useful marker for identifying patients with coronary artery disease. *Arterioscler Thromb Vasc Biol* 2001;21: 844–848.
166. Suzuki T, Kohno H, Hasegawa A, et al: Diagnostic implications of circulating oxidized low-density lipoprotein levels as a biochemical risk marker of coronary artery disease. *Clin Biochem* 2002;35:347–353.
167. Toshima S, Hasegawa A, Kurabayashi M, et al: Circulating oxidized low-density lipoprotein levels: A biochemical risk marker for coronary heart disease. *Arterioscler Thromb Vasc Biol* 2000;20:2243–2247.
168. Holvoet P, Harris TB, Tracy RP, et al: Association of high coronary heart disease risk status with circulating oxidized LDL in the well-functioning elderly: findings from the health, aging, and body composition study. *Arterioscler Thromb Vasc Biol* 2003;23:1444–1448.
169. Tsimikas S, Brilakis ES, Miller ER, et al: Oxidized phospholipids, Lp(a) lipoprotein, and coronary artery disease. *N Engl J Med* 2005;353:46–57.
170. Tsimikas S, Bergmark C, Beyer RW, et al: Temporal increases in plasma markers of oxidized low-density lipoprotein strongly

reflect the presence of acute coronary syndromes. *J Am Coll Cardiol* 2003;41:360–370.
171. Tsimikas S, Lau HK, Han KR, et al: Percutaneous coronary intervention results in acute increases in oxidized phospholipids and lipoprotein(a): short-term and long-term immunologic responses to oxidized low-density lipoprotein. *Circulation* 2004;109:3164–3170.
172. Tsimikas S, Witztum JL, Miller ER, et al: High-dose atorvastatin reduces total plasma levels of oxidized phospholipids and immune complexes present on apolipoprotein B-100 in patients with acute coronary syndromes in the MIRACL trial. *Circulation* 2004;110:1406–1412.
173. Tsimikas S, Kiechl S, Willeit J, et al: Oxidized phospholipids predict the presence and progression of carotid and femoral atherosclerosis and symptomatic cardiovascular disease: five-year prospective results from the Bruneck study. *J Am Coll Cardiol* 2006;47:2219–2228.
174. Edelstein C, Pfaffinger D, Hinman J, et al: Lysine-phosphatidylcholine adducts in kringle V impart unique immunological and potential pro-inflammatory properties to human apolipoprotein(a). *J Biol Chem* 2003;278:52841–52847.
175. Ehara S, Ueda M, Naruko T, et al: Elevated levels of oxidized low-density lipoprotein show a positive relationship with the severity of acute coronary syndromes. *Circulation* 2001;103: 1955–1960.
176. Holvoet P, Vanhaecke J, Janssens S, et al: Oxidized LDL and malondialdehyde-modified LDL in patients with acute coronary syndromes and stable coronary artery disease. *Circulation* 1998;98:1487–1494.
177. Holvoet P, Collen D, van de Werf F: Malondialdehyde-modified LDL as a marker of acute coronary syndromes. *JAMA* 1999;281:1718–1721.
178. Hayashida K, Kume N, Murase T, et al: Serum soluble lectin-like oxidized low-density lipoprotein receptor-1 levels are elevated in acute coronary syndrome: a novel marker for early diagnosis. *Circulation* 2005;112:812–818.
179. Cominacini L, Anselmi M, Garbin U, et al: Enhanced plasma levels of oxidized low-density lipoprotein increase circulating nuclear factor-kappa B activation in patients with unstable angina. *J Am Coll Cardiol* 2005;46:799–806.
180. Nishi K, Itabe H, Uno M, et al: Oxidized LDL in carotid plaques and plasma associates with plaque instability. *Arterioscler Thromb Vasc Biol* 2002;22:1649–1654.
181. Crisby M, Nordin-Fredriksson G, Shah PK, et al: Pravastatin treatment increases collagen content and decreases lipid content, inflammation, metalloproteinases, and cell death in human carotid plaques: Implications for plaque stabilization. *Circulation* 2001;103:926–933.
182. Segev A, Strauss BH, Witztum JL, et al: Relationship of a comprehensive panel of plasma oxidized low-density lipoprotein markers to angiographic restenosis in patients undergoing percutaneous coronary intervention for stable angina. *Am Heart J* 2005;150:1007–1014.
183. Naruko T, Ueda M, Ehara S, et al: Persistent high levels of plasma oxidized low-density lipoprotein after acute myocardial infarction predict stent restenosis. *Arterioscler Thromb Vasc Biol* 2006;26:877–883.
184. Braun S, Ndrepepa G, von Beckerath N, et al: Lack of association between circulating levels of plasma oxidized low-density lipoproteins and clinical outcome after coronary stenting. *Am Heart J* 2005;150:550–556.
185. Kiechl S, Willeit J, Mayr M, et al: Oxidized phospholipids, lipoprotein(a), lipoprotein-associated phospholipase A2 activity and 10-year cardiovascular outcomes: prospective results from the Bruneck study. *Arterioscler Thromb Vasc Biol* 2007;27:1788–1795.
186. Shimada K, Mokuno H, Matsunaga E, et al: Circulating oxidized low-density lipoprotein is an independent predictor for cardiac event in patients with coronary artery disease. *Atherosclerosis* 2004;174:343–347.
187. Holvoet P, Kritchevsky SB, Tracy RP, et al: The metabolic syndrome, circulating oxidized LDL, and risk of myocardial infarction in well-functioning elderly people in the health, aging, and body composition cohort. *Diabetes* 2004;53: 1068–1073.
188. Meisinger C, Baumert J, Khuseyinova N, et al: Plasma oxidized low-density lipoprotein, a strong predictor for acute coronary heart disease events in apparently healthy, middle-aged men from the general population. *Circulation* 2005;112:651–657.
189. Tsimikas S, Willerson JT, Ridker PM: C-Reactive protein and other emerging blood biomarkers to optimize risk stratification of vulnerable patients. *J Am Coll Cardiol* 2006;47:C19–C31.
190. Walldius G, Erikson U, Olsson AG, et al: The effect of probucol on femoral atherosclerosis: the Probucol Quantitative Regression Swedish Trial (PQRST). *Am J Cardiol* 1994;74:875–883.
191. Lonn E, Yusuf S, Dzavik V, et al: Effects of ramipril and vitamin E on atherosclerosis: The study to evaluate carotid ultrasound changes in patients treated with ramipril and vitamin E (SECURE). *Circulation* 2001;103:919–925.
192. Brown BG, Zhao XQ, Chait A, et al: Simvastatin and niacin, antioxidant vitamins, or the combination for the prevention of coronary disease. *N Engl J Med* 2001;345:1583–1592.
193. Sawayama Y, Shimizu C, Maeda N, et al: Effects of probucol and pravastatin on common carotid Atherosclerosis in patients with asymptomatic hypercholesterolemia: Fukuoka Atherosclerosis Trial (FAST). *J Am Coll Cardiol* 2002;39: 610–616.
194. Fang JC, Kinlay S, Beltrame J, et al: Effect of vitamins C and E on progression of transplant-associated arteriosclerosis: a randomised trial. *Lancet* 2002;359:1108–1113.
195. Hodis HN, Mack WJ, LaBree L, et al: Alpha-tocopherol supplementation in healthy individuals reduces low-density lipoprotein oxidation but not atherosclerosis: the Vitamin E Atherosclerosis Prevention Study (VEAPS). *Circulation* 2002;106:1453–1459.
196. Tardif JC, Gregoire J, Schwartz L, et al: Effects of AGI-1067 and probucol after percutaneous coronary interventions. *Circulation* 2003;107:552–558.
197. Salonen RM, Nyyssonen K, Kaikkonen J, et al: Six-year effect of combined vitamin C and E supplementation on atherosclerotic progression: the Antioxidant Supplementation in Atherosclerosis Prevention (ASAP) Study. *Circulation* 2003;107: 947–953.
198. Magliano D, McNeil J, Branley P, et al: The Melbourne Atherosclerosis Vitamin E Trial (MAVET): a study of high dose vitamin E in smokers. *Eur J Cardiovasc Prev Rehabil* 2006;13: 341–347.
199. Tardif JC, Cote G, Lesperance J, et al: Probucol and multivitamins in the prevention of restenosis after coronary angioplasty. Multivitamins and Probucol Study Group. *N Engl J Med* 1997;337:365–372.
200. Yokoi H, Daida H, Kuwabara Y, et al: Effectiveness of an antioxidant in preventing restenosis after percutaneous transluminal coronary angioplasty: the Probucol Angioplasty Restenosis Trial. *J Am Coll Cardiol* 1997;30:855–862.
201. Serruys PW, Foley DP, Hofling B, et al: Carvedilol for prevention of restenosis after directional coronary atherectomy: final results of the European carvedilol atherectomy restenosis (EUROCARE) trial. *Circulation* 2000;101:1512–1518.
202. Beta Carotene Cancer Prevention Study Group The Alpha-Tocopherol. The Effect of Vitamin E and Beta Carotene on the Incidence of Lung Cancer and Other Cancers in Male Smokers. *N Engl J Med.* 1994;330:1029–1035.
203. Stephens NG, Parsons A, Schofield PM et al: Randomised controlled trial of vitamin E in patients with coronary disease: Cambridge Heart Antioxidant Study (CHAOS). *Lancet* 1996;347: 781–786.
204. Dietary supplementation with n-3 polyunsaturated fatty acids and vitamin E after myocardial infarction: results of the GISSI-Prevenzione trial. *Lancet* 1999;354:447–455.
205. The Heart Outcomes Prevention Evaluation Study Investigators. Vitamin E Supplementation and Cardiovascular Events in High-Risk Patients. *N Engl J Med* 2000;342:154–160.
206. Boaz M, Smetana S, Weinstein T et al: Secondary prevention with antioxidants of cardiovascular disease in endstage renal disease (SPACE): randomised placebo-controlled trial. *Lancet* 2000;356:1213–1218.
207. Roncaglioni MC. Low-dose aspirin and vitamin E in people at cardiovascular risk: a randomised trial in general practice. *Lancet* 2001;357:89–95.
208. MRC/BHF Heart Protection Study of cholesterol lowering with simvastatin in 20,536 high-risk individuals: a randomised placebo-controlled trial. *Lancet* 2002;360:7–22.

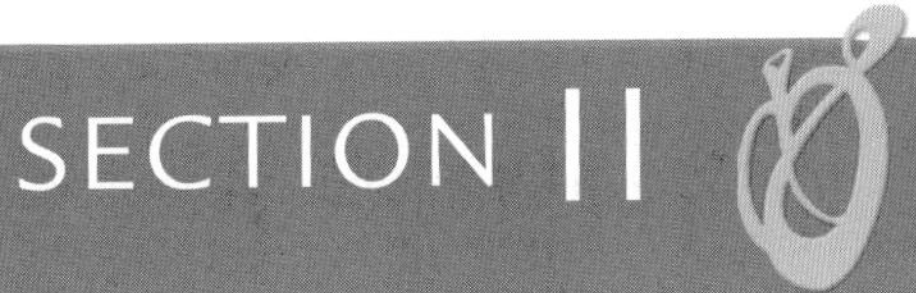

SECTION II

Risk Assessment

CHAPTER 9

Cholesterol: Concentration, Ratio, and Particle Number

Ngoc-Anh Le and Peter W. F. Wilson

ABSTRACT

Atherosclerosis is a chronic disease associated with excess deposition of cholesterol along the arterial walls of blood vessels. The initiation and rate of progression of atherosclerotic disease depends on multiple factors, and cholesterol is one of the key parameters. In plasma, cholesterol is distributed among several classes of lipoproteins, each with distinct effect on the disease process. Having a single cholesterol number for a management goal is a useful way to simplify the message to the layperson and the busy clinician. Low-density lipoprotein (LDL) cholesterol, which accounts for 60% of the cholesterol in plasma, has been the preferred index for many years. More recently, there is increasing evidence that the protective effect of high-density lipoprotein (HDL) cholesterol, as well as the atherogenic impact of triglyceride (TG)-rich lipoproteins, should be taken into account. There has also been some interest over the years in the use of protein concentrations as an alternative to cholesterol levels for risk assessment. Until recently, standardization of immunoassays for protein quantitation has been difficult, especially in view of the different analytic methods available, including radioimmunoassay, enzyme-linked immunosorbent assay (ELISA), and nephlometric, immunoturbidimetric, and immunobead methods. This chapter reviews epidemiologic and clinical evidence in support of newer indices for cholesterol metabolism as it is related to cardiovascular risk.

PLASMA AND LIPOPROTEIN CHOLESTEROL

Atherosclerosis is a complex disease that develops over several decades of life and depends on environmental and genetic factors.[1] Different hypotheses have been forwarded to explain the initiation and rate of progression of atherosclerotic disease, and the key component in the formation of atherosclerotic plaques is cholesterol.[2] In plasma, most of the cholesterol is transported in spherical particles ranging in diameter from 800 to 1000 Å.[3] Of the total cholesterol in fasting plasma, 60% is associated with LDL, 30% with HDL, and 10% with very-low-density lipoproteins (VLDL). The concentration of chylomicrons, which are present only during the postabsorptive state, may range from 10 to 25 mg/dL, depending on the cholesterol content of recent meals. In spite of the relatively low concentrations in plasma, chylomicrons are responsible for the transport of the entire dietary cholesterol load, which may range from 200 mg/day to 500 mg/day, depending on individual dietary habits.

CHOLESTEROL AND CARDIOVASCULAR DISEASE

From a screening and follow-up study of 356,222 men between the ages of 35 and 57 years who were free of history of hospitalization for myocardial infarction (MI), the Multiple Risk Factor Intervention Trial (MRFIT) investigators reported that for each 5-year age group, the relationship between serum cholesterol and coronary heart disease (CHD) death rate was continuous, graded, and highly significant.[4] The investigators also reported that the age-adjusted risk of CHD death for the highest quintile of cholesterol (≥240 mg/dL, or 6.34 mmol/L) was 3.4-fold greater than that of the lowest quintile (cholesterol 182–202 mg/dL, or 4.71–5.22 mmol/L). Of all CHD deaths, 46% were estimated to be excess deaths attributable to serum cholesterol levels of 180 mg/dL (4.65 mmol/L) or greater.[4] This finding is consistent with the hypothesis advanced by Keys in his survey of cholesterol levels and mortality in different populations around the world[5] as well as with the data from the Framingham Heart Study[6] and the Pooling Project Research Group.[7]

Although the analytical method for the chemical analysis of various lipoprotein fractions has been well documented since 1967, the first population data to highlight the importance of LDL cholesterol did not appear until the Lipid Research Clinics Program report was released in 1979.[8] In fact, results from the Lipid Research Clinics Coronary Primary Prevention Trial have been central in demonstrating that reductions in total cholesterol and LDL cholesterol were associated with reduction in CHD risk. It was reported that a 25% reduction in cholesterol or a 35% reduction in LDL cholesterol resulted in a 49% decrease in CHD risk.[9,10] There are three different estimates available for LDL cholesterol:

- LDL cholesterol = CHOL − HDL cholesterol – TG/5, commonly known as the Friedewald formula.[11] From the cholesterol contents in VLDL isolated by ultracentrifugation, investigators demonstrated that VLDL cholesterol can be approximated by dividing total plasma TG by 5. This is a very good approximation of LDL cholesterol when TG is less than 400 mg/dL.
- BQ_{LDLC} = Bottom Cholesterol − HDL cholesterol. This is known as the beta-quantitation method standardized by the Lipid Research Clinics Program.[12] In this instance, bottom cholesterol corresponds to the cholesterol content in the supernate after the removal of the TG-rich lipoproteins by ultracentrifugation at density 1.006 g/mL. This approach can be used for TG greater than 400 mg/dL, but it is time consuming and requires a highly standardized procedure to minimize loss during the ultracentrifugation.
- Direct LDL cholesterol. Homogeneous methods have been implemented that allow the direct determination of LDL cholesterol from plasma/serum after the precipitation of HDL and TG-rich lipoproteins. The advantage of these newer LDL cholesterol kits is that all of the steps can be completed automatically.

CHOLESTEROL RATIOS AND CARDIOVASCULAR DISEASE

The first indication that there may be other lipid risk factors for CHD besides elevated total cholesterol may be credited to the work of Barr and coworkers in 1951.[13] Using a series of extraction steps, different fractions of plasma were isolated and characterized for protein and cholesterol contents. Patients with atherosclerosis, diabetes, or nephrotic syndrome tended to have higher cholesterol levels compared with normal men and women, and the percentage of total cholesterol in specific lipid fraction of plasma was variable.[13] This situation was demonstrated for alphalipoproteins, or HDL, and the need to incorporate HDL cholesterol as part of the "lipoprotein profile" in the prediction of CHD risk was asserted by Ancel Keys in 1983.[14] The role of HDL in reverse cholesterol transport was first reported by Stender and Hjelms.[15] From the injection of autologous plasma containing either radiolabeled free cholesterol or radiolabeled cholesteryl esters into nonatherosclerotic patients prior to a scheduled surgical procedure, the investigators were able to demonstrate that the influx of cholesteryl esters into the aorta was too high to explain the measured cholesteryl ester contents in the intima–media layer of the ascending aortic wall. They concluded that there must be cholesterol efflux from the arterial wall. In a subset of individuals, direct specific activity data in LDL and HDL suggested that HDL may be involved in cholesterol efflux, a hypothesis that was later confirmed in animal studies.[16,17] The contribution of low HDL cholesterol in the prediction of CHD risk is well documented by subsequent epidemiologic studies.[18]

Attempts to incorporate information regarding HDL cholesterol into the risk assessment have been varied. Investigators from the Framingham Heart Study used bivariate cross tabulations of LDL cholesterol, HDL cholesterol, and VLDL cholesterol to demonstrate that the joint consideration of different lipoprotein cholesterol patterns provides information that could not be appreciated by univariate analysis and may be important in assessing CHD risk.[19]

The two most common approaches to incorporate HDL cholesterol information into risk assessment has been CHOL/HDL cholesterol ratio[20–22] and nonHDL cholesterol = CHOL − HDL cholesterol.[23] In the Scandinavian Simvastatin Survival Study (4S), CHOL/HDL cholesterol ratio had the strongest association with risk.[23] After 1 year of treatment with simvastatin, each 1% decrease in CHOL/HDL cholesterol ratio was associated with a 1.3% reduction in CHD risk.[23] In the Air Force/Texas Coronary Atherosclerosis Prevention study (*AFCAPS/Tex CAPS*)[24] the LDL cholesterol/HDL cholesterol ratio at baseline was also found to be associated with the risk of a first acute major coronary event. The appropriateness of the LDL cholesterol/HDL cholesterol ratio, however, has been questioned by some, because until recently LDL cholesterol was a calculated value which depended on HDL cholesterol. Thus in this ratio, the value for HDL cholesterol is reflected in both the numerator and the denominator. The same circular reason would be applicable to the use of nonHDL cholesterol/HDL cholesterol ratio.

Data from 4S also indicated that baseline nonHDL cholesterol was strongly associated with CHD risk.[23] Because the value calculated as nonHDL cholesterol would include cholesterol associated with other apolipoprotein B (apoB)–containing lipoproteins that may be as atherogenic as LDL, this parameter has been favored by some. In fact, nonHDL cholesterol has been recommended as a secondary therapeutic target (after LDL cholesterol) in individuals with elevated TG concentrations.[25]

APOLIPOPROTEINS AND CARDIOVASCULAR DISEASE

Total cholesterol level is minimally affected by postprandial lipemia, but the distribution of cholesterol among the various lipoprotein fractions may be affected by activities of cholesteryl ester transfer protein (CETP) and lecithin:cholesterol acyltransferase (LCAT) (Figure. 9-1). LCAT is responsible for the conversion of unesterified cholesterol on nascent HDL to cholesteryl esters, which can potentially be exchanged to TG-rich lipoproteins for TG. During postprandial lipemia with the presence of high TG substrate, the net result would be a transient redistribution of cholesteryl esters from HDL to VLDL—a net reduction in HDL cholesterol. The redistribution of cholesterol from HDL to LDL and VLDL can also be d emonstrated *in vitro* as the plasma is exposed to room temperature for an extended period of time. Figure 9-2, *A,* illustrates the redistribution of cholesterol from HDL to apoB-containing lipoproteins as whole plasma was incubated at 37°C for 4 hours before fractionation by FPLC.[26] There was concomitant movement of TG from VLDL to LDL- and HDL-sized particles (Fig. 9-2*B*). This redistribution was inhibited by the addition of a specific inhibitor of CETP to whole plasma during the incubation (Figure 9-2, *C*). Similar redistribution of cholesterol and TG can be demonstrated with plasma kept at room temperature for 8 hours. The extent of this redistribution depends on the lipid concentrations in the respective lipoprotein substrates and the activity of CETP present in the plasma. Because of this potential source of biologic variability, the concentrations of the structural proteins for the various lipoprotein fractions have been used as indices of cholesterol transport.[27–29] ApoB is the key structural protein for the TG-rich lipoproteins, non fasting chylomicrons, and fasting VLDL, as well as for LDL. ApoA-I is considered a key protein for HDL particles. In fact, Mao and coworkers were among the first investigators to suggest that apoA-I levels may be a better marker of angiographically assessed CHD.[30–31]

Several large prospective studies have demonstrated that apoB measurements are superior to any of the cholesterol-based indices with respect to CHD risk. The Québec Cardiovascular Study showed that apoB was the strongest predictor of risk for CHD in 2155 men followed for 5.5 years.[32] After controlling for TG, HDL cholesterol, and CHOL/HDL cholesterol ratio, the relationship between apoB and CHD risk remained statistically significant. In fact, when data from the long-term 13-year follow-up were available, apoB remained a strong correlate with CHD risk.[33] The Apolipoprotein-related Mortality Risk (AMORIS) study, based on 177,533 Swedish men and women, also found that apoB was superior to the cholesterol indices in predicting risk for the entire cohort as well as for all major subgroups.[34] Of particular interest in AMORIS was the difference associated with age and gender. Levels of LDL cholesterol were predictive only in participants younger than age 70, and apoB was strongly predictive in both age groups. Although LDL cholesterol was only weakly predictive in women, apoB was strongly predictive in both sexes. It should be noted that in AMORIS, LDL cholesterol was calculated using a formula that is different from the Friedewald calculation. In the Northwick Park Heart Study in 2508 healthy, middle-aged men followed for 6 years, apoB was superior to LDL cholesterol in identifying coronary events.[25] ApoB was found to be superior to LDL cholesterol in identifying cardiovascular risk for women participating in the Nurses' Health Study,[35] in patients who had experienced MI in the Thrombogenic Factors and Recurrent Coronary Events (THROMBO) study,[36] in patients with type 2 diabetes mellitus in the Health Professionals' Follow-up Study,[37] and in the Women's Health Study.[38] Figure 9-3 summarizes the key results from AMORIS with respect to the advantage of apoB/apoA-I ratio as compared to CHOL/HDL cholesterol ratio. After adjustment for age, the odds ratio for the risk of fatal MI based on 1-SD change in each variable was found to be 1.53 for men and 1.43 for women using the apoB/apoA-I ratio (Figure 9-3, *A*). The odds ratio did not differ from 1.00 when other ratios, including LDL cholesterol/HDL cholesterol, CHOL/HDL cholesterol, and non-HDL cholesterol/HDL cholesterol, were used.[39] Furthermore, the age-adjusted odds ratio for the risk of fatal MI was also found to be dose dependent across quintiles of the apoB/apoA-I ratio (Figure 9-3, *B*).[39] In fact, among men in the lowest quintile (Q1) of apoB/apoA-I ratio, 72.9% had CHOL/HDL cholesterol in Q1 and 23.4% had CHOL/HDL cholesterol in the second quintile (Q2). This concordance was 71.5% for men in the highest quintile (Q5) of apoB/apoA-I. The concordance between apoB/apoA-I ratio and CHOL/HDL cholesterol ratio in women

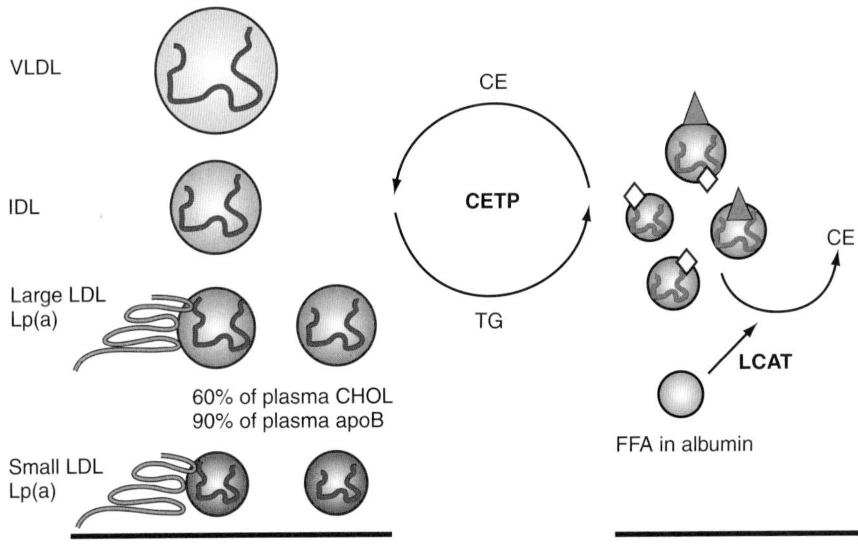

FIGURE 9-1 Dynamic equilibration of plasma lipids among the major lipoprotein classes. Cholesterol and TG levels in each lipoprotein fraction are in a quasi-steady state. While values can be obtained for each metabolite in the different lipoprotein classes, the lipoproteins are constantly under remodeling, and redistribution of the lipid molecules is ongoing all of the time.

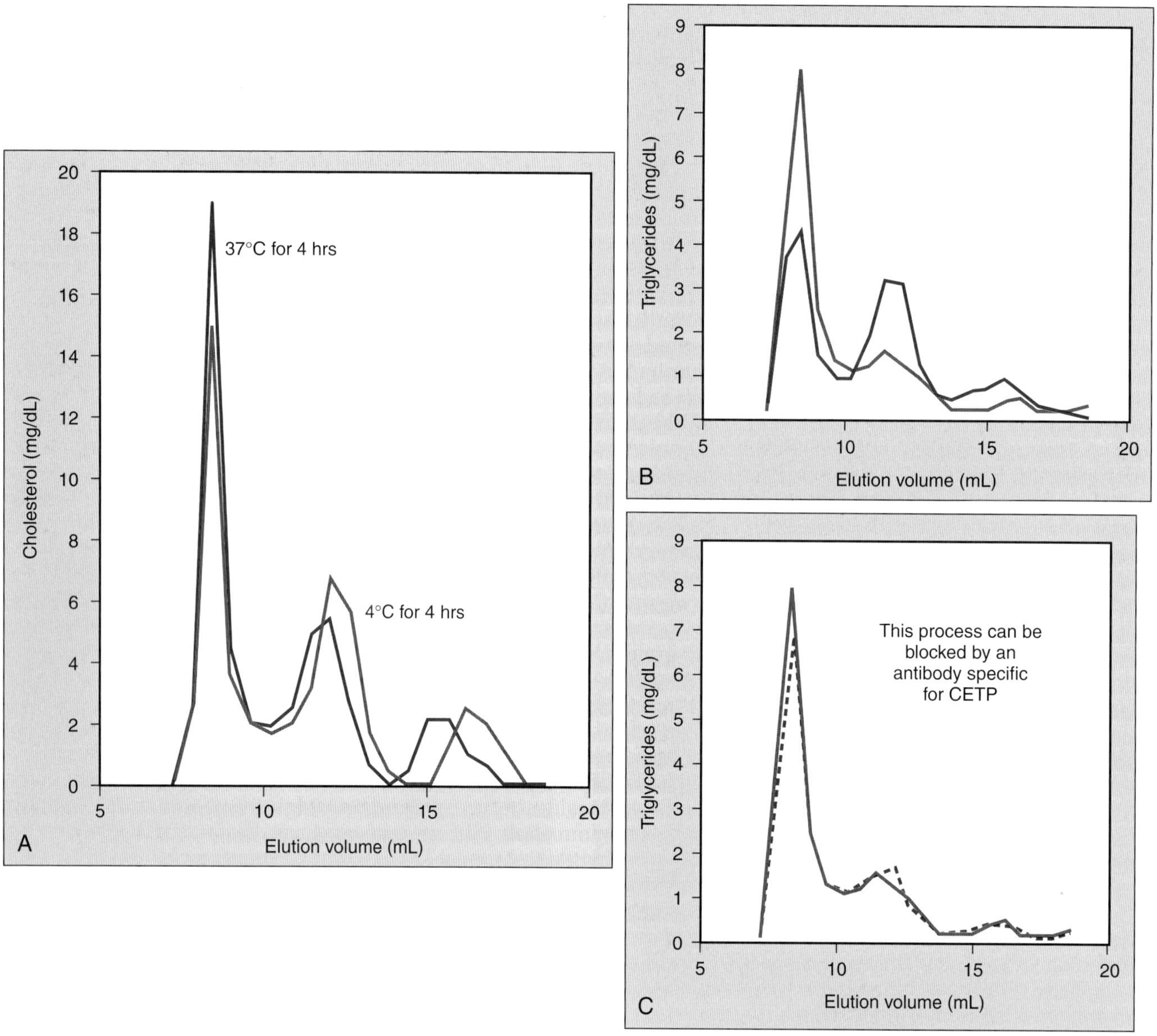

FIGURE 9-2 Effect of CETP on cholesterol and TG distribution *in vitro*. Unless the plasma specimen is handled properly, artifactual changes in the cholesterol and TG distribution among plasma lipoproteins can occur spontaneously. *A,* The net result is lower values for both HDL cholesterol and LDL cholesterol, while VLDL cholesterol is increased. *B,* TG contents of LDL and HDL could be significantly increased. *C,* This *in vitro* redistribution results from the activity of CETP present in whole plasma.

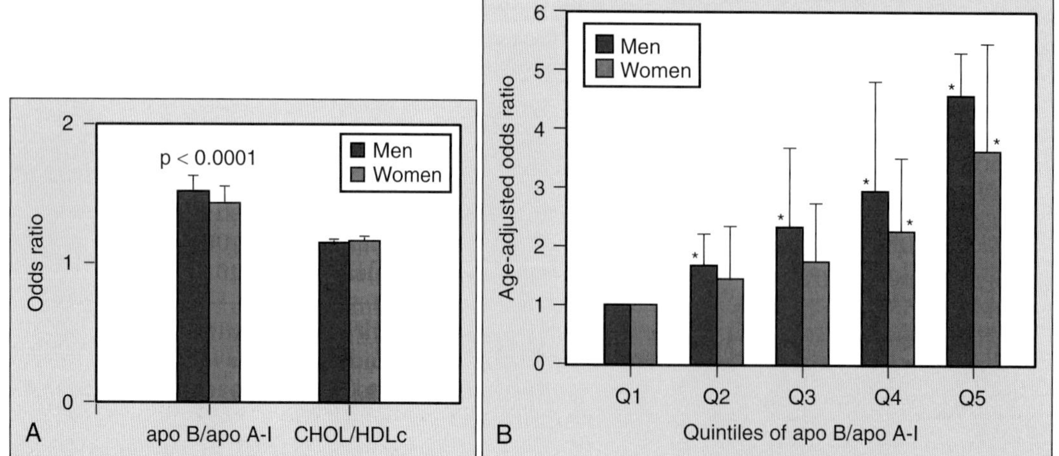

FIGURE 9-3 *A,* Adjusted odds ratio for future cardiovascular disease events in men and women from AMORIS using either the apoB/apoA-I ratio or CHOL/HDL cholesterol ratio. *B,* The adjusted odds ratio can be shown to be graded over the entire range of apoB/apoA-I values.

was 73% and 78% for Q1 and Q5, respectively. For the intermediate quintiles, however, the concordance was quite poor. For instance, among men in the third quintile (Q3) of apoB/apoA-I ratio, 24.3%, 42.2%, and 27.9% would be classified as Q2, Q3 and Q4, respectively, for CHOL/HDL cholesterol. In other words, 52.2% would be incorrectly classified using CHOL/HDL cholesterol ratio. For women, 50.8% in Q3 of apoB/apoA-I would be incorrectly classified if CHOL/HDL cholesterol ratio was used. In both men and women of AMORIS, the risk of fatal MI was additive in relation to increasing plasma glucose and increasing apoB/apoA-I ratio (Figure 9-4, *A* and *B*).[34,40] Data from numerous clinical trials with statins, which can significantly reduce CHOL, LDL cholesterol, and apoB, have also been used to assess the importance of on-treatment lipid values as a guide to lipid-lowering therapy. Most studies have reported that residual risk was more strongly related to apoB than LDL cholesterol or nonHDL cholesterol.[28] In the Leiden Heart Study, a group of 848 patients with angiographically documented CHD achieved a mean reduction in CHOL of 30% with statin therapy. The age-adjusted Cox regression analysis showed no significant association between either on-treatment LDL cholesterol or on-treatment nonHDL cholesterol and subsequent events.[41] By contrast, on-treatment apoB was predictive of MI and all-cause mortality.[41] In this study, the apoB/apoA-I ratio was even an even stronger predictor of future events, with an age-adjusted hazard ratio of 7.22 ($p < 0.0001$).[41] In the THROMBO study in 1045 patients who had recovered from MI, higher apoB and lower apoA-I levels were independently associated with the risk for recurrent events, whereas the traditional lipid parameters (HDL cholesterol, LDL cholesterol, and TG) were not.[36] In 4S on-treatment LDL cholesterol and apoB were both predictive of major coronary events.[23] In a subgroup analysis using data from 4S, it was noted that the risk for major coronary events for participants in the hypertriglyceridemic, hyperapobetalipoproteinemic group on placebo was significantly greater than in those with normal TG and elevated LDL cholesterol. Using the 1-year on-treatment values, investigators in the AFCAPS/TexCAPS reported that only apoB/apoA-I ratio was predictive of future events.[24] In the Long-Term Intervention with Prevastatin in Ischemia Disease (LIPID) trial, the unadjusted 1-year on-treatment LDL cholesterol was not predictive of vascular outcomes, but the adjusted 1-year on-treatment LDL cholesterol level did predict vascular events (hazard ratios (HR) of 1.08 and 1.20, respectively).[42] On-treatment apoB levels, both unadjusted and adjusted, were also predictive of future events with higher HR (1.49 and 2.10, respectively). The unadjusted on-treatment CHOL/HDL cholesterol ratio was modestly predictive of subsequent events (HR, 1.03, $p < 0.03$), and the unadjusted apoB/apoA-I ratio was strongly associated with future events (HR, 1.43, $p < 0.002$).

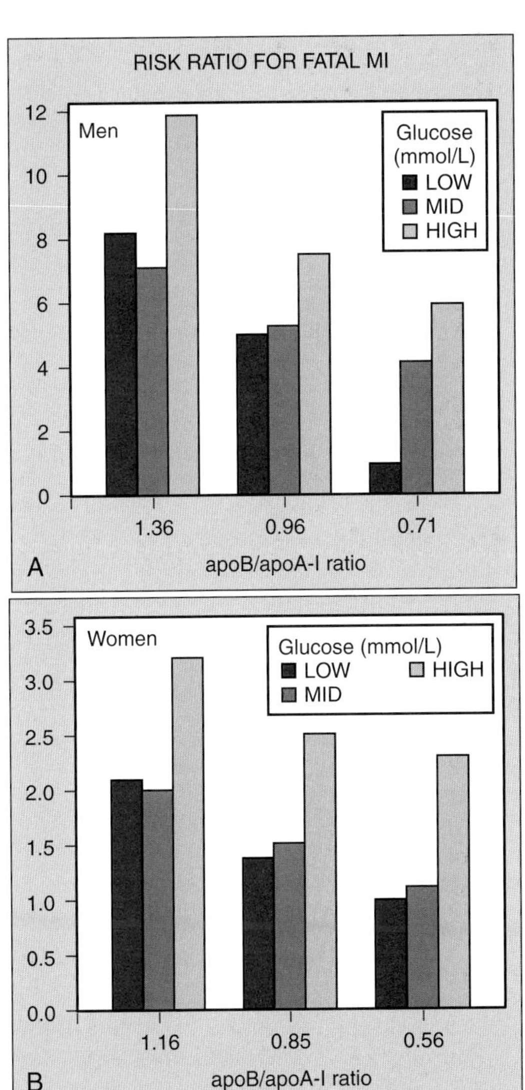

FIGURE 9-4 Synergistic effect of glucose and apoB/apoA-I ratio in the risk for fatal MI among the men *(A)* and women *(B)* of AMORIS. *Reprinted from Ref. 40, with permission.*

PARTICLE SIZE, PARTICLE NUMBER, AND CARDIOVASCULAR DISEASE

In the past 20 years, there has been increasing interest in the use of LDL particle size as an additional risk factor. In a series of papers, Fisher and coworkers were among the first to suggest that there might be considerable heterogeneity within the class of cholesterol-carrying lipoproteins known as LDL (plasma density of 1.019–1.063 g/mL).[43,44] It was reported that patients with type IV or type IIb (familial combined hyperlipidemia) were more likely to have polydisperse LDL as compared with normolipidemic and type IIa (familial hypercholesterolemia).[45,46] Sniderman and coworkers[47] demonstrated that type IIa patients with deficiency in LDL receptor and patients with documented CHD have comparable cholesterol levels, but the CHD patients had higher protein content in LDL. Using nondenaturing gradient polyacrylamide gels, Krauss and coworkers were able to characterize the presence of small dense LDL in whole plasma,[48,49] which was called *LDL phenotype B*. Subsequent case–control and prospective studies have linked the presence of small dense LDL with increased risk for cardiovascular events[50–52] and diabetes.[53–55] Although LDL phenotype B has been reported to be an independent risk factor in some studies, the predictive value for this measure is significantly reduced or even lost after adjustment for traditional risk factors.[56] It would appear that LDL particle size can contribute to risk assessment only after LDL cholesterol has been taken into consideration. The biochemistry of LDL is such that once therapy has been

initiated to reduce LDL to less than 100 or 75 mg/dL, it is difficult to have large buoyant LDL in the circulation because lipid concentrations are not sufficient to make large LDL particles.[57] Nuclear magnetic resonance (NMR) technology was initially introduced as an alternative to gradient gel technology for the assessment of lipoprotein particle size.[58] The characteristic spectroscopic signal from the clustering of the methyl groups in various lipids can be resolved into individual subclass signal amplitudes by deconvolution.[59] For the deconvolution process, a library of approximately 30 NMR spectra representative of individual lipoprotein subfractions isolated by ultracentrifugation and/or column chromatography has been compiled and characterized.[58] LDL particle sizes determined by gradient gel electrophoresis and by NMR spectroscopy have been reported to be highly correlated (r = 0.946). NMR-derived LDL sizes are, however, uniformly smaller by 5 to 6 nm compared with those obtained by gradient gel electrophoresis.[60,61]

More recently, NMR analysis has focused on the concept of particle concentrations or particle number. This is consistent with the concept that LDL particle size must be used in conjunction with LDL cholesterol levels to yield optimal information with respect to the characteristics of the circulating LDL particles. From the signal amplitudes, another series of calculations was performed to convert the NMR subclass concentrations to particle concentrations (nmoles of particles per liter).[62] This calculation is based on previously published data on the relations among lipoprotein particle diameter, core lipid volume, and mass.[60,62]

In a prospective, nested, case–control study among healthy, middle-aged women, the median LDL particle number (LDLp) was higher (1597 vs. 1404 nmol/L, p <0.0001) among women who subsequently had cardiovascular events, defined as MI, stroke, or death of CHD.[63] LDL particle size (LDLs) was also smaller among women who developed cardiovascular disease events (21.5 vs. 21.8 nm, p <0.046).[63] The relative risk for the highest quartile of LDLp as compared to the lowest quartile was 4.17 (95% confidence interval [CI], 1.96–8.87). This was higher than the relative risk of 3.11 (95% CI, 1.55–6.26) obtained for the CHOL/HDL cholesterol ratio. The predictive power of LDLp was also demonstrated in several other major studies including the Framingham Heart Study,[64] the Veterans Affairs HDL Intervention Trial (VA-HIT) study,[65] the Insulin Resistance Atherosclerosis Study,[66] the EPIC-Norfolk Prospective Population Study,[67] the DCCT/EDIC cohort,[68] and the Multi-Ethnic Study of Atherosclerosis.[69]

FUTURE DIRECTIONS

Measurement of lipids is a dynamic field. Newer lipid measurements are constantly being assessed, and greater efficacy in lipid treatments is also changing expectations of clinicians and their patients. We have moved beyond assessing only total cholesterol and total TG and now regularly use HDL cholesterol information. The uptake on using either non-HDL cholesterol or apoB has been slow but the evidence is strong that these measures equal or surpass LDL cholesterol as predictors of cardiac risk. Additionally, information on lipid particles is increasingly available. The greatest interest in the past was LDL particle size, but research is now emphasizing that an increased LDL particle number may be especially important. Finally, we are just beginning to develop databases that can assess the role of lipid levels on treatment as predictors of vascular disease risk. Only greater experience with these newer measures in this situation will help us to more effectively guide preventive care to lower the risk of cardiovascular events.

REFERENCES

1. Wilcox JN and Harker LA: Molecular and cellular mechanisms of atherogenesis: Studies of human lesions linked with animal modeling. In Haemostasis and Thrombosis. Bloom AL, Forbes CD, and Thomas DP, editors. Churchill Livingstone, Edinburgh 1993. 1139–1152.
2. Ross R: The pathogenesis of atherosclerosis: A perspective for the 1990's. *Nature* 1993;362:801–809.
3. Fredrickson DS, Levy RI, and Lees RS: Fat transport in lipoproteins: An integrated approach to mechanisms and disorders. *N Engl J Med* 1967;276:34–44.
4. Stamler J, Wentworth D, and Neaton JD: Is relationship between serum cholesterol and risk of premature death from CHD continuous and graded? Findings in 356,222 primary screenees of the MRFIT. *JAMA* 1986;256:2823–2828.
5. Keys A: Prediction and possible prevention of coronary disease. *Am J Public Health* 1953;43:1399–1407.
6. Kannel WB, Castelli WP, and Gordon T: Cholesterol in the prediction of atherosclerotic disease: New perspectives based on the Framingham Heart Study. *Ann Intern Med* 1979;90:85–91.
7. The Pooling Project Research Group: Relationship of blood pressure, serum cholesterol, smoking habit, relative weight and ECG abnormalities to incidence of major coronary events. Final report of the Pooling Project. *J Chronic Dis* 1978;31:201–306.
8. The LRC Program Epidemiology Committee: Plasma lipid distribution in selected North American populations. The Lipid Research Clinics Program Prevalence Study. *Circulation* 1979;60:427–439.
9. Lipid Research Clinics Program: The LRC-CPPT results: I. Reduction in incidence of coronary heart disease. *JAMA* 1984;251: 351–364.
10. Lipid Research Clinics Program: The LRC-CPPT results: II. The relationship of reduction in incidence of coronary heart disease to cholesterol lowering. *JAMA* 1984;251:365–374.
11. Friedewald WT, Levy RI, and Fredrickson DS: Estimation of the concentration of low-density lipoprotein cholesterol in plasma, without the use of the preparative ultracentrifuge. *Clin Chem* 1972;18:499–502.
12. Lipid Research Clinics Program: Manual of Laboratory Operations: I. Lipid and Lipoprotein Analysis. US Department of Health, Education and Welfare. Bethesda, MD, NIH 1974; 75-628.
13. Barr DP, E.R. and Eder HA: Protein-lipid relationships in human plasma. *Am J Med* 1951;11:480–493.
14. Keys A: Lipoprotein profile — its value in prediction. *Preventive Med* 1983;12:25–31.
15. Stender S and Hjelms E: *In vivo* influx of free and esterified plasma cholesterol into human aortic tissue without atherosclerotic lesions. *J Clin Invest* 1984;74:1871–1881.
16. Miller NE, La Ville A, and Crook D: Direct evidence that reverse cholesterol is mediated by highdensity lipoproteins in rabbit. *Nature* 1985;314:109–111.
17. Pittman RC and Steinberg D: Sites and mechanisms of uptake and degradation of high-density and low-density lipoproteins. *J Lipid Res* 1984;25:1577–1585.
18. Gordon DJ, Probstfield JL, Garrison RJ, et al: High-density lipoprotein cholesterol and cardiovascualr disease. Four prospective American studies. *Circulation* 1989;79:8–15.
19. Abbott RD, Garrison RJ, Wilson PWF, et al: Joint distribution of lipoprotein cholesterol classes. The Framingham Study. *Arteriosclerosis* 1983;3:260–272.
20. Castelli WP: Cholesterol and lipids in the coronary artery disease — the Framingham Heart Study. *Can J Cardiology* 1988;4 (Suppl A):5A–10A.

21. Kinosian B, Glick H, and Garland G: Cholesterol and coronary artery disease: Predicting risks by levels and ratios. *Ann Intern Med* 1994;121:641–647.
22. Rader DJ, Davidson M, Caplan RJ, and Pears JS: Lipid and apolipoprotein ratios: Association with CAD and effects of rosuvastatin compared with atorvastatin, pravastatin and simvastatin. *Am J Cardiol* 2003;91(Suppl):20C–24C.
23. Pederson TR, Olsson AG, Faergemen O, et al: Lipoprotein changes and reduction in the incidence of major coronary heart disease events in the Scandinavian Simvastatin Survival Study (4S). *Circulation* 1998;97:1453–1460.
24. Gotto Jr., AM, Whitney E, Stein EA, et al: Relation between baseline and on-treatment lipid parameters and first acute major coronary events in the Air Force/Texas Coronary Atherosclerosis Prevention Study (AFCAPS/TexCAPS). *Circulation* 2000; 101:484.
25. Talmud PJ, Hawe E, Miller GJ, and Humphries SE: Nonfasting apoB and triglyceride levels as a useful predictor of CHD risk in middle-aged UK men. *Arterioscl Thromb Vasc Biol* 2003;22: 1918–1923.
26. Innis-Whitehouse W, Li X, Brown WV, and Le N-A: An efficient chromatographic system for lipoprotein fractionation using whole plasma. *J Lipid Res* 1998;39:679–690.
27. Rader DJ, Hoeg JM, and Brewer Jr, HB: Quantitation of plasma apolipoproteins in the primary and secondary prevention of coronary artery disease. *Ann Intern Med* 1994;120:1012–1025.
28. Sniderman AD, Furberg CD, Keech A, et al: Apolipoproteins versus lipids as indices of coronary risk and as targets for statin therapy treatment. *Lancet* 2003;361:777–780.
29. Sniderman AD and Marcovina SM: Apolipoprotein A-I and B. *Clin Lab Med* 2006;26:733–750.
30. Maciejko JJ, Holmes DR, Kottke BA, et al: ApoA-I as a marker of angiographically assessed coronary artery disease. *N Engl J Med* 1983;309:385–389.
31. Kottke BA, Zinmeister AR, Holmes DR, et al: Apolipoproteins and coronary artery disease. *Mayo Clin Proc* 1986;61:313–320.
32. Lamarche B, Moorjani S, Lupien PJ, et al: Apolipoprotein A1 and B levels and the risk of ischemic heart disease during a 5 year follow-up of men in the Quebec Cardiovascular Study. *Circulation* 1996;94:273–278.
33. St Pierre A, Cantin B, Dagenais GR, et al: Low-density lipoprotein subfractions and the long-term risk of ischemic heart disease in men. 13-year follow-up data from the Quebec Cardiovascular Study. *Arterioscl Thromb Vasc Biol* 2005;25:553–559.
34. Walldius G, Jungner I, Holmes I, et al: High apoB, low apoA-I, and improvement in the prediction of fatal myocardial infarction (AMORIS study): a prospective study. *Lancet* 2001;358: 2026–2033.
35. Shai I, Rimm EB, Hankinson SE, et al: Multivariate assessment of lipid parameters as predictors of coronary heart disease among postmenopausal women. Potential implications for clinical guidelines. *Circulation* 2004;110:2824–2830.
36. Moss AJ, Goldstein RE, Marder VJ, et al: Thrombogenic factors and recurrent coronary events. *Circulation* 1999;99: 2517–2522.
37. Jiang R, Schulze MB, Li T, et al: Non-HDL cholesterol and apoB predict cardiovascular disease events among men with type 2 diabetes. *Diabetes Care* 2004;27:1991–1997.
38. Ridker PM, Rifai N, Cook NR, et al: NonHDL cholesterol, apolipoproteins A-I, and B100, standard lipid measures, lipid ratios, and CRP as risk factors for cardiovascular disease in women. *JAMA* 2005;294:326–333.
39. Sniderman AD, Junger I, Holme I, et al: Errors that result from using the TC/HDL cholesterol ratio rather than the apoB/apoA-I ratio to identify the lipoprotein-related risk of vascular disease. *J Internal Med* 2006;259:455–461.
40. Walldius G and Junger I: The apoB.apoA-I ratio: a strong, new risk factor for cardiovascular disease and a target foe lipid-lowering therapy — a review of the evidence. *J Internal Med* 2006;259:493–519.
41. Roeters van Lennep JE, Westerveld HT, Roeters van Lennep HWO, et al: Apolipoprotein concentrations during treatment and recurrent CAD events. *Arterioscl Thromb Vasc Biol* 2000;20:2048–2013.
42. Simes RJ, Marschner IC, Hunt D, et al: Relationship between lipid levels and clinical outcome in the Long-Term Intervention with Pravastatin in Ischemic Disease (LIPID) trial. *Circulation* 2002;105:1162–1169.
43. Hammond MG and Fisher WR: The characterization of a discrete series of LDL in the disease hyperprebeta-lipoproteinemia. *J Biol Chem* 1971;246:5454–5465.
44. Fisher WR, Hammond MG, and Warmke GL: Measurements of the molecular weight variability of plasma LDL among normal and subjects with hyper-beta-lipoproteinemia. Demonstration of macromolecular heterogeneity. *Biochemistry* 1972;11: 519–525.
45. Hammond MG, Mengel MC, Warmke GL, and Fisher WR: Macromolecular dispension of human LDL in hyperlipoproteinemia. *Metabolism* 1977;26:1231–1242.
46. Fisher WR: Heterogeneity of plasma LDL: Manifestations of the physiologic phenemonen in man. *Metabolism* 1983;32: 283–291.
47. Sniderman A, Shapiro S, Marpole D, et al: Association of coronary atherosclerosis with hyperapobetalipoproteinemia [increased protein but normal cholesterol levels in human plasma low-density (beta) lipoproteins]. *Proc Natl Acad Sci USA* 1980;77:604–608.
48. SHen MMS, Krauss RM, Lindgren FT, and Forte TM: Heterogeneity of serum LDL in normal human subjects. *J Lipid Res* 1981;22:236–244.
49. Krauss RM and Burke DJ: Identification of multiple subclasses of plasma LDL in normal humans. *J Lipid Res* 1982;23: 97–104.
50. Austin MA, Breslow JL, Hennekens CH, et al: LDL subclass patterns and risk of myocardial infarction. *JAMA* 1988;260: 1917–1921.
51. Campos H, Genest JJ, Blijlevens E, et al: LDL particle size and coronary artery disease. *Arterioscl Thromb* 1992;12:187–195.
52. Lamarche B, Tchernof A, Moorjani S, et al: Small dense LDL particles as a prodictor of the risk of ischemic heart disease in me: prospective results from the Quebec Cardiovascular Study. *Circulation* 1997;95:69–75.
53. Lamarche B, A Tchernof, Mauriege P, et al: Fasting insulin and apoB levels and LDL particle size as risk factors for ischemic heart disease. *JAMA* 1998;279:1955–1961.
54. Haffner SM, Mykkanen L, Valdez RA, et al: Low-density lipoprotein size and subclass pattern in a biethnic population. *Arterioscl Thromb* 1993;13:1623–1630.
55. Selby JV, Austin MA, Newman B, et al: LDL subclass pattern and the insulin resistance syndrome in women. *Circulation* 1993;88:381–387.
56. Junger I, Sniderman AD, Furberg C, et al: Does LDL size add to atherogenic particle number in predicting the risk of fatal myocardial infarction? *Am J Cardiol* 2006;97:943– 946.
57. Le NA: Small, dense low-density lipoprotein: Risk or myth. *Current Atherosclerosis Reviews* 2003;5:22–28.
58. Otvos JD, Jeyarajah EJ, Bennett DW, and Krauss RM: Development of a proton nuclear magnetic resonance spectroscopic method for determining plasma lipoprotein concentrations and subspecies distributions from a single, rapid measurement. *Clin Chem* 1992;38:1632–1638.
59. Jeyarajah EJ, Cromwell WC, and Otvos JD: Lipoprotein particle analysis by NMR spectroscopy. *Clin Lab Med* 2006;26: 847–870.
60. Tall AR, Small DM, and Atkinson D: Studies of LDL isolated from Macaca Fascicularis fed an atherogenic diet. *J Clin Invest* 1978;62:1354–1363.
61. Friedman DS, Otvos JD, Jeyarajah EJ, et al: Relation of lipoprotein subclasses as measured by proton NMR spectroscopy to coronary artery disease. *Arterioscl Thromb Vasc Biol* 1998;18: 1046–1053.
62. Otvos JD: Measurement of lipoprotein subclass profiles by NMR spectroscopy. In Handbook of Lipoprotein Testing. N Rifai, GR Warnick, and MH Domoniczak, editors. AACC Press, Washington DC 2000;609–623.
63. Blake GJ, Otvos JD, Rifai N, et al: LDL particle concentration and size as determined by NMR spectroscopy as predictors of cardiovascular disease in women. *Circulation* 2002;106: 1930–1937.
64. Kathiresan S, Otvos JD, Sullivan LM, et al: Increased small LDL particle number: a prominent feature of the metabolic syndrome in the Framingham Heart Study. *Circulation* 2006;113:20–29.
65. Otvos JD, Collins D, Friedman DS, et al: LDL and HDL particle subclasses predict coronary events and are favorably changed by gemfibrozil therapy in the VA-HIT. *Circulation* 2006;113: 1556–1563.

66. Festa A, Williams K, Hanley AJ, et al: NMR lipoprotien abnormalities in prediabetic subjects in the Insulin Resistance Atherosclerosis Study. *Circulation* 2005;111:3465–3472.
67. El Harchaoui K, van der Steeg WA, Stroes ESG, et al: Value of LDL particle number and size as predictors of CAD in apparently healthy men and women: the EPIC-Norfolk Prospective Population Study. *J Am Coll Cardiol* 2007;49:547–553.
68. Lyons TJ, Jenkins AJ, Zheng D, et al: NMR-determined lipoprotein subclass profile in the DCCT/EDIC cohort: associations with carotid intima-media thickness. *Diabetic Med* 2006;23: 955–966.
69. Mora S, Szklo M, Otvos JD, et al: LDL particle subclasses, LDL particle size and carotid atherosclerosis in the Multi-Ethnic Study of Atherosclerosis (MESA). *Atherosclerosis* 2007;192:211–217.

CHAPTER 10

High-Density Lipoprotein Cholesterol in Coronary Heart Disease Risk Assessment

Michael Miller

In 1975, Norman and George Miller[1] proposed that a low level of high-density lipoprotein (HDL) cholesterol was associated with an increased risk for vascular disease and coronary atherosclerosis. This insight reflected, in part, pioneering studies by Glomset,[2] who demonstrated that -HDL played a pivotal role in the transfer of cholesterol from the periphery to the liver. Clinical proof for this concept was subsequently borne out in prospective studies conducted in Tromso, Norway,[3] Framingham, Massachusetts,[4] and Münster, Germany,[5] where an inverse association between HDL cholesterol and coronary heart disease (CHD) was consistently demonstrated. This chapter focuses on the epidemiology of HDL cholesterol as an independent predictor of CHD, highlights the prognostic impact of reduced HDL cholesterol when accompanied by increases in low-density lipoprotein (LDL) cholesterol or triglycerides (TGs) or both, and assesses the clinical relevance of the extreme HDL phenotype.

HIGH-DENSITY LIPOPROTEIN CHOLESTEROL AS A PREDICTOR OF CORONARY HEART DISEASE

Epidemiologic Studies

Observational studies conducted in the United States, Europe, and Scandinavia during the 1970s and early 1980s identified an inverse relation between HDL cholesterol and CHD.[3–7] In the Framingham Heart Study (FHS), low HDL cholesterol was associated with an increased risk for incident CHD events even in the absence of increased LDL cholesterol levels[4,8] (Fig. 10-1). Overall, for each 5-mg/dL decrement less than median HDL cholesterol (i.e., 45 mg/dL in men and 55 mg/dL in women), an approximate 25% increased risk for CHD was observed. Conversely, increases greater than the median percentile of HDL cholesterol corresponded to a reduced risk for initial CHD events (Table 10-1).[4] Other studies also identified low HDL cholesterol as predictive of initial CHD event rates. For example, in the 5-year prospective Israeli Ischemic Heart Disease Study, the inverse association between HDL cholesterol and incident myocardial infarction (MI) in men aged 50 years and older remained statistically significant after controlling for cigarette smoking, blood pressure, weight, and diabetes.[7] Similarly, in the Münster Heart Study (Prospective Cardiovascular Münster [PROCAM] study), low HDL cholesterol, defined as less than 35 mg/dL, conferred a 2.5-fold increase in incident CHD with total cholesterol (TC) levels less than 200 mg/dL and a 5-fold increase at greater TC levels (i.e., 200–300 mg/dL).[5] Studies evaluating the prevalence of low HDL and CHD in the absence of hypercholesterolemia (e.g., TC levels <200 mg/dL) also identified low HDL cholesterol to be highly prevalent[9–16] and predictive of primary and recurrent CHD events.[17,18] Overall, data from the Multiple Risk Factor Intervention Trial (MRFIT),[19] the Lipid Research Clinics (LRC) follow-up trial,[20] the placebo arm of the Coronary Primary Prevention Trial (CPPT),[21] and the Physicians' Health Study (PHS)[22] found that for each 1-mg/dL increment in HDL cholesterol, there was an approximate 3% reduction in CHD risk (Table 10-2).

Nonetheless, not all studies have concluded that HDL cholesterol is inversely correlated with CHD.[23,24] Notably, in the Minnesota Prospective Study, low HDL cholesterol was not associated with a statistically significant greater risk for CHD death in men

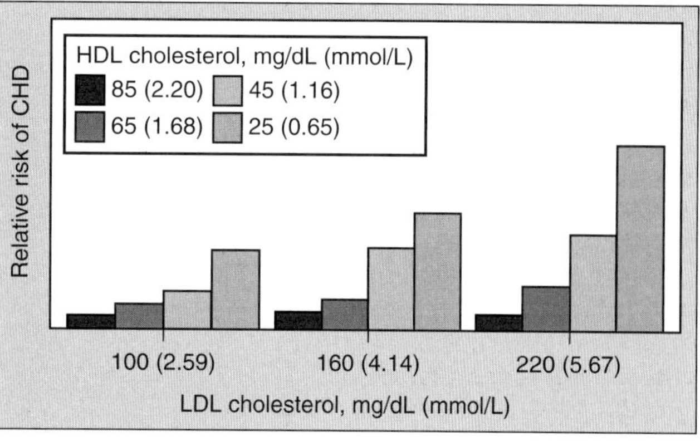

FIGURE 10-1 Risk for coronary heart disease (CHD) by high-density lipoprotein (HDL) cholesterol and low-density lipoprotein (LDL) cholesterol levels. *(From Ref. 8, with permission.)*

over a 25-year follow-up period.[24] Subsequently, Keys and colleagues[25] extended these findings to a Finnish cohort that after a 24-year follow-up period did not demonstrate a statistically significant relation between baseline HDL cholesterol levels and CHD death, thereby raising the suggestion that short (e.g., 3- to 5-year) follow-up periods may be insufficient to adequately address the inverse relation between HDL cholesterol and CHD.

Angiographic and Clinical Trials

Coronary arteriographic studies lasting 2 to 5 years have also demonstrated the greatest rate of progression in native and saphenous grafts among patients with low HDL cholesterol as illustrated in the Lipoprotein and Coronary Atherosclerosis Study (LCAS)[26] (Fig. 10-2) and Post Coronary Artery By pass Graft study (Post-CABG)[27] (Fig. 10-3). Similarly, randomized clinical trials that used statin therapy have consistently found subjects treated with placebo with the lowest levels of HDL cholesterol to be at the greatest risk for future CHD events.[28,29] Importantly, treatment with statins was effective in patients with low HDL cholesterol by reducing the excess risk to that observed in subjects treated with placebo with normal HDL cholesterol (Fig. 10-4). Despite the relatively modest HDL cholesterol–increasing effect (e.g., 5–10%), statins appear to be a particularly effective therapy in patients with low HDL cholesterol by reducing atherogenic lipids and lipoproteins accompanying a proinflammatory milieu.[30,31]

LOW LEVEL OF HIGH-DENSITY LIPOPROTEIN AS A BIOMARKER OF CORONARY HEART DISEASE

Although there is consensus that HDL cholesterol is inversely correlated with CHD,[32] what remains less established is the extent to which low HDL may directly

TABLE 10-1 Relative Risk for Coronary Heart Disease for Each 5-mg/dL Change beyond Median High-Density Lipoprotein Cholesterol in the Framingham Heart Study

High-Density Lipoprotein Cholesterol (mg/dL)	Men	Women
30	1.82	–
35	1.49	–
40	1.22	1.94
45	1.00	1.55
50	0.82	1.25
55	0.67	1.00
60	0.55	0.80
65	0.45	0.64
70	–	0.52

TABLE 10-2 Relation of High-Density Lipoprotein Cholesterol and Coronary Heart Disease Risk in Several Large American Prospective Studies

Study Population	N	Age (yr)	Follow-up (yr)	CHD Decrease, (%)	
				Men	Women
FHS	704	49+	10.3	1.9	3.2
MRFIT	5792	35–57	7	2	
LRCF	4152	35+	8.4	4.2	3.7
CPPT	1900	35–59	7	2.3	
PHS	14,916	40–84	5	3.5	

Each 1-mg/dL increment in high-density lipoprotein cholesterol was associated with percentage coronary heart disease (CHD) reduction after adjustment for other covariates. Adjustment included age, systolic blood pressure, cigarette smoking, and body mass index.

CPPT, Coronary Primary Prevention Trial (placebo arm); FHS, Framingham Heart Study; LRCF, Lipid Research Clinics follow-up trial; MRFIT, Multiple Risk Factor Intervention Trial; PHS, Physicians' Health Study. Adapted from references 19–22.

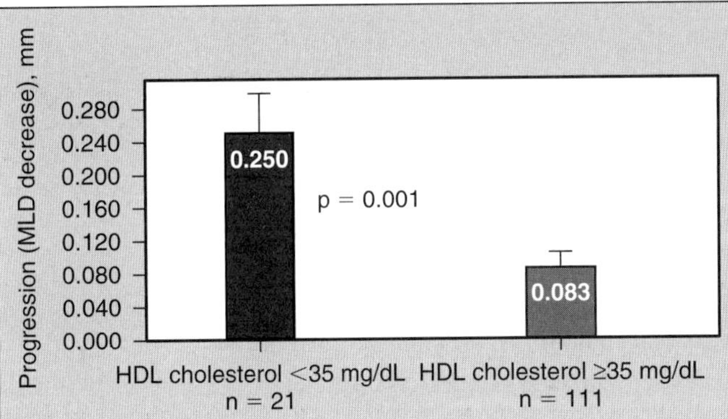

FIGURE 10-2 Comparison of 2.5-year minimum lumen diameter (MLD) change (mean ± standard error) among placebo-only patients showed significantly more coronary artery disease progression in patients with low high-density lipoprotein (HDL) cholesterol than in patients with greater HDL cholesterol levels. *(From Ref. 26, with permission.)*

promote atherothrombosis. It has been recognized that in addition to reduced efficiency of reverse cholesterol transport (RCT) (see chapters 4, 5, and 45), low HDL may also produce a proinflammatory and pro-oxidative state.[33,34] Others have suggested that low HDL cholesterol reflects metabolic alterations associated with visceral adiposity, hypertriglyceridemia, and insulin resistance.[35,36] Under this guise, low HDL cholesterol level may serve more appropriately as a biomarker rather than as an inciter of disease. As discussed later, compelling data demonstrate that a low HDL cholesterol level becomes most clinically noteworthy when accompanied by these metabolic or environmental (e.g., smoking) abnormalities. However, what remains less well established is whether an "isolated" low HDL cholesterol level promotes an atherogenic state and, conversely, whether a high level of HDL cholesterol is cardioprotective, especially when accompanied by other CHD risk factors.

LOW LEVEL OF HIGH-DENSITY LIPOPROTEIN WITH INCREASED TRIGLYCERIDE OR LOW-DENSITY LIPOPROTEIN CHOLESTEROL LEVEL OR BOTH

An inverse correlation between HDL cholesterol and TG concentration is well established (Fig. 10-5).[35] Moreover, at least three observational studies have suggested that the link between low HDL cholesterol level and CHD is, in part, contributed to by associated increases in TG, LDL cholesterol, or both. For example, in the FHS, CHD risk was accentuated twofold when low HDL cholesterol level was accompanied by increased TG levels (i.e., levels exceeding 150 mg/dL) even after adjustment for other covariates that included age, hypertension, cigarette smoking, obesity, and left ventricular hypertrophy.[37] As well, TG levels greater than the median (138 mg/dL) conferred an approximate twofold increased risk for initial CHD events at every tertile of TC/HDL in the Québec Cardiovascular Study (Fig. 10-6). Amplification of CHD risk was also demonstrated in the PROCAM study, in which the combination of high LDL cholesterol (>160 mg/dL) and TG levels (≥200 mg/dL) resulted in a sixfold greater risk for incident CHD compared with lower LDL cholesterol (<135 mg/dL) and TG levels (<150 mg/dL) in middle-aged men with HDL cholesterol levels less than 45 mg/dL (Fig. 10-7).[38] Finally, in the Helsinki Heart Study, the combination of a high LDL/HDL cholesterol ratio and high TG level (e.g., >200 mg/dL) coincided with the greatest risk for incident CHD in patients treated with placebo (Fig. 10-8).[39] Taken together, these data support the concept that the atherogenic risk imposed by low HDL cholesterol is most pronounced when accompanied by increases in LDL cholesterol or TG-rich lipoproteins, or both. Unfortunately, none of these studies addressed the potential

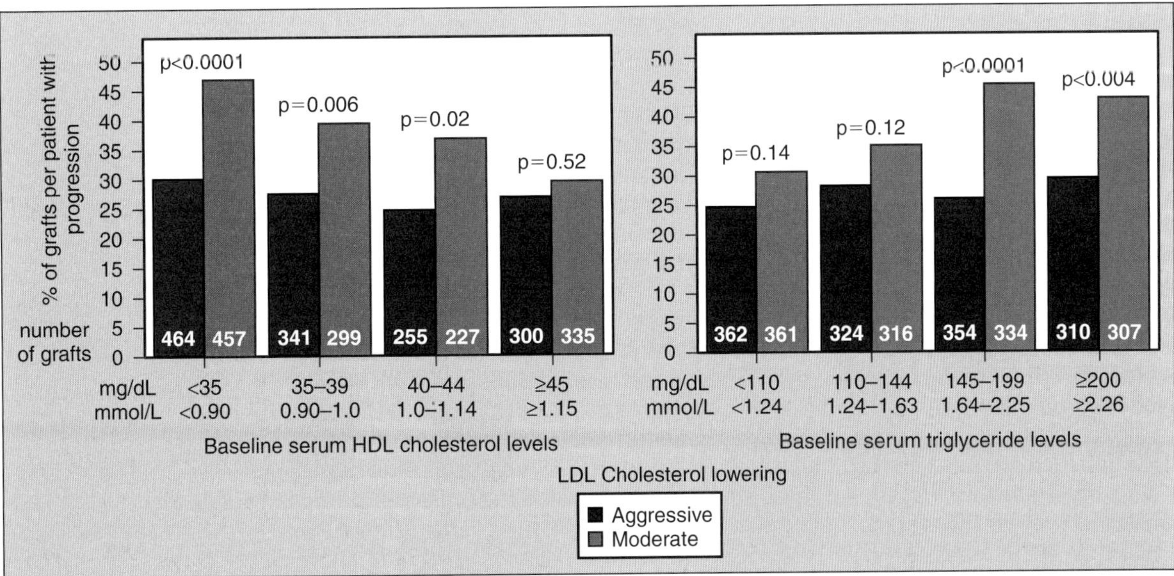

FIGURE 10-3 Probability of progression of saphenous vein coronary bypass graft atherosclerosis after aggressive *(red bars)* compared with moderate *(gray bars)* low-density lipoprotein (LDL) cholesterol lowering with respect to baseline high-density lipoprotein (HDL) cholesterol and serum triglyceride levels. *(From Ref. 27, with permission.)*

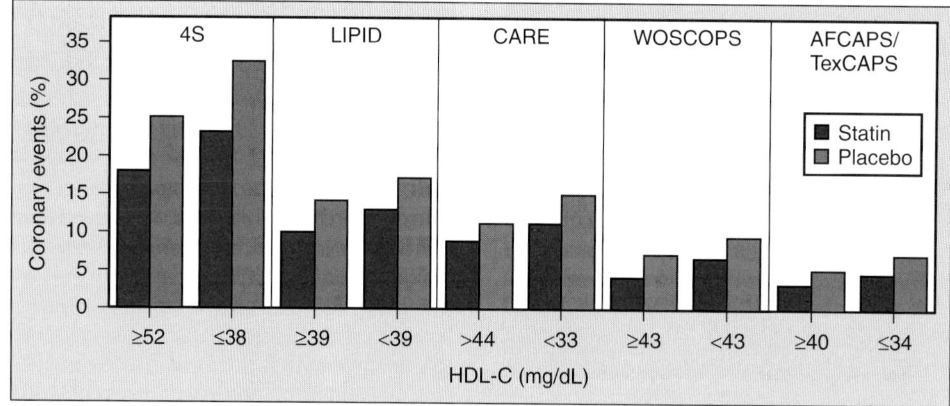

FIGURE 10-4 Event reduction with statin therapy in patients with low versus high high-density lipoprotein (HDL) cholesterol levels. In all five trials, patients with low HDL cholesterol levels on placebo had the greatest event rate, and therapy with statin in patients with lower HDL cholesterol levels consistently reduced coronary event rates to approximately those of patients with higher HDL cholesterol levels receiving placebo. Comparisons are the highest versus lowest quartile for HDL cholesterol levels in the Scandinavian Simvastatin Survival Study (4S), the Long-Term Intervention with Pravastatin in Ischaemic Disease (LIPID) and the Cholesterol and Recurrent Events trial (CARE); at or above the median versus below the median in the West of Scotland Coronary Prevention Study (WOSCOPS); and the highest versus lowest tertile for HDL cholesterol levels in the Air Force/Texas Coronary Atherosclerosis Prevention Study (AFCAPS/TexCAPS). *(From Ref. 28, with permission.)*

atherogenicity imposed by an isolated low HDL cholesterol level or the relative cardioprotection afforded by a high HDL cholesterol level.

CAUSES OF LOW AND HIGH LEVELS OF HIGH-DENSITY LIPOPROTEIN CHOLESTEROL

The causes of low and high levels of HDL cholesterol are outlined in Table 10-3. During illness or hospitalization, increases in acute-phase proteins, such as serum amyloid A, may displace apolipoprotein A-I (apoA-I) and accelerate the clearance of HDL particles.[40] Likewise, release of endotoxins (e.g., lipopolysaccharide) and cytokines reduce lecithin:cholesterol acyltransferase (LCAT) and lipoprotein lipase (LPL) activity that, in turn, may contribute to a transient hypertriglyceridemic low HDL phenotype.[41–43] Similarly, metabolic conditions such as insulin resistance promote free fatty acid release from adipocytes that, in turn, stimulates hepatic secretion of very-low-density lipoprotein (VLDL). The exchange of TG for cholesteryl ester mediated by the cholesteryl ester transfer protein (CETP) results in TG-enriched HDL particles that are subsequently catabolized by lipases to form small, cholesterol-depleted HDL particles.[44] Among the common lifestyle-related factors contributing to reduced HDL cholesterol are cigarette smoking[45] and very low-fat diets,[46] the former reflecting reduced LCAT activity whereas the latter associated with decreased apoA-I production. Genetic factors account for approximately 10% of cases of low HDL cholesterol in the general population,[47] and molecular

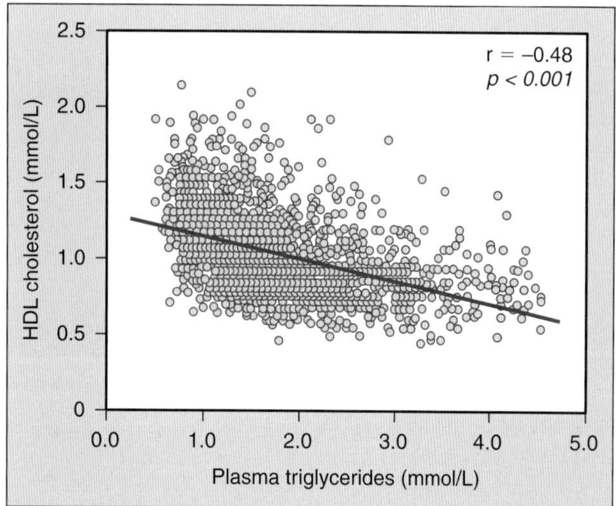

FIGURE 10-5 Relation between plasma high-density lipoprotein (HDL) cholesterol and triglyceride concentrations in the sample of 2103 men of the Québec Cardiovascular Study. $r = -0.48$. $P < 0.001$. *(From Ref. 35, with permission.)*

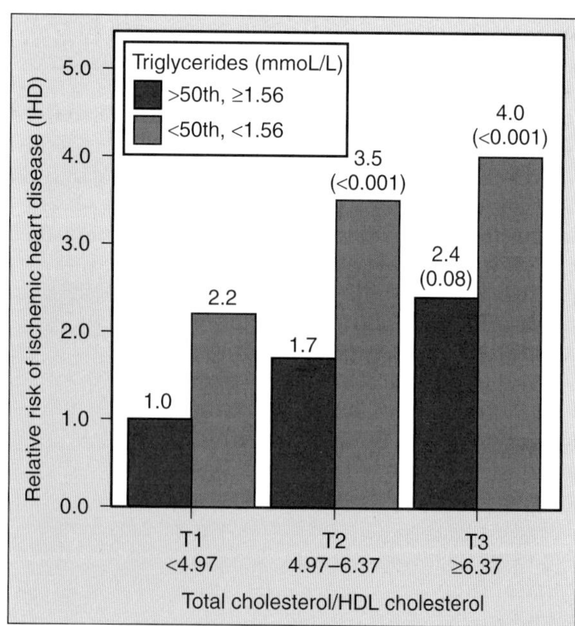

FIGURE 10-6 Relative risk of ischemic heart disease (IHD) over a 5-year follow-up period among men of the Québec Cardiovascular Study stratified into tertiles of the total cholesterol/high-density lipoprotein (HDL) cholesterol ratio and the 50th percentile of fasting triglyceride levels. Numbers above bars indicate the "fold" relative risk compared with the first tertile of total cholesterol/HDL cholesterol ratio combined with low triglyceride levels. *P* values are indicated in parentheses. *(From Ref. 35, with permission.)*

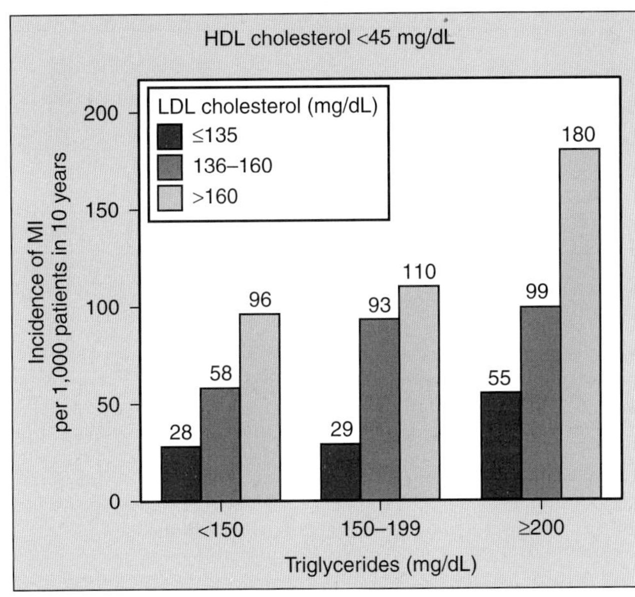

FIGURE 10-7 Incidence of myocardial infarction (MI) in 10 years according to baseline triglyceride level and low-density lipoprotein (LDL) cholesterol level in patients with a low level of high-density lipoprotein (HDL) cholesterol (<45 mg/dL) in the Prospective Cardiovascular Münster study. There were 206 coronary events in 2490 men aged 35 to 65 years. *(From Ref. 38, with permission.)*

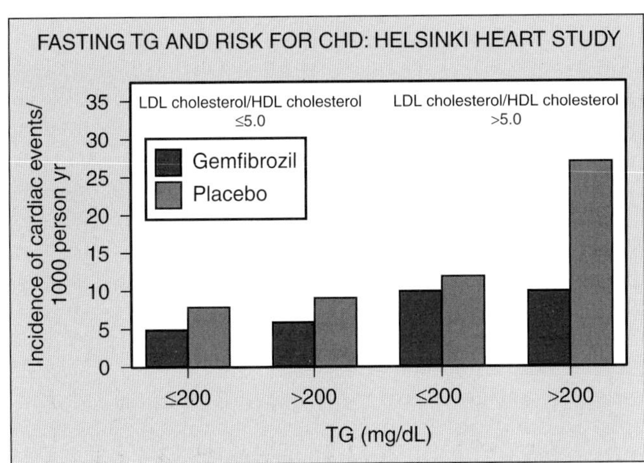

FIGURE 10-8 Fasting triglyceride (TG) and risk for coronary heart disease: Helsinki Heart Study. HDL, high-density lipoprotein; LDL, low-density lipoprotein. *Red bars* represent gemfibrozil; *gray bars* represent placebo. *(From Ref. 39 with permission.)*

variation is most commonly observed in *ABCA1* followed by *LCAT* and *APOA1*.[48–50] Several inborn errors of metabolism detected during childhood have been associated with low HDL cholesterol levels.[51–53] Androgenic medications such as danazol[54,55] are potent HDL cholesterol–lowering agents, and anabolic steroid use may be the basis for low HDL cholesterol levels in professional athletes.[56] Other iatrogenic causes of low HDL cholesterol levels include β-blockers[57] and probucol.[58] Finally, celiac sprue has also been linked to very low HDL cholesterol levels.[59] In contrast, considerably fewer causes or ways to increase HDL cholesterol are known. Increased levels of HDL cholesterol and reduced TG are commonly observed with aerobic conditioning[60] and weight reduction. However, these effects are most pronounced when baseline levels of HDL cholesterol are high before the intervention.[61] The most common

TABLE 10-3 Causes of Low and High Levels of High-Density Lipoprotein Cholesterol

	Low HDL	High HDL
General	Acute illness[40]	
Lifestyle	Cigarette smoking[45] Very-low-fat diet[46]	Aerobic activity[60] Alcohol consumption[65]
Genetic	ABCA1[47,49] apoA-I[50] LCAT[48]	CETP[62] Hepatic lipase [63] Endothelial lipase[64]
Metabolic	Visceral obesity[44] Insulin resistance[44] Diabetes mellitus[44]	
Inborn errors of metabolism	Gaucher disease[52] Glycogen storage disease[53] Niemann-Pick disease[51]	
Medications	Anabolic steroids[54,55] β-blockers[57] Probucol[58]	Estrogenic compounds[65] Corticosteroids[66] Antiseizure medications[70,71] β_2-agonists [69] Niacin[68] Fibrates[67]
Miscellaneous	Celiac sprue[59] Lymphoma[73]	Paraproteinemia[72]

ABCA1, ATP-binding cassette transporter A1; apoA-I, apolipoprotein A-I; CETP, cholesteryl ester transfer protein; HDL, high-density lipoprotein; LCAT, lecithin: cholesterol acyltransferase.

genetic cause of increased HDL cholesterol level is deficiency in CETP.[62] Other potential genetic causes include polymorphisms or mutations in the hepatic lipase or endothelial lipase genes.[63,64] Estrogen,[65] corticosteroids,[66] and alcohol use[65] are associated with greater HDL cholesterol levels; however, they may also be accompanied by an increase in TG concentration. In addition to nicotinic acid and fibrates,[67,68] other medications that increase HDL cholesterol levels include β_2-agonists, phenytoin, and phenobarbital.[69–71] Finally, paraproteinemia has been linked to artificial increases in HDL cholesterol levels.[72]

EXTREME HIGH-DENSITY LIPOPROTEIN PHENOTYPES

The Isolated Low High-Density Lipoprotein Cholesterol Syndrome

In the absence of other CHD risk factors and associated dyslipidemia (i.e., increased LDL cholesterol and TG levels), less convincing data exist that isolated low HDL cholesterol per se poses an increased risk for

CHD. That is, although subjects with low HDL cholesterol consistently exhibit a greater prevalence of CHD than those with greater HDL cholesterol levels, it is within the purview of increased LDL cholesterol or TG levels or both. For example, in the Cooperative Lipoprotein Phenotyping Study,[74] the lower limit of LDL cholesterol evaluated was less than 140 mg/dL. In other studies, either TG concentration was not included in the low HDL analysis,[17,75] or the combination of low HDL cholesterol, low TG, and low LDL cholesterol levels was too rare to permit adequate assessment of incident CHD.[4] Therefore, it is not surprising that several of the most influential epidemiologic studies, FHS, PROCAM, and the Quebec Cardiovascular Study, did not evaluate incident CHD in the cohort with *isolated* low HDL cholesterol levels.

That the impact of *isolated* low HDL cholesterol level on incident CHD has not been well adjudicated is also attested to by its relatively low prevalence. For example, whereas low HDL cholesterol levels (i.e., less than the 10th percentile) are commonly observed in families with premature CHD (33%), nearly 90% of these patients also have concomitant increases in TG or LDL cholesterol levels or both, leaving an estimated 4% with low HDL cholesterol as the sole lipid abnormality.[76] In the United States, the prevalence of low HDL cholesterol level, defined as less than 40 mg/dL,[77] is illustrated in Fig. 10-9. Based on the National Health and Nutrition Examination Survey (NHANES) III, approximately one of seven adult women and one of three adult men have low HDL cholesterol levels.[78] However, such sex-related differences become obscured when the metabolic syndrome criteria are used to define low HDL cholesterol level in women (i.e., less than 50mg/dL rather than less than 40 mg/dL), as the prevalence of the low HDL phenotype increases to one in three women. Similarly, whereas low HDL cholesterol level is common in the U.S. adult population, *isolated* low HDL cholesterol level is relatively rare except in young adults. Specifically, in NHANES III, the prevalence of low HDL cholesterol level (less than 40 mg/dL in men and 50 mg/dL in women) in association with low TG concentration (i.e., less than 100 mg/dL) was greater in men and women between the ages of 20 and 34 years compared with older adults (aged 35 years and older). Conversely, a greater prevalence of the hypertriglyceridemic (i.e., TG concentration greater than 200 mg/dL) low HDL phenotype was observed in middle and older aged men and women[79] (Table 10-4). Further examination of low HDL cholesterol levels in

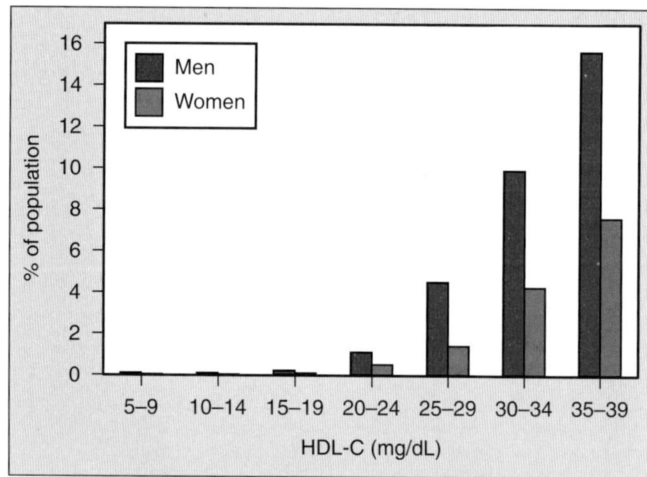

FIGURE 10-9 Distribution of low levels of high-density lipoprotein cholesterol (HDL cholesterol) in 16,988 adult participants of National Health and Nutrition Examination Survey (NHANES) III. *Red bars* represent men; *gray bars* represent women. *(From Ref. 78, with permission.)*

the setting of normal TG levels (less than 150 mg/dL) reveals similar prevalence rates in men (12.9–14.9%) across the adult age ranges. However, in women, prevalence rates of normotriglyceridemic low HDL cholesterol levels are 1.5- to 3 fold greater in young premenopausal women (younger than 45 years) compared with women older than 45 years. With additional refinement of the *isolated* low HDL phenotype to include normal LDL cholesterol levels (e.g., less than 100 mg/dL), the result is an uncommon lipoprotein pattern identified in only 1 in 40 young adult men (aged 20–34 years) to 1 in 80 middle-aged men (aged 55–64 years). Although low HDL cholesterol levels in combination with normal TG (less than 150 mg/dL) and LDL levels (less than 100 mg/dL) was common in women younger than 35 years (8.8%), much lower prevalence rates were observed in women aged 45 years and older (Table 10-5). Thus, the rarity of this phenotype illustrates the difficulty in gauging the predictive risk for CHD imposed by *isolated* low HDL cholesterol level.

Notwithstanding the aforementioned epidemiologic constraints, a number of cases of premature CHD have been reported in association with very low levels of HDL cholesterol (Table 10-6). As noted previously, the most common link between HDL cholesterol deficiency and accelerated CHD is the presence of other CHD risk factors.[80–92] In contrast, few, if any, cases have been reported of CHD in association with HDL cholesterol

TABLE 10-4 Prevalence of Low Levels of High-Density Lipoprotein Cholesterol (<40 mg/dL in Men and <50 mg/dL in Women) with Low (<100 mg/dL) or High (≥200 mg/dL) Triglyceride Levels in National Health and Nutrition Examination Survey III

	Low HDL and Low TG Levels				Low HDL and High TG Levels			
Age (yr)	Men	n	Women	n	Men	n	Women	n
20–34	7.4%*	1405	20%†	1642	6.9%*	1405	4.7%*	1642
35+	4.8%	2937	8.7%	3297	12.7%	2937	12.6%	3297

*$P < 0.0001$, †$P < 0.0005$, by χ^2 analysis (between ages 20-34 and 35+).
HDL, high-density lipoprotein; TG, triglycerides.
Adapted from Ref. 79, with permission.

TABLE 10-5 Age-Related Prevalence of Low Levels of High-Density Lipoprotein Cholesterol with Normal Triglyceride (<150 mg/dL) and Low-Density Lipoprotein Cholesterol (<100 mg/dL) Levels in National Health and Nutrition Examination Survey III

Age	N	TG <150 mg/dL	TG <150 mg/dL, LDL <100 mg/dL
Men with HDL cholesterol level <40 mg/dL			
20–34	1405	14.9%	2.5%
35–44	759	13.7%	2.2%
45–54	511	14.3%	1.6%
55–64	549	12.9%	1.3%
65–74	584	13.5%	1.7%
75+	534	13.5%	2.4%
Women with HDL cholesterol level <50 mg/dL			
20–34	1642	31.2%	8.8%
35–44	962	33.2%	5.5%
45–54	565	19.1%	1.6%
55–64	584	18.0%	2.1%
65–74	559	10.6%	1.1%
75+	627	13.1%	1.0%

HDL, high-density lipoprotein; LDL, low-density lipoprotein; TG, triglycerides.

levels less than 40 mg/dL, untreated LDL cholesterol and TG levels less than 100 mg/dL and 150 mg/dL, respectively, and the absence of other traditional risk factors. Although uncommon in societies galvanized by affluence, sedentary lifestyle, and dietary fat, distinct cohorts exist in whom such a phenotype predominates. This is most evident in developing countries, present hunter-gatherer societies, and a vegetarian lifestyle where despite reduced levels of HDL cholesterol, the overall risk for CHD remains low. Examples include the Maasai tribe of Southern Kenya,[93] Bantu villagers in Tanzania,[94] Melanesians of Papua New Guinea,[95] Tarahumara Indians of Mexico,[96] and Yanomamo nomadics of the Amazon[97] (Table 10-7).

In contrast with the delayed clearance of atherogenic remnants commonly found in subjects with low HDL cholesterol and high fasting TG levels,[98,99] a normal postprandial response to a fat load is observed with low HDL cholesterol and normal TG levels (less than 150 mg/dL).[100,101] Associated hypertriglyceridemia also accompanies the insulin resistance syndrome observed in low HDL cholesterol states.[102,103] That TG enrichment

TABLE 10-6 Selected Cases of Premature Coronary Disease (Age <55 years) in Association with Low Levels of High-Density Lipoprotein Cholesterol

CHD	Sex	TC mg/dL	HDL mg/dL	TG mg/dL	LDL mg/dL	ApoA-I mg/dL	ApoB mg/dL	CHD RF	Reference
48	F	260	3	290	134	2	125	NR	80
37	M	159	29	108	105	—	—	S	81
45	F	111	1	62	106	—	105	FH/BSO	82
31	F	130	0	31	124	—	106	NR	83
52	F	154	0	84	147	—	—		84
46	M	92	5	229	41	4.5	—	NR	85
42	M	142	7	131	118	37	108	S, HTN	86
43	M	214	0	142	186	3	—	BMI: 26.6	87
34	F	210	4	97	200	—	149	S	88
35	M	222	6	165	182	25	177	S	89
44	M	120	13	263	84	49	93	S	90
48	M	141	5	224	91*	23	114	S, HTN	91
44	M	115	6	95	90*	24	101	FH	92

One family member per affected pedigree reported.

*Statin treated.

apo, apolipoprotein; BMI, body mass index; BSO, bilateral salpingo-oophorectomy; CHD, coronary heart disease; F, female; FH, family history; HDL, high-density lipoprotein; HTN, hypertension; LDL, low-density lipoprotein; M, male; NR, not reported; RF, risk Factor; S, cigarette smoker; TC, total cholesterol; TG, triglyceride.

TABLE 10-7 Selected Lipids and Lipoproteins in Societies with Low Prevalence of Coronary Heart Disease

Country	Number	Male %	Mean Age (yr)	BMI	TC	HDL	TG	LDL
Kenya[93]	57	100	—	—	185	41	—	—
Tanzania[94]								
Fish diet	618	41	38.0	20.5	134	33	81	85
Vegetarian	645	44	46.7	20.6	137	38	118	75
Papua New Guinea[95]	93 men		46.5	21.8	166	34	104	109
	95 women		45.0	20.7	174	37	107	113
Tarahumara[96]	257	58	19-70	23.1	136	25	126	87
Yanomamo[97]	41 men		36.8	20.4	122	34	112	68
	21 women		35	21.3	143	40	110	78

BMI, body mass index; HDL, high-density lipoprotein; LDL, low-density lipoprotein; TC, total cholesterol; TG, triglyceride.

of HDL particles may adversely affect RCT[104,105] lends further credence to the concept that compositional changes in HDL particles play a more important role *vis-à-vis* HDL functionality than the mere presence of reduced HDL cholesterol.[106,107] Therefore, it is conceivable that subjects with isolated low HDL cholesterol levels may, in effect, exhibit greater -HDL functionality as compared with hypertriglyceridemic low HDL cholesterol levels because of potential impairment of RCT and/or other cardioprotective indices attributable to HDL.

THE HIGH HIGH-DENSITY LIPOPROTEIN CHOLESTEROL PHENOTYPE

In 1993, the Adult Treatment Panel of the National Cholesterol Education Program added high HDL cholesterol levels (defined as 60 mg/dL or greater) to counteract a CHD risk factor based on the epidemiologic data described earlier that, in part, reflected the relative cardioprotection conferred even in the setting of increased LDL cholesterol levels (see Fig. 10-1). Additional data suggested that families with high HDL cholesterol were afforded cardioprotection and longevity.[108] Whether the putatively inherent cardioprotection of HDL cholesterol elevation reflects greater efficiency of RCT, reduced thrombotic tendency via stabilization of prostacyclin,[109] or HDL-mediated attenuation of inflammation and oxidation[110] remains speculative. In the United States, HDL cholesterol levels of 60 mg/dL or greater occur in approximately one of every three adult women and one in six men. However, very high HDL cholesterol level (more than 100 mg/dL) is rare and found in only 1% of women and 0.65% of men (Table 10-8). Within this context, surprisingly few data evaluate the extent to which very high HDL cholesterol levels may be associated with longevity.

The most common molecular basis for high levels of HDL cholesterol is genetic alteration in CETP. Variation in *CETP* may result in a dysfunctional protein with minimal or no activity, thereby preventing transfer of cholesteryl ester from HDL to lower density lipoproteins (e.g., VLDL, LDL) in exchange for TG. Although one consequence of CETP deficiency is an increase in the level of HDL cholesterol, the functionality of cholesteryl ester–enriched HDL particles *vis-à-vis* RCT remains unclear. That is, although these particles are poor acceptors of free cholesterol from ABCA1,[111,112] they interact with ABCG1 to accept cholesterol for ultimate disposal mediated via apoE-mediated uptake in hepatocytes.[113,114] In rabbits, artificial CETP inhibition was associated with greater cholesterol efflux and reduced aortic atherosclerosis compared with controls.[115]

However, recent data using the CETP inhibitor torcetrapib failed to demonstrate significant changes in atheromatous lesion progression in either the carotid or coronary arteries, despite significant increases in HDL cholesterol.[116,117]

Other studies evaluating mutations in *CETP* and hepatic lipase (i.e., *LIPC*) have not consistently

TABLE 10-8 Prevalence of High Levels of High-Density Lipoprotein Cholesterol in National Health and Nutrition Examination Survey III

HDL Range (mg/dL)	Men (%)[n]	Women (%)[n]
<60	84% [6686]	68% [6102]
60-64	5.6% [443]	9.9% [893]
65-69	3.6% [289]	7.3% [659]
70-74	2.2% [177]	5.0% [448]
75-79	1.6% [130]	3.8% [343]
80-84	0.9% [72]	2.2% [198]
85-89	0.7% [53]	1.7% [156]
90-94	0.4% [33]	0.9% [84]
95-99	0.3% [26]	0.6 % [51]
100-119	0.5% [37]	0.7% [66]
120-149	0.2% [14]	0.2% [17]
≥150	0.01% [1]	0.1% [10]
≥100	0.65% [52]	1.0% [93]

HDL, high-density lipoprotein.

From National Center for Health Statistics. Available at: http://www.cdc.gov/nchs/nhanes.htm. Accessed July 31, 2007 demonstrated cardioprotection or increased life span,[118–121] unless accompanied by low LDL cholesterol levels.[122] Therefore, the identification of novel gene regions associated with HDL cholesterol levels[123,124] is likely to provide new insights into HDL metabolism and RCT.[124]

CONCLUSIONS

Low levels of HDL cholesterol are inversely correlated with CHD, and the low HDL phenotype is frequently encountered in CHD populations that extend to coronary care units, progressive care units, and outpatient cardiology clinics. The combination of increased LDL cholesterol and TG levels markedly increases atherothrombotic event rates, whereas statin therapy attenuates the excess risk imposed by low HDL cholesterol levels. In contrast, isolated low HDL cholesterol level, defined as normal LDL cholesterol (i.e., untreated and arbitrarily defined as less than 100 mg/dL) and TG levels (i.e., untreated, less than 150 mg/dL), is uncommon (generally less than 2%) in middle-aged men and women in the U.S. general population. However, in contrast with hyperlipidemic low HDL cholesterol level, isolated low HDL cholesterol level unaccompanied by other CHD risk factors offers little evidence for accelerated CHD. A high level of HDL cholesterol (i.e., greater than 60 mg/dL) has been defined as cardioprotective, although clinical studies evaluating CETP-deficient states have not demonstrated immunity from CHD. Further studies aimed at better defining the genetic basis of high HDL cholesterol in association with longevity and the development of assays that provide an accurate assessment of HDL functionality as it relates to RCT, inflammation, and oxidation will provide new insights into the clinical utility of this complicated lipoprotein.

REFERENCES

1. Miller GJ, Miller NE: Plasma-high-density-lipoprotein concentration and development of ischaemic heart-disease. *Lancet* 1975;1:16–19.
2. Glomset JA: The plasma lecithins:cholesterol acyltransferase reaction. *J Lipid Res* 1968;9:155–167.
3. Miller NE, Thelle DS, Forde OH, Mjos OD: The Tromso heart-study. High-density lipoprotein and coronary heart-disease: A prospective case–control study. *Lancet* 1977;1:965–968.
4. Gordon T, Castelli WP, Hjortland MC, et al: High-density lipoprotein as a protective factor against coronary heart disease. The Framingham Study. *Am J Med* 1977;62:707–714.
5. Assmann G, Cullen P, Schulte H: The Munster Heart Study (PROCAM). Results of follow-up at 8 years. *Eur Heart J* 1998;19: A2–A11.
6. Rhoads GG, Gulbrandsen CL, Kagan A: Serum lipoproteins and coronary heart disease in a population study of Hawaii Japanese men. *N Engl J Med* 1976;294:293–298.
7. Goldbourt U, Medalie JH: High-density lipoprotein cholesterol and incidence of coronary 1 heart disease—the Israeli Ischemic Heart Disease Study. *Am J Epidemiol* 1979;109:296–308.
8. Harper CR, Jacobson TA: New perspectives on the management of low levels of high-density lipoprotein cholesterol. *Arch Intern Med* 1999;159:1049–1057.
9. Miller M, Mead LA, Kwiterovich PO Jr, Pearson TA: Dyslipidemias with desirable plasma total cholesterol levels and angiographically demonstrated coronary artery disease. *Am J Cardiol* 1990;65:1–5.
10. Ginsburg GS, Safran C, Pasternak RC: Frequency of low serum high-density lipoprotein cholesterol levels in hospitalized patients with "desirable" total cholesterol levels. *Am J Cardiol* 1991;68:187–192.
11. Hong MK, Romm PA, Reagan K, et al: Usefulness of the total cholesterol to high-density lipoprotein cholesterol ratio in predicting angiographic coronary artery disease in women. *Am J Cardiol* 1991;68:1646–1650.
12. Genest JJ, McNamara JR, Salem DN, Schaefer EJ: Prevalence of risk factors in men with premature coronary artery disease. *Am J Cardiol* 1991;67:1185–1189.
13. French JK, Elliott JM, Williams BF, et al: Association of angiographically detected coronary artery disease with low levels of high-density lipoprotein cholesterol and systemic hypertension. *Am J Cardiol* 1993;71:505–510.
14. Glueck CJ, Sanghvi VR, Laemmle P, et al: Lack of concordance in classification of coronary heart disease risk: High-risk HDL cholesterol less than 35 mg/dL in subjects with desirable total serum cholesterol, less than 200 mg/dl. *J Lab Clin Med* 1990;116: 377–385.
15. Romm PA, Green CE, Reagan K, Rackley CE: Relation of serum lipoprotein cholesterol levels to presence and severity of angiographic coronary artery disease. *Am J Cardiol* 1991;67:479–483.
16. Agmon J, Behar S, Brunner D, et al: Lipids and lipoproteins in symptomatic coronary heart disease. Distribution, intercorrelations, and significance for risk classification in 6,700 men and 1,500 women. The Bezafibrate Infarction Prevention (BIP) Study Group, Israel. *Circulation* 1992;86:839–848.
17. Abbott RD, Wilson PW, Kannel WB, Castelli WP: High-density lipoprotein cholesterol, total cholesterol screening, and myocardial infarction. The Framingham Study. *Arteriosclerosis* 1988;8:207–211.
18. Miller M, Seidler A, Kwiterovich PO, Pearson TA: Long-term predictors of subsequent cardiovascular events with coronary artery disease and 'desirable' levels of plasma total cholesterol. *Circulation* 1992;86:1165–1170.
19. Watkins LO, Neaton JD, Kuller LH: Racial differences in high-density lipoprotein cholesterol and coronary heart disease incidence in the usual-care group of the Multiple Risk Factor Intervention Trial. *Am J Cardiol* 1986;57:538–545.
20. Gordon DJ, Knoke J, Probstfield JL, et al: High-density lipoprotein cholesterol and coronary heart disease in hypercholesterolemic men: The Lipid Research Clinics Coronary Primary Prevention Trial. *Circulation* 1986;74:1217–1225.
21. Gordon DJ, Probstfield JL, Garrison RJ, et al: High-density lipoprotein cholesterol and cardiovascular disease. Four prospective American studies. *Circulation* 1989;79:8–15.
22. Stampfer MJ, Sacks FM, Salvini S, et al. A prospective study of cholesterol, apolipoproteins, and the risk of myocardial infarction. *N Engl J Med* 1991;325:373–381.
23. Wiklund O, Wilhelmsen L, Elmfeldt D, et al: Alpha-lipoprotein cholesterol concentration in relation to subsequent myocardial infarction in hypercholesterolemic men. *Atherosclerosis* 37: 47–53, 1980.
24. Keys A: Alpha lipoprotein (HDL) cholesterol in the serum and the risk of coronary heart disease and death. *Lancet* 1980;2:603–606.
25. Keys A, Karvonen MJ, Punsar S, et al: HDL serum cholesterol and 24-year mortality of men in Finland. *Int J Epidemiol* 1984;13:428–435.
26. Ballantyne CM, Herd JA, Ferlic LL, et al: Influence of low HDL on progression of coronary artery disease and response to fluvastatin therapy. *Circulation* 1999;99:736–743.
27. Campeau L, Hunninghake DB, Knatterud GL, et al: Aggressive cholesterol lowering delays saphenous vein graft atherosclerosis in women, the elderly, and patients with associated risk factors. NHLBI Post Coronary Artery Bypass Graft clinical trial. Post CABG Trial Investigators. *Circulation* 1999;99:3241–3247.
28. Ballantyne CM, Rangaraj GR: The evolving role of high-density lipoprotein in reducing cardiovascular risk. *Prev Cardiol* 2001;4:65–72.
29. Heart Protection Study Collaborative Group. MRC/BHF Heart Protection Study of cholesterol lowering with simvastatin in 20,536 high-risk individuals: A randomised placebo-controlled trial. *Lancet* 2002;360:7–22.
30. Rezaie-Majd A, Prager GW, Bucek RA, et al. Simvastatin reduces the expression of adhesion molecules in circulating monocytes from hypercholesterolemic patients. *Arterioscler Thromb Vasc Biol* 2003;23:397–403.

31. Calabresi L, Gomaraschi M, Villa B, Omoboni L, et al: Elevated soluble cellular adhesion molecules in subjects with low HDL cholesterol. *Arterioscler Thromb Vasc Biol* 2002;22:656–661.
32. Gotto AM Jr, Brinton EA: Assessing low levels of high-density lipoprotein cholesterol as a risk factor in coronary heart disease: A working group report and update. *J Am Coll Cardiol* 2004;43:717–724.
33. Barter PJ, Nicholls S, Rye KA, et al: Antiinflammatory properties of HDL. *Circ Res* 2004;95:764–772.
34. Lewis GF, Rader DJ: New insights into the regulation of HDL metabolism and reverse cholesterol transport. *Circ Res* 2005;96: 1221–1232.
35. Despres JP, Lemieux I, Dagenais GR, et al: HDL cholesterol as a marker of coronary heart disease risk: The Québec Cardiovascular Study. *Atherosclerosis* 2000;153:263–272.
36. Karhapaa P, Malkki M, Laakso M: Isolated low HDL cholesterol. An insulin–resistant state. *Diabetes* 1994;43:411–417.
37. Castelli WP: Lipids, risk factors and ischaemic heart disease. *Atherosclerosis* 1996;124l:S1–S9.
38. Assmann G: Pro and con: High-density lipoprotein, triglycerides, and other lipid subfractions are the future of lipid management. *Am J Cardiol* 2001;87:2B–7B.
39. Manninen V, Tenkanen L, Koskinen P, et al: Joint effects of serum triglyceride and LDL cholesterol and HDL cholesterol concentrations on coronary heart disease risk in the Helsinki Heart Study. Implications for treatment. *Circulation* 1992;85:37–45.
40. Van Lenten BJ, Reddy ST, Navab M, Fogelman AM: Understanding changes in high-density lipoproteins during the acute phase response. *Arterioscler Thromb Vasc Biol* 2006;26:1687–1688.
41. Auerbach BJ, Parks JS: Lipoprotein abnormalities associated with lipopolysaccharide-induced lecithin:cholesterol acyltransferase and lipase deficiency. *J Biol Chem* 1989;264:10264–10270.
42. Hardardóttir I, Grünfeld C, Feingold KR: Effects of endotoxin and cytokines on lipid metabolism. *Curr Opin Lipidol* 1994;5: 207–215.
43. Kitchens RL, Thompson PA, Munford RS, O'Keefe GE: Acute inflammation and infection maintain circulating phospholipid levels and enhance lipopolysaccharide binding to plasma lipoproteins. *J Lipid Res* 2003;44:2339–2348.
44. Smith SC Jr: Multiple risk factors for cardiovascular disease and diabetes mellitus. *Am J Med* 2007;120:S3–S11.
45. McCall MR, van den Berg JJ, Kuypers FA, et al: Modification of LCAT activity and HDL structure. New links between cigarette smoke and coronary heart disease risk. *Arterioscler Thromb* 1994;14:248–253.
46. Sacks FM, Katan M: Randomized clinical trials on the effects of dietary fat and carbohydrate on plasma lipoproteins and cardiovascular disease. *Am J Med* 2002;113:13S–24S.
47. Frikke-Schmidt R, Nordestgaard BG, Jensen GB, Tybjaerg-Hansen A: Genetic variation in ABC transporter A1 contributes to HDL cholesterol in the general population. *J Clin Invest* 2004;114: 1343–1353.
48. Kuivenhoven JA, Pritchard H, Hill J, et al: The molecular pathology of lecithin:cholesterol acyltransferase (LCAT) deficiency syndromes. *J Lipid Res* 1997;38:191–205.
49. Miller M, Rhyne J, Hamlette S, et al: Genetics of HDL regulation in humans. *Curr Opin Lipidol* 2003;14:273–279.
50. Cohen JC, Kiss RS, Pertsemlidis A, et al: Multiple rare alleles contribute to low plasma levels of HDL cholesterol. *Science* 2004;305:869–872.
51. Viana MB, Giugliani R, Leite VH, et al: Very low levels of high-density lipoprotein cholesterol in four sibs of a family with non-neuropathic Niemann-Pick disease and sea-blue histiocytosis. *J Med Genet* 1990;28:499–504.
52. Ginsberg H, Grabowski GA, Gibson JC, et al: Reduced plasma concentrations of total, low-density lipoprotein and high-density lipoprotein cholesterol in patients with Gaucher type I disease. *Clin Genet* 1984;26:109–116.
53. Keddad K, Razavian SM, Baussan C, et al: Blood lipids and rheological modifications in glycogen storage disease. *Clin Biochem* 1996;29:73–78.
54. Wu FC, von Eckardstein A: Androgens and coronary artery disease. *Endocr Rev* 2003;24:183–217.
55. Fahraeus L, Larsson-Cohn U, Ljungberg S, et al: Plasma lipoproteins during and after danazol treatment. *Acta Obstet Gynecol Scand Suppl* 1984;123:133–135.
56. Cantwell JD: Serum lipid levels in a major league baseball team. *Am J Cardiol* 2002;90:1395–1397.
57. Grimm RH Jr: Antihypertensive therapy: Taking lipids into consideration. *Am Heart J* 1991;122:910–918.
58. Buckley MM, Goa KL, Price AH, Brogden RN: Probucol. A reappraisal of its pharmacological properties and therapeutic use in hypercholesterolaemia. *Drugs* 1989;37:761–800.
59. Brar P, Kwon GY, Holleran S, et al: Change in lipid profile in celiac disease: Beneficial effect of gluten-free diet. *Am J Med* 2006;119:786–790.
60. Wood PD, Haskell WL: The effect of exercise on plasma high-density lipoproteins. *Lipids* 1979;14:417–427.
61. Williams PT: The relationships of vigorous exercise, alcohol, and adiposity to low and high high-density lipoprotein-cholesterol levels. *Metabolism* 53:700–709, 2004.
62. Tall AR, Jiang X, Luo Y, Silver D: 1999 George Lyman Duff memorial lecture: Lipid transfer proteins, HDL metabolism, and atherogenesis. *Arterioscler Thromb Vasc Biol* 2000;20: 1185–1188.
63. Goldberg IJ, Mazlen RG, Rubenstein A, et al: Plasma lipoprotein abnormalities associated with acquired hepatic triglyceride lipase deficiency. *Metabolism* 1985;34:832–835.
64. Badellino KO, Rader DJ: The role of endothelial lipase in high-density lipoprotein metabolism. *Curr Opin Cardiol* 2004;19: 392–395.
65. Lamon-Fava S: High-density lipoproteins: Effects of alcohol, estrogen, and phytoestrogens. *Nutr Rev* 2002;60:1–7.
66. Ettinger WH Jr, Hazzard WR: Prednisone increases very-low-density lipoprotein and high-density lipoprotein in healthy men. *Metabolism* 1988;37:1055–1058.
67. Despres JP, Lemieux I, Robins SJ: Role of fibric acid derivatives in the management of risk factors for coronary heart disease. *Drugs* 2004;64:2177–2198.
68. Miller M: Niacin as a component of combination therapy for dyslipidemia. *Mayo Clin Proc* 2003;78:735–742.
69. Maki KC, Skorodin MS, Jessen JH, Laghi F: Effects of oral albuterol on serum lipids and carbohydrate metabolism in healthy men. *Metabolism* 1996;45:712–717.
70. Calandre EP, Rodriquez-Lopez C, Blazquez A, Cano D: Serum lipids, lipoproteins and apolipoproteins A and B in epileptic patients treated with valproic acid, carbamazepine or phenobarbital. *Acta Neurol Scand* 1991;83:250–253.
71. Miller M, Burgan RG, Osterlund L, et al: A prospective, randomized trial of phenytoin in nonepileptic subjects with reduced HDL cholesterol. *Arterioscler Thromb Vasc Biol* 1995;15:2151–2156.
72. Goldberg RB, Mendez AJ: Case 40-2006: Anemia and low HDL cholesterol. *N Engl J Med* 2007;356:1893–1895.
73. Blackman JD, Cabana VG, Mazzone T: The acute-phase response and associated lipoprotein abnormalities accompanying lymphoma. *J Intern Med* 1993;233:201–204.
74. Castelli WP, Doyle JT, Gordon T, et al: HDL cholesterol and other lipids in coronary heart disease. The Cooperative Lipoprotein Phenotyping Study. *Circulation* 1977;55:767–772.
75. Goldbourt U, Yaari S, Medalie JH: Isolated low HDL cholesterol as a risk factor for coronary heart disease mortality. A 21-year follow-up of 8000 men. *Arterioscler Thromb Vasc Biol* 1997;17:107–113.
76. Genest JJ, Martin-Munley SS, McNamara JR, et al: Familial lipoprotein disorders in patients with premature coronary artery disease. *Circulation* 1992;85:2025–2033.
77. Expert Panel on Detection, Evaluation, and Treatment of High Blood Cholesterol in Adults. Executive Summary of the Third Report of The National Cholesterol Education Program (NCEP) Expert Panel on Detection, Evaluation, And Treatment of High Blood Cholesterol In Adults (Adult Treatment Panel III). *JAMA* 2001;285:2486–2497.
78. Miller M, Zhan M: Genetic determinants of low high-density lipoprotein cholesterol. *Curr Opin Cardiol* 2004;19:380–384.
79. Miller M, Zhan M: Factors influencing coronary risk in low HDL syndromes. Atherosclerosis 2003;169:347–348.
80. Gustafson A, McConathy WJ, Alaupovic P, et al: Identification of lipoprotein families in a variant of human plasma apolipoprotein A deficiency. Scand J Clin Lab Invest 1979;39:377–387.
81. Vergani C, Bettale G: Familial hypo-alpha-lipoproteinemia. Clin Chim Acta 1981;114:45–52.
82. Schaefer EJ, Heaton WH, Wetzel MG, Brewer HB Jr: Plasma apolipoprotein A-1 absence associated with a marked reduction of high-density lipoproteins and premature coronary artery disease. Arteriosclerosis 1982;2:16–26.

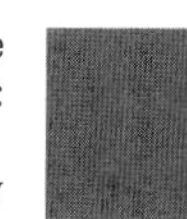

83. Norum RA, Lakier JB, Goldstein S, et al: Familial deficiency of apolipoproteins A-I and C-III and precocious coronary-artery disease. N Engl J Med 1982;306:1513–1519.
84. Matsunaga T, Hiasa Y, Yanagi H, et al: Apolipoprotein A-I deficiency due to a codon 84 nonsense mutation of the apolipoprotein A-I gene. Proc Natl Acad Sci U S A 1991;88:2793–2797.
85. Emmerich J, Verges B, Tauveron I, et al: Familial HDL deficiency due to marked hypercatabolism of normal apoA-I. Arterioscler Thromb 1993;13:1299–1306.
86. Marcil M, Boucher B, Krimbou L, et al: Severe familial HDL deficiency in French-Canadian kindreds. Clinical, biochemical, and molecular characterization. Arterioscler Thromb Vasc Biol 1995;15:1015–1024.
87. Miccoli R, Bertolotto A, Navalesi R, et al: Compound heterozygosity for a structural apolipoprotein A-I variant, apo A-I(L141R)Pisa, and an apolipoprotein A-I null allele in patients with absence of HDL cholesterol, corneal opacifications, and coronary heart disease. Circulation 1996;94:1622–1628.
88. Ng DS, Leiter LA, Vezina C, et al: Apolipoprotein A-I Q[-2]X causing isolated apolipoprotein A-I deficiency in a family with analphalipoproteinemia. J Clin Invest 1994;93:223–229.
89. Miller M, Aiello D, Pritchard H, et al: Apolipoprotein A-$I_{Zavallo}$ (Leu159→Pro): HDL cholesterol deficiency in a kindred associated with premature coronary artery disease. Arterioscler Thromb Vasc Biol 1998;18:1242–1247.
90. Hong SH, Riley W, Rhyne J, et al: Lack of association between increased carotid intima–media thickening and decreased HDL cholesterol in a family with a novel ABCA1 variant, G2265T. Clin Chem 2002;48:2066–2070.
91. Hong SH, Rhyne J, Zeller K, Miller M: $ABCA1_{Alabama}$: A novel variant associated with HDL deficiency and premature coronary artery disease. Atherosclerosis 2002;164:245–250.
92. Hong SH, Rhyne J, Miller M: Novel polypyrimidine variation (IVS46: del T -39...-46) in ABCA1 causes exon skipping and contributes to HDL cholesterol deficiency in a family with premature coronary disease. Circ Res 2003;93:1006–1012.
93. Robinson D, Williams P, Day J: High-density-lipoprotein cholesterol in the Maasai of East Africa: A cautionary note. Br Med J 1979;1:1249.
94. Pauletto P, Puato M, Caroli MG, et al: Blood pressure and atherogenic lipoprotein profiles of fish-diet and vegetarian villagers in Tanzania: The Lugalawa study. Lancet 1996;348:784–788.
95. Hodge AM, Dowse GK, Erasmus RT, et al: Serum lipids and modernization in coastal and highland Papua New Guinea. Am J Epidemiol 1996;144:1129–1142.
96. Connor WE, Cerqueira MT, Connor RW, et al: The plasma lipids, lipoproteins, and diet of the Tarahumara indians of Mexico. Am J Clin Nutr 1978;31:1131–1142.
97. Mancilha-Carvalho JJ, Crews DE: Lipid profiles of Yanomamo Indians of Brazil. Prev Med 1990;19:66–75.
98. Ooi TC, Simo IE, Yakichuk JA: Delayed clearance of postprandial chylomicrons and their remnants in the hypoalphalipoproteinemia and mild hypertriglyceridemia syndrome. Arterioscler Thromb 1992;12:1184–1190.
99. Karpe F, Bard JM, Steiner G, et al: HDLs and alimentary lipemia. Studies in men with previous myocardial infarction at a young age. Arterioscler Thromb 1993;13:11–22.
100. Cohen JC, Grundy SM: Normal postprandial lipemia in men with low plasma HDL concentrations. Arterioscler Thromb 1992;12:972–975.
101. Miller M, Kwiterovich PO Jr, Bachorik PS, Georgopoulos A: Decreased postprandial response to a fat meal in normotriglyceridemic men with hypoalphalipoproteinemia. Arterioscler Thromb 1993;13:385–392.
102. Tai ES, Emmanuel SC, Chew SK, et al: Isolated low HDL cholesterol: An insulin-resistant state only in the presence of fasting hypertriglyceridemia. Diabetes 1999;48:1088–1092.
103. Al-Mahmood A, Ismail A, Rashid F, Mohamed W: Isolated hypertriglyceridemia: An insulin-resistant state with or without low HDL cholesterol. J Atheroscler Thromb 2006;13:143–148.
104. Greene DJ, Skeggs JW, Morton RE: Elevated triglyceride content diminishes the capacity of high-density lipoprotein to deliver cholesteryl esters via the scavenger receptor class B type I (SR-BI). J Biol Chem 2001;276:4804–4811.
105. Skeggs JW, Morton RE: LDL and HDL enriched in triglyceride promote abnormal cholesterol transport. J Lipid Res 2002;43:1264–1274.
106. Rader DJ, Ikewaki K, Duverger N, et al: Very low high-density lipoproteins without coronary atherosclerosis. Lancet 1993;342:1455–1458.
107. Miller M, Rhyne J, Hong SH, et al: Do mutations causing low HDL cholesterol promote increased carotid intima-media thickness? Clin Chim Acta 2007;377:273–275.
108. Glueck CJ, Gartside P, Fallat RW, et al: Longevity syndromes: Familial hypobeta and familial hyperalpha lipoproteinemia. J Lab Clin Med 1976;88:941–957.
109. Pirich C, Efthimiou Y, O'Grady J, Sinzinger H: Hyperalphalipoproteinemia and prostaglandin I2 stability. Thromb Res 1997;88:41–47.
110. Pirro M, Siepi D, Lupattelli G, et al: Plasma C-reactive protein in subjects with hypo/hyperalphalipoproteinemias. *Metabolism* 2003;52:432–436.
111. Asztalos BF, Horvath KV, Kajinami K, et al: Apolipoprotein composition of HDL in cholesteryl ester transfer protein deficiency. J Lipid Res 2004;45:448–455.
112. Rye KA, Barter PJ: Formation and metabolism of prebeta-migrating, lipid-poor apolipoprotein A-I. Arterioscler Thromb Vasc Biol 2004;24:421–428.
113. Mahley RW, Huang Y, Weisgraber KH: Putting cholesterol in its place: apoE and reverse cholesterol transport. J Clin Invest 2006;116:1226–1229.
114. Matsuura F, Wang N, Chen W, et al: HDL from CETP-deficient subjects shows enhanced ability to promote cholesterol efflux from macrophages in an apoE- and ABCG1-dependent pathway. J Clin Invest 2006;116:1435–1442.
115. Morehouse LA, Sugarman ED, Bourassa PA, et al: Inhibition of CETP activity by torcetrapib reduces susceptibility to diet-induced atherosclerosis in New Zealand White rabbits. J Lipid Res 2007;48:1263–1272.
116. Nissen SE, Tardif JC, Nicholls SJ, et al: Effect of torcetrapib on the progression of coronary atherosclerosis. N Engl J Med 2007;356:1304–1316.
117. Kastelein JJ, van Leuven SI, Burgess L, et al: Effect of torcetrapib on carotid atherosclerosis in familial hypercholesterolemia. N Engl J Med 2007;356:1620–1630.
118. Hirano K, Yamashita S, Nakajima N, et al: Genetic cholesteryl ester transfer protein deficiency is extremely frequent in the Omagari area of Japan. Marked hyperalphalipoproteinemia caused by CETP gene mutation is not associated with longevity. Arterioscler Thromb Vasc Biol 1997;17:1053–1059.
119. Barzilai N, Atzmon G, Schechter C, et al: Unique lipoprotein phenotype and genotype associated with exceptional longevity. JAMA 2003;290:2030–2040.
120. Arai Y, Hirose N, Yamamura K, et al: Deficiency of cholesteryl ester transfer protein and gene polymorphisms of lipoprotein lipase and hepatic lipase are not associated with longevity J Mol Med 2003;81:102–109.
121. Cellini E, Nacmias B, Olivieri F, et al: Cholesteryl ester transfer protein (CETP) I405V polymorphism and longevity in Italian centenarians. Mech Ageing Dev 2005;126:826–828.
122. Rhyne J, Ryan MJ, White C, et al: The two novel CETP mutations Gln87X and Gln165X in a compound heterozygous state are associated with marked hyperalphalipoproteinemia and absence of significant coronary artery disease. J Mol Med 2006;84:647–650.
123. Canizales-Quinteros S, Aguilar-Salinas CA, Reyes-Rodriguez E, et al: Locus on chromosome 6p linked to elevated HDL cholesterol serum levels and to protection against premature atherosclerosis in a kindred with familial hypercholesterolemia. Circ Res 2003;92:569–576.
124. Heid IM, Boes E, Müller M, et al: A genome-wide association analysis of HDL cholesterol in the population-based KORA study sheds new light on intergenic regions. *Circ Cardiovasc Genet* (in press).

CHAPTER 11

Lipoprotein(a)

Marlys L. Koschinsky and Santica M. Marcovina

Although numerous studies since the 1960s have identified increased plasma concentrations of lipoprotein(a) [Lp(a)] as a risk factor for coronary heart disease (CHD), the pathophysiologic and physiologic roles of Lp(a), as well as its potential use in clinical risk assessment, remain elusive. Lp(a) is a challenging lipoprotein to study because it has a complex structure consisting of a low-density lipoprotein (LDL)–like moiety to which is covalently attached the unique glycoprotein moiety apolipoprotein(a) [apo(a)]. Apo(a) contains multiply repeated kringle motifs that are similar to a sequence found in the fibrinolytic proenzyme plasminogen; differing numbers of kringle sequences in apo(a) create Lp(a) isoform size heterogeneity. In addition to increased plasma concentrations of Lp(a), small apo(a) isoform size has been identified as a risk factor for CHD, although further studies to define the latter relationship are required. The similarity of Lp(a) to LDL and plasminogen provides an enticing potential link between the processes of atherosclerosis and thrombosis. Clearly, Lp(a) is a risk factor for both atherothrombotic and purely thrombotic events; a plethora of mechanisms to explain these clinical findings has been provided by both *in vitro* studies and animal models for Lp(a). However, the relative resistance of Lp(a) to standard lipid-lowering strategies has prevented key studies aimed at evaluating the effect of prospective reduction of plasma Lp(a) concentrations on cardiovascular endpoints.

As a result of the size heterogeneity of Lp(a), significant challenges are associated with the measurement of this lipoprotein. This, in turn, has complicated the interpretation of clinical studies and has posed major obstacles for the development of a standardized method for Lp(a) measurement in the clinic. Despite these challenges, Lp(a) measurement can be useful in informing the treatment of patients at high risk for CHD.

Since its initial identification by Berg[1] as an antigenic variant of human LDL, Lp(a) has been studied extensively with respect to basic research investigations into the mechanism of action of this unique lipoprotein or atherothrombosis, as well as epidemiologic studies of the association of increased Lp(a) concentrations with a variety of vascular diseases. Lp(a) contains a lipoprotein moiety that is highly similar to LDL both in lipid composition and the presence of apoB-100. In the Lp(a) particle, the unique glycoprotein apo(a), which is synthesized and secreted from the liver,[2] is covalently attached to the apoB-100 component of LDL by a single disulfide bond[3]; as such, Lp(a) particles contain apo(a) and apoB-100 in a 1:1 molar ratio[4] (Fig 11-1). A large body of evidence has demonstrated that Lp(a) particle assembly occurs outside the hepatocytes[3,5] and involves initial lysine-dependent noncovalent interactions between apo(a) and apoB-100, which precede disulfide bond formation between the two molecules.[5]

It is well accepted that the apo(a) component of Lp(a) renders many of the defining properties attributable to Lp(a). For example, the presence of apo(a) appears to inhibit catabolism of Lp(a) by the LDL receptor *in vivo* (see Lipoprotein(a) Catabolism later in this chapter). As such, attention has focused on characterization of the structure and function of apo(a).

In a seminal study, McLean and coworkers[6] reported that the sequence of apo(a) (obtained from analysis of a human liver complementary DNA sequence) bears a striking similarity to the serine protease zymogen plasminogen; plasmin, which is the active form of this zymogen, is a key enzyme in the fibrinolytic cascade. Specifically, apo(a) contains a number of repeated copies of a sequence that is similar to plasminogen kringle IV, followed by sequences that are homologous to the kringle V and protease domains of plasminogen[6] (Fig 11-2). Kringle domains are tri-looped

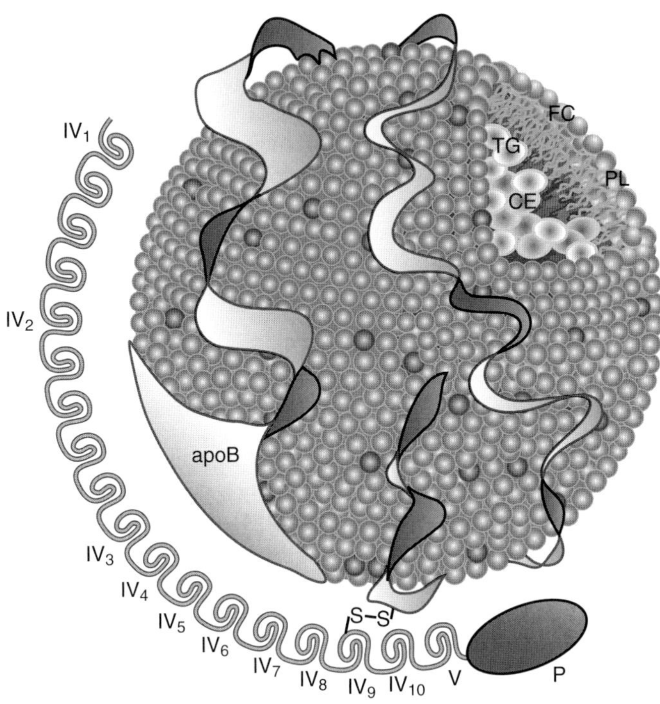

FIGURE 11-1 Lipoprotein [Lp(a)] consists of an low-density lipoprotein (LDL)–like moiety covalently linked to apolipoprotein(a) [apo(a)]. The LDL-like moiety is composed of a central core of triglycerides (TG) and cholesteryl esters (CE) surrounded by phospholipids (PL), free cholesterol (FC), and a single molecule of apoB. Apo(a) contains 10 different types of plasminogen kringle IV–like repeats, as well as regions homologous to the kringle V and protease (P) regions of plasminogen. The kringle IV type 2 domain (IV_2) is present in multiply-repeated copies that differ in number between apo(a) isoforms. Apo(a) is joined to apoB by a single disulfide bond involving an unpaired cysteine residue in kringle IV type 9. Also depicted is the noncovalent interaction between apoB and apo(a) kringle IV types 7 and 8 that plays a role in Lp(a) assembly. Reprinted from Ref. 5, with permission.

protein structural motifs that are characterized by the presence of three invariant disulfide bonds, and that are present in a number of proteins involved in both blood coagulation and fibrinolysis. The apo(a) kringle IV–like sequences can be grouped into 10 types on the basis of amino acid sequence (designated KIV_1 to KIV_{10}; see Fig. 11-2).[6] All kringle IV types are present in a single copy in the apo(a) molecule[7,8] with the exception of kringle IV type 2, which is represented in a variable number of identically repeated copies ranging from 3 to more than 30.[9] This identically repeated domain forms the molecular basis of Lp(a) isoform size heterogeneity which is a hallmark of this lipoprotein. Unique functions have been ascribed to some of the other KIV domains. For example, KIV types 5 to 8 each contain a weak lysine-binding site; in the noncovalent step of Lp(a) formation, the weak lysine binding sites in KIV types 7 and 8 mediate noncovalent, lysine-dependent interactions with two lysine residues in the amino terminus of apoB-100.[10] This interaction precedes disulfide bond formation between the unpaired cysteine in apo(a) KIV type 9[3] with an unpaired cysteine residue in the C terminus of apoB-100.[11] KIV type 10 is characterized by the presence of a strong lysine-binding site that likely mediates the interaction of apo(a) with biological substrates such as fibrin(ogen).[12]

The presence of LDL-like and plasminogen-like moieties in Lp(a) have led investigators to hypothesize that Lp(a) constitutes a unique link between atherosclerosis (contributed largely by the LDL component) and attendant thrombotic events (contributed by the plasminogen-like apo(a) moiety).[13] Indeed, both atherogenic and thrombotic mechanisms for Lp(a) have been reported (see Proposed Mechanisms of Lipoprotein(a) Action later in this chapter). However, it is important to note that a number of mechanisms proposed for Lp(a) pathogenicity, in fact, correspond to unique properties of this lipoprotein (i.e., are not directly related to its similarity to either LDL or plasminogen). This may reflect, for example, the extreme glycosylation modification of apo(a) (~28% of the molecule by weight)[14] compared with plasminogen, the consequences of which have been largely unexplored.

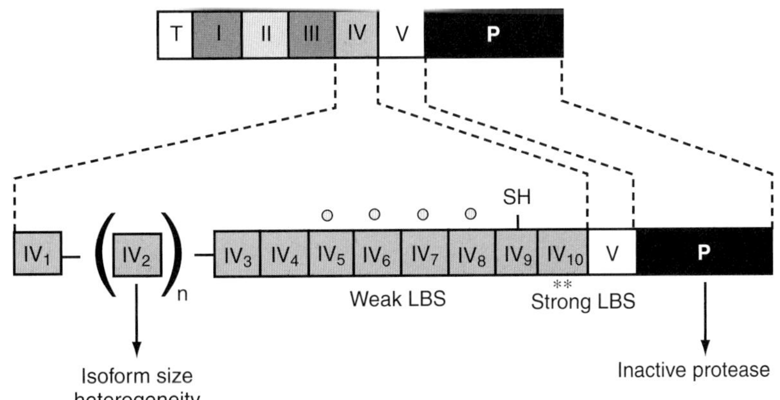

FIGURE 11-2 Relationship between apolipoprotein(a) [apo(a)] and plasminogen. Plasminogen consists of an amino-terminal tail region *(T)* followed by five different kringle domains (denoted by the Roman numerals I to V) and a trypsin-like protease domain *(P)*. Apo(a) lacks the tail region and kringles I to III, and consists of multiple copies of a sequence resembling plasminogen kringle IV, followed by domains analogous to the kringle V and protease domains of plasminogen. There are 10 different types of apo(a) kringle IV that differ in amino acid sequence. Of the 10 different kringle IV types in apo(a), types 1 and 3 to 10 are each present in a single copy in all apo(a) isoforms. Apo(a) kringle IV type 2 is present in a variable number of repeated copies, which is the molecular basis of Lp(a) isoform heterogeneity. Kringle IV type 10 has been shown to harbor strong lysine binding sites *(LBS),* whereas weaker LBS are present in kringle IV types 5 to 8. A single unpaired cysteine present in kringle IV type 9 has been shown to mediate disulfide bond formation with apoB to form covalent Lp(a) particles. The apo(a) protease-like domain cannot be cleaved by plasminogen activators because of a substitution at the cryptic cleavage site and is thus inactive; the domain also contains a critical 10–amino acid deletion compared with plasminogen.

DETERMINATION OF PLASMA LIPOPROTEIN(a) CONCENTRATIONS

Lp(a) concentrations in plasma vary more than 1000-fold in the human population—ranging from undetectable to greater than 100 mg/dL—and primarily reflect differences in Lp(a) production rather than catabolism of the particle.[15] In white populations, variability in Lp(a) concentrations can be largely explained at the level of the gene (~90%), with size of the gene (reflecting the size of the repeated kringle IV type 2 domain) contributing approximately 60% of the variation.[16] The strong genetic control of Lp(a) concentrations explains why there is little modulation of plasma concentrations of this lipoprotein by environmental factors, and why Lp(a) concentrations are relatively resistant to pharmacologic interventions including statin therapy[17-19] (see Strategies for Modulation of Plasma Lipoprotein(a) Concentrations later in this chapter). It is, therefore, not feasible currently to perform prospective studies aimed at evaluating the effect of therapeutic reduction of Lp(a) concentrations on clinical outcomes.

A general inverse correlation has been demonstrated between apo(a) isoform size and plasma Lp(a) concentrations[20]; this may result from the less efficient secretion of larger apo(a) isoforms from hepatocytes,[21] reflecting, at least in part, longer retention times in the endoplasmic reticulum and subsequent quality control–mediated degradation associated with this intracellular compartment.[22] The potential impact of the relationship between apo(a) isoform size and transcript stability, translational efficiency, and the efficiency of Lp(a) particle assembly on the inverse correlation has not been studied. Notably, however, the relationship between isoform size and corresponding Lp(a) concentrations is not absolute. Indeed, there are marked differences in this relationship in certain ethnic populations. For example, black individuals have greater Lp(a) concentrations associated with midsized apo(a) isoform sizes compared with white individuals.[23] Although the molecular basis of this observation remains to be completely determined, a new study suggests that the apoE genotype affects allele-specific apo(a) levels for large apo(a) isoform sizes in black individuals.[24] Another study has reported that three single-nucleotide polymorphisms in *LPA* can explain the majority of increased Lp(a) concentrations (nearly twofold) in black versus white populations.[25]

It has been reported that in individuals heterozygous for apo(a) isoform sizes, the small apo(a) allele is not consistently dominant; this appears to depend on the size of the larger isoform, particularly in white individuals.[26] Interesting evidence is also emerging that within individuals, each allele size affects not only the level of that allele, but also the level of the other allele.[27] Taken together, these findings argue strongly for the measurement of allele-specific Lp(a) concentrations; this involves determining the ratio of intensity of apo(a) isoform sizes in a gel-based assay, and the multiplication of this ratio by plasma Lp(a) concentrations to assign the relative contributions of each isoform to total Lp(a) concentrations. Elegant studies by Paultre and colleagues[28] have demonstrated the predictive value of computing allele-specific Lp(a) values to assess Lp(a) as a risk factor in black individuals. In this study, these investigators demonstrated that increased concentrations of Lp(a) associated with small apo(a) isoform sizes independently predict CHD risk in black and white men. This clearly demonstrates the value of determining allele-specific Lp(a) concentrations, because neither measure alone predicts Lp(a) risk in the black population.

LIPOPROTEIN(a) CATABOLISM

Despite many studies aimed at addressing this question, the metabolic fate of Lp(a) remains largely undetermined. However, clearance of Lp(a) does not appear to involve the LDL component of the particle, which, in turn, has been postulated to underscore the lack of responsiveness of plasma Lp(a) concentrations to LDL-lowering strategies.[18] Studies in patients with renal failure have pointed to a possible role for the kidney in Lp(a) catabolism[29,30]; Frischmann and colleagues'[31] kinetic study has specifically determined that Lp(a) catabolism, rather than production, is impaired in hemodialysis patients. However, other studies have reported that the kidney does not constitute a major route of clearance for Lp(a) in normal physiology[32,33]; a number of studies have provided evidence that the liver is the major organ responsible for Lp(a) catabolism.[32,34] Several candidate receptors for Lp(a) catabolism by the liver have been suggested based on their ability to bind and internalize apoB-100–containing lipoproteins; these include the LDL receptor and the LDL receptor–related protein, although the data demonstrating a role for both the LDL receptor[35-39] and the LDL receptor–related protein[40] in Lp(a) catabolism have been challenged.[32,41] More recently, a role for the asialoglycoprotein receptor in apo(a)-mediated clearance of Lp(a) by the liver has been suggested,[34] although this finding has been challenged by Cain and colleagues[32] using a mouse model system to study Lp(a) clearance. At least some of the controversial findings in this area may stem from the use of heterologous animal models versus the use of human kinetic studies or cultured cell models to study apo(a)/Lp(a) catabolism. Because apo(a) is not expressed in species other than Old World monkeys and humans,[42] caution needs to be exercised in the interpretation of results obtained from studying the clearance of human apo(a)/Lp(a) in other animals such as mice. Clearly, additional studies are required to determine conclusively the liver receptor(s) that are involved in the removal of Lp(a) from the circulation and the relative role of the kidney in Lp(a) catabolism.

LIPOPROTEIN(a) AS A RISK FACTOR FOR CORONARY HEART DISEASE: EVIDENCE FROM CLINICAL STUDIES

Based on the National Cholesterol Education Program Adult Treatment Panel III (NCEP ATP III) guidelines, Lp(a) is currently classified as an "emerging" lipid risk factor for cardiovascular disease.[43] Increased plasma Lp(a) concentrations (>30 mg/dL in many studies) have been identified as a risk factor for a variety of atherosclerotic disorders including peripheral vascular disease,[44,45] ischemic stroke,[46,47] aortic aneurysm,[48] and premature CHD, the last of which corresponds to the majority of the studies performed to date (reviewed in Anuurad and colleagues,[18] Koschinsky,[49] and Marcovina and coworkers[19]). Notably, Lp(a) excess is the most common inherited lipid disorder in patients with premature CHD,[50] which drives interest in understanding the mechanism of action of Lp(a) in atherogenesis.

The clinical significance of Lp(a) in CHD has been consistently confirmed in numerous retrospective case–control studies performed during the past three decades.[18,19,49] In essentially all studies of this design, plasma Lp(a) concentrations are increased in patients with existing CHD compared with matched control subjects. These types of studies have been criticized in that patients are selected with existing CHD, which favors the inclusion of subjects with other CHD risk factors. In addition, retrospective case–control studies cannot distinguish a causative role for Lp(a) from the possibility that Lp(a) may merely be a marker for CHD, or that plasma Lp(a) concentrations may increase as a consequence of CHD.

A smaller number of prospective studies have been performed to assess more directly the contribution of plasma Lp(a) to the future development of CHD. The results from prospective studies have yielded conflicting results, however, ranging from a strong positive association between Lp(a) and CHD,[51-55] to a weak association,[56] to no association whatsoever.[57,58] The discrepant results may be attributable to variations in study design such as study population composition with respect to sex and ethnicity, collection and storage of samples, and methods used for statistical analysis. In addition, the structural heterogeneity of Lp(a) (see later) can greatly affect the accuracy of Lp(a) measurement.[18,19,49] Clearly, however, the majority of prospective studies performed over the past decade have demonstrated that increased plasma Lp(a) concentrations are a predictor of CHD. Meta-analysis of 12 prospective studies performed between 1991 and 1997 indicates that plasma Lp(a) concentrations are an independent risk factor in both men and women; in the majority of these studies, there was a dose–response relationship between plasma Lp(a) concentrations and CHD risk.[59] Most recently, meta-analysis of 27 prospective studies corresponding to 5436 CHD cases observed during a mean follow-up time of 10 years indicated that individuals in the general population with Lp(a) concentrations in the top third of baseline measurements are at approximately 70% increased risk for CHD compared with individuals in the bottom third.[60]

The predictive strength of Lp(a) concentrations for CHD was evaluated in the Atherosclerosis Risk in Communities (ARIC) study, with a 10-year follow-up period and 725 CHD events[61]; Lp(a) concentrations were found to be associated with modest risk ratios. In terms of population differences, the ARIC study results suggest that Lp(a) concentrations confer less risk in black than in white individuals. A recent prospective study[62] examined a cohort of 1216 patients with a mean follow-up time of 6.7 years, with total mortality and mortality because of cardiovascular disease used as outcome variables. In this study, Lp(a) concentrations in excess of 30 mg/dL were present in 30% of the study population and were found to be an independent predictor of death. On this basis, the authors suggested that Lp(a) concentration in excess of 30 mg/dL is associated with a poor prognosis, and may serve to identify patients who would benefit from aggressive secondary prevention programs.

Although there is little or no correlation between plasma concentrations of Lp(a) and other vascular risk factors, evidence has been provided from a number of studies to suggest that the risk attributable to increased Lp(a) concentrations is dependent on the concomitant presence of other such risk factors. In the Familial Atherosclerosis Treatment Study (FATS), Lp(a) concentrations were a strong predictor of events at baseline, but they lost their predictive value when LDL cholesterol level was reduced to less than 100 mg/dL in the treatment group.[63] More recently, in the Prospective Epidemiological Study of Myocardial Infarction (PRIME) study,[64] Lp(a) concentrations were investigated as a CHD risk factor using a prospective cohort of 9133 French and Northern Irish men aged 50 to 59 years without a history of CHD. Increased Lp(a) concentrations increased the risk for myocardial infarction (MI) and angina pectoris, and the effect was most pronounced in men with a high LDL cholesterol concentration. The results of the Québec Cardiovascular Study suggest that Lp(a) is, in fact, not an independent risk factor for ischemic heart disease in men, but it does increase the risk associated with increased apoB and total cholesterol levels, and appears to attenuate the beneficial effects of increased HDL level.[65] Similar interactions of increased Lp(a) concentrations with other risk factors were found in the Münster Heart study. Specifically, a high concentration of Lp(a) further increased the risk for MI in men with high or moderately increased estimated global risk (i.e., risk for a coronary event >10% in 10 years) but not in men with a low estimated global risk.[66]

Baseline Lp(a) concentrations were measured in a large, prospective study of 27,791 initially healthy women in the Women's Health Study, who had been followed up for 10 years. The findings indicated that extremely increased Lp(a) concentrations (greater than the 90th percentile) were associated with increased cardiovascular risk, especially in women with high LDL concentrations.[67] Interestingly, no risk gradient was observed in individuals with lower plasma Lp(a) concentrations. This raises the possibility that previous studies that did not evaluate for thresholds may have missed relationships between Lp(a) and risk, and further suggest that the current risk threshold for Lp(a) (>30 mg/dL, as previously defined[68]) may be too low, especially in some populations.

RELATIONSHIP BETWEEN APOLIPOPROTEIN(a) ISOFORM SIZE AND CARDIOVASCULAR DISEASE RISK

A number of studies since the late 1990s have sought to define the role of apo(a) isoform size, independent of plasma Lp(a) concentrations, in CHD risk. For example, in the Bruneck study, it was shown that small apo(a) sizes are an independent risk factor for advanced carotid atherosclerosis, although risk is further increased in conjunction with increased Lp(a) concentrations.[69] On the other hand, these investigators reported that plasma

Lp(a) concentrations, but not small apo(a) isoform sizes, were predictive of risk for early atherosclerosis, and that this association was present only when LDL cholesterol concentrations were also increased. Although a relationship between cardiovascular disease and Lp(a) concentrations associated with small apo(a) isoform sizes in both white and black men has been documented,[28] this association has not been consistently observed in women.[28,70,71] Interestingly, conflicting data also have been reported regarding whether increased Lp(a) concentrations in women are[72,73] or are not[74,75] associated with increased risk for cerebrovascular or cardiovascular diseases; one study suggests that Lp(a) risk in women is applicable only to those with extremely increased concentrations in conjunction with increased LDL concentrations.[67] Further studies on the role of Lp(a) concentrations and apo(a) isoform size as risk factors for vascular disease in women are clearly necessary.

Results of Wu and coworkers'[76] study suggest that small apo(a) isoform size (<22 kringle IV repeats) is associated with lower endothelium-dependent, flow-mediated dilation of the brachial artery regardless of plasma Lp(a) concentrations. In addition, Emanuele and coworkers[77] report that the percentage of subjects with at least one small apo(a) isoform was significantly greater in those patients who presented with acute MI versus those with unstable angina; small apo(a) isoform size, but not increased Lp(a) concentration, was an independent predictor of acute MI versus unstable angina pectoris in a multivariate logistic regression model. Evidence for a role of apo(a) isoform size and risk for the development of angina was also provided by Rifai and colleagues.[78] In this study, it was demonstrated that although both Lp(a) concentrations and small apo(a) isoforms were associated with risk for angina, only the association between apo(a) size and risk remained significant in a multivariate model.

PROPOSED MECHANISMS OF LIPOPROTEIN(a) ACTION

Despite a plethora of studies designed to investigate the basis of the pathogenicity associated with increased plasma Lp(a) concentrations, the role of Lp(a) in the development and progression of CHD remains poorly understood. It has been documented, however, that Lp(a) is present in the arterial wall at the sites of atherosclerotic lesions, and that it accumulates at these sites to an extent that is proportional to plasma Lp(a) concentrations.[79] Lp(a) is preferentially retained in this milieu, likely by virtue of its ability to bind to a number of arterial wall components including fibrinogen/fibrin, fibronectin, and glycosaminoglycans (Fig 11-3).[5] The localization of

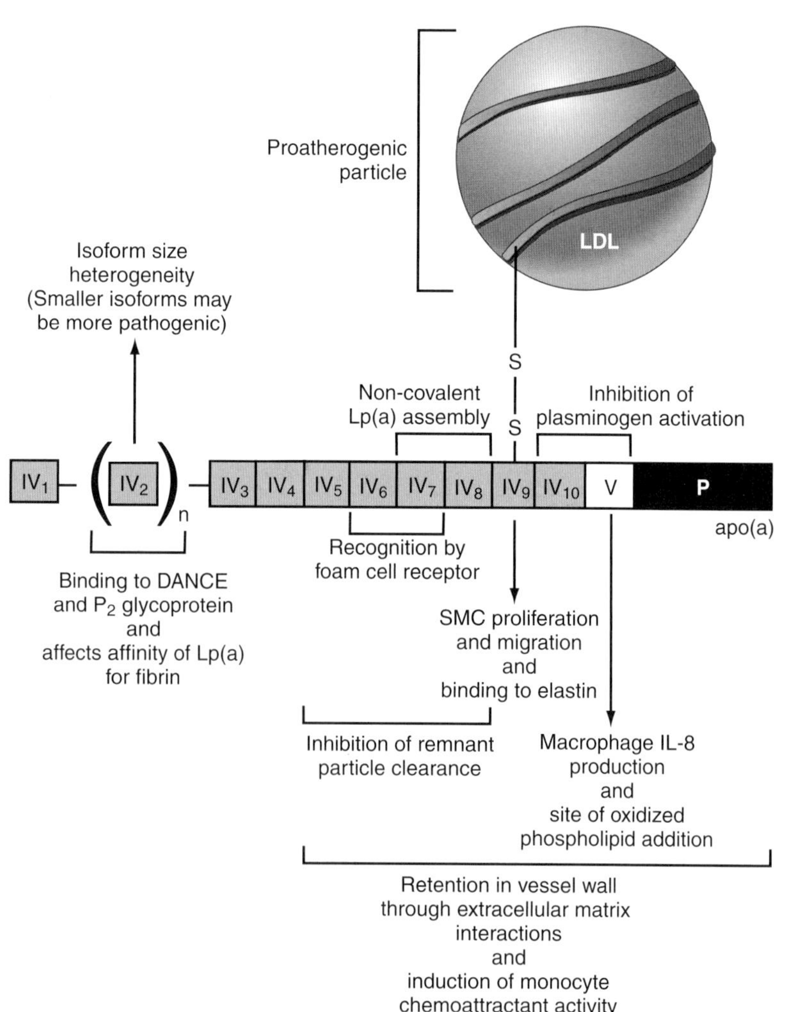

FIGURE 11-3 Specific functions have been mapped to discrete structural units in lipoprotein(a) [Lp(a)]. Using a combination of expression of recombinant forms of apolipoprotein(a) [apo(a)] and elastase cleavage of apo(a)/Lp(a), functional domains in apo(a) have been identified. These domains are potentially involved in promotion of atherosclerosis and inflammation, inhibition of angiogenesis and fibrinolysis, and Lp(a) assembly. The low-density lipoprotein (LDL)–like moiety promotes foam cell formation by virtue of the interaction of apo(a) kringle 4 types 6 and 7 with a specific receptor expressed on foam cells. DANCE, developmental arteries and neural crest epidermal growth factor–like; IL-8, P, protease-like domain in apo(a); interleukin-8; SMC, smooth muscle cells.

Lp(a) within the arterial wall implies a direct causative role for Lp(a) in the initiation or progression, or both, of atherosclerosis.

Insights into possible roles for Lp(a) in vascular disease have been gained through *in vitro* studies and animal models; both proatherosclerotic and prothrombotic roles for Lp(a) have been postulated based on these studies (Table 11-1). Many *in vitro* studies have probed structure–function relationships involving different kringle modules of apo(a).[5] These studies, which have been greatly facilitated by the use of recombinant variants of apo(a), have helped to delineate unique contributions of specific kringle domains, and suggest that many functions of apo(a) reside within the C-terminal half of the molecule (see Fig 11-3).[5] Analysis of apo(a)/Lp(a) function *in vitro* has revealed the potential for Lp(a) to inhibit fibrinolysis,[80] likely through the ability of apo(a) to interfere with the efficient activation of plasminogen to plasmin (reviewed by Marcovina and Koschinsky[81]), and to affect the function of arterial smooth muscle cells. With respect to the latter, O'Neil and colleagues'[82] study reports that the apo(a) component of Lp(a) can stimulate the migration and proliferation of aortic smooth muscle cells; this effect appears to be mediated by the apo(a) kringle IV type 9 domain and involves the inhibition of activation of transforming growth factor–β as was reported previously by several other groups. The stimulatory effect of Lp(a) on smooth muscle cell migration and proliferation may underscore, in part, correlations that have been reported between Lp(a) concentrations and rapid restenosis rates in coronary vessels after percutaneous transluminal coronary angioplasty and vein grafts of coronary artery bypasses.[83,84]

In addition to the ability of Lp(a) to interfere with the efficient formation of plasmin, a study has reported that Lp(a) may alter the architecture of fibrin clots, thereby decreasing their permeability and susceptibility to breakdown.[85] In addition, direct prothrombotic effects of apo(a)/Lp(a) have been reported in *in vitro* studies through its ability to inhibit tissue factor pathway inhibitor[86] and to enhance platelet responsiveness.[87]

A study using human vascular endothelial cells has shown that both apo(a) and Lp(a) can elicit cytoskeletal rearrangements.[88] This, in turn, renders the endothelial cells more permeable, which may contribute to a dysfunctional endothelium *in vivo*. Given that endothelial dysfunction is an early event in the atherosclerotic process, it is interesting to speculate that consistent with the Bruneck study,[69] Lp(a) concentrations in conjunction with increased LDL concentrations may potentiate endothelial dysfunction. Specifically, the increased permeability of endothelial cells, mediated by Lp(a), could facilitate the deposition of LDL in the arterial wall. This process would be enhanced by increased plasma LDL concentrations, which may explain the dependence of Lp(a) risk in early atherosclerosis on concomitant increases of plasma LDL and Lp(a), but not apo(a) isoform size, as reported in the Bruneck study. Data suggesting that Lp(a) may contribute to a dysfunctional endothelium *in vitro* (e.g., by stimulating endothelial cell adhesion molecule expression[89] and increasing endothelial cell permeability)[88] are supported by a number of studies that demonstrate that increased plasma Lp(a) concentrations contribute to endothelial dysfunction *in vivo*.[90]

Some studies have suggested a link between Lp(a) and oxidized phospholipids. Specifically, it has been shown that in human plasma, oxidized phospholipids are preferentially associated with Lp(a) compared with free LDL.[91] More recently, it has been demonstrated that percutaneous coronary intervention results in acute increases of both oxidized LDL and oxidized Lp(a), and that oxidized phospholipid is rapidly transferred to and becomes predominantly associated with Lp(a) compared with other apoB-containing lipoproteins.[92] This is in keeping with Edelstein and colleagues' report that demonstrated that the kringle V domain in apo(a) itself contains oxidized phospholipids covalently bound to lysine residues present in this kringle. Interestingly, the kringle V domain was also implicated in stimulation of the production and secretion of interleukin-8 from cultured human THP-1 macrophages[93]; a link with the presence of oxidized phospholipids in apo(a) kringle V in mediating this effect remains to be determined.

Several animal models have been used to probe the function of apo(a)/Lp(a) in a more physiologic setting.[94] However, these studies have been generally complicated by the unusual species distribution of this lipoprotein (present only in humans and Old World monkeys).[42] This has called into question the applicability of using animals such as mice and rabbits as models for Lp(a) pathogenicity given that the gene encoding apo(a) is absent in these species. However, the balance of opinion is that single- and double-transgenic animals (i.e., overexpressing both human apo(a) and LDL) can be useful tools to understand the role of Lp(a) in atherosclerosis. Indeed, transgenic apo(a) mouse and rabbit models have been used to study processes such as Lp(a) assembly, structure–function relationships in Lp(a), regulation of the expression of the gene encoding apo(a), and mechanisms of Lp(a) involvement in the

TABLE 11-1 Proposed Mechanisms of Lipoprotein(a) Pathogenicity

Prothrombotic	Proatherogenic
↓Plasmin formation (fibrin)	↑Smooth muscle cell proliferation/migration
↓Plasmin formation (pericellular)	↑Endothelial cell permeability
↓TFPI activity	↑Endothelial cell adhesion molecule expression
↑Platelet aggregation	Carrier of oxidized phospholipids
Alteration of fibrin clot architecture	Selective retention in arterial intima
↓EC PAI-1 activity/expression	↑Foam cell formation
	↑Proinflammatory expression in macrophages
	↑Lesion calcification
	↑EC monocyte chemotaxis and trans EC migration

EC, endothelial cell; PAI-1, plasminogen activator inhibitor-1; TFPI, tissue factor pathway inhibitor.

cause of atherosclerosis (see later for a more detailed discussion).[94]

Studies using apo(a) transgenic rabbits are in agreement with data from transgenic mice in that apo(a) deposition in both models was coincident with the presence of accumulated intimal smooth muscle cells and decreased active transforming growth factor–β.[95] The possibility that Lp(a) might modulate smooth muscle cell phenotype by promoting dedifferentiation was suggested by the enhanced staining for markers of activated or immature smooth muscle cells in this study.[95] A somewhat different effect of Lp(a) on smooth muscle cell phenotype was reported in transgenic apo(a) rabbits constructed on the Watanabe heritable hyperlipidemic (WHHL) rabbit background.[96] The advanced, complex lesions observed in the transgenic animals showed notable calcification, unlike the less advanced lesions in the nontransgenic WHHL rabbits; examination of advanced human lesions also showed association of Lp(a) deposition with areas of calcification.[96] Interestingly, it was shown that Lp(a) promotes calcification of cultured smooth muscle cells, as evidenced by stimulation of calcium uptake, promotion of an osteogenic pattern of protein expression, and promotion of an osteoblast-like phenotype (i.e., upregulated osteoblast-specific factor–2 and alkaline phosphatase activity).[96] The role of apo(a) in aortic calcification remains unclear, however, particularly in light of several recent reports that suggest no relationship between coronary calcium and either Lp(a) concentrations or apo(a) isoform sizes.[97]

Several studies have been published using transgenic apo(a) mice that may shed light on the role of Lp(a) *in vivo*. In the first study, mice expressing low and high concentrations of apo(a) (~35 mg/dL and 700 mg/dL, respectively) in a transgenic human apoB background were used.[98] It was reported that high levels of oxidized phospholipids were present in Lp(a) from the high apo(a)-expressing mice but not in LDL from mice with human apoB alone. This likely results from preferential transfer of oxidized phospholipids to Lp(a) as has been previously suggested to occur in human plasma (see earlier). The significance of this finding in the context of how Lp(a) contributes to atherosclerosis is unclear. However, it is tempting to speculate that the deposition of Lp(a) containing these oxidized phospholipids in the developing lesion may contribute to both proatherosclerotic and proinflammatory processes; such an effect would be magnified by the preferential retention of Lp(a) in this milieu. This study is the first to report the use of transgenic mice expressing high concentrations of Lp(a); apo(a) and Lp(a) concentrations in previous transgenic models have been more than an order of magnitude lower.

In the second study, Devlin and colleagues[99] reported the overexpression of a fragment of apo(a) (containing kringle IV types 5–8, each containing a weak lysine-binding site; see Fig 11-2 and 11-3). Compared with control animals, these mice had greatly enhanced atherosclerosis and markedly increased non-HDL cholesterol. Accordingly, these investigators found by using a perfused mouse liver model that this four-kringle apo(a) species, as well as full-length apo(a), inhibited the clearance of cholesterol-rich remnant particles. The molecular basis of this observation is the subject of ongoing study and may help to shed light on our understanding of the effect of Lp(a) on the catabolism of other lipoproteins.

A report using the same WHHL rabbit line expressing human apo(a) described earlier[96] has further shown that Lp(a) in the context of a hypercholesterolemia setting enhances coronary artery lesion size; the increased coronary atherosclerosis in these animals was associated with a greater incidence of chronic ischemia and MI.[100] This study underscores the ability of Lp(a) to further contribute to the burden of atherosclerosis in hypercholesterolemic animals.

Based on our knowledge of the potential roles of Lp(a) to date, what might be the mechanism(s) underlying a pathogenic role for apo(a) isoform size independent of plasma Lp(a) concentrations? Surprisingly, few mechanistic studies have considered the role of apo(a) size. The exception to this is the effect of apo(a) isoform size on fibrin binding and plasminogen activation to plasmin. In this regard, recent studies indicate that smaller Lp(a) isoforms bind more avidly to fibrin[101] and inhibit plasmin formation to greater extents.[102] However, contradictory evidence has been provided: larger isoforms of Lp(a) (as well as larger isoforms of free apo(a)) were reported to be more effective in reducing plasmin formation on fibrin.[103] Clearly, more studies are required to understand the molecular mechanism(s) by which small apo(a) isoform size can confer risk independently of plasma Lp(a) concentrations. Interesting recent data suggest that small apo(a) isoforms may be preferentially retained in the intima of atherosclerotic lesions relative to large isoform sizes, irrespective of corresponding plasma Lp(a) concentrations.[104] The molecular basis for this intriguing observation may help in our understanding of the pathogenic nature of small apo(a) isoforms.

CHALLENGES IN LIPOPROTEIN(a) MEASUREMENT

For increased plasma Lp(a) concentration to be considered a "major" risk factor (i.e., in the same category as cigarette smoking, increased LDL cholesterol level, etc.), it has to meet the following criteria: (1) robust predictive power for cardiovascular disease; (2) high prevalence of Lp(a) concentrations greater than an arbitrary risk threshold in the general population; (3) ready availability of clinical samples and a widely available, standardized, inexpensive means to measure Lp(a); and (4) evidence for a benefit of reducing Lp(a) concentrations.[19] For these reasons, it is essential to define stringent criteria for Lp(a) assay standardization because the predictive power of Lp(a) can be fully explored only if measurements are made with methods that have been evaluated for their ability to produce accurate Lp(a) values.

Measurement of Lp(a) in plasma samples has almost exclusively relied on immunologic methods including enzyme-linked immunosorbent assay (ELISA), nephelometry, and immunoturbidimetry. The high degree of size heterogeneity of apo(a) derived from the variable number of KIV type 2 sequences, the association of apo(a) with apoB-100 in the Lp(a) particle, and the high degree of sequence similarity between apo(a) and plasminogen all constitute challenges to the measurement of Lp(a) using these methods. Unfortunately, the interpretation of results from clinical studies addressing the role of Lp(a) as a risk factor for CHD has been complicated by the lack of standardization of Lp(a) measurement. As such, approaches to achieve standardization of Lp(a) measurement have represented a major focus of recent study.

The largest challenge in Lp(a) measurement is the presence of a variable number of identical epitopes (specifically, the variable size of the identically repeated KIV type 2 domain underlying apo(a)/Lp(a) isoform size heterogeneity) that may interact with the antibodies used in immunoassays to measure the concentration of Lp(a) in serum or plasma. If this is the case, then the antibodies in the assay will not possess the same immunoreactivity per particle if the apo(a) isoform size of the sample and calibrator are not the same. Indeed, the choice of apo(a) size in the calibrator is arbitrary and, irrespective of the choice, the size would not be representative of the size of apo(a) in most of the samples. As such, the immunoassays using antibodies sensitive to apo(a) isoform size tend to underestimate Lp(a) concentrations in samples with apo(a) sizes smaller than the size of the apo(a) calibrator, whereas Lp(a) concentrations in samples with larger apo(a) isoforms overestimated.

Another major factor that constitutes a challenge for the accurate measurement of Lp(a) is differences in the properties of Lp(a) assays from different manufacturers. Assay kits may vary in terms of antibody properties, assay precision, and sensitivity of the assays to sample handling and storage conditions. An international standard reference material for assay calibration is required to allow different assays to be appropriately optimized with respect to these factors. Significant progress in the development of such a standard has been made.[105,106] Nonetheless, it is clear that no reference material can eliminate differences in Lp(a) values obtained by methods that are affected by apo(a) size heterogeneity or are not properly optimized, or both.

PROGRESS IN THE STANDARDIZATION OF LIPOPROTEIN(a) MEASUREMENT

In a study designed to document the impact of apo(a) size on the accuracy of Lp(a) measurements, Marcovina and colleagues[107] generated and characterized a variety of monoclonal antibodies (mAbs) directed to different apo(a) epitopes. A mAb directed to an epitope present in KIV type 2 (whose immunoreactivity per particle would vary depending on apo(a) size) and another mAb specific for a unique epitope located in apo(a) KIV type 9 were used to develop two ELISA methods to measure Lp(a) in a large number of samples.[107] Both assays were calibrated with the same serum containing an apo(a) species with a total of 21 KIV-like motifs. The Lp(a) protein value was assigned to the assay calibrator using a primary preparation, and the values were expressed in nanomoles per liter (nmol/L) to reflect the number of Lp(a) particles in plasma. As expected, highly comparable values were obtained by the two ELISA methods in the samples with the same apo(a) size as that of the assay calibrator, whereas Lp(a) values measured using the apo(a) KIV type 2–specific antibody were either underestimated or overestimated in samples with apo(a) containing less than 21 or more than 21 KIV repeats, respectively, compared with values obtained by the KIV type 9–specific mAb. The KIV type 9 mAb-based ELISA has been carefully validated in a large number of individuals and has been used as a reference method for the standardization of Lp(a) measurement.

Extensive work has been conducted on the development of a reference material for the purpose of achieving comparability of values among different Lp(a) assays. Based on analyses performed by the International Federation of Clinical Chemistry and Laboratory Medicine (IFCC) Working Group on Lp(a), a lyophilized serum pool preparation was selected as a secondary reference material for Lp(a).[106] As a collaboration between the recipients of a National Institutes of Health (NIH)/National Heart, Lung, and Blood Institute contract and the IFCC Working Group on Lp(a), a consensus reference method using the ELISA employing the MAb against apo(a) KIV type 9, as described earlier, and calibrated with two purified Lp(a) preparations was used to assign a target value to the IFCC secondary reference material.[105] The IFCC preparation has been shown to have excellent stability and commutability properties, and has been accepted by the World Health Organization (WHO) Expert Committee on Biological Standardization as the "First WHO/IFCC International Reference Reagent for Lipoprotein(a) for Immunoassay."[108] This represents the achievement of a worldwide consensus on the calibration of Lp(a) test systems and will allow the determination of threshold values for increased risk for CHD in different populations to be determined based on a molar concentration of Lp(a), as has been recommended.[19] The issue of isoform-size bias in different assay methodologies still needs to be addressed; this may necessitate the development of a range of Lp(a) isoform sizes for use as assay calibrators to correct for the inherent bias in a particular assay (see later).

To evaluate the performance of commercially available methods for Lp(a) immunoassay, the authors used the IFCC reference preparation to transfer an accuracy-based value to the various immunoassay calibrators.[105] Among the 22 Lp(a) test systems evaluated, 10 were turbidimetric, 6 were nephelometric, 2 were fluorescence based, 1 was an electroimmunodiffusion assay, and 1 was ELISA based. Most methods used polyclonal antibodies against apo(a) to measure Lp(a). After uniformity of calibration was demonstrated in the 22 evaluated systems, Lp(a) was measured in 30 fresh-frozen samples covering a wide range of Lp(a) concentrations and apo(a) sizes with values assigned by the reference method. A significant apo(a) size–dependent bias was observed for all the evaluated systems. Three systems showed a minimal extent of bias, and of these, only one displayed a high level of concordance with the reference method over the full range of apo(a) sizes.[105] As such, despite the use of a common reference preparation, no harmonization in Lp(a) values among the different methods was achieved. This clearly indicates that the impact of apo(a) isoform size on Lp(a) concentrations varies among the different methods as a function of the apo(a) size of the assay calibrators.

Studies have been conducted to determine how to overcome the problem of isoform-size dependence in Lp(a) measurement methods. Instead of using serial dilutions of a single calibrator, five fresh-frozen samples with a range of apo(a) sizes and suitable Lp(a) concentrations were used to calibrate a turbidimetric assay affected by apo(a) size variation.[19] Analyses were performed in parallel using the original assay calibrator and the five-sample calibrator on a large number of samples. A consistent apo(a) size-dependent bias was observed with the original assay calibrator. In contrast, good comparability was observed between the observed values and the values obtained by the reference method (the ELISA used the mAb directed against apo(a) KIV type 9; see earlier) when the five independent samples were used to calibrate the assay.[19] Although this approach appears promising for reducing assay inaccuracy, it may not be equally effective in all methods or in all samples. Therefore, its potential use for assay standardization will require further evaluation using multiple methods and a large number of samples with a good representation of single and double apo(a) isoforms.

Progress has also been made in establishing a primary reference standard for Lp(a). In particular, Edelstein and colleagues[109] and Scanu and colleagues[110] have examined the effects of freezing and lyophilization of Lp(a) on its immunologic properties, and have described methods for preserving purified Lp(a) in a form suitable for a primary reference material. When isolated Lp(a) was lyophilized in the presence of suitable cryopreservatives and then reconstituted, it was found to be indistinguishable from the starting material with respect to chemical and biological properties. Moreover, the reconstituted products exhibited unchanged immunochemical properties and thus appeared to have all of the requisites to be used as a primary reference material.[110]

NONIMMUNOLOGICALLY BASED METHODS FOR LIPOPROTEIN(a) MEASUREMENT

A potential approach to bypass the problems of immunochemical determination of Lp(a) concentrations involves quantification of Lp(a) by measuring its cholesterol content. Early methods used continuous flow analysis of lipoprotein classes separated by ultracentifugation[111] or by lectin affinity chromatography to separate Lp(a) from other lipoproteins[112]; Lp(a) cholesterol was then measured by enzymatic assay. A more recent method involves plasma electrophoresis followed by detection of Lp(a) cholesterol by *in situ* enzymatic assay and densitometry.[113] Importantly, it was found that an ultracentrifugation step intended to eliminate β–very-low-density lipoprotein that might overlap with Lp(a) on the gels did not materially affect the outcome of the assays.[113] Further studies are required to compare the clinical significance of Lp(a) cholesterol with that of Lp(a) mass.

IMPACT OF LIPOPROTEIN(a) METHOD INACCURACY ON THE INTERPRETATION OF LIPOPROTEIN(a) VALUES

In the majority of clinical studies, Lp(a) concentrations have been determined by methods affected by apo(a) size heterogeneity. Therefore, for the conclusions of these studies to be valid, the assumption has to be made that the distribution of apo(a) isoforms was similar between cases and control subjects, thus minimizing the potential that method-dependent overestimation or underestimation of Lp(a) values contributed to the observed difference or lack thereof between cases and control subjects. Despite the importance of this topic, few studies have been performed to evaluate the impact of method inaccuracy on the interpretation of clinical data.

Marcovina and coworkers[19] determined Lp(a) concentrations (using the reference method described earlier) and apo(a) isoform sizes in 2940 samples from the participants in the Framingham study collected during the fifth cycle. During the same cycle, Lp(a) concentrations were also determined in other laboratories in 2556 of the samples by a turbidimetric method and in 2662 of the samples by a commercially available ELISA. Depending on the assay used, 5% to 15% of the subjects were misclassified as being at greater risk (false positive), whereas approximately 1% were misclassified as being not at risk (false negative). Most of the misclassifications observed by the turbidimetric method were explained by the overestimation or underestimation of Lp(a) values based on the apo(a) size in the samples; this, in turn, was attributable to the small apo(a) size in the assay calibrator and by the high frequency of samples in the general population with apo(a) sizes larger than that in the calibrator. In contrast, the large number of false-positive values generated by the ELISA method was not explained by the apo(a) sizes in these samples. In fact, a high degree of variability in Lp(a) values was observed with this ELISA method. In addition, the values obtained from frozen samples were generally greater than those from fresh samples, but the magnitude of the increase was sample dependent. These findings clearly indicate that assay standardization can be achieved only if each assay is properly optimized in addition to being evaluated for its sensitivity to apo(a) size heterogeneity.[19]

In a separate study, Marcovina and coworkers[19] directly compared the ability of the ELISA reference method and a commercially available latex-based nephelometric method to predict future angina pectoris in men participating in the Physicians' Health Study.[78] Apo(a) isoform size was determined and plasma Lp(a) concentration was simultaneously measured by the ELISA reference method and in a different laboratory by the nephelometric method. Analyses were performed in samples from 195 study participants who subsequently developed of angina and from paired control subjects, matched for age and smoking, who remained free of reported vascular disease. The baseline median concentration of Lp(a) in cases, as determined by the reference method, was approximately 35% greater ($P = 0.02$) than that in control subjects. In addition, Lp(a) was associated with increased relative risk for angina, and this association was strengthened after controlling for lipid risk factors. However, the median Lp(a) concentration determined by the commercial method was not statistically different between cases and control subjects, and the association with angina was also not significant. Very high Lp(a) values obtained by the nephelometric assay (>95th percentile of control subjects) were a significant predictor of angina, even though the relative risk was not as strong as that ascertained using the reference method. These results clearly indicate the importance of using suitable and standardized methods for risk assessment and for the interpretation of clinical outcomes.

STRATEGIES FOR MODULATION OF PLASMA LIPOPROTEIN(a) CONCENTRATIONS

Compared with plasma LDL, Lp(a) concentrations are relatively resistant to alteration by traditional pharmacologic and nonpharmacologic approaches. This follows from the large contribution of the gene encoding apo(a) to Lp(a) concentrations that has been reported previously (see Determination of Plasma Lipoprotein(a) Concentrations earlier in this chapter). However, there are reports of several interventions and disease conditions such as renal disease and poorly controlled diabetes mellitus that significantly increase plasma Lp(a) concentrations (for a review, see Marcovina and Koschinsky[114]). The most effective method to decrease Lp(a) concentrations by 50% or more is by LDL- or Lp(a)-apheresis procedures.[115,116] However, these procedures are costly and are generally reserved for patients with extreme forms of familial hypercholesterolemia.

Several agents have been reported to reduce Lp(a) concentrations, including niacin in high doses,[117] L-carnitine at a dose of 2 g/day,[118] and ascorbic acid (3 g/day), together with L-lysine monohydrochloride (3 g/day).[119] The moderate Lp(a)-lowering effect of niacin is relatively consistent, and the use of niacin therapy is becoming more feasible because of the recent availability of slow-release preparations that maintain efficacy of the drug whereas reducing problematic side effects including flushing and hepatotoxicity.[120]

A variety of different hormones has also been shown to modulate plasma Lp(a) concentrations. Androgens, such as danazol and tibolone, were reported to significantly reduce Lp(a) concentrations,[121–123] whereas estrogen treatment was reported to decrease Lp(a) concentrations by 50%.[124] Both tamoxifen and estrogen have been shown to reduce Lp(a) concentrations significantly in postmenopausal women.[125]

Contradictory findings have been reported concerning the effect of statins on Lp(a) concentrations. A modest increase in Lp(a) concentrations was found in patients with increased cholesterol levels receiving simvastatin,[126] and a 36% increase in plasma Lp(a) concentrations was reported in patients receiving atorvastatin.[127] Results from the Comparative Effects on Lipid Levels (COMPELL) study have also demonstrated that treatment with simvastatin/ezetimibe or rosuvastatin significantly increased Lp(a) concentrations over the course of a 12-week study; either rosuvastatin or atorvastatin in combination with niacin reduced Lp(a) concentrations.[128] Other studies have reported that the use of pravastatin did not influence Lp(a) concentrations,[129] whereas fluvastatin was found to significantly reduce Lp(a) concentrations.[130] In a study using a large patient cohort, both atorvastatin and simvastatin therapy for 6 weeks resulted in a modest but significant reduction in Lp(a) concentrations.[131] Clearly, the effect of statins on Lp(a) concentrations requires further analysis using large cohorts to define the roles of baseline Lp(a) concentration and apo(a) isoform size on the magnitude of the statin effect. In addition, mechanistic studies need to be performed to identify the molecular basis for the potential modulation of Lp(a) concentrations by statin therapy.

Aspirin therapy (81 mg/day) has been reported to reduce serum Lp(a) concentrations in a study of 70 patients with atherosclerotic disease.[132] Interestingly, the magnitude of the decrease in Lp(a) concentrations was larger in patients with high Lp(a) concentrations, regardless of apo(a) isoform size. This has been speculated to result from a greater reduction by aspirin of apo(a) gene transcription in patients with high baseline transcriptional activity of the gene. Clearly, these intriguing results need to be confirmed with a larger patient population, and the mechanism underlying the effect of aspirin on apo(a) gene transcription requires further analysis.

In contrast with plasma LDL concentrations, Lp(a) concentrations are relatively resistant to alteration by diet and exercise. However, in a study of obese women with high baseline Lp(a) concentrations, a low-calorie diet with concomitant weight loss resulted in a significant reduction in Lp(a) concentrations.[133] In terms of specific dietary effects, a randomized crossover study has reported that almonds, which are rich in monounsaturated fat, significantly reduced Lp(a) concentrations.[134] Ginsberg and coworkers[135] reported a significant increase in Lp(a) concentrations in individuals who reduced their intake of saturated fat. Therefore, the results of these two studies support the notion that fat intake may affect Lp(a) concentrations. Interestingly, Meinertz and colleagues[136] demonstrated that alcohol-extracted (but not intact) soy protein markedly reduced Lp(a) concentrations. Notably, the interventions described also had beneficial effects on LDL cholesterol and triglyceride concentrations; identification of agents capable of specifically reducing plasma Lp(a) concentrations has the potential to provide a study design in which the consequences of Lp(a) reduction can be evaluated prospectively. This will allow a direct assessment of the contribution of Lp(a) concentration to atherosclerotic risk.

For the measurement of Lp(a) in population studies, as well as in clinical practice, the NIH Working Group has established a number of guidelines (summarized in Table 11-2) that will help to compare results from one study with another and to obtain the level of rigor required to use Lp(a) measurement in the clinic (see next section).

TABLE 11-2 Guidelines for the Measurement of Lipoprotein(a) in Population Studies and in Clinical Practice

• Assays for measuring Lp(a) levels in clinical and epidemiologic studies must be validated for their ability to produce accurate values independently of apo(a) isoform size values in the samples.
• Because of the potential impact on Lp(a) measurement, stringent conditions for blood collection and storage must be developed and followed. Effects of collection/storage on individual assays must be determined.
• Lp(a) values should not be measured in terms of mass (which reflects the contributions of lipid and carbohydrate), but rather in terms of nmol/L of Lp(a) protein. This will allow direct comparison of data from different studies.
• The WHO-approved IFCC secondary reference material with the assigned value of 107 nmol/L should be used as a point of reference for assay calibration.
• If methods sensitive to isoform size are used for risk assessment, samples with values > 50 nmol/L should be remeasured by referral laboratories using validated methods. This should minimize the chance of misclassification because of method inaccuracy.

apo, apolipoprotein; IFCC, International Federation of Clinical Chemistry and Laboratory Medicine; Lp(a), lipoprotein(a); WHO, World Health Organization.

SUGGESTED USE OF LIPOPROTEIN(a) IN CLINICAL PRACTICE

Currently, Lp(a) is not an established cardiovascular risk factor, and there are no guidelines recommending intervention or defining a suitable clinical target for Lp(a) reduction.[19,43] Our current level of understanding does suggest, however, that Lp(a) reduction might be beneficial in some subgroups of patients with high Lp(a) concentrations, but sufficient details remain lacking on how to define such subgroups with respect to Lp(a) concentrations, apo(a) size, and presence of other risk factors. Moreover, a well-characterized therapeutic agent capable of adequately reducing plasma Lp(a) concentrations long term does not currently exist.[18,19] Clearly, the lack of knowledge of Lp(a) metabolism particularly with respect to the pathway for its catabolism raises considerable challenges in devising strategies to reduce Lp(a) concentrations. Because apo(a) production is of major importance in regulating Lp(a) concentrations, inhibition of Lp(a) particle formation at the step of the extracellular particle assembly from apo(a) and apoB-100 may offer intervention possibilities.[3,137] Furthermore, studies in transgenic animals and cultured cell systems have suggested a hepatic elimination pathway for Lp(a) that might be a fruitful target (see Cain and colleagues[32] and references therein). However, caution must be exercised in the extrapolation of these findings to Lp(a) catabolism in humans.

It has been suggested that emerging risk factors such as Lp(a) as defined in the NCEP ATP III treatment guidelines[43] may be useful in refinement of patient risk classification.[138] Although screening for Lp(a) concentration increases in the general population is not suggested at this time, measurement of Lp(a) concentration is recommended in individuals with an increased risk for CHD, particularly in those with borderline-high LDL cholesterol or high apoB levels, and in individuals who exhibit poor responses to statins with respect to LDL cholesterol reduction; these individuals may be poor responders because of increased Lp(a) concentrations (Table 11-3). Individuals with high (>30 mg/dL or 75 nmol/L; i.e., >80th percentile) Lp(a) concentrations should be managed more aggressively with respect to modifiable risk factors.

TABLE 11-3 Identification of Individuals for Lipoprotein(a) Measurement

• Individuals at high risk for CHD with:
• Increased apolipoprotein B or LDL cholesterol levels
• Family history of CHD
• Premature myocardial infarction with otherwise normal risk profile
• Individuals who respond poorly to statins for LDL cholesterol reduction

CHD, coronary heart disease; LDL, low-density lipoprotein.

REFERENCES

1. Berg K: A new serum type system in man: The Lp system. *Acta Pathol Microbiol Scand* 1963;59:362–382.
2. Kraft HG, Menzel HJ, Hoppichler F, et al: Changes of genetic apolipoprotein phenotypes caused by liver transplantation. Implications for apolipoprotein synthesis. *J Clin Invest* 1989;83:137–142.
3. Koschinsky ML, Côté GP, Gabel BR, van der Hoek YY: Identification of the cysteine residue in apolipoprotein(a) that mediates extracellular coupling with apolipoprotein B-100. *J Biol Chem* 1993;268:19819–19825.
4. Albers JJ, Kennedy H, Marcovina SM: Evidence that Lp(a) contains one molecule of apo(a) and one molecule of apo B: Evaluation of amino acid analysis data. *J Lipid Res* 1996;37:192–196.
5. Koschinsky ML, Marcovina SM: Structure-function relationships in apolipoprotein(a): Insights into lipoprotein(a) assembly and pathogenicity. *Curr Opin Lipidol* 2004;15:167–174.
6. McLean JW, Tomlinson JE, Kuang WJ, et al: cDNA sequence of human apolipoprotein(a) is homologous to plasminogen. *Nature* 1987;330:132–137.
7. Lackner C, Cohen JC, Hobbs HH: Molecular definition of the extreme size polymorphism in apolipoprotein(a). *Hum Mol Genet* 1993;2:933–940.
8. van der Hoek YY, Wittekoek ME, Beisiegel U, et al: The apolipoprotein(a) kringle IV repeats which differ from the major repeat kringle are present in variably sized isoforms. *Hum Mol Genet* 1993;2:361–366.
9. Marcovina SM, Hobbs HH, Albers JJ: Relation between number of apolipoprotein(a) kringle 4 repeats and mobility of isoforms in agarose gel: Basis for a standardized isoform nomenclature. *Clin Chem* 1996;42:436–439.
10. Becker L, Cook PM, Wright TG, Koschinsky ML: Quantitative evaluation of the contribution of weak lysine-binding sites present within apolipoprotein(a) kringle IV types 6-8 to lipoprotein(a) assembly. *J Biol Chem* 2004;279:2679–2688.
11. Callow MJ, Rubin EM: Site-specific mutagenesis demonstrates that cysteine 4326 of apolipoprotein B is required for covalent linkage with apolipoprotein(a) *in vivo*. *J Biol Chem* 1995;270: 23914–23917.
12. Sangrar W, Marcovina SM, Koschinsky ML: Expression and characterization of apolipoprotein(a) kringle IV types 1, 2 and 10 in mammalian cells. *Protein Eng* 1993;7:723–731.

13. Scanu AM: Lipoprotein(a). A potential bridge between the fields of atherosclerosis and thrombosis. *Arch Pathol Lab Med* 1988;112:1045–1047.
14. Fless GM, ZumMallen ME, Scanu AM: Physicochemical properties of apolipoprotein(a) and lipoprotein(a) derived from the dissociation of human plasma lipoprotein(a). *J Biol Chem* 1986;261:8712–8718.
15. Rader DJ, Cain W, Ikewaki K, et al: The inverse association of plasma lipoprotein(a) concentrations with apolipoprotein(a) isoform size is not due to differences in Lp(a) catabolism but to differences in production rate. *J Clin Invest* 1994;93: 2758–2763.
16. Boerwinkle E, Leffert CC, Lin J, et al: Apolipoprotein(a) gene accounts for greater than 90% of the variation in plasma lipoprotein(a) concentrations. *J Clin Invest* 1990;90:52–60.
17. Angelin B: Therapy for lowering lipoprotein (a) levels. *Curr Opin Lipidol* 1997;8:337–341.
18. Anuurad E, Boffa MB, Koschinsky ML, Berglund L: Lipoprotein(a): A unique risk factor for cardiovascular disease. *Clin Lab Med* 2006;26:751–772.
19. Marcovina SM, Koschinsky ML, Albers JJ, Skarlatos S: Report of the National Heart, Lung, and Blood Institute Workshop on Lipoprotein(a) and Cardiovascular Disease: Recent advances and future directions. *Clin Chem* 2003;49:1785–1796.
20. Utermann G, Menzel HJ, Kraft HG, et al: Lp(a) glycoprotein phenotypes. Inheritance and relation to Lp(a)-lipoprotein concentrations in plasma. *J Clin Invest* 1987;80:458–465.
21. Brunner C, Lobentanz EM, Petho-Schramm A, et al: The number of identical kringle IV repeats in apolipoprotein(a) affects its processing and secretion by HepG2 cells. *J Biol Chem* 1996;271: 32403–32410.
22. White AL, Rainwater DL, Lanford RE: Intracellular maturation of apolipoprotein(a) and assembly of lipoprotein(a) in primary baboon hepatocytes. *J Lipid Res* 1993;34:509–517.
23. Marcovina SM, Albers JJ, Wijsman et al: Differences in Lp(a) concentrations and apo(a) polymorphs between black and white Americans. *J Lipid Res* 1996;37:2569–2585.
24. Anuurad E, Lu G, Rubin J, et al: ApoE genotype affects allele-specific apo[a] levels for large apo[a] sizes in African Americans: The Harlem-Basset Study. *J Lipid Res* 2007;48:693–698.
25. Chretien JP, Coresh J, Berthier-Schaad Y, et al: Three single-nucleotide polymorphisms in LPA account for most of the increase in lipoprotein(a) level elevation in African Americans compared with European Americans. *J Med Genet* 2006;43: 917–923.
26. Rubin J, Paultre F, Tuck CH, et al: Apolipoprotein(a) genotype influences isoform dominance pattern differently in African Americans and Caucasians. *J Lipid Res* 2002;43:234–244.
27. Berglund L, Ramakrishnan R: Lipoprotein(a). An elusive cardiovascular risk factor. *Arterioscler Thromb Vasc Biol* 2004;24: 2219–2226.
28. Paultre F, Pearson TA, Weil HF, et al: High levels of Lp(a) with a small apo(a) isoform are associated with coronary artery disease in African American and White men. *Arterioscler Thromb Vasc Biol* 2000;20:2619–2624.
29. Kostner KM, Clodi M Bodlaj G, et al: Decreased urinary apolipoprotein(a) excretion in patients with impaired renal function. *Eur J Clin Invest* 1998;28:447–452.
30. Sechi LA, Zingaro L, De Carli S, et al: Increased serum lipoprotein(a) levels in patients with early renal failure. *Ann Intern Med* 1998;129:457–461.
31. Frischmann ME, Kronenberg F, Trenkwalder E, et al: *In vivo* turnover study demonstrates diminished clearance of lipoprotein(a) in hemodialysis patients. *Kidney Int* 2007;71: 1036–1043.
32. Cain WJ, Millar JS, Himebauch AS, et al: Lipoprotein [a] is cleared from the plasma primarily by the liver in a process mediated by apolipoprotein [a]. *J Lipid Res* 2005;46:2681–2691.
33. Kostner KM, Maurer G, Huber K, et al: Urinary excretion of apo(a) fragments. Role in apo(a) catabolism. *Arterioscler Thromb Vasc Biol* 1996;16:905–911.
34. Hrzenjak A, Frank S, Wo X, et al: Galactose-specific asialoglycoprotein receptor is involved in lipoprotein (a) catabolism. *Biochem J* 2003;376:765–771.
35. Floren CH, Albers JJ, Bierman EL: Uptake of Lp (a) lipoprotein by cultured fibroblasts. *Biochem Biophys Res Commun* 1981;102:636–639.
36. Havekes L, Vermeer BJ, Brugman T, Emeis J: Binding of LP(a) to the low-density lipoprotein receptor of human fibroblasts. *FEBS Lett* 1981;132:169–173.
37. Krempler F, Kostner GM, Roscher A, et al: Studies on the role of specific cell surface receptors in the removal of lipoprotein (a) in man. *J Clin Invest* 1983;71:1431–1441.
38. Mbewu AD, Bhatnagar D, Durrington PN, et al: Serum lipoprotein(a) in patients heterozygous for familial hypercholesterolemia, their relatives, and unrelated control populations. *Arterioscler Thromb* 1991;11:940–946.
39. Utermann G, Hoppichler F, Dieplinger H, et al: Defects in the low-density lipoprotein receptor gene affect lipoprotein (a) levels: Multiplicative interaction of two gene loci associated with premature atherosclerosis. *Proc Natl Acad Sci USA* 1989;86: 4171–4174.
40. Marz W, Beckmann A, Scharnagl H, et al: Heterogeneous lipoprotein (a) size isoforms differ by their interaction with the low-density lipoprotein receptor and the low-density lipoprotein receptor-related protein/alpha 2-macroglobulin receptor. *FEBS Lett* 1993;325:271–275.
41. Rader DJ, Mann WA, Cain W, et al: The low-density lipoprotein receptor is not required for normal catabolism of Lp(a) in humans. *J Clin Invest* 1995;95:1403–1408.
42. Lawn RM: How often has Lp(a) evolved? *Clin Genet* 1996;49:167–174.
43. Expert Panel on Detection, Evaluation, and Treatment of High Blood Cholesterol in Adults:: Executive Summary of the Third Report of The National Cholesterol Education Program (NCEP) Expert Panel on Detection, Evaluation, and Treatment of High Blood Cholesterol in Adults (Adult Treatment Panel III). *JAMA* 2001;285:2486–2497.
44. Aboyans V, Criqui MH, Denenberg JO, et al: Risk factors for progression of peripheral arterial disease in large and small vessels. *Circulation* 2006;113:2623–2639.
45. Cheng SW, Ting AC, Wong J: Lipoprotein(a) and its relationship to risk factors and severity of atherosclerotic peripheral vascular disease. *Eur Vasc Endovasc Surg* 1997;14:17–23.
46. Ohira T, Schreiner PJ, Morrisett JD, et al: Lipoprotein(a) and incident ischemic stroke: The Atherosclerosis Risk in Communities (ARIC) study. *Stroke* 2006;37:1407–1412.
47. Peng DQ, Zhao SP, Wang JL: Lipoprotein(a) and apolipoprotein E epsilon 4 as independent risk factors for ischemic stroke. *J Cardiovasc Risk* 1999;6:1–6.
48. Jones GT, van Rij AM, Cole J, et al: Plasma lipoprotein(a) indicates risk for 4 distinct forms of vascular disease. *Clin Chem* 2007;53:679–685.
49. Koschinsky ML: Lipoprotein(a) and atherosclerosis: New perspectives on the mechanism of action of an enigmatic lipoprotein. *Curr Atheroscler Rep* 2005;7:389–395.
50. Genest J Jr, Jenner JL, McNamara JR, et al: Prevalence of lipoprotein (a) [Lp(a)] excess in coronary artery disease. *Am J Cardiol* 1991;67:1039–1145.
51. Assmann G, Schulte H, von Eckardstein A: Hypertriglyceridemia and elevated lipoprotein(a) are risk factors for major coronary events in middle-aged men. *Am J Cardiol* 1996;77:1179–1184.
52. Bostom AG, Gagnon DR, Cupples LA, et al: A prospective investigation of elevated lipoprotein (a) detected by electrophoresis and cardiovascular disease in women. The Framingham Heart Study. *Circulation* 1994;90:1688–1695.
53. Bostom AG, Cupples LA, Jenner JL, et al: Elevated plasma lipoprotein(a) and coronary heart disease in men aged 55 years and younger. A prospective study. *JAMA* 1996;276:544–548.
54. Sigurdsson G, Baldursdottir A, Sigvaldason H, et al: Predictive value of apolipoproteins in a prospective survey of coronary artery disease in men. *Am J Cardiol* 1992;69:1251–1254.
55. Wald NJ, Law M, Watt HC, et al: Apolipoproteins and ischaemic heart disease: Implications for screening. *Lancet* 1994;343:75–79.
56. Schaefer EJ, Lamon-Fava S, Jenner JL, et al: Lipoprotein(a) levels and risk of coronary heart disease in men. The Lipid Research Clinics Coronary Primary Prevention Trial. *JAMA* 1996;271:999–1003.
57. Jauhiainen M, Koskinen P, Ehnholm C, et al: Lipoprotein (a) and coronary heart disease risk: A nested case–control study of the Helsinki Heart Study participants. *Atherosclerosis* 1991;89:59–67.
58. Ridker PM, Hennekens CH, Stampfer MJ: A prospective study of lipoprotein(a) and the risk of myocardial infarction. *JAMA* 1993;270:2195–2199.

59. Craig WY, Neveux LM, Palomaki GE, et al: Lipoprotein(a) as a risk factor for ischemic heart disease: Meta-analysis of prospective studies. *Clin Chem* 1998;44:2301–2306.
60. Danesh J, Collins R, Peto R: Lipoprotein(a) and coronary heart disease. Meta-analysis of prospective studies. *Circulation* 2000;102:1082–1085.
61. Sharrett AR, Ballantyne CM, Coady SA, et al: Coronary heart disease prediction from lipoprotein cholesterol levels, triglycerides, lipoprotein(a), apolipoproteins A-I and B, and HDL density subfractions: The Atherosclerosis Risk in Communities (ARIC) Study. *Circulation* 2001;104:1108–1113.
62. Glader CA, Birgander LS, Stenlund H, Dahlen GH: Is lipoprotein(a) a predictor for survival in patients with established coronary artery disease? Results from a prospective patient cohort study in northern Sweden. *J Intern Med* 2002;252:27–35.
63. Maher VM, Brown BG, Marcovina SM, et al: Effects of lowering elevated LDL cholesterol on the cardiovascular risk of lipoprotein(a). *J Am Med Assoc* 1995;274:1771–1774.
64. Luc G, Bard JM, Arveiler D, et al: Lipoprotein (a) as a predictor of coronary heart disease: The PRIME Study. *Atherosclerosis* 2002;163:377–384.
65. Cantin B, Gagnon F, Moorjani S, et al: Is lipoprotein(a) an independent risk factor for ischemic heart disease in men? The Quebec Cardiovascular Study. *J Am Coll Cardiol* 1998;31: 519–525.
66. von Eckardstein A, Schulte H, Cullen P, Assmann G: Lipoprotein(a) further increases the risk of coronary events in men with high global cardiovascular risk. *J Am Coll Cardiol* 2001;37:434–439.
67. Suk Danik J, Rifai N, Buring JE, Ridker PM: Lipoprotein(a), measured with an assay independent of apolipoprotein(a) isoform size, and risk of future cardiovascular events among initially healthy women. *JAMA* 2006;296:1363–1370.
68. Dahlen GH, Guyton JR, Attar M, et al: Association of levels of lipoprotein Lp(a), plasma lipids, and other lipoproteins with coronary artery disease documented by angiography. *Circulation* 1986;74:758–765.
69. Kronenberg F, Kronenberg MF, Kiechl S, et al: Role of lipoprotein(a) and apolipoprotein(a) phenotype in atherogenesis: Prospective results from the Bruneck study. *Circulation* 1999;100:1154–1160.
70. Paultre F, Tuck CH, Boden-Albala B, et al: Relation of apo(a) size to carotid atherosclerosis in an elderly multiethnic population. *Arterioscler Thromb Vasc Biol* 2002;22:141–146.
71. Wild SH, Fortmann SP, Marcovina SM: A prospective case–control study of lipoprotein(a) levels and apo(a) size and risk of coronary heart disease in Stanford Five-City Project participants. *Arterioscler Thromb Vasc Biol* 1997;17:239–245.
72. Orth-Gomer K, Mittleman MA, Schenck-Gustafsson K, et al: Lipoprotein(a) as a determinant of coronary heart disease in young women. *Circulation* 1997;95:329–334.
73. Shai I, Rimm EB, Hankinson SE, et al: Lipoprotein (a) and coronary heart disease among women: Beyond a cholesterol carrier? *Eur Heart J* 2005;26:1633–1639.
74. Ariyo AA, Thach C, Tracy R: Lp(a) lipoprotein, vascular disease, and mortality in the elderly. *N Engl J Med* 2003;349: 2108–2115.
75. Ridker PM, Hennekens CH, Buring JE, Rifai N: C-reactive protein and other markers of inflammation in the prediction of cardiovascular disease in women. *N Engl J Med* 2000;342: 836–843.
76. Wu HD, Berglund L, Dimayuga C, et al: High lipoprotein(a) levels and small apolipoprotein(a) sizes are associated with endothelial dysfunction in a multiethnic cohort. *J Am Coll Cardiol* 2004;43:1828–1833.
77. Emanuele E, Peros E, Minoretti P, et al: Significance of apolipoprotein(a) phenotypes in acute coronary syndromes: Relation with clinical presentation. *Clin Chim Acta* 2004;350: 159–165.
78. Rifai N, Ma J, Sacks FM, et al: Apolipoprotein(a) size and lipoprotein(a) concentrations and future risk of angina pectoris with evidence of severe coronary atherosclerosis in men: The Physician's Health Study. *Clin Chem* 2004;50:1364–1371.
79. Rath M, Niendorf A, Reblin T, et al: Detection and quantification of lipoprotein(a) in the arterial wall of 107 coronary bypass patients. *Arteriosclerosis* 1989;9:579–592.
80. Sangrar W, Bajzar L, Nesheim ME, Koschinsky ML: Antifibrinolytic effect of recombinant apolipoprotein(a) *in vitro* is primarily due to attenuation of tPA-mediated Glu-plasminogen activation. *Biochemistry* 1995;34:5151–5157.
81. Marcovina SM, Koschinsky ML: Evaluation of lipoprotein(a) as a prothrombotic factor: Progress from bench to bedside. *Curr Opin Lipidol* 2003;14:361–366.
82. O'Neil CH, Boffa MB, Hancock MA, et al: Stimulation of vascular smooth muscle cell proliferation and migration by apolipoprotein(a) is dependent on inhibition of transforming growth factor-beta activation and on the presence of kringle IV type 9. *J Biol Chem* 2004;279:55187–55195.
83. Desmarais RL, Sarembock IJ, Ayers CR, et al: Elevated serum lipoprotein(a) is a risk factor for clinical recurrence after coronary balloon angioplasty. *Circulation* 1995;91:1403–1409.
84. Pokrovsky SN, Ezhov MV, Il'ina LN, et al: Association of lipoprotein(a) excess with early vein graft occlusions in middle-aged men undergoing coronary artery bypass surgery. *J Thorac Cardiovasc Surg* 2003;126:1071–1075.
85. Undas A, Stepien E, Tracz W, Szczeklik A: Lipoprotein(a) as a modifier of fibrin clot permeability and susceptibility to lysis. *J Thromb Haemost* 2006;4:973–975.
86. Caplice NM, Panetta C, Peterson TE, et al: Lipoprotein (a) binds and inactivates tissue factor pathway inhibitor: A novel link between lipoproteins and thrombosis. *Blood* 2001;98:2980–2987.
87. Rand ML, Sangrar W, Hancock MA, et al: Apolipoprotein(a) enhances platelet responses to the thrombin receptor-activating peptide SFLLRN. *Arterioscler Thromb Vasc Biol* 1998;18:1393–1399.
88. Pellegrino M, Furmaniak-Kazmierczak E, LeBlanc JC, et al: The apolipoprotein(a) component of lipoprotein(a) stimulates actin stress fiber formation and loss of cell-cell contact in cultured endothelial cells. *J Biol Chem* 2004;279:6526–6533.
89. Allen S, Khan S, Tam S-P, et al: Expression of adhesion molecules by Lp(a): A potential novel mechanism for its atherogenicity. *FASEB J* 1998;12:1765–1776.
90. Schachinger V, Halle M, Minners J, et al: Lipoprotein(a) selectively impairs receptor-mediated endothelial vasodilator function of the human coronary circulation. *J Am Coll Cardiol* 1997;30:927–934.
91. Tsimikas S, Bergmark C, Beyer RW, et al: Temporal increases in plasma markers of oxidized low-density lipoprotein strongly reflect the presence of acute coronary syndromes. *J Am Coll Cardiol* 2003;41:360–370.
92. Tsimikas S, Lau HK, Han KR, et al: Percutaneous coronary intervention results in acute increases in oxidized phospholipids and lipoprotein(a): Short-term and long-term immunologic responses to oxidized low-density lipoprotein. *Circulation* 2004;109:3164–3170.
93. Edelstein C, Pfaffinger D, Hinman J, et al: Lysine-physphatidylcholine adducts in kringle V impart unique immunological and protein pro-inflammatory properties to human apolipoprotein(a). *J Biol Chem* 2003;278:52841–52847.
94. Boffa MB, Marcovina SM, Koschinsky ML: Lipoprotein(a) as a risk factor for atherosclerosis and thrombosis: Mechanistic insights from animal models. *Clin Biochem* 2004;37:333–343.
95. Fan J, Shimoyamada H, Sun H, et al: Transgenic rabbits expressing human apolipoprotein(a) develop more extensive atherosclerotic lesion in response to a cholesterol-rich diet. *Arterioscler Thromb Vasc Biol* 2001;21:88–94.
96. Sun H, Unoki H, Wang X, et al. Lipoprotein(a) enhances advanced atherosclerosis and vascular calcification in WHHL transgenic rabbits expressing human apolipoprotein(a). *J Biol Chem* 2002;277:47486–47492.
97. Guerra R, Yu Z, Marcovina S, et al: Lipoprotein(a) and apolipoprotein(a) isoforms: No association with coronary artery calcification in the Dallas Heart Study. *Circulation* 2005;111: 1471–1479.
98. Schneider M, Witztum JL, Young SG, et al: High-level lipoprotein(a) expression in transgenic mice: Evidence for oxidized phospholipids in lipoprotein(a) but not in low-density lipoproteins. *J Lipid Res* 2005;46:769–778.
99. Devlin CM, Lee SJ, Kuriakose G, et al: An apolipoprotein(a) peptide delays chylomicron remnant clearance and increases plasma remnant lipoproteins and atherosclerosis *in vivo*. *Arterioscler Thromb Vasc Biol* 2005;25:1704–1710.

100. Kitajima S, Jin Y, Koike T, et al: Lp(a) enhances coronary atherosclerosis in transgenic Watanabe heritable hyperlipidemic rabbits. *Atherosclerosis* 2007;193:269–276.
101. Kang C, Dominguez M, Loyau S, et al: Lp(a) particles mold fibrin-binding properties of apo(a) in size-dependent manner: A study with different-length recombinant apo(a), native Lp(a), and monoclonal antibody. *Arterioscler Thromb Vasc Biol* 2002;22:1232–1238.
102. Anglés-Cano E, de la Peña Díaz A, Loyau S: Inhibition of fibrinolysis by lipoprotein(a). *Ann N Y Acad Sci* 2001;936: 261–275.
103. Knapp JP, Herrmann W: *In vitro* inhibition of fibrinolysis by apolipoprotein(a) and lipoprotein(a) is size- and concentration-dependent. *Clin Chem Lab Med* 2004;42:1013–1019.
104. Baldo G, Giunco S, Kontothanassis D, et al: Different apoprotein(a) isoform proportions in serum and carotid plaque. *Atherosclerosis* 2007;193:177–185.
105. Marcovina SM, Albers JJ, Scanu AM, et al: Use of a reference material proposed by the International Federation of Clinical Chemistry and Laboratory Medicine to evaluate analytical methods for the determination of plasma lipoprotein(a). *Clin Chem* 2000;46:1956–1967.
106. Tate JR, Berg K, Couderc R, et al: International Federation of Clinical Chemistry and Laboratory Medicine (IFCC) Standardization Project for the Measurement of Lipoprotein(a). Phase 2: selection and properties of a proposed secondary reference material for lipoprotein(a). *Clin Chem Lab Med* 1999;37: 949–958.
107. Marcovina SM, Albers JJ, Gabel B, et al: Effect of the number of apolipoprotein(a) kringle 4 domains on immunochemical measurements of lipoprotein(a). *Clin Chem* 1995;41: 246–255.
108. Dati F, Tate JR, Marcovina SM, Steinmetz A: First WHO/IFCC International Reference Reagent for Lipoprotein(a) for Immunoassay—Lp(a) SRM 2B. *Clin Chem Lab Med* 2004;42: 670–676.
109. Edelstein C, Hinman J, Marcovina S, Scanu AM: Properties of human free apolipoprotein(a) and lipoprotein(a) after either freezing or lyophilization in the presence and absence of cryopreservatives. *Anal Biochem* 2001;288:201–208.
110. Scanu AM, Hinman J, Pfaffinger D, Edelstein C: Successful utilization of lyophilized lipoprotein(a) as a biological reagent. *Lipids* 2004;39:589–593.
111. Kulkarni KR, Garber DW, Marcovina SM, Segrest JP: Quantification of cholesterol in all lipoprotein classes by the VAP-II method. *J Lipid Res* 1994;35:159–168.
112. Seman LJ, Jenner JL, McNamara JR, Schaefer EJ: Quantification of lipoprotein(a) in plasma by assaying cholesterol in lectin-bound plasma fraction. *Clin Chem* 1994;40:400–403.
113. Baudhuin LM, Hartman SJ, O'Brien JF, et al: Electrophoretic measurement of lipoprotein(a) cholesterol in plasma with and without ultracentrifugation: Comparison with an immunoturbidimetric lipoprotein(a) method. *Clin Biochem* 2004;37: 481–488.
114. Marcovina SM, Koschinsky ML: Lipoprotein(a): Structure, measurement and clinical significance. In Rifai N, Warnick GR, Dominiczak MH (eds): Handbook of Lipoprotein Testing, 2nd ed. Washington, DC, AACC Press, 2000, pp 345–385.
115. Armstrong VW, Schleef J, Thiery J, et al: Effect of HELP-LDL-apheresis on serum concentrations of human lipoprotein(a): Kinetic analysis of the post-treatment return to baseline levels. *Eur J Clin Invest* 1989;19:235–240.
116. Pokrovsky SN, Adamova I, Afanasieva OY, Benevolenskaya GF: Immunosorbent for selective removal of lipoprotein(a) from human plasma: *in vitro* study. *Artif Organs* 15:136–140, 1991.
117. Crouse JR III: New developments in the use of niacin for treatment of hyperlipidemia: New considerations in the use of an old drug. *Coron Artery Dis* 1996;7:321–326.
118. Sirtori CR, Calabresi L, Ferrara S, et al: L-carnitine reduces plasma lipoprotein(a) levels in patients with hyper Lp(a). *Nutr Metab Cardiovasc Dis* 2000;10:247–251.
119. Dalessandri KM: Multiple methods for reduction of lipoprotein(a). *Atherosclerosis* 2002;163:409–410.
120. McCormack PL, Keating GM: Prolonged-release nicotinic acid: A review of its use in the treatment of dyslipidaemia. *Drugs* 2005;65:2719–2740.
121. Crook D, Sidhu M, Seed M, et al: Lipoprotein Lp(a) levels are reduced by danazol, an anabolic steroid. *Atherosclerosis* 1992;92:41–47.
122. Haenggi W, Riesen W, Birkhaeuser MH: Postmenopausal hormone replacement therapy with tibolone decreases serum lipoprotein(a). *Eur J Clin Chem Clin Biochem* 1993;31: 645–650.
123. Rymer J, Crook D, Sidhu M, et al: Effects of tibolone on serum concentrations of lipoprotein(a) in postmenopausal women. *Acta Endocrinol* 1993;128:259–262.
124. Henriksson P, Angelin B, Berglund L: Hormonal regulation of serum Lp(a) levels. Opposite effects after estrogen treatment and orchidectomy in males with prostatic carcinoma. *J Clin Invest* 1992;89:1166–1171.
125. Shewmon DA, Stock JL, Rosen CJ, et al: Tamoxifen and estrogen lower circulating lipoprotein(a) concentrations in healthy postmenopausal women. *Arterioscler Thromb* 1994;14:1586–1593.
126. Plenge JK, Hernandez TL, Weil KM, et al: Simvastatin lowers C-reactive protein within 14 days: An effect independent of low-density lipoprotein cholesterol reduction. *Circulation* 2002;106:1447–1452.
127. Dujovne CA, Harris WS, Altman R, et al: Effect of atorvastatin on hemorheologic-hemostatic parameters and serum fibrinogen levels in hyperlipidemic patients. *Am J Cardiol* 2000;85: 350–353.
128. McKenney JM, Jones PH, Bays HE, et al: Comparative effects on lipid levels of combination therapy with a statin and extended-release niacin or ezetimibe versus a statin alone (the COMPELL study). *Atherosclerosis* 2007;192:432–437.
129. Cobbaert C, Jukema JW, Zwinderman AH, et al: Modulation of lipoprotein(a) atherogenicity by high-density lipoprotein cholesterol levels in middle-aged men with symptomatic coronary artery disease and normal to moderately elevated serum cholesterol. Regression Growth Evaluation Statin Study (REGRESS) Study Group. *J Am Coll Cardiol* 1997;30:1491–1499.
130. Duriez P, Dallongeville J, Fruchart JC: Lipoprotein(a) as a marker for coronary heart disease. *Br J Clin Pract* 1996;77A: 54–61.
131. Gonbert S, Malinsky S, Sposito AC, et al: Atorvastatin lowers lipoprotein(a) but not apolipoprotein(a) fragment levels in hypercholesterolemic subjects at high cardiovascular risk. *Atherosclerosis* 2002;164:305–311.
132. Akaike M, Azuma H, Kagawa A, et al: Effect of aspirin treatment on serum concentrations of lipoprotein(a) in patients with atherosclerotic diseases. *Clin Chem* 2002;48:1454–1459.
133. Kiortsis DN, Tzotzas T, Giral P, et al: Changes in lipoprotein(a) levels and hormonal correlations during a weight reduction program. *Nutr Metab Cardiovasc Dis* 2001;11:153–157.
134. Jenkins DJ, Kendall CW, Marchie A, et al: Dose response of almonds on coronary heart disease risk factors: Blood lipids, oxidized low-density lipoproteins, lipoprotein(a), homocysteine, and pulmonary nitric oxide: A randomized, controlled, crossover trial. *Circulation* 2002;106:1327–1332.
135. Ginsberg HN, Kris-Etherton P, Dennis B, et al: Effects of reducing dietary saturated fatty acids on plasma lipids and lipoproteins in healthy subjects: The DELTA Study, protocol 1. *Arterioscler Thromb Vasc Biol* 1998;18:441–449.
136. Meinertz H, Nilausen K, Hilden J: Alcohol-extracted, but not intact, dietary soy protein lowers lipoprotein(a) markedly. *Arterioscler Thromb Vasc Biol* 2002;22:312–316.
137. White AL, Lanford RE: Biosynthesis and metabolism of lipoprotein(a). *Curr Opin Lipidol* 1995;6:75–80.
138. Assmann G, Cullen P, Fruchart JC, et al: Implications of emerging risk factors for therapeutic intervention. International Task Force for Prevention of Coronary Heart Disease. *Nutr Metab Cardiovasc Dis* 2005;15:373–381.

CHAPTER 12

Clinical Evaluation for Genetic and Secondary Causes of Dyslipidemia

Neil J. Stone

When a patient presents with abnormal total cholesterol, triglyceride (TG), and high-density lipoprotein (HDL) cholesterol concentrations, a genetic or familial cause should be considered, and secondary causes should be ruled out at the initial visit (Table 12-1).

Certainly an underlying genetic lipid/lipoprotein disorder should be suspected in those patients with premature coronary heart disease (CHD) or recurrent pancreatitis. Situations in which suspicion for a secondary cause for abnormal lipids should be strong include[1]:

- New-onset or progressive lipid abnormalities with no family history of lipid disorders
- Worsening lipid profile in a patient whose lipid disorder has been controlled
- Refractory lipid disorder
- Acute severe exacerbation in a previously mild lipid disorder

Confirmation of an inherited lipid abnormality does not mean that the clinician should avoid seeking an acquired or secondary cause of hyperlipidemia as well. Indeed, a combination of an inherited lipid disorder and an acquired cause of abnormal lipids can result in strikingly severe lipid abnormalities with risk for not only CHD, but also in those with disorders of TG-rich lipoproteins, acute recurrent pancreatitis[2] (Table 12-2).

The following case study provides an example of how diet, drugs, and diseases interact. A man with type 2 diabetes mellitus (DM) presented to the emergency department with abdominal discomfort and a TG level of 2240 mg/dL. His diabetic control had been poor (a recent nemoglobin A1c was 9%), and his primary care physician had recently started a bile acid–binding resin because the patient reported myalgias when he had been given a statin for his abnormal lipids. He had stigmata of the metabolic syndrome with a body mass index (BMI) of 32 kg/m^2, a waist circumference of 42 inches, and borderline hypertension. He admitted to a sedentary lifestyle with poor eating habits and recent weight gain in the last 2 years. Although the patient was prescribed a fibrate and put on a strict diet for the strikingly increased TG level, the influence of his high-calorie, high-sugar, high–saturated fat and *high–trans* fat diet, poor control of his type 2 DM, and the bile acid resin administration was considerable. The patient was asked to work with a dietitian, started on insulin therapy to control his blood sugar, and taken off the bile acid resin with marked improvement in his lipids and clinical status.

It should be noted that bile acid resins, such as colestipol and cholestyramine, should be used to reduce low-density lipoprotein (LDL) cholesterol levels only and are contraindicated in patients with TG concentration higher than 500 mg/dL because these drugs increase TG concentrations. A point worth stressing is that the marked increase in TG concentration actually makes an accompanying LDL cholesterol level increase less likely. One study found that only 5% of those with TG concentration greater than 500 mg/dL and 0% of those with TG concentration greater than 1000 mg/dL had significant LDL cholesterol increases.[3] This emphasizes that, in individuals with increased TG concentration, most of the cholesterol is in the very-low-density lipoprotein (VLDL) and chylomicron fractions, and therapy with a focus on diet, lifestyle, fibrates, fish oil, and/or niacin should be favored over LDL cholesterol–lowering therapy such as statins and resins. Statins are the drugs of choice for increased LDL cholesterol levels, but in patients with TG concentrations greater than 800 mg/dL, statins should not be considered first-line medications.

What is often less well appreciated is that, in certain situations, diet and drugs used to improve lipids can paradoxically make the lipid profile worse. For example, when dietary fat intake is less than 25% of total energy, careful

TABLE 12-1 Considerations before Starting Treatment When Hyperlipidemia Is Present

A. Inherited? Consider whether lipid/lipoproteins are markedly abnormal (upper or lower 5th percentile especially); screen the family 1. Excess LDL cholesterol disorders a. Monogenic* b. Polygenic
2. Excess TG disorders†
3. Low/abnormal HDL cholesterol level‡
4. Severe TG elevation (chylomicronemia)†
B. Presence of secondary causes? (the 4 Ds) 1. Diet: saturated fats, *trans* fats, dietary cholesterol, excess (>60%) carbohydrates, alcohol, weight gain
2. Drugs (not a complete list): glucocorticoids, estrogens, progestins, anabolic steroids, protease inhibitors, retinoic acid, tamoxifen, cyclosporine, sirolimus, atypical antipsychotics, or lipid drugs with unwanted effects (fish oil, fibrates increasing LDL cholesterol, resins, increasing TG concentration; thiazolidinediones, and a fibrates lowering HDL cholesterol
3. Diseases: obstructive liver disease, nephrosis, chronic renal disease, human immunodeficiency virus disorder; rarely, systemic lupus erythematosus
4. Disorders (metabolic): hypothyroidism, diabetes (type 2 diabetes mellitus), pregnancy, metabolic syndrome, menopause
C. Combination of inherited and secondary causes?

*May have tendon xanthomas; may have eruptive/tuberous xanthomas.
†May have lipemia retinalis, eruptive xanthomas, hepatos plenomegaly.
‡Not all low HDL cholesterol levels are pathogenic (e.g., apolipoprotein A1 Milano).
HDL cholesterol, high-density lipoprotein cholesterol; LDL cholesterol, low-density lipoprotein cholesterol; TG, triglyceride.

feeding studies show increases in TG concentration and reduced HDL cholesterol level.[4] Thus, the National Cholesterol Education Program Adult Treatment Panel III (NCEP ATP III) in 2001 recommended that dietary fat should be in the 25% to 35% range and not lower.[5] In patients with combined increases of cholesterol and TG, fibrates and fish oil capsules used to reduce TG concentration can lead to increased LDL cholesterol levels. As noted earlier, bile acid resins (cholestyramine and colestipol) should be avoided in high TG states because they can exacerbate hypertriglyceridemia. Finally, a fibrate and a thiazolidine either alone or in combination in a patient with hypertriglyceridemia with type 2 DM can rarely cause a markedly low level of HDL cholesterol, which requires the offending drugs to be stopped.[6] Thus, negative aspects of diet and drug therapy should be considered carefully in those with lipid disorders who are not responding well to therapy.

The patient history and physical examination may help to explain abnormal lipoprotein levels. Basic laboratory measures should also be performed in patients who require drug treatment for hyperlipidemia to be sure that no treatable secondary cause is lurking (see Table 12-3 for a useful checklist).

Now we consider the 4 Ds. This is a useful mnemonic for remembering the secondary causes of hyperlipidemia.[1] The Ds represent:

- Diet
- Drugs
- Disorders of metabolism
- Diseases

TABLE 12-2 Clinical Conditions That May Develop When Inherited and Secondary Causes Occur Together

Inherited Disorder	Secondary Cause	Clinical Condition
Familial hypercholesterolemia	Hypothyroidism	Difficult to treat low-density lipoprotein cholesterol; increased risk for statin-induced myositis
Familial dysbetalipoproteinemia (type III hyperlipidemia)	Hypothyroidism, obesity	Metabolic cause brings out the clinical picture in patients with apolipoprotein E_2/E_2 homozygosity
Familial hypertriglyceridemia	Hormone therapy (estrogen) after hysterectomy alcohol excess, high-fat diet, and weight gain	Chylomicronemia syndrome and acute pancreatitis

TABLE 12-3 Laboratory Workup to Identify Secondary Causes

Laboratory Test	Secondary Disorder	Lipid, Lipoproteins	Comments
TSH	Hypothyroidism	Increased LDL cholesterol level, increased TG concentration, type III pattern in patients with apolipoprotein E_2/E_2 phenotype, or chylomicron excess	Hypothyroidism is crucial to rule out before drug treatment of lipid disorders because it affects both LDL receptor regulation and TG-rich lipoprotein metabolism
Urine analysis	Nephrotic syndrome	Increased LDL cholesterol	Nephrotic syndrome should be considered in edematous patients with increased blood pressure
FBS	Type 2 DM	Atherogenic dyslipidemia with high TG concentration, reduced levels of HDL cholesterol, and small dense LDL	Consider a 2-hour glucose tolerance test if increased fasting glucose (100–125 mg/dL) to determine whether glucose at 120 minutes indicates impaired glucose tolerance (>140 mg/dL) or diabetes (>200 mg/dL)
Liver panel		Obstructive liver disease	Increased alkaline phosphatase/bilirubin levels are markers for obstruction/cholestasis; also, liver panel is a useful baseline for lipid drugs

DM, diabetes mellitus; FBS, fasting blood sugar; HDL, high-density lipoprotein LDL, low-density lipoprotein; TG, triglycerides; TSH, thyroid-stimulating hormone.

Tables 12-4 through 12-6 show the 4 Ds and their effects on LDL cholesterol, TG, and HDL cholesterol levels.

DIETARY FACTORS AS SECONDARY CAUSES OF LIPID/LIPOPROTEIN ABNORMALITIES

Dietary Factors That Cause Increased Low-Density Lipoprotein Cholesterol Levels

Diets high in saturated fats and *trans* fatty acids increase LDL cholesterol levels.[5] Weight gain is associated with increased LDL cholesterol, although when it results in insulin resistance, the dominant lipid/lipoprotein change is an increase in TG concentration together with a decreased HDL cholesterol level (see next section). Individuals who have diets rich in beans, legumes, nuts, seeds, whole grains, fruits, and vegetables have lower cholesterol values.[7] (For a more complete discussion, see Chapter 19.)

Dietary/Lifestyle Factors That Worsen Triglyceride/High-Density Lipoprotein Cholesterol Levels

Major causes of high TG concentrations in the general population include overweight and obesity, physical inactivity, cigarette smoking, very-high-carbohydrate diets (>60% of energy), and excess alcohol intake.[6] All of these, except for excess alcohol, also depress HDL cholesterol levels at the same time.[8] In many individuals, decreased levels of HDL cholesterol correlate with increases in TG concentration and remnant lipoproteins; moreover, the low HDL cholesterol level is often associated with small dense LDL particles.[5,9] This triad of increased TGs, low HDL cholesterol, and small dense LDL cholesterol has been called *atherogenic dyslipidemia* and is commonly seen in individuals with other metabolic risk factors.[5] It is important to recognize because LDL cholesterol levels can be normal or only slightly increased in these persons who are at increased risk for CHD because of their metabolic risk factors. Indeed, in this setting, an increased TG/HDL cholesterol ratio can be seen as a sign of insulin resistance,[10] although this relation does not hold for black patients with similar ratios.[11]

As the global population has become more obese, the emergence of the metabolic syndrome and an increased prevalence of type 2 DM has led experts to reconsider both the amount and quality of carbohydrates in the diet.[12] Because excess carbohydrates reduce HDL cholesterol levels as well, a sensible approach to carbohydrates in the diet calls for reductions in low-fiber, refined-carbohydrate foods, added sugars, and high-fructose corn syrup–sweetened foods, with an emphasis on fruits, vegetables, whole grains, and nonfat dairy products instead. Data from the large Nurses' Health Study based on a food-frequency questionnaire showed that a high glycemic load was associated with an increased CHD risk.[13] The authors concluded that, in women, diets lower in carbohydrate and higher in protein and fat are not associated with increased CHD risk, advocating vegetable sources of fat and protein to keep total carbohydrates lower.

Weight loss obtained by both diet and exercise changes can result in a mild to moderate decrease in TG levels and a significant increase in HDL cholesterol and HDL_2 levels with a decrease in the small dense LDL fraction.[14] In the Diabetes Prevention Program study, in which intensive lifestyle intervention was more effective than metformin therapy in preventing diabetes, reductions in serum TG levels were accompanied by concomitant increases in HDL cholesterol levels and LDL size in the intensive lifestyle intervention group. Importantly, benefit with lifestyle change was maintained over the course of the study.[15]

Aerobic exercise of moderate intensity with high frequency (30 minutes of exercise 5–7 days/week) has been associated with maintenance of improved cardiorespiratory fitness.[16] Weight loss induced by increased daily physical activity without caloric restriction substantially reduces obesity (particularly abdominal obesity) and insulin resistance in men. Exercise without weight loss reduces abdominal fat and prevents further weight gain.[17] The emphasis should be on losing visceral fat, because liposuction of subcutaneous fat is not associated with improvement of metabolic markers such as lipids, hypertension, and measures of glycemia.[18]

TABLE 12-4 Acquired Causes for Increased Low-Density Lipoprotein Cholesterol Levels*

LDL Cholesterol Levels	Acquired Traits/Habits	Diseases	Drugs
Mild elevation	Increased intake of saturated fat Increased intake of *trans* fatty acids Weight gain	Subclinical hypothyroidism Anorexia (paradoxical increase in cholesterol levels)	Cyclosporine Rosiglitazone Fibrates† Omega-3 fatty acids† Amiodarone High-dose chlorthalidone Hydrochlorothiazide
Moderate to severe increases (>280 mg/dL)	Some individuals can be quite diet sensitive and LDL cholesterol can increase levels to ≥100 mg/dL	Pregnancy (greater each trimester, maximal in third trimester) Hypothyroidism Obstructive liver disease Nephrosis	Cyclosporine

*There may be more examples than listed; this is meant to be useful to the practicing physician.

†Paradoxical increase in low-density lipoprotein (LDL) cholesterol occurs when an individual has combined hyperlipidemia and is given these lipid drugs that reduce triglycerides (very-low-density lipoprotein).

TABLE 12-5 Acquired Causes for High Triglycerides*

TG Levels	Acquired Traits/Habits	Diseases	Drugs
Borderline high (150–199 mg/dL)	Overweight, obesity Physical inactivity Cigarette smoking Excess alcohol intake High carbohydrate intake (≥60% of energy)	See below	See below
High (200–499 mg/dL)	Same	Diabetes, chronic renal failure, nephrotic syndrome, Cushing disease, lipodystrophy, systemic lupus erythematosus (rarely) HIV Pregnancy (increased each trimester)	Oral estrogens (not transcutaneous) tamoxifen, corticosteroids, β-blockers (including eye preparations), retinoids, protease inhibitors for AIDS (especially ritonavir), bile acid resins, sirolimus
Very high (≥500 mg/dL)	Same (not enough by themselves usually; require drugs/diseases or genetic fault as well)	Above diseases and T-cell lymphoma–related panniculitis	Above diseases plus individual with inherited lipid abnormality Asparaginase plus prednisone treatment of leukemia

* There may be more examples than listed; this is meant to be useful to the practicing physician.
AIDS, acquired immunodeficiency syndrome; HIV human immunodeficiency virus. TG, triglyceride.

TABLE 12-6 Acquired Causes for Low Levels of High-Density Lipoprotein Cholesterol*

HDL Cholesterol Levels	Acquired Traits/Habits	Diseases	Drugs
<50 mg/dL in women; <40 mg/dL in men	Overweight, obesity Physical inactivity Cigarette smoking High carbohydrate intake (≥60% of energy)	See below	Progestins, androgens, β-blockers (including eye preparations)
<30 mg/dL		Usually heterozygous forms of inherited low HDL cholesterol levels	
<10 mg/dL		Usually homozygous forms of inherited low HDL cholesterol levels	Androgens, paradoxical response of fenofibrate and thiazolidinediones

* There may be more examples than listed; this is meant to be useful to the practicing physician.
HDL, high-density lipoprotein.

Dietary Factors for Patients with Severe Hypertriglyceridemia

Patients with severe TG excess most likely have an underlying genetic condition that can be exacerbated by either a high-fat diet or alcohol, or, especially, both. If these patients present with the chylomicronemia syndrome (lipemia retinalis, eruptive xanthomas, and TGs that usually exceed 2500 mg/dL), they are at high risk for pancreatitis and may require hospitalization, especially if abdominal discomfort is present. An important caveat is that pancreatitis can be present in the face of a normal amylase level in such patients, and computed tomography or magnetic resonance imaging may be required to detect pancreatitis.[1]

DISEASES THAT CAUSE LIPID/LIPOPROTEIN ABNORMALITIES

Insulin Resistance and Diabetes Mellitus

Patients who have "atherogenic dyslipidemia" as defined earlier have increased levels of apolipoprotein B (apoB)–containing lipoproteins, including VLDL remnants and small LDL particles, and reduced levels of HDL cholesterol.[19] This is seen commonly in states of insulin resistance and is associated with increased synthesis of fatty acids from glucose, as well as increased TG concentration from lipolysis of adipose tissue TG leading to overproduction of large VLDL particles from the liver.[20] This leads to increased plasma TG concentration that, by means of an exchange process mediated by cholesteryl ester transfer protein (CETP), results in reduced levels of HDL cholesterol and apoA-I, and an increase in small dense LDL particles. Typically, reduced plasma HDL levels in type 2 diabetes are manifest as reductions in the HDL_{2b} subspecies and relative or absolute increases in smaller denser HDL_{3b} and HDL_{3c}.[21]

Major causes of insulin resistance include both a genetic predisposition and environmental influences such as sedentary lifestyle and obesity.[22] Although insulin resistance is seen in individuals with increased waist circumference and hypertriglyceridemia,[23] there are important exceptions. For example, South Asian women with atherogenic dyslipidemia may not have increased waist circumference, even though they have insulin resistance, underscoring the strong genetic contribution to insulin resistance.[24] Also, black patients with TG in the range of 110 to 149 mg/dL (considered reference range by NCEP ATP III) had insulin resistance, as measured by the insulin clamp, that was believed to be equivalent to that of nonblack individuals with TG concentrations of 150 mg/dL or more.[25]

Thus, a reasonable approach to patients presenting with hyperlipidemia would be to screen them for metabolic syndrome and type 2 DM with measurements of waist circumference, blood pressure, and fasting blood sugar. Although statins potently reduce elevated LDL cholesterol levels, drug therapy for metabolic syndrome risk factors need not pre-empt emphasis on lifestyle change. Indeed, in those with metabolic risk factors, especially in the prediabetic stage, lifestyle therapy is even more potent than the drug metformin in preventing type 2 DM. In the Diabetes Prevention Program study of subjects with impaired glucose tolerance, TG levels declined significantly more with intensive lifestyle intervention than with placebo or metformin. Although LDL cholesterol levels were similar among the treatment groups, intensive lifestyle intervention significantly increased the HDL cholesterol level and reduced the small dense LDL pattern. At 3 years of follow-up, the lifestyle therapy group required significantly less pharmacologic therapy to achieve goals for hypertension (27–28%) and hyperlipidemia (25% less) as compared with placebo and metformin groups.[15] Of course, statin therapy to get LDL cholesterol to target level is recommended for both primary and secondary prevention in the patient with diabetes.[6]

Hypothyroidism

Hypothyroidism is a common condition in the general population, and it is at least twice as common in lipid clinics.[26] Hypothyroidism causes increases of cholesterol, and the severity of the abnormality depends on the degree of hypothyroidism and the underlying genetics of the patient. Thyroid hormone most likely results in downregulation of the LDL receptor, and thyroid-stimulating hormone (TSH) levels greater than 20 mIU/L usually result in increased total and LDL cholesterol levels. NCEP ATP III suggests that TSH be measured in all patients with LDL cholesterol levels greater than 160 mg/dL.[6]

Hypothyroidism can provide the metabolic trigger that causes the expression of the characteristic dyslipidemia of type III hyperlipidemia in individuals who have apoE_2 homozygosity.[27,28] Although the E_2/E_2 genotype is necessary, it appears that secondary causes such as type 2 DM, hypothyroidism, or obesity are necessary for the type III pattern to be expressed. Although palmar xanthomas are important clues to type III hyperlipidemia, this is another important reason to check a TSH level in a person who presents with significant increases of total cholesterol or TG that are roughly equivalent. Finally, thyroid replacement in hypothyroidism is reported to reduce lipoprotein(a) [Lp(a)].[29]

Controversy exists, however, about the wisdom of treating "subclinical" hypothyroidism (SCH) with mildly increased TSH and normal free T_4 level, as improvements in lipids are not invariably seen. Indeed, a MEDLINE search of controlled clinical trials was unable to show that treatment with thyroid replacement would improve the quality of life in otherwise healthy patients who meet the criteria for SCH.[30] Reasons exist, however, to consider treatment of those with SCH. A 12-week trial of 100 μm L-thyroxine versus placebo in 100 subjects with mean TSH levels of 6.6 mIU/L showed that L-thyroxine treatment reduced LDL cholesterol from 142.9 to 131.3 mg/dL and significantly improved waist-to-hip ratio and brachial artery flow-mediated dilatation.[31] Thus, in certain patients, treating SCH may help patients get to their LDL cholesterol goals. L-thyroxine also reduces non-HDL cholesterol in patients with SCH, as well as in those with primary hypothyroidism.[32] Finally, case reports of statin-induced myositis suggest that it is prudent to diagnose and treat hypothyroidism before starting statin therapy.[33,34] Because thyroid hormone replacement appears to produce LDL lowering in relation to the initial LDL cholesterol level, some argue that those with significantly increased LDL cholesterol and SCH may benefit more than those with LDL cholesterol in the reference range.[35]

Nephrotic Syndrome

Patients with nephrotic syndrome present with hypercholesterolemia, hypertension, and edema. Low levels of serum albumin and marked proteinuria complete the clinical picture that can be missed unless there is a high index of suspicion and a urine sample is taken. With increasing levels of proteinuria, the initial increased LDL cholesterol level becomes accompanied by an excess of TG-rich lipoproteins as well.[36] Thus, the severity of the hypoalbuminemia explains the degree of change in the plasma lipoproteins. In patients with nondiabetic nephrotic syndrome, it is not uncommon for the total cholesterol level to be 300 mg/dL or greater.[37]

The increased LDL cholesterol level results from increased production of LDL, but the increased VLDL in patients with nephrotic syndrome results from a decreased catabolism.[38] HDL cholesterol levels are usually normal to low. A potential mechanism is via CETP, which influences the distribution of cholesterol among LDL, VLDL, and HDL.[39] This mechanism explains increased levels of LDL and VLDL that are unusually enriched in cholesteryl ester. Although not surprising, apoB levels are increased in nephrotic syndrome, and apoA-I and apoA-II levels are usually normal.

Statin therapy reverses the abnormalities seen in apoB-containing lipoproteins (LDL and VLDL) by reducing input rates for LDL and enhancing VLDL catabolism.[40] ApoB kinetics, however, are different depending on whether there is only hypercholesterolemia or combined cholesterol and TG excess.[41] HDL, but not apoA-I, is excreted in the urine and likely explains the lipiduria seen. In nondiabetic patients with nephrotic syndrome, Lp(a) concentrations are substantially increased (either because of the proteinuria or an acute-phase response) compared with controls with the same apo(a) isoform, and concentrations are substantially reduced when remission of the nephrotic syndrome is induced.[42] In the face of a considerable increase in Lp(a), the calculated LDL cholesterol level may not be as responsive to statin therapy as one might expect.[43,44] Indeed, Lp(a) values may respond to specific treatment for the nephrosis in both white and black patients.[45]

Chronic Kidney Disease

The spectrum of lipid abnormalities in patients with chronic kidney disease (CKD) and dialysis patients involves all lipoprotein classes, including Lp(a), but varies depending on the severity of the kidney function and also whether intercurrent illnesses such as diabetes or nephrotic syndrome are also present. The Third National Health and Nutrition Examination Survey reports that adults with CKD (an estimated glomerular filtration rate <60 mL/min per 1.73 m^2 based on the abbreviated Modification of Diet in Renal Disease study formula) have lower apoA-I levels and greater homocysteine, Lp(a), fibrinogen, and C-reactive protein levels than adults without CKD.[46] Each of these differences increases the risk for subsequent cardiovascular disease.

In chronic renal insufficiency and end-stage renal disease, there are both quantitative and qualitative abnormalities in serum lipoproteins, with moderately severe hypertriglyceridemia caused by a defect in TG lipolysis and remnant clearance, and reduced levels of HDL cholesterol.[47] Findings in children with CKD largely parallel those found in adults. Moderate hypertriglyceridemia, increased TG-rich lipoproteins, and reduced HDL cholesterol levels are the most often seen, whereas total and LDL cholesterol levels remain normal or modestly increased. Measures of lipoprotein lipase and hepatic lipase activity are reduced, and concentrations of apoC-III are markedly increased.[48] One investigator has noted that although there are differences, there are many similarities to the abnormalities seen with the metabolic syndrome.[49]

In end-stage renal disease and uremia, the kind of lipid abnormalities noted is strongly influenced by the type of renal replacement therapy: hemodialysis or continuous ambulatory peritoneal dialysis (CAPD).[50] Patients undergoing both types of therapy have increased TG and reduced HDL cholesterol levels, as well as oxidized LDL and increased Lp(a) levels. Those receiving CAPD have more small dense LDL particles and increased levels of apoB. Not surprisingly, patients receiving CAPD have overproduction of VLDL as contrasted with the presence of TG-rich VLDL in those receiving hemodialysis. Differences exist in LDL cholesterol levels as well. LDL cholesterol levels were greater than 100mg/dL in 55.7% of patients receiving hemodialysis versus 73.2% of those receiving CAPD.[51] Because most CKD patients have a 10-year risk for CHD events greater than 20%,[52] this makes them a coronary risk equivalent according to the NCEP ATP III guidelines.[6] After kidney transplantation, LDL cholesterol levels are most often increased, but this may be caused, at least in part, by the effects of weight gain and the medications used (prednisone, cyclosporine, sirolimus).

Lipid abnormalities may also depend on the treatment given for CKD. Statin treatment in clinical trials in patients with cardiovascular disease appears to reduce proteinuria modestly and results in a small reduction in the rate of kidney function loss.[53] Analysis of clinical trial data that included subjects with up to stage 3 of CKD indicates that these patients derive considerable cardiovascular benefit from statin-induced reduction of LDL cholesterol level.[54,55] In the Assessment of Lescol in Renal Transplantation (ALERT) trial, the use of fluvastatin in patients with renal transplants was found to decrease coronary events and cardiovascular mortality rates by an extent similar to that observed in patients without kidney disease, although no significant decrease was seen in all-cause mortality.[56]

The available evidence supporting statin use in end-stage renal disease is not strong. Die Devtsche Diabetes Dialyse Studie (4D) in diabetic patients receiving dialysis failed to show a statistically significant effect of atorvastatin on the composite end point of death from cardiac causes, fatal stroke, nonfatal myocardial infarction (MI), or nonfatal stroke.[57] The use of atorvastatin did decrease the number of cardiovascular events (fatal and nonfatal) significantly (risk ratio [RR], 0.82; 95% confidence interval [CI], 0.68–0.99; $P = 0.03$), but the impact on all-cause mortality was not significant in comparison with placebo (RR, 0.93; 95% CI, 0.79–1.08; $P = 0.33$). This suggests that, in end-stage kidney disease, the ability of statins to favorably affect the course of the disease remains unproved.

Obstructive Liver Disease

Biliary obstruction may be associated with severe hypercholesterolemia that is resistant to conventional cholesterol-lowering drugs. An example is obstructive liver disease caused by graft-versus-host disease.[58] The only effective therapy is treatment of the underlying liver or biliary tract disease. When high cholesterol levels are seen in patients (usually middle-aged women) with clinical features of obstructive liver disease, the diagnosis of primary biliary cirrhosis should be strongly considered. These patients have marked increases of free cholesterol because of a special lipoprotein called *lipoprotein X* (Lp-X) and exhibit planar xanthomas, which are among those most clinically recognizable characteristics of secondary hyperlipidemia.[59] Patients usually describe unremitting pruritus that is responsive to bile acid resins such as cholestyramine or colestipol. Those with early-stage primary biliary cirrhosis have mild increases of LDL and VLDL levels and increased HDL cholesterol level, whereas HDL cholesterol level is lower in the later stages.[60] Some physicians believe that associated low levels of Lp(a) may protect against early atherosclerosis.[61,62] Unfortunately, this chronic, progressive cholestatic liver disease of unknown cause eventually leads to liver failure and the need for liver transplantation.

Lp-X, an abnormal form of LDL, has a vesicular structure that appears in rouleaux formation under the electron microscope.[63] It is virtually specific for cholestasis and familial lecithin:cholesterol acyltransferase (LCAT) deficiency. Some propose that Lp-X has *anti*atherogenic properties and may reduce atherosclerotic risk.[64] Notably, few studies have examined atherosclerotic coronary events in primary biliary cirrhosis, and none has sufficient sample size or follow-up to determine accurately CHD risk.

When patients with cholestasis have hypertriglyceridemia, the excess TG concentration is to be found predominantly in two LDL fractions rather than in VLDL. Not surprisingly, HDL differs in composition and in quantity in disorders of cholestasis. In extrahepatic obstruction, HDL and its major apolipoproteins, apoA-I and apoA-II, are frequently reduced, whereas in all but the latest stages of chronic intrahepatic cholestasis caused by primary biliary cirrhosis, HDL, especially HDL_2, concentrations, are increased, probably because of the presence of a circulating inhibitor of hepatic lipase. In acute hepatocellular disease, such as alcoholic or viral hepatitis, patients may exhibit a cholestatic phase, and many of the same lipoprotein changes described earlier may be seen. For cirrhosis without cholestasis, patients are not markedly hyperlipidemic, and in advanced cases, cholesterol and apoB levels may be reduced.

Human Immunodeficiency Virus Disorder

Lipid abnormalities occur in human immunodeficiency virus (HIV) even before treatment with highly active retroviral therapy (HAART).[65] Low levels of cholesterol are seen during the early stages of HIV-1 infection and are associated with specific alterations in immune function. Changes occur that are characteristic of insulin resistance with increased TG and lower HDL cholesterol levels.[66] Not surprisingly, there are also increased levels of small dense LDL.[67] These changes are shown to occur before the more profound clinical and lipid changes seen with protease inhibitors (PIs) are noted (see Drugs section later in chapter).

Cushing Syndrome

A controlled study of women with Cushing syndrome (CS) showed increased lipids, including increased VLDL cholesterol, LDL cholesterol, and HDL cholesterol levels. All lipid and lipoprotein abnormalities were completely abolished after successful surgery. The authors concluded that hypercortisolism stimulates the hepatic production of VLDL particles.[68] Despite similar BMI values, in patients with subclinical CS and nonfunctioning adenomas, the occurrence of diabetes and abnormal lipids levels was greater than in patients with adenomas without subclinical CS (50% vs. 26% and 50% vs. 21%, respectively). The difference was even greater for hypertension, which occurred in 91.8% of patients with subclinical CS and in 34% of the remaining patients.[69]

Monoclonal Antibodies Causing Type III Hyperlipidemia

An acquired form of the type III hyperlipidemia phenotype may rarely be associated with myeloma and immunoglobulin (Ig)–lipoprotein complexes. In one informative case, a workup for malignancy showed monoclonal IgA gammopathy, and immunostaining confirmed IgA antibodies complexed to the patient's VLDL. Strikingly, lipid-lowering therapy for type III hyperlipidemia did not correct the hyperlipidemia, but when chemotherapy for the patient's myeloma reduced his IgA, improvements in cholesterol and TG, as well as xanthomas, were seen.[70]

Anorexia Nervosa

Studies of biochemical abnormalities in women in an eating disorders clinic showed hypercholesterolemia was more common in anorexia nervosa, and abnormal liver enzymes were more common in bulimia.[71]

Acute Intermittent Porphyria

Reports are inconsistent as to whether LDL cholesterol level is increased in asymptomatic acute porphyria, but there does seem to be an increase in HDL cholesterol and apoA-I. The favorable changes in HDL cholesterol and apoA-I may attenuate CHD risk for those in whom LDL cholesterol level is increased.[72,73]

Acute or Chronic Severe Inflammatory Disease

Low HDL cholesterol level has numerous causes including androgens, progestins, cigarette smoking, obesity, a low-fat diet, and drugs such as β-blockers, isotretinoin, PIs, and sirolimus. Yet some may consider the most frequent cause of a low level of HDL cholesterol in hospitalized patients as an acute or chronic severe inflammatory disease with a marked acute-phase reaction. Together with albumin and transferrin, HDL cholesterol level declines and returns to reference within days after the end of the acute-phase reaction. This was confirmed in a study of high-school-aged children at boarding school with standardized activity and food service where a decline in HDL cholesterol level was seen after an acute illness when contrasted with values when the children were healthy.[74–77]

Paraproteinemia

Paraproteinemia can be a cause of very low levels of HDL cholesterol through either acquired or artifactual means. The mechanism for severe HDL deficiency and its resolution with chemotherapy of the paraproteinemia may relate to monoclonal IgG paraproteins binding to HDL, perhaps through an interaction with apoA-I, causing these complexes to be rapidly removed.[78] Direct assays of HDL cholesterol may be susceptible to error as contrasted with the older precipitation methods, although these artifactual effects may, in some cases, obscure a true paraprotein-associated HDL cholesterol deficiency.

Polycystic Ovary Syndrome

Polycystic ovary syndrome (PCOS) is seen in women with hyperinsulinemia and insulin resistance. Abnormalities of HDL are more common than TGs, with the HDL_2 cholesterol fraction reduced in both obese and thin women with PCOS.[79] Metformin therapy and diet in women with PCOS effectively and safely reduced weight and LDL cholesterol levels while increasing HDL cholesterol levels, and maintained these outcomes stably over 4 years.[80]

DRUGS THAT CAUSE ABNORMAL LIPID/LIPOPROTEIN LEVELS

The most important drug–lipid interactions are those that cause severe exacerbations of increased TG levels. A useful list of drugs that have been reported to cause severe hypertriglyceridemia (with excess levels of chylomicrons, VLDL, or both) and pancreatitis when given to a susceptible individual (usually with familial forms of hypertriglyceridemia) includes estrogen, cholestyramine or colestipol, oral contraceptives containing "second-generation" progestins, danazol, tamoxifen, clomiphene, β-blockers, thiazide diuretics, cyclosporine, isotretinoin PIs, atypical antipsychotics, and glucocorticoids.[1,81,82] Although sometimes genetic hyperlipidemia may not be uncovered, careful investigations most often disclose an underlying inherited lipid problem. All drug effects are not harmful with respect to the lipid profile. For example, α-blocking agents, estrogens, hormone replacement therapy, combined oral contraceptives containing "third-generation" progestins, selective estrogen receptor modulators, growth hormone, and valproic appear to benefit the lipid profile.[77]

Antihypertensive Drugs

Most antihypertensive drugs, with the exception of the calcium-channel blockers, have effects on lipids and lipoproteins.[83] Thiazide diuretics are recommended as either initial therapy or as part of a multidrug regimen.[84] They have dose-related effects on cholesterol that are greater with high doses and worse in black individuals.[79] Low doses of diuretics, however, barely increase cholesterol levels, so this should not be considered a reason not to use them.[85] Data from the 3- and 4-year follow-up of a subset of Systolic Hypertension in the Elderly Program (SHEP) participants indicate that low-dose diuretic therapy had modest and no progressive effects on levels of fasting glucose, total cholesterol, and HDL cholesterol.[86] Larger effects were seen on TG, uric acid, and potassium in this study. The effects of loop diuretics are similar to those of thiazides with increases in LDL cholesterol levels, whereas HDL cholesterol levels are generally lower in individuals taking furosemide.[6] Data regarding indapamide are inconclusive, but it is considered to have neutral effects on lipids.[87] Although α_1-adrenergic blockers and centrally acting α_2-receptor agonists have a slight beneficial effect on blood lipids by decreasing LDL cholesterol levels, this should not be the basis for using these medications over thiazides. It should be noted that in patients with diabetes and those with metabolic syndrome, thiazides will be needed at least as a second drug to counteract the increased sodium reabsorption and volume expansion that invariably accompanies the high circulating insulin levels (at least 80%) in patients with metabolic syndrome and type 2 DM.

Asparaginase

Asparaginase is a recognized treatment in acute lymphocytic leukemia. In a systematic appraisal of asparaginase therapy, 67% of patients were found to have increased TG levels.[88] This was attributed to an overproduction of VLDL particles because there was an associated increase in apoB-100 levels. Although about 20% had TG concentrations greater than 1000 mg/dL, none of these individuals developed acute pancreatitis in this small series. The authors stressed that close clinical monitoring is required, though, when TG levels exceed 2000 mg/dL, because risk for pancreatitis is present and conventional markers such as serum amylase are not usually helpful for early detection.

β-Blockers

In general, β-blockers without intrinsic sympathomimetic activity (ISA) or α-blocking properties tend to reduce HDL cholesterol and increase serum TG concentrations. These effects are modest and should not play a role in the selection of specific antihypertensive agents. In a study contrasting patients with CHD with matched control subjects from the offspring cohort of Framingham, β-blockers were associated with a reduced prevalence of intermediate LDL particles and increased prevalence of small and very small LDL.[89] This was believed to be an important confounding factor when comparisons of healthy subjects and patients with CHD were made. Indeed, in the placebo arm of the Helsinki trial, men who received antihypertensive therapy had reduced CHD incidence despite adverse effects on HDL cholesterol and TG concentrations[90] (most were treated with thiazides, β-blockers, or both).

β-blockers with ISA and the β-blocker labetalol (which has α_1-adrenergic–blocking properties) produce no appreciable changes in lipid levels.[80] Carvedilol and metoprolol are both widely used for patients with dilated cardiomyopathy. In both individuals without diabetes[91] and those with type 2 DM,[92] carvedilol treatment resulted in improved parameters of glycemia and insulin action as contrasted with either atenolol or metoprolol. In a trial of subjects with diabetes receiving renin–angiotensin system blockade, insulin sensitivity improved and progression to microalbuminuria was significantly less frequent with carvedilol, but not metoprolol, despite similar blood pressure between groups.[93]

Protease Inhibitor–Induced Dyslipidemia

Treatment of HIV with PIs was a striking clinical success, yet some PIs have direct effects on glucose and lipid metabolism.[94] The hallmarks of the clinical syndrome seen with PIs are[95]:

- Hypertriglyceridemia and low HDL cholesterol level
- Central fat distribution
- Insulin resistance
- Peripheral lipodystrophy

The lower body fat seen in these patients is independently associated with longer duration of PI therapy and lower body weight before therapy. More severe lipodystrophy was seen with greater previous and current TG and C-peptide concentrations, and a more central fat distribution.[96] Impaired glucose tolerance occurred in 16% of patients treated with a PI, and type 2 DM occurred in 7%; in all but three patients, these abnormalities were detected on 2-hour postglucose load values.

PIs are associated with a small, but increased CHD risk as compared with non-nucleoside reverse-transcriptase inhibitors (NNRTIs).[97] Some, but not all, of the increased CHD risk may be caused by the adverse lipid profile.[98] The atherogenic dyslipidemia becomes increasingly notable early after the initiation of HAART, and the level of abnormalities peaks during the second or third year. Low HDL cholesterol levels persisted in the majority of men. In a cross-sectional study of men with HIV infection, patients being treated with a PI had greater total cholesterol and TG levels than patients receiving no therapy ($P < 0.05$ for each). Patients in the NNRTI group had greater TG and LDL cholesterol levels and lower HDL cholesterol levels than patients receiving no therapy ($P < 0.05$ for each). Both PI and NNRTI therapy resulted in increased levels of TG and greater apoC-III levels in apoB-containing lipoproteins.[99] In contrast, in antiretroviral naive patients, NNRTI increased levels of total and HDL cholesterol.[100] The increase in HDL cholesterol may help explain why in the Data Collection on Adverse Events of Anti-HIV Drugs (DAD) follow-up study, there was a documented increased risk for MI associated with the use of PIs but not NNRTIs after adjustments. Nonetheless, this increased risk with PI therapy was not fully explained by the lipid changes induced by the drugs in this class.[93]

Lifestyle changes are always a mainstay of therapeutic recommendations for patients with HIV with lipid abnormalities. Drug therapy should follow guidelines of the NCEP ATP III but must be prescribed with several caveats in mind.[101,102] Statins are the drugs of choice for reducing LDL cholesterol level, but simvastatin and lovastatin are best avoided because of CYP 3A4 interactions that boost blood levels of these agents and increases the risk for rhabdomyolysis. Atorvastatin levels increase, but low doses can be used. Fibrates may be especially useful to prevent the occurrence of acute pancreatitis associated with severe hypertriglyceridemia. Niacin can be used safely, but there are concerns about its increasing insulin resistance. Omega-3 fatty acid capsules can also help treat hypertriglyceridemia. In contrast, bile acid sequestrants could bind needed HIV drugs and should not be used.

Hormonal Drugs

Estrogens reduce LDL cholesterol and increase both HDL cholesterol and TG levels.[103] Progestins oppose these effects. Postmenopausal estrogen replacement increases apoA-I levels and production rate, but when progestin is added to estrogen, it opposes these effects by reducing the production of apoA-I.[104] When using continuous 0.625 mg conjugated equine estrogen (CEE) plus 2.5 mg medroxyprogesterone acetate (or in hysterectomized women, 0.625 mg CEE), Turkish investigators confirmed reductions in LDL cholesterol, apoB, and Lp(a) levels, with the greatest reductions in Lp(a) seen in those women having the highest Lp(a) level.[105] Although estrogen causes approximately a 15% reduction in LDL cholesterol level, the Heart and Estrogen Replacement Study (HERS) did not show a beneficial effect of hormone replacement therapy in postmenopausal women with CHD.[106] Nonetheless, this double-blind, randomized trial showed that Lp(a) is an independent risk factor for recurrent CHD in such women, and that treatment with combination oral estrogen and progestin reduced Lp(a) levels.[107] Of note, combination hormonal therapy had a more favorable effect (relative to placebo) in study participants with high initial Lp(a) levels than in those with low levels.

However, in some women with baseline hypertriglyceridemia, oral estrogen therapy can cause markedly increased serum TG concentrations and pancreatitis that requires discontinuation of therapy.[108,109] Progestins increase LDL cholesterol but reduce TGs and HDL cholesterol, the opposite one would expect from estrogenic hormones. Some combination regimens for menopausal symptoms may have less adverse lipid profiles. Estradiol/dydrogesterone and CEE/norgestrel were given in a double-blind, randomized trial to 193 women and found to be similarly effective for climacteric symptoms, but the estradiol/dydrogesterone combination showed advantages in terms of lipid profile and incidence of bleeding.[110]

As an alternative to oral estrogen therapy, the estrogen patch does not increase TG and can be used in women who become markedly hypertriglyceridemic with oral estrogen. Tamoxifen can cause marked hypertriglyceridemia and has been associated with chylomicronemia syndrome and pancreatitis.[111] Raloxifene reduces LDL cholesterol similarly to estrogen, but in patients with a history of hypertriglyceridemia with oral estrogen, raloxifene can be associated with severe hypertriglyceridemia. Therefore, patients should have serum TG concentrations monitored after beginning raloxifene therapy and may even require fibrate therapy before taking raloxifene.[112] Thus, a fasting lipid panel should be considered in women who are about to start any hormonal therapies.

Oral contraceptives have variable effects on lipids that usually reflect progestin androgenicity or a progestin-estrogen interaction.[113] Those that combine C21 progestins and certain C19 progestin derivatives with estrogen have little or no effect on HDL_2. Combined oral contraceptives with progestins that give a marked androgenic effect are more likely to reduce HDL cholesterol and HDL_2 levels.

A special consideration is pregnancy. During pregnancy, estrogen and progesterone levels are extremely high, resulting in increased cholesterol and TG levels. LDL cholesterol level gradually increases to a maximum value at term of 50% greater than the nonpregnant level, and total HDL and HDL_2 concentrations also increase. In subjects with a physiologic lipid increase during pregnancy, postpartum TG returned to baseline within 6 weeks. In contrast, LDL cholesterol level exhibited a slow postpartum decline and was still increased at 20 weeks after birth.[114] Women whose lipid levels during pregnancy exceed the 95th percentile are, not unexpectedly, at greater risk for hyperlipidemia with aging. HDL cholesterol levels are increased during pregnancy but decline to baseline by 20 weeks after birth. These physiologic changes in lipoproteins are not associated with increased atherosclerosis.

On the other hand, for those women with an underlying genetic lipid disorder who begin pregnancy with increased TG concentrations, substantial clinical problems may occur during the third trimester, when an acceleration of TG values can be seen. When TG concentrations exceed 2000 mg/dL, these women are at substantial risk for the chylomicronemia syndrome and acute pancreatitis, and careful management is required to prevent serious comorbidity or death.[115] Hospitalization, intravenous feeding, and if required, plasma exchange have been utilized to prevent and/or treat this complication.

Anabolic Steroids

When hypogonadal men receive intramuscular administration of testosterone esters, there is a small, dose-dependent decrease in HDL cholesterol and concomitant declines in total cholesterol and LDL cholesterol levels.[116] This is not seen with transdermal administration of testosterone.[117] For hypogonadal men who require testosterone supplementation, no adverse effect on insulin sensitivity or C-reactive protein has been shown except at the highest doses. At 600 mg/week testosterone, there is a reduction in plasma HDL cholesterol and apoA-I levels.[118] Given to elderly eugonadal men, intramuscular testosterone is a potent stimulator of hepatic lipase activity, with decreases in HDL cholesterol, HDL_2, and HDL_3 levels, as well as increasing small dense LDL.[119] The lowest HDL cholesterol values encountered in subjects taking androgenic agents occur in weight lifters taking high doses of multiple androgenic agents, typically combinations of testosterone with several anabolic steroids, which produce dramatic declines in HDL cholesterol levels that occur within 1 to 2 weeks of beginning therapy and resolve slowly when these therapy is discontinued.[120]

Glucocorticoids

Glucocorticoids increase LDL cholesterol level, but they also increase TG and HDL cholesterol levels. These effects are especially seen with prolonged use after transplantation (see Transplant Drugs). In survivors of heart transplantation, stepwise multiple linear regression analysis demonstrated cumulative prednisone exposure to be the strongest predictor of both total cholesterol and LDL cholesterol levels. Glucocorticoids, like estrogens and tamoxifen, can be associated with the chylomicronemia syndrome if given to patients with underlying genetic hypertriglyceridemia.[121]

Atypical Antipsychotic Drugs

Drugs of the atypical antipsychotic class can increase weight markedly during the first few months of therapy. Clozapine and olanzapine have been considered to be associated with the greatest weight gain and also the greatest occurrence of diabetes and dyslipidemia.[121a] Olanzapine therapy with its known metabolic side effects was believed to exacerbate a patient's underlying lipoprotein disorder, causing an expression of the type III hyperlipidemia phenotype in a patient with the rare $apoE_2/E_2$ (arginine 145 to cysteine) mutation.[122]

Transplant Drugs

Drugs given to prevent organ rejection in transplant recipients are associated with significant lipid abnormalities. Cyclosporine is a widely used immunosuppressive agent that increases LDL cholesterol level[123] and is involved with drug–drug interactions.[124] Most important, cyclosporine interacts with the statins, and its levels should be monitored when initiating lipid therapy. Patients treated with cyclosporine have higher blood statin levels with all statins, with the least increase seen with fluvastatin.[125] Thus, using a lower dose of statins in patients taking cyclosporine produces a treatment effect similar to that seen with greater statin dosages in those not taking cyclosporine. Tacrolimus does not increase cholesterol values as cyclosporine does. Yet, switching to another immunosuppressive therapy such as tacrolimus may not be the answer. A recent study showed that atorvastatin was more efficient in reducing LDL cholesterol levels than conversion from cyclosporine to tacrolimus.[126]

Acne Drugs

Isotretinoin (13-*cis*-retinoic acid; Accutane) is a natural metabolite of vitamin A that is used for severe acne and other dermatologic conditions. Increased TG concentrations are seen frequently. A large population-based trial with 12,049 subjects noted that 10% had TG levels of 400 mg/dL or greater. Although isotretinoin increases TG concentration in healthy individuals by impairing TG clearance, it does not impair insulin-mediated antilipolysis or glucose disposal.[127] HDL cholesterol level declines in patients with underlying genetic problems, with no change in apoA-I, suggesting cholesterol depletion of the HDL particle.[128]

In some individuals, exposure to isotretinoin produces TG concentration increases so severe that pancreatitis is seen. Those at risk for these TG concentration increases include overweight subjects, who are six times more likely to experience significant increases in TG concentrations, and individuals with increased baseline TG concentration, who are 4.3 times more likely to have significant TG increases.[129] A cross-sectional study in young adults with 6 months of therapy noted that isotretinoin-induced hypertriglyceridemia identified those who 4 years later had stigmata of the metabolic syndrome, with hyperlipidemia, truncal obesity, and hyperinsulinemia. The lipid response was closely associated with the apoE phenotype ($apoE_2$ or $apoE_4$) and the presence of dyslipidemia.[130] Plasma lipid and lipoprotein levels returned to baseline by 8 weeks after treatment.[131] For most patients, mild liver and lipid abnormalities rarely necessitate dosage reduction, but patients given isotretinoin should benefit from counseling on how to lose excess weight, increase physical activity, and avoid excess calories from carbohydrates and especially from simple sugars and high-fructose corn syrup.

CONCLUSIONS

Diet, drugs, diseases, and disorders of metabolism frequently cause abnormal levels of lipids and lipoproteins. Acquired causes can increase LDL cholesterol levels, necessitating drug therapy that can be avoided or minimized if the acquired causes are dealt with appropriately. When acquired lipid abnormalities are mild, it may be possible to have the patient improve diet, increase physical activity, and lose excess weight to minimize this adverse change. In cases with an underlying genetic TG abnormality, the abnormal lipids and/or lipoproteins that are produced can increase the risk for CHD, pancreatitis, or both. If the potential for severe lipid changes is present such as with pregnancy, the clinician can use this knowledge for appropriate prenatal counseling to avoid pregnancy until TG levels have been reduced through appropriate lifestyle change and thus markedly reduce the risks associated with a strongly hyperlipidemic pregnancy. Thus, a review of potential secondary causes of hyperlipidemia is as important as taking a careful family history and often remarkably helpful in providing optimal clinical care.

REFERENCES

1. Stone NJ, Blum C: Management of Lipids in Clinical Practice, 6th ed. Caddo, OK, Professional Communications, Inc., 2006.
2. Brunzell JD, Schrott HG: The interaction of familial and secondary causes of hypertriglyceridemia: Role in pancreatitis. *Trans Assoc Am Physicians* 1973;86:245–254.
3. Crouse JR: Hypertriglyceridemia: A contraindication to the use of bile acid binding resins. *Am J Med* 1987;83:243–248.
4. Knopp RH, Walden CE, Retzlaff BM, et al: Longterm cholesterol-lowering effects of 4 fat-restricted diets in hypercholesterolemic and combined hyperlipidemic men. The Dietary Alternatives Study. *JAMA* 1998;279:1345–1346.
5. Goldberg RB, Mendez AJ: Case 40-2006: Anemia and low HDL cholesterol. *N Engl J Med* 2007;356:1893–1895.
6. Third report of the National Cholesterol Education Program (NCEP) Expert Panel on Detection, Evaluation, and Treatment of High Blood Cholesterol in Adults (Adult Treatment Panel III): Final report. *Circulation* 2002;106:3143–3421.
7. Gardner CD, Coulston A, Chatterjee L, et al: The effect of a plant-based diet on plasma lipids in hypercholesterolemic adults: A randomized trial. *Ann Intern Med* 2005;142: 725–733.
8. Phillips NR, Havel RJ, Kane JP: Levels and interrelationships of serum and lipoprotein cholesterol and triglycerides: Association with adiposity and the consumption of ethanol, tobacco, and beverages containing caffeine. *Arteriosclerosis* 1981;1:13–24.
9. Schaefer EJ, Lamon-Fava S, Ordovas JM, et al: Factors associated with low and elevated plasma high-density lipoprotein cholesterol and apolipoprotein A-I levels in the Framingham Offspring Study. *J Lipid Res* 1994;35:871–882.
10. McLaughlin T, Abbasi F, Cheal K, et al: Use of metabolic markers to identify overweight individuals who are insulin resistant. *Ann Intern Med* 2003;139:802–809.
11. Sumner AE: Fasting triglyceride and the TG/HDL ratio are not markers of insulin resistance in African Americans. *Arch Intern Med* 2005;165:1395–1400.
12. Griel AE, Ruder EH, Kris-Etherton PM: The changing roles of dietary carbohydrates: From simple to complex. *Arterioscler Thromb Vasc Biol* 2005;26;1958–1965.
13. Halton TL, Willett WC, Stampfer MJ, et al: Low-carbohydrate-diet score and the risk of coronary heart disease in women. *N Engl J Med* 2006;355:1991–2002.
14. Purnell JQ, Kahn SE, Albers JJ, et al: Effect of weight loss with reduction of intra-abdominal fat on lipid metabolism in older men. *J Clin Endocrinol Metab* 2000;85:977–982.
15. Ratner R, Goldberg R, Haffner S, et al; Diabetes Prevention Program Research Group. Impact of intensive lifestyle and metformin therapy on cardiovascular disease risk factors in the diabetes prevention program. *Diabetes Care* 2005;28:888–894.
16. Slentz CA, Duscha BD, Johnson JL, et al: Effects of the amount of exercise on body weight, body composition, and measures of central obesity: STRRIDE—a randomized controlled study. *Arch Intern Med* 1994;164:31–39.
17. Ross R, Dagnone D, Jones PJH, et al: Reduction in obesity and related comorbid conditions after diet-induced weight loss or exercise-induced weight loss in men: A randomized, controlled trial. *Ann Intern Med* 2000;133:92–103.
18. Klein S, Fontana L, Young VL, et al: Absence of an effect of liposuction on insulin action and risk factors for coronary heart disease. *N Engl J Med* 2004;350:2549–2557.
19. Grundy SM: Atherogenic dyslipidemia associated with metabolic syndrome and insulin resistance. *Clin Cornerstone* 2006;8(suppl 1):S21–S27.
20. Ginsberg HN, Zhang YL, Hernandez-Ono A: Regulation of plasma triglycerides in insulin resistance and diabetes. *Arch Med Res* 2005;36:232–240.
21. Krauss RM: Lipids and lipoproteins in patients with type 2 diabetes. *Diabetes Care* 2004;27:1496–1504.
22. Kashyap SR, Defronzo RA: The insulin resistance syndrome: Physiological considerations. *Diab Vasc Dis Res* 2007;4:13–19.
23. Lemieux I, Pascot A, Couillard C, et al: Hypertriglyceridemic waist: A marker of the atherogenic metabolic triad (hyperinsulinemia; hyperapolipoprotein B; small dense LDL) in men? *Circulation* 2000;102:179–184.
24. Palaniappan LP, Kwan AC, Abbasi F, et al: Lipoprotein abnormalities are associated with insulin resistance in South Asian Indian women. *Metabolism* 2007;56:899–904.
25. Stein E, Kushner H, Gidding S, Falkner B: Plasma lipid concentrations in nondiabetic African American adults: Associations with insulin resistance and the metabolic syndrome. *Metabolism* 2007;56:954–960.
26. Diekman T, Lansberg PJ, Kastelein JJ, Wiersinga WM: Prevalence and correction of hypothyroidism in a large cohort of patients referred for dyslipidemia. *Arch Intern Med* 1995;155:1490–1495.
27. Retnakaran R, Connelly PW, Goguen J: Unmasking of type III hyperlipoproteinemia by hypothyroidism: A dramatic illustration of altered lipoprotein metabolism in a postpartum woman. *Endocr Pract* 2005;(11):394–398.
28. Crook MA, Mukherjee A, Marshall K: Unusual presentations to a lipid clinic. *Postgrad Med J* 1999;75:633–634.
29. Yildirimkaya M, Ozata M, Yilmaz K, et al: Lipoprotein(a) concentration in subclinical hypothyroidism before and after levothyroxine therapy. *Endocr J* 1996;43:731–736.
30. Helfand M: Screening for subclinical thyroid dysfunction in nonpregnant adults: A summary of the evidence for the U.S. Preventive Services Task Force. *Ann Intern Med* 2004;140: 128–141.
31. Razvi S, Ingoe L, Keeka G, et al: The beneficial effect of L-thyroxine on cardiovascular risk factors, endothelial function, and quality of life in subclinical hypothyroidism: Randomized, crossover trial. *J Clin Endocrinol Metab* 2007;92:1715–1723.
32. Ito M, Arishima T, Kudo T, et al: Effect of levo-thyroxine replacement on non-high-density lipoprotein cholesterol in hypothyroid patients. *J Clin Endocrinol Metab* 2007;92:608–611.
33. Hamilton CI: Statin-associated myopathy. *Med J Aust* 2001;175: 486–489.
34. Bar SL, Holmes DT, Frohlich J: Asymptomatic hypothyroidism and statin-induced myopathy. *Can Fam Physician* 2007;53: 428–431.
35. Danese MD, Ladenson PW, Meinert CL, Powe NR: Clinical review 115: Effect of thyroxine therapy on serum lipoproteins in patients with mild thyroid failure: A quantitative review of the literature. *J Clin Endocrinol Metab* 2000;85:2993–3001.
36. Joven J, Villabona C, Vilella E, et al: Abnormalities of lipoprotein metabolism in patients with the nephrotic syndrome. *N Engl J Med* 1990;323:579–584.

37. Kronenberg F, Lingenhel A, Lhotta K, et al: Lipoprotein(a)- and low-density lipoprotein-derived cholesterol in nephrotic syndrome: Impact on lipid-lowering therapy? *Kidney Int* 2004;66:348–354.
38. de Sain-van der Velden MG, Kaysen GA, Barrett HA, et al: Increased VLDL in nephrotic patients results from a decreased catabolism while increased LDL results from increased synthesis. *Kidney Int* 1998;53:994–1001.
39. Moulin P, Appel GB, Ginsberg HN, Tall AR: Increased concentration of plasma cholesteryl ester transfer protein in nephrotic syndrome: Role in dyslipidemia. *J Lipid Res* 1992;33: 1817–1822.
40. Vega GL, Grundy SM: Lovastatin therapy in nephrotic hyperlipidemia: Effects on lipoprotein metabolism. *Kidney Int* 1988;33:1160–1168.
41. Vega GL, Toto RD, Grundy SM: Metabolism of low-density lipoproteins in nephrotic dyslipidemia: Comparison of hypercholesterolemia alone and combined hyperlipidemia. *Kidney Int* 1995;47:579–586.
42. Wanner C, Rader D, Bartens W, et al: Elevated plasma lipoprotein(a) in patients with the nephrotic syndrome. *Ann Intern Med* 1993;119:263–269.
43. Kronenberg F: Dyslipidemia and nephrotic syndrome: Recent advances. *J Ren Nutr* 2005:195–203.
44. Scanu A: Lipoprotein(a), Friedewald formula, and NCEP guidelines. National Cholesterol Education Program. *Am J Cardiol* 2001;87:608–609, A9.
45. Schlueter W, Keilani T, Batlle DC: Metabolic effects of converting enzyme inhibitors: Focus on the reduction of cholesterol and lipoprotein(a) by fosinopril. *Am J Cardiol* 1993;72:37H–44H.
46. Muntner P, Hamm LL, Kusek JW, et al: The prevalence of nontraditional risk factors for coronary heart disease in patients with chronic kidney disease. *Ann Int Med* 2004;140:9–17.
47. Quaschning T, Krane V, Metzger T, Wanner C: Abnormalities in uremic lipoprotein metabolism and its impact on cardiovascular disease *Am J Kidney Dis* 2001;38(4 suppl 1):S14–S19.
48. Saland JM, Ginsberg HN: Lipoprotein metabolism in chronic renal insufficiency. *Pediatr Nephrol* 2007;22:1095–1112.
49. Kaysen GA: Metabolic syndrome and renal failure: Similarities and differences. *Panminerva Med* 2006;48:151–164.
50. Prichard SS: Impact of dyslipidemia in end-stage renal disease. *J Am Soc Nephrol* 2003;14:S315–S320.
51. National Kidney Foundation: K/DOQI clinical practice guidelines for managing dyslipidemias in chronic kidney disease. *Am J Kidney Dis* 2003;41(suppl 3):S1–S92.
52. Farbakhsh K, Kasiske BL: Dyslipidemias in patients who have chronic kidney disease. *Med Clin N Am* 2005;89:689–699.
53. Sandhu S, Wiebe N, Fried LF, Tonelli M: Statins for improving renal outcomes: A meta-analysis. *J Am Soc Nephrol* 2006;17: 2006–2016.
54. Molitch ME: Management of dyslipidemias in patients with diabetes and chronic kidney disease. *Clin J Am Soc Nephrol* 2006;1:1090–1099.
55. Navaneethan SD, Pansini F, Strippoli GFM: Statins in patients with chronic kidney disease: Evidence from systematic reviews and randomized clinical trials. *PLoS Med* 2006;3:e123.
56. Holdaas H, Fellstrom B, Jardine AG, et al: Effect of fluvastatin on cardiac outcomes in renal transplant recipients: A multicentre, randomised, placebo-controlled trial. *Lancet* 2003;14:2024–2031.
57. Wanner C, Krane V, Marz W, et al: Atorvastatin in patients with type 2 diabetes mellitus undergoing hemodialysis. *N Engl J Med* 2005;353:238–248.
58. Turchin A, Wiebe DA, Seely EW, et al: Graft-versus-host disease severe hypercholesterolemia mediated by lipoprotein X in patients with chronic graft-versus-host disease of the liver. *Bone Marrow Transplantation* 2005;35:85–89.
59. Kaplan MM: Primary biliary cirrhosis. *N Engl J Med* 1996;335; 1570–1580.
60. Jahn CE, Schaefer EJ, Taam LA, et al: Lipoprotein abnormalities in primary biliary cirrhosis: Association with hepatic lipase inhibition as well as altered cholesterol esterification. *Gastroenterology* 1985;89:1266–1278.
61. Crippin JS, Lindor KD, Jorgensen R, et al: Hypercholesterolemia and atherosclerosis in primary biliary cirrhosis: What is the risk? *Hepatology* 1992;15:858–862.
62. Gregory WL, Game FL, Farrer M, et al: Reduced serum lipoprotein(a) levels in patients with primary biliary cirrhosis. *Atherosclerosis* 1994;105:43–50.
63. Miller JP: Dyslipoproteinaemia of liver disease. *Baillieres Clin Endocrinol Metab* 1990;(4):807–832.
64. Thompson PD: Risk in primary biliary cirrhosis. *Atherosclerosis* 2007;194:293–299.
65. Riddler SA, Li X, Chu H, et al: Longitudinal changes in serum lipids among HIV-infected men on highly active antiretroviral therapy. *HIV Med* 2007;(5):280–287.
66. Dube MP, Stein JH, Aberg JA, et al: Guidelines for the evaluation and management of dyslipidemia in human immunodeficiency virus (HIV)-infected adults receiving antiretroviral therapy: Recommendations of the HIV Medical Association of the Infectious Disease Society of America and the Adult AIDS Clinical Trials Group. *Clin Infect Dis* 2003;37: 613–627.
67. Feingold KR, Krauss RM, Pang M, et al: The hypertriglyceridemia of acquired immunodeficiency syndrome is associated with an increased prevalence of low-density lipoprotein subclass pattern B. *J Clin Endocrinol Metab* 1993;76:1423–1427.
68. Taskinen MR, Nikkilä EA, Pelkonen R, Sane T: Plasma lipoproteins, lipolytic enzymes, and very low-density lipoprotein triglyceride turnover in Cushing's syndrome. *J Clin Endocrinol Metab* 1983;57:619–626.
69. Rossi R, Tauchmanova L, Luciano A, et al: Subclinical Cushing's syndrome in patients with adrenal incidentaloma: Clinical and biochemical features. *J Clin Endocrinol Metab* 2000;85:1440–1448.
70. Burnside NJ, Alberta L, Robinson-Bostom L, Bostom A: Type III hyperlipoproteinemia with xanthomas and multiple myeloma. *J Am Acad Dermatol* 2005;53(5 suppl 1):S281–S284.
71. Mira M, Stewart PM, Vizzard J, Abraham S: Biochemical abnormalities in anorexia nervosa and bulimia. *Ann Clin Biochem* 1987;24:29–35.
72. Fernandez-Miranda C, De La Calle M, Larumbe S, et al: Lipoprotein abnormalities in patients with asymptomatic acute porphyria. *Clin Chim Acta* 2000;294(1-2):37–43.
73. Mustajoki P, Nikkila EA: Serum lipoproteins in asymptomatic acute porphyria: No evidence for hyperbetalipoproteinemia. *Metabolism* 1984;33:266–269.
74. Van Lenten BJ, Reddy ST, Navab M, Fogelman AM: Understanding changes in high-density lipoproteins during the acute phase response. *Arterioscler Thromb Vasc Biol* 2006;26:1687–1688.
75. Khovidhunkit W, Memon RA, Feingold KR, Grunfeld C: Infection and inflammation-induced proatherogenic changes of lipoproteins. *J Infect Dis* 2000;181(suppl 3):S462–S472.
76. Goldberg R: Acquired low HDL. *J Clin Lipidol* 2007;1:32–34.
77. Gidding SS, Stone NJ, Bookstein LC, et al: Month-to-month variability of lipids, lipoproteins, and apolipoproteins and the impact of acute infection in adolescents. *J Pediatr* 1998;133: 242–246.
78. Mendez AJ, Goldberg RB, Arnold PI, Schultz DR: Acquired HDL deficiency associated with apolipoprotein A-I reactive monoclonal immunoglobulins. *Arterioscler Thromb Vasc Biol* 2002;22:1740–1741.
79. Robinson S, Henderson AD, Gelding SV, et al: Dyslipidaemia is associated with insulin resistance in women with polycystic ovaries. *Clin Endocrinol (Oxf)* 1996;44:277–284.
80. Glueck CJ, Aregawi D, Agloria M, et al: Sustainability of 8% weight loss, reduction of insulin resistance, and amelioration of atherogenic-metabolic risk factors over 4 years by metformin-diet in women with polycystic ovary syndrome. *Metabolism* 2006;55:1582–1589.
81. Henkin Y, Como JA, Oberman A: Secondary dyslipidemia. Inadvertent effects of drugs in clinical practice. *JAMA* 1992;267:961–968.
82. Mantel-Teeuwisse AK, Kloosterman JM, Maitland-van der Zee AH, et al: Drug-induced lipid changes: A review of the unintended effects of some commonly used drugs on serum lipid levels. *Drug Saf* 2001;24:443–456.
83. Kasiske BL, Ma JZ, Kalil RS, Louis TA: Effects of antihypertensive therapy on serum lipids. *Ann Intern Med* 1995;122: 133–141.
84. Chobanian AV, Bakris GL, Black HR, et al: The Seventh Report of the Joint National Committee on Prevention, Detection, Evaluation, and Treatment of High Blood Pressure: The JNC 7 Report. *JAMA, May* 2003;289:2560–2571.
85. Freis ED: The efficacy and safety of diuretics in treating hypertension. *Ann Intern Med* 1995;122:223–226.

86. Savage PJ, Pressel SL, Curb JD, et al, for the SHEP Cooperative Research Group. Influence of long-term, low-dose, diuretic-based, antihypertensive therapy on glucose, lipid, uric acid, and potassium levels in older men and women with isolated systolic hypertension: The Systolic Hypertension in the Elderly Program. *Arch Intern Med* 1998;158:741–751.
87. Ames RP: A comparison of the blood lipid and blood pressure responses during the treatment of systemic hypertension with indapamide and with thiazides. *Am J Cardiol* 1996;77:12b–16b.
88. Parsons SK, Skapek SX, Neufeld EJ, et al: Asparaginase-associated lipid abnormalities in children with acute lymphoblastic leukemia. *Blood* 1997;89:1886–1895.
89. Campos H, Genest J, Blijlevens E, et al: Low-density lipoprotein particle size and coronary artery disease. *Arteriosclerosis* 1992;12:187–195.
90. Manttari M, Tenkanen L, Manninen V, et al: Antihypertensive therapy in dyslipidemic men: Effects on coronary heart disease incidence and total mortality. *Hypertension* 1995;25:47–52.
91. Jacob S, Rett K, Wicklmayr M, et al: Differential effect of chronic treatment with two beta blocking agents on insulin sensitivity: The carvedilol-metoprolol study. *J Hypertens* 1996;14:489–494.
92. Giugliano D, Acampora R, Marfella R, et al: Metabolic and cardiovascular effects of carvedilol and atenolol in non-insulin-dependent diabetes mellitus and hypertension: A randomized, controlled trial. *Ann Intern Med* 1997;126:955–959.
93. Bakris GL, Fonseca V, Katholi, RE, et al, for the GEMINI Investigators. Metabolic effects of carvedilol vs. metoprolol in patients with type 2 diabetes mellitus and hypertension: A randomized controlled trial. *JAMA* 2004;292:2227–2236.
94. Ranganathan S, Kern PA: The HIV protease inhibitor saquinavir impairs lipid metabolism and glucose transport in cultured adipocytes. *J Endocrinol* 2002;172:155–162.
95. Carr A, Samaras K, Burton S, et al: A syndrome of peripheral lipodystrophy, hyperlipidaemia and insulin resistance in patients receiving HIV protease inhibitors. *AIDS* 1998;12: F51–F58.
96. Carr A, Samaras K, Thorisdottir A, et al: Diagnosis, prediction, and natural course of HIV-1 protease-inhibitor-associated lipodystrophy, hyperlipidaemia, and diabetes mellitus: A cohort study. *Lancet* 1999;353:2093–2099.
97. The DAD Study Group: Class of antiretroviral drugs and the risk of myocardial infarction. *N Engl J Med* 2007;356:1723–1735.
98. Riddler SA, Li X, Chu H, et al: Longitudinal changes in serum lipids among HIV-infected men on highly active antiretroviral therapy. *HIV Med* 2007;(5):280–287.
99. Rimland D, Guest JL, Hernández I, et al: Antiretroviral therapy in HIV-positive men is associated with increased apolipoprotein CIII in triglyceride-rich lipoproteins. *HIV Med* 2005;6: 326–333.
100. van Leth F, Phanuphak P, Stroes E, et al: Nevirapine and efavirenz elicit different changes in lipid profiles in antiretroviral-therapy-naïve patients infected with HIV-1. *PLoS Med* 2004;1:e19.
101. Dube MP, Stein JH, Aberg JA, et al, Adult AIDS Clinical Trials Group Cardiovascular Subcommittee; HIV Medical Association of the Infectious Disease Society of America: Guidelines for the evaluation and management of dyslipidemia in human immunodeficiency virus (HIV)-infected adults receiving antiretroviral therapy: Recommendations of the HIV Medical Association of the Infectious Disease Society of America and the Adult AIDS Clinical Trials Group. *Clin Infect Dis* 2003;37:613–627.
102. Tungsiripat M, Aberg J: Dyslipidemia in HIV patients. *Cleve Clin J Med* 2005;72:1113–1120.
103. The Writing Group for the PEPI Trial: Effects of estrogen or estrogen/progestin regimens on heart disease risk factors in postmenopausal women. The Postmenopausal Estrogen/Progestin Interventions (PEPI) Trial. *JAMA* 1995;273:199–208.
104. Lamon-Fava S, Postfai B, Diffenderfer M, et al: Role of the estrogen and progestin in hormonal replacement therapy on apolipoprotein A-I kinetics in postmenopausal women. *Arterioscler Thromb Vasc Biol* 2006;26:385–391.
105. Bayrak A, Aldemir DA, Bayrak T, et al: The effect of hormone replacement therapy on the levels of serum lipids, apolipoprotein AI, apolipoprotein B and lipoprotein (a) in Turkish postmenopausal women. *Arch Gynecol Obstet* 2006;274: 289–296.
106. Hulley S, Grady D, Bush T, et al: Randomized trial of estrogen plus progestin for secondary prevention of coronary heart disease in postmenopausal women. Heart and Estrogen/progestin Replacement Study (HERS) Research Group. *JAMA* 1998;280: 605–613.
107. Shlipak MG, Simon JA, Vittinghoff E, et al: Estrogen and progestin, lipoprotein(a), and the risk of recurrent coronary heart disease events after menopause. *JAMA* 2000;283:1845–1855.
108. Glueck CJ, Lang J, Hamer T, Tracy T: Severe hypertriglyceridemia and pancreatitis when estrogen replacement therapy is given to hypertriglyceridemic women. *J Lab Clin Med* 1994;123: 59–64.
109. Stone NJ: Estrogen-induced pancreatitis: A caveat worth remembering. *J Lab Clin Med* 1994;123:18–19.
110. Cieraad D, Conradt C, Jesinger D, Bakowski M: Clinical study comparing the effects of sequential hormone replacement therapy with oestradiol/dydrogesterone and conjugated equine oestrogen/norgestrel on lipids and symptoms. *Arch Gynecol Obstet* 2006;274:74–80.
111. Love RR, Newcomb PA, Wiebe DA, et al: Effects of tamoxifen therapy on lipid and lipoprotein levels in postmenopausal patients with node-negative breast cancer. *J Natl Cancer Inst* 1990;82:1327–1332.
112. Carr MC, Knopp RH, Brunzell JD, et al: Effect of raloxifene on serum triglycerides in women with a history of hypertriglyceridemia while on oral estrogen therapy. *Diabetes Care* 2005;28: 1555–1561.
113. Knopp RH: Cardiovascular effects of endogenous and exogenous sex hormones over a woman's lifetime. *Am J Obstet Gynecol* 1988;158(6 pt 2):1630–1643.
114. Montes A, Walden CE, Knopp RH, et al: Physiologic and supraphysiologic increases in lipoprotein lipids and apoproteins in late pregnancy and postpartum. Possible markers for the diagnosis of "prelipemia." *Arteriosclerosis* 1984;4: 407–417.
115. Sanderson SL, Iverius PH, Wilson DE: Successful hyperlipemic pregnancy. *JAMA* 1991;265:1858–1860.
116. Whitsel EA, Boyko EJ, Matsumoto AM, et al: Intramuscular testosterone esters and plasma lipids in hypogonadal men: A meta-analysis. *Am J Med* 2001;111:261–299.
117. Snyder PJ, Peachey H, Berlin JA, et al: Effect of transdermal testosterone treatment on serum lipid and apolipoprotein levels in men more than 65 years of age. *Am J Med* 2001;111: 255–260.
118. Singh AB, Hsia S, Alaupovic P, et al: The effects of varying doses of testosterone on insulin sensitivity, plasma lipids apolipoproteins, and C-reactive protein in healthy young men. *J Clin Endocrinol Metab* 2002;87:136–143.
119. Herbst KL, Amory JK, Brunzell JD, et al: Testosterone administration to men increases hepatic lipase activity and decreases HDL and LDL size in 3 wk. *Am J Physiol Endocrinol Metab* 2003;284:112–118.
120. Alen M, Rahkila P, Marniemi J: Serum lipids in power athletes self-administering testosterone and anabolic steroids. *Int J Sports Med* 1985;6:139–144.
121. Bagdade JD, Porte D Jr, Bierman EL: Steroid-induced lipemia. A complication of high-dosage corticosteroid therapy. *Arch Intern Med* 1970;125:129–134.
121a. American Diabetes Association; American Psychiatric Association; American Association of Clinical Endocrinologists; North American Association for the Study of Obesity: Consensus development conference on antipsychotic drugs and obesity and diabetes. *Diabetes Care.* 2004;27(2):596–601
122. Sinnott BP, Mazzone T: Tuberous xanthomas associated with olanzapine therapy and hypertriglyceridemia in the setting of a rare apolipoprotein E mutation. *Endocr Pract* 2006;12: 183–187.
123. Ballantyne CM, Podet EJ, Patsch WP, et al: Effects of cyclosporine therapy on plasma lipoprotein levels. *JAMA* 1989;262:53–56.
124. Launay-Vacher V, Izzedine H, Deray G: Statins' dosage in patients with renal failure and cyclosporine drug-drug interactions in transplant recipient patients. *Int J Cardiol* 2005;101:9–17.
125. Ballantyne CM, Corsini A, Davidson MH, et al: Risk for myopathy with statin therapy in high-risk patients. *Arch Intern Med* 2003;163:553–564.
126. Wissing KM, Unger P, Ghisdal L, et al: Effect of atorvastatin therapy and conversion to tacrolimus on hypercholesterol-

emia and endothelial dysfunction after renal transplantation. *Transplantation* 2006;82:771–778.
127. Stoll D, Binnert C, Mooser V, Tappy L: Short-term administration of isotretinoin elevates plasma triglyceride concentrations without affecting insulin sensitivity in healthy humans. *Metabolism* 2004;53:4–10.
128. O'Leary TJ, Simo IE, Kanigsberg N, et al: Changes in serum lipoproteins and high-density lipoprotein composition during isotretinoin therapy. *Clin Invest Med* 1987;10: 355–360.
129. McElwee NE, Schumacher MC, Johnson SC, et al: An observational study of isotretinoin recipients treated for acne in a health maintenance organization. *Arch Dermatol* 1991;127:341–346.
130. Rodondi N, Darioli R, Ramelet AA, et al: High risk for hyperlipidemia and the metabolic syndrome after an episode of hypertriglyceridemia during 13-cis retinoic acid therapy for acne: pharmacogenetic study. *Ann Intern Med* 2002;136:582–589.
131. Bershad S, Rubinstein A, Paterniti JR, et al: Changes in plasma lipids and lipoproteins during isotretinoin therapy for acne. *N Engl J Med* 1985;313:981–985.

CHAPTER 13

Use of High-Sensitivity C-Reactive Protein for Risk Assessment

Catherine Y. Campbell, Kiran Musunuru, Samia Mora, and Roger S. Blumenthal

More than 800,000 individuals suffer a myocardial infarction annually in the United States, and another 700,000 have a stroke.[1] Of these events, at least 50% occur in patients with no overt evidence of hyperlipidemia, and 15% to 20% occur in patients with none of the major traditional risk factors.[2,3] Improving risk classification is the basis for current preventive strategies. Despite adoption in national prevention guidelines and widespread use in clinical practice, the National Cholesterol Education Program Adult Treatment Panel III (NCEP ATP III) global risk score is an imperfect tool for estimating cardiovascular disease (CVD) risk. Only about 5% of asymptomatic men and less than 1% of asymptomatic women in the United States without coronary heart disease are classified as high risk using the NCEP ATP III global risk score.[4,5] In contrast, the lifetime risk for CVD is 1 in 2 for women and 2 in 3 for men after the age of 40 years.[1] This "detection gap" in cardiovascular risk assessment[6] highlights the need for improved risk evaluation in asymptomatic individuals, particularly those at intermediate risk.

According to National Health and Nutrition Examination Survey III data, about 4% of women and 30% of men have a 10-year absolute risk rate of 10% to 20%.[5] Using a 10-year absolute risk rate of 6% to 20% as the definition of intermediate risk places 10% and 40% of asymptomatic women and men, respectively, in the intermediate-risk category.[5] With these proportions, about 8 million women and 27 million men in the United States have a 10-year absolute risk rate of 5% to 20%.[5] With a focus on targeting preventive strategies to the level of risk, millions of men and women would benefit from more accurate coronary risk assessment. Novel tools are needed to improve risk classification beyond the standard risk assessment models.

Multiple avenues of research ranging from basic experimental evidence to population-based observational studies have led to the recognition that CVD is, in large part, a systemic inflammatory process.[7] Large epidemiologic studies conducted in diverse populations have repeatedly documented the association between high-sensitivity C-reactive protein (hsCRP), an indicator of inflammation, and CVD outcomes, independent of traditional cardiovascular risk factors.[8–24] In addition, hsCRP adds prognostic information across a full range of NCEP ATP III risk scores, improves risk detection for patients with metabolic syndrome and diabetes, and assists with targeting of lifestyle modification.[23–26] However, it remains uncertain whether therapies that specifically reduce CRP levels would also result in lower cardiovascular event rates.

BIOLOGY OF C-REACTIVE PROTEIN

Inflammation contributes to all stages of the atherosclerotic process (initiation, growth, plaque rupture).[27–29] T lymphocytes and macrophages predominate in the fatty streak and, accompanied by mast cells, eventually accumulate in atheroma. These cells produce proteolytic enzymes and cytokines that weaken the fibrous cap, thus converting a stable plaque into a "vulnerable" plaque more susceptible to rupture. Given the interactions between inflammation and atherosclerosis, it is not surprising that increased levels of inflammatory markers predict greater CVD risk.

CRP, which is produced predominantly by the liver and is found in atherosclerotic plaque,[30] is a nonspecific inflammatory marker and acute-phase reactant that influences numerous proatherogenic and proinflammatory pathways (Figure 13-1). Many of its effects

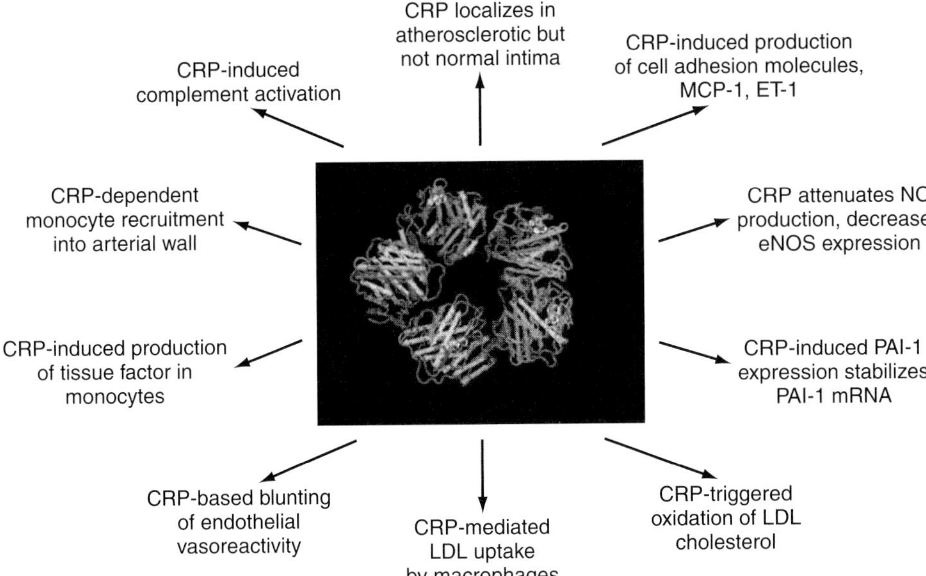

FIGURE 13-1 C-reactive protein (CRP) is likely more than just a marker for atherosclerosis, playing an active role in the pathogenesis of atherosclerosis. eNOS = endothelial nitric oxide synthase; ET-1 = endothelin-1; LDL = low-density lipoprotein; MCP-1 = monocyte chemoattractant protein–1; mRNA = messenger ribonucleic acid; NO = nitric oxide; PAI-1 = plasminogen activator inhibitor–1. *(Reprinted from Ref. 31, with permission.)*

are mediated through activation of the classic complement pathway. It increases cytokine and adhesion molecule production, inhibits the survival and function of endothelial progenitor cells, induces endothelial cell apoptosis, decreases nitric oxide production, increases endothelin-1 levels, and inhibits fibrinolysis through its effects on tissue plasminogen activator and plasminogen activator inhibitor–1.[31] Given the influence of inflammation on plaque instability, hsCRP may more accurately reflect plaque "vulnerability" rather than total plaque burden.[26]

PRIMARY PREVENTION

More than 20 prospective cohort studies have demonstrated that hsCRP predicts future CVD risk independent of other risk factors (Table 13-1).[8–24] hsCRP provides independent prognostic information for CVD risk after controlling for Framingham risk score factors and/or diabetes and obesity[17–24]; indeed, it appears to have a predictive value similar to that of tobacco use, systolic blood pressure, or low-density lipoprotein (LDL) cholesterol level. hsCRP levels of less than 1, 1 to 3, and more than 3 mg/L correspond to low, intermediate, and high relative risks (RRs) of CVD, respectively. In a meta-analysis of 22 prospective studies, the overall odds ratio (OR) for coronary heart disease in the highest versus the lowest tertiles of hsCRP levels was 1.6 (95% confidence interval [CI] = 1.5–1.7) after adjusting for traditional risk factors.[32]

hsCRP can be added to standard risk assessment models for more accurate CVD risk assessment. In the Women's Health Study, the addition of hsCRP to the NCEP ATP III global risk score resulted in reclassification of about 40% of women at intermediate risk into a lower or higher risk category.[33] Measurement of hsCRP levels also results in improved prediction using Framingham risk score in elderly women at high risk and elderly men at intermediate risk.[34]

The Reynolds risk score is a new risk prediction algorithm for women that adds two new variables—hsCRP and parental family history of premature coronary heart disease—to the existing variables in the NCEP ATP III global risk score.[35] The Reynolds model predicts CVD risk in women more accurately than the existing NCEP ATP III global risk score. This algorithm demonstrates the benefits of incorporating additional variables such as hsCRP into risk prediction models. One caveat is that the cohort on which the Reynolds model is based comprises mainly white individuals, and further data are needed to validate it in other groups. A user-friendly calculator for the Reynolds Risk Score is available online at: http://www.reynoldsriskscore.org.

hsCRP levels are the most useful for risk assessment in patients at intermediate risk. Although hsCRP has good predictive value in all risk categories,[23,24] the patients at intermediate risk are most likely to benefit from more accurate risk assessment. hsCRP testing is not recommended for patients at low risk, because even a doubling or tripling of risk in this group is not likely to influence patient or physician behavior. Similarly, hsCRP testing is not recommended for risk prediction in patients at high risk because these patients should receive aspirin and lipid-lowering therapy and undertake therapeutic lifestyle changes regardless of their hsCRP levels, although hsCRP may be used for targeting the level of therapy (see Secondary Prevention later in this chapter). hsCRP screening is most appropriate for patients at intermediate risk (NCEP ATP III score of 5–20%). In these patients, reclassification to a greater or lower cardiovascular risk should influence preventive strategies, that is, the addition or withholding of aspirin and lipid-lowering therapy. In women at intermediate risk by NCEP ATP III, the Reynolds risk score can be used to more accurately assess the need for preventive strategies. A suggested algorithm for hsCRP screening is outlined in Figure 13-2.

Measurement of hsCRP is cost-effective for screening in the primary prevention setting.[36] Measurement of hsCRP at the time of lipid evaluation may be reasonable in patients at intermediate risk, if these patients do not already qualify for lipid-lowering and aspirin therapies. Because hsCRP testing is inexpensive, this

TABLE 13-1 Multivariate Adjusted Odds Ratios for Studies Evaluating High-Sensitivity C-Reactive Protein as a Predictor of Cardiovascular Events in Asymptomatic Men and Women

Study	Year	Population	End Point	Adjusted Risk
MRFIT[10]	1996	Men	CHD death	2.8 (1.4–5.4) (OR)*
PHS[16]	1997	Men	First MI	2.9 (1.8–4.6) (RR)*
BRHS[12]	2000	Men	MI, CHD death	2.13 (1.38–3.28) (OR)†
WHS[23]	2002	Postmenopausal women	MI, stroke, revascularization procedure, CV death	2.3 (1.6–3.4) (RR)‡
WHI[11]	2002	Postmenopausal women	MI, CHD death	2.1 (1.1–4.1) (OR)*
Helsinki[13]	2000	Dyslipidemic men	MI, CHD death	3.56 (1.93–6.57) (OR)§
HHS[15]	2002	Men	MI	1.6 (1.1–2.2) (OR)*
Rotterdam Study[95]	2003	Men and women >55 years old	MI	1.2 (0.6–2.2) (OR)*
MONICA[24]	2004	Men	Fatal/nonfatal MI, sudden cardiac death	2.21 (1.49–3.27) (HR)¶
Reykjavik Study[32]	2004	Men and women	CHD death, nonfatal MI	1.45 (1.25–1.68) (OR)†
Framingham Offspring Study[14]	2004	Men and women	New-onset angina, MI, CVA, TIA, HF, claudication	1.9 (1.2–2.9) (HR)*
CHS[34]	2005	Men and women >65 years old	MI, CHD death	1.45 (1.14–1.86) (RR)¶
FHS[22]	2005	Men and women	MI, CHD death, stroke	1.22 (0.90–1.66) (RR)¶
ARIC[9]	2004	Men and women	Incident CHD	2.53 (1.88–3.40) (HR)¶
EPIC-Norfolk[21]	2006	Men and women	Incident CHD	1.66 (1.31–2.12) (OR)*

*Quartile extremes.
†Tertile extremes.
‡Quintile extremes.
§Fourth quartile compared with combined 1st and 2nd quartiles.
¶Greater than 3 mg/L.
ARIC, Atherosclerosis Risk in Communities; BRHS, British Regional Heart Study; CHD, coronary heart disease; CHS, Cardiovascular Health Study; CV, cardiovascular; CVA, cerebrovascular accident; EPIC-Norfolk: European Prospective Investigation into Cancer and Nutrition; FHS, Framingham Heart Study; HELSINKI, Helsinki Heart Study; HF, heart failure; HHS, Honolulu Heart Study; HR, hazard ratio; MI, myocardial infarction; MONICA, Monitoring Trends and Determinents in Cardiovascular Disease; MRFIT, Multiple Risk Factor Intervention Trial; OR, odds ratio; PHS, Physicians' Health Study; RR, relative risk; TIA, transient ischemic attack; WHI, Women's Health Initiative; WHS, Women's Health Study.

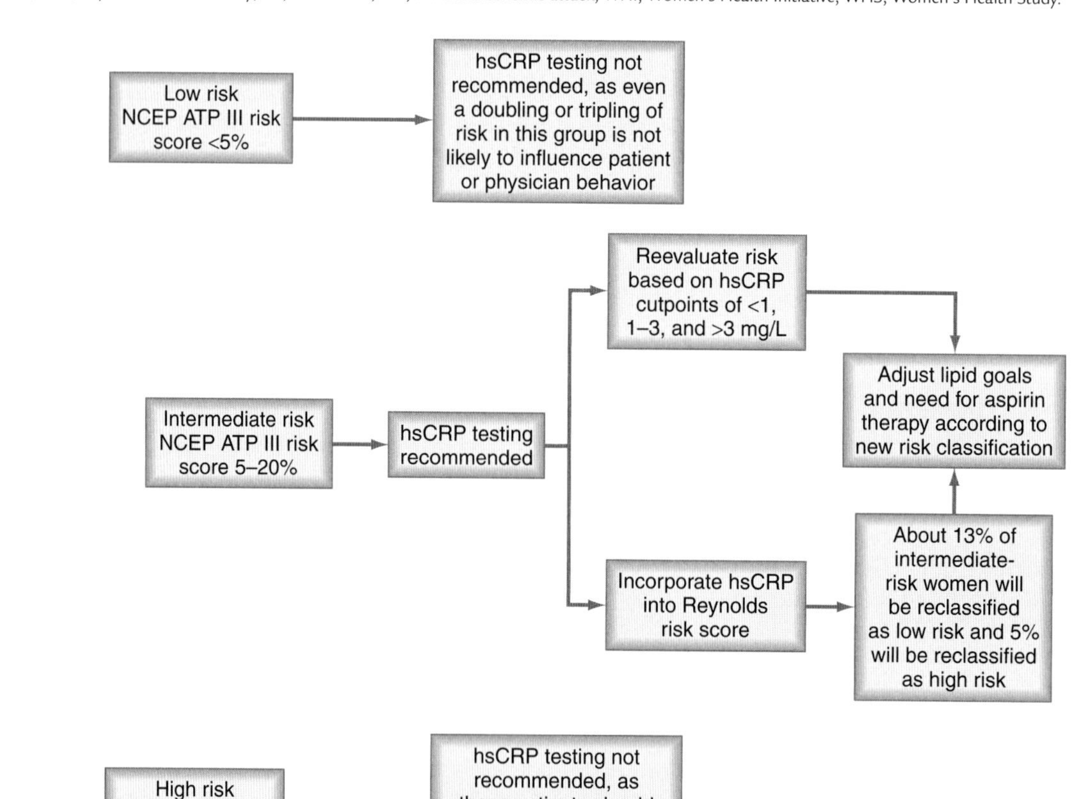

FIGURE 13-2 Algorithm for hsCRP screening. hsCRP, high-sensitivity C-reactive protein; NCEP ATP III, National Cholesterol Education Program Adult Treatment Panel III.

approach may be more efficient than arranging phlebotomy and a second physician visit after lipid results are obtained. Furthermore, isolated hsCRP level increase may reflect increased cardiovascular risk even in a patient with normal lipid values.[37]

High levels of hsCRP are associated with increased risk for development of type 2 diabetes.[38–47] Furthermore, among individuals with diabetes or the metabolic syndrome, hsCRP levels further stratify cardiovascular risk.[26] Increased hsCRP levels in patients with the metabolic syndrome should prompt more vigorous efforts to implement lifestyle modifications such as diet and exercise. hsCRP levels also correlate with risk for stroke,[18,20,48–55] with the RR associated with hsCRP ranging from 1.5 to 2.0, greater than that for LDL cholesterol. Thus, hsCRP measurement should be considered as a risk assessment tool in the primary prevention of stroke.

THE JUPITER TRIAL

The potential benefit of statin therapy in asymptomatic patients with high hsCRP levels and low LDL cholesterol levels is being evaluated in a recently completed clinical trial, the Justification for the Use of statins in Primary prevention: an Intervention Trial Evaluating Rosuvastatin (JUPITER). A total of 17,802 subjects with LDL cholesterol levels less than 130 mg/dL and hsCRP of 2 mg/L or greater were randomized to rosuvastatin (20 mg/day) or placebo.[56,57] The design of the JUPITER trial is outlined in Figure 13-3, and the baseline characteristics of the study participants are described in Table 13-2. JUPITER is unique in its use of hsCRP to stratify individuals. The patient population enrolled in the JUPITER study is thus quite different from the patient populations enrolled in previous primary prevention and secondary prevention statin trials (Table 13-3). AstraZeneca has announced that the trial was stopped early, apparently because rosuvastatin was more beneficial than expected in reducing CVD morbidity and mortality when compared with placebo, and it was believed to be unethical to withhold rosuvastatin from the group assigned to placebo.[58]

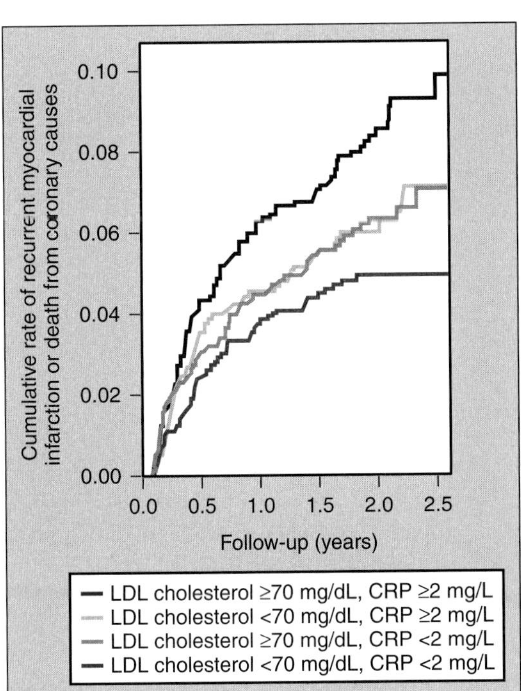

FIGURE 13-3 Cumulative incidence of recurrent myocardial infarction or death from coronary causes, according to the achieved levels of both LDL cholesterol and CRP in the Pravastatin or Atorvastatin Evaluation and Infection Therapy–Thrombolysis in Myocardial Infarction 22 (PROVE IT–TIMI 22) study. *(Reprinted from Ref. 70, with permission.)*

SECONDARY PREVENTION

hsCRP levels have strong prognostic value in patients with coronary heart disease. hsCRP levels predict recurrent cardiovascular events in patients with stable coronary artery disease and acute coronary syndromes.[59–64] hsCRP levels also predict coronary artery bypass graft failure and in-stent restenosis.[65,66] For such patients, the best long-term clinical outcomes are observed among those with low levels of LDL cholesterol (<70 mg/dL) and of hsCRP (<2 mg/L). Similarly, in patients with coronary heart disease receiving statin therapy, low levels of both LDL cholesterol and hsCRP predict the best outcomes.[26,63,67,68] Indeed, those individuals with increased hsCRP levels receive the greatest benefit from statin therapy.[67] In the Pravastatin or Atorvastatin Evaluation and Infection Therapy–Thrombolysis in Myocardial Infarction 22 (PROVE IT–TIMI 22) and Aggrastat to Zocor (A to Z) trials, hsCRP level less than 2 mg/L was just as important as LDL cholesterol level less than 70 mg/dL for improving survival and reducing future coronary events (Figure 13-4).[63,67] In patients with coronary disease, lower achieved hsCRP levels are also associated with a smaller risk for stroke.[69] Thus, greater lifestyle changes should be encouraged in individuals with an hsCRP level of 2 mg/L or more.

VARIATION IN HIGH-SENSITIVITY C-REACTIVE PROTEIN LEVELS

Analysis in the Women's Heath Study cohort determined the hsCRP cutpoints of less than 1, 1 to 3, and more than 3 mg/L for low, intermediate, and high RR for CVD, respectively.[11] Studies in the United States, Europe, and Asia have also used these cutpoints. Data to support the use of these hsCRP cutpoints in minority populations are sparse, though the available data appear relatively consistent across most minority subgroups.[8]

Numerous genetic and environmental factors, such as physical fitness,[70] obesity,[71–73] and smoking,[74] influence hsCRP levels. Behavioral and lifestyle factors (hormone replacement therapy, smoking, alcohol intake), sociodemographic factors (age, education, location), diabetes, and abdominal and total obesity account for 22% of the interindividual CRP variability in women and 30% of the variability in men.[75] Genetic differences are thought to account for the remaining variability in hsCRP levels. The median hsCRP levels vary by sex and across different ethnic populations. For example, black individuals may have greater hsCRP levels than white and Asian individuals.[76,77] Furthermore, levels may be greater in women compared with men, but further data are needed.[5,78]

TABLE 13-2 Baseline Characteristics of JUPITER

Baseline Characteristics	Screened Cohort (*N* = 90,000)	Randomized Cohort (*N* = 17,802)
Age (yr)	65.7 (60.2–71.0)	66.3 (60.9–71.8)
Women (%)	37.2	38.2
Race (%)*		
White	76.8	71.3
Black	8.1	12.5
Asian	1.9	1.6
Hispanic	11.1	12.7
Other	2.1	2.0
Education (%)		
High school	NA	59.4
Some college	NA	17.7
College graduate	NA	14.5
Postgraduate	NA	8.4
Body mass index (kg/m^2)	NA	28.4 (25.3–32.0)
Blood pressure (mm Hg)		
Systolic	NA	134 (124–145)
Diastolic	NA	80 (75–87)
Current smoker (%)	NA	15.8
Family history of CHD (%)	NA	11.5
Metabolic syndrome (%)	NA	32.1
Aspirin use (%)		
Any report	NA	15.3
Prophylactic	NA	14.0
Total cholesterol (mg/dL)	204 (182–226)	185 (169–200)
LDL cholesterol (mg/dL)	124 (105–143)	108 (94–119)
HDL cholesterol (mg/dL)	51 (43–62)	49 (40–60)
Non-HDL cholesterol (mg/dL)	150 (129–172)	134 (118–147)
Triglycerides (mg/dL)	116 (84–163)	118 (85–169)
hsCRP (mg/L)†	1.9 (1.0–4.1)	4.3 (2.8–7.1)
Glucose concentration (mg/dL)	NA	94 (88–102)
Hemoglobin A1c (%)	NA	5.7 (5.5–5.9)

All values are percentage or median (interquartile range) except high-sensitivity C-reactive protein (hsCRP). Data are current as of July 27, 2007.

*For 11,894 subjects of the screened cohort, race data are misssing.

†For hsCRP, values for the randomized cohort are the mean of the screening and randomization visits.

CHD, coronary heart disease; HDL, high-density lipoprotein; JUPITER, Justification for the Use of statins in Primary prevention: an Intervention Trial Evaluating Rosuvastatin; LDL, low-density lipoprotein; NA, not available.

Adapted from Ref. 57, with permission.

LABORATORY TESTING OF HIGH-SENSITIVITY C-REACTIVE PROTEIN

Fasting is not required for hsCRP testing. Intraindividual variation of hsCRP levels is similar to that of cholesterol levels. Thus, measuring hsCRP values twice may improve the predictive value of hsCRP levels. CVD risk increases in a linear fashion across the full range of hsCRP levels. Even mild increases in hsCRP (>1 mg/L) suggest increased CVD risk.[79] The cutpoints of less than 1, 1 to 3, and more than 3 mg/L are recommended, though using five categories of hsCRP levels (<0.5, 0.5–1.0, 1.0–3.0, 3.0–5.0, and >5.0 mg/L) may improve risk discrimination.[80] Because hsCRP levels may be falsely increased during an acute-phase response, patients should be metabolically stable at the time of hsCRP measurement, and hsCRP values greater than 5 mg/L should prompt repeat testing. Persistently increased hsCRP levels greater than 10 mg/L suggest

TABLE 13-3 Comparison of the JUPITER Population to Previous Statin Trials of Primary Prevention or High-Risk Patients

	Primary Prevention Trials			High-Risk Patient Trials			
	JUPITER*	WOSCOPS	AFCAPS	HPS	ALL-HAT	ASCOT	PROSPER
Sample size *(N)*	17,802	6,595	6,605	20,536	10,355	10,305	5,804
Women *(N)*	6,801	0	997	5,082	5,051	1,942	3,000
Duration (yr)	Ongoing	4.9	5.2	5	4.8	3.3	3.2
Previous CVD or CHD (%)	0	0	0	65	14	14	44
Diabetes (%)	0	1	6	29	35	25	11
Baseline lipids (mg/dL)							
Total cholesterol	183	272	221	228	224	213	221
LDL cholesterol	104	192	150	132	146	132	147
HDL cholesterol	51	44	36–40	41	48	50	50
Triglycerides	138	164	158	124	152	152	158
hsCRP (mg/L)	≥2	NA	NA	NA	NA	NA	NA
Intervention	Rosuvastatin 20 mg	Pravastatin 40 mg	Lovastatin 20–40 mg	Simvastatin 40 mg	Pravastatin 20–40 mg	Atorvastatin 10 mg	Pravastatin 40 mg

Baseline lipid levels are mean values.

*Justification for the Use of statins in Primary prevention: an Intervention Trial Evaluating Rosuvastatin (JUPITER) data are current as of July 27, 2007.

AFCAPS, Air Force/Texes Coronary Atherosclerosis Prevention Study; ALLHAT, Antihypertensive and Lipid-Lowering Treatment to Prevent Heart Attack; ASCOT, Anglo-Scandinavian Cardiac Outcome Trial; CHD, coronary heart disease; CVD, cardiovascular disease; HDL, high-density lipoprotein; HPS, Heart Protection Study; hsCRP, high-sensitivity C-reactive protein; LDL, low-density lipoprotein; PROSPER, PROspective Study of Pravastatin in the Elderly at Risk; WOSCOPS, West of Scotland Coronary Prevention Study.

Adapted from Ref. 57, with permission.

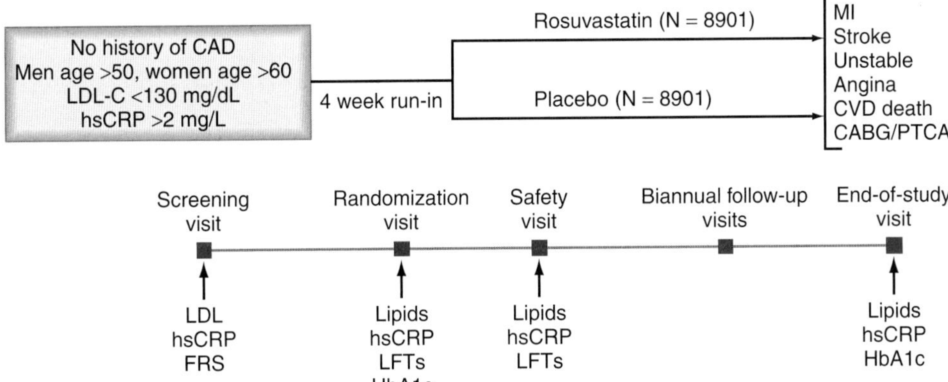

FIGURE 13-4 Diagram of the basic trial design for the JUPITER study. CABG/PTCA, coronary artery bypass graft surgery/percutaneous transluminal coronary angioplasty; CAD, coronary artery disease; CVD, cardiovascular disease; FRS, Farmingham Risk Score; HbA1c= hemoglobin A1c; LDL, low-density lipoprotein; LDL-C, low-density lipoprotein cholesterol; low-density lipoprotein cholesterol; LFTs, liver function tests; MI, myocardial infarction. (Adapted from Ref. 59, with permission.)

even greater CVD risk,[80] even in the presence of collagen vascular disease or other underlying chronic systemic inflammatory diseases.

Many outpatient and hospital-based laboratories offer both regular CRP testing for rheumatologic assessment and hsCRP testing for cardiovascular assessment. Thus, when ordering an hsCRP test to evaluate vascular risk, an "hsCRP" or "cardiac CRP" test should be specified. Multiple commercial hsCRP assays are available and have been standardized for outpatient and inpatient settings.[26] hsCRP levels are most useful for patients at intermediate risk by NCEP ATP III. Given potential genetic influences on hsCRP levels,[75] those with a family history of premature atherosclerosis may also benefit from hsCRP screening. Initial evaluation with hsCRP in individuals between the ages of 20 and 40 years may be appropriate. Although increased hsCRP levels in teenagers predict increased CVD risk,[37] screening should be considered in teenagers on an individual basis.

STATISTICAL ANALYSIS

The accuracy of risk prediction models can be assessed using model calibration or discrimination. Model calibration denotes how well the predicted probability using the model agrees with the actual risk observed over time. Model discrimination (as determined by the c-statistic) denotes the relative ranking of patients; those who do not develop of CVD have a lower predicted risk than those who do of CVD. The clinical setting determines whether discrimination or calibration is more important.[81] If the aim is to compare an individual's chance of an event relative to that of other individuals, then discrimination is more important. However, if the aim is to predict the likelihood that a patient will have a CVD event during the follow-up period, calibration is more important.[82]

Most studies that have investigated the prognostic value of hsCRP compared with traditional risk factors have reported either the OR and multivariable-adjusted RR or the receiver operating characteristic curve (c-statistic). The c-statistic is appropriate for diagnostic testing or retrospective case–control studies when the outcome has already been determined[82]; however, because it is based only on ranks, it is not appropriate for risk prediction models.[83] Moreover, reliance on the c-statistic would exclude lipids and blood pressure from risk prediction models, because these factors do not significantly improve or only modestly improve the c-statistic. Instead, calibration is more appropriate in evaluating the accuracy of predicted probabilities compared with the actual risk observed.

For risk prediction, the most important issue is reclassification of risk level compared with NCEP ATP III and whether that reclassification is accurate. Adding hsCRP to the NCEP ATP III global risk score reclassifies about 40% of intermediate-risk women into higher or lower risk categories.[33] This reclassification using the hsCRP level is considerably more accurate compared with the NCEP ATP III global risk score alone.[33] Similar data on the benefits of reclassification using hsCRP have been reported in the elderly[34] and in men,[23] particularly for patients in the intermediate-risk group. The Reynolds risk score has incorporated hsCRP and parental history of coronary artery disease into a new model for risk prediction in women that is more accurate than NCEP ATP III alone.[35]

FUTURE DIRECTIONS

Although the correlation between hsCRP levels and CVD risk is well established, it is unclear whether CRP itself directly contributes to the pathophysiology of CVD. Supporting data for a role for CRP in atherothrombosis remains limited to *in vitro* studies and experiments in animal models.[31] The presence of CRP in atherosclerotic lesions is suggestive but does not confirm a causative role for the protein.[30] Recent data from Pepys and colleagues[84] show that specific inhibition of CRP is feasible, with a small-molecule synthetic compound (1,6 bis(phosphocholine)-hexane), and resulted in smaller infarct size in rats.

Genetic evidence appears to support a role for CRP in at least the acute setting of atherothrombotic disease. Polymorphisms in the CRP gene locus have been shown to account for some interindividual variability in plasma CRP levels[85–89]; a genome-wide association study found that CRP levels are also associated with a number of polymorphisms near genes that influence insulin resistance, diabetes, weight gain, early atherogenesis, and β-cell function.[89] Specific CRP polymorphisms appear to be associated with increased risk for death from CVD events.[90] These data suggest that variability in either CRP levels or CRP function, or both, is directly linked to CVD pathogenesis. One explanation is that transient increase of CRP levels, as part of the acute-phase reactant response in the setting of myocardial infarction,[91,92] may, in turn, up-regulate inflammatory mediators that increase myocardial damage, inhibit myocardial remodeling, or predispose to recurrent atherothrombotic events.[93] Genetically determined interindividual variation in the degree of acute CRP level increase or CRP function may thereby influence clinical outcomes for patients suffering acute coronary syndromes. In the future, genotyping of CRP polymorphisms in individuals at risk for CVD may possibly identify those at greatest risk for poor outcomes and in whom CRP-targeting therapy may be of most benefit.

CONCLUSIONS

In summary, hsCRP is an inexpensive and validated test that improves model calibration and helps to provide a more accurate prediction of CVD risk than standard risk prediction models alone. Its predictive value has been confirmed in both the primary prevention and secondary prevention settings. In the primary prevention setting, it is most useful for patients at intermediate risk, for reclassifying patients into a higher or lower risk category and appropriately targeting preventive therapies. The recent announcement of the early termination of the JUPITER trial because of benefit suggests that statin therapy may reduce CVD events in individuals with increased hsCRP and normal or low levels of LDL cholesterol, although trial publication of the trial results is forthcoming. In the secondary prevention setting, hsCRP may be selectively used for further risk stratification in addition to LDL cholesterol, with the best outcomes observed among those with low levels of both LDL cholesterol (<70 mg/dL) and hsCRP (<2 mg/L).

REFERENCES

1. Rosamond W, Flegal K, Friday G, et al: Heart disease and stroke statistics—2007 update: A report from the American Heart Association Statistics Committee and Stroke Statistics Subcommittee. *Circulation* 2007;115:e69–e171.
2. Khot UN, Khot MB, Bajzer CT, et al: Prevalence of conventional risk factors in patients with coronary heart disease. *JAMA* 2003;290:898–904.
3. Greenland P, Knoll MD, Stamler J, et al: Major risk factors as antecedents of fatal and nonfatal coronary heart disease events. *JAMA* 2003;290:891–897.
4. Ajani UA, Ford ES: Has the risk for coronary heart disease changed among U.S. adults? *J Am Coll Cardiol* 2006;48:1177–1182.
5. Ford ES, Giles WH, Mokdad AH: The distribution of 10-year risk for coronary heart disease among US adults: Findings from the National Health and Nutrition Examination Survey III. *J Am Coll Cardiol* 2004;43:1791–1796.
6. Pasternak RC, Abrams J, Greenland P, et al: 34th Bethesda Conference: Task force #1—Identification of coronary heart disease risk: Is there a detection gap? *J Am Coll Cardiol* 2003;41:1863–1874.
7. Libby P, Ridker PM, Maseri A: Inflammation and atherosclerosis. *Circulation* 2002;105:1135–1143.
8. Ridker PM: Clinical application of C-reactive protein for cardiovascular disease detection and prevention. *Circulation* 2003;107:363–369.
9. Ballantyne CM, Hoogeveen RC, Bang H, et al: Lipoprotein-associated phospholipase A2, high-sensitivity C-reactive protein, and risk for incident coronary heart disease in middle-aged men and women in the Atherosclerosis Risk in Communities (ARIC) study. *Circulation* 2004;109:837–842.
10. Kuller LH, Tracy RP, Shaten J, et al: Relation of C-reactive protein and coronary heart disease in the MRFIT nested case–control study. *Am J Epidemiol* 1996;144:537–547.
11. Pradhan AD, Manson JE, Rossouw JE, et al: Inflammatory biomarkers, hormone replacement therapy, and incident coronary heart disease: Prospective analysis from the Women's Health Initiative Observational Study. *JAMA* 2002;288:980–987.
12. Danesh J, Whincup P, Walker M, et al: Low grade inflammation and coronary heart disease: Prospective study and updated meta-analyses. *BMJ* 2000;321:199–204.

13. Roivainen M, Viik-Kajander M, Palosuo T, et al: Infections, inflammation, and the risk of coronary heart disease. *Circulation* 2000;101:252–257.
14. Rutter MK, Meigs JB, Sullivan LM, et al: C-reactive protein, the metabolic syndrome, and prediction of cardiovascular events in the Framingham Offspring Study. *Circulation* 2004;110: 380–385.
15. Sakkinen P, Abbott RD, Curb JD, et al: C-reactive protein and myocardial infarction. *J Clin Epidemiol* 2002;55:445–451.
16. Ridker PM, Cushman M, Stampfer MJ, et al: Inflammation, aspirin, and the risk of cardiovascular disease in apparently healthy men. *N Engl J Med* 1997;336:973–979.
17. Tsimikas S, Willerson JT, Ridker PM: C-reactive protein and other emerging blood biomarkers to optimize risk stratification of vulnerable patients. *J Am Coll Cardiol* 2006;47:C19–C31.
18. Curb JD, Abbott RD, Rodriguez BL, et al: C-reactive protein and the future risk of thromboembolic stroke in healthy men. *Circulation* 2003;107:2016–2020.
19. Laaksonen DE, Niskanen L, Nyyssonen K, et al: C-reactive protein in the prediction of cardiovascular and overall mortality in middle-aged men: A population-based cohort study. *Eur Heart J* 2005;26:1783–1789.
20. Wakugawa Y, Kiyohara Y, Tanizaki Y, et al: C-reactive protein and risk of first-ever ischemic and hemorrhagic stroke in a general Japanese population: The Hisayama Study. *Stroke* 2006;37: 27–32.
21. Boekholdt SM, Hack CE, Sandhu MS, et al: C-reactive protein levels and coronary artery disease incidence and mortality in apparently healthy men and women: The EPIC-Norfolk prospective population study 1993-2003. *Atherosclerosis* 2006;187: 415–422.
22. Wilson PW, Nam BH, Pencina M, et al: C-reactive protein and risk of cardiovascular disease in men and women from the Framingham Heart Study. *Arch Intern Med* 2005;165:2473–2478.
23. Ridker PM, Rifai N, Rose L, et al: Comparison of C-reactive protein and low-density lipoprotein cholesterol levels in the prediction of first cardiovascular events. *N Engl J Med* 2002;347: 1557–1565.
24. Koenig W, Lowel H, Baumert J, Meisinger C: C-reactive protein modulates risk prediction based on the Framingham Score: Implications for future risk assessment: Results from a large cohort study in southern Germany. *Circulation* 2004;109:1349–1353.
25. Pradhan AD, Manson JE, Rifai N, et al: C-reactive protein, interleukin 6, and risk of developing type 2 diabetes mellitus. *JAMA* 2001;286:327–334.
26. Ridker PM, Wilson PW, Grundy SM: Should C-reactive protein be added to metabolic syndrome and to assessment of global cardiovascular risk? *Circulation* 2004;109:2818–2825.
27. Ross R: Atherosclerosis—an inflammatory disease. *N Engl J Med* 1999;340:115–126.
28. Hansson GK: Inflammation, atherosclerosis, and coronary artery disease. *N Engl J Med* 2005;352:1685–1695
29. Libby P, Ridker PM: Inflammation and atherothrombosis from population biology and bench research to clinical practice. *J Am Coll Cardiol* 2006;48:A33–A46.
30. Yasojima K, Schwab C, McGeer EG, McGeer PL: Generation of C-reactive protein and complement components in atherosclerotic plaques. *Am J Pathol* 2001;158:1039–1051.
31. Scirica BM, Morrow DA, Verma S, et al: Is C-reactive protein an innocent bystander or proatherogenic culprit? *Circulation* 2006;113:2128–2151.
32. Danesh J, Wheeler JG, Hirschfield GM, et al: C-reactive protein and other circulating markers of inflammation in the prediction of coronary heart disease. *N Engl J Med* 2004;350:1387–1397.
33. Cook NR, Buring JE, Ridker PM: The effect of including C-reactive protein in cardiovascular risk prediction models for women. *Ann Intern Med* 2006;145:21–29.
34. Cushman M, Arnold AM, Psaty BM, et al: C-reactive protein and the 10-year incidence of coronary heart disease in older men and women: The Cardiovascular Health Study. *Circulation* 2005;112:25–31.
35. Ridker PM, Buring JE, Rifai N, Cook NR: Development and validation of improved algorithms for the assessment of global cardiovascular risk in women: The Reynolds risk score. *JAMA* 2007;297:611–619.
36. Blake GJ, Ridker PM, Kuntz KM: Potential cost-effectiveness of C-reactive protein screening followed by targeted statin therapy for the primary prevention of cardiovascular disease among patients without overt hyperlipidemia. *Am J Med* 2003;114:485–494.
37. Zieske AW, Tracy RP, McMahan CA, et al: Elevated serum C-reactive protein levels and advanced atherosclerosis in youth. *Arterioscler Thromb Vasc Biol* 2005;25:1237–1243.
38. Festa A, D'Agostino R Jr, Tracy RP, Haffner SM: Elevated levels of acute-phase proteins and plasminogen activator inhibitor-1 predict the development of type 2 diabetes: The insulin resistance atherosclerosis study. *Diabetes* 2002;51:1131–1137.
39. Barzilay JI, Abraham L, Heckbert SR, et al: The relation of markers of inflammation to the development of glucose disorders in the elderly: The Cardiovascular Health Study. *Diabetes* 2001;50: 2384–2389.
40. Freeman DJ, Norrie J, Caslake MJ, et al: C-reactive protein is an independent predictor of risk for the development of diabetes in the West of Scotland Coronary Prevention Study. *Diabetes* 2002;51:1596–1600.
41. Thorand B, Lowel H, Schneider A, et al: C-reactive protein as a predictor for incident diabetes mellitus among middle-aged men: Results from the MONICA Augsburg cohort study, 1984-1998. *Arch Intern Med* 2003;163:93–99.
42. Spranger J, Kroke A, Mohlig M, et al: Inflammatory cytokines and the risk to develop type 2 diabetes: Results of the prospective population-based European Prospective Investigation into Cancer and Nutrition (EPIC)-Potsdam Study. *Diabetes* 2003;52: 812–817.
43. Duncan BB, Schmidt MI, Pankow JS, et al: Low-grade systemic inflammation and the development of type 2 diabetes: The Atherosclerosis Risk in Communities Study. *Diabetes* 2003;52:1799–1805.
44. Hu FB, Meigs JB, Li TY, et al: Inflammatory markers and risk of developing type 2 diabetes in women. *Diabetes* 2004;53: 693–700.
45. Laaksonen DE, Niskanen L, Nyyssonen K, et al: C-reactive protein and the development of the metabolic syndrome and diabetes in middle-aged men. *Diabetologia* 2004;47:1403–1410.
46. Malik S, Wong ND, Franklin S, et al: Cardiovascular disease in U.S. patients with metabolic syndrome, diabetes, and elevated C-reactive protein. *Diabetes Care* 2005;28:690–693.
47. Dehghan A, Kardys I, de Maat MP, et al: Genetic variation, C-reactive protein levels, and incidence of diabetes. *Diabetes* 2007;56:872–878.
48. Gussekloo J, Schaap MC, Frolich M, et al: C-reactive protein is a strong but nonspecific risk factor of fatal stroke in elderly persons. *Arterioscler Thromb Vasc Biol* 2000;20:1047–1051.
49. Ford ES, Giles WH: Serum C-reactive protein and self-reported stroke: Findings from the Third National Health and Nutrition Examination Survey. *Arterioscler Thromb Vasc Biol* 2000;20: 1052–1056.
50. Rost NS, Wolf PA, Kase CS, et al: Plasma concentration of C-reactive protein and risk of ischemic stroke and transient ischemic attack: The Framingham Study. *Stroke* 2001;32:2575–2579.
51. Cao JJ, Thach C, Manolio TA, et al: C-reactive protein, carotid intima-media thickness, and incidence of ischemic stroke in the elderly: The Cardiovascular Health Study. *Circulation* 2003;108: 166–170.
52. Cesari M, Penninx BWJH, Newman AB, et al: Inflammatory markers and onset of cardiovascular events: Results from the Health ABC study. *Circulation* 2003;108:2317–2322.
53. Ballantyne CM, Hoogeveen RC, Bang H, et al: Lipoprotein-associated phospholipase A2, high-sensitivity C-reactive protein, and risk for incident ischemic stroke in middle-aged men and women in the Atherosclerosis Risk in Communities (ARIC) study. *Arch Intern Med* 2005;165:2479–2484.
54. Bos MJ, Schipper CM, Koudstaal PJ, et al: High serum C-reactive protein level is not an independent predictor for stroke: The Rotterdam Study. *Circulation* 2006;114:1591–1598.
55. Everett BM, Kurth T, Buring JE, Ridker PM: The relative strength of C-reactive protein and lipid levels as determinants of ischemic stroke compared with coronary heart disease in women. *J Am Coll Cardiol* 2006;48:2235–2242.
56. Ridker PM, on behalf of the JUPITER Study Group: Rosuvastatin in the primary prevention of cardiovascular disease among patients with low levels of low-density lipoprotein cholesterol

and elevated high-sensitivity C-reactive protein: Rationale and design of the JUPITER trial. *Circulation* 2003;108:2292–2297.

57. Ridker PM, Fonseca F, Genest J, et al: Baseline characteristics of participants in the JUPITER trial, a randomized placebo-controlled primary prevention trial of statin therapy among individuals with low low-density lipoprotein cholesterol and elevated high-sensitivity C-reactive protein. *Am J Cardiol* 2007;100:1659–1664.
58. AstraZeneca: Crestor outcomes study JUPITER closes early due to unequivocal evidence of benefit [press release]. March 31, 2008. Available at: http://www.astrazeneca.com/pressrelease/5385.aspx.
59. Liuzzo G, Biasucci LM, Gallimore JR, et al: The prognostic value of C-reactive protein and serum amyloid A protein in severe unstable angina. *N Engl J Med* 1994;331:417–424.
60. Haverkate F, Thompson SG, Pyke SD, et al: Production of C-reactive protein and risk of coronary events in stable and unstable angina. European Concerted Action on Thrombosis and Disabilities Angina Pectoris Study Group. *Lancet* 1997;349: 462–466.
61. Morrow DA, Rifai N, Antman EM, et al: C-reactive protein is a potent predictor of mortality independently of and in combination with troponin T in acute coronary syndromes: A TIMI 11A substudy. Thrombolysis in Myocardial Infarction. *J Am Coll Cardiol* 1998;31:1460–1465.
62. Lindahl B, Toss H, Siegbahn A, et al: Markers of myocardial damage and inflammation in relation to long-term mortality in unstable coronary artery disease. FRISC Study Group. Fragmin during Instability in Coronary Artery Disease. *N Engl J Med* 2000;343:1139–1147.
63. Morrow DA, de Lemos JA, Sabatine MS, et al: Clinical relevance of C-reactive protein during follow-up of patients with acute coronary syndromes in the Aggrastat-to-Zocor Trial. *Circulation* 2006;114:281–288.
64. Sabatine MS, Morrow DA, de Lemos JA, et al: Multimarker approach to risk stratification in non-ST elevation acute coronary syndromes: Simultaneous assessment of troponin I, C-reactive protein, and B-type natriuretic peptide. *Circulation* 2002;105: 1760–1763.
65. Kangasniemi OP, Biancari F, Luukkonen J, et al: Preoperative C-reactive protein is predictive of long-term outcome after coronary artery bypass surgery. *Eur J Cardiothorac Surg* 2006;29: 983–985.
66. Hong YJ, Jeong MH, Lim SY, et al: Relation of soft plaque and elevated preprocedural high-sensitivity C-reactive protein levels to incidence of in-stent restenosis after successful coronary artery stenting. *Am J Cardiol* 2006;98:341–345.
67. Ridker PM, Cannon CP, Morrow D, et al: C-reactive protein levels and outcomes after statin therapy. *N Engl J Med* 2005;352:20–28.
68. Nissen SE, Tuzcu EM, Schoenhagen P, et al: Statin therapy, LDL cholesterol, C-reactive protein, and coronary artery disease. *N Engl J Med* 2005;352:29–38.
69. Mega JL, Morrow DA, Cannon CP, et al: Cholesterol, C-reactive protein, and cerebrovascular events following intensive and moderate statin therapy. *J Thromb Thrombolysis* 2006;22:71–76.
70. LaMonte MJ, Durstine JL, Yanowitz FG, et al: Cardiorespiratory fitness and C-reactive protein among a tri-ethnic sample of women. *Circulation* 2002;106:403–406.
71. Greenfield JR, Samaras K, Jenkins AB, et al: Obesity is an important determinant of baseline serum C-reactive protein concentration in monozygotic twins, independent of genetic influences. *Circulation* 2004;109:3022–3028.
72. Mora S, Lee IM, Buring JE, Ridker PM: Association of physical activity and body mass index with novel and traditional cardiovascular biomarkers in women. *JAMA* 2006;295:1412–1419.
73. Visser M, Bouter LM, McQuillan GM, et al: Elevated C-reactive protein levels in overweight and obese adults. *JAMA* 1999. 282:2131–2135.
74. Tracy RP, Psaty BM, Macy E, et al: Lifetime smoking exposure affects the association of C-reactive protein with cardiovascular disease risk factors and subclinical disease in healthy elderly subjects. *Arterioscler Thromb Vasc Biol* 1997;17:2167–2176.
75. Pankow JS, Folsom AR, Cushman M, et al: Familial and genetic determinants of systemic markers of inflammation: The NHLBI family heart study. *Atherosclerosis* 2001;154:681–689.
76. Albert MA, Glynn RJ, Buring J, Ridker PM: C-reactive protein levels among women of various ethnic groups living in the United States (from the Women's Health Study). *Am J Cardiol* 2004;93:1238–1242.
77. Albert MA, Ridker PM: C-reactive protein as a risk predictor: Do race/ethnicity and gender make a difference? *Circulation* 2006;114:e67–e74.
78. Lakoski SG, Cushman M, Criqui M, et al: Gender and C-reactive protein: Data from the Multiethnic Study of Atherosclerosis (MESA) cohort. *Am Heart J* 2006;152:593–598.
79. Sabatine MS, Morrow DA, Jablonski KA, et al: Prognostic significance of the Centers for Disease Control/American Heart Association high-sensitivity C-reactive protein cut points for cardiovascular and other outcomes in patients with stable coronary artery disease. *Circulation* 2007;115:1528–1536.
80. Ridker PM, Cook NR: Clinical utility of very high and very low levels of C-reactive protein across the full range of Framingham risk scores. *Circulation* 2004;109:1955–1959.
81. Justice AC, Covinsky KE, Berlin JA: Assessing the generalizability of prognostic information. *Ann Intern Med* 1999;130: 515–524.
82. Gail MH, Pfeiffer RM: On criteria for evaluating models of absolute risk. *Biostatistics* 2005;6:227–239.
83. Cook NR: Use and misuse of the receiver operating characteristic curve in risk prediction. *Circulation* 2007;115:928–935.
84. Pepys MB, Hirschfield GM, Tennent GA, et al: Targeting C-reactive protein for the treatment of cardiovascular disease. *Nature* 2006;440:1217–1221.
85. Carlson CS, Aldred SF, Lee PK, et al: Polymorphisms within the C-reactive protein (CRP) promoter region are associated with plasma CRP levels. *Am J Hum Genet* 2005;77:64–77.
86. Szalai AJ, Wu J, Lange EM, et al: Single-nucleotide polymorphisms in the C-reactive protein (CRP) gene that affect transcription factor binding, alter transcriptional activity, and associate with differences in baseline CRP level. *J Mol Med* 2005;83: 440–447.
87. Miller DT, Zee RY, Suk Danik J, et al: Association of common CRP gene variants with CRP levels and cardiovascular events. *Ann Hum Genet* 2005;69:623–638.
88. Kathiresan S, Larson MG, Vasan RS, et al: Contribution of clinical correlates and 13 C-reactive protein gene polymorphisms to interindividual variability in serum C-reactive protein level. *Circulation* 2006;113:1415–1423.
89. Ridker PM, Guillaume P, Parker A, et al: Loci related to metabolic-syndrome pathways including *LEPR, HNF1A, IL6R*, and *GCKR* associate with plasma C-reactive protein: The Women's Genome Health Study. *Am J Hum Genet* 2008;82:1–8.
90. Lange LA, Carlson CS, Hindorff LA, et al: Association of polymorphisms in the CRP gene with circulating C-reactive protein levels and cardiovascular events. *JAMA* 2006;296:2703–2711.
91. Kushner I, Broder ML, Karp D: Control of the acute phase response: Serum C-reactive protein kinetics after acute myocardial infarction. *J Clin Invest* 1978;61:235–242.
92. De Beer FC, Hind CR, Fox KM, et al: Measurement of serum C-reactive protein concentration in myocardial ischaemia and infarction. *Br Heart J* 1982;47:239–243.
93. Griselli M, Herbert J, Hutchinson WL, et al: C-reactive protein and complement are important mediators of tissue damage in acute myocardial infarction. *J Exp Med* 1999;190:1733–1740.
94. Mora S, Ridker PM: Justification for the use of statins in primary prevention: An intervention trial evaluating rosuvastatin (JUPITER)—Can C-reactive protein be used to target statin therapy in primary prevention? *Am J Cardiol* 2006;97: 33a–41a.
95. van der Meer IM, de Maat MP, Killiaan AJ, et al: The value of C-reactive protein in cardiovascular risk prediction: The Rotterdam Study. *Arch Intern Med* 2003;163:1323–1328.

CHAPTER 14

Role of Lipoprotein-Associated Phospholipase A_2 in Vascular Disease

Chris J. Packard

Lipoprotein-associated phospholipase A_2 (Lp-PLA_2; platelet-activating factor acetyl hydrolase [PAF-AH]) is an emerging biomarker for vascular disease. The enzyme is produced by cells of the monocyte/macrophage series under the control of inflammatory mediators. It circulates in association with lipoproteins; about 80% is bound to low-density lipoprotein (LDL) and 15% to high-density lipoprotein (HDL). The relationship of Lp-PLA_2 to atherosclerosis is ambiguous because potentially it has both proatherogenic and antiatherogenic properties. However, epidemiologic studies in the general population and in individuals with established vascular disease reveal a positive association of Lp-PLA_2 mass and activity to risk for a coronary event. Evidence also exists that plasma levels of the enzyme are linked to stroke and heart failure.

How measurement of Lp-PLA_2 fits into coronary heart disease (CHD) risk prediction and into improved treatment strategies is not as yet clear. It is a moderately strong risk factor that makes a contribution similar to that of C-reactive protein (CRP) and other markers of inflammation. Further information will be gleaned from genotype–phenotype investigations and from larger pooling projects that aggregate the data from many studies. Potential exists for the enzyme to be a novel drug target in its own right given its role in the pathogenic sequence leading from LDL oxidation to vascular wall inflammation.

Inflammation of the arterial wall is believed to be central to the pathogenesis of atherosclerosis. Interplay between various components of the innate immune system and endothelial and smooth muscle cells results in the initiation and growth of plaque at susceptible sites.[1] The trigger for these events is not yet clear, but mounting evidence suggests that oxidized lipids play an important part.[2] The source of these altered lipids currently is unclear, but it is likely that many are derived from the lipid components of plasma lipoproteins. Epidemiologic studies show a strong positive relationship between circulating levels of LDL and the rate of progression of disease, and clinical trials in which LDL levels are reduced demonstrate a reduction in risk for acute coronary events, indicating a cause-and-effect relationship.[3] A great deal of research focuses currently on the early consequences of LDL accumulation in the subendothelial space of the artery wall. The lipoprotein binds to extracellular matrix components such as proteoglycan and is retained long enough to become damaged by free radical attack.[1,4] The resultant oxidized LDL is a strong candidate for the initiator of the inflammatory process through endothelial cell activation, monocyte recruitment, and cytokine release.

Phospholipases present in the circulation and in the artery wall are responsible for the generation and breakdown of bioactive lipid products. Each enzyme has its particular pathophysiologic relevance depending on location, activity, and substrate specificity. Two members of the growing superfamily of PLA_2 enzymes have been identified as relevant to atherosclerosis and heart disease risk. One is secretory PLA_2,[5] and the other, the subject of this chapter, is Lp-PLA_2, commonly known also as PAF-AH.[6–8] A_2 phospholipases exist within cells and in extracellular compartments, and catalyze the hydrolysis of the fatty acid at the *sn*-2 position of the phospholipid molecule, yielding fatty acid and lysophosphatidyl choline. This hydrolytic step converts a hydrophobic membrane or lipoprotein constituent to two components of increased water solubility that have an array of biological activities; for example, lysophosphatidyl choline has profound effects on endothelial cells and is considered a pro-proatherogenic entity.[9]

The preferred substrate for secretory PLA_2 is intact phospholipid, and its action generates lipoprotein particles that are smaller and more susceptible to oxidation.[10] High circulating levels of secretory PLA_2 have been linked to increased risk for CHD in healthy subjects[11] and in patients with established cardiovascular disease.[12] Lp-PLA_2, in contrast, acts primarily on oxidized lipid when the fatty acid at the *sn*-2 position has been altered by free radical attack. PAF is also a substrate; this molecule is associated with thrombogenesis and hence, theoretically, increased CHD risk. Conceptually, Lp-PLA_2 has an ambiguous effect on atherothrombosis; on the one hand, removal of PAF and oxidized phospholipid reduces risk for an acute coronary event, but on the other hand, generation of short-chain, oxidized fatty acids and lysophosphatidyl choline is potentially detrimental. These opposing actions may help explain some of the apparently paradoxical findings relating to the role of Lp-PLA_2 in cardiovascular disease in animal models and in humans.

Currently, an intensive search is ongoing for biomarkers that help predict risk for disease. In the atherosclerosis field, a number of candidates have been explored recently, particularly those associated with chronic inflammation. CRP, white blood cell count, and the levels of proinflammatory cytokines such as interleukin-6 (IL-6) have all been evaluated for their ability to improve prediction of CHD risk.[13,14] Lp-PLA_2 is a further promising possibility because it is produced by cells of the monocyte/macrophage series and is found in significant quantity in atherosclerotic plaque. Further, the enzyme sits in the putative pathogenic sequence leading from LDL oxidation to endothelial activation and monocyte recruitment, and thus is of interest as a target for pharmacotherapy. The discussion that follows elaborates what is known of the biology and epidemiology of Lp-PLA_2 and how it may contribute to tailoring therapy in those at risk for CHD. The effects of lipid-lowering drugs on the plasma levels of the enzyme are explored together with its potential as a new drug target.

BIOLOGY OF LIPOPROTEIN-ASSOCIATED PHOSPHOLIPASE A_2

Lp-PLA_2 is produced mainly by monocytes, macrophages, T lymphocytes, and mast cells. It is a 50-kD, Ca^{2+}-independent phospholipase (EC 3.1.1.47) and a member of the superfamily of A_2 phospholipases.[7,9] Initially, the enzyme was termed *PAF-AH* because of its ability to degrade and inactivate PAF. However, its association with lipoproteins in plasma and recognition of its broader substrate specificity has led to Lp-PLA_2 becoming the more widely used nomenclature. Early investigations report that inflammatory mediators such as interferon-γ and bacterial polysaccharide (lipopolysaccharide [LPS]) regulated production of Lp-PLA_2.[15] For a period, it was unclear whether LPS stimulated or inhibited production of the enzyme, and it now appears likely that the direction of response depends on cell type within the hematopoietic lineage[16] and the state of differentiation.[17] The role of hematopoietic cells as the primary source of Lp-PLA_2 was confirmed by Asano and colleagues[16] in studies of bone marrow transplant recipients with varying Lp-PLA_2 genotype.

It has been found recently that exposure of human and murine macrophages to LPS increases Lp-PLA_2 synthesis via the p38 mitogen-activated protein kinase pathway.[17] Studies of atherosclerotic plaque containing large numbers of activated macrophages show the presence of high levels of the enzyme,[18,19] and Shi and coworkers[20] observed a marked increase in Lp-PLA_2 messenger RNA in the peripheral blood mononuclear cells of pigs rendered as having diabetes or hypercholesterolemia. Production of Lp-PLA_2 in these animal models was accompanied by leukocyte activation and was stimulated *in vitro* by LPS and tumor necrosis factor–α. Thus, it appears that increased Lp-PLA_2 expression is a component of generalized monocyte/macrophage activation in conditions associated with accelerated atherogenesis. The reasons underlying this are not clear but may be linked to the need in such conditions to hydrolyze and inactivate substances such as PAF and oxidized lipids. However, in this process, the action of the enzyme can lead to adverse effects, particularly in the walls of arteries where the products of the reaction are themselves potent inflammatory mediators (Figure 14-1).

Lp-PLA_2 on entering the circulation binds to lipoproteins. About 80% of the circulating enzyme is found on LDL because of a specific protein–protein interaction between the N terminus of Lp-PLA_2 and the C-terminal portion of apolipoprotein B-100 (apoB-100), the major protein in LDL.[21] Of the remainder, most (about 15%) is bound to HDL[22,23] in an association that is dependent on the extent of N-linked glycosylation of Lp-PLA_2.[24] Further work has revealed that the enzyme has a propensity to bind to small dense LDL, a structural variant of the lipoprotein that is commonly found in subjects with increased plasma triglyceride levels (i.e., >1.5 mmol/L).[8,23] It is likely that the altered conformation of apoB in small versus normal-sized LDL favors binding of the enzyme, but this has yet to be confirmed experimentally. A minor plasma species, electronegative LDL, has been reported to have the greatest relative proportion of Lp-PLA_2 per particle[25] and is enriched in the products of PLA_2 activity. Both small dense and electronegative LDL are believed to be highly atherogenic; whether this is due, in part, to the presence of increased amounts of Lp-PLA_2 per particle currently is conjecture. Other animal species (e.g., rodents, dog, and rabbit) have no Lp-PLA_2 on LDL because of sequence changes in the enzyme or apoB that disrupt the physical association.[9]

Hyperlipidemic states are associated with an altered disposition of Lp-PLA_2. Tsimihodimos and coauthors[23] report that in individuals with heterozygous or homozygous familial hypercholesterolemia (FH), there was not only an increase in circulating enzyme levels because of the large increase in LDL particle number but also a 50% increase in average Lp-PLA_2 activity per particle. In these patients, Lp-PLA_2 was found preferentially in dense LDL despite the fact that in FH most of the LDL increase is in normal-sized particles. The observations may be explained by altered LDL structure in FH or by the presence of atherosclerotic or generalized inflammation as in the pig model described earlier.[17] In contrast, HDL-associated Lp-PLA_2 was similar in abundance in control subjects and subjects with FH.

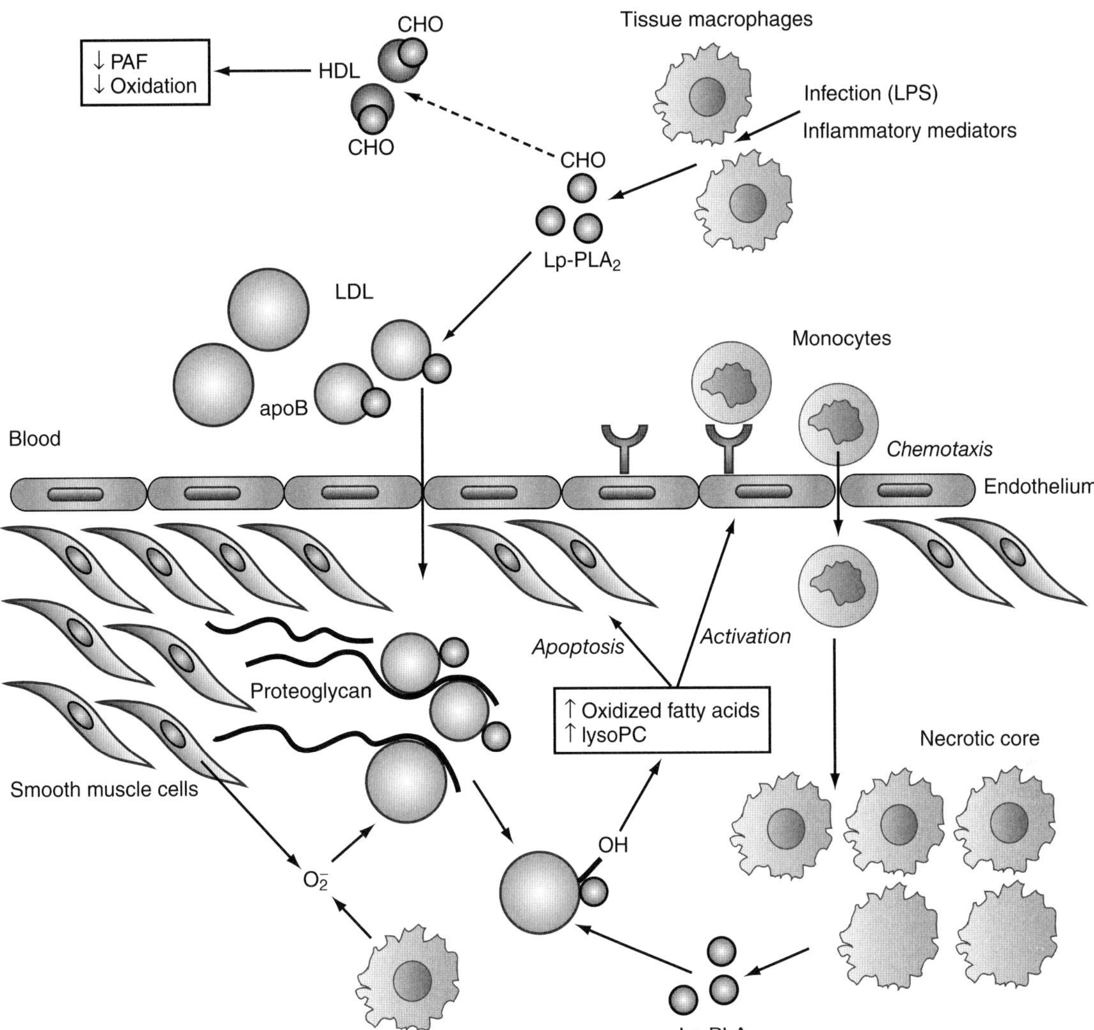

FIGURE 14-1 Role of lipoprotein-associated phospholipase A_2 (Lp PLA_2) in atherosclerosis. In this putative scheme, Lp-PLA_2 is secreted throughout the body by cells of the monocyte/macrophage series. The rate of production is regulated by inflammatory mediators and the presence of bacterial lipopolysaccharide (LPS). Lp-PLA_2 binds mainly to apolipoprotein B (apoB) via a protein–protein interaction but associates also with high-density lipoprotein (HDL). Small dense low-density lipoprotein (LDL) *(smaller circles)* has a greater affinity for the enzyme than normal-sized lipid particles. Lp-PLA_2: LDL complexes penetrate the subendothelial space and are retained there by extracellular proteoglycans. Cells of the arterial wall release free radicals such as superoxide, and these cause oxidative damage to lipid and protein components of lipoproteins. Lp-PLA_2 releases oxidized fatty acids from damaged LDL, and the resultant lysophosphatidyl choline (lysoPC) is water soluble and desorbs from the particle. Both products of enzyme action have potential biological effects that are proatherogenic. For example, they are capable of promoting endothelial activation so that cellular adhesion molecules are expressed; also, they can act as chemoattractants for monocytes. Monocyte recruitment and conversion to macrophages lead to further expression at the site of the atherosclerotic lesion. CHO, carbohydrate; PAF, platelet-activating factor.

Lp-PLA_2 carried on LDL may contribute differently to atherogenesis from that bound to HDL. As described later, it is now clear that plasma levels of Lp-PLA_2 (reflecting principally the amount of enzyme in LDL) are positively related to atherosclerosis and to risk for a vascular event. That is, Lp-PLA_2 on LDL is believed to be proatherogenic. It is relatively straightforward to envisage a scenario in which Lp-PLA_2 released throughout the body from monocyte/macrophages, possibly under the influence of proinflammatory cytokines, enters the circulation and becomes bound to LDL, which acts as a reservoir of the enzyme (see Figure 14-1). LDL: Lp-PLA_2 complexes penetrate the artery wall and become trapped in the subendothelial space as the lipoprotein is retained by extracellular proteoglycans.[4] In the milieu of the artery wall, LDL is subject to bombardment by free radicals including nitric oxide and superoxide ion, and oxidation of its contained lipid ensues. Lp-PLA_2 is then in prime position to release from the lipoprotein oxidized short-chain fatty acids and lysophosphatidyl choline, which are highly inflammatory, affecting endothelial cell function and promoting the recruitment of monocytes to the area.[8,9] These monocytes themselves on entering the growing lesion become activated and release further Lp-PLA_2. In support of this concept, it has been shown that Lp-PLA_2 is expressed by macrophages in human and rabbit atherosclerotic lesions,[18] and that Lp-PLA_2 is most abundant in the necrotic cores and thin fibrous caps of lesions in coronary segments taken from patients who suffered sudden coronary death.[19] Lp-PLA_2 activity has also been linked to the preponderance of oxidized LDL in plasma.[26]

A different view emerges in animal models of atherosclerosis in which the Lp-PLA_2 level has been manipulated by gene therapy. Introduction of the human Lp-PLA_2 gene *(PLA2G7)* via an adenoviral rector to apoE-deficient mice increased plasma and HDL-associated

Lp-PLA$_2$ (mouse LDL does not bind Lp-PLA$_2$), and led to a reduction in the mean thickness of the artery wall and less spontaneous atherosclerosis.[27,28] It was shown further that this maneuver protected all lipoprotein classes against oxidation, and HDL-associated Lp-PLA$_2$ inhibited foam cell formation and enhanced cholesterol efflux from macrophages.[29] These findings support the view that, in certain circumstances, especially when present on HDL, Lp-PLA$_2$ has beneficial effects. Thus, future research needs to study the distribution of the enzyme between LDL and HDL, and cognizance must be taken of the potential beneficial actions of Lp-PLA$_2$ when designing novel therapies based on inhibition of the enzyme.

EPIDEMIOLOGY OF LIPOPROTEIN-ASSOCIATED PHOSPHOLIPASE A$_2$

Since the first reports appeared in 2000,[22,30] a series of studies have demonstrated positive associations between plasma levels of Lp-PLA$_2$ and risk for an acute coronary event in asymptomatic individuals and in those with established CHD. Interpretation of this relationship is complex: in biological terms, because of ambiguity in pathogenic mechanisms, and in statistical terms, because of the strong association of Lp-PLA$_2$ with LDL and the potential confounding this causes in multivariate models. From the properties of the enzyme described earlier, it is conceivable that the relationship of Lp-PLA$_2$ to CHD is indirect in that it is a surrogate marker of the abundance of small dense LDL,[31] or it is an indicator of a generalized increase in systematic inflammation, or it is reporting the presence of activated macrophages in atherosclerotic lesions. Alternatively, the enzyme may have a direct involvement in promoting endothelial dysfunction and lesion instability. These various possibilities are explored in this section, which discusses the findings of epidemiologic surveys. First, however, it is useful to note the characteristics of the assay systems used to determine Lp-PLA$_2$.

Measurement of Lipoprotein-Associated Phospholipase A$_2$ in Plasma

The enzyme was identified first by its ability to hydrolyze PAF, and use of labeled PAF as substrate has remained the principle of the activity assay.[7] In any activity-based method, there are theoretical limitations with regard to the uniformity with which enzyme molecules are detected particularly because the conformation of Lp-PLA$_2$, and hence the accessibility of its active site, may differ according to whether it is associated with LDL or HDL. Gazi and colleagues[31] examined the specific activity (activity per unit mass) of Lp-PLA$_2$ in LDL, HDL, and their subfractions, and reported variation that may be attributable to differential binding of the enzyme protein to lipoproteins, or to the presence of inactive Lp-PLA$_2$; for example, the specific activity of the enzyme on HDL was one eighth of that seen on LDL.

Measuring protein mass in theory overcomes many of the problems associated with activity-based estimation of enzyme levels. An "in-house" enzyme-linked immunoassay was used in early epidemiologic studies,[22] but a commercially available kit has been produced.[32] The latter utilizes two highly specific monoclonal antibodies and a recombinant Lp-PLA$_2$ standard. Possibly as a result of calibration differences, observed values differ between the original and the commercial mass assays. In most studies in which both Lp-PLA$_2$ activity and mass have been measured, the correlation is not strong ($r = 0.5$), and questions remain as to what precisely is being detected by these two methods.[33,34] Currently, it is too early to decide which is the superior predictor of risk because in some investigations mass shows the stronger independent association with CHD risk, whereas in others the opposite is the case.

Lipoprotein-Associated Phospholipase A$_2$ and Risk in Subjects without Coronary Heart Disease

The West of Scotland Coronary Prevention Study (WOSCOPS) was the first large-scale study to report an association of Lp-PLA$_2$ with risk for a coronary event. In a nested case–control design,[30] it was found that a 1–standard deviation (SD) increase in plasma Lp-PLA$_2$ mass caused a 20% increase (odds ratio, 1.20; 95% confidence interval [CI], 1.08–1.35) in risk for fatal myocardial infarction (MI) or sudden cardiac death. Those with Lp-PLA$_2$ in the top quintile for this population of hypercholesterolemic, middle-aged men had a twofold greater risk compared with those in the bottom (referent) quintile. A similar increment in risk was observed using coronary revascularization as the endpoint. Other inflammatory markers were examined in the study (CRP, white blood cell count, and fibrinogen), and all were related to risk. However, Lp-PLA$_2$ did not correlate strongly with these (Table 14-1), and their inclusion in multivariate models did not attenuate the strength of the association of Lp-PLA$_2$ mass with risk. Indeed, the relationship of the enzyme to CHD was found to be independent of classic risk factors (age, blood pressure, smoking status), lipoprotein fractions (triglyceride, LDL cholesterol, HDL cholesterol) or a combination of inflammatory markers (Figure 14-2).

Four further studies of the general population followed this initial publication. In the Women's Health Study,[35] it was found that plasma Lp-PLA$_2$ mass showed a trend toward a positive association with risk for a nonfatal MI, sudden coronary death, or stroke. The relative risk in quartile 4 versus quartile 1 of Lp-PLA$_2$ distribution was 1.73 ($P = 0.14$). However, in contrast with the findings in WOSCOPS, the association was attenuated considerably when LDL cholesterol and HDL cholesterol levels were included in the statistical model (relative risk of 1.08 for quartile 4 vs. 1). Also noted in this investigation was that hormone replacement therapy affected Lp-PLA$_2$ levels, reducing them about 20% ($P < 0.0001$). In the Atherosclerosis Risk in Communities (ARK) study, the relationship of Lp-PLA$_2$ to incident CHD was examined for both sexes. Ballantyne and colleagues[36] reported a hazard ratio of 1.78 (95% CI, 1.33–2.38) for tertile 3 versus tertile 1 of enzyme mass, compared with a hazard ratio of 2.53 for tertile 3 versus tertile 1 of CRP. Lp-PLA$_2$ correlated positively with LDL

TABLE 14-1 Relationship of Lipoprotein-Associated Phospholipase A_2 to Risk Factors and Inflammatory Markers

Variable	WOSCOPS[30]	MONICA[34]	Rotterdam[47]	Ludwigshafen[48]
Age	0.013	0.12*	0.025	
Male sex			0.16*	
Body mass index	−0.034	−0.06	0.074†	
Systolic BP	−0.008	0.02	0.07†	
Cholesterol	0.17†	0.30*	0.42*	0.57*
Triglyceride	−0.048			0.24*
LDL cholesterol	0.21*			0.52*
HDL cholesterol	0.044	0.09†	−0.28*	−0.17*
Fibrinogen	0.086†			−0.018
White blood cell count	0.023		0.06†	0.074*
CRP	0.019	0.06	−0.01	0.001
SAA				−0.068*

Pearson (MONItoring of trends and determinants in CArdiovascular diseases [MONICA])-Augsburg or Spearman's rank (West of Scotland Coronary Prevention study [WOSCOPS], Rotterdam, Ludwigshafen) correlation coefficients.

$*P < 0.001$; $^{\dagger}P < 0.05$.

BP, blood pressure; LDL, low-density lipoprotein; HDL, high-density lipoprotein; CRP, C-reactive protein; SAA, serum amyloid.

Data from Koenig W, Khuseyinova N, Lowel H, et al: Lipoprotein-associated phospholipase A_2 adds to risk prediction of incident coronary events by C-reactive protein in apparently healthy middle-aged men from the general population: Results from the 14-year follow-up of a large cohort from southern Germany. Circulation 2004;110:1903–1908; Oei HH, van der Meer IM, Hofman A, et al: Lipoprotein-associated phospholipase A_2 activity is associated with risk of coronary heart disease and ischemic stroke: The Rotterdam Study. Circulation 2005;111:570–575; Packard CJ, O'Reilly DS, Caslake MJ, et al: Lipoprotein-associated phospholipase A_2 as an independent predictor of coronary heart disease. West of Scotland Coronary Prevention Study Group. N Engl J Med 2000;343:1148–1155; and Winkler K, Winkelmann BR, Scharnagl H, et al: Platelet-activating factor acetylhydrolase activity indicates angiographic coronary artery disease independently of systemic inflammation and other risk factors: The Ludwigshafen Risk and Cardiovascular Health Study. Circulation 2005;111:980–987.

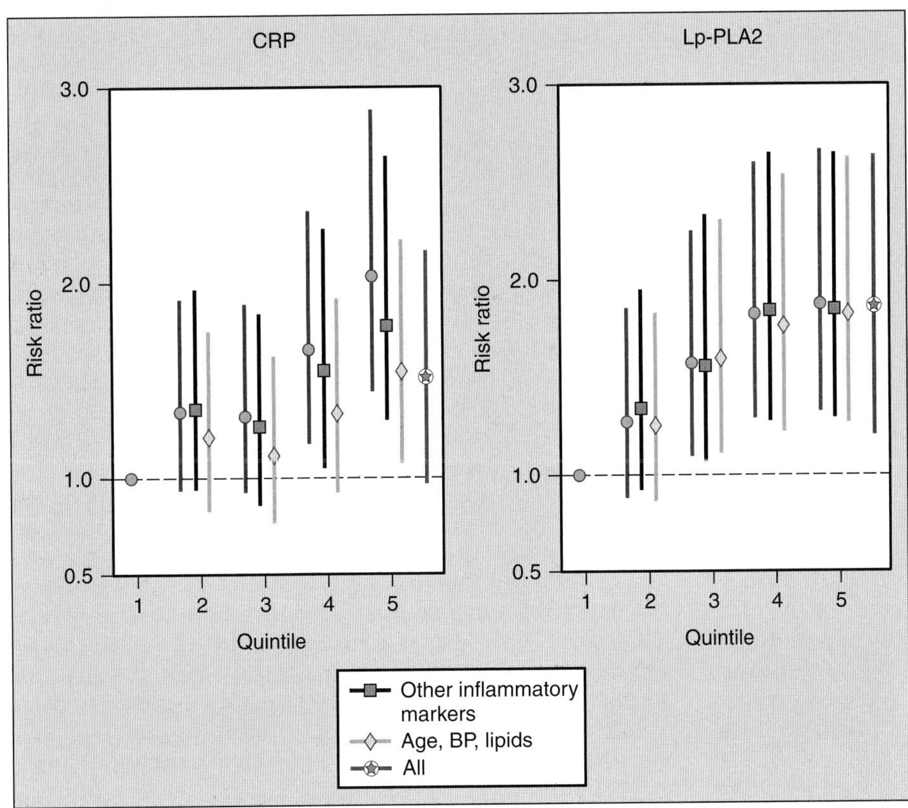

FIGURE 14-2 Relationship of C-reactive protein (CRP) and lipoprotein-associated phospholipase A_2 (Lp-PLA_2) to risk for a vascular event in the West of Scotland Coronary Prevention Study (WOSCOPS). The WOSCOPS population of middle-aged men was divided into quintiles of Lp-PLA_2 mass at baseline. Risk for an event (myocardial infarction or revascularization) was estimated over the follow-up period of 5 years and risk ratios presented relative to quintile 1. Univariate association is given for CRP and Lp-PLA_2 (*solid circles* plus 95% confidence interval). Models were then constructed to include the variable of interest plus other inflammatory markers *(squares)*, classic risk factors *(diamonds)*, and a combination of these *(stars)*. *(Redrawn from Packard and colleagues,[30] by permission).*

cholesterol ($r = 0.36$) and negatively with HDL cholesterol ($r = -0.33$). Inclusion of lipoprotein levels in the model reduced substantially the hazard ratio in tertile 3 (vs. tertile 1) to 1.16 (95% CI, 0.82–1.65), so that the association was no longer significant. Lp-PLA_2 mass was found to be 24% greater in men than in women and 15% greater in white subjects compared with black subjects. It was noted that if a subgroup analysis was performed in subjects with LDL levels less than 130 mg/dL, then Lp-PLA_2 retained a significant association with CHD. The Monitoring of trends and Determinants of Cardiovascular Diseases (MONICA)–Augsburg study published in 2004[37] found that in men over a 14-year follow-up period, Lp-PLA$_2$ mass was related to greater risk for MI or sudden coronary death; the hazard ratio for a 1-SD increase was 1.37 (95% CI, 1.16–1.62) in univariate analysis and 1.23 (95% CI, 1.02–1.47) in a model adjusting for classic risk factors including lipoproteins. More recently, Oei and coworkers[38] observed in the Rotterdam study of 7983 men and women older than 55 years a strong association of Lp-PLA$_2$ activity with CHD. The hazard ratio for those in quartile 4 versus quartile 1 of enzyme activity was 2.36 (95% CI, 1.58–3.52), and this was independent of other risk factors including lipoprotein levels.

On the basis of these surveys, it can be concluded that the Lp-PLA$_2$ mass is a moderately strong predictor of CHD risk in the general population. Plasma levels are affected by sex and hormone therapy, and are correlated positively with LDL cholesterol. The last observation is predictable given the known physical association of the enzyme with this lipoprotein class. Notably, although plasma triglyceride is linked to the concentration of small dense LDL, Lp-PLA$_2$ levels do not show a strong association with triglyceride (see Table 14-1). The biological association of Lp-PLA$_2$ with LDL cholesterol renders statistical models that include both variables difficult to interpret because they may "overcorrect" the relationship between the enzyme and risk.

Lipoprotein-Associated Phospholipase A$_2$ in Subjects with Established Coronary Heart Disease

After a series of reports, it is now clear that Lp-PLA$_2$ is a risk factor for recurrent CHD. Blankenberg and researchers[39] found in a case–control study a 1.8-fold increased risk for CHD in those subjects with the highest versus lowest quartile of Lp-PLA$_2$ activity (P = 0.048), a risk ratio that increased to 3.9-fold (P < 0.0001) when individuals receiving statin or an angiotensin-converting enzyme inhibitor were excluded from the analysis. This association was independent of other risk factors and of plasma lipoproteins. As in the studies in the general population, Lp-PLA$_2$ activity did not show strong correlations (r < 0.2) with other inflammatory markers such as IL-6, fibrinogen, and CRP, indicating separate regulation of this enzyme even in subjects with the exacerbation of chronic inflammation associated with established CHD (see Table 14-1). Brilakis and coworkers[40] examined Lp-PLA$_2$ mass in subjects undergoing angiography and reported a hazard ratio of 1.28 (95% CI, 1.06–1.54) for a 1-SD change in plasma level. Lp-PLA$_2$ in this investigation correlated with the extent of angiographically defined disease at baseline in univariate but not in multivariate analysis.

In a comprehensive study of more than 1000 patients with CHD, Koenig and colleagues[33] measured mass and activity of plasma Lp-PLA$_2$. Both variables gave similar results with respect to correlation with other risk factors and association with future cardiovascular events. About 5% of the patients in the bottom tertile of Lp-PLA$_2$ mass or activity had a coronary event compared with 11% in the top tertile (P < 0.03 for mass; P < 0.01 for activity). Not only was this relationship independent of traditional risk factors, but it was also not attenuated by CRP, cystatin C, creatinine clearance, or plasma brain natruretic peptide levels. This demonstrated the usefulness of the marker in the presence of other indices of inflammation, or of indicators of renal disease or hemodynamic stress. Lp-PLA$_2$ association with subsequent coronary events, revascularization, and stroke was examined in the large Pravastatin Or atorvastatin Evaluation and Infection Trial (PROVE-IT) study.[34] Plasma Lp-PLA$_2$ activity and mass were tested at baseline (i.e., at enrollment within 10 days of the index event) and again at 30 days into the follow-up period. No significant association was observed between baseline levels and risk for a subsequent event (P = 0.88). However, the 30-day activity levels (on average, 12.7% less than those seen at baseline) did predict risk for recurrent cardiovascular disease; 26.4% of those in the highest quintile versus 17.7% of those in the lowest had an event (P = 0.0002). This was independent of achieved LDL cholesterol (all patients in the PROVE IT study were taking pravastatin 40 mg or atorvastatin 80 mg) or achieved CRP. Although there was no formal statistical evidence of an interaction between the prescribed statin and relationship of Lp-PLA$_2$ to risk, the association appeared attenuated with high-dose atorvastatin. When Lp-PLA$_2$ mass was tested, this variable showed less impressive associations with risk that were not significant after adjustment for achieved LDL cholesterol and other clinical risk factors (hazard ratio, 0.98; 95% CI, 0.76–1.25 for highest vs. lowest quintile). In a third study,[41] it was observed in post-MI patients that Lp-PLA$_2$ activity was the strongest predictor of a risk for recurrent events supplanting even apoB in multivariate models. To this striking observation must be added the caution that this was a relatively small survey of 766 patients.

In contrast with Koenig and colleagues,[33] Oldgren and coauthors[42] reported in subjects enrolled to two major clinical trials of short-term intervention a lack of association of Lp-PLA$_2$ mass with risk for mortality or ischemic events over a 1-year follow-up period. These seemingly discordant results may be explained by the fact that the blood sample was drawn in the period immediately after the index event. Although the authors observed no evidence of a marked acute-phase response in Lp-PLA$_2$, the findings of the PROVE IT study indicate that sampling should be delayed until at least 1 month after an acute episode. Thus, the relationship of Lp-PLA$_2$ to a coronary event appears to be as strong in those with established CHD as in those without; that is, the hazard ratios for a 1-SD increase in plasma levels appear to be approximately equal in the primary and secondary prevention scenarios, although the concentrations are generally greater than in those with disease in the general population. The question remains whether activity or mass provides the better prediction of risk.

Lipoprotein-Associated Phospholipase A_2 and Heart Failure

The potential role of Lp-PLA$_2$ in cardiovascular pathology was explored further in the Rotterdam study,[43] which linked the enzyme to risk for heart failure. Lp-PLA$_2$ activity was measured in a random population of 1820 subjects free of established CHD or heart failure at baseline. Follow-up was for 6.7 years, on average, and 94 heart failure cases were identified; those with an MI during follow-up were excluded from the analysis. It was observed that both plasma Lp-PLA$_2$ activity and CRP predicted incident heart failure independent of other risk factors. The hazard ratio for heart failure adjusted for potential confounding factors in this cohort was 2.33 (95% CI, 1.21–1.49) for quartile 4 of Lp-PLA$_2$ relative to quartile 1. This is a surprising result given the differing causative factors of MI and heart failure; the pathology of the latter is complex, and formation of atherosclerotic plaque is not believed to play a significant part. It is likely that it was the influence of chronic inflammation, as reflected in increased Lp-PLA$_2$ and CRP levels, on ventricular remodeling that was responsible for the association. These provocative findings need to be replicated in other larger studies.

Lipoprotein-Associated Phospholipase A_2 and Stroke

Stroke is often included in a composite endpoint in epidemiologic studies or clinical trials to give an overall assessment of vascular risk, despite inherent differences in the pathogenesis of cerebrovascular and cardiovascular disease. Several studies, however, have reported separately the relationship of plasma Lp-PLA$_2$ to risk for stroke and CHD. For example, in ARIC,[44] it was found that in addition to the traditional factors such as hypertension, diabetes, age, and race, Lp-PLA$_2$ and CRP were independent predictors of ischemic stroke. For Lp-PLA$_2$ mass, the hazard ratio for the top versus bottom tertile was 1.91 (95% CI, 1.15–3.18) in a fully adjusted model that included lipids and antihypertensive medication; CRP showed a similar hazard ratio of 1.87 (95% CI, 1.13–3.10). Individuals with high CRP and high Lp-PLA$_2$ levels had 11 times the risk for stroke compared with those with the lowest levels of these two variables. Oei and coworkers[38] described a similar result in the Rotterdam study. In this population of men and women 55 years or older, 110 cases were compared with 1820 control Subjects selected from the cohort. Over 6.4 years of follow-up, risk for ischemic stroke was 1.97 (95% CI, 1.03–3.79) greater in those in the top compared with the bottom quartile of the Lp-PLA$_2$ activity distribution. Again, the association was independent of classic risk factors, other inflammatory markers, and CHD status at baseline.

The PROVE IT study, in contrast, found no evidence for a relationship of Lp-PLA$_2$ activity and mass with stroke in a cohort with pre-existing heart disease.[34] The adjusted hazard ratio for Lp-PLA$_2$ activity measured at 30 days was 0.97 (not significant) comparing quintiles 5 and 1. Likewise, in unpublished data from the Prospective Study of Pravastatin in the Elderly at Risk (PROSPER), we found that Lp-PLA$_2$ mass and activity were related to incident CHD but not stroke. PROSPER recruits were male and female subjects 70 years or older who had had a vascular event or were at high risk because of hypertension, smoking, or diabetes (M. J. Caslake and C. J. Packard, unpublished data).

Thus, in distinction to the relatively uniform observations relating Lp-PLA$_2$ to CHD, controversy exists whether the enzyme predicts risk for ischemic stroke. It appears to do so in population surveys but not in individuals who have had a vascular event. Because LDL is not a risk factor for stroke, the finding that Lp-PLA$_2$ exhibits a positive relationship to this outcome may, as Ballantyne and colleagues[44] suggest, provide part of the explanation of why statins reduce stroke risk, that is, by decreasing circulating levels of the enzyme (see later).

Lipoprotein-Associated Phospholipase A_2 and Atherosclerosis

Lp-PLA$_2$ is enriched in atherosclerotic plaques and may play a pivotal role in the release of proatherogenic moieties into the growing lesion. Thus, the enzyme may be related more strongly to the burden of atherosclerosis in an individual than to risk for a coronary event that follows plaque rupture and clot formation. Early studies of the association of Lp-PLA$_2$ levels with angiographic evidence of CHD involved a small number of subjects and gave mixed results. In some cross-sectional analyses, a link was reported,[22,39,45] whereas in others, it was not apparent.[40,46] When larger studies were performed, clearer evidence was obtained that indicated that Lp-PLA$_2$ was related to the degree of atherosclerosis.

Iribarren and researchers[47] in the Coronary Artery Disease in Young Adults (CARDIA) study demonstrated in 266 cases and an equal number of matched control subjects that greater levels of Lp-PLA$_2$ mass and activity were associated with the presence of disease (Figure 14-3). The odds ratios for the presence of calcified plaque detected by computed tomography in the top compared with bottom tertile were 2.15 (95% CI, 1.36–3.42) for mass and 2.40 (95% CI, 1.52–3.81) for activity. With adjustment for other risk factors, the association was attenuated, and for that activity became nonsignificant. The problems in interpreting cross-sectional angiographic studies was highlighted by Winkler and coauthors,[48] who found significant influences of a host of cardiovascular drugs on Lp-PLA$_2$ (including statins, aspirin, β-blockers, and digitalis). In their study, crude odds ratios for all subjects showed no association of Lp-PLA$_2$ activity with presence of disease. However, in those not taking lipid-lowering drugs, Lp-PLA$_2$ correlated clearly with the severity of CHD; risk for disease was 1.94 (95% CI, 1.34–2.82) in the top compared with the bottom quartile in fully adjusted models.

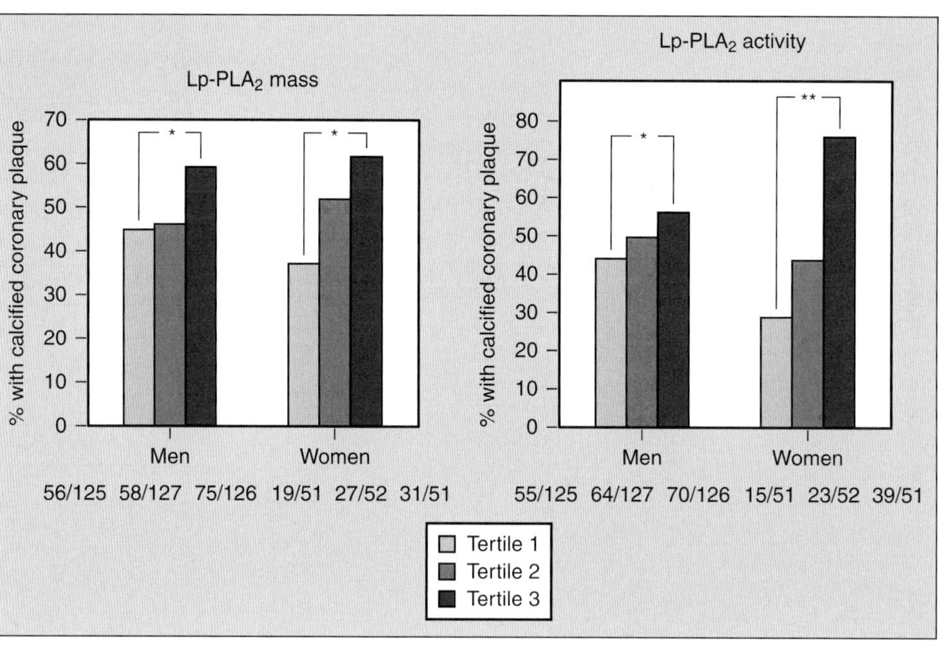

FIGURE 14-3 Lipoprotein-associated phospholipase A_2 (Lp-PLA_2) and calcified coronary plaque in the Coronary Artery Risk Development in Young Adults (CARDIA) study. The proportion of cases with calcified coronary plaque is presented by tertile of Lp-PLA_2 mass or activity for men and women. The overall proportion of cases in each sex is 50% because of the matched design. Significant Cochrane–Armitage test: $^*P < 0.05$; $^{**}P < 0.01$. *(Redrawn from Iribarren and colleagues,[47] by permission.)*

GENETICS OF LIPOPROTEIN-ASSOCIATED PHOSPHOLIPASE A_2

It has been known for some time that functional mutations exist in the gene coding for Lp-PLA_2. Stafforini and researchers[49] located the 12-exon gene for the enzyme, *PLA2G7,* on chromosome 6 region p12 to p21.1, and showed in the Japanese population that a G-to-T substitution in exon 9 at position 994, which results in a valine-to-phenylalanine change at residue 279 (V279F), causes deficiency of the enzyme in the circulation. This mutation is common in Japan, with 27% of the population being heterozygotes with about a 50% decrease in activity and 4% being homozygotes with complete absence of Lp-PLA_2. The amino acid substitution results in failure to secrete the protein from cells, and as a consequence, the misfolded Lp-PLA_2 is retained. This may have deleterious effects on monocyte/macrophage function and may complicate interpretation of the impact of the mutation on CHD.[9] Studies of Japanese subjects with the reside 279 mutation indicate that the 279F variant is linked to greater risk for vascular disease and stroke,[50,51] a finding that at face value contradicts the observations in the general population because it leads to lower plasma Lp-PLA_2. Many of the reports are based on small numbers, however, and there was no distinction in risk between those with partial and complete deficiency. A report in Korean men (who are genetically related to the Japanese) helps to clarify the situation. Jang and coworkers[52] found in a case–control study a smaller risk for cardiovascular disease in those heterozygous for phenylalanine at position 279; the odds ratio for 279F compared with 279V was 0.683 (95% CI, 0.512–0.911) after adjustment for other risk factors. Enzyme activity was 23% lower in heterozygotes versus V/V control subjects, and intriguingly, the decrement in Lp-PLA_2 level was associated with a reduced plasma concentration of malondialdehyde (a marker of lipid oxidation).

A second mutation replacing valine for alanine at residue 379 (A379V) was found in Europeans and causes reduced affinity of the enzyme for PAF.[53] Homozygotes for the 379V allele were reported to have a reduced risk for MI in a European multicenter study.[54] This was confirmed in the AtheroGene cohort,[55] in whom inheritance of a 379V allele was associated with an odds ratio of 0.74 (95% CI, 0.60–0.91) for cardiovascular disease in the cross-sectional study at baseline, and a reduced incidence of risk during follow-up. Paradoxically, in AtheroGene, possession of the 379V allele was linked to increased Lp-PLA_2 activity, suggesting a protective action of the enzyme. However, because there are clear qualitative differences in the nature of Lp-PLA_2 in 379V versus 379A subjects, it is premature to draw conclusions as to the net effect of perturbed activity on risk. In contrast with the above observations, no association of A379V with CHD risk was seen in Korean men[52] and in a U.K. cohort.[26]

The existence of polymorphisms in *PLA2G7* that cause reduced circulating levels of Lp-PLA_2 or generation of dysfunctional enzyme offers the opportunity for new insight into the pathobiology of the protein. More comprehensive studies of the V279F and A379V mutations are needed to cast further light on the association with vascular disease (using, for example, Mendelian randomization approaches in a similar manner to that applied to CRP[56]) and on the metabolic consequences of variation in enzyme properties.

EFFECTS OF DRUGS ON PLASMA LIPOPROTEIN-ASSOCIATED PHOSPHOLIPASE A_2

Because Lp-PLA_2 is transported in the circulation bound to lipoproteins, it is to be expected that lipid-lowering drugs will alter the plasma levels of the enzyme. Statins, inhibitors of 3-hydroxy-3 methylglutaryl–coenzyme A reductase, reduce LDL cholesterol concentrations by 20% to 50% depending on the type of agent and the dose used. In an early study in 21 patients, lovastatin 40 mg/day was shown to reduce Lp-PLA$_2$ by 30% to 40%, in line with the decrement in LDL cholesterol.[57] Likewise, Tsimihodimos and coauthors[23] reported that atorvastatin 20 mg/day reduced Lp-PLA$_2$ activity by 28% to 42% in patients with types IIa and IIb hyperlipidemia. The reduction in enzyme levels correlated with the decline in LDL cholesterol, and a preferential decrease was observed in the amount of enzyme present in small dense LDL. In theory, statins reduce plasma Lp-PLA$_2$ levels through a combination of two effects, by reducing the LDL "reservoir" to which the enzyme is bound and by decreasing the overall level of systemic inflammation, as reflected in the impact of statin treatment on CRP levels.[58] Kom and coauthors[59] have reported on the effects of atorvastatin 40 mg/day on lipoprotein concentrations and the activities of secretory PLA$_2$ and LpPLA$_2$. Treatment decreased Lp-PLA$_2$ in proportion to the LDL reduction but had no effect on secretory PLA$_2$ or, in this small study, on CRP. The findings indicate that the primary influence of these agents on the plasma enzyme is via LDL reduction. In Tsimihodimos and coauthors,[23] study, the authors noted that HDL-associated PLA$_2$ was not altered by statin therapy and that there was a relative increase in the amount of enzyme carried in this density range.

Fibrates reduce plasma triglyceride, shift the LDL size distribution toward larger species, and increase HDL levels. The effects of these drugs on Lp-PLA$_2$ have been examined in a number of clinical trials. Treatment with fenofibrate 200 mg for 3 months has been shown to decrease plasma Lp-PLA$_2$ levels in subjects with types IIa, IIb, and IV hyperlipidemia.[60] Total activity was reduced by 22% to 28%, and in hypercholesterolemic patients, the decrease was proportional to the decline in LDL level, but in patients with type IV hyperlipidemia, the strongest correlation was with the decrease in plasma apoE ($r = 0.45$; $P = 0.05$). In patients with initially high plasma triglyceride levels (types IIb and IV), there was with fibrate an increase in relative, and in absolute, levels of HDL-associated Lp-PLA$_2$, whereas in type IIa patients, there was no effect of treatment on enzyme activity in the HDL fraction. As with statins, the greatest change across the lipoprotein spectrum was seen in small dense LDL. Filippatos and coauthors[61] reported the effects of fenofibrate alone and in combination with orlistat (a lipase inhibitor used as an antiobesity drug) in obese patients with metabolic syndrome. Total plasma Lp-PLA$_2$ was reduced by each drug given as monotherapy, and the combination was more effective than fenofibrate alone, producing a 35% decline in activity. HDL-associated PLA$_2$ increased by about 40% with fenofibrate therapy, and the increment was proportional to the decline in plasma triglyceride ($r = 0.39$; $P < 0.0001$). If the enzyme present on HDL has antiatherogenic properties, this increase with fibrate may contribute to the benefits of therapy.[62]

INHIBITION OF LIPOPROTEIN-ASSOCIATED PHOSPHOLIPASE A$_2$ AS A DRUG TARGET

The putative role of Lp-PLA$_2$ in the pathogenic sequence leading from LDL oxidation to inflammation in, and monocyte recruitment to, the artery wall makes it an attractive target for intervention with inhibitors. Potent agents have been described and tested that reduce plasma activity of the enzyme by more than 95%.[9] In model systems, inhibitors have been used to abolish the enhanced chemoattractant activity of oxidized LDL,[63] and in the Watanabe rabbit, Lp-PLA$_2$ inhibition was associated with a reduction in plaque development.[64] Current work has focused on pyrimidines as orally active competitive inhibitors of the enzyme, and candidate compounds such as SB-480848 are currently in clinical trials.[9]

LIPOPROTEIN-ASSOCIATED PHOSPHOLIPASE A$_2$ AND RISK ASSESSMENT

Global risk assessment is a key step in guiding the aggressiveness of intervention strategies in asymptomatic individuals. Tools such as the equations developed by the Framingham Heart Study[65] are used to predict risk for a vascular event and hence to tailor treatment algorithms to clinical need. Individuals with a predicted risk greater than 3% per year are deemed at high risk, and the recommendation is to use aggressive treatment including lipid-lowering drugs. People with a low risk of less than 1% per year are directed toward healthy lifestyle choices.[66] It is the intermediate range, in which a significant proportion of the population lies, that presents a major challenge for guideline writers and the primary care physician. As new biomarkers of cardiovascular disease emerge, they are tested for their ability to improve risk prediction. CRP is the variable most thoroughly evaluated in this regard, although D-dimer, B-type natruretic peptide, and others have also been examined.[13] Lp-PLA$_2$ measurement in the general population was reported by Folsom and colleagues[67] to add only modestly to the area under the receiver operating characteristic curve, a commonly used indication of predictive accuracy. Others have argued that Lp-PLA$_2$ offers incremental information in risk assessment and may be a useful addition in recategorizing individuals at intermediate risk on the basis of a Framingham Risk Score.[37,68] It is probably too early to draw firm conclusions, and the place of Lp-PLA$_2$ mass or activity measurement may become clear only once outputs from a large collaboration in which it is planned to pool virtually all available data are published.[69]

Acknowledgment

I gratefully acknowledge the excellent secretarial help of Shelley Wilkie in the preparation of this chapter.

REFERENCES

1. Libby P, Theroux P: Pathophysiology of coronary artery disease. *Circulation* 2005;111:3481–3488.
2. Berliner JA, Watson AD: A role for oxidized phospholipids in atherosclerosis. *N Engl J Med* 2005;353:9–11.
3. Baigent C, Keech A, Kearney PM, et al: Efficacy and safety of cholesterol-lowering treatment: Prospective meta-analysis of data from 90 056 participants in 14 randomised trials of statins. *Lancet* 2005;366:1267–1278.
4. Skalen K, Gustafsson M, Rydberg EK, et al: Subendothelial retention of atherogenic lipoproteins in early atherosclerosis. *Nature* 2002;417:750–754.
5. Rosengren B, Jonsson-Rylander AC, Peilot H, et al: Distinctiveness of secretory phospholipase A_2 group IIA and V suggesting unique roles in atherosclerosis. *Biochim Biophys Acta* 2006;1761: 1301–1308.
6. Macphee CH, Nelson J, Zalewski A: Role of lipoprotein-associated phospholipase A_2 in atherosclerosis and its potential as a therapeutic target. *Curr Opin Pharmacol* 2006;6:154–161.
7. Stafforini DM, McIntyre TM, Zimmerman GA, et al: Platelet-activating factor acetylhydrolases. *J Biol Chem* 1997;272: 17895–17898.
8. Tselepis AD, John Chapman M: Inflammation, bioactive lipids and atherosclerosis: Potential roles of a lipoprotein-associated phospholipase A2, platelet activating factor-acetylhydrolase. *Atherosclerosis* 2002;(suppl 3):57–68.
9. Zalewski A, Macphee C: Role of lipoprotein-associated phospholipase A2 in atherosclerosis: Biology, epidemiology, and possible therapeutic target. *Arterioscler Thromb Vasc Biol* 2005;25:923–931.
10. Hurt-Camejo E, Camejo G, Sartipy P: Phospholipase A_2 and small, dense low-density lipoprotein. *Curr Opin Lipidol* 2000;11:465–471.
11. Boekholdt SM, Keller TT, Wareham NJ, et al: Serum levels of type II secretory phospholipase A_2 and the risk of future coronary artery disease in apparently healthy men and women: The EPIC-Norfolk Prospective Population Study. *Arterioscler Thromb Vasc Biol* 2005;25:839–846.
12. Kugiyama K, Ota Y, Takazoe K, et al: Circulating levels of secretory type II phospholipase A(2) predict coronary events in patients with coronary artery disease. *Circulation* 1999;100: 1280–1284.
13. Koenig W, Khuseyinova N: Biomarkers of atherosclerotic plaque instability and rupture. *Arterioscler Thromb Vasc Biol* 2007;27: 15–26.
14. Libby P, Ridker PM: Inflammation and atherosclerosis: Role of C-reactive protein in risk assessment. *Am J Med 2004*;116 (suppl 6A):9S–16S.
15. Cao Y, Stafforini DM, Zimmerman GA, et al: Expression of plasma platelet-activating factor acetylhydrolase is transcriptionally regulated by mediators of inflammation. *J Biol Chem* 1998;273:4012–4020.
16. Asano K, Okamoto S, Fukunaga K, et al: Cellular source(s) of platelet-activating-factor acetylhydrolase activity in plasma. *Biochem Biophys Res Commun* 1999;261:511–514.
17. Wu X, Zimmerman GA, Prescott SM, et al: The p38 MAPK pathway mediates transcriptional activation of the plasma platelet-activating factor acetylhydrolase gene in macrophages stimulated with lipopolysaccharide. *J Biol Chem* 2004;279: 36158–36165.
18. Hakkinen T, Luoma JS, Hiltunen MO, et al: Lipoprotein-associated phospholipase A(2), platelet-activating factor acetylhydrolase, is expressed by macrophages in human and rabbit atherosclerotic lesions. *Arterioscler Thromb Vasc Biol* 1999;19:2909–2917.
19. Kolodgie FD, Burke AP, Skorija KS, et al: Lipoprotein-associated phospholipase A_2 protein expression in the natural progression of human coronary atherosclerosis. *Arterioscler Thromb Vasc Biol* 2006;26:2523–2529.
20. Shi Y, Zhang P, Zhang L, et al: Role of lipoprotein-associated phospholipase A_2 in leukocyte activation and inflammatory responses. *Atherosclerosis* 2007;191:54–62.
21. Stafforini DM, Tjoelker LW, McCormick SP, et al: Molecular basis of the interaction between plasma platelet-activating factor acetylhydrolase and low-density lipoprotein. *J Biol Chem* 1999;274:7018–7024.
22. Caslake MJ, Packard CJ, Suckling KE, et al: Lipoprotein-associated phospholipase A(2), platelet-activating factor acetylhydrolase: A potential new risk factor for coronary artery disease. *Atherosclerosis* 2000;150:413–419.
23. Tsimihodimos V, Karabina SA, Tambaki AP, et al: Atorvastatin preferentially reduces LDL-associated platelet-activating factor acetylhydrolase activity in dyslipidemias of type IIA and type IIB. *Arterioscler Thromb Vasc Biol* 2002;22:306–311.
24. Tselepis AD, Karabina SA, Stengel D, et al: N-linked glycosylation of macrophage-derived PAF-AH is a major determinant of enzyme association with plasma HDL. *J Lipid Res* 2001;42: 1645–1654.
25. Gaubatz JW, Gillard BK, Massey JB, et al: Dynamics of dense electronegative low-density lipoproteins and their preferential association with lipoprotein phospholipase A(2). *J Lipid Res* 2007;48:348–357.
26. Wootton PT, Stephens JW, Hurel SJ, et al: Lp-PLA2 activity and PLA2G7 A379V genotype in patients with diabetes mellitus. *Atherosclerosis* 2006;189:149–156.
27. Hase M, Tanaka M, Yokota M, et al: Reduction in the extent of atherosclerosis in apolipoprotein E-deficient mice induced by electroporation-mediated transfer of the human plasma platelet-activating factor acetylhydrolase gene into skeletal muscle. *Prostaglandins Other Lipid Mediat* 2002;70:107–118.
28. Quarck R, De Geest B, Stengel D, et al: Adenovirus-mediated gene transfer of human platelet-activating factor-acetylhydrolase prevents injury-induced neointima formation and reduces spontaneous atherosclerosis in apolipoprotein E-deficient mice. *Circulation* 2001;103:2495–2500.
29. Noto H, Hara M, Karasawa K, et al: Human plasma platelet-activating factor acetylhydrolase binds to all the murine lipoproteins, conferring protection against oxidative stress. *Arterioscler Thromb Vasc Biol* 2003;23:829–835.
30. Packard CJ, O'Reilly DS, Caslake MJ, et al: Lipoprotein-associated phospholipase A2 as an independent predictor of coronary heart disease. West of Scotland Coronary Prevention Study Group. *N Engl J Med* 2000;343:1148–1155.
31. Gazi I, Lourida ES, Filippatos T, et al: Lipoprotein-associated phospholipase A_2 activity is a marker of small dense LDL particles in human plasma. *Clin Chem* 2005;51:2264–2273.
32. Dada N, Kim NW, Wolfert RL: Lp-PLA2: An emerging biomarker of coronary heart disease. *Expert Rev Mol Diagn* 2002;2:17–22.
33. Koenig W, Twardella D, Brenner H, et al: Lipoprotein-associated phospholipase A_2 predicts future cardiovascular events in patients with coronary heart disease independently of traditional risk factors, markers of inflammation, renal function, and hemodynamic stress. *Arterioscler Thromb Vasc Biol* 2006;26: 1586–1593.
34. O'Donoghue M, Morrow DA, Sabatine MS, et al: Lipoprotein-associated phospholipase A2 and its association with cardiovascular outcomes in patients with acute coronary syndromes in the PROVE IT-TIMI 22 (PRavastatin Or atorVastatin Evaluation and Infection Therapy–Thrombolysis In Myocardial Infarction) trial. *Circulation* 2006;113:1745–1752.
35. Blake GJ, Dada N, Fox JC, et al: A prospective evaluation of lipoprotein-associated phospholipase A(2) levels and the risk of future cardiovascular events in women. *J Am Coll Cardiol* 2001;38:1302–1306.
36. Ballantyne CM, Hoogeveen RC, Bang H, et al: Lipoprotein-associated phospholipase A_2, high-sensitivity C-reactive protein, and risk for incident coronary heart disease in middle-aged men and women in the Atherosclerosis Risk in Communities (ARIC) study. *Circulation* 2004;109:837–842.
37. Koenig W, Khuseyinova N, Lowel H, et al: Lipoprotein-associated phospholipase A_2 adds to risk prediction of incident coronary events by C-reactive protein in apparently healthy middle-aged men from the general population: Results from the 14-year follow-up of a large cohort from southern Germany. *Circulation* 2004;110:1903–1908.
38. Oei HH, van der Meer IM, Hofman A, et al: Lipoprotein-associated phospholipase A_2 activity is associated with risk of coronary heart disease and ischemic stroke: The Rotterdam Study. *Circulation* 2005;111:570–575.
39. Blankenberg S, Stengel D, Rupprecht HJ, et al: Plasma PAF-acetylhydrolase in patients with coronary artery disease: Results of a cross-sectional analysis. *J Lipid Res* 2003;44:1381–1386.

40. Brilakis ES, McConnell JP, Lennon RJ, et al: Association of lipoprotein-associated phospholipase A_2 levels with coronary artery disease risk factors, angiographic coronary artery disease, and major adverse events at follow-up. *Eur Heart J* 2005;26: 137–144.
41. Corsetti JP, Rainwater DL, Moss AJ, et al: High lipoprotein-associated phospholipase A_2 is a risk factor for recurrent coronary events in postinfarction patients. *Clin Chem* 2006;52: 1331–1338.
42. Oldgren J, James SK, Siegbahn A, et al: Lipoprotein-associated phospholipase A_2 does not predict mortality or new ischaemic events in acute coronary syndrome patients. *Eur Heart J* 2007;28:699–704.
43. van Vark LC, Kardys I, Bleumink GS, et al: Lipoprotein-associated phospholipase A_2 activity and risk of heart failure: The Rotterdam study. *Eur Heart J* 2006;27:2346–2352.
44. Ballantyne CM, Hoogeveen RC, Bang H, et al: Lipoprotein-associated phospholipase A_2, high-sensitivity C-reactive protein, and risk for incident ischemic stroke in middle-aged men and women in the Atherosclerosis Risk in Communities (ARIC) study. *Arch Intern Med* 2005;165:2479–2484.
45. May HT, Horne BD, Anderson JL, et al: Lipoprotein-associated phospholipase A_2 independently predicts the angiographic diagnosis of coronary artery disease and coronary death. *Am Heart J* 2006;152:997–1003.
46. Shohet RV, Anwar A, Johnston JM, et al: Plasma platelet-activating factor acetylhydrolase activity is not associated with premature coronary atherosclerosis. *Am J Cardiol* 1999;83:109–111, A108–109.
47. Iribarren C, Gross MD, Darbinian JA, et al: Association of lipoprotein-associated phospholipase A_2 mass and activity with calcified coronary plaque in young adults: The CARDIA study. *Arterioscler Thromb Vasc Biol* 2005;25:216–221.
48. Winkler K, Winkelmann BR, Scharnagl H, et al: Platelet-activating factor acetylhydrolase activity indicates angiographic coronary artery disease independently of systemic inflammation and other risk factors: The Ludwigshafen Risk and Cardiovascular Health Study. *Circulation* 2005;111:980–987.
49. Stafforini DM, Satoh K, Atkinson DL, et al: Platelet-activating factor acetylhydrolase deficiency. A missense mutation near the active site of an anti-inflammatory phospholipase. *J Clin Invest* 1996;97:2784–2791.
50. Hiramoto M, Yoshida H, Imaizumi T, et al: A mutation in plasma platelet-activating factor acetylhydrolase (Val279→Phe) is a genetic risk factor for stroke. *Stroke* 1997;28:2417–2420.
51. Yamada Y, Ichihara S, Fujimura T, et al: Identification of the G994→T missense in exon 9 of the plasma platelet-activating factor acetylhydrolase gene as an independent risk factor for coronary artery disease in Japanese men. *Metabolism* 1998;47: 177–181.
52. Jang Y, Kim OY, Koh SJ, et al: The Val279Phe variant of the lipoprotein-associated phospholipase A_2 gene is associated with catalytic activities and cardiovascular disease in Korean men. *J Clin Endocrinol Metab* 2006;91:3521–3527.
53. Kruse S, Mao XQ, Heinzmann A, et al: The Ile198Thr and Ala379Val variants of plasmatic PAF-acetylhydrolase impair catalytical activities and are associated with atopy and asthma. *Am J Hum Genet* 2000;66:1522–1530.
54. Abuzeid AM, Hawe E, Humphries SE, et al: Association between the Ala379Val variant of the lipoprotein associated phospholipase A_2 and risk of myocardial infarction in the north and south of Europe. *Atherosclerosis* 2003;168:283–288.
55. Ninio E, Tregouet D, Carrier JL, et al: Platelet-activating factor-acetylhydrolase and PAF-receptor gene haplotypes in relation to future cardiovascular event in patients with coronary artery disease. *Hum Mol Genet* 2004;13:1341–1351.
56. Casas JP, Shah T, Cooper J, et al: Insight into the nature of the CRP-coronary event association using Mendelian randomization. *Int J Epidemiol* 2006;35:922–931.
57. Kudolo GB, Bressler P, DeFronzo RA: Plasma PAF acetylhydrolase in non-insulin dependent diabetes mellitus and obesity: Effect of hyperinsulinemia and lovastatin treatment. *J Lipid Mediat Cell Signal* 1997;17:97–113.
58. Ray KK, Cannon CP: Pathological changes in acute coronary syndromes: The role of statin therapy in the modulation of inflammation, endothelial function and coagulation. *J Thromb Thrombolysis* 2004;18:89–101.
59. Kom GD, Schwedhelm E, Maas R, et al: Impact of atorvastatin treatment on platelet-activating factor acetylhydrolase and 15-F(2trans)-isoprostane in hypercholesterolaemic patients. *Br J Clin Pharmacol* 2007;63:672–679.
60. Tsimihodimos V, Kakafika A, Tambaki AP, et al: Fenofibrate induces HDL-associated PAF-AH but attenuates enzyme activity associated with apoB-containing lipoproteins. *J Lipid Res* 2003;44:927–934.
61. Filippatos TD, Gazi IF, Liberopoulos EN, et al: The effect of orlistat and fenofibrate, alone or in combination, on small dense LDL and lipoprotein-associated phospholipase A_2 in obese patients with metabolic syndrome. *Atherosclerosis* 2007;193: 428–437.
62. Eisaf M, Tselepis AD: Effect of hypolipidemic drugs on lipoprotein-associated platelet activating factor acetylhydrolase. Implication for atherosclerosis. *Biochem Pharmacol* 2003;66:2069–2073.
63. MacPhee CH, Moores KE, Boyd HF, et al: Lipoprotein-associated phospholipase A_2, platelet-activating factor acetylhydrolase, generates two bioactive products during the oxidation of low-density lipoprotein: Use of a novel inhibitor. *Biochem J* 1999;338:479–487.
64. Macphee CH: Lipoprotein-associated phospholipase A_2: A potential new risk factor for coronary artery disease and a therapeutic target. *Curr Opin Pharmacol* 2001;1:121–125.
65. Wilson PW: Established risk factors and coronary artery disease: The Framingham Study. *Am J Hypertens* 7:7S–12S, 1994.
66. Grundy SM, Bazzarre T, Cleeman J, et al: Prevention Conference V: Beyond secondary prevention: Identifying the high-risk patient for primary prevention: Medical office assessment: Writing Group I. *Circulation* 2000;101:E3–E11.
67. Folsom AR, Chambless LE, Ballantyne CM, et al: An assessment of incremental coronary risk prediction using C-reactive protein and other novel risk markers: The atherosclerosis risk in communities study. *Arch Intern Med* 2006;166:1368–1373.
68. Caslake MJ, Packard CJ: Lipoprotein-associated phospholipase A_2 as a biomarker for coronary disease and stroke. *Nat Clin Pract Cardiovasc Med* 2005;2:529–535.
69. Ballantyne C, Cushman M, Psaty B, et al: Collaborative meta-analysis of individual participant data from observational studies of Lp-PLA2 and cardiovascular diseases. *Eur J Cardiovasc Prev Rehabil* 2007;14:3–11.

CHAPTER 15

Emerging Assays

Ron C. Hoogeveen and Christie M. Ballantyne

INTRODUCTION

Despite the proven efficacy of plasma lipid profiles in the assessment of cardiovascular risk, many individuals who are considered to be at low risk for cardiovascular disease according to U.S. National Cholesterol Education Program Adult Treatment Panel III guidlines[1] have cardiovascular events. Over the last two decades, it has become increasingly clear that inflammation, endothelial dysfunction, and oxidative stress play a key role in the pathogenesis of atherosclerosis. Evidence from numerous *in vitro* studies as well as *in vivo* studies in animals and humans points to a key role for inflammation in the initiation and development of atherosclerotic lesions (see reviews[2,3]). Inflammatory cytokines mediate the activation of endothelial adhesion molecules and stimulate the production of acute-phase reactants, such as C-reactive protein.[4] These processes lead to the recruitment and transmigration of leukocyte-derived macrophages into the vascular wall in the initial step in the formation of atherosclerotic lesions, also called fatty streaks.[5] Specific enzymes that are released by activated leukocytes catalyze the formation of reactive oxygen species, which promote lipid peroxidation of potential targets, including low-density lipoprotein.[6]

The recent progress in our understanding of the underlying pathways in the development of cardiovascular disease has led to the emergence of a large number of potential novel biomarkers for cardiovascular risk prediction (beyond the traditional risk factors) that may be useful in risk stratification, in monitoring response to therapy, or as targets of therapy. To address all the emerging biomarkers for atherosclerosis would be beyond the scope of this review. Therefore, we will focus on recent technological approaches that facilitate the discovery and validation of emerging biomarkers.

BIOMARKERS AS CLINICAL TOOLS

From a clinical perspective, biomarkers can be of use in risk assessment for a variety of factors related to health or disease, such as exposure to environmental factors, genetic exposure or susceptibility, markers of subclinical or clinical disease, or surrogate endpoints, to evaluate safety and efficacy of different therapies.[7] Therefore, biomarkers are generally classified according to different stages in the development of a disease: screening biomarkers are markers used for screening of patients who have no apparent disease, diagnostic biomarkers can assist in the care of patients who are suspected to have disease, and prognostic biomarkers are used in patients with overt disease to aid in the categorization of disease severity and prediction of future disease course, including recurrence and monitoring of treatment efficacy.[8] Because prevention of cardiovascular events in patients at increased risk is likely to have a significant impact on the overall public health burden, the development of novel biomarkers for screening is currently an active area of investigation. Identification of biomarkers to monitor the efficacy of new treatments for atherosclerosis is emerging as a critical priority to enhance translational research in atherosclerosis drug development.

TECHNICAL ASPECTS FOR BIOMARKER DEVELOPMENT

It is important to consider a number of issues that influence the clinical utility of potential novel biomarkers for cardiovascular risk assessment. One of the major considerations is whether a novel biomarker can improve the cardiovascular risk prediction that can be attained with existing well-established cardiovascular risk markers. To this end, a potential marker needs to exhibit sufficient sensitivity and specificity to allow for risk classification. The receiver operating characteristic (ROC) curve is typically used to evaluate the clinical utility of a biomarker for both diagnostic and prognostic purposes.[9] More specifically, evaluation of a novel biomarker is generally based on its capability to improve the area under the ROC curve (AUC).[10] However, even strong independent risk predictors can have a very limited impact on the AUC. Therefore, calibration (i.e., measuring how well the predicted probability agrees with the observed proportions in a population) is essential in the assessment of the accuracy of prediction models.[11] Reclassification can directly compare the clinical impact of two prediction models by determining how many individuals would be reclassified into clinically relevant risk strata (e.g., low, intermediate, or high), which may form the basis for treatment decisions. The percent reclassified can thus be used as a measure of the clinical impact of a new marker when added to an existing prediction model.

A number of aspects related to the biophysical and/or structural features of a specific biomarker can also greatly influence its utility. For example, it is important to understand how circulating levels of a particular marker are influenced by factors such as diet, diurnal variation, day-to-day variation within an individual, half-life in circulation, and dynamic range within a population. Biomarkers that have a relatively long half-life in circulation (i.e., at least several hours) and a relatively small intraindividual variation in circulating levels compared with the dynamic range within a population are better suited as potential markers for risk prediction.

In addition, it is highly desirable that a proposed marker can be measured accurately using standardized and cost-effective methods in a routine clinical laboratory setting. Although methods for most well-established risk factors are eventually adapted so that these biomarkers can be measured using standardized assays on specialized automated chemistry analyzers in routine clinical laboratories, enzyme-linked immunosorbent assay (ELISA) methods are most commonly used to evaluate emerging risk factors. ELISA methodology generally provides sufficient sensitivity, is relatively cost-effective, does not require advanced instrumentation, and can be performed in routine laboratories.[12] However, ELISA methods are notoriously difficult to standardize, even when monoclonal antibodies are used, and can be subject to interfering factors such as antibody-specific cross-reactivity, the complexity of the sample matrix, autoantibodies, and genetic mutations or polymorphisms that can alter epitope recognition by monoclonal antibodies. In contrast, methods based on the combination of chromatography and mass spectrometry techniques (e.g., gas chromatography–mass spectrometry [GC-MS] and liquid chromatography–tandem mass spectroscopy [LC-MS/MS]) are generally considered the "gold standard" because they are not affected by the same interfering factors as ELISA methods. However, GC-MS and LC-MS are generally less cost-effective and, because they require a higher level of operator expertise, are generally not well suited for routine clinical laboratories. The recent advancement in GC-MS and LC-MS technologies may improve their clinical utility in the near future.

Specialized sample processing and storage requirements can also affect the clinical utility of a biomarker. In particular, the effect of long-term storage on biomarker stability varies greatly among analytes and is dependent on storage conditions, sample matrix, and the addition of specific preservatives. Large prospective epidemiological studies are ideally suited to assess the predictive value of novel risk factors. However, because most epidemiological studies measure biomarkers in biological samples that have been stored for long time periods, it is currently not clear what impact long-term storage has on the field of biomarker research.

Finally, issues related to the need for a causal relationship between a marker and the pathogenesis of a certain disease remain a controversial topic among biomarker researchers. Markers that have proven to be valuable in risk assessment without a clear causal relationship as well as markers that are established mediators of disease but fail to predict risk for disease have been described.

GENETIC MARKERS AND GENOMICS APPROACH FOR THE DEVELOPMENT OF NOVEL CARDIOVASCULAR BIOMARKERS

The completion of the Human Genome Project[13] and the HapMap Project[14] in conjunction with the development of microarrays, nanotechnology, and recent advances in bioinformatics provide new possibilities to generate and analyze a tremendous amount of data to facilitate the discovery of highly informative novel cardiovascular biomarkers. Current technology in genetics research allows us to examine hundreds of thousands of single-nucleotide polymorphisms (SNPs) and investigate their associations with disease. Typically, the association strategy evaluates the relation of common genetic variants in unrelated individuals to the presence or absence of disease. The scientific rationale behind association studies is that common genetic variants with modest effects contribute to the overall variation of complex disease in the population (Table 15-1).[15] Although there

TABLE 15-1 Comparison of Association and Linkage Studies for Genetics Research

Area of Study	Association	Linkage
Human material	Families or case-control	Families
Gene effect	Genes of small to modest effect	Genes of modest to large effect
Candidate genes	Markers must be in linkage disequilibrium; haplotype approach optimal	Any marker, optimally highly polymorphic
Genome-wide	Thousands to millions of genetic markers required	Hundreds of genetic markers required

From Ref. 15, with permission.

have been numerous reports of associations between genetic variants in candidate genes and cardiovascular disease (see Gibbons et al.[15] for review), in many cases these associations were not reproducible in subsequent studies.[16,17] The availability of dense SNP maps of the humane genome has spurred the recent proliferation of a number of genome-wide association studies (GWAS), that have been successful in some cases in revealing novel pathways associated with cardiovascular diseases.[18–20] A different analysis approach is used in genetic linkage studies, which involve a genome-wide scan in related family members to identify potential genes related to disease susceptibility (see Table 15-1). Although the genetic linkage approach has been successful in the detection of genes for single-gene disorders with large genetic effects, it has been less successful for investigations of complex genetic traits such as cardiovascular disease.

PROTEOMICS-BASED DEVELOPMENT OF CARDIOVASCULAR BIOMARKERS

Despite the considerable progress that has been made through genetics and genomics research, it is clear that the complexity of cardiovascular disease requires a more complete understanding of the role of gene expression in the pathogenesis of cardiovascular disease. This can be achieved in part through characterization of proteins, the products of gene expression that are the essential biological determinants of disease phenotype. Proteins are the major constituents of cellular structures and are the mediators for most cellular functions, either directly or indirectly through their actions on other molecules. The recent advent of novel multiplexing methods and proteomic approaches allows for a more systematic investigation of complex human diseases and provides new tools for biomarker development.

Although a number of different proteomic approaches have been applied to identify new biomarkers for cardiovascular diseases, the principle underlying all proteomic approaches is the comparative analysis of protein expression profiles in normal versus diseased tissues. Several recent studies have used proteomic analysis of different types of tissues, including vascular cells, atherosclerotic plaques, heart, and blood, to identify potential novel protein biomarkers associated with the pathogenesis of cardiovascular disease.[21–25] Furthermore, the Human Proteome Organization (www.HUPO.org) initiatives have been created to aid in the development of a human protein reference database derived from different biological compartments, including plasma, urine, brain, heart, and liver.

Tools Used in Proteomics

The human proteome is far more complex than the human genome because of the intricacy of a number of specific protein features such as post-transcriptional modification, intracellular compartmentalization, and interactions with other molecules (Figure 15-1).[26] Therefore, unlike genomics research, which uses a common technological approach, proteomics relies on a vast number of different technologies that often focus on a specific protein subset isolated from a specific tissue, cell type, or intracellular compartment (see Mayr et al.[27] for review).

Mass spectrometry is the most common technology used in proteomics research because of its unique ability to identify proteins in a nonbiased manner. The mass-to-charge (m/z) ratio of a molecule is the principal measurement obtained from mass spectrometry analysis, and data from a specific sample are usually displayed as a "spectrum," which is a plot of the m/z ratio on the x-axis versus the level of intensity on the y-axis. Currently a number of different instruments are being manufactured that use mass spectrometry, sometimes in combination with a chromatographic technique to aid in the separation of molecules in a complex sample matrix. The two most common chromatographic techniques used in combination with mass spectrometry are liquid chromatography and gas chromatography. With the use of liquid chromatography combined with LC-MS/MS, captured ions are subjected to sequential ionization, and fragmented products of these ions can be analyzed, which allows for the identification of different peptides. A large number of different methods for sample preparation and protein separation and identification have been described (see Figure 15-2 for overview) and have been the topic of a number of recent reviews.[28] Generally, proteomic methods involve a number of critical steps that need to be optimized according to the specific aims of a study (Figure 15-3).[28] These steps include sample collection, sample processing, protein separation, and protein identification. Sample collection is a critical step in proteomic analysis and must be compatible with the subsequent separation and quantification methods. Furthermore, the complexity of the sample matrix needs

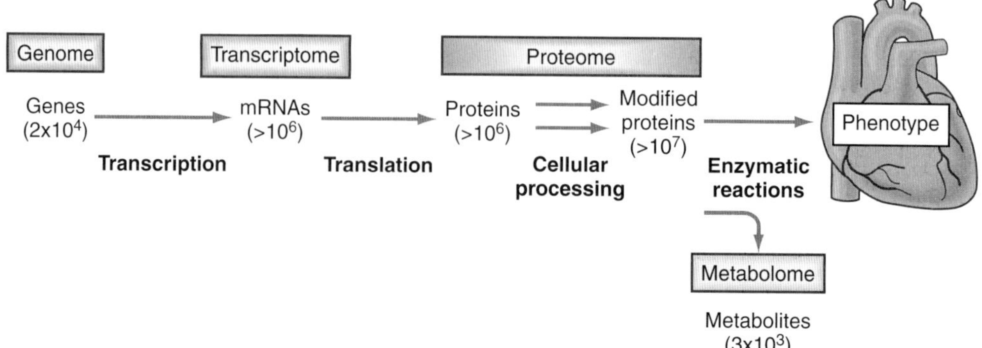

FIGURE 15-1 Increasing complexity of the human proteome compared with the human genome. *(From Ref. 26, with permission.)*

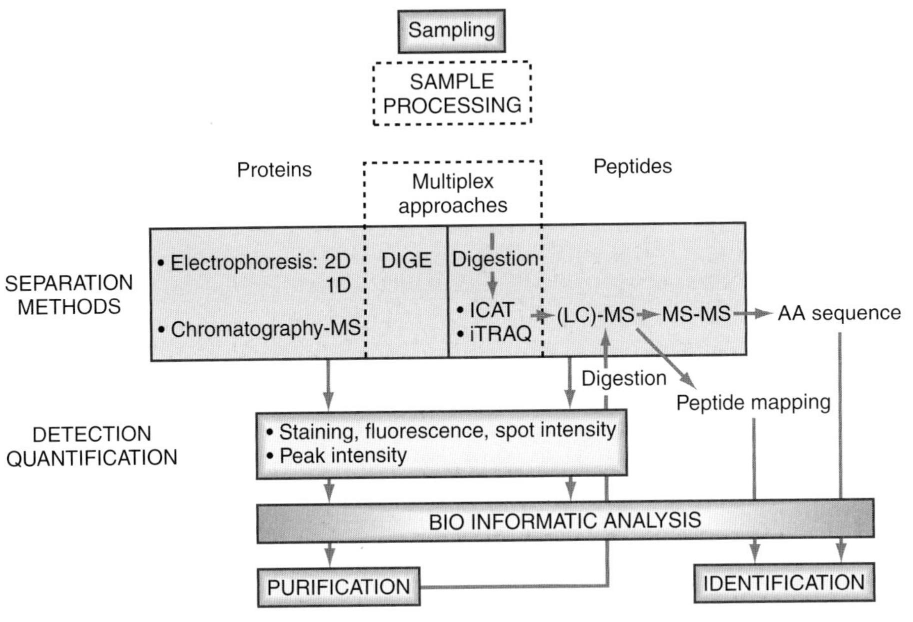

FIGURE 15-2 Methods for sample preparation and protein separation and identification for proteomic analysis. DIGE, differential gel electrophoresis; ICAT, isotrope-coded affinity tag. *(From Ref. 28, with permission.)*

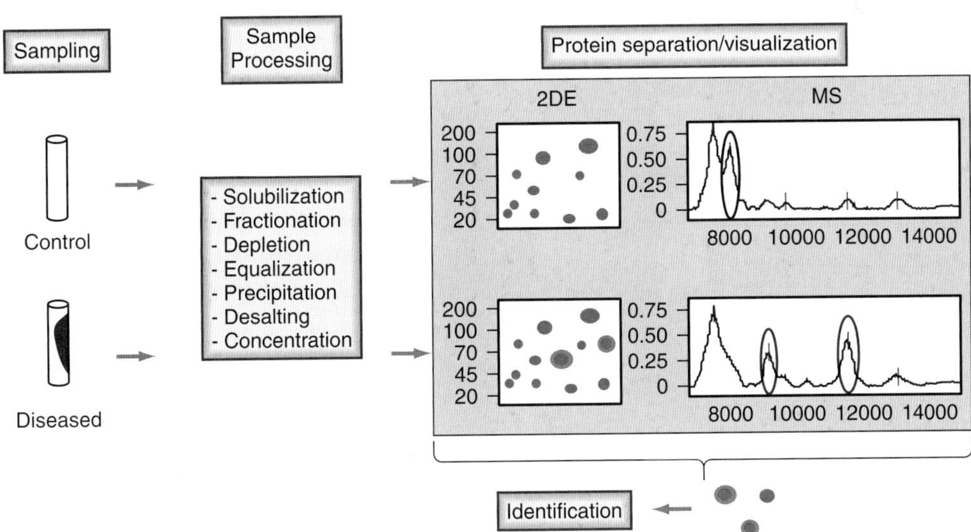

FIGURE 15-3 Proteomic methods. *(From Ref. 28, with permission.)*

to be taken into consideration because the wide range of protein expression levels in biological samples can greatly influence the identification of potential biomarkers that are present at extremely low concentrations.[29] Sample processing usually includes protocols to solubilize proteins in chaotropic agents (e.g., urea) or nonionic detergents (e.g., 3-[(3-cholamido-propyl) dimethylammonio]-1-propanesulfonate [CHAPS]). These types of reagents do not substantially alter protein charge, which affects the chromatographic properties of proteins during fractionation. Furthermore, protocols to concentrate low-abundance proteins and the removal of high-abundance, constitutively expressed proteins are generally included in sample processing techniques.

A large number of different proteomic research techniques have been described for the separation of proteins in complex sample matrices. However, the most widely used technique for proteomic protein separation is two-dimensional electrophoresis (2-DE).[30,31] Proteins are amphoteric molecules that carry a negative, positive, or zero net charge that is determined by their amino acid composition and the pH of their environment (molecular charge). In 2-DE, proteins are first separated based on their differences in molecular charge, a process known as isoelectric focusing. The proteins are then separated according to their molecular weight by sodium dodecyl sulfate–polyacrylamide gel electrophoresis (SDS-PAGE) in the second dimension. Following separation by 2-DE, the proteins can be visualized via a number of different techniques, such as staining, radiolabeling, and immunodetection. The final step in the proteomic analysis is protein identification, which almost always involves some form of mass spectrometry, as mentioned before.

Although 2-DE and mass spectrometry have been the methods of choice for proteomic analysis, other methodologies are currently being developed. Protein microarray technology generally uses a platform for capturing proteins by immobilizing potential ligands (binding partners) on a solid surface, followed by the detection and identification of the bound protein.[32] Potential ligands include antibodies and nucleic acids, among other molecules. A specific example of microarray technology has been developed by the Luminex Corporation (Austin, TX). The Luminex xMAP system is a multiplexed microsphere-based suspension array platform for high-throughput protein and nucleic acid detection.[33] This platform is unique because it combines flow cytometry with conventional ELISA technology, which makes it relatively cost-effective and accessible to routine laboratories. Several recent studies have demonstrated its use as an efficient tool for both genetic and proteomic biomarker discovery.[33–36] Multiplex analysis can be very useful for examining the effects of an intervention on numerous biomarkers in clinical research studies, particularly when there may be a small sample volume of stored plasma or serum.[34] However, some multiplex assays may require validation before selection in a clinical research protocol because low assay sensitivity and relatively poor correlation to conventional ELISA methods may be problematic, particularly for some analytes with very low plasma concentrations.[34] Other proteomic approaches under development include microfluidic in-solution assay systems and yeast two-hybrid systems.

"SYSTEMS BIOLOGY": AN INTEGRATED APPROACH TO FUTURE BIOMARKER DISCOVERY

In an attempt to capture the full complexity of disease phenotypes, several other areas of "-omics" research are being explored. These include the fields of transcriptomics, which explores the analysis of universal gene expression through cellular mRNA expression profiles, and metabolomics, which aims to identify and measure the time-related concentration, activity, and flux of endogenous small molecules or metabolites (<2 kD, e.g., carbohydrates, peptides, and lipids) in various cell types, tissues, and biofluids.

Transcriptomics has been successfully used to identify molecular signatures based on specific gene expression profiles and has led to the development of molecular signature–based biomarkers in oncology. In cardiovascular research, transcriptomics has been used as a tool to identify specific gene expression profiles for the differentiation between ischemic and nonischemic cardiomyopathy[37] and to improve the diagnosis of transplant rejection in cardiac allograft recipients.[38]

It is estimated that the human metabolome comprises approximately 3000 small molecules, and efforts are currently underway to record the complete human plasma metabolome.[39] Examination of the human metabolome, which is significantly smaller in comparison with the genome, transcriptome, and proteome, may allow for a more efficient approach to gaining in-depth understanding of disease phenotypes. However, this remains purely speculative at this time, because there are insufficient data available from metabolomics studies.

Recently, investigators have attempted to use an integrated approach, also known as "systems biology" or "integromics," to systematically assess variations in genes, RNA, proteins, and metabolites.[40] Most likely, future technological advances in systems biology will continue to drive the development of new tools for biomarker development and improve our understanding of the pathogenesis of human diseases. However, for the field of systems biology to contribute significantly to our current understanding of cardiovascular disease phenotypes, it is paramount that generally accepted standards for biomarker discovery and validation be established.

SUMMARY/CONCLUSIONS

Identification of individuals at increased risk for cardiovascular events is a key concept used to determine which individuals require the initiation of lipid-modifying therapy as well as the intensity of therapy. The use of multiple new biomarkers has shown promise for assessing risk for coronary heart disease and stroke.[41–43] Accurate identification of individuals at increased risk for cardiovascular disease events will allow clinical trials in primary prevention to be performed with smaller and more manageable sample sizes and shorter durations of follow-up, therefore reducing the cost of research.[44] In addition, the identification of populations who do not meet the treatment criteria of the current guidelines will allow for the use of a placebo control group, as in Justification for the Use of Statins in Primary Prevention: an Intervention Trial Evaluating Rosuvastatin (JUPITER),[45,46] which was stopped early because of clear benefit.[47]

However, the development of "personalized" medicine and the successful clinical development of novel therapies for atherosclerosis will require much greater advances in biomarker discovery and validation, as there are currently no validated assays that quantitatively assess either the burden or activity of atherosclerosis in humans.

REFERENCES

1. Expert Panel on Detection, Evaluation, and Treatment of High Blood Cholesterol in Adults: Executive summary of the third report of the National Cholesterol Education Program (NCEP) Expert Panel on Detection, Evaluation, and Treatment of High Blood Cholesterol in Adults (Adult Treatment Panel III). *JAMA* 2001;285:2486–2497.
2. Ross R: Atherosclerosis—an inflammatory disease. *N Engl J Med* 1999;340:115–126.
3. Packard RR, Libby P: Inflammation in atherosclerosis: From vascular biology to biomarker discovery and risk prediction. *Clin Chem* 2008;54:24–38.
4. Libby P, Ridker PM, Maseri A: Inflammation and atherosclerosis. *Circulation* 2002;105:1135–1143.
5. Stary HC, Chandler AB, Glagov S, et al: A definition of initial, fatty streak, and intermediate lesions of atherosclerosis: A report from the Committee on Vascular Lesions of the Council on Arteriosclerosis, American Heart Association. *Circulation* 1994;89:2462–2478.
6. Podrez EA, Schmitt D, Hoff HF, Hazen SL: Myeloperoxidase-generated reactive nitrogen species convert LDL into an atherogenic form *in vitro*. *J Clin Invest* 1999;103:1547–1560.
7. Vasan RS: Biomarkers of cardiovascular disease: Molecular basis and practical considerations. *Circulation* 2006;113:2335–2362.
8. Biomarkers Definitions Working Group: Biomarkers and surrogate endpoints: Preferred definitions and conceptual framework. *Clin Pharmacol Ther* 2001;69:89–95.
9. Zou KH, O'Malley AJ, Mauri L: Receiver-operating characteristic analysis for evaluating diagnostic tests and predictive models. *Circulation* 2007;115:654–657.

10. Hanley JA, McNeil BJ: The meaning and use of the area under a receiver operating characteristic (ROC) curve. *Radiology* 1982;143:29–36.
11. Cook NR: Statistical evaluation of prognostic versus diagnostic models: Beyond the ROC curve. *Clin Chem* 2008;54:17–23.
12. Oellerich M: Enzyme-immunoassay: A review. *J Clin Chem Clin Biochem* 1984;22:895–904.
13. International Human Genome Sequencing Consortium: Finishing the euchromatic sequence of the human genome. *Nature* 2004;431:931–945.
14. International HapMap Consortium: The International HapMap Project. *Nature* 2003;426:789–796.
15. Gibbons GH, Liew CC, Goodarzi MO, et al: Genetic markers: Progress and potential for cardiovascular disease. *Circulation* 2004;109:IV47–IV58.
16. Tabor HK, Risch NJ, Myers RM: Candidate-gene approaches for studying complex genetic traits: Practical considerations. *Nat Rev Genet* 2002;3:391–397.
17. Hirschhorn JN, Lohmueller K, Byrne E, Hirschhorn K: A comprehensive review of genetic association studies. *Genet Med* 2002;4:45–61.
18. Samani NJ, Erdmann J, Hall AS, et al: Genomewide association analysis of coronary artery disease. *N Engl J Med* 2007;357: 443–453.
19. McPherson R, Pertsemlidis A, Kavaslar N, et al: A common allele on chromosome 9 associated with coronary heart disease. *Science* 2007;316:1488–1491.
20. Helgadottir A, Thorleifsson G, Manolescu A, et al: A common variant on chromosome 9p21 affects the risk of myocardial infarction. *Science* 2007;316:1491–1493.
21. Jang WG, Kim HS, Park KG, et al: Analysis of proteome and transcriptome of tumor necrosis factor alpha stimulated vascular smooth muscle cells with or without alpha lipoic acid. *Proteomics* 2004;4:3383–3393.
22. Donners MM, Verluyten MJ, Bouwman FG, et al: Proteomic analysis of differential protein expression in human atherosclerotic plaque progression. *J Pathol* 2005;206:39–45.
23. Knecht M, Regitz-Zagrosek V, Pleissner KP, et al: Characterization of myocardial protein composition in dilated cardiomyopathy by two-dimensional gel electrophoresis. *Eur Heart J* 1994;15 Suppl D:37–44.
24. Jungblut P, Otto A, Zeindl-Eberhart E, et al: Protein composition of the human heart: The construction of a myocardial two-dimensional electrophoresis database. *Electrophoresis* 1994;15: 685–707.
25. Mateos-Caceres PJ, Garcia-Mendez A, Lopez Farre A, et al: Proteomic analysis of plasma from patients during an acute coronary syndrome. *J Am Coll Cardiol* 2004;44:1578–1583.
26. Gerszten RE, Wang TJ: The search for new cardiovascular biomarkers. *Nature* 2008;451:949–952.
27. Mayr M, Zhang J, Greene AS, et al: Proteomics-based development of biomarkers in cardiovascular disease: Mechanistic, clinical, and therapeutic insights. *Mol Cell Proteomics* 2006;5: 1853–1864.
28. Blanco-Colio LM, Martin-Ventura JL, Vivanco F, et al: Biology of atherosclerotic plaques: What we are learning from proteomic analysis. *Cardiovasc Res* 2006;72:18–29.
29. Anderson NL, Anderson NG: The human plasma proteome: History, character, and diagnostic prospects. *Mol Cell Proteomics* 2002;1:845–867.
30. O'Farrell PH: High resolution two-dimensional electrophoresis of proteins. *J Biol Chem* 1975;250:4007–4021.
31. Klose J: Protein mapping by combined isoelectric focusing and electrophoresis of mouse tissues. A novel approach to testing for induced point mutations in mammals. *Humangenetik* 1975;26:231–243.
32. Kingsmore SF: Multiplexed protein measurement: Technologies and applications of protein and antibody arrays. *Nat Rev Drug Discov* 2006;5:310–320.
33. Dunbar SA: Applications of Luminex xMAP technology for rapid, high-throughput multiplexed nucleic acid detection. *Clin Chim Acta* 2006;363:71–82.
34. Liu MY, Xydakis AM, Hoogeveen RC, et al: Multiplexed analysis of biomarkers related to obesity and the metabolic syndrome in human plasma, using the Luminex-100 system. *Clin Chem* 2005;51:1102–1109.
35. Binder SR, Hixson C, Glossenger J: Protein arrays and pattern recognition: New tools to assist in the identification and management of autoimmune disease. *Autoimmun Rev* 2006;5: 234–241.
36. Tozzoli R: Recent advances in diagnostic technologies and their impact in autoimmune diseases. *Autoimmun Rev* 2007;6:334–340.
37. Kittleson MM, Ye SQ, Irizarry RA, et al: Identification of a gene expression profile that differentiates between ischemic and nonischemic cardiomyopathy. *Circulation* 2004;110:3444–3451.
38. Morgun A, Shulzhenko N, Perez-Diez A, et al: Molecular profiling improves diagnoses of rejection and infection in transplanted organs. *Circ Res* 2006;98:e74–e83.
39. Wishart DS, Tzur D, Knox C, et al: HMDB: The Human Metabolome Database. *Nucleic Acids Res* 2007;35:D521–D526.
40. Thomas CE, Ganji G: Integration of genomic and metabonomic data in systems biology—are we 'there' yet? *Curr Opin Drug Discov Devel* 2006;9:92–100.
41. Wang TJ, Gona P, Larson MG, et al: Multiple biomarkers for the prediction of first major cardiovascular events and death. *N Engl J Med* 2006;355:2631–2639.
42. Zethelius B, Berglund L, Sundstrom J, et al: Use of multiple biomarkers to improve the prediction of death from cardiovascular causes. *N Engl J Med* 2008;358:2107–2116.
43. Ballantyne CM, Hoogeveen RC, Bang H, et al: Lipoprotein-associated phospholipase A_2, high-sensitivity C-reactive protein, and risk for incident ischemic stroke in middle-aged men and women in the Atherosclerosis Risk in Communities (ARIC) study. *Arch Intern Med* 2005;165:2479–2484.
44. Brune K, Katus HA, Moecks J, et al: The concentration of N-terminal pro-B-type natriuretic peptide predicts the risk of cardiovascular adverse events from antiinflammatory drugs: A pilot trial. *Clin Chem* 2008;54:1149–1157.
45. Ridker PM: Rosuvastatin in the primary prevention of cardiovascular disease among patients with low levels of low-density lipoprotein cholesterol and elevated high-sensitivity C-reactive protein: Rationale and design of the JUPITER trial. *Circulation* 2003;108:2292–2297.
46. Ridker PM, Fonseca FA, Genest J, et al: Baseline characteristics of participants in the JUPITER trial, a randomized placebo-controlled primary prevention trial of statin therapy among individuals with low low-density lipoprotein cholesterol and elevated high-sensitivity C-reactive protein. *Am J Cardiol* 2007;100:1659–1664.
47. U.S. National Institutes of Health: JUPITER—Crestor 20mg Versus Placebo in Prevention of Cardiovascular (CV) Events. Available at http://clinicaltrials.gov/ct2/show/NCT00239681. Accessed 21 May 2008.

CHAPTER 16

Noninvasive Assessments of Atherosclerosis for Risk Stratification

Patrick J. Devine and Allen J. Taylor

INTRODUCTION

Although mortality from coronary heart disease (CHD) has declined significantly over the past three decades, CHD remains the leading cause of death in adults. It is estimated that the lifetime risk of CHD in asymptomatic patients at 40 years of age is 49% in men and 32% in women.[1] In light of this, there is considerable interest in identifying heightened risk for CHD at an early, presymptomatic stage so that appropriate preventive therapy can be offered.

The concepts of risk assessment and reduction remain the cornerstones of preventive cardiology practice. To achieve this, the Framingham Risk Score (FRS) remains a widely used clinical tool that has guided the delivery of preventive cardiology over the past 30 years.[2,3] It has moderate accuracy for the prediction of incident CHD over modest time periods, but it is limited by its lack of inclusion of all contributory factors for CHD (e.g., lifestyle factors and family history), has reduced applicability in multiracial ethnic populations and select age groups (particularly the old and the young), assigns a large group of middle-aged patients to an intermediate–CHD risk category whose treatments and targets are less informed by guidelines, and does not accurately discriminate lifelong risk for CHD. Subsequently, many patients are not identified as candidates for preventive therapy with medications such as statins and aspirin because they are deemed "low or intermediate" risk for incident CHD. Presymptomatic testing through detection of subclinical atherosclerosis refines the assessment of global risk, specifically in those subjects classified as "intermediate risk" by the FRS. Through the assessment of subclinical atherosclerosis, either anatomically with carotid ultrasound, coronary computed tomography, and magnetic resonance imaging or functionally with brachial flow-mediated dilation (FMD), a patient's individual cardiovascular risk can be better defined.

RATIONALE FOR SCREENING

The first clinical manifestation of CHD can range from stable angina to unstable angina, acute myocardial infarction, and even sudden cardiac death.[4] Such catastrophic consequences can surface without previous warning signs in the asymptomatic patient. By screening for the early detection of CHD during the subclinical stage of disease, subjects at increased risk for an adverse cardiac event can be identified and offered appropriate preventive therapy and education for behavioral change. Thus, the risk stratification of asymptomatic patients and identification of high-risk patients are critical initial steps in preventing future adverse cardiac events such as myocardial infarction and sudden cardiac death.

THE FRAMINGHAM RISK SCORE: APPLICATION, LIMITATIONS

The FRS is a well-characterized risk assessment tool recommended as a first step in coronary risk assessment. By including risk factors of gender, age, total cholesterol, high-density lipoprotein (HDL) cholesterol, systolic blood pressure, and cigarette use, a patient's 10-year risk for myocardial infarction and cardiac death can be easily estimated. The clinical importance of the FRS is underscored by its inclusion in guideline-based publications such as the National Cholesterol Education Program Adult Treatment Panel III (NCEP ATP III) guidelines released in 2001.[5] These guidelines continue to support the panel's previous recommendations for intensive management of low-density lipoprotein (LDL) in individuals known to have CHD or CHD risk equivalents, while providing a new focus of intensive management of LDL cholesterol for primary prevention in individuals with multiple risk factors. Individuals with two or more risk factors are recommended to have their FRS calculated. Individuals with a 10-year predicted CHD risk of 20% or higher (high risk) are considered to have CHD risk equivalents and are urged to maintain an LDL cholesterol level of <100 mg/dL. For those with an FRS of 10% to 20% (intermediate risk), an LDL cholesterol goal of <130 mg/dL is advised. Low-risk patients have an FRS of <10% (Figure 16-1).

The NCEP ATP III guidelines were recently applied to 13,769 participants in the Third National Health and Nutrition Examination Survey.[6] Extrapolating these results to the U.S. population ages 20 to 79 years revealed that approximately 81.7% (140 million adults) fell into the low-risk group, 15.5% (23 million adults) fell into the intermediate-risk group, while only 2.9% (4 million adults) fell into the high-risk group. Thus, only 2.9% of the population would be defined as having CHD equivalents and therefore be recommended for intensive lipid therapy according to the NCEP ATP III guidelines. Clearly this represents a gross underestimation of overall lifetime cardiovascular risk by the FRS and underestimates the size of the intermediate-risk group among middle-aged individuals.

While the Framingham Heart Study has been a rich source of information regarding risk assessment for cardiovascular diseases, there are several limitations that need to be considered when applying the FRS to an individual patient. Young patients were underrepresented and had few coronary events in the Framingham Heart Study cohort. Because of the dominant effect of age as a primary risk factor for cardiovascular disease (reflecting age-related incidence of coronary risk factors and accounting for duration of exposure), there is a low likelihood of identifying young patients with a high lifetime risk using the FRS. In fact, one study suggested that almost 70% of young men and women (defined as men ages ≤55 years and women ages ≤65 years) who presented with acute myocardial infarction as their first manifestations of CHD were classified as low risk by FRS.[7] As a 10-year model, the FRS is ideal for identifying patients who are at increased short-term risk for future incident coronary events but does not accurately reflect the effect of risk factor exposure over time and the overall lifetime risk of coronary disease, particularly among young patients. This is illustrated by a study from the Framingham cohort in which the lifetime rate of development of CHD was compared with the 10-year prediction rates for various age groups.[8] It was found that younger subjects in the lower-risk groups who had a very low 10-year risk for CHD still had a substantial lifetime risk for CHD. As an example, 50-year-old men in the lowest risk tertile had a 10-year cumulative risk of 1 in 25 but had a lifetime risk of 44%, which was similar to that observed in high-risk patients (54%).

The FRS is also limited by its lack of inclusion of other potential risk predictors of coronary disease, such as family history of premature coronary disease. A family history of premature coronary disease is a widely accepted risk factor for the development of coronary disease. In an analysis of the Framingham cohort by Lloyd-Jones et al., a validated positive family history of premature coronary disease conveyed a two-fold increased risk for future coronary events in men and a 70% increase in women.[9] Lastly, because of the relatively homogenous demographics of the Framingham cohort (predominantly a white, middle-class population), the results of the FRS are most applicable to whites and may be inaccurate when applied to other ethnic groups.[10–12] While the FRS performed well for white and black men and women, one study showed that FRS overestimated the cardiac event rate for Japanese American men, Hispanic men, and Native American women.[13]

Because the FRS underestimates the lifetime incidence of CHD, a new refined risk assessment model would be helpful to guide aggressive primary prevention while limiting unnecessary therapy. Presymptomatic testing using noninvasive cardiovascular imaging has emerged as a potential tool to add incremental

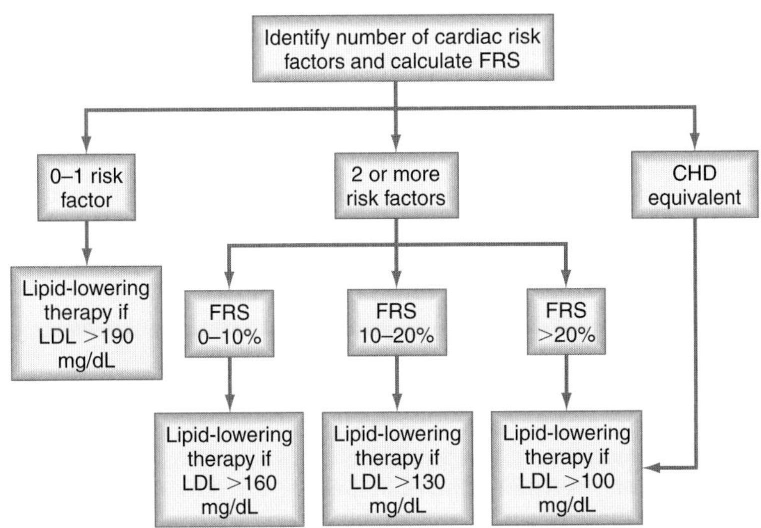

FIGURE 16-1 Using the Framingham Risk Score (FRS) in the identification of asymptomatic patients for lipid-lowering therapy. Cardiac risk factors include cigarette smoking, hypertension (blood pressure >140/90 mm Hg or taking antihypertensive medication), family history of premature coronary heart disease (CHD; CHD in first-degree male relative <55 years of age or CHD in female first-degree relative <65 years of age), age (men, ≥45 years; women, ≥55 years), and low high-density lilpoprotein (HDL) cholesterol (< 40 mg/dL). CHD equivalents include diabetes mellitus and the presence of any noncoronary atherosclerotic disease such as stroke, transient ischemic attack, peripheral vascular disease or abdominal aortic aneurysm.

prognostic value beyond that provided by standard cardiovascular risk factors.

CORONARY ARTERY CALCIUM SCORING

The association between vascular calcification and vascular disease has long been appreciated by pathologists. Calcification of the coronary arteries is part of the atherosclerotic process, occurring in small amounts in early atherosclerotic lesions and found more frequently with advanced lesions and older age. The origins of radiographic detection of calcified coronary atherosclerosis began with cardiac fluoroscopy, which was primarily a qualitative technique. The development of electron beam computed tomography (EBCT) in 1984 permitted noninvasive quantification of coronary artery calcium (CAC). Coronary calcium deposits have a high x-ray density that is approximately 2- to 10-fold higher than the low-density adjacent noncalcified tissue and surrounding fat tissue. The area/density method of CAC quantitation, originally known as the Agatston score, is the most widely adopted method of quantifying CAC. This unitless measurement is derived from the product of the area of calcification (mm^2) and its x-ray coefficient, a measure of maximal density that is measured in Hounsfield units (Figure 16-2). During the scan, approximately 40 axial slices, 3 mm in thickness, are obtained within seconds, delivering a relatively low dose of radiation estimated at less than 1 mSv. Although the advantage of EBCT is its temporal resolution, lower spatial resolution limits this scanner for cardiac CT applications beyond CAC quantitation. Subsequently, rapid developments in multislice computed tomography (MSCT) leading to improved temporal and spatial resolution allowed for its use as an alternative to EBCT for quantification of epicardial CAC. Presently, based on similar results in CAC scoring with these two methods (though most studies examining the prognostic implications of CAC have been conducted with EBCT), it is implied that MSCT-generated CAC scores have similar significance.[14]

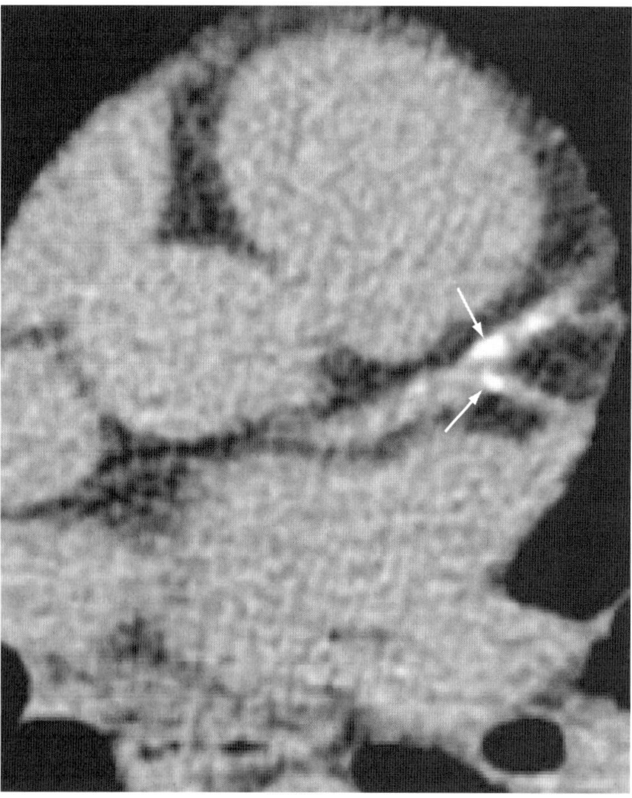

FIGURE 16-2 The Agatston method of calculating coronary artery calcium. For each coronary artery, a region of interest (ROI) is drawn around each calcified lesion. The area, *A*, of the ROI is determined. A weighting factor, *w*, is assigned based on the degree of attenuation as assessed by hounsfield units (HU). The Agatston score, *S*, is computed as the product of the weighting factor and the area: $S = w \times A$. The score for all lesions in all coronary arteries is summed to determine the total calcium burden. $W = 1$ if 130 to < 200 HU; 2 if 200 to < 300 HU; 3 if 300 to < 400 HU; and 4 if ≥ 400 HU.

Rationale of Coronary Artery Calcium Scoring for Risk Assessment

Although CAC is observed more extensively in atherosclerotic plaques associated with stable angina pectoris, patients with elevated CAC have higher incident rates of myocardial infarction and cardiac death.[15] This paradox can be readily explained by the fact that patients with a high burden of calcified plaque are also more likely to have noncalcified plaque that is more prone to rupture and thrombosis, and pathologic data suggest that prior subclinical plaque ruptures presage subsequent plaque calcification during healing. Although CAC detection does not specifically predict a stenotic or rupture-prone lesion,[16,17] its correlation with overall atherosclerotic disease burden has been well established.[18,19]

The ability to detect and quantify CAC as an early marker for subclinical atherosclerosis is the cornerstone of its role as a risk stratification tool in preventive cardiology. The limited ability of the FRS to identify patients at high risk for CHD was illustrated in a report of 1611 asymptomatic subjects who underwent CAC screening. Using the NCEP ATP III recommendations for lipid-lowering therapy, 59% of subjects with a CAC score greater than 400 and 73% with a score >75th percentile would not have qualified for pharmacotherapy.[20]

Prognostic Value of Coronary Artery Calcium

Multiple prospective studies have shown that high CAC scores are independently associated with increased risk for adverse coronary events. In a meta-analysis by Pletcher et al., it was found that the CAC score was associated with an increase in future CHD risk.[21] CAC scores were reported in one of four categories: no detectable CAC, low risk with a score of 1 to 100, medium risk with a score of 101 to 400, and high risk with a score of greater than 400. Figure 16-3 shows the adjusted odds ratios comparing the three positive groups with those with no detectable CAC. Increasing CAC scores carry progressively higher odds ratios, with scores greater than 400 having an odds ratio that is

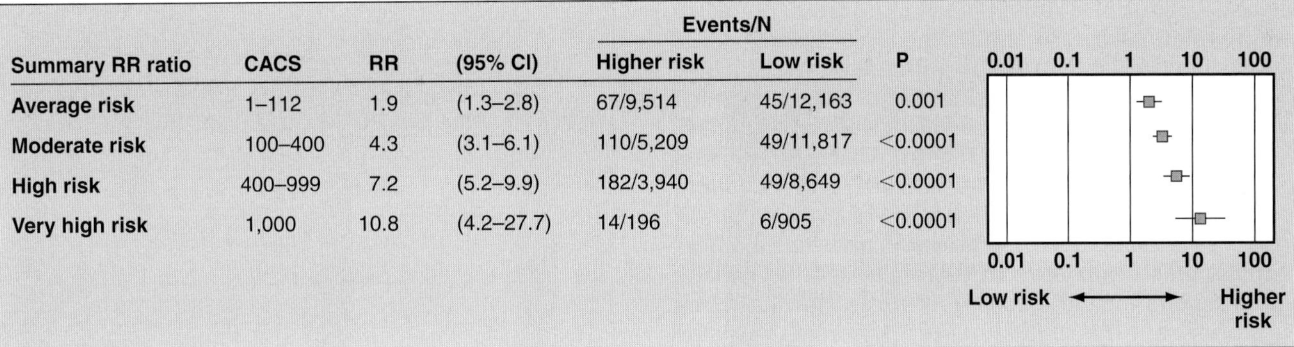

Summary RR ratio	CACS	RR	(95% CI)	Events/N Higher risk	Events/N Low risk	P
Average risk	1–112	1.9	(1.3–2.8)	67/9,514	45/12,163	0.001
Moderate risk	100–400	4.3	(3.1–6.1)	110/5,209	49/11,817	<0.0001
High risk	400–999	7.2	(5.2–9.9)	182/3,940	49/8,649	<0.0001
Very high risk	1,000	10.8	(4.2–27.7)	14/196	6/905	<0.0001

FIGURE 16-3 Adjusted relative risk (RR) comparing risk of a coronary heart disease event in persons with low (1–100), medium (101–400), and high (>400) coronary artery calcium scores (CACS) with those of persons without calcification. Error bars indicate a 95% confidence interval (CI). From Ref. 30.

10 times higher than those found in the normal group. The authors further found that the relative risks reported by the four studies were between 4.3 and 17.0 in those individuals with high CAC score (>400) (Table 16-1). These relative risks are generally higher than those of standard risk factors, such as the presence of diabetes, use of tobacco, extreme values of LDL cholesterol or HDL cholesterol, or blood pressure, that individually confer a relative risk of 1.5 to 3.4.

Early controversy about whether CAC predicted hard cardiovascular events (myocardial infarction or cardiac death) has dissipated with the publication of higher-quality studies in larger patient cohorts.[22–25] The largest observational series to date more than 25,000 consecutive asymptomatic patients referred for CAC scanning confirmed these findings.[26] With a mean follow-up of 6.8 years, this study showed that CAC is an independent estimator of all-cause mortality and that patients without CAC had an extremely low event rate, with a 12-year survival rate of 99.4%. Conversely, patients with CAC scores of greater than 1000 had a 12-year survival rate of 76.9%.

Most studies evaluating the predictive value of CAC have used absolute values of the calcium score, although few asymptomatic patients who undergo screening have calcium scores in the range that is most predictive of future cardiac events. In one series, for example, only 7% of a screening population of 632 patients had calcium scores greater than 400.[27] Alternatively, a calcium score above the 75th percentile for age and gender may be a better predictor of future cardiac events. Table 16-1 displays the percentile strata of CAC for both men and women across different age groups.[28] For any given CAC score, a greater number of calcified coronary vessels predicts worse cardiovascular outcomes.[26]

The Clinical Application of Coronary Artery Calcium Scoring in the Asymptomatic Patient

Bayesian theory relates the post-test likelihood to the pretest probability for the particular patient undergoing a given test with defined test operating characteristics. For example, CAC in a low-risk (as assessed by the FRS) patient would not significantly affect post-test prediction for future events in the short term. Conversely, a negative calcium scan in an otherwise high-risk patient would not reduce the risk to a level at which preventive measures would be withheld. The value of CAC assessment appears to be in patients with an intermediate pretest probability as predicted by the FRS. In the South Bay Heart Watch study, Greenland et al. concluded that a high CAC score was predictive of high risk among patients with a FRS greater than 10% (intermediate risk) but not in patients with an FRS less than 10% (low risk).[29] Furthermore, recent data from additional reports provide further support that CAC scoring adds incremental prognostic value for patients with intermediate risk according to the FRS. As seen in Figure 16-3, intermediate-risk patients with CAC score greater than 400 would be expected to have event rates similar to those of patients with CHD risk equivalent (10-year risk of >20%). In the recent American College of Cardiology Foundation (ACCF)/American Heart Association (AHA) consensus document, the task force concluded that it was reasonable to consider CAC measurement in patients with intermediate risk by FRS with the assumption that such patients with high CAC would be reclassified to a "high" risk status and be treated with aggressive preventive therapy accordingly.[30] The task force did not recommend the use of CAC scoring in

TABLE 16-1 Distribution of Coronary Artery Calcium Scores for Women and Men Across Different Age Groups

	Age Groups													
	40–44		45–49		50–54		55–59		60–64		65–69		≥70	
	Women	Men	Women	Men	Women	Men	Women	Men	Women	Men	Women	Men	Women	Men
Median	0	0	0	2	0	16	0	47	2	121	15	205	35	295
75th Percentile	0	11	1	29	3	94	20	222	59	453	122	672	195	794
90th Percentile	9	56	17	142	48	321	155	671	202	1026	527	1333	645	1571

low- and high-risk populations. Figure 16-4 offers an example of an algorithm employing CAC scoring in the risk stratification of patients asymptomatic for CHD.

Serial CAC testing is presently not recommended because of the lack of understanding of the independent relationship to CHD outcomes. Preliminary data suggest that a CAC score progression of 15% or greater per year may be associated with a worse prognosis.[31–33] Further work is needed in this area. The use of cardiac CT imaging as a surrogate in therapeutic drug trials to identify agents that lead to CAC stabilization has been disappointing. Most notably statin therapy[34] and the intensity of statin treatment[35] have not been associated with slowed CAC progression. These data further limit the value of serial CAC scanning as a surrogate to tailor individual patient treatment.

Coronary Artery Calcium and Future Challenges

Despite the potential benefits of CAC screening, there are a few limitations that challenge its widespread adoption in the risk assessment of CHD. First, it has not been proven that instituting pharmacologic therapy in asymptomatic patients with CAC ultimately improves outcomes. However, data from the Prospective Army Coronary Calcium study showed that statin and aspirin use are strongly influenced by coronary calcium within a screening cohort under community-based care.[36] Among 1620 men followed for up to 6 years after CAC screening, the use of statin and aspirin were both significantly increased by 3.5-fold in subjects with CAC independent of other coronary risk factors. Furthermore, the use of aspirin and statin combined was sevenfold more likely (Figure 16-5). Interestingly, CAC also influenced the prescription of statins in subjects relative to NCEP ATP III guidelines such that statins were more commonly provided in all patients, regardless of whether the LDL cholesterol was above or below target. These data provide the first indication that community-based preventive cardiology management can be meaningfully altered by the use of CAC scoring. Whether CAC scanning can be reasonably extended to low-risk patients to refine lifetime risk of CHD is an area of active study. Lastly, the cost-effectiveness of presymptomatic testing with coronary atherosclerosis imaging has not been well defined, but it is likely to be more dependent on the subsequent therapeutic decisions and medical adherence than on the test itself.

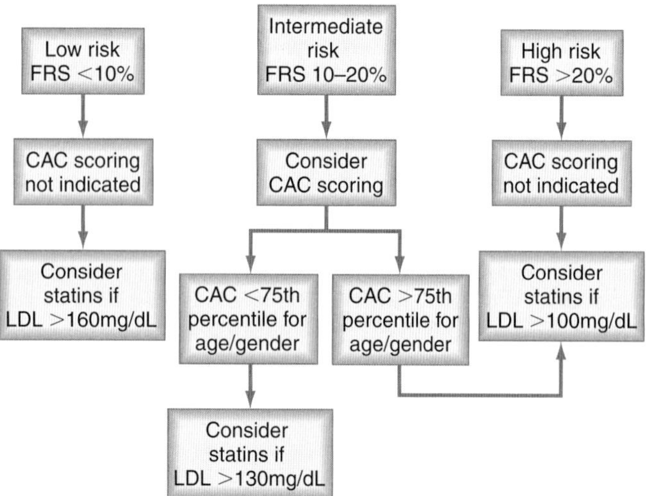

FIGURE 16-4 Implementing coronary artery calcium (CAC) in risk stratifying asymptomatic patients for lipid therapy. FRS, Framigham Risk Score; LDL, low-density lipoprotein.

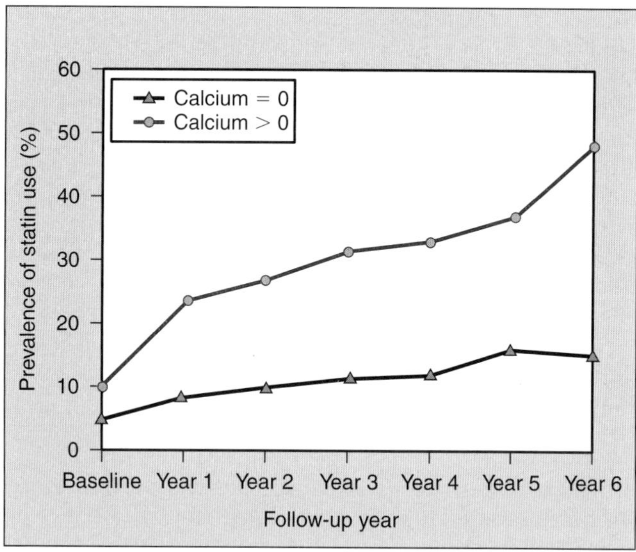

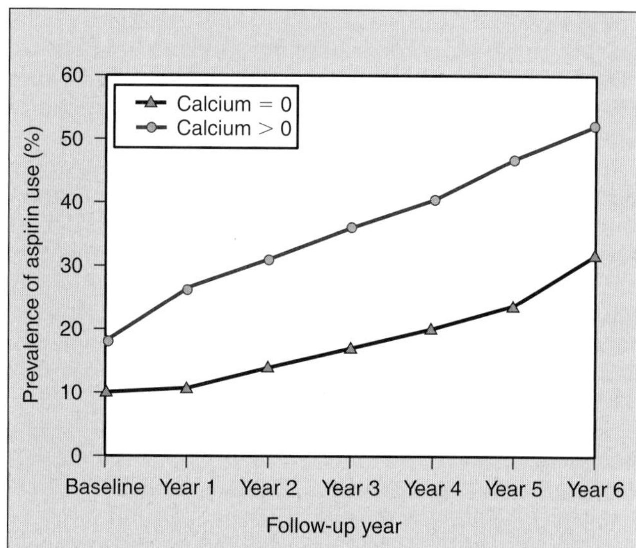

FIGURE 16-5 Prevalence of provision of statin and aspirin over 6 years of community-based follow-up among 1620 male participants of the Prospective Army Coronary Calcium Project. From Ref. 36.

Atherosclerotic disease burden often varies from a patient's chronological age, leading to the concept of identifying vascular age as an alternative for integration of CAC with the FRS. Shaw et al. used CAC to estimate the number of life years lost (calcium-adjusted age) in 10,377 asymptomatic individuals referred for EBCT screening who were followed for 5 years for all-cause mortality.[37] In linear prediction models, a calcium score less than 10 resulted in a reduction in observed age of 10 years in subjects older than 70 years, while a calcium score geater than 400 added as much as 30 years of age to younger patients. Furthermore, using calcium adjustments to age, 55% of those with a previous low-risk FRS were escalated to intermediate risk ($P < 0.0001$) while 45% of those with an unadjusted intermediate FRS were reclassified as high risk ($P < 0.0001$). CAC-adjusted age was a better predictor of mortality than observed age, leading to the conclusion that an integrated risk scoring system using an individual's biological age as determined by CAC instead of chronological age would likely refine the risk assessment process.

CORONARY MULTISLICE COMPUTED TOMOGRAPHY ANGIOGRAPHY

The presence of CAC is associated with increased plaque burden and increased cardiovascular risk. A potential concern, however, is the presence of isolated noncalcified plaques in the setting of a CAC score of zero. Theoretically, the identification of patients with noncalcified plaques could possibly improve or refine risk stratification (Figure 16-6). With the advent of MSCT contrast angiography, direct visualization of coronary plaque is now possible. This has stimulated interest in the angiographic evaluation of coronary plaque as a potential tool for risk assessment in CHD.

The occurrence of isolated noncalcified plaque was recently estimated in a cohort of 161 asymptomatic patients with intermediate risk by FRS.[38] In this study, 6.2% of patients had noncalcified plaques as their only manifestation of coronary atherosclerosis. Knez et al. studied 2115 consecutive symptomatic patients who underwent both EBCT and coronary angiography.[39] No calcium was found in 7 of 872 (0.7%) men and 1 of 383 (0.03%) women who had significant luminal stenosis. Seven of these eight patients were younger than

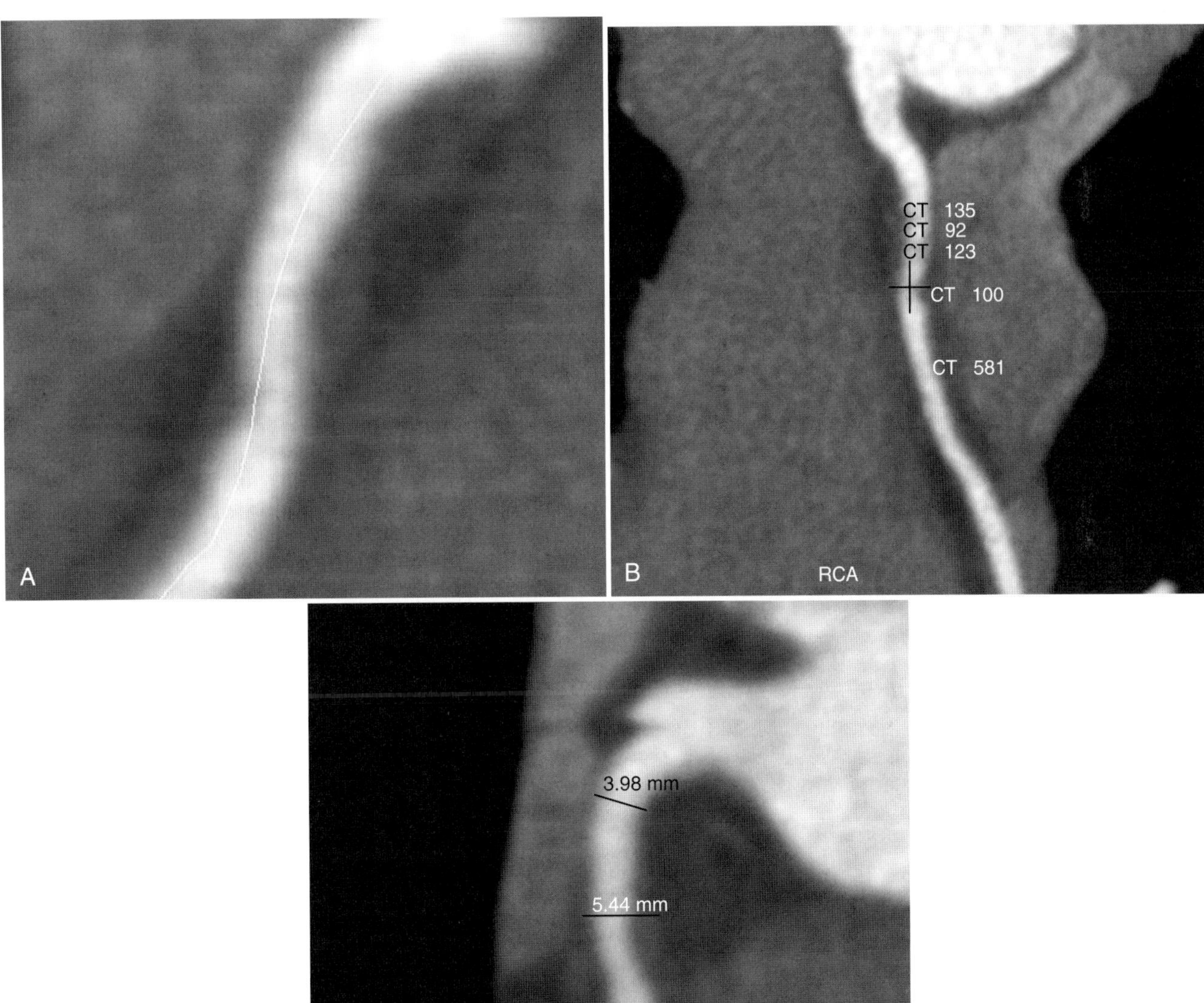

FIGURE 16-6 Coronary computed tomography (CT) angiography images of noncalcified plaque from the proximal right coronary artery (RCA) *(panel* **A***)*. The CT density of the plaque was >90 HU, consistent with fibrous plaque *(panel* **B***)*. Outward arterial remodeling was seen, with a remodeling index (comparison of proximal arterial diameter and lesion arterial diameter) of 1.37 *(panel* **C***)*.

45 years of age. Several other reports indicate that CAC scoring is not sensitive in patients younger than 45 years of age, leading to the hypothesis that MSCT, particularly among select subgroups (i.e., young patients, intermediate-risk patients with no evidence of CAC), may be useful. However, it should be noted that a CAC score of zero is associated with an extremely low risk (0.2% per year) of cardiovascular events over 3 to 5 years.[26] Thus, the clinical value of detection of noncalcified plaque remains unknown.

Methods of quantitation of noncalcified plaque are in development, with the requirement for high spatial and temporal resolution. Leber et al. compared the assessment of total coronary plaque volume by 64-slice MSCT with intravascular ultrasound (IVUS), considered the gold standard for plaque quantification.[40] Although MSCT underestimated plaque relative to IVUS (54/65 plaques correctly identified), correlation for determination of overall plaque volume was good ($R^2 = 0.69$). The major obstacle for plaque identification and quantification is the edge definition of the outer vessel boundary, which makes it difficult to distinguish between plaque and soft tissue. Even with the later-generation scanners such as 64-slice scanners, the limited spatial resolution prevents an exact separation of lumen, plaque, and vessel wall and the subsequent detection of very early stages of coronary atherosclerosis. Furthermore, limits of temporal resolution create the potential for false-positive findings resulting from motion artifact/blurring.

Further characterization of noncalcified plaques is proposed as an additional risk stratification method. Because of the different x-ray density profiles of the various plaque components, MSCT can potentially distinguish unstable, and presumably lipid-laden, coronary plaques from more stable, fibrous plaques. Fibrous plaques are proposed to display mean attenuation values of approximately 90 Hounsfield units, whereas plaques with large lipid-rich cores have lower attenuation patterns (30–50 Hounsfield units).[41] However, substantial overlap of the CT densities of fibrous and soft plaques limits their consistent differentiation. Beyond CT density of plaque, other findings suggestive of high-risk morphological features of coronary plaques include the presence of outward remodeling of the vessel wall or spotty calcifications.[42] To date, there is no evidence that plaque characterization by either Hounsfield units or by the presence of high-risk features with MSCT has any meaningful impact on risk stratification or patient management beyond the detection of CAC alone.

Several features of MSCT limit enthusiasm for its use as a cardiovascular risk assessment tool in asymptomatic individuals. Increased clarity of images provided by new-generation scanners requires radiation doses which can range from 4.8 to 21.6 mSv.[43] Other issues to consider are the need for intravenous contrast and the potential for needless follow-up radiographic studies for incidental findings.[44] Furthermore, there is the potential that physicians may prescribe statins to asymptomatic patients based solely on the "presence of plaque," ignoring more extensively studied and validated parameters of risk assessment such as CAC. Given these limitations, in the 2006 ACCF/AHA consensus document, the task force concluded that asymptomatic patients should not undergo routine screening with coronary MSCT angiography.[30]

CAROTID INTIMA–MEDIA THICKNESS

Carotid intima–media thickness (CIMT) is associated with known cardiovascular risk factors and accurately detects the presence and extent of atherosclerosis. This relationship allows for its use as a noninvasive marker of early, preclinical atherosclerosis. CIMT is related to CHD risk factors, future cardiovascular events, and atherosclerosis elsewhere in the vascular system. Although it is primarily used as a research tool in epidemiologic trials and in clinical trials assessing the therapeutic effect of antiatherosclerotic drugs, it has the potential as a simple, low-cost, safe test to have a clinical role in the primary prevention of CHD. Specific imaging advantages of CIMT include its noninvasive nature without a requirement for ionizing radiation or intravenous contrast and the low likelihood of incidental scan findings.

Definition and Measurement of Carotid Intima–Media Thickness

The arterial wall consists of three layers—the intima, the media, and the adventitia. Clinically detectable atherosclerosis initially consists of the gradual thickening of the intima and media. Through direct visualization of the wall of a superficial artery such as the carotid artery, B-mode ultrasound can measure this thickening as the combined thickness of the intima and media because these two layers cannot be reliably distinguished using ultrasound. The intima–media thickness, defined as the thickness between the intima–lumina and the media–adventitia interfaces, is measured (Figure 16-7).

Sonograms are generally obtained with the patient in the supine position and his or her head turned

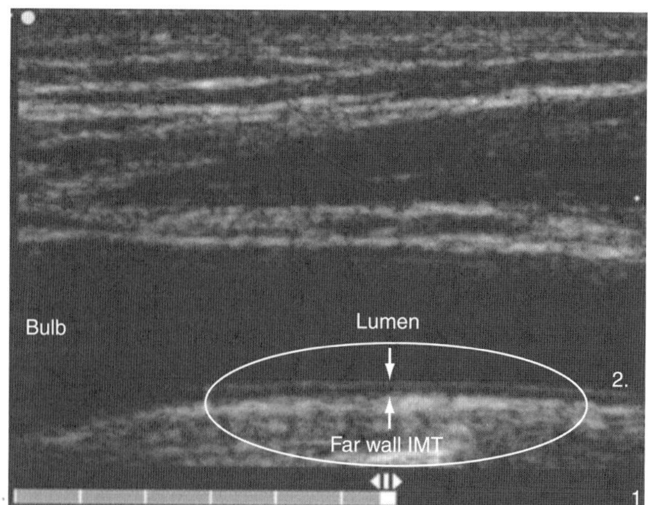

FIGURE 16-7 Carotid ultrasound image (10 MHz) of the distal common carotid artery. The two arrows represent the intima–lumina and media–adventitia interfaces which collectively border the carotid intima–media thickness (CIMT). In this example, CIMT was reported as the mean thickness over the distal 1 cm of the far wall of the common carotid artery.

slightly to the contralateral side. Longitudinal images of the carotid artery focusing on the imaging target of interest (e.g., far wall of the common carotid artery) are acquired with linear digital ultrasound probes at high frequency (≥10 to 13 MHz). Because of systolic arterial expansion and the resultant CIMT thinning, digital images are acquired from an end-diastolic frame of the cine-loop recording, electronically stored, and transferred to a workstation for quantification. The intimal–luminal and medial–adventitial borders can be manually or automatically traced (using edge-detection software) to measure the CIMT (Figure 16-6). Measurement of the far wall of the distal 1 cm of the common carotid artery is preferred over measurement of other segments, such as the carotid bulb or internal carotid artery, because of its greater reproducibility and the completeness of the evaluation. CIMT in different segments is equally predictive of future cardiovascular events.[45–49] Several studies have verified the reproducibility of CIMT measurements. Most of the measurement variability in CIMT is caused by differences among observers whereas the within-observer variability over time appears to be very small.[50]

Normal CIMT values have been defined based on their distribution within a general, healthy population and have been classified according to age and gender.[51,52] CIMT increases with age and, on average, is slightly greater in men than in women. Slight racial differences have also been reported for CIMT, with thickness being highest in African Americans, the least in Hispanics, and intermediate in whites.[46,53,54] The definition of the upper limit of normal is arbitrary but is frequently set at the 75th percentile of CIMT distribution (Figure 16-8) for the determination of increased relative CHD risk. Alternatively, epidemiologic studies suggest that a CIMT of 1 mm or greater is associated with a significantly increased absolute risk of CHD.[51] Reliance on a single absolute threshold abnormality will result in underdetection of disease in younger individuals and overdetection in older individuals.

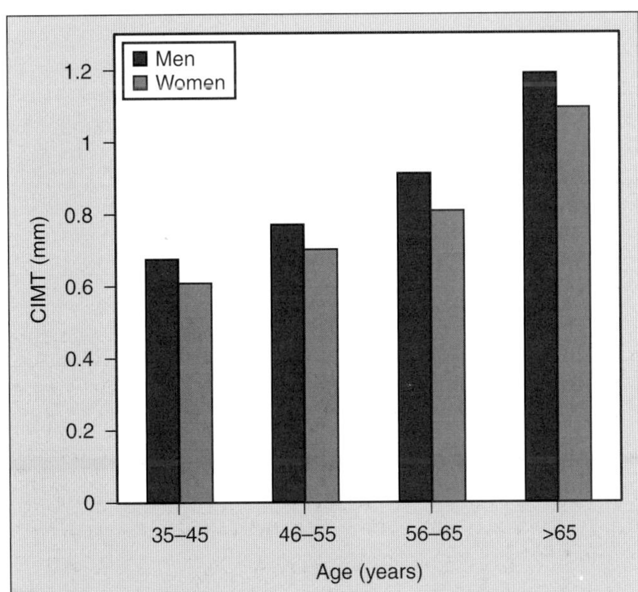

FIGURE 16-8 Approximate 75th percentile values for the common carotid intima–media thickness (CIMT) by age and gender.

Surrogate Marker for Atherosclerosis Risk

The Muscatine study followed 725 individuals from childhood to early adulthood (33–42 years of age) and found that CIMT was associated with the childhood presence of cardiovascular risk factors, especially total and LDL cholesterol in both genders and diastolic blood pressure in women.[55] Raitakari et al. also confirmed an association between childhood cardiovascular risk factors (namely, LDL cholesterol, systolic blood pressure, and smoking) and CIMT measured 21 years later.[56] In this study, adolescents with these cardiac risk factors had an approximately 0.1 mm greater CIMT as adults compared with those without risk factors. In the Bogalusa Heart Study, metabolic syndrome during childhood was associated with a 2.5-fold increased likelihood of having a CIMT in the highest quintile.[57] In addition to reflecting an individual's past exposure to cardiovascular risk factors, CIMT is associated with prevalent cardiovascular disease and future cardiovascular risk. The Atherosclerosis Risk In Communities (ARIC) study demonstrated a 5% prevalence of myocardial infarction in individuals in the highest quartile of CIMT.[58] In the Cardiovascular Health Study (CHS), the odds ratio for symptomatic CHD was 2.8 when comparing the highest with the lowest quartile of CIMT.[59]

The relationship between CIMT and incident CHD events first became evident in the Kuopio Ischemic Heart Disease Risk Factor Study (KIHD), in which, for every 0.1-mm increment of CIMT, the risk of future myocardial infarction in Finnish men increased by 11%.[60] For CIMT values greater than 1 mm, there was a twofold greater risk for acute myocardial infarction over 3 years. The ARIC study provided further support, noting that for every 0.19-mm increment in CIMT, the risk of death or myocardial infarction increased by 36% in middle-aged patients (45–65 years of age).[51] The CHD risk was almost twofold greater in men with mean CIMT greater than 1 mm and even greater in women (risk ratio of 5). Not all studies, however, have shown gender differences in the predictive value of CIMT. For example, the Rotterdam study found that the risk of CHD events and CIMT was similar among men and women.[61] The association between CIMT and incidence of myocardial infarction and stroke has been noted in older populations as well. In CHS, the adjusted relative risk for myocardial infarction was 3.6, holding true for both individuals with and without known cardiovascular disease (Table 16-2).[62]

Because CIMT testing at any given moment reflects the integrated effect of cumulative risk factor exposure, it is primarily a reliable predictor of future CHD risk in patients whose risk factor status (including lifestyle behavior) is stable. However, in patients undergoing risk factor modification, CIMT testing likely will not accurately reflect current risk factor burden and consequently may be a poor predictor of outcome. It has been proposed that CIMT *progression* in such individuals might be a better index of risk for future CHD.[63] In the Cholesterol Lowering Atherosclerosis Study (CLAS), men who had undergone previous coronary artery bypass graft surgery were treated with colestipol and niacin.[64] An annual CIMT increase >0.033 mm per year was associated with a 2.8-fold increased risk of myocardial infarction, death, or need for revascularization over

TABLE 16-2 Summary of Prospective Trials Evaluating Carotid Intima–Media Thickness and Incident Coronary Events in Patients without Known Coronary Heart Disease

			Patient Details				
Study	**CIMT Measurement**	**Clinical Events**	**Follow-up (y)**	**Age (y)**	**Gender**	**CIMT Increment (mm)**	**Odds Ratio (CI)**
KIHD[60]	CCA/carotid bifurcation*	Fatal/nonfatal MI	1 m–3 y	42–60	Men	0.1	1.11 (1.06–1.16)
ARIC[58]	CCA/ICA/carotid bifurcation†	Coronary death and MI	4–7	45–64	Men Women	0.19 0.19	1.36 (1.23–1.51) 1.69 (1.50–1.90)
CHS[62]	CCA/ICA††	MI/stroke	6.2	>65	Men and women	0.2	1.46 (1.33–1.60)‡,§
Rotterdam Study[61]	CCA¶	MI/stroke	2.7	>55	Men Women	0.163 0.163	1.56 (1.12–2.18)‖ 1.44 (1.00–2.08)‖

*Mean carotid intime-media thickness (CIMT).
†Mean far wall, internal carotids, and bifurcation.
††Mean of common carotid artery (CCA) and internal carotid artery (ICA).
‡The odds ratio stated is risk for myocardial infarction (MI) and coronary death only. The odds ratio for MI and stroke was 1.47 (1.37–1.67).
§CCA CIMT.
¶Mean CCA.
‖The odds ratio stated is for risk of MI only.

7 years. CIMT and progression of CIMT predicted CHD risk beyond that predicted by measurements of coronary atherosclerosis by angiography and lipid measurements.[65] The strategy of using serial CIMT studies as a surrogate of atherosclerosis effects has been used in multiple clinical lipid trials (Table 16-3). In a placebo-controlled study of statin monotherapy (Regression Growth Evaluation Statin Study [REGRESS]), a 0.05-mm annual reduction in mean carotid and femoral artery intima–media thickness led to an absolute risk reduction of 10% over 2 years in the incidence of cardiac events.[66] It should be noted that because of the relatively high interscan variability of CIMT (>0.02 mm) relative to the annual progression rate (typically ≥0.01 mm/year), the serial use of CIMT for individual patient assessments is difficult unless performed after an extended time interval to permit the discrimination of true CIMT progression from measurement variability.

Ultrasound plaque composition, determined by using gray-scale and integrated backscatter within carotid ultrasound images, has been correlated with the extent of lipid deposition within plaques.[67] Individuals with stable CHD and low-intensity (lipid-rich) carotid plaques are predicted to have a higher risk of subsequent recurrent CHD events.[68] Standardized methods of determining ultrasonic plaque composition are needed.

TABLE 16-3 Summary of Trials Demonstrating the Effects of Lipid Therapy on Carotid Intima–Media Thickness in Patients with Known Coronary Heart Disease

				Mean Change in CIMT (mm/y)		
Trial	**Patients Randomized**	**Length of Study (y)**	**Intervention**	**Treatment**	**Placebo**	***P* value**
PLAC II[65]*	151 patients with CAD and elevated LDL cholesterol	3	Pravastatin 10-40 mg/day	+0.0295*	+0.0456*	0.03
REGRESS[66]	255 male patients with CAD and normal to moderately elevated total cholesterol	2	Pravastatin 40 mg/day	−0.05†	0†	0.0085
MARS[65]†	188 patients with CAD and moderately elevated total cholesterol	2	Lovastatin 80 mg/day	−0.038*,§	+0.019*,§	<0.001
LIPID[65]‡	522 patients with CAD and moderately elevated total cholesterol	4	Pravastatin 40 mg/day	−0.014‡,§	+0.048‡,§	<0.001
CLAS[64]	188 male patients who had undergone coronary artery bypass surgery	4	Colestipol and niacin	−0.026‡	+0.018‡	<0.05
ARBITER[65]§	161 patients with CAD and who met NCEP-II criteria for statin therapy	1	Atorvastatin 80 mg/day	−0.034*	+0.025*,¶	0.03
ARBITER 2[65]¶	167 patients with CAD already taking statins	1	Extended-release niacin	+0.014*	+0.044*	0.08

*Carotid Intime-Media Thickness (CIMT) of the Common Carotid Artey.
†Mean intima-media thickness of femoral and carotid arteries.
‡CIMT of the right CCA.
§Mean change in CIMT during study period.
¶Pravastatin 40 mg served as comparison group.
CAD, coronary artery disease.

Role of Carotid Intima–Media Thickness in Risk Assessment

CIMT has favorable characteristics as a CHD screening tool. It is noninvasive and quantitative, and it correlates with clinical outcomes. Furthermore, it is repeatable and demonstrates satisfactory interscan and interobserver reproducibility that may allow for assessment of atherosclerotic progression over time.[69] Because CAC may be absent in young individuals, for whom the concerns about radiation exposure are heightened, CIMT testing may offer specific advantages in the young.

Many patients, particularly young adults, are classified as low to intermediate risk despite the presence of metabolic syndrome, which has been shown to be clearly associated with increased CIMT and risk for atherosclerotic progression. This was assessed by Baldassarre et al., who investigated whether CIMT could be combined with the FRS to improve the predictability of cardiovascular events in dyslipidemic patients who are at low or intermediate risk.[70] Both FRS and CIMT proved to be independent outcome predictors, with a hazard ratio of 6.7 in patients with an FRS of 10% to 20% and elevated CIMT (>60th percentile for men or >80th percentile for women). This category of patients, who currently are not aggressively treated based on current guidelines, proved to have similar risk as patients with an FRS of 20% to 30%.

Stein et al. further explored the effect of age on the calculated FRS. By substituting CIMT-determined "vascular age" for chronological age, they reclassified cardiovascular risk according to FRS in patients without known CHD.[71] The substitution of "vascular age" for chronological age increased the Framingham 10-year risk score from 6.5% to 8.0% ($P < 0.001$). Of the subjects initially deemed to be intermediate risk, 35.7% were reclassified as higher risk when the CIMT-determined "vascular age" was applied. Although interesting, this strategy has not been tested in a large trial with hard clinical endpoints. Nevertheless, the findings of these studies are consistent with recommendations from Prevention Conference V, which stated that CIMT measurement can be considered for further clarification of CHD risk.[72]

MAGNETIC RESONANCE IMAGING

Cardiovascular magnetic resonance (CMR) imaging offers the ability to detect subclinical arterial and coronary plaque.[73,74] Instead of using ionizing radiation, CMR uses proton excitation with a radiofrequency pulse in the setting of a high local magnetic field, usually around 1.5 Tesla. Beyond identification and quantitation of plaque, a specific potential advantage of CMR plaque assessment is the differentiation of the tissue content within atheroma on the basis of magnetic properties of protons in water, by use of a range of imaging algorithms to optimize contrast and proton density. By using a multicontrast approach with high-resolution black blood spin-echo– and fast spin-echo–based CMR sequences, the blood flow signal can be rendered black, allowing characterization of the adjacent vessel wall and differentiation of fibrocellular, lipid-rich, and calcified regions of atherosclerotic plaque.[75,76] Furthermore, the quantification of plaque size and the detection of fibrous cap integrity and the presence of lipid cores are possible.[77–79]

Presently, limitations to the spatial and temporal resolution of CMR limits its application to large-vessel pathology such as aortic, carotid, and peripheral artery disease.[80,81] The ability of CMR to potentially serve as a tool in risk assessment was first seen in the offspring cohort of the Framingham Heart Study who underwent T2-weighted black-blood thoracoabdominal aortic CMR scanning.[82] Plaque prevalence and all measures of plaque burden increased by age group and were greater in the abdomen than in the thorax for both sexes and across all age groups. Furthermore, it was significantly correlated with the FRS in both men and women.

The composition of atherosclerotic plaques governs their vulnerability to rupture and hence their propensity to cause cardiovascular events. Because of its putative ability to characterize plaque content, CMR may have important implications for the understanding and modification of atherosclerosis. It was recently demonstrated that gadolinium-based contrast agents enhance the identification of the fibrous cap of atherosclerotic plaques, possibly through a greater distribution of the agent in the neovascularized areas of the cap.[83] The identification of high-risk atherosclerotic plaque with CMR may be aided in the future by the detection of specific molecular plaque components through targeted CMR contrast agents *in vivo*.[84] CMR may potentially add prognostic value of qualitative (e.g., the presence of a "thin" fibrous cap) beyond quantitative (e.g., plaque thickness) atherosclerotic measures, although further research is needed in this area.

The characterization of the coronary epicardial vessels with coronary artery magnetic resonance angiography (CMRA) remains challenging. Despite numerous ongoing technical improvements, difficulties in coronary imaging include smaller vessel caliber, cardiac and respiratory motion artifacts, vessel tortuosity, and limited temporal resolution. A large multicenter trial of patients who underwent CMRA and traditional coronary angiography revealed that primarily the proximal 3 to 5 cm of the major coronary vessels were deemed interpretable.[85] Currently, CMR is used clinically in the evaluation of large vessel pathology and in the research setting to assess vascular response to antiatherosclerotic therapy (Figure 16-9) as a clinical surrogate with high reproducibility. Further improvements in temporal and spatial resolution may enable coronary arterial wall imaging.

BRACHIAL ARTERY FLOW-MEDIATED DILATION

Most noninvasive risk assessment tools are based on anatomical measures of atherosclerosis such as plaque burden or plaque composition. In contrast, brachial artery reactivity testing (BART) is a functional assessment of the arteries. An increase in shear stress on the surface of the endothelial cells results in activation of nitric oxide synthase and an increase in available nitric oxide, the predominant vasodilator in the arterial system. Nitric oxide plays a critical role in the atherosclerotic process, including platelet adhesion and aggregation,

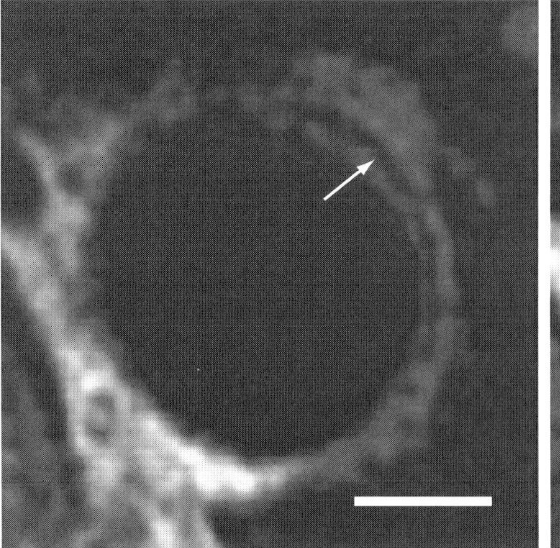

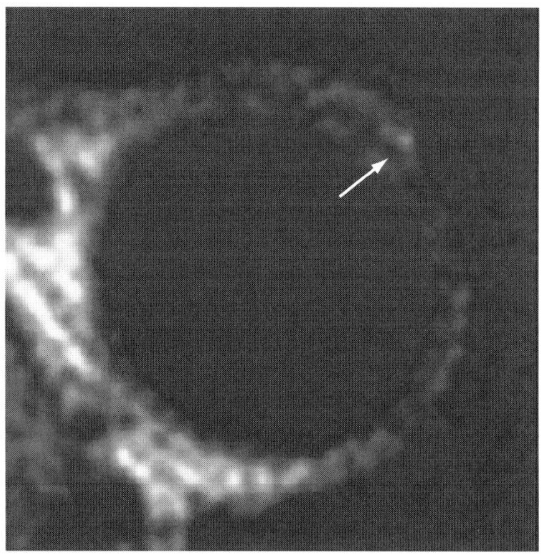

FIGURE 16-9 T2-weighted magnetic resonance (MR) images of descending aorta at baseline and after 24 months of patient treatment with statin therapy.[109] After 24 months of lipid lowering therapy, there is a reduction in the hypodense signal *(arrows),* suggestive of plaque reduction of the lipid-laden component. Because of its ability to quantify and characterize plaque without ionizing radiation, MR may emerge as a powerful noninvasive imaging tool for serial evaluation of progression and therapy-induced regression of atherosclerotic plaques.

smooth muscle proliferation, and LDL uptake.[86] It is postulated that the degree of arterial vasodilation in the setting of a flow-mediated increase in shear stress acts as a surrogate for endothelial cell function, namely the ability to produce and release nitric oxide. Endothelial dysfunction is characterized by a reduction of the bioavailability of nitric oxide and an impairment of endothelium-dependent vasodilation. Given the relationship between endothelial dysfunction and atherosclerosis, it is likely that the status of endothelial function may reflect the propensity of an individual to develop atherosclerotic disease, and thus, the presence of endothelial dysfunction may serve as a marker of an unfavorable cardiovascular prognosis.

In BART, endothelial function of the peripheral artery is assessed by applying an increased hemodynamic shear stress during reactive hyperemia as a stimulus for the release of nitric oxide. During BART, a sphygmomanometric cuff is placed around the arm, just above the antecubital fossa, of a resting patient. Baseline ultrasound images of the brachial artery are acquired using high-frequency ultrasound with a vascular transducer and built-in ECG capabilities. After inflation of the cuff to approximately 50 mm Hg above the resting systolic blood pressure for 5 minutes, the cuff is released and ultrasound images are again obtained, assessing the degree of vasodilation of the brachial artery 1 minute later during the reactive hyperemic phase. Clear visualization of the lumina–intima interface of both the near and far walls of the brachial artery is essential. After identifying these boundaries with edge calipers, the operator can determine the diameter of the vessel by using specialized software packages. The response of brachial artery reactivity is generally measured as the change in poststimulus diameter as a percentage of the baseline diameter. It is critical that patients are instructed not to smoke or eat for at least 12 hours before testing and that testing is conducted in a quiet, temperature-controlled room. Several factors have been identified that can affect flow-mediated vascular response, including recent fat and caffeine digestion, drugs, temperature, and sympathetic stimuli.[87,88] A vasodilator response is generally considered normal when there is at least a 10% increase in the diameter of the brachial artery during the reactive hyperemic phase relative to baseline.[89] The response, however, tends to be significantly attenuated in men older than 40 years and women older than 50 years of age. The vasodilator response is also inversely dependent on the baseline brachial artery diameter.[90]

Because the endothelium may be a target that integrates the damaging effects of traditional risk factors, it may serve as a potential indicator of cardiovascular risk. Endothelial dysfunction has been linked to dyslipidemia, hypertension, diabetes mellitus, smoking, aging, menopause, family history of premature atherosclerosis, and hyperhomocysteinemia.[91–93] Endothelial dysfunction represents an early stage in the atherosclerotic process, preceding the anatomical features of subclinical disease.[94] Thus, BART may be particularly useful in the risk stratification of younger populations for whom the sensitivity of other tests such as CAC is reduced.

Emerging evidence suggests that brachial artery FMD may be an independent predictor of outcomes.[95–97] It is essential, however, to realize that the data correlating brachial artery FMD to coronary endothelial function and to cardiovascular outcomes are derived primarily from studies in individuals with manifest cardiovascular disease or at high risk for cardiovascular disease, with very limited information on low- and moderate-risk groups. Gokce et al. preoperatively examined brachial artery vasodilation in 187 patients undergoing vascular surgery.[95] Preoperative endothelium-dependent FMD was significantly lower in patients with a cardiovascular event (4.9 ± 3.1%) than in those without an event (7.3 ± 5%; $P < 0.001$) within the first 30 days of the postoperative period.

The major limitation of BART is the short-term biologic variability of the measurement. Because of the effects of dietary changes and the phase of the menstrual cycle on BART, patient preparation is critical. Furthermore, protocols for assessing BART vary among laboratories and are operator-dependent, decreasing the feasibility of this noninvasive tool to serve as a valuable screening tool for endothelial dysfunction in clinical practice.[86,98] Unlike other noninvasive assessments like CIMT, there is no proof that therapeutic improvement in endothelial function translates into lower cardiovascular morbidity and mortality, and further prospective trials are required to determine the suitability of BART to serve as a primary therapeutic endpoint. Currently, BART is used as a research tool but has limited clinical application.

MOTIVATIONAL EFFECTS OF ATHEROSCLEROSIS IMAGING

Atherosclerosis imaging has been postulated to motivate patient behavioral change. However, despite anecdotal and logical plausibility, the evidence to date fails to suggest a long-term, durable motivational effect of atherosclerosis imaging. Several survey studies using either EBCT for the detection of coronary calcium[99,100] or carotid ultrasonography for the detection of intima–media thickness or plaque[101] have suggested that survey respondents among primarily referred populations report being motivated for healthy behavioral change with a common theme of increased perception of risk. In contrast, studies of actual behavioral change have yielded conflicting results. Although a study of carotid ultrasonography showed improved success at smoking cessation in smokers shown ultrasound evidence of carotid plaque,[102] in general, biomedical aids to enhance smoking cessation have not been shown to be effective.[103] Two randomized trials of CAC assessment have also shown imaging to be ineffective in motivating behavioral change. In studies of CAC screening among healthy middle-aged military personnel (the Prospective Army Coronary Calcium Study)[104] and of postmenopausal women,[105] there was no relationship between imaging and behavioral change or motivation after 1 year. These findings parallel the limited motivational impact that even definite cardiac events such as myocardial infarction have on long-term patient behavior. Notably, within the factorial design of the Prospective Army Coronary Calcium Project randomized trial, a randomization arm of a nurse-based case management approach to behavioral change was successful in stabilizing coronary risk, reducing the incidence of metabolic syndrome, and increasing patient motivation for change.[104,106] Thus, while the available data suggest against a large and directly attributable effect of atherosclerosis imaging on patient motivation, incorporating these data into a recurring clinical patient/physician relationship could lead to behavioral modification.[107]

CONCLUSION

Standard CHD risk assessment with the FRS is imprecise and leaves a large proportion of patients classified as "intermediate" risk, effectively underestimating the actual lifetime risk of CHD in a large group of patients. It is logical to conclude that using one or more of these noninvasive techniques in addition to the risk models previously discussed could improve the predictive power of the FRS with enhancements in sensitivity and specificity. An improved model could help to identify individuals whose lifetime risk of CHD may be underrepresented by the standard FRS as well as improve the risk stratification of the large population in the intermediate-risk category.

Currently, plaque burden has been the most extensively studied variable of subclinical atherosclerosis. However, different imaging modalities have been proven to be inconsistent in the identification of high degrees of plaque burden and demonstrate poor correlation. For example, in a comparison of the overlap across CMR aortic plaque, CAC, and CIMT in the offspring cohort of the Framingham study, only 4% of men and 16% of women were classified as having a high level of atherosclerosis on all three measurements.[108] Nevertheless, CAC scoring and CIMT measurement remain the most accepted means of improving risk stratification from an evidence-based approach, while MSCT angiography, CMR, and BART await validation as measures of cardiovascular risk in prospective trials. Screening for subclinical atherosclerosis has been advocated for individuals at intermediate global risk for CHD. There is a need for an improved integrated risk-scoring system with biological age determined by CIMT and/or CAC replacing chronological age in the FRS. Future studies assessing outcome improvement and cost-effectiveness of these primary prevention efforts are warranted.

REFERENCES

1. Lloyd-Jones DM, Larson MG, Beiser A, Levy D: Lifetime risk of developing coronary heart disease. *Lancet* 1999;353:89–92.
2. Wilson PW, D'Agostino RB, Levy D, et al.: Prediction of coronary heart disease using risk factor categories. *Circulation* 1998;97:1837–1847.
3. D'Agostino RB, Russell MW, Huse DM, et al.: Primary and subsequent coronary risk appraisal: New results from the Framingham study. *Am Heart J* 2000;139:272–281.
4. Lerner DJ, Kannel WB: Patterns of coronary heart disease morbidity and mortality in the sexes: A 26-year follow-up of the Framingham population. *Am Heart J* 1986;111:383–390.
5. Expert Panel: Executive Summary of The Third Report of The National Cholesterol Education Program (NCEP) Expert Panel on Detection, Evaluation, and Treatment of High Blood Cholesterol in Adults (Adult Treatment Panel III). *JAMA* 2001;285:2486–2497.
6. Ford ES, Giles WH, Mokdad AH: The distribution of 10-year risk for coronary heart disease among US adults: Findings from the National Health and Nutrition Examination Survey III. *J Am Coll Cardiol* 2004;43:1791–1796.
7. Akosah KO, Schaper A, Cogbill C, Schoenfeld P: Preventing myocardial infarction in the young adult in the first place: How do the National Cholesterol Education Panel III guidelines perform? *J Am Coll Cardiol* 2003;41:1475–1479.
8. Lloyd-Jones DM, Wilson PW, Larson MG, et al.: Framingham risk score and prediction of lifetime risk for coronary heart disease. *Am J Cardiol* 2004;94:20–24.
9. Lloyd-Jones DM, Nam BH, D'Agostino RB Sr, et al.: Parental cardiovascular disease as a risk factor for cardiovascular disease in middle-aged adults: A prospective study of parents and offspring. *JAMA* 2004;291:2204–2211.
10. Brindle P, Emberson J, Lampe F, et al.: Predictive accuracy of the Framingham coronary risk score in British men: Prospective cohort study. *BMJ* 2003;327:1267.
11. Empana JP, Ducimetiere P, Arveiler D, et al.: Are the Framingham and PROCAM coronary heart disease risk functions applicable to different European populations? The PRIME Study. *Eur Heart J* 2003;24:1903–1911.
12. Marrugat J, D'Agostino R, Sullivan L, et al.: An adaptation of the Framingham coronary heart disease risk function to European Mediterranean areas. *J Epidemiol Community Health* 2003;57:634–638.

13. D'Agostino RB Sr, Grundy S, Sullivan LM, Wilson P: Validation of the Framingham coronary heart disease prediction scores: Results of a multiple ethnic groups investigation. *JAMA* 2001;286:180–187.
14. Horiguchi J, Yamamoto H, Akiyama Y, et al.: Coronary artery calcium scoring using 16-MDCT and a retrospective ECG-gating reconstruction algorithm. *AJR Am J Roentgenol* 2004;183:103–108.
15. Schmermund A, Erbel R: Unstable coronary plaque and its relation to coronary calcium. *Circulation* 2001;104:1682–1687.
16. Haberl R, Becker A, Leber A, et al.: Correlation of coronary calcification and angiographically documented stenoses in patients with suspected coronary artery disease: Results of 1,764 patients. *J Am Coll Cardiol* 2001;37:451–457.
17. Rumberger JA, Brundage BH, Rader DJ, Kondos G: Electron beam computed tomographic coronary calcium scanning: A review and guidelines for use in asymptomatic persons. *Mayo Clin Proc* 1999;74:243–252.
18. Rumberger JA, Simons DB, Fitzpatrick LA, et al.: Coronary artery calcium area by electron-beam computed tomography and coronary atherosclerotic plaque area. A histopathologic correlative study. *Circulation* 1995;92:2157–2162.
19. Sangiorgi G, Rumberger JA, Severson A, et al.: Arterial calcification and not lumen stenosis is highly correlated with atherosclerotic plaque burden in humans: A histologic study of 723 coronary artery segments using nondecalcifying methodology. *J Am Coll Cardiol* 1998;31:126–133.
20. Nasir K, Michos ED, Blumenthal RS, Raggi P: Detection of high-risk young adults and women by coronary calcium and National Cholesterol Education Program Panel III guidelines. *J Am Coll Cardiol* 2005;46:1931–1936.
21. Pletcher MJ, Tice JA, Pignone M, Browner WS: Using the coronary artery calcium score to predict coronary heart disease events: A systematic review and meta-analysis. *Arch Intern Med* 2004;164:1285–1292.
22. Arad Y, Goodman KJ, Roth M, et al.: Coronary calcification, coronary disease risk factors, C-reactive protein, and atherosclerotic cardiovascular disease events: The St. Francis Heart Study. *J Am Coll Cardiol* 2005;46:158–165.
23. Greenland P, LaBree L, Azen SP, et al.: Coronary artery calcium score combined with Framingham score for risk prediction in asymptomatic individuals. *JAMA* 2004;291:210–215.
24. Taylor AJ, Bindeman J, Feuerstein I, et al.: Coronary calcium independently predicts incident premature coronary heart disease over measured cardiovascular risk factors: Mean three-year outcomes in the Prospective Army Coronary Calcium (PACC) project. *J Am Coll Cardiol* 2005;46:807–814.
25. Vliegenthart R, Oudkerk M, Song B, et al.: Coronary calcification detected by electron-beam computed tomography and myocardial infarction. The Rotterdam Coronary Calcification Study. *Eur Heart J* 2002;23:1596–1603.
26. Budoff MJ, Shaw LJ, Liu ST, et al.: Long-term prognosis associated with coronary calcification: Observations from a registry of 25,253 patients. *J Am Coll Cardiol* 2007;49:1860–1870.
27. Raggi P, Callister TQ, Cooil B, et al.: Identification of patients at increased risk of first unheralded acute myocardial infarction by electron-beam computed tomography. *Circulation* 2000;101:850–855.
28. Hoff JA, Chomka EV, Krainik AJ, et al.: Age and gender distributions of coronary artery calcium detected by electron beam tomography in 35,246 adults. *Am J Cardiol* 2001;87:1335–1339.
29. Greenland P, LaBree L, Azen SP, et al.: Coronary artery calcium score combined with Framingham score for risk prediction in asymptomatic individuals. *JAMA* 2004;291:210–215.
30. Greenland P, Bonow RO, Brundage BH, et al.: ACCF/AHA 2007 clinical expert consensus document on coronary artery calcium scoring by computed tomography in global cardiovascular risk assessment and in evaluation of patients with chest pain: A report of the American College of Cardiology Foundation Clinical Expert Consensus Task Force (ACCF/AHA Writing Committee to Update the 2000 Expert Consensus Document on Electron Beam Computed Tomography) developed in collaboration with the Society of Atherosclerosis Imaging and Prevention and the Society of Cardiovascular Computed Tomography. *J Am Coll Cardiol* 2007;49:378–402.
31. Raggi P, Cooil B, Shaw LJ, et al.: Progression of coronary calcium on serial electron beam tomographic scanning is greater in patients with future myocardial infarction. *Am J Cardiol* 2003;92:827–829.
32. Raggi P, Callister TQ, Shaw LJ: Progression of coronary artery calcium and risk of first myocardial infarction in patients receiving cholesterol-lowering therapy. *Arterioscler Thromb Vasc Biol* 2004;24:1272–1277.
33. Raggi P, Cooil B, Ratti C, et al.: Progression of coronary artery calcium and occurrence of myocardial infarction in patients with and without diabetes mellitus. *Hypertension* 2005;46:238–243.
34. Arad Y, Spadaro LA, Roth M, et al.: Treatment of asymptomatic adults with elevated coronary calcium scores with atorvastatin, vitamin C, and vitamin E: The St. Francis Heart Study randomized clinical trial. *J Am Coll Cardiol* 2005;46:166–172.
35. Raggi P, Davidson M, Callister TQ, et al.: Aggressive versus moderate lipid-lowering therapy in hypercholesterolemic postmenopausal women: Beyond Endorsed Lipid Lowering with EBT Scanning (BELLES). *Circulation* 2005;112:563–571.
36. Taylor AJ, Bindeman J, Feuerstein I, et al.: Community-based provision of statin and aspirin after the detection of coronary artery calcium within a community-based screening cohort. *J Am Coll Cardiol* 2008;51:1337–1341.
37. Shaw LJ, Raggi P, Berman DS, Callister TQ: Coronary artery calcium as a measure of biologic age. *Atherosclerosis* 2006;188:112–119.
38. Hausleiter J, Meyer T, Hadamitzky M, et al.: Prevalence of noncalcified coronary plaques by 64-slice computed tomography in patients with an intermediate risk for significant coronary artery disease. *J Am Coll Cardiol* 2006;48:312–318.
39. Knez A, Becker A, Leber A, et al.: Relation of coronary calcium scores by electron beam tomography to obstructive disease in 2,115 symptomatic patients. *Am J Cardiol* 2004;93:1150–1152.
40. Leber AW, Knez A, von Ziegler F, et al.: Quantification of obstructive and nonobstructive coronary lesions by 64-slice computed tomography: A comparative study with quantitative coronary angiography and intravascular ultrasound. *J Am Coll Cardiol* 2005;46:147–154.
41. Leber AW, Knez A, Becker A, et al.: Accuracy of multidetector spiral computed tomography in identifying and differentiating the composition of coronary atherosclerotic plaques: A comparative study with intracoronary ultrasound. *J Am Coll Cardiol* 2004;43:1241–1247.
42. Ehara S, Kobayashi Y, Yoshiyama M, et al.: Spotty calcification typifies the culprit plaque in patients with acute myocardial infarction: An intravascular ultrasound study. *Circulation* 2004;110:3424–3429.
43. Zanzonico P, Rothenberg LN, Strauss HW: Radiation exposure of computed tomography and direct intracoronary angiography: Risk has its reward. *J Am Coll Cardiol* 2006;47:1846–1849.
44. Onuma Y, Tanabe K, Nakazawa G, et al.: Noncardiac findings in cardiac imaging with multidetector computed tomography. *J Am Coll Cardiol* 2006;48:402–406.
45. O'Leary DH, Polak JF, Wolfson SKJ, et al.: Use of sonography to evaluate carotid atherosclerosis in the elderly. The Cardiovascular Health Study. CHS Collaborative Research Group. *Stroke* 1991;22:1155–1163.
46. Howard G, Sharrett AR, Heiss G, et al.: Carotid artery intimal-medial thickness distribution in general populations as evaluated by B-mode ultrasound. ARIC Investigators. *Stroke* 1993;24:1297–1304.
47. Crouse JR III, Craven TE, Hagaman AP, Bond MG: Association of coronary disease with segment-specific intimal-medial thickening of the extracranial carotid artery. *Circulation* 1995;92:1141–1147.
48. Stensland-Bugge E, Bonaa KH, Joakimsen O: Reproducibility of ultrasonographically determined intima–media thickness is dependent on arterial wall thickness. The Tromso Study. *Stroke* 1997;28:1972–1980.
49. del Sol AI, Moons KG, Hollander M, et al.: Is carotid intima–media thickness useful in cardiovascular disease risk assessment? The Rotterdam Study. *Stroke* 2001;32:1532–1538.
50. Kanters SD, Algra A, van Leeuwen MS, Banga JD: Reproducibility of *in vivo* carotid intima–media thickness measurements: A review. *Stroke* 1997;28:665–671.
51. Chambless LE, Heiss G, Folsom AR, et al.: Association of coronary heart disease incidence with carotid arterial wall thickness and major risk factors: The Atherosclerosis Risk in Communities (ARIC) Study, 1987-1993. *Am J Epidemiol* 1997;146:483–494.
52. O'Leary DH, Polak JF, Kronmal RA, et al.: Carotid-artery intima and media thickness as a risk factor for myocardial infarction

and stroke in older adults. Cardiovascular Health Study Collaborative Research Group. *N Engl J Med* 1999;340:14–22.
53. Urbina EM, Srinivasan SR, Tang R, et al.: Impact of multiple coronary risk factors on the intima–media thickness of different segments of carotid artery in healthy young adults (The Bogalusa Heart Study). *Am J Cardiol* 2002;90:953–958.
54. D'Agostino RB Jr, Burke G, O'Leary D, et al.: Ethnic differences in carotid wall thickness. The Insulin Resistance Atherosclerosis Study. *Stroke* 1996;27:1744–1749.
55. Davis PH, Dawson JD, Riley WA, Lauer RM: Carotid intimal-medial thickness is related to cardiovascular risk factors measured from childhood through middle age: The Muscatine Study. *Circulation* 2001;104:2815–2819.
56. Raitakari OT, Juonala M, Kahonen M, et al.: Cardiovascular risk factors in childhood and carotid artery intima–media thickness in adulthood: The Cardiovascular Risk in Young Finns Study. *JAMA* 2003;290:2277–2283.
57. Tzou WS, Douglas PS, Srinivasan SR, et al.: Increased subclinical atherosclerosis in young adults with metabolic syndrome: The Bogalusa Heart Study. *J Am Coll Cardiol* 2005;46:457–463.
58. Burke GL, Evans GW, Riley WA, et al.: Arterial wall thickness is associated with prevalent cardiovascular disease in middle-aged adults. The Atherosclerosis Risk in Communities (ARIC) Study. *Stroke* 1995;26:386–391.
59. O'Leary DH, Polak JF, Kronmal RA, et al.: Distribution and correlates of sonographically detected carotid artery disease in the Cardiovascular Health Study. The CHS Collaborative Research Group. *Stroke* 1992;23:1752–1760.
60. Salonen JT, Salonen R: Ultrasound B-mode imaging in observational studies of atherosclerotic progression. *Circulation* 1993;87:II56–II65.
61. Bots ML, Hoes AW, Koudstaal PJ, et al.: Common carotid intima–media thickness and risk of stroke and myocardial infarction: The Rotterdam Study. *Circulation* 1997;96:1432–1437.
62. O'Leary DH, Polak JF, Kronmal RA, et al.: Carotid-artery intima and media thickness as a risk factor for myocardial infarction and stroke in older adults. Cardiovascular Health Study Collaborative Research Group. *N Engl J Med* 1999;340:14–22.
63. Crouse JR III: Predictive value of carotid 2-dimensional ultrasound. *Am J Cardiol* 2001;88:27E–30E.
64. Cashin-Hemphill L, Mack WJ, Pogoda JM, et al.: Beneficial effects of colestipol-niacin on coronary atherosclerosis. A 4-year follow-up. *JAMA* 1990;264:3013–3017.
65. Hodis HN, Mack WJ, LaBree L, et al.: The role of carotid arterial intima–media thickness in predicting clinical coronary events. *Ann Intern Med* 1998;128:262–269.
65a Crouse JR III, Byington RP, Bond MG, et al.: Pravastatin, lipids, and atherosclerosis in the carotid arteries (PLAC-II). *Am J Cardiol* 1995;75:455–459.
65b. Hodis HN, Mack WJ, LaBree L, et al.: Reduction in carotid arterial wall thickness using lovastatin and dietary therapy: a randomized controlled clinical trial. *Ann Intern Med* 1996;124:548–556.
65c. MacMahon S, Sharpe N, Gamble G, et al.: Effects of lowering average of below-average cholesterol levels on the progression of carotid atherosclerosis: results of the LIPID Atherosclerosis Substudy. *Circulation* 1998;97:1784–1790.
65d. Taylor AJ, Kent SM, Flaherty PJ, et al.: ARBITER: Arterial Biology for the Investigation of the Treatment Effects of Reducing Cholesterol: a randomized trial comparing the effects of atorvastatin and pravastatin on carotid intima medial thickness. *Circulation* 2002;106:2055–2060.
65e. Taylor AJ, Sullenberger LE, Lee HJ, et al.: Arterial Biology for the Investigation of the Treatment Effects of Reducing Cholesterol (ARBITER) 2: a double-blind, placebo-controlled study of extended-release niacin on atherosclerosis progression in secondary prevention patients treated with statins. *Circulation* 2004;110:3512–3517.
66. de Groot E, Jukema JW, van Boven AJ, et al.: Effect of pravastatin on progression and regression of coronary atherosclerosis and vessel wall changes in carotid and femoral arteries: A report from the Regression Growth Evaluation Statin Study. *Am J Cardiol* 1995;76:40C–46C.
67. Gronholdt ML, Nordestgaard BG, Wiebe BM, et al.: Echo-lucency of computerized ultrasound images of carotid atherosclerotic plaques are associated with increased levels of triglyceride-rich lipoproteins as well as increased plaque lipid content. *Circulation* 1998;97:34–40.
68. Honda O, Sugiyama S, Kugiyama K, et al.: Echolucent carotid plaques predict future coronary events in patients with coronary artery disease. *J Am Coll Cardiol* 2004;43:1177–1184.
69. Tang R, Hennig M, Thomasson B, et al.: Baseline reproducibility of B-mode ultrasonic measurement of carotid artery intima–media thickness: The European Lacidipine Study on Atherosclerosis (ELSA). *J Hypertens* 2000;18:197–201.
70. Baldassarre D, Amato M, Pustina L, et al.: Measurement of carotid artery intima–media thickness in dyslipidemic patients increases the power of traditional risk factors to predict cardiovascular events. *Atherosclerosis* 2007;191:403–408.
71. Stein JH, Fraizer MC, Aeschlimann SE, et al.: Vascular age: Integrating carotid intima–media thickness measurements with global coronary risk assessment. *Clin Cardiol* 2004;27:388–392.
72. Greenland P, Abrams J, Aurigemma GP, et al.: Prevention Conference V: Beyond secondary prevention: Identifying the high-risk patient for primary prevention: Noninvasive tests of atherosclerotic burden: Writing Group III. *Circulation* 2000;101:E16–E22.
73. Fayad ZA, Fuster V: Clinical imaging of the high-risk or vulnerable atherosclerotic plaque. *Circ Res* 2001;89:305–316.
74. Fayad ZA, Fuster V, Nikolaou K, Becker C: Computed tomography and magnetic resonance imaging for noninvasive coronary angiography and plaque imaging: Current and potential future concepts. *Circulation* 2002;106:2026–2034.
75. Itskovich VV, Samber DD, Mani V, et al.: Quantification of human atherosclerotic plaques using spatially enhanced cluster analysis of multicontrast-weighted magnetic resonance images. *Magn Reson Med* 2004;52:515–523.
76. Worthley SG, Helft G, Fuster V, et al.: Noninvasive *in vivo* magnetic resonance imaging of experimental coronary artery lesions in a porcine model. *Circulation* 2000;101:2956–2961.
77. Yuan C, Beach KW, Smith LH, Jr, Hatsukami TS: Measurement of atherosclerotic carotid plaque size *in vivo* using high resolution magnetic resonance imaging. *Circulation* 1998;98:2666–2671.
78. Corti R, Fayad ZA, Fuster V, et al.: Effects of lipid-lowering by simvastatin on human atherosclerotic lesions: A longitudinal study by high-resolution, noninvasive magnetic resonance imaging. *Circulation* 2001;104:249–252.
79. Hatsukami TS, Ross R, Polissar NL, Yuan C: Visualization of fibrous cap thickness and rupture in human atherosclerotic carotid plaque *in vivo* with high-resolution magnetic resonance imaging. *Circulation* 2000;102:959–964.
80. Fayad ZA, Nahar T, Fallon JT, et al.: *In vivo* magnetic resonance evaluation of atherosclerotic plaques in the human thoracic aorta: A comparison with transesophageal echocardiography. *Circulation* 2000;101:2503–2509.
81. Coulden RA, Moss H, Graves MJ, et al.: High resolution magnetic resonance imaging of atherosclerosis and the response to balloon angioplasty. *Heart* 2000;83:188–191.
82. Jaffer FA, O'Donnell CJ, Larson MG, et al.: Age and sex distribution of subclinical aortic atherosclerosis: A magnetic resonance imaging examination of the Framingham Heart Study. *Arterioscler Thromb Vasc Biol* 2002;22:849–854.
83. Yuan C, Kerwin WS, Ferguson MS, et al.: Contrast-enhanced high resolution MRI for atherosclerotic carotid artery tissue characterization. *J Magn Reson Imaging* 2002;15:62–67.
84. Sirol M, Fuster V, Fayad ZA: Plaque imaging and characterization using magnetic resonance imaging: Towards molecular assessment. *Curr Mol Med* 2006;6:541–548.
85. Kim WY, Danias PG, Stuber M, et al.: Coronary magnetic resonance angiography for the detection of coronary stenoses. *N Engl J Med* 2001;345:1863–1869.
86. Corretti MC, Anderson TJ, Benjamin EJ, et al.: Guidelines for the ultrasound assessment of endothelial-dependent flow-mediated vasodilation of the brachial artery: A report of the International Brachial Artery Reactivity Task Force. *J Am Coll Cardiol* 2002;39:257–265.
87. Celermajer DS, Sorensen KE, Georgakopoulos D, et al.: Cigarette smoking is associated with dose-related and potentially reversible impairment of endothelium-dependent dilation in healthy young adults. *Circulation* 1993;88:2149–2155.
88. Harris CW, Edwards JL, Baruch A, et al.: Effects of mental stress on brachial artery flow-mediated vasodilation in healthy normal individuals. *Am Heart J* 2000;139:405–411.
89. Vogel RA: Coronary risk factors, endothelial function, and atherosclerosis: A review. *Clin Cardiol* 1997;20:426–432.

90. Herrington DM, Fan L, Drum M, et al.: Brachial flow-mediated vasodilator responses in population-based research: Methods, reproducibility and effects of age, gender and baseline diameter. *J Cardiovasc Risk* 2001;8:319–328.
91. Cai H, Harrison DG: Endothelial dysfunction in cardiovascular diseases: The role of oxidant stress. *Circ Res* 2000;87:840–844.
92. Bonetti PO, Lerman LO, Lerman A: Endothelial dysfunction: A marker of atherosclerotic risk. *Arterioscler Thromb Vasc Biol* 2003;23:168–175.
93. Vita JA, Treasure CB, Nabel EG, et al.: Coronary vasomotor response to acetylcholine relates to risk factors for coronary artery disease. *Circulation* 1990;81:491–497.
94. Schachinger V, Britten MB, Zeiher AM: Prognostic impact of coronary vasodilator dysfunction on adverse long-term outcome of coronary heart disease. *Circulation* 2000;101:1899–1906.
95. Gokce N, Keaney JF Jr, Hunter LM, et al.: Risk stratification for postoperative cardiovascular events via noninvasive assessment of endothelial function: A prospective study. *Circulation* 2002;105:1567–1572.
96. Chan SY, Mancini GB, Kuramoto L, et al.: The prognostic importance of endothelial dysfunction and carotid atheroma burden in patients with coronary artery disease. *J Am Coll Cardiol* 2003;42:1037–1043.
97. Mancini GB: Vascular structure versus function: Is endothelial dysfunction of independent prognostic importance or not? *J Am Coll Cardiol* 2004;43:624–628.
98. Anderson TJ: Assessment and treatment of endothelial dysfunction in humans. *J Am Coll Cardiol* 1999;34:631–638.
99. O' Malley PG, Rupard EJ, Jones DL, et al.: Does the diagnosis of coronary calcification with electron beam computed tomography motivate behavioral change in smokers? *Mil Med* 2002;167:211–214.
100. Wong ND, Detrano RC, Diamond G, et al.: Does coronary artery screening by electron beam computed tomography motivate potentially beneficial lifestyle behaviors? [see comments]. *Am J Cardiol* 1996;78:1220–1223.
101. Shahab L, Hall S, Marteau T: Showing smokers with vascular disease images of their arteries to motivate cessation: A pilot study. *Br J Health Psychol* 2007;12:275–283.
102. Bovet P, Perret F, Cornuz J, et al.: Improved smoking cessation in smokers given ultrasound photographs of their own atherosclerotic plaques. *Prev Med* 2002;34:215–220.
103. Bize R, Burnand B, Mueller Y, Cornuz J: Biomedical risk assessment as an aid for smoking cessation. *Cochrane Database Syst Rev* 2005;CD004705.
104. O'Malley PG, Feuerstein IM, Taylor AJ: Impact of electron beam tomography, with or without case management, on motivation, behavioral change, and cardiovascular risk profile: A randomized controlled trial. *JAMA* 2003;289:2215–2223.
105. Lederman J, Ballard J, Njike VY, et al.: Information given to postmenopausal women on coronary computed tomography may influence cardiac risk reduction efforts. *J Clin Epidemiol* 2007;60:389–396.
106. O'Malley PG, Kowalczyk C, Bindeman J, Taylor AJ: A randomized trial assessing the impact of cardiovascular risk factor case-management on the metabolic syndrome. *J Cardiometabolic Syndrome* 2006;1:6–12.
107. Vale MJ, Jelinek MV, Best JD, et al.: Coaching patients On Achieving Cardiovascular Health (COACH): A multicenter randomized trial in patients with coronary heart disease. *Arch Intern Med* 2003;163:2775–2783.
108. Kathiresan S, Larson MG, Keyes MJ, et al.: Assessment by cardiovascular magnetic resonance, electron beam computed tomography, and carotid ultrasonography of the distribution of subclinical atherosclerosis across Framingham risk strata. *Am J Cardiol* 2007;99:310–314.
109. Corti R, Fayad ZA, Fuster V, et al.: Effects of lipid-lowering by simvastatin on human atherosclerotic lesions: A longitudinal study by high-resolution, noninvasive magnetic resonance imaging. *Circulation* 2001;104:249–252.

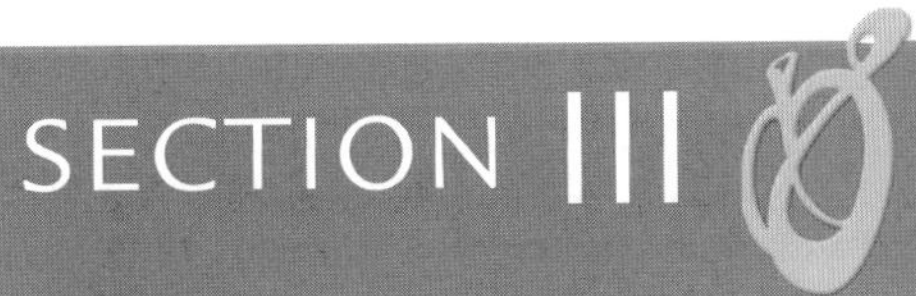

SECTION III Therapy

CHAPTER 17

Overview of General Approach to Management of Elevated Low-Density Lipoprotein Cholesterol and Mixed Dyslipidemia, High Triglycerides, and Low High-Density Lipoprotein Cholesterol

Christie M. Ballantyne, and Peter H. Jones

This chapter provides a general overview of treatment approaches for dyslipidemias commonly encountered in clinical practice. Specific treatment guidelines are reviewed in Chapter 18, individual therapies are discussed in Chapters 19 through 31, and considerations in treating special patient populations are presented in Chapters 37 through 43. While these recommendations are intended as a practical guide for clinicians, clinical judgment is required to determine an individual's absolute risk and therefore the need for and optimal intensity of therapy. For all patients, management should also include assessment for and, if possible, treatment of causes of secondary dyslipidemias (see Chapter 12) as well as reduction of other modifiable risk factors to decrease overall risk. Lifestyle modifications (see Chapters 19 through 21) are an essential component of therapy for lipid disorders, either alone or in conjunction with drug therapy.

ELEVATED LOW-DENSITY LIPOPROTEIN CHOLESTEROL

The association between low-density lipoprotein (LDL) cholesterol and cardiovascular disease has been well established in observational epidemiologic studies and interventional clinical trials, and LDL cholesterol remains the primary target of therapy in the U.S. National Cholesterol Education Program Adult Treatment Panel III (NCEP ATP III)[1] and other major guidelines (see Chapter 18). Absolute risk assessment is used to determine the need for and intensity of lipid-regulating therapy. At highest risk are individuals with known coronary heart disease (CHD) or CHD risk equivalents (other atherosclerotic vascular disease, diabetes, 10-year absolute risk >20%), and within this category, the NCEP ATP III update identifies a subgroup with very high risk, defined as individuals with CHD or CHD risk equivalent in addition to multiple major risk factors, severe and poorly controlled risk factors, metabolic syndrome, or acute coronary syndromes.[2] For individuals without CHD or CHD risk equivalent, absolute risk is assessed by risk factor counting in conjunction with Framingham Risk Score (see Chapter 18). To refine risk assessment in intermediate-risk individuals, measurement of biomarkers (see Chapter 15), such as C-reactive protein[3] (see Chapter 13) and lipoprotein-associated phospholipase A_2 (see Chapter 14), and noninvasive imaging (see Chapter 16) may be helpful.

The most aggressive LDL cholestrol treatment goals are for individuals at highest CHD risk. The NCEP ATP III guidelines recommend an LDL cholesterol goal of less than 100 mg/dL for high-risk individuals with CHD,[1] and the ATP III update establishes an optional goal of less than 70 mg/dL for individuals with very high risk.[2] For individuals with high or moderately high risk, the ATP III update recommends that therapy be of sufficient intensity to reduce LDL cholesterol by 30% to 40%.[2] The American Heart Association/American College of Cardiology Guidelines for Secondary Prevention establish an LDL cholesterol goal of less than 100 mg/dL but consider an LDL cholesterol goal of less than 70 mg/dL "reasonable" for all patients with cardiovascular disease, with an alternative of reducing LDL cholesterol by more than 50% if the lower goal of less than 70 mg/dL cannot be achieved.[4] In primary prevention, the ATP III update sets an optional LDL cholesterol goal of less than 100 mg/dL in moderately high-risk patients (≥2 risk factors with 10-year risk of 10%–20%),[2] whereas the goals for patients with moderate (≥2 risk factors with 10-year risk of <10%) and lower (<2 risk factors with 10-year risk of <10%) risk remain less than 130 and <160 mg/dL, respectively, as in the original NCEP ATP III report.

Statins are the first choice of therapy for LDL cholesterol lowering in most patients (see Chapter 22). Other agents that reduce LDL cholesterol include bile acid sequestrants (see Chapter 23), ezetimibe (see Chapter 24), niacin (see Chapter 25), fibrates (see Chapter 26), and certain dietary components such as soluble fiber and plant sterols and stanols (see Chapters 19 and 31). Combination treatment with statins and these other drugs, as well as nonstatin combinations, can be used to lower LDL cholesterol (see Chapter 29). In the most severe hypercholesterolemias, such as homozygous and heterozygous familial hypercholesterolemia, LDL apheresis can be used (see Chapter 30).

MIXED DYSLIPIDEMIA

Mixed dyslipidemia is the combination of elevated LDL cholesterol and triglyceride and decreased High-density liproprotein (HDL) Cholesterol, and may occur with certain genetic disorders (familial combined hyperlipidemia, familial dysbetalipoproteinemia [also known as type III hyperlipoproteinemia]), diabetes mellitus, the metabolic syndrome, or the use of drugs such as immunosuppressive agents or protease inhibitors. Patients with mixed dyslipidemia have increased numbers of triglyceride-rich remnant lipoproteins, including very-low-density lipoprotein (VLDL) remnants and intermediate-density lipoproteins (IDLs), as well as increased numbers of small dense LDL particles. VLDL cholesterol is typically increased, and most VLDL cholesterol is in smaller VLDL remnants.

Non-HDL cholesterol is a useful measure of both triglyceride-rich and cholesterol-rich particles. It can be calculated easily from the standard lipid profile by subtracting HDL cholesterol from total cholesterol, and reflects the combined cholesterol in all apolipoprotein (apo) B–containing (i.e., atherogenic) lipoproteins, including VLDL, IDL, LDL, and lipoprotein(a) [Lp(a)]. In the NCEP ATP III guidelines, non-HDL cholesterol is a secondary therapeutic target (after the primary target of LDL cholesterol is achieved) in patients with triglycerides ≥200 mg/dL.[1] ApoB targets of less than 90 mg/dL in high-risk patients[5,6] and less than 80 mg/dL in highest-risk patients[6] have also been suggested.

Treatment should begin with lifestyle modification therapy, including diet, weight reduction, and increased physical activity. Statins decrease LDL cholesterol, non-HDL cholesterol, and triglycerides, reduce apoB and LDL particle number, and modestly increase HDL cholesterol. Additional therapies to achieve reductions in non-HDL cholesterol and apoB include ezetimibe, bile acid–binding resins (which may, however, increase triglycerides), niacin, fibrates, and omega-3 fatty acids. The most effective therapies for additional triglyceride reduction are niacin, fibrates, and omega-3 fatty acids. Niacin, fibrates, and omega-3 fatty acids also improve LDL particle size, and niacin substantially increases HDL cholesterol and reduces Lp(a).

SEVERE ELEVATIONS OF TRIGLYCERIDES

Triglycerides may become elevated with obesity, physical inactivity, high-carbohydrate diet, cigarette smoking, alcohol, diseases such as diabetes and renal failure, drugs including estrogen and corticosteroids, and genetic disorders (familial hypertriglyceridemia, familial combined hyperlipidemia, and familial dysbetalipoproteinemia). Evaluation of secondary causes of dyslipidemia (see Chapter 12) is especially important in hypertriglyceridemic patients. In patients with very high triglycerides (≥500 mg/dL), the initial goal of therapy is to prevent acute pancreatitis. Therapy should include very-low-fat diet (≤15% of total calories as fat), weight

TABLE 17-1 Classification and Treatment of Hypertriglyceridemia in Adult Treatment Panel III Guidelines[1]

TG, mg/dL	ATP III Classification	Primary Target of Therapy	Treatment Recommendations
<150	Normal		
150–199	Borderline high	LDL cholesterol goal	Weight reduction, increased physical activity
200–499	High	LDL cholesterol goal	Weight reduction, increased physical activity; consider drug therapy to achieve non-HDL cholesterol goal (intensify LDL cholesterol lowering with statin or lower VLDL cholesterol by adding niacin or fibrate)
≥500	Very high	Reduce TG to prevent acute pancreatitis	Very-low-fat diet (fat ≤15% of total calories), weight reduction, increased physical activity, and drug therapy with niacin or fibrate

ATP III, U.S. National Cholesterol Education Program Adult Treatment Panel III; LDL, low-density lipoprotein; non-HDL, non–high-density lipoprotein; TG, triglycerides; VLDL, very-low-density lipoprotein.

reduction, increased physical activity, and drug therapy with niacin, fibrates, or omega-3 fatly acids (Table 17-1). When triglycerides are reduced to less than 500 mg/dL, LDL cholesterol becomes the primary therapeutic target according to the NCEP ATP III guidelines, and non-HDL cholesterol is a secondary therapeutic target. Combination therapy (see Chapter 29) is usually required to manage dyslipidemia in patients with severe elevations of triglycerides. Lifestyle modification, including reduction or cessation of alcohol (see Chapter 19), weight loss (see Chapter 21), and glycemic control (see Chapter 37) are all critical for successful treatment of these patients.

LOW HIGH-DENSITY LIPOPROTEIN CHOLESTEROL

In the NCEP ATP III guidelines, low HDL cholesterol is defined as less than 40 mg/dL in the algorithm for risk factor counting, and HDL cholesterol less than 40 mg/dL in men or less than 50 mg/dL in women is a diagnostic criterion for the metabolic syndrome.[1] Low HDL cholesterol can be caused by elevated triglycerides, diabetes, obesity, physical inactivity, high-carbohydrate diet, cigarette smoking, drugs such as β-blockers and anabolic steroids, and rare genetic disorders.

HDL cholesterol can be increased with increased physical activity and weight reduction. Niacin is the most efficacious HDL cholesterol–raising drug; fibrates also increase HDL cholesterol substantially, and statins provide modest increases in HDL cholesterol. Although estrogen increases HDL cholesterol, estrogen did not reduce cardiovascular risk in the Women's Health Initiative[7] and the Heart and Estrogen/Progestin Replacement Study (HERS)[8] and therefore is not recommended for this purpose. In the NCEP ATP III guidelines, drug therapy to raise HDL cholesterol is recommended for consideration primarily in high-risk patients,[1] although the selection of agents to reduce LDL cholesterol and non-HDL cholesterol to NCEP ATP III targets should consider their effect on HDL cholesterol. The NCEP ATP III guidelines do not establish a treatment goal for HDL cholesterol.[1] In contrast, the American Diabetes Association guidelines recommend that HDL cholesterol be greater than 40 mg/dL and suggest the use of fibrate or niacin to raise isolated low HDL cholesterol,[9] and the American Heart Association guidelines for women recommend that HDL cholesterol be greater than 50 mg/dL, to be achieved with lifestyle modification in all women and as a secondary target of therapy in high-risk women (also to be considered for women at moderately high risk), for whom the guidelines recommend the use of fibrate or niacin therapy.[10]

ELEVATED LIPOPROTEIN(A)

Lp(a) and considerations about measuring Lp(a) are discussed in depth in Chapter 11. Although elevated Lp(a) is an independent risk factor for cardiovascular disease, the level at which risk increases has not been established; Lp(a) levels of 75 nmol/L or greater are generally considered elevated. The optimal treatment approach for elevated Lp(a) is not known. Lifestyle modifications do not affect Lp(a) level. Niacin and estrogen reduce Lp(a), but effects with statins and fibrates are variable. Lp(a) is also removed with LDL apheresis. For patients with elevated Lp(a), an alternative to reducing Lp(a) is to lower LDL cholesterol more aggressively, for example, with intensive statin therapy.

REFERENCES

1. Expert Panel on Detection Evaluation and Treatment of High Blood Cholesterol in Adults: Executive summary of the third report of the National Cholesterol Education Program (NCEP) Expert Panel on Detection, Evaluation, and Treatment of High Blood Cholesterol in Adults (Adult Treatment Panel III). JAMA 2001;285:2486–2497.
2. Grundy SM, Cleeman JI, Bairey Merz CN, et al: Implications of recent clinical trials for the National Cholesterol Education Program Adult Treatment Panel III guidelines. Circulation 2004;110:227–239.
3. Pearson TA, Mensah GA, Alexander RW, et al: Markers of inflammation and cardiovascular disease: Application to clinical and public health practice: A statement for healthcare professionals from the Centers for Disease Control and Prevention and the American Heart Association. Circulation 2003;107:499–511.
4. Smith SC Jr, Allen J, Blair SN, et al: AHA/ACC guidelines for secondary prevention for patients with coronary and other atherosclerotic vascular disease: 2006 update. Endorsed by the National Heart, Lung, and Blood Institute. Circulation 2006;113:2363–2372.
5. Grundy SM: Low-density lipoprotein, non-high-density lipoprotein, and apolipoprotein B as targets of lipid-lowering therapy. Circulation 2002;106:2526–2529.
6. Brunzell JD, Davidson M, Furberg CD, et al: Lipoprotein management in patients with cardiometabolic risk: Consensus conference report from the American Diabetes Association and the American College of Cardiology Foundation. J Am Coll Cardiol 2008;51:1512–1524.
7. Manson JE, Hsia J, Johnson KC, et al: Estrogen plus progestin and the risk of coronary heart disease. N Engl J Med 2003;349: 523–534.
8. Grady D, Herrington D, Bittner V, et al: Cardiovascular disease outcomes during 6.8 years of hormone therapy: Heart and Estrogen/Progestin Replacement Study Follow-up (HERS II). JAMA 2002;288:49–57.
9. American Diabetes Association: Standards of medical care in diabetes—2008. Diabetes Care 2008;31(Suppl 1):12–54.
10. Mosca L, Banka CL, Benjamin EJ, et al: Evidence-based guidelines for cardiovascular disease prevention in women: 2007 update. Circulation 2007;115:1481–1501.

CHAPTER 18

Treatment Guidelines Overview

C. Noel Bairey Merz and Donna Polk

A plethora of data over the last two decades demonstrates not only reduction in atherosclerosis progression, but actually atherosclerosis reversal with aggressive medical and lifestyle management. Four classes of drugs (lipid-lowering agents, antiplatelet agents, β-blockers, and angiotensin-converting enzyme [ACE]/ angiotensin receptor blockers [ARB]), and three lifestyle components (cigarette smoking cessation, nutrition, and physical activity) provide lifesaving reductions in cardiovascular risk by modulation of atherosclerosis and cardiovascular disease (CVD) pathophysiology.

Lipid-lowering therapy reduces CVD risk in patients with established CVD as well as in at-risk patients, reducing event rates by approximately 30% to 50%.[1] Aspirin, an over-the-counter, inexpensive treatment, has a large body of evidence documenting its utility for risk reduction in patients with established CVD,[2] with an overall magnitude of risk reduction in terms of death and nonfatal myocardial infarction (MI) of approximately 25%.[3] More than 20 randomized controlled trials demonstrate the efficacy of β-blocker therapy for the reduction of adverse events in CVD patients and in at-risk patients undergoing surgery and anesthesia.[4] In the setting of post-MI, unstable angina, and congestive heart failure, the overall risk reduction with β-blocker therapy is 25%.[5] Data supports strong consideration of ACE inhibitor use in established CVD patients, independent of hypertensive status, suggesting also that these be used as first line medications in post-MI patients and in patients with heart failure, high CVD risk, diabetes, and chronic kidney disease, as well as for recurrent stroke prevention.[6] The overall magnitude of risk reduction in terms of death and nonfatal MI with ACE inhibitor therapy is on the order of 25%.

Comprehensive lifestyle change clearly can reduce cardiovascular risk. Specifically, cigarette smoking cessation,[7] nutrition,[8] and physical activity[9] reduce risk of adverse events, typically to a greater magnitude than medication, ranging from 50% risk reduction for smoking cessation and nutrition changes, to 20% to 25% risk reduction for increased exercise in controlled trials. Summary studies document the potent utility of combining these three effective therapies for maximal cardiovascular risk reduction. Mukerjee and coworkers observed a more than 90% reduction in risk for death and recurrent events in the year following an acute coronary syndrome/MI among patients prescribed a statin, aspirin, β-blocker, and ACE/ ARB.[10] Despite these compelling data, national survey data indicate that only a minority of patients eligible by guidelines for these therapies receive them.

Translation of the aforementioned efficacies into clinical practice is our most critical need to address the burgeoning epidemic of CVD. A number of treatment guidelines have been established to address this need and put our clinical trial evidence into practice.[1,5,6] This text addresses the lipid treatment components of these guidelines, describing the guidelines themselves as well as the rationales behind them.

ADULT TREATMENT PANEL III

The 1987 launch of lovastatin, the first approved hydroxy-methylglutaryl – coenzyme A (HMG-CoA) reductase inhibitor, and subsequent introduction of more powerful and therapeutically effective statins have revolutionized not only the treatment of patients with frank hyperlipidemia, but also the treatment of at-risk patients in general. A solid body of evidence demonstrates that statins reduce the risk of cardiovascular events in patients with established CVD and in patients at risk for CVD because of cardiac risk factors or concomitant vascular disease.

The National Cholesterol Education Program Adult Treatment Panel on Detection, Evaluation, and Treatment of High Blood Cholesterol in Adults (NCEP ATP) addressed sequentially these studies, publishing NCEP ATP I, NCEP ATP II,[11] and most recently NCEP ATP III.[1] The executive summary of NCEP ATP III was published in May 2001.[12] The full report of NCEP ATP III was published in December 2002.[1]

NCEP ATP III provided evidence-based recommendations on the management of high blood cholesterol and related disorders. For development of its recommendations, NCEP ATP III placed primary emphasis on large, randomized, controlled clinical trials. Other lines of evidence, including prospective epidemiologic studies and smaller clinical trials, provided additional evidence for the recommendations. The full NCEP ATP III document is an evidenced-based and extensively referenced report that provides the scientific rationale for the recommendations contained in the executive summary. The guidelines were written to inform, not replace, the physician's judgment, in order to best determine patient treatment. Finally, the NCEP ATP III guidelines reiterated that low-density lipoprotein (LDL) cholesterol remains the primary target of lipid-lowering therapy and classifies optimal, near or above optimal, borderline high, high, and very high LDL cholesterol (Table 18-1).

Risk Assessment and Treatment

According to the NCEP ATP III algorithm, persons are categorized into three risk categories: (1) established coronary heart disease (CHD) and CHD risk equivalents, (2) multiple (two or more) risk factors, and (3) zero to one risk factors (Table 18-2). CHD risk equivalents include noncoronary forms of clinical atherosclerotic disease, diabetes, and multiple (two or more) CHD risk factors with 10-year risk for CHD of greater than 20%. All persons with CHD or CHD risk equivalents can be called *high risk*. The goal for LDL-lowering therapy in high-risk patients is an LDL cholesterol level of less than 100 mg/dL. According to ATP III, for a baseline or on-treatment LDL cholesterol of less than 100 mg/dL, no

TABLE 18-1 Adult Treatment Panel III Classification of Low-Density Lipoprotein, Total, and High-Density Lipoprotein Cholesterol (mg/dL)

LDL Cholesterol	
<100	Optimal
100–129	Near or above optimal
130–159	Borderline high
160–189	High
≥190	Very high
Total Cholesterol	
<200	Desirable
200–239	Borderline high
≥240	High
HDL Cholesterol	
<40	Low
≥60	High

ATP, Adult Treatment Panel; HDL, high-density lipoprotein; LDL, low-density lipoprotein. *Reprinted from Ref. 12, with permission.*

TABLE 18-2 Three Categories of Risk That Modify Low-Density Lipoprotein Cholesterol Goals

Risk Category	LDL Goal (mg/dL)
CHD and CHD risk equivalents	<100
Multiple (2+) risk factors*	<130
0–1 risk factor*	<160

*Risk factors that modify low-density lipoprotein (LDL) goal are listed in Table 18-4. CHD, coronary heart disease. *Reprinted from Ref. 12, with permission.*

further LDL-lowering therapy was recommended. For all high-risk patients with LDL cholesterol levels ≥100 mg/dL, LDL-lowering dietary therapy should be initiated. When baseline LDL cholesterol is ≥130 mg/dL, an LDL-lowering drug should be started simultaneously with dietary therapy (see Table 18-3). However, LDL-lowering drugs were not stipulated if the baseline LDL cholesterol level is in the range of 100 to 129 mg/dL; in this range, NCEP ATP III suggested several therapeutic options. Dietary therapy should be intensified, whereas adding or intensifying an LDL-lowering drug was said to be optional. Alternatively, if the patient has elevated triglyceride or low HDL, a drug that targets these abnormalities can be added.

NCEP ATP III recommended that Framingham risk scoring be carried out in individuals with at least two risk factors so as to classify them into three levels of 10-year risk for hard CHD events (MI + CHD death): greater than 20%, 10% to 20%, and less than 10% (Table 18-4).[13,19] Persons with a 10-year risk greater than 20% were elevated to the high-risk category; for them, the LDL cholesterol goal is less than 100 mg/dL. For persons with two or more risk factors and a 10-year risk of 20% or less, the LDL cholesterol goal is less than 130 mg/dL. LDL-lowering dietary therapy is universally advocated for patients with an LDL cholesterol above the goal level. If the 10-year risk is 10% to 20%, drug therapy should be considered if the LDL cholesterol level is above the goal level (i.e., ≥130 mg/dL) after a trial of dietary therapy. When 10-year risk is less than 10%, an LDL-lowering drug may be considered if the LDL cholesterol level is ≥160 mg/dL on maximal dietary therapy (see Table 18-3).

Finally, most persons with zero to one risk factor have a 10-year risk of less than 10%. For these individuals, clinical management and dietary therapy is recommended when the LDL cholesterol level is 160 mg/dL or greater. The goal is to lower LDL cholesterol concentrations to less than 160 mg/dL. If the LDL cholesterol is 190 mg/dL or greater after an adequate trial of dietary therapy, the guidelines suggested consideration of adding a lipid-lowering drug. When serum LDL cholesterol ranges from 160 to 189 mg/dL, use of a lipid-lowering drug is a therapeutic option in appropriate circumstances, such as when a severe risk factor is present.

Therapeutic Lifestyle Change

NCEP ATP III placed major emphasis on therapeutic lifestyle change (TLC) as an essential modality in clinical management for persons at risk for CHD (Table 18-5). The TLC approach of NCEP ATP III was

TABLE 18-3 Low-Density Lipoprotein Cholesterol Goals and Cutpoints for Therapeutic Lifestyle Changes and Drug Therapy in Different Risk Categories

Risk Category	LDL Goal (mg/dL)	LDL Level at Which to Initiate Therapeutic Lifestyle Changes (mg/dL)	LDL Level at Which to Consider Drug Therapy (mg/dL)
CHD or CHD risk equivalents (10-year risk >20%)	<100	≥100	≥130 (100–129: drug optional)*
2+ Risk factors (10-year risk ≤20%)	<130	≥130	10-year risk 10%-20%: ≥130 10-year risk <10%: ≥160
0–1 Risk factor†	<160	≥160	≥190 (160–189: LDL-lowering drug optional)

*Some authorities recommend use of low-density lipoprotein (LDL)-lowering drugs in this category if an LDL cholesterol level of less than 100 mg/dL cannot be achieved by therapeutic lifestyle changes. Others prefer use of drugs that primarily modify triglycerides and high-density lipoprotein (HDL), such as nicotinic acid or fibrate. Clinical judgment also may call for deferring drug therapy in this subcategory.
†Almost all people with zero to one risk factor have a 10-year risk of less than 10%; thus, 10-year risk assessment in people with zero to one risk factor is not necessary.
CHD, coronary heart disease.
Reprinted from Ref. 12, with permission.

TABLE 18-4 Major Risk Factors (Exclusive of LDL Cholesterol) that Modify LDL Goals*

- Cigarette smoking
- Hypertension (blood pressure ≥140/90 mm Hg or on antihypertensive medication)
- Low HDL cholesterol (<40 mg/dL)†
- Family history of premature CHD (CHD in male first-degree relative <55 years; CHD in female first-degree relative <65 years)
- Age (men ≥45 years; women ≥55 years)

*Diabetes is regarded as a coronary heart disease (CHD) equivalent.
†High-density lipoprotein (HDL) cholesterol ≥60 mg/dL counts as a "negative" risk factor; its presence removes one risk factor for the total count.
LDL, low-density lipoprotein.
Reprinted from Ref. 12, with permission.

TABLE 18-5 Nutrient Composition of the Therapeutic Lifestyle Changes Diet

Nutrient	Recommended Intake
Saturated fat*	<7% of total calories
Polyunsaturated fat	Up to 10% of total calories
Monounsaturated fat	Up to 20% of total calories
Total fat	25%–35% of total calories
Carbohydrate†	50%–60% of total calories
Fiber	20–30 g/d
Protein	Approximately 15% of total calories
Cholesterol	<200 mg/d
Total calories‡	Balance energy intake and expenditure to maintain desirable body weight/prevent weight gain

**Trans* fatty acids are another low-density lipoprotein (LDL)-raising fat that should be kept at a low intake.
†Carbohydrates should be derived predominantly from foods rich in complex carbohydrates including grains, especially whole grains, fruits, and vegetables.
‡Daily energy expenditure should include at least moderate physical activity (contributing approximately 200 kcal/d).
Reprinted from Ref. 12, with permission.

designed to achieve risk reduction through both LDL cholesterol lowering and metabolic syndrome management (Fig. 18-1). Therefore when the implications of additional post–NCEP ATP III LDL-lowering drug trials are considered, the guidelines emphasized that the results do not in any way diminish the importance of lifestyle change for CHD risk reduction.

Drug Therapy to Achieve Low-Density Lipoprotein Cholesterol Goals

Medications for lipid lowering are listed in Table 18-6. NCEP ATP III stated that when medication is prescribed, TLC should be maintained and reinforced.

Benefit Beyond Low-Density Lipoprotein Lowering: the Metabolic Syndrome as a Secondary Target

The metabolic syndrome represents a constellation of lipid and nonlipid risk factors of metabolic origin. Closely linked with insulin resistance, in which the normal actions of insulin are impaired, the metabolic syndrome may be secondary to abdominal obesity, physical inactivity, or genetic predisposition. Criteria for clinical identification of the metabolic syndrome are listed in Table 18-7. It is noteworthy that for the first time, the guidelines listed separate thresholds for women and men for high-density lipoprotein (HDL) cholesterol and waist circumference.

Special Issues

A number of special issues are addressed by the ATP III. *Very high LDL cholesterol* (≥190 mg/dL) is usually a genetic form of hypercholesterolemia and should prompt family testing; it typically requires combined drug therapy such as statin and bile acid agents or niacin to achieve the LDL goals. *Elevated serum triglycerides* were identified as an independent risk factor for CHD and a marker of atherogenic remnant lipoproteins, most easily measured as very-low-density lipoprotein (VLDL) cholesterol. NCEP ATP III identified the sum of LDL plus VLDL cholesterol as non-HDL cholesterol (calculated as total cholesterol minus HDL cholesterol) and as a secondary target of therapy in persons with elevated triglycerides above 200 mg/dL. The goal for non-HDL cholesterol was set at 30 mg/dL above the LDL cholesterol goal (Table 18-8). In addition to treatment with TLC, the non-HDL cholesterol goal can be achieved by intensifying LDL cholesterol–lowering medication and adding niacin or fibrate to the medication regimen. *Very low HDL cholesterol* was

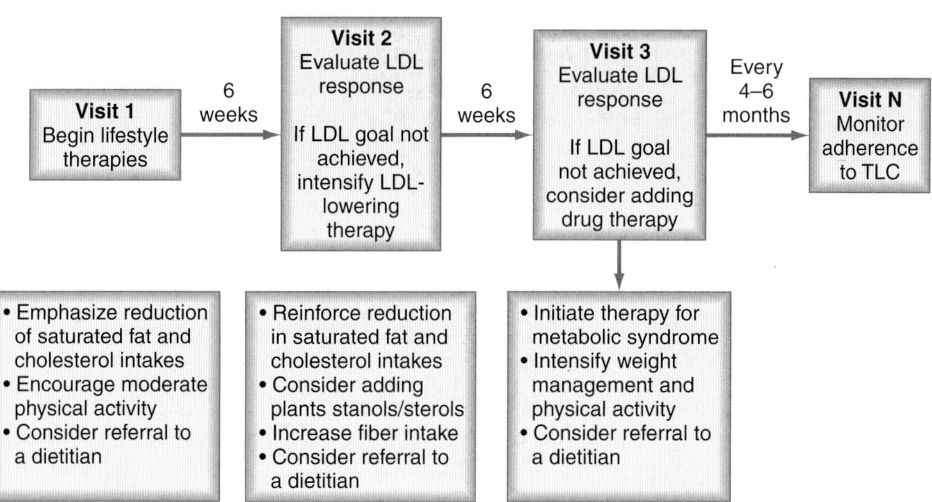

FIGURE 18-1 Model of steps in therapeutic lifestyle changes (TLC). LDL, low-density lipoprotein. *Reprinted from Ref. 12, with permission.*

TABLE 18-6 Drugs Affecting Lipoprotein Metabolism

Drug Class, Agents, and Daily Doses	Lipid/Lipoprotein Effects	Side Effects	Contraindications	Clinical Trial Results
HMG-CoA reductase inhibitors (statins)*	LDL ↓ 18%–55% HDL ↑ 5%–15% TG ↓ 7%–30%	Myopathy; increased liver enzymes	Absolute: active or chronic liver disease Relative: concomitant use of certain drugs†	Reduced major coronary events, CHD deaths, need for coronary procedures, stroke, and total mortality
Bile acid sequestrants‡	LDL ↓ 15%–30% HDL ↑ 3%–5% TG no change or increase	Gastrointestinal distress; constipation; decreased absorption of other drugs	Absolute: dysbetalipoproteinemia; TG >400 mg/dL Relative:TG >200 mg/dL	Reduced major coronary events and CHD deaths
Nicotinic acid§	LDL ↓ 5%–25% HDL ↑ 15%–35% TG ↓ 20%–50%	Flushing; hyperglycemia; hyperuricemia (or gout); upper gastrointestinal distress; hepatotoxicity	Absolute: chronic liver disease; severe gout Relative: diabetes; hyperuricemia; peptic ulcer disease	Reduced major coronary events, and possibly total mortality
Fibric acids‖	LDL ↓ 5%–20% (may be increased in patients with high TG) HDL ↑ 10%–20% TG ↓ 20%–50%	Dyspepsia; gallstones; myopathy; unexplained non-CHD deaths in WHO study	Absolute: severe renal disease; severe hepatic disease	Reduced major coronary events

*Lovastatin (20–80 mg), pravastatin (20–40 mg), simvastatin (20–80 mg), fluvastatin (20–80 mg), and atorvastatin (10–80 mg).
‡Cholestyramine (4–16 g), colestipol (5–20 g), and colesevelam (2.6–3.8 g).
†Cyclosporine, macrolide antibiotics, various antifungal agents, and cytochrome P-450 inhibitors (fibrates and niacin should be used with appropriate caution).
§Immediate-release (crystalline) nicotinic acid (1.5–3 g), extended-release nicotinic acid (1–2 g), and sustained-release nicotinic acid (1–2 g).
‖Gemfibrozil (600 mg twice daily), fenofibrate (130 or 145 mg), and clofibrate (1000 mg twice daily).
HMG-CoA, 3-hydroxy-3-methylglutaryl-coenzyme A; LDL, low-density lipoprotein; HDL, high-density lipoprotein; TG, triglycerides; ↓, decrease; ↑, increase; CHD, coronary heart disease.
Reprinted from Ref. 12, with permission.

addressed similarly, although NCEP ATP III reserved medication treatment for subjects with established CHD or CHD risk equivalents. *Diabetic dyslipidemia* was addressed by reiterating that diabetes is a CHD risk equivalent and therefore the treatment goal for LDL cholesterol less than 100 mg/dL. NCEP ATP III further indicated that the guidelines were relevant across a wide range of subjects, ages, and racial/ethnic groups and that statin therapy was preferable to hormone replacement therapy in older women.

Adherence to Low-Density Lipoprotein-Lowering Therapy

Recognizing the importance and challenge of maintaining compliance to TLC and medication over time as necessary to combat atherosclerosis and CHD, NCEP ATP III recommended multidisciplinary methods for the patient, clinician, and health care system to achieve guideline effectiveness.

ADULT TREATMENT PANEL III UPDATE

Following the publication of NCEP ATP III, subsequent clinical trials strongly suggested that modifications to the guidelines should be made, resulting in the NCEP ATP III guidelines update in 2004 (ATP III Update).[14]

New Clinical Trials

The update reviewed the results of five major clinical trials with statin therapy available at the time, including the Heart Protection Study (HPS),[15] Prospective Study of Pravastatin in the Elderly at Risk (PROSPER),[16] Antihypertensive and Lipid-Lowering Treatment to

TABLE 18-7 Clinical Identification of the Metabolic Syndrome

Risk Factor	Defining Level
· Abdominal obesity* (waist circumference)†	
Men	>102 cm (>40 in)
Women	>88 cm (>35 in)
· Triglycerides	≥150 mg/dL
· High-density lipoprotein cholesterol	
Men	<40 mg/dL
Women	<50 mg/dL
· Blood pressure	≥130/≥85 mm Hg
· Fasting glucose	≥110 mg/dL

*Overweight and obesity are associated with insulin resistance and the metabolic syndrome. However, the presence of abdominal obesity is more highly correlated with the metabolic risk factors than is an elevated body mass index. Therefore, the simple measure of waist circumference is recommended to identify the body weight component of the metabolic syndrome.

†Some male patients can develop multiple metabolic risk factors when the waist circumference is only marginally increased, e.g., 94–102 cm (37–40 in). Such patients may have strong genetic contribution to insulin resistance, and they should benefit from changes in life habits, similarly to men with categoric increases in waist circumference.

Reprinted from Ref. 12, with permission.

TABLE 18-8 Comparison of Low-Density Lipoprotein Cholesterol and Non-High-Density Lipoprotein Cholesterol Goals for Three Risk Categories

Risk Category	LDL Goal (mg/dL)	Non-HDL Goal (mg/dL)
CHD and CHD risk equivalent (10-year risk for CHD >20%)	<100	<130
Multiple (2+) risk factors and 10-year risk ≤20%	<130	<160
0–1 Risk factor	<160	<190

CHD, coronary heart disease; LDL, low-density lipoprotein; non-HDL, non-high-density lipoprotein

Reprinted from Ref. 12, with permission.

Prevent Heart Attack Trial–Lipid Lowering Trial (ALLHAT-LLT),[17] Anglo-Scandinavian Cardiac Outcomes Trial–Lipid Lowering Arm (ASCOT-LLA),[18] and Pravastatin or Atorvastatin Evaluation and Infection–Thrombolysis in Myocardial Infarction 22 (PROVE IT–TIMI 22) trial.[19] These trials addressed issues that had not been adequately addressed in previous statin trials, addressed NCEP ATP III treatment thresholds, and had important implications for the management of patients with lipid disorders, particularly for high-risk patients. The report also reviewed relevant published findings of other, smaller trials and subgroup analyses of major trials that had been published.

Expanded Efficacy in Diabetes and the Elderly

The ATP III Update reiterated that TLC remains an essential modality in clinical management of dyslipidemia. The reviewed newer trials confirmed the benefit of cholesterol-lowering therapy in high-risk patients and supported the NCEP ATP III treatment goal of LDL cholesterol of less than 100 mg/dL. They also supported identifying patients with diabetes as high risk by confirming the benefits of LDL-lowering therapy in these patients. They further confirmed that older persons benefit from therapeutic lowering of LDL cholesterol. The new clinical trial data also supported that recommendations should not be modified on the basis of ethnicity.

New Treatment Goals

The major recommendations for modifications to the previous NCEP ATP III treatment algorithm include the following:

1. In *high-risk persons*, the recommended LDL cholesterol goal is less than 100 mg/dL. When risk is *very high*, an LDL cholesterol goal of less than 70 mg/dL is a therapeutic option, that is, a reasonable clinical strategy based on available clinical trial evidence. This therapeutic option extends also to patients at very high risk who have a baseline LDL cholesterol of less than 100 mg/dL.
2. When a high-risk patient has high triglyceride or low HDL cholesterol, consideration can be given to combining a fibrate or nicotinic acid with an LDL-lowering drug.
3. For *moderately high risk persons* (two or more risk factors and 10-year risk of 10% to 20%), the recommended LDL cholesterol goal is less than 130 mg/dL, but an LDL cholesterol goal of less than 100 mg/dL is a therapeutic option based on recent trial evidence, and the latter option extends also to moderately high risk persons with a baseline LDL cholesterol of 100 to 129 mg/dL.
4. When LDL-lowering drug therapy is employed in high-risk or moderately high risk persons, it is advised that intensity of therapy be sufficient to achieve at least a 30% to 40% reduction in LDL cholesterol levels.
5. Any person at high risk or moderately high risk who has lifestyle-related risk factors (e.g., obesity, physical inactivity, elevated triglyceride, low HDL cholesterol, or metabolic syndrome) is a candidate for TLC to modify these risk factors regardless of LDL cholesterol level.
6. For people in lower-risk categories, recent clinical trials do not modify the goals and cutpoints of therapy. These revised recommendations and rationale from the ATP III Update are outlined in Tables 18-9 and 18-10.

Very-High-Risk Patients

Probably the most significant modification in the ATP III Update is the "lower is better" approach to lipid lowering, stating that an LDL cholesterol goal of less than 70 mg/dL is a reasonable therapeutic strategy in patients at very high cardiac risk, such as those with known CHD and diabetes, the metabolic syndrome, or a recent cardiac event. High risk was further defined

TABLE 18-9 Adult Treatment Panel III Low-Density Lipoprotein-Cholesterol Goals and Cutpoints for Therapeutic Lifestyle Changes and Drug Therapy in Different Risk Categories and Proposed Modifications Based on Recent Clinical Trial Evidence

Risk Category	LDL Cholesterol Goal	Initiate Therapeutic Lifestyle Changes	Consider Drug Therapy*
CHD† or CHD risk equivalents‡ (10-year risk >20%) *High risk*	<100 mg/dL (optional goal: <70 mg/dL)¶	≥100 mg/dL§	≥100 mg/dL‖ (<100 mg/dL: consider drug options)*
2+ Risk factors# (10-year risk 10%–20%) *Moderately high risk*	<130 mg/dL**	≥130 mg/dL§	≥130 mg/dL (100–129 mg/dL; consider drug options)††
2+ Risk factors# (10-year risk <10%) *Moderate risk*	<130 mg/dL	≥130 mg/dL	>160 mg/dL
0–1 Risk factor‡‡	<160 mg/dL	≥160 mg/dL	≥190 mg/dL (160–189 mg/dL: LDL-lowering drug optional)

*When LDL-lowering drug therapy is used, it is advised that intensity of therapy be sufficient to achieve at least a 30% to 40% reduction in LDL cholesterol levels.

†Coronary heart disease (CHD) includes history of myocardial infarction, unstable angina, stable angina, coronary artery procedures (angioplasty or bypass surgery), or evidence of clinically significant myocardial ischemia.

‡CHD risk equivalents include clinical manifestations of noncoronary forms of atherosclerotic disease (peripheral artery disease, abdominal aortic aneurysm, and carotid artery disease [transient ischemic attack or stroke of carotid origin or more than 50% obstruction of a carotid artery]), diabetes, and at least two risk factors with 10-year risk for hard CHD events greater than 20%.

§Any person at high risk or moderately high risk who has lifestyle-related risk factors (e.g., obesity, physical inactivity, elevated triglyceride, low HDL cholesterol, or metabolic syndrome) is a candidate for therapeutic lifestyle changes to modify these risk factors regardless of LDL cholesterol level.

‖If baseline LDL cholesterol is less than 100 mg/dL, institution of an LDL-lowering drug is a therapeutic option based on available clinical trial results. If a high-risk person has high triglycerides or low HDL cholesterol, combining a fibrate or nicotinic acid with an LDL-lowering drug can be considered.

¶Very high risk favors the optional low-density lipoprotein (LDL) cholesterol goal of less than 70 mg/dL.

#Risk factors include cigarette smoking, hypertension (blood pressure ≥140/90 mm Hg or on antihypertensive medication), low high-density lipoprotein (HDL) cholesterol (<40 mg/dL), family history of premature CHD (CHD in male first-degree relative younger than 55 years; CHD in female first-degree relative younger than 65 years), and age (men ≥45 years; women ≥55 years)

**Optional LDL cholesterol goal of less than 100 mg/dL.

††For moderately high-risk persons, when LDL cholesterol level is 100 to 129 mg/dL, at baseline or on lifestyle therapy, initiation of an LDL-lowering drug to achieve an LDL cholesterol level less than 100 mg/dL is a therapeutic option based on available clinical trial results.

‡‡Almost all people with zero to one risk factor have a 10-year risk of less than 10%, and 10-year risk assessment in people with zero to one risk factor is thus not necessary.

Reprinted from Ref. 12, with permission.

TABLE 18-10 Recommendations for Modifications to Footnote the Adult Treatment Panel III Treatment Algorithm for Low-Density Lipoprotein-Cholesterol

- In high-risk persons, the recommended LDL cholesterol goal is <100 mg/dL.
  - An LDL cholesterol goal of <70 mg/dL is a therapeutic option based on available clinical trial evidence, especially for patients at very high risk.
  - If LDL cholesterol is ≥100 mg/dL, an LDL-lowering drug is indicated simultaneously with lifestyle changes.
  - If baseline LDL cholesterol is <100 mg/dL, institution of an LDL-lowering drug to achieve an LDL cholesterol level of <70 mg/dL is a therapeutic option based on available clinical trial evidence.
  - If a high-risk person has high triglycerides or low HDL cholesterol, consideration can be given to combining a fibrate or nicotinic acid with an LDL-lowering drug.
- For moderately high risk persons (two or more risk factors and 10-year risk of 10%–20%), the recommended LDL cholesterol goal is <130 mg/dL; an LDL cholesterol goal of <100 mg/dL is a therapeutic option based on available clinical trial evidence. When LDL cholesterol level is 100–129 mg/dL, at baseline or on lifestyle therapy, initiation of an LDL-lowering drug to achieve an LDL cholesterol level of <100 mg/dL is a therapeutic option based on available clinical trial evidence.
- Any person at high risk or moderately high risk who has lifestyle-related risk factors (e.g., obesity, physical inactivity, elevated triglyceride, low HDL cholesterol, or metabolic syndrome) is a candidate for therapeutic lifestyle changes to modify these risk factors regardless of LDL cholesterol level.
- When LDL-lowering drug therapy is used in high risk or moderately high risk persons, it is advised that intensity of therapy be sufficient to achieve at least a 30%–40% reduction in LDL cholesterol levels.
- For people in lower-risk categories, recent clinical trials do not modify the goals and cutpoints of therapy.

HDL, high-density lipoprotein; LDL, low-density lipoprotein.

Reprinted from Ref. 12, with permission.

as the presence of established CVD plus (1) multiple major risk factors (especially diabetes); (2) severe and poorly controlled risk factors (especially continued cigarette smoking); (3) multiple risk factors of the metabolic syndrome (especially elevated triglyceride ≥ 200 mg/dL plus non-HDL cholesterol ≥130 mg/dL with low HDL cholesterol [<40 mg/dL]); (4) patients with acute coronary syndromes. The ATP III Update also indicates that when a high-risk patient has high triglyceride or low HDL cholesterol, consideration can be given to combining a fibrate or nicotinic acid with an LDL-lowering drug.

Low–Baseline Low-Density Lipoprotein Cholesterol Patients

The ATP III Update further modified treatment initiation thresholds for LDL cholesterol, supporting the concept "treat high risk, including low baseline levels." The newer clinical trials were consistent with prior data that indicated that for every 1% reduction in LDL cholesterol levels, relative risk for major CHD events is reduced by approximately 1%. The new data further demonstrated that this relationship holds for baseline LDL cholesterol levels even below 100 mg/dL, expanding the number of high-risk patients who would benefit from LDL cholesterol treatment. For high-risk or moderately high-risk persons, the ATP III Update indicates that intensity of therapy be sufficient to achieve at least a 30% to 40% reduction in LDL cholesterol levels.

Drug Dosing and Low-Density Lipoprotein Cholesterol–Lowering Safety

The ATP III Update listed the statin doses available to produce reductions in LDL cholesterol of 30% to 40% (Table 18-11) and noted that similar reductions can be attained by combining lower doses of statins with other medications or products (e.g., bile acid sequestrants, nicotinic acid, ezetimibe, plant stanol/sterols). Because of the availability of a variety of relatively safe LDL-lowering options, when medication therapy should be considered, the ATP III Update suggested that it is reasonable to use doses adequate to achieve a reduction in risk for major coronary events of 30% to 40%. To use minimal medication therapy to produce a small LDL cholesterol reduction is not a prudent use of medication. The ATP III Update also reiterated the safety of lipid treatment in clinical trials and the absence of adverse effects even among patients treated to very low LDL cholesterol levels.

AMERICAN HEART ASSOCIATION/ AMERICAN COLLEGE OF CARDIOLOGY GUIDELINES FOR SECONDARY PREVENTION: 2006 UPDATE

The 2006 update of the American Heart Association (AHA)/American College of Cardiology (ACC) consensus statement on secondary prevention included important evidence from clinical trials that further supported and broadened the merits of aggressive risk-reduction therapies for patients with established coronary and other atherosclerotic vascular disease, including peripheral artery disease, atherosclerotic aortic disease, and carotid artery disease, including lipid management (Table 18-12).[20] Using partial adaptation of other guideline statements and reports and supplemental literature searches, the findings from additional lipid reduction trials involving more than 50,000 patients resulted in new optional therapeutic targets, as outlined in the 2004 ATP III Update. The 2006 AHA/ACC Update made extensive reference to the ATP III Update and identified two additional trials that demonstrated cardiovascular benefit for lipid lowering significantly below current cholesterol goal levels for patients with chronic CHD. These new trials allowed for alterations in guidelines, such that LDL cholesterol should be less than 100 mg/dL for all patients with CHD and other clinical forms of atherosclerotic disease but, in addition, it is reasonable to treat to LDL cholesterol of less than 70 mg/dL in all such patients. When the target of less than 70 mg/dL chosen, it may be prudent to increase statin therapy in a graded fashion to determine a patient's response and tolerance. If it is not possible to attain LDL cholesterol of less than 70 mg/dL because of a high baseline LDL cholesterol, it generally is possible to achieve LDL cholesterol reductions of greater than 50% with either statins or LDL cholesterol–lowering drug combinations. The 2006 AHA/ACC update emphasized that a reasonable cholesterol level of less than 70 mg/dL does not apply to other types of lower-risk individuals who do

TABLE 18-11 Doses of Currently Available Statins Required to Attain a Low-Density Lipoprotein Approximate 30% to 40% Reduction of LDL Cholesterol Levels (Standard Doses)*

Drug	Dose (mg/day)	LDL Reduction (%)
Atorvastatin	10†	39
Lovastatin	40†	31
Pravastatin	40†	34
Simvastatin	20-40†	35-41
Fluvastatin	40-80	25-35
Rosuvastatin	5-10‡	39-45

*Estimated low-density lipoprotein (LDL) reductions were obtained from Food and Drug Administration (FDA) package inserts for each drug.

†All of these are available at doses up to 80 mg. For every doubling of the dose above standard dose, an approximate 6% decrease in LDL cholesterol level can be obtained [45].

‡For rosuvastatin, doses are available up to 40 mg; the efficacy for 5 mg is estimated by subtracting 6% from the FDA-reported efficacy at 10 mg [45].

TABLE 18-12 American Heart Association/American College of Cardiology Secondary Prevention for Patients with Coronary and Other Vascular Disease: 2006 Update

	Intervention Recommendations with Class of Recommendation and Level of Evidence
SMOKING: Goal Complete cessation. No exposure to environmental tobacco smoke.	• Ask about tobacco use status at every visit. **I (B)** • Advise every tobacco user to quit. **I (B)** • Assess the tobacco user's willingness to quit. **I (B)** • Assist by counseling and developing a plan for quitting. **I (B)** • Arrange follow-up, referral to special programs, or pharmacotherapy (including nicotine replacement and bupropion). **I (B)** • Urge avoidance of exposure to environmental tobacco smoke at work and home. **I (B)**
BLOOD PRESSURE CONTROL: Goal <140/90 mm Hg or <130/80 mm Hg if patient has diabetes or chronic kidney disease	**For all patients:** • Initiate or maintain lifestyle modification–weight control; increased physical activity; alcohol moderation; sodium reduction; and emphasis on increased consumption of fresh fruits, vegetables, and low-fat dairy products. **I (B)** **For patients with blood pressure ≥140/90 mm Hg (or ≥130/80 mm Hg for individuals with chronic kidney disease or diabetes):** • As tolerated, add blood pressure medication, treating initially with β-blockers and/or ACE inhibitors, with addition of other drugs such as thiazides as needed to achieve goal blood pressure. **I (A)**
LIPID MANAGEMENT: Goal LDL cholesterol <100 mg/dL If triglycerides are ≥200 mg/dL, non-HDL cholesterol should be <130 mg/dL	**For all patients:** • Start dietary therapy. Reduce intake of saturated fats (to <7% of total calories), *trans* fatty acids, and cholesterol (to <200 mg/d). **I (B)** • Adding plant stanol/sterols (2 g/d) and viscous fiber (>10 g/d) will further lower LDL cholesterol. • Promote daily physical activity and weight management. **I (B)** • Encourage increased consumption of omega-3 fatty acids in the form of fish or in capsule form (1 g/d) for risk reduction. For treatment of elevated triglycerides, higher doses are usually necessary for risk reduction. **IIb (B)** **For lipid management:** Assess fasting lipid profile in all patients, and within 24 hours of hospitalization for those with an acute cardiovascular or coronary event. For hospitalized patients, initiate lipid-lowering medication as recommended below before discharge according to the following schedule: • LDL cholesterol should be <100 mg/dL. **I (A), and** • Further reduction of LDL cholesterol to <70 mg/dL is reasonable. **IIa (A)** • If baseline LDL cholesterol is ≥100 mg/dL, initiate LDL-lowering drug therapy.**I (A)** • If on-treatment LDL cholesterol is ≥100 mg/dL, intensify LDL-lowering drug therapy (may require LDL-lowering drug combination. **I (A)** • If baseline LDL cholesterol is 70–100 mg/dL, it is reasonable to treat to LDL cholesterol <70 mg/dL. **IIa (B)** • If triglycerides are 200–499 mg/dL, non-HDL cholesterol should be <130 mg/dL. **I (B), and** • Further reduction of non-HDL cholesterol to <100 mg/dL is reasonable. **IIa (B)** • Therapeutic options to reduce non-HDL cholesterol are: ⇒ More intense LDL cholesterol–lowering therapy. **I (B), or** ⇒ Niacin (after LDL cholesterol–lowering therapy). **IIa (B), or** ⇒ Fibrate therapy (after LDL cholesterol–lowering therapy). **IIa (B)** • If triglycerides are ≥500 mg/dL, therapeutic options to prevent pancreatitis are fibrate or niacin before LDL-lowering therapy; and treat LDL cholesterol to goal after triglyceride-lowering therapy. Achieve non-HDL cholesterol <130 mg/dL if possible. **I (C)**
PHYSICAL ACTIVITY: Goal 30 minutes, 7 days per week (minimum 5 days per week)	• For all patients, assess risk with a physical activity history and/or an exercise test, to guide prescription. **I (B)** • For all patients, encourage 30 to 60 minutes of moderate-intensity aerobic activity, such as brisk walking, on most, preferably all, days of the week, supplemented by an increase in daily lifestyle activities (e.g., walking breaks at work, gardening, household work). **I (B)** • Encourage resistance training 2 days per week. **IIb (C)** • Advise medically supervised programs for high-risk patients (e.g., recent acute coronary syndrome or revascularization, heart failure). **I (B)**

Continued

TABLE 18-12 American Heart Association/American College of Cardiology Secondary Prevention for Patients with Coronary and Other Vascular Disease: 2006 Update—cont'd

WEIGHT MANAGEMENT:	• Assess body mass index and/or waist circumference on each visit and consistently encourage weight maintenance/reduction through an appropriate balance of physical activity, caloric intake, and formal behavioral programs when indicated to maintain/achieve a body mass index between 18.5 and 24.9 kg/m². **I (B)**
Goal Body mass index: 18.5 to 24.9 kg/m² Waist circumference: men <40 inches, women <35 inches	• If waist circumference (measured horizontally at the iliac crest) is ≥35 inches in women and ≥40 inches in men, initiate lifestyle changes and consider treatment strategies for metabolic syndrome as indicated. **I (B)** • The initial goal of weight loss therapy should be to reduce body weight by approximately 10% from baseline. With success, further weight loss can be attempted if indicated through further assessment. **I (B)**

ACE, angiotensin-converting enzyme; LDL, low-density lipoprotein; non-HDL, non-high-density lipoprotein.
Reprinted from Ref. 20, with permission.

not have CHD or other forms of atherosclerotic disease; in such cases, recommendations contained in the 2004 ATP III Update still pertain.

EVIDENCE-BASED GUIDELINES FOR CARDIOVASCULAR DISEASE PREVENTION IN WOMEN

CVD is the leading cause of death in women, and because women are often a small minority in randomized trials, an expert panel was formed to review available data and create a gender-specific set of cardiovascular guidelines for women.[21] In the United States, more than 500,000 women each year die of CVD, mostly CHD, more than that in men.[22] More women die without previously recognized symptoms, have higher post-MI mortality at ages younger than 75 years, and have atypical symptoms at presentation.[22-24] Because of the enormous potential for prevention of CVD among women, this set of guidelines sought to aggressively identify and target appropriate therapies for at-risk women.

Because of the limited data available for women, the expert panel was challenged with evaluating the gender-specific data and, when such was not available, how well the existing data could be extrapolated to females. In addition to determining the strength of the evidence and hence the recommendation (class I, IIa, IIb, or III) and the level of evidence (A, sufficient from multiple randomized trials; B, limited evidence from single randomized trial or other nonrandomized studies; C, based on expert opinion, case studies, or standard of care), the experts also determined the likelihood that data available only in men would generalize to women (1, very likely; 2, somewhat likely; 3, unlikely; 0, unable to project). Almost 7000 articles and abstracts were identified, and nearly 400 were included in the final evaluation.

With the increasing awareness that CVD is a continuum of disease, women were identified as being at high risk (20% 10-year absolute CHD risk), intermediate risk (10%–20%), lower risk (<10%), and optimal risk (<10%). Of note, women were not identified as low risk or no risk, but rather the knowledge that women have a high lifetime risk of CVD was incorporated into the risk assessment to help promote preventive measures. The high-risk group included those with established disease and those with CVD risk equivalents including cerebrovascular disease, peripheral artery disease, and diabetes. Because of the growing evidence of the risk of CVD in patients with chronic kidney disease, these women were also included in the high-risk category. Women with evidence of subclinical disease (e.g., coronary calcification), women with a strong family history of CVD, as well as some high-risk women with metabolic syndrome were considered to be at intermediate 10-year risk for CHD. This risk stratification also takes into account the individual variation in risk, with some individuals with a markedly elevated single risk factor included in the intermediate-risk category and some women with multiple risk factors considered lower risk. The following are specific recommendations from this consensus guideline.

Lifestyle Interventions

Lifestyle interventions formed the basis for class I recommendations in each of the risk groups of women (Table 18-13). These interventions include smoking cessation, including avoidance of environmental tobacco, a minimum of 30 minutes of moderate-intensity physical activity on most or all days of the week, cardiac rehabilitation in appropriate cases, and the maintenance of a healthy weight with body mass index between 18.5 and 24.9 and waist circumference of less than 35 inches. A "heart-healthy" diet, including a varied eating plan with low-fat or nonfat dairy, fish, legumes, limited saturated fat (<10% calories), limited *trans* fatty acids, and limited cholesterol (<300 mg/day), as well as a variety of fruits and vegetables, is the recommended dietary plan for all women. In addition, identification and treatment of women with CVD and symptoms of depression was a class IIa recommendation. Recommended supplements included omega-3 fatty acids in high-risk women (class IIb, level B). The initial recommendation for folic acid supplementation in high-risk women was revised in the 2007 update.[25]

TABLE 18-13 Priorities for Prevention of Cardiovascular Disease in women in Practice According to Risk Group

High-Risk Women (>20% risk) ***Class I recommendations:*** • Smoking cessation
• Physical activity/cardiac rehabilitation
• Diet therapy
• Weight maintenance/reduction
• Blood pressure control
• Lipid control/statin therapy
• Aspirin therapy
• β-blocker therapy
• ACE inhibitor therapy (ARBs if contraindicated)
• Glycemic control in diabetics
Class IIa recommendation: • Evaluate/treat for depression
Class IIb recommendations: • Omega-3 fatty acid supplementation
• Folic acid supplementation
Intermediate-Risk Women (10%–20% risk) ***Class I recommendations:*** • Smoking cessation
• Physical activity
• Heart-healthy diet
• Weight maintenance/reduction
• Blood pressure control
• Lipid control
Class IIa recommendations: • Aspirin therapy
Lower-Risk Women (<10% risk) ***Class I recommendations:*** • Smoking cessation
• Physical activity
• Heart-healthy diet
• Weight maintenance/reduction
• Treat individual CVD risk factors as indicated
Stroke Prevention among Women with Atrial Fibrillation ***Class I recommendations:*** • High-intermediate risk of stroke: warfarin therapy
• Low risk of stroke (<1%/yr) or contraindication to warfarin: aspirin therapy

ACE, angiotensin-converting enzyme; ARB, angiotensin receptor blocker.
Reprinted from Ref. 21, with permission.

Major Risk Factor Interventions

Blood pressure control through lifestyle with the addition of pharmacotherapy in women whose blood pressure exceeds 140/90 mm Hg is considered fundamental for CVD prevention. Blood pressure goals lower than this target are appropriate for individuals with diabetes or other blood pressure–mediated target organ damage. Lifestyle and pharmacotherapy are a class I intervention in diabetics to maintain HbA1c of less than 7%. In all women, the optimal LDL cholesterol level should be less than 100 mg/dL, HDL cholesterol should be greater than 50 mg/dL, triglycerides should be less than 150 mg/dL, and non-HDL cholesterol should be less than 130 mg/dL. Achieving these levels through lifestyle modifications should be encouraged in all women. In women at high risk, a more restricted diet should be prescribed, with saturated fat being less than 7% of intake and dietary cholesterol less than 200 mg/dL in order to achieve these goals. High-risk women should receive LDL cholesterol–lowering therapy, usually with a statin, if their levels are 100 mg/dL or more (class I, level A) and all high-risk women with LDL cholesterol less than 100 mg/dL should receive a statin unless contraindicated (class I, level B). The threshold for initiation of pharmacologic treatment in intermediate-risk women is an LDL cholesterol level of 130 mg/dL or greater; in those with multiple risk factors, at an LDL cholesterol level of 160 mg/dL or greater, and in those women at lower risk with 0 or 1 risk factor, an LDL cholesterol level of 190 mg/dL or greater. In all women, regardless of their risk, secondary targets such as non-HDL cholesterol and HDL cholesterol should also be treated with lifestyle, fibrates, and niacin therapy.

Class III Interventions

In light of data from the Heart and Estrogen/Progestin Replacement Study (HERS) and the Women's Health Initiative, combined estrogen and progestin is not an appropriate strategy for cardiovascular prevention in postmenopausal women.[26,27] Evidence also does not support the use of antioxidant supplements for the prevention of CVD.

EVIDENCE-BASED GUIDELINES FOR CARDIOVASCULAR DISEASE PREVENTION IN WOMEN: 2007 UPDATE

Several significant studies published after the initial guidelines in 2004 prompted re-review of the literature and revision of the guidelines.[25] A better understanding of the average lifetime risk of CHD in women and the underestimation of disease in some populations prompted a simplification of the risk stratification into women at high risk, women at risk, and women at optimal risk (Table 18-14). Recommendations regarding cigarette smoking, physical activity, cardiac rehabilitation, diet, weight management, and depression are similar to the previous guidelines. For weight loss or maintenance of weight loss, an extended period of physical activity of 60 to 90 minutes on most or all days of the week was included in the new set of guidelines. In addition, more specific dietary recommendations included limitation of alcohol intake to no more than one drink per day, limitation of dietary sodium intake to 2.3 g/day, and the inclusion of fish (especially oily fish) at least two times per week. Omega-3 fatty acid supplementation (850 to 1000 mg

TABLE 18-14	Classification of Cardiovascular Disease Risk in Women
Risk Status	**Criteria**
High risk	Established coronary heart disease
	Cerebrovascular disease
	Peripheral artery disease
	Abdominal aortic aneurysm
	End-stage or chronic renal disease
	Diabetes mellitus
	10-Year Framingham global risk >20%*
At risk	≥1 major risk factors for CVD, including:
	Cigarette smoking
	Poor diet
	Physical inactivity
	Obesity, especially central adiposity
	Family history of premature CVD (CVD at <55 years of age in male relative and <65 years of age in female relative)
	Hypertension
	Dyslipidemia
	Evidence of subclinical vascular disease (eg, coronary calcification)
	Metabolic syndrome
	Poor exercise capacity on treadmill test and/or abnormal heart rate recovery after stopping exercise
Optimal risk	Framingham global risk <10% and a healthy lifestyle, with no risk factors

*Or at high risk on the basis of another population-adapted tool used to assess global risk.

CVD, cardiovascular disease.

Reprinted from Ref. 21, with permission.

of EPA and DHA) can be considered in women with CHD and in higher doses as treatment for hypertriglyceridemia. An algorithm for CVD prevention in women is shown in Figure 18-2.

Major Risk Factor Interventions

In addition to lifestyle modifications, pharmacotherapy for lipid management in high-risk women should achieve LDL cholesterol levels of less than 100 mg/dL and an optional target of LDL cholesterol less than 70 mg/dL in very-high-risk women. These very-high-risk women are those with established CHD and multiple major risk factors, severe and poorly controlled risk factors, or diabetes. The intensity of lipid-lowering pharmacotherapy in those at-risk women should be based on the degree of risk. Those with multiple risk factors and a 10-year absolute risk of 10% to 20%, therapy should be initiated to lower LDL cholesterol levels if the level is 130 mg/dL or greater. Women with multiple risk factors and 10-year risk of less than 10% should receive lipid-lowering therapy if their LDL cholesterol is 160 mg/dL or greater because of the high lifetime risk for the progression of atherosclerosis. In all other at-risk women, therapy should be initiated if LDL cholesterol is 190 mg/dL or greater. HDL cholesterol and non-HDL cholesterol should be targeted after LDL cholesterol goals are met with niacin or fibrate therapy in high-risk women, and should be considered in at-risk women with multiple risk factors and 10-year absolute risk of 10% to 20%.

Preventive Drug Interventions

Aspirin therapy (75–325 mg/day) should be initiated in all high-risk women unless contraindicated. For women 65 years of age and older, the individual benefits and risks of aspirin therapy for cardiovascular and ischemic stroke prevention should be reviewed and low-dose aspirin (81 mg/day or 100 mg every other day) should be instituted if there is adequate blood pressure control. In women younger than 65, low-dose aspirin therapy should be considered for stroke prevention if the benefits outweigh the risks of therapy.

Class III Interventions

Hormone therapy and selective estrogen-receptor modulators are not useful or may be harmful for the primary or secondary prevention of CVD in women. Additionally, antioxidant supplements including folic acid should not be used as primary or secondary prevention. Because of results of the Women's Health Initiative, aspirin for the primary prevention of MI in women younger than age 65 years is not recommended.

DYSLIPIDEMIA MANAGEMENT IN ADULTS WITH DIABETES

Published in 2004, the American Diabetes Association (ADA) position statement on dyslipidemia management in adult diabetics focused on aggressive management of dyslipidemia in this population to reduce CVD risk.[28] Diabetic subjects have a twofold to fourfold increased risk of developing CHD compared with nondiabetic subjects.[29-31] Two thirds of all diabetic subjects die of CVD, and CVD is often unrecognized in diabetic subjects with as many as half manifesting silent ischemia.[32] Aggressive treatment of dyslipidemia with LDL cholesterol goals of less than 100 mg/dL or a reduction of greater than 30%, HDL cholesterol levels greater than 40 mg/dL, and triglycerides less than 150 mg/dL through lifestyle interventions and pharmacotherapy including combination therapy constitute the recommendations of the ADA position statement.[28]

Dyslipidemia in Type 2 Diabetic Subjects

The pattern of dyslipidemia seen most commonly in diabetic subjects is an increased level of triglycerides and decreased HDL cholesterol levels. The LDL cholesterol levels are often not elevated in comparison to those in nondiabetic subjects, but LDL particles are often small

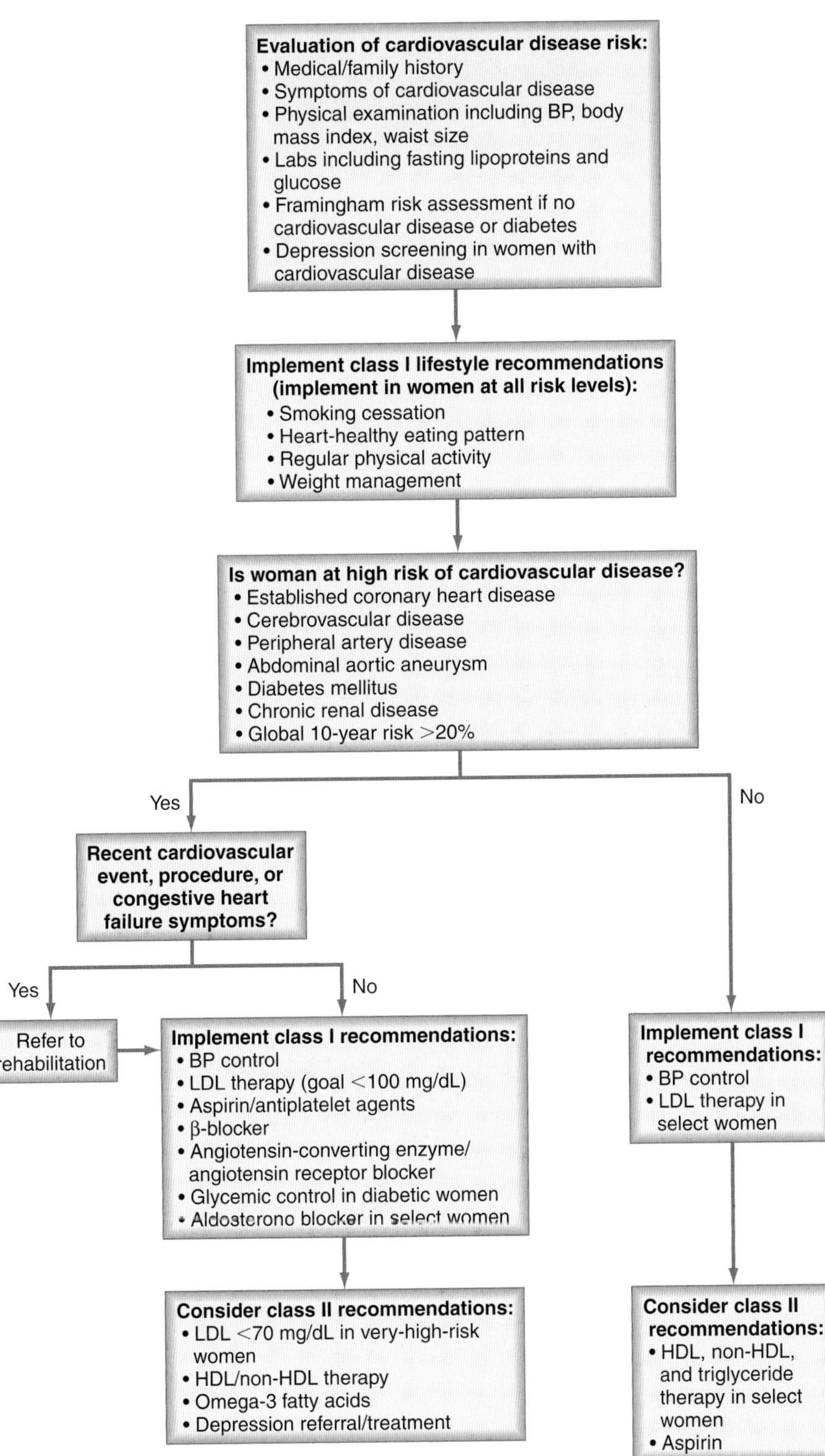

FIGURE 18-2 Evaluation of cardiovascular disease risk in women. BP, blood pressure; HDL, high-density lipoprotein; LDL, low-density lipoprotein. *Reprinted from Ref. 25, with permission.*

and dense and are considered more atherogenic and more prone to oxidation. The prevalence of hypertriglyceridemia and low HDL cholesterol levels is more pronounced in women.[33] The dyslipidemia of diabetes mellitus can be worsened by the presence of other disease states, such as renal disease or hypothyroidism or the ingestion of alcohol or estrogen.

Clinical Trials of Lipid-Lowering in Diabetic Subjects

Several large primary and secondary prevention trials included a substantial number of diabetic subjects, allowing for adequate information regarding effectiveness in individuals with diabetes. The Heart Protection Study included 20,536 men and women, of whom 5963 were diabetic and were randomized to a fixed dose of 40 mg of simvastatin.[34] Among the diabetic population, major vascular events were reduced by 22% ($P < .0001$). Diabetic subgroups who showed benefit included women and men, those older and younger than age 65, those with and without a previous history of CHD, and those with an entry level of LDL cholesterol of less than 116 mg/dL. In the secondary prevention Veterans Affairs High-Density Lipoprotein Cholesterol Intervention Trial (VA-HIT), 2431 (25% diabetic) men with predominantly low HDL cholesterol levels (<40 mg/dL) were randomized to the fibrate gemfibrozil.[35] Although the study was not adequately powered for subgroup analysis, there was a statistically significant 24% risk reduction in the combined endpoint of death due to CHD, nonfatal MI, and stroke in the diabetic population.

Modifications of Lipoproteins by Medical Nutrition Therapy and Physical Activity

Recommendations for physical activity and medical nutrition therapy should be included for all diabetic subjects. Moderate activity for at least 30 minutes most days of the week should be encouraged.[36] In diabetic subjects with hyperlipidemia, reducing saturated fat to less than 7% to 10% of calories and limiting *trans* fats can improve LDL cholesterol. For diabetic subjects who are overweight, lifestyle interventions (limiting saturated fat to less than 7% of total calories, limiting dietary cholesterol to less than 200 mg/day, including 10 to 25 g/day of soluble fiber, losing weight, increasing activity, and including plant stanol/sterols) can improve HDL cholesterol and triglyceride levels and to a lesser extent LDL cholesterol level.[37]

Treatment Goals for Lipoprotein Therapy

Because of the high risk of CVD in diabetics, the goals of therapy are an LDL cholesterol level less than 100 mg/dL, HDL cholesterol level greater than 40 mg/dL in men and greater than 50 mg/dL in women, and triglyceride level less than 150 mg/dL. The initial approach should include intensive lifestyle interventions followed by pharmacotherapy, except in diabetic patients with documented CHD, who should receive lipid-lowering therapy simultaneously with lifestyle recommendations. For diabetic patients without documented CHD, pharmacologic therapy should be started when the LDL cholesterol level is 130 mg/dL or greater. The treatment strategy for diabetic dyslipidemia recommended in the ADA guidelines is shown in Table 18-15.

Hypertriglyceridemia in diabetic patients should be targeted with lifestyle interventions including weight loss, exercise, and reduced fat and carbohydrate intake, as well as glycemic control. The addition of a fibrate, nicotinic acid, or higher-dose statin should be considered when adequate glycemic control is achieved. Targeting low HDL cholesterol levels often requires pharmacologic treatment with fibrates or nicotinic acid in addition to lifestyle interventions such as smoking cessation, increased physical activity, and weight loss. The use of nicotinic acid may worsen glucose control, and thus potential benefit in the lipid profile must be weighed against mild increases in plasma glucose. Another pharmacologic consideration in the treatment of diabetics is the increased risk of myositis with the use of gemfibrozil in combination with statins or nicotinic acid.

TABLE 18-15 Order of Priorities for Treatment of Diabetic Dyslipidemia in Adults

I. LDL cholesterol lowering
Lifestyle interventions
Preferred : HMG CoA reductase inhibitor (statin)
Others: bile acid binding resin, cholesterol absorption inhibitor, fenofibrate, or niacin
II. HDL cholesterol raising
Lifestyle interventions
Nicotinic acid or fibrates
III. Triglyceride lowering
Lifestyle interventions
Glycemic control
Fibric acid derivative (gemfibrozil, fenofibrate)
Niacin
high-dose statins (in those who also have high LDL cholesterol)
IV. Combined hyperlipidemia
First choice: improved glycemic control plus high-dose statin
Second choice: improved glycemic control plus statin plus fibric acid derivative
Third choice: improved glycemic control plus statin plus nicotinic acid

Decision for treatment of high low-density lipoprotein (LDL) before elevated triglyceride is based on clinical trial data indicating safety as well as efficacy of the available agents. The combination of statins with nicotinic acid, fenofibrate, and especially gemfibrozil may carry an increased risk of myositis.

Reprinted from Ref. 28, with permission.

Recommendations for Lipid Screening in Adults with Diabetes Mellitus

For adults with diabetes, at least annual screening of lipids is recommended, and if at low risk (LDL cholesterol <100 mg/dL, HDL cholesterol >50 mg/dL, and triglycerides <150 mg/dL), every 2 years.

TREATMENT RECOMMENDATIONS AND GOALS

- Lifestyle modification should include reduction in dietary saturated fat and cholesterol, weight loss, increased physical activity, and smoking cessation.
- Pharmacologic therapy is recommended for patients not at goal with lifestyle modifications.
- Primary goal of therapy is LDL cholesterol less than 100 mg/dL.
- Lowering LDL cholesterol with a statin is associated with lower cardiovascular events.
- In diabetics older than 40 years of age and with an LDL cholesterol level greater than 135 mg/dL,

initiation of statin therapy to reduce LDL cholesterol by at least 30% should be considered.

- Dietary therapy and medications if necessary should be used in children and adolescents with diabetes to achieve LDL cholesterol levels less than 100 mg/dL.
- Targeting triglycerides to achieve levels less than 150 mg/dL and HDL cholesterol to achieve levels greater than 50 mg/dL in women and greater than 40 mg/dL in men should be considered in all diabetic patients.
- The use of fibrate therapy to lower triglycerides and raise HDL cholesterol in patients with CVD, low HDL cholesterol, and near-normal levels of LDL cholesterol is associated with a reduction of cardiovascular events.
- Combination therapy may be necessary to achieve lipid goals.

SUMMARY

Clinical trials subsequent to the ATP III Update have provided further support for these guideline recommendations, specifically for the "lower is better" and "treat high risk including low baseline levels" recommendations.[38] A new position statement or "ATP IV" has not been issued by the NCEP. Accordingly, the NCEP has directed attention to the large treatment gaps in lipid-lowering treatment, resulting in widespread undertreatment in eligible subjects in clinical practice.[39] The 2004 ADA statement and the 2007 Updated guidelines for women are consistent with the ATP III Update thresholds and strategies, and are aimed at closing treatment gaps in these large groups of patients.

Given the large body of clinical trial evidence documenting the utility of aggressive medical management both to prevent and to reverse CVD, the existing lipid lowering treatment gaps have enormous implications for the need and utilization of guidelines-based strategies. It is clear from clinical translation programs such as the AHA's "Get with the Guidelines" and ACC's "Guidelines in Practice" that strategies that improve adherence to guidelines can be achieved and result in improved patient cardiovascular outcomes.[40-42] Furthermore, recent studies[43,44] comparing aggressive lipid-lowering treatment to revascularization strategies suggest superiority of the preventive approach to interventional revascularization in appropriately selected patients. It is clear that cardiovascular care must evolve to emphasize an aggressive preventive approach. Guidelines-based lipid-lowering treatment is a cornerstone of effective cardiovascular risk reduction.

REFERENCES

1. National Cholesterol Education Program (NCEP) Expert Panel on Detection, Evaluation, and Treatment of High Blood Cholesterol in Adults (Adult Treatment Panel III): Third report of the National Cholesterol Education Program (NCEP) Expert Panel on Detection, Evaluation, and Treatment of High Blood Cholesterol in Adults (Adult Treatment Panel III) final report. *Circulation.* 2002;106:3143–3421.
2. Antiplatelet Trialist's Collaboration: Secondary prevention of vascular disease by prolonged antiplatelet treatment. *BMJ* 1983;296:320–331.
3. Eidelman RS, Hebert PR, Weisman SM, et al: An update on aspirin in the primary prevention of cardiovascular disease. *Arch Intern Med* 2003;163:2006–2010.
4. The Beta-Blocker Pooling Project Research Group: The Beta-Blockers Pooling Project (BBPP): Subgroup findings from randomized trials in post infarction patients. *Eur Heart J* 1988;9:8–16.
5. Smith SC Jr, Blair SN, Criqui MH, et al: AHA Consensus Panel Statement. Preventing heart attack and death in patients with coronary disease. The Secondary Prevention Panel. *J Am Coll Cardiol* 1995;26:292–294.
6. National High Blood Pressure Education Program: The seventh report of the Joint National Committee on prevention, detection, evaluation, and treatment of high blood pressure. *JAMA* 2003;289:2560–2572.
7. Wilhemsson C, Elmfeldt D, Vedin JA, Tibblin G: Smoking and myocardial infarction. *Lancet* 1975;i:415–419.
8. Lorgeril M, Renaud S, Nicole M, et al: Mediterranean alpha-linolenic acid-rich diet in secondary prevention of coronary heart disease. *Lancet* 1994;343:1454–1459.
9. O'Connor GT, Buring JE, Yusuf S, et al: An overview of randomized trials of rehabilitation with exercise after myocardial infarction. *Circulation* 1989;80:234–244.
10. Mukerjee D, Fang J, Chetcuti S, et al: Impact of combination evidence-based medical therapy on mortality in patients with acute coronary syndromes. *Circulation* 2004;109:745–749.
11. National Cholesterol Education Program. Second Report of the Expert Panel on Detection, Evaluation, and Treatment of High Blood Cholesterol in Adults (Adult Treatment Panel II). *Circulation.* 1994;89:1333–1445.
12. Expert Panel on Detection, Evaluation, and Treatment of High Blood Cholesterol in Adults: Executive summary of the third report of The National Cholesterol Education Program (NCEP) Expert Panel on Detection, Evaluation, and Treatment of High Blood Cholesterol In Adults (Adult Treatment Panel III). *JAMA.* 2001;285:2486–2497.
13. D'Agostino RB Sr, Sullivan LM, Levy D: MI and coronary death risk prediction. National Cholesterol Education Program Adult Treatment Panel III (risk estimator). Available at http://hin.nhlbi.nih.gov/atpiii/riskcalc.htm.
14. Grundy SM, Cleeman JI, Bairey Merz CN, et al: Implications of recent clinical trials for the National Cholesterol Education Program Adult Treatment Panel III Guidelines. *Circulation* 2004;110:227–239.
15. Heart Protection Study Collaborative Group: MRC/BHF Heart Protection Study of cholesterol lowering with simvastatin in 20,536 high-risk individuals: A randomised placebo-controlled trial. *Lancet.* 2002;360:7–22.
16. Shepherd J, Blauw GJ, Murphy MB, et al, the PROSPER study group: PROspective Study of Pravastatin in the Elderly at Risk. Pravastatin in elderly individuals at risk of vascular disease (PROSPER): A randomised controlled trial. *Lancet* 2002;360:1623–1630.
17. ALLHAT Officers and Coordinators for the ALLHAT Collaborative Research Group: The Antihypertensive and Lipid-Lowering Treatment to Prevent Heart Attack Trial. Major outcomes in moderately hypercholesterolemic, hypertensive patients randomized to pravastatin vs usual care: The Antihypertensive and Lipid-Lowering Treatment to Prevent Heart Attack Trial (ALLHAT-LLT). *JAMA* 2002;288:2998–3007.
18. Sever PS, Dahlof B, Poulter NR, et al: Prevention of coronary and stroke events with atorvastatin in hypertensive patients who have average or lower-than-average cholesterol concentrations, in the Anglo-Scandinavian Cardiac Outcomes Trial—Lipid Lowering Arm (ASCOT-LLA): A multicentre randomised controlled trial. *Lancet* 2003;361:1149–1158.
19. Cannon CP, Braunwald E, McCabe CH, et al: Comparison of intensive and moderate lipid lowering with statins after acute coronary syndromes. *N Engl J Med* 2004;350:1495–1504.
20. Smith SC Jr, Allen J, Blair SN, et al: AHA/ACC guidelines for secondary prevention for patients with coronary and other atherosclerotic vascular disease: 2006 update: endorsed by the National Heart, Lung, and Blood Institute. *Circulation* 2006;11:2363–2367.
21. Mosca L, Appel LJ, Benjamin EJ, et al: Evidence-based guidelines for cardiovascular disease prevention in women. *J Am Coll Cardiol* 2004;43:900–921.
22. Rosamond W, Flegal K, Friday G, et al: Heart disease and stroke statistics—2007: A report from the American Heart Association

Statistics Committee and Stroke Statistics Subcommittee. *Circulation* 2007;115:a69–e171.
23. Vaccarino V, Parsons L, Every NR, et al: Sex-based differences in early mortality after myocardial infarction. National Registry of Myocardial Infarction 2 Participants. *N Engl J Med* 1999;341: 217–225.
24. McSweeney JC, Cody M, O'Sullivan P, et al: Women's early warnings symptoms of acute myocardial infarction. *Circulation* 2003;108;2619–2623.
25. Mosca L, Banka CL, Benjamin EJ, et al: Evidence-based guidelines for cardiovascular disease prevention in women: 2007 update. *Circulation* 2007;114:1481–1501.
26. Hulley S, Grady D, Bush T, et al: Randomized trial of estrogen plus progestin for secondary prevention of coronary heart disease in postmenopausal women. Heart and Estrogen/Progestin Replacement Study (HERS) Research Group. *JAMA* 1998;280: 605–613.
27. Manson JE, Hsia J, Johnson KC, et al: Estrogen plus progestin and the risk of coronary heart disease. *N Engl J Med* 2003;349:523–534.
28. American Diabetes Association: Dyslipidemia management in adults with diabetes. *Diabetes Care* 2004;27:S68–S71.
29. Jacoby RM, Nesto RW: Acute myocardial infarction in the diabetic patient: pathophysiology, clinical course and prognosis. *J Am Coll Cardiol* 1992;20:736–744.
30. Kannel WB, McGee DL: Diabetes and glucose tolerance as risk factors for cardiovascular disease: The Framingham study. *Diabetes Care* 1979;2:120–126.
31. Granger CB, Califf RM, Young S, et al: Outcome of patients with diabetes mellitus and acute myocardial infarction treated with thrombolytic agents. The Thrombolysis and Angioplasty in Myocardial Infarction (TAMI) Study Group. *J Am Coll Cardiol* 1993;21:920–925.
32. Kannel WB, Abbott RD: Incidence and prognosis of unrecognized myocardial infarction. An update on the Framingham experience. *Am Heart J* 1990;120:672–676.
33. Roeters van Lennep JE, Westerveld HT, Erkelens DW, et al: Risk factors for coronary heart disease: Implications of gender. *Cardiovasc Res* 2002;53:538–549.
34. Heart Protection Study Collaborative Group. MRC/BHF Heart Protection Study of cholesterol-lowering with simvastatin in 5963 people with diabeties: A randomised placebo-controlled trial. *Lancet* 2003;361:2005–2006.
35. Rubins HB, Robins SJ, Collins D, et al: Gemfibrozil for the secondary prevention of coronary heart disease in men with low levels of high-density lipoprotein cholesterol. *N Engl J Med* 1999;341:410–418.
36. American Diabetes Association: Physical activity/exercise and diabetes: Position statement. *Diabetes Care* 2004;27:S58–S62.
37. American Diabetes Association: Nutrition principles and recommendations in diabetes: Position statement. *Diabetes Care* 2004;27:S36–S46.
38. LaRosa JC, Grundy SM, Waters DD, et al: Intensive lipid lowering with atorvastatin in patients with stable coronary disease. *N Engl J Med* 2005;352:1425–1435.
39. Meyers CD, McCarren M, Wong ND, et al: Baseline achievement of lipid goals and usage of lipid medications in patients with diabetes mellitus (from the Veterans Affairs Diabetes Trial). *Am J Cardiol* 2006;98:63–65.
40. Smaha L: The American Heart Association Get with the Guidelines program. *Am Heart J* 2004;148:S46–S48.
41. Montoye CK, Eagle KA, Michigan ACC-GAP Investigators: ACC-GAP Steering Committee. American College of Cardiology. An organizational framework for the AMI ACC-GAP Project. *J Am Coll Cardiol* 2005;46:S1–S29.
42. Eagle KA. Montoye CK, Riba AL, et al: Guideline-based standardized care is associated with substantially lower mortality in Medicare patients with acute myocardial infarction: The American College of Cardiology's Guidelines Applied in Practice (GAP) Projects in Michigan. *J Am Coll Cardiol* 2005;46:1242–1248.
43. Schwartz GG, Olsson AG, Ezekowitz MD, et al: Effects of atorvastatin on early recurrent ischemic events in acute coronary syndromes: The MIRACL study: A randomized controlled trial. *JAMA* 2001;285:1711–1718.
44. Boden WE, O'Rourke RA, Teo KK, et al: The evolving pattern of symptomatic coronary artery disease in the United States and Canada: Baseline characteristics of the Clinical Outcomes Utilizing Revascularization and Aggressive DruG Evaluation (COURAGE) trial. *Am J Cardiol* 2007;99:208–212.
45. Jones P, Kafonek S, Laurora I, Hunninghake D: Comparative dose efficacy study of atorvastatin versus simvastatin, pravastatin, lovastatin, and flurastatin in patients with hypercholesterol emia (The CURVES Study). *Am J Cordiol* 1998;81: 582–587.

CHAPTER 19

Dietary Patterns for the Prevention and Treatment of Cardiovascular Disease

Penny M. Kris-Etherton, Melissa Ohlson, Deborah Bagshaw, and Neil J. Stone

Healthy lifestyle practices are the foundation of prevention and treatment efforts to reduce cardiovascular disease (CVD) morbidity and mortality. Diet is a key lifestyle practice that continues to be the cornerstone of CVD risk management. A large evidence-based study has convincingly demonstrated beneficial effects of several dietary patterns on multiple risk factors for CVD, including major risk factors: lipids and lipoproteins, blood pressure, insulin sensitivity, body weight and fatness, as well as emerging risk factors.[1-3] Of note is that impressive strides have been made in lowering coronary heart disease (CHD) mortality between 1980 and 2000; 44% of the decrease was attributable to a reduction in major risk factors (i.e., reductions in total cholesterol, systolic blood pressure [SBP], smoking prevalence, and physical inactivity), and 47% was due to a number of medical therapies.[4] These findings are important because they demonstrate the significance of healthy lifestyle behaviors to reduce CVD risk. Thus healthy diet and lifestyle practices that decrease total cholesterol and SBP, together with smoking cessation and increased physical activity, are the key to ongoing CVD risk reduction efforts. Diet and lifestyle practices that also target other CVD risk factors offer the potential of moving us closer to the goal of essentially eradicating CVD that is attributable to risk burden due to modifiable causes.

There is great interest in decreasing multiple risk factors to reduce CVD risk. A dietary pattern approach that targets many CVD risk factors through numerous nutrition interventions has become the gold standard for achieving maximal CVD risk reduction. Several dietary patterns have been defined that currently are implemented in clinical practice. These include the Dietary Approaches to Stop Hypertension (DASH)/ DASH Sodium diet,[5,6] diets higher in protein and unsaturated fat (the OmniHeart study[7]), the Portfolio diet,[8] and Mediterranean-type diets,[9-11] all of which are discussed in this chapter. In addition, the evidence that supports the beneficial effects on CVD risk factors of the nutrients and dietary factors that comprise the different dietary patterns are reviewed. Strategies for implementing healthy dietary patterns to decrease CVD risk are discussed. In addition, key resources for clinicians to use in practice for the dietary management of CVD risk factors are presented. Collectively, this information benefits clinicians in managing CVD risk status in patients using a dietary pattern approach.

Because elevated low-density lipoprotein (LDL) cholesterol and total cholesterol are the primary targets for intervention, dietary patterns that achieve maximal reductions are discussed first. Strategies for managing atherogenic dyslipidemia (elevated triglyceride [TG] and low high-density lipoprotein [HDL] cholesterol levels), elevated blood pressure, high glucose levels, and overweight and obesity, all of which are components of the metabolic syndrome, also are discussed.

DIETARY PATTERNS TO LOWER TOTAL AND LOW-DENSITY LIPOPROTEIN CHOLESTEROL

Therapeutic Lifestyle Changes Diet

Therapeutic lifestyle changes (TLC) are the foundation for the clinical management of elevated LDL cholesterol levels. New clinical trial evidence supports the relationship between marked cholesterol lowering and CHD risk reduction in high-risk and very-high-risk patients.[12] The Adult Treatment Panel III of the National Cholesterol Education Program (NCEP ATP III) recommends a TLC diet for lowering LDL cholesterol in individuals who are above the LDL cholesterol goal to reduce risk of CHD[13] (Table 19-1). The TLC diet together with other LDL cholesterol–lowering options has been shown to reduce LDL cholesterol levels by as much as 24% to 37% (Table 19-2).

The TLC diet is low in saturated fatty acids (SFA; <7% of calories) and cholesterol (<200 mg/day), emphasizes unsaturated fat in a moderate-fat diet (25% to 35% of calories from total fat), and includes 20 to 30 g/day of dietary fiber (see Table 19-1). Therapeutic options to enhance LDL cholesterol lowering are increased viscous (soluble) fiber (10–25 g/day) and plant sterols/stanols (2 g/day). The effectiveness of this dietary pattern on LDL cholesterol lowering is based on a large body of research that has evaluated diet response in both controlled settings as well as in free-living cohorts on self-selected diets. This research has provided important information about the maximal efficacy of a cholesterol-lowering dietary pattern compared with what is achievable in individuals given dietary guidance. The Portfolio diet,[8,14] the Lifestyle Heart Program,[15-17] and the DASH Diet[5,6,18,19] all evaluated the maximum response achievable with very similar dietary patterns on LDL cholesterol lowering, as well as what can be attained in a "real world" setting.

TABLE 19-1 Nutrient Composition of Therapeutic Lifestyle Changes in Adult Treatment Panel III

Nutrient	Recommended Intake
Saturated fat (lower *trans* fat)	<7% of total calories
Polyunsaturated fat	Up to 10% of total calories
Monounsaturated fat	Up to 20% of total calories
Total fat	25%–35% of total calories
Carbohydrate (emphasize complex sources)	50%–60% of total calories
Fiber	20–30 g per day
Protein	Approximately 15% of total calories
Cholesterol	<200 mg/day
Total calories (energy)	Balance energy intake and output to maintain healthy body weight and prevent weight gain

TABLE 19-2 Cumulative Low-Density Lipoprotein Cholesterol Reduction By Dietary Modification

Dietary Component	Dietary Change	Approximate LDL Reduction
Saturated fat	<7% of calories	8%–10 %
Trans fat	<1% of calories	1%–2 %
Dietary cholesterol	<200 mg/day	3%–5 %
Weight reduction	Lose 10 lb	5%–8 %
Soy protein		3%–5 %
Other LDL-lowering options		
Viscous fiber	5 to 10 g/day	3%–5 %
Plant sterol/stanol esters	2 g/day	6%–15 %
Cumulative estimate		24%–37 %

LDL, low-density lipoprotein.

Portfolio Diet

The Portfolio diet is comprised of four cholesterol-lowering components: plant sterols (1.0 g/1000 calories), soy protein (21.4 g/1000 calories), viscous fiber (9.8 g/1000 calories), and almonds (14 g/1000 calories).[8] It is primarily a vegetarian diet that provides 30% of calories from total fat, 6.3% of calories from saturated fat, and 54 mg of cholesterol per day. Sources of viscous fiber include oats, barley, psyllium, eggplant, and okra. Soy milk and soy meat analogues were sources of soy protein. After 1 month of the Portfolio diet, subjects had a 28.6% reduction in LDL cholesterol compared with their self-reported diet low in saturated fat (7%–8% of calories) and dietary cholesterol (<200 mg/day). In this study, the control diet tested was low in saturated fat (4.5% of calories) and dietary cholesterol (128 mg/day) and elicited an 8% reduction in LDL cholesterol compared with the baseline standard cholesterol-lowering diet that subjects had been following. Thus the "portfolio" of cholesterol-lowering foods markedly augmented the LDL cholesterol–lowering response of a traditional cholesterol-lowering diet.

In a longer-term study with subjects following a self-selected Portfolio diet for 1 year, LDL cholesterol was reduced by 12.8%, a response that is appreciably less than that observed after the 1-month metabolic diet.[14] Nonetheless, 32% of the participants (n = 21 of 66) had LDL cholesterol reductions of greater than 20% at 1 year, a reduction that was not significantly different from that observed after the metabolically controlled Portfolio diet was consumed for 1 month. The authors reported satisfactory compliance (on the basis of amount consumed compared to the prescribed amount) for the almond component of the diet, that is, there was 78% compliance with the recommendation to consume 23 g/1000 calories, and for plant sterol–enriched margarine, compliance was 67%. However, viscous fiber compliance was 55% and soy protein compliance was 51%, both considered as less than adequate by the study authors. At 1 year, only two subjects were following a vegan diet and five were following a lacto-ovo-vegetarian diet. The remaining subjects were following an omnivorous diet. These results are important because they convey the difficulty in following a habitual plant-based diet that maximizes LDL cholesterol lowering. Nonetheless, this study provides important information about what is realistically achievable in a free-living situation: an LDL cholesterol–lowering response that is clinically significant. Importantly, for individuals who can adopt and adhere to a habitual Portfolio dietary pattern, the LDL cholesterol–lowering response is most impressive and would be equivalent to two doublings of an initial dose of a statin.

Delta Study, Dash Trial

The Dietary Effects on Lipoproteins and Thrombogenic Activity (DELTA) study was a multicenter, randomized, crossover-design trial conducted to assess the effects of reducing dietary saturated fat on plasma lipids and lipoproteins in 103 healthy adults 22 to 67 years old.[20] The study compared three diets— an average American diet (AAD), a Step 1 diet (28.6% of calories from fat and 9.0% of calories from SFA), and a low-SFA diet (Low-Sat) 25.3% of calories from fat and 6.1% of calories from SFA) which were fed for 8 weeks. Dietary cholesterol was constant (275 mg cholesterol/day). Compared with AAD, total cholesterol fell 5% on Step 1 and 9% on Low-Sat. LDL cholesterol was 7% lower on Step 1 and 11% lower on Low-Sat than on the AAD. HDL cholesterol fell 7% on the Step 1 and 11% on Low-Sat diets. Plasma TG levels increased approximately 9% between AAD and Step 1 but did not increase further from Step 1 to the Low-Sat diet.

The DASH trial was a landmark study that evaluated the effects of a dietary pattern on blood pressure, as well as on lipids and lipoproteins.[5] The DASH dietary pattern is low in saturated fat (7% of calories) and cholesterol (141 mg/day), reduced in total fat (27% of calories), and rich in fruits and vegetables (8–10 servings per day), whole grains, low-fat dairy products (2–3 servings per day), and dietary fiber (approximately 30 g/day of fiber, of which approximately 9 g is soluble). The DASH study was a randomized, controlled, outpatient feeding trial conducted in four field centers with a total of 436 participants.[5] Compared to the average Western diet, which is high in saturated fat, total fat, and cholesterol and low in dietary fiber, the DASH diet reduced total, LDL and HDL cholesterol by 9.5%, 9.1%, and 9.2%, respectively, with no change in TG levels.[21]

Collectively, the DELTA study and the DASH trial provide information that is a useful benchmark of the extent of LDL cholesterol lowering in response to dietary patterns that are consistent with contemporary dietary guidance for saturated fat and cholesterol.[1,13] As would be expected, the decrease in saturated fat elicits a decrease in HDL cholesterol along with decreases in total and LDL cholesterol. In both studies, the total cholesterol/HDL cholesterol ratio was unchanged. To elicit a decrease in this ratio would necessitate further reductions in LDL cholesterol via therapeutic options such as including viscous fiber and plant stanols/sterols. The DELTA study reported an increase in TGs with a reduction in total fat, whereas TGs were unchanged in response to the DASH diet, which may be due to the higher dietary fiber content of the DASH diet. This is supported by a recent review[22] that presented a number of reduced fat, high-fiber diet studies that demonstrated no TG-raising response.

Low-Fat Dietary Pattern

Women's Health Initiative Dietary Modification Trial

The Women's Health Initiative Dietary Modification Trial is a randomized controlled trial of 48,835 postmenopausal women ranging in age from 50 to 79 years who were assigned to a low-fat diet intervention or a comparison group.[23] The target intervention was 20% of calories from total fat, 5 servings per day of vegetables and fruits, and 6 servings per day of grains. An intensive behavior modification program was implemented that involved 18 group sessions in year 1, and quarterly maintenance sessions thereafter, led by qualified nutritionists. By year 6 of an 8.1-year follow-up, mean fat intake had decreased by 8.2% in the intervention versus the control group (baseline for intervention = 37.8% of calories from fat; after year 6 = 28.8%) with decreases in saturated fat (2.9%), monounsaturated fat (3.3%), and polyunsaturated fat (1.5%). Vegetable and fruit intake increased by 1.1 servings per day and grain intake increased by 0.5 serving per day. LDL cholesterol, diastolic blood pressure (DBP), and factor VIIc decreased significantly by 3.6 mg/dL, 0.31 mm Hg, and 4.3%, respectively, in the intervention versus comparison groups. Women in the treatment group also lost 2.2 kg during the first year of the intervention and maintained a slightly lower weight (−0.4 kg) than control women after 7.5 years of follow-up.[24]

Mediterranean-Style Dietary Patterns

Predimed Study

The Prevencion con Dieta Mediterranea (Predimed) Study is a large (n = 9000 high-risk participants) parallel-group multicenter, randomized, controlled 4-year clinical trial that is being conducted in Spain to evaluate the effects of the Mediterranean diet on the primary prevention of CVD (www.predimed.org). The study is ongoing with a completion date of 2010. Three diets are being studied: a "low-fat" (fat modified, i.e., low in saturated fat and cholesterol) diet (that met American Heart Association guidelines), and two Mediterranean-style diets, with one providing virgin olive oil (15 L = 1 L/wk for 15 weeks) and one providing sachets of walnuts, hazelnuts, and almonds (1350 g walnuts = 15 g/day; 675 g hazelnuts = 7.5 g/day, and 675 g almonds = 7.5 g/day, alloted for 90 days), together with instructions about their use.

A subgroup of 772 asymptomatic subjects ranging in age from 55 to 80 years was followed up for 3 months.[11] There was no significant difference in LDL cholesterol among treatments. The Mediterranean diet with nuts decreased total cholesterol by 6.2 mg/dL compared to the low-fat diet. Both Mediterranean diets increased HDL cholesterol, 2.9 mg/dL versus 1.6 mg/dL for the olive oil and nuts diets, respectively versus the low-fat diet. TGs were lower in subjects on the nuts diet (−13 mg/dL) compared to the low-fat diet. The total cholesterol HDL cholesterol ratio decreased on the two Mediterranean-style diets. In addition, the Mediterranean diets reduced plasma glucose levels by an average of 6.2 mg/dL. Moreover, SBP decreased by about 6.5 mm Hg, and DBP decreased by 2.1 mm Hg.

Medi-RIVAGE Study

The Mediterranean Diet, Cardiovascular Risks and Gene Polymorphisms (Medi-RIVAGE) Study is another interventional trial conducted in France that compared a Mediterranean-type diet with a low-fat (prudent, i.e., low in saturated fat, and cholesterol) diet.[10] The Mediterranean-type diet had a total fat goal of 35% to 38% of calories with emphasis on monounsaturated fat (50% of total fat) and polyunsaturated fat (25% of total fat). The low-fat diet had a total fat goal of 30% of calories with equal contributions from the three fatty acid classes. Subjects were provided with nutritional recommendations by a physician or dietitian and received a booklet that described the diet to be followed. After a 3-month dietary intervention, both groups decreased total fat, saturated fat, and cholesterol similarly, with the consequent outcome that the only difference between the diets was intake of monounsaturated fat (15.6% vs. 13.4% on the Mediterranean vs. the low-fat diet, respectively). LDL cholesterol decreased by 11.4% on the Mediterranean diet and by 5% in the low-fat group. When averaged over both diet groups, there were decreases in plasma TGs, glucose, and insulin versus baseline; however, there was no diet effect. This is not surprising because the two diets were similar compositionally after the initial intervention, which underscores the challenges of implementation of a dietary pattern that achieves target nutrient goals.

Lyon Diet Heart Study

The Lyon Diet Heart Study, a randomized controlled trial with free-living subjects, tested the effectiveness of a Mediterranean-type diet on composite measures of recurrent cardiovascular events after a first myocardial infarction.[9] Experimental subjects were provided a test margarine that was compositionally similar to olive oil but higher in linolenic acid (16.4% vs. 8.6% of kcal) and α-linolenic acid (4.8% vs. 0.6% of kcal).

Subjects in the control group consumed a diet that included approximately 34% of calories from fat, 12% from saturated fat, 11% from monounsaturated fat, 6% from polyunsaturated fat, and 312 mg/day of cholesterol. Subjects on the Mediterranean-style diet averaged 30% of calories from fat, 8% from saturated fat, 13% from monounsaturated fat, 5% from polyunsaturated fat, and 203 mg/day of cholesterol. These subjects consumed more α-linolenic acid (0.84% vs. 0.29% of kcal) and dietary fiber.

After 46 months, 204 control and 219 experimental subjects participated in the final examination. Despite similar plasma lipids and lipoproteins (and SBP and DBP, body mass index, and smoking status), subjects following the Mediterranean-style diet had a 50% to 70% lower risk of recurrent heart disease, as measured by different combinations of outcome measures.

The findings from the Lyon Diet Heart Study illustrate the potential importance of a dietary pattern that emphasizes fruits, vegetables, breads and cereals, and fish, as well as α-linolenic acid, within the context of a blood cholesterol–lowering diet. The clinical findings from the Lyon Diet Heart Study implicate other risk factors beyond lipids and lipoproteins, which have historically been primary targets of intervention.

Very-Low-Fat or High PUFA Dietary Patterns

Lifestyle Diet Heart Program

The Lifestyle Diet Heart Program consists of a plant-based, whole foods diet, rich in fruits, vegetables, grains, legumes, nonfat dairy products (1 cup per day), and egg whites.[15,16] This diet only contributes 10% of calories from total fat and provides 75% of calories from complex carbohydrates. The program promotes other intensive lifestyle changes, for example, aerobic exercise, stress management, smoking cessation, and group psychological support (two meetings weekly).[15] In a small study with 48 patients with moderate to severe CHD, 20 (of 28) subjects in the experimental group had a 37% reduction in LDL cholesterol after 1 year and a 20% reduction after 5 years versus the usual care group.[16] For subjects in the control group, LDL cholesterol decreased by 1.2% at year 1 and by 19.3% after 5 years. In the intervention group, there was an average 3.1–percentage point decrease in percent diameter stenosis versus baseline and an 11.8–percentage point increase in the control group after 5 years. In addition, there were fewer cardiac events in the intervention group (25 versus 45). Atherosclerosis regression was related to adherence to the Lifestyle Diet Heart Program. Approximately one third of the subjects were most adherent, one third were medium adherent, and one third were least adherent, indicating that adherence to this program is challenging for some individuals. A more recent study[17] reported a lower LDL cholesterol–lowering response in individuals on the Lifestyle Diet Heart Program. In this short-term (3 months) intervention study, 869 nonsmoking CHD patients enrolled in the health insurance–based Multisite Cardiac Lifestyle Intervention Program. Patients attended an onsite program twice weekly for 3 months for a total of 104 hours. After 3 months, LDL cholesterol decreased by 14% in women (n = 275) and 17% in men (n = 554), a lesser response than previously reported for the Lifestyle Diet Heart Program. Although the authors reported that 74% of the subjects adhered to the dietary fat recommendation after 3 months, this program is challenging to follow, and it will be important to determine if this level of adherence can be maintained long term.

High Polyunsaturated Fatty Acid Diets

Four randomized clinical trials tested the effect of high–Polyunsaturated Fatty Acid (PUFA) diets (using soy and other unhydrogenated vegetable oils) on cholesterol lowering and CVD events.[25-28] The diets provided 15% to 21% of calories from PUFA, and total fat ranged from 34% to 46% of calories. In all four studies, total cholesterol was decreased by 13% to 15% over a 4- to 8-year period. CVD events were significantly reduced (by 25%–43%) in three of the studies.[25,26,28]

DIETARY PATTERNS TO MANAGE ATHEROGENIC DYSLIPIDEMIA

Therapeutic Lifestyle Changes Diet

Atherogenic dyslipidemia is characterized principally by elevated TG and low HDL cholesterol levels. Often these patients present with the metabolic syndrome, characterized by three of the following five clinical criteria: (1) abdominal obesity (waist circumference greater than 40 inches for men and greater than 35 inches for women), (2) TG 150 mg/dL or greater, (3) HDL cholesterol less than 40 mg/dL in men and less than 50 mg/dL in women, (4) blood pressure 130/85 mm Hg or higher, and (5) fasting glucose 100 mg/dL or greater. As noted by NCEP ATP III,[13] treatment strategies for atherogenic dyslipidemia and metabolic syndrome include the TLC diet with emphasis on weight loss (if needed). Guidelines for recommended weight loss can be found In the National Heart, Lung, and Blood Institute Clinical Guidelines for the Identification, Evaluation and Treatment of Overweight and Obesity in Adults from the Obesity Education Initiative.[29,30] The 2005 Dietary Guidelines for Americans[31] recommends aiming for a slow, steady weight loss by decreasing calorie intake while maintaining an adequate nutrient intake and increasing physical activity (http://www.health.gov/dietaryguidelines/dga2005/document/html/chapter3.htm). Increased physical activity is recommended for weight loss. Up to 60 minutes of moderate- to vigorous-intensity physical activity per day may be needed to prevent weight gain; however, 60 to 90 minutes of moderate-intensity physical activity per day is recommended to sustain weight loss for previously overweight people (http://www.health.gov/dietaryguidelines/dga2005/document/html/chapter3.htm).

For treatment of atherogenic dyslipidemia, total fat intake at the upper range is recommended (i.e., 35% of calories), and dietary carbohydrate at the lower range of that recommended (50% of calories). A strategy to achieve this recommendation is to replace calories from SFA and carbohydrate with unsaturated fat; typically monounsaturated fat is used. Replacing dietary carbohydrate with monounsaturated fatty acids (MUFA) will decrease TG and increase HDL cholesterol.[32] A meta-analysis of 60 controlled trials showed that the replacement of carbohydrate with MUFA resulted in significant decrease in LDL cholesterol and the total cholesterol/HDL cholesterol ratio, and increase in HDL cholesterol.[33] Thus very-high-carbohydrate diets are not recommended for the management of low HDL cholesterol and high TG.

OmniHeart Study

The OmniHeart study was a large (n = 164 subjects with prehypertension or stage 1 hypertension) crossover, controlled-feeding study that compared the effects of three blood cholesterol–lowering diets high in carbohydrate (58% of calories), protein (25% of calories, of which about 50% came from plant protein sources), or unsaturated fat (31% of calories, primarily monounsaturated fat), on lipids, lipoproteins, and blood pressure.[7] The diet high in unsaturated fat lowered TG by 9.6 mg/dL, increased HDL cholesterol by 1.1 mg/dL, and decreased LDL cholesterol similarly (13.1 vs. 11.6 mg/dL) compared to the high-carbohydrate diet. Compared to the high-carbohydrate diet, the high-protein diet decreased TG by 15.7 mg/dL and decreased HDL cholesterol by 1.3 mg/dL; the LDL cholesterol decrease was similar. Interestingly, the high-protein diet elicited the greatest TG-lowering effect among all the diets (−16.4 mg/dL vs. −9.3 mg/dL for high unsaturated fat vs. 0.1 mg/dL for high carbohydrate). LDL cholesterol lowering was similar among all three diets (11.6, 14.2, and 13.1 mg/dL for high carbohydrate, protein, and unsaturated fat, respectively).

All diets decreased SBP and DBP compared with baseline (SBP = −8.2 mm Hg, −9.5 mm Hg, −9.3 mm Hg for high carbohydrate, protein, unsaturated fat), respectively; DBP- (−4.1 mm Hg, −5.2 mm Hg, −4.8 mm Hg for high carbohydrate, protein, unsaturated fat, respectively). The high-protein versus high-carbohydrate diet significantly lowered SBP (−0.9 mm Hg) and DBP (−0.9 mm Hg) in participants with prehypertension. Likewise, in subjects with hypertension, the high-protein versus high-carbohydrate diet significantly lowered SBP (−3.5 mm Hg) and DBP (−2.4 mm Hg) in participants with hypertension. In addition, the high–unsaturated fat versus high-carbohydrate diet significantly lowered SBP (−2.9 mm Hg) and DBP (−1.9 mm Hg) in participants with hypertension.

The OmniHeart Study is important because it clearly demonstrates that dietary protein (principally plant-derived) and unsaturated fat are preferred macronutrient substitutes to use rather than dietary carbohydrate for decreasing saturated fat in the diet. Further studies are needed to resolve the optimal proportion of protein and unsaturated fat to use in blood cholesterol–lowering diets for maximal CVD risk factor reduction in different patient cohorts.

Dietary Effects on Lipoproteins and Thrombogenic Activity Study

Protocol 2 of the DELTA study sought to determine whether replacement of dietary saturated fat with monounsaturated fat, as opposed to carbohydrate, would result in a better overall risk factor profile in nondiabetic individuals with one or more of the following: low HDL cholesterol, high TG, or high insulin levels.[34] Fifty-two men and 33 women were randomly assigned to a 7-week randomized, crossover design diet study that compared an AAD (36% of energy from fat), and two additional diets in which 7% of energy from saturated fat was replaced with either carbohydrate or monounsaturated fat.

Compared to the AAD, LDL cholesterol was lower on both the carbohydrate and monounsaturated fat diets (−7% and −6.3%), whereas the decrease in HDL cholesterol was less during the monounsaturated fat diet (−4.3%) versus the carbohydrate diet (−7.2%). Plasma TC tended to be lower on the monounsaturated fat diet compared to the AAD (−4.9%; $P < .03$); TG levels were significantly higher on the carbohydrate diet when compared to either the AAD (+6.5%) or the monounsaturated fat diet (+11.4%) ($P < .01$ for each comparison). The DELTA study demonstrated that in a dyslipidemic population, monounsaturated fat rather than carbohydrate is a preferable replacement for saturated fat to provide the greatest lipid risk factor reduction.

DIETARY PATTERNS TO MANAGE HYPERTENSION

Healthy lifestyles are recommended for the prevention and treatment of high blood pressure.[35] Table 19-3 presents the impact of various lifestyle behaviors on blood pressure. Even a small weight loss of as little as 10 lb (4.5 kg) reduces blood pressure and/or prevents hypertension. The DASH eating plan along a dietary sodium restriction (<2.3 g/day, with the goal of 1.5 g/day)[1] will decrease blood pressure markedly. In addition, regular

TABLE 19-3 Joint National Committee 7 Report—Lifestyle Modifications to Prevent and Manage Hypertension

Modification	Recommendations	Approximate SBP Reduction (range)
Weight reduction	Maintain normal body weight (BMI 18.5–24.9 kg/m^2)	5–20 mm Hg/10 kg
Adopt DASH eating plan	Consume a diet rich in fruits, vegetables, and low-fat dairy products with a reduced content of saturated and total fat	8–14 mm Hg
Dietary sodium restriction	Reduce sodium intake to no more than 100 m Eq/L (2.4 g sodium or 6 g sodium chloride)	2–8 mm Hg
Physical activity	Engage in regular aerobic physical activity such as brisk walking (at least 30 min/day, most days)	4–9 mm Hg
Moderation of alcohol consumption	Limit consumption to no more than 2 drinks (e.g., 24 oz beer, 10 oz wine, 3 oz 80-proof whiskey) per day in most men, no more than 1 drink per day in women and lighter-weight men	2–4 mm Hg

From Ref. 35, with permission.

aerobic physical activity such as brisk walking at least 30 minutes per day most days of the week is recommended for blood pressure control. Alcohol should be limited, and moderation is recommended for those who choose to consume alcohol.

Dietary and Approaches to Stop Hypertension-Sodium Studies

The DASH[5] and DASH-Sodium[6] trials were seminal studies designed to test effects of modifying dietary patterns, including sodium restriction, in individuals with DBP of 80 to 95 mm Hg and SBP of less than 160 mm Hg.

In the DASH trial, three diets were fed for 8 weeks: a control diet, a fruits and vegetables diet, or a combination diet.[5] The fruits and vegetables diet provided approximately 10 servings of fruits and vegetables per day and was similar to the control diet in macronutrient content. The combination diet was high in fruits and vegetables (approximately 9 servings), low-fat dairy products, whole grains, fish, poultry, and nuts, and was low in fat, red meat, and sweets. The combination diet was reduced in saturated fat, total fat, and cholesterol, and was moderately high in protein, calcium, potassium, and magnesium. All three diets contained about 3000 mg of sodium per day, and body weight was maintained throughout the study.

Both intervention diets reduced blood pressure compared to the control diet. The DASH diet significantly lowered SBP by 5.5 mm Hg and DBP by 3 mm Hg compared to the control diet.[5] Although to a lesser degree, the fruits and vegetables diet also significantly lowered blood pressure by 2.8/1.1 mm Hg compared to the control diet. In subjects with stage 1 hypertension (140/90 to 159/95 mm Hg, 29% of the total sample), the combination diet decreased SBP by 11.6 mm Hg and DBP by 5.3 mm Hg.[36] Normotensive subjects had a significant reduction in blood pressure but to a much lesser extent (3.5/2.2 mm Hg). Hypertensive African Americans had the most robust response to the combination diet, reducing blood pressure by 13.2/6.1 mm Hg compared to the control diet.[36]

To evaluate the effect of sodium reduction in the context of the combination diet, the DASH-Sodium trial was conducted.[6] There were three levels of sodium intake: high level of 3300 mg/day, which is similar to the average U.S. intake; intermediate level of 2400 mg/day, which is the upper level of current recommendations; and low level of 1500 mg/day.

Reduction in sodium intake reduced blood pressure (from high sodium to low sodium, a decrease of 3.0/1.6 mm Hg on the combination diet and 6.7/3.5 mm Hg on the control diet).[6] Compared to the combination diet, the sodium-related decrease in blood pressure was greater in the control diet. The greatest blood pressure reduction was achieved in subjects consuming the combination diet at the lowest level of sodium (Fig. 19-1). The hypotensive effects were significant in all subgroups, although hypertensive individuals, those older than 45 years of age, women, and African Americans appeared to derive the greatest benefit from the combined interventions.[37,38] The DASH-Sodium trial demonstrated hypotensive benefits of the DASH dietary pattern over a range of sodium intakes, and the combined effects of the DASH diet and sodium restriction elicited the greatest blood pressure–lowering effect.

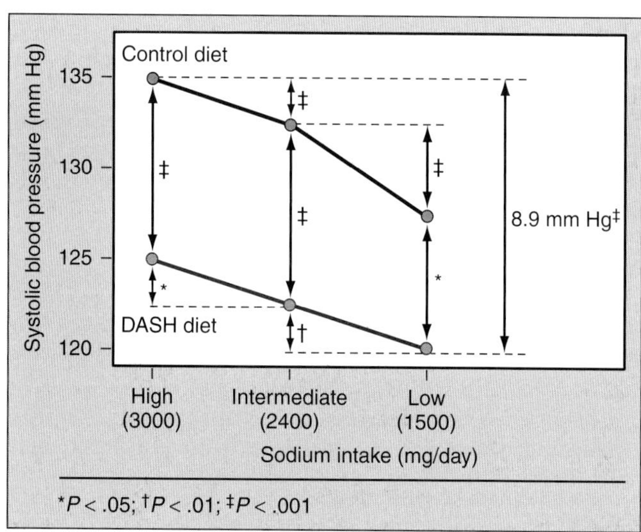

FIGURE 19-1 Reduction in systolic blood pressure in the Dietary Approaches to Stop Hypertension (DASH)-Sodium study. Participants were randomized to a control diet or the DASH diet; within each group, each participant rotated through three sodium intake levels (3000, 2400, and 1500 mg/day). *Adapted from Ref. 6, with permission.*

PREMIER Study

Because the DASH trials were controlled-feeding studies, the PREMIER study was conducted to test the implementation of the DASH dietary pattern under free-living conditions after 6 or 18 months of follow-up.[18,19] Food was not provided, and blood pressure response was evaluated in three groups of subjects with above-optimal blood pressure: (1) advice only—participants were given a single counseling session and printed handouts, (2) established recommendations—participants participated in 18 sessions of behavioral counseling, and (3) established recommendations plus instructions for the DASH diet. The counseling sessions dealt with weight loss (when indicated), moderate-intensity physical activity, dietary sodium, and alcohol guidance. Subjects were 800 men and women with SBP of 120 to 159 mm Hg and DBP of 80 to 95 mm Hg. After 6 months, both groups that received the established recommendations, with and without the DASH diet, lost substantial weight (5–6 kg). The effects attributed to the DASH diet were less than in previous studies and were not significantly different from the established recommendation group. However, hypertension was best controlled in the established recommendations plus DASH group; 77% of participants with stage 1 hypertension ended the study with blood pressure lower than 140/90 mm Hg.

In the 19-month follow-up of the PREMIER study,[19] relative to the advice-only group, the odds ratio for hypertension were 0.83 (95% confidence internal (CI), 0.67–1.04) for the established recommendations group and 0.77 (95% CI, 0.62–0.97) for the established plus DASH group. At 18 months, the mean SBP and DBP had decreased from baseline in participants in every treatment group. These reductions were greater for the established recommendations and the established recommendations plus DASH group than for the advice-only group (by 0.9 and 1.9 mm SBP respectively); however, the treatments did not differ statistically. Thus, people can make healthful behavior changes to reduce high blood pressure, but the 18-month follow-up of the PREMIER study points out the challenges of eliciting multiple behavior changes in a sustained manner.

FOOD-BASED DIETARY RECOMMENDATIONS FOR HEART HEALTH

Food-based dietary recommendations have been made for the implementation of healthful dietary patterns to decrease CVD risk.[1] The American Heart Association Diet and Lifestyle Recommendations Revision 2006 present food-based recommendations for implementation of the TLC diet and the DASH diet.[1] These are summarized in Table 19-4. The scientific basis for these specific food-based recommendations is discussed herein.

Fruits and Vegetables

The Nurses' Health Study and the Health Professionals, Follow-up Study reported that persons in the highest quintile of fruit and vegetable intake (≥ 8 servings/day) had a relative risk of CHD of 0.80 (95% CI, 0.69–0.93) compared with persons in the lowest quintile of intake (<3 servings/day).[39] Green leafy vegetables and vitamin C–rich fruits and vegetables were the strongest protectors of heart health. In addition, an inverse association between CVD risk and fruit and vegetable intake was noted in the Women's Health Study.[40] After multiple statistical adjustments, the relative risk of CVD was 0.45 (95% CI, 0.22–0.91) when comparing the highest to lowest quintiles of fruit and vegetable intake. The risk for myocardial infarction also was lower when comparing extreme quintiles. Similar results were found in the Physicians' Health Study, which followed more than 22,000 physicians over 12 years.[41] Men who consumed at least 2 servings per day of vegetables had a 22% lower risk of CHD than men who ate less than 1 serving per day (relative risk [RR], 0.77; 95% CI, 0.60–0.98). For each additional serving per day of vegetables, the risk of

TABLE 19-4 Two Examples of Daily Dietary Patterns That Are Consistent with American Heart Association Diet Lifestyle Recommendations Revision 2006

Eating Pattern	DASH	TLC	Serving Size
Grains	6–8 sv/day	7 sv/day	1 slice bread, 1 oz dry cereal, ½ c cooked rice, pasta
Vegetables	4–5 sv/day	5 sv/day	1 c raw leafy vegetables, ½ c cut-up raw or cooked vegetables, ½ c vegetable juice
Fruits	4–5 sv/day	4 sv/day	1 medium fruit, ¼ c dried fruit, ½ c fresh, frozen canned fruit, ½ c fruit juice
Fat-free or low-fat milk products	2–3 sv/day	2–3 sv/day	1 c milk, 1 c yogurt, 1/5 oz cheese
Lean meats, poultry, fish	<6 oz/day	≤5 oz/day	1 oz cooked
Nuts, seeds, legumes	4–5 sv/day	Counted in vegetable servings	1/3 ; 2 Tbsp peanut butter or seeds, ½ c dry beans or peas
Fats and oils	2–3 sv/day	Amount Depends on daily calorie level	1 tsp soft margarine, 1 Tbsp mayonnaise, 1 tsp vegetable Oil, 2 Tbsp salad dressing
Sweets and added sugars	≤5 sv/week	No recommendation	1 Tbsp sugar, jelly, jam; ½ c sorbet; 1 c lemonade

Adapted from Ref. 1, with permisssion.

CHD decreased by 17% (RR, 0.83; 95% CI, 0.71–0.98). Using the National Health and Nutrition Examination Survey (NHANES) Epidemiologic Follow-up Study, Bazzano and colleagues[42] reported that consuming fruits and vegetables three or more times daily versus less than once daily was associated with a 27% and 24% lower mortality from CVD and ischemic heart disease, respectively. Stroke mortality and incidence also decreased by 42% and 27%, respectively.

Whole Grains

Whole grains include wheat, brown rice, corn, oats, rye, barley, triticale, sorghum, bulgur, kasha, couscous, and millet. In addition to being rich in fiber, whole grains provide minerals, vitamins, phenols, phytoestrogens, α-linolenic acid, and resistant starch. In a recent meta-analysis of seven prospective cohort studies of whole grain intake and CVD outcomes, greater whole grain intake (2.5 servings/day vs. 0.2 serving/day) was associated with a 21% lower risk of CVD events (odds ratio [OR], 0.79, 95% CI, 0.73–0.85).[43] Similar associations were reported for other CVD outcomes (heart disease, stroke, fatal CVD). In the Insulin Resistance Atherosclerosis Study in 1178 participants, whole grain intake was inversely associated with common carotid artery intima–media thickness (beta ± SE, −0.043 ± 0.013; $P = .005$) and intima–media progression (beta ± SE, −0.019 ± 0.011; $P = .09$).[44]

Fish

Many epidemiologic and controlled interventional studies have reported beneficial effects of omega-3 fatty acid consumption, whether marine or plant derived, on many CVD endpoints, including all CVD, defined as all CHD, fatal and nonfatal myocardial infarction, and stroke; sudden cardiac death; and all-cause mortality (reviewed in reference 45). Collectively, CVD benefits have been found with consumption of modest amounts of omega-3 fatty acids provided by an average intake of 25 to 57 g (1–2 oz) of fish consumed daily or an intake of an equivalent amount consumed in one or more meals weekly or even monthly. Increasing fish consumption decreases risk in a dose-dependent manner. A meta-analysis of 13 cohort studies found a gradual beneficial effect of increasing fish dose and CHD mortality.[45] Fish consumption five times per week decreased CHD mortality by 38%. There is evidence, albeit limited, that α-linolenic acid also has cardioprotective effects.

Reduced-Fat/Skim-Milk Dairy Products

The Coronary Artery Risk Development in Young Adults (CARDIA) Study, a population-based, prospective study of 3157 black and white adults ranging in age from 18 to 30 years, reported an inverse association with 10-year cumulative incidence of insulin resistance syndrome among individuals who were overweight (body mass index ≥25 kg/m²) at baseline but not among leaner individuals (body mass index <25 kg/m²).[46] Each daily occasion of dairy consumption was associated with 21% lower odds of insulin resistance syndrome (OR, 0.79; 95% CI, 0.70–0.88) for blacks and whites and for men and women. In the Caerphilly Prospective Study, an inverse association was reported for milk and dairy product consumption and metabolic syndrome.[47] Adjusted odds ratios were 0.38 (95% CI, 0.18–0.78) for men who drank a pint or more daily of milk and 0.44 (95% CI, 0.21–0.91) for dairy product consumption.

Other Foods—Nuts, Seeds, and Legumes

A recent review summarized the epidemiologic and clinical studies of nut consumption and CHD risk and risk factors.[48] A pooled analysis of four U.S. epidemiologic studies showed that subjects in the highest intake group for nut consumption (about 5 servings/week) had about a 35% reduced risk of CHD incidence. Clinical studies have evaluated the effects of many different nuts and peanuts on lipids, lipoproteins, and various CHD risk factors, including oxidation, inflammation, and vascular reactivity. Evidence from these studies consistently shows a beneficial effect on these CHD risk factors. A summary of studies conducted to date demonstrates that tree nuts reduce LDL cholesterol by 3% to 19% compared with Western and lower-fat diets. The LDL cholesterol–lowering response of nut and peanut studies is greater than expected on the basis of blood cholesterol–lowering equations that are derived from changes in the fatty acid profile of the diet, and appears to be due to other bioactive compounds.

Alcohol

Although clinical trial data are lacking, moderate intake of alcoholic beverages (½ to 1 per day on average for women and 1 to 2 per day on average for men) is associated with a reduced risk of CHD in various populations.[49]

This observational data on a beneficial effect for alcohol ingestion is based on comparisons of those who drink modestly as above versus those who are teetotalers and those who drink more heavily. Interestingly, in a large observational study of men, in those already at low risk on the basis of body mass index, physical activity, smoking, and diet, moderate alcohol intake is associated with lower risk for myocardial infarction.[50] Genetic (a relationship with the polymorphism for alcohol dehydrogenase) and metabolic (improved HDL cholesterol) mechanisms support a causal relationship between alcohol and CHD prevention with no strong evidence that one beverage is superior to the others.[51]

STRATEGIES FOR IMPLEMENTATION OF HEALTHFUL DIETARY PATTERNS

Providing patients with practical, ready-to-use nutritional guidelines that can fit into their busy lifestyles is the key to risk factor management. Although most patients, particularly those presenting with multiple risk factors, would benefit from a referral to a registered dietitian trained in CVD, the cardiologist plays a unique role in facilitating lifestyle change. Regardless of motivation level, ongoing reinforcement, education, and appropriate follow-up to measure risk factor status is essential.

This section aims to provide the physician with first-line nutrition strategies to present to patients. Although there are subtle differences in the eating patterns discussed in this chapter's previous section, a nutritional theme among the dietary approaches exists. The foundation of maximal CVD risk reduction by diet includes the DASH, Mediterranean, Portfolio, and OmniHeart eating plans, all of which provide similar guidance. The following list of six steps, equipped with tables and instructive suggestions, highlights principal dietary strategies that patients should implement to achieve optimal CVD risk factor status.

Step 1: Substitute Fats in a Heart-Friendly Manner

In the United States, consumption of saturated fat continues to exceed recommended guidelines. Saturated fat should be limited to no more than 7% of total daily calories for patients with an increased risk of developing CVD, existing coronary disease, or elevated LDL cholesterol. Because percentages are difficult to decipher in real world situations, Table 19-5 illustrates the saturated fat recommendation in grams for various calorie levels and Figure 19-2 shows major sources of SFAs in the diet.

Patients should become familiar with foods high in saturated fat and encouraged to reduce overall consumption. Saturated fat reduction can be achieved in two ways: (1) Reduce the portion size, choose leaner versions of foods (e.g., meats and dairy products), or eliminate saturated fat–rich foods. (2) Substitute saturated fat calories with unsaturated fat sources (e.g., replacing butter with *trans*-free tub margarine). The former is ideal for patients with caloric excess who would benefit from weight loss. However, removing food sources of saturated fat in the diet completely can backfire, because these calories are often replaced with refined carbohydrate food sources. Replacing carbohydrates for fat can yield small reductions in total and LDL cholesterol. However, when carbohydrates are not chosen wisely, they can also yield reductions in HDL cholesterol and elevations in blood TG. Ideally, unsaturated fats should be substituted for saturated fats while keeping total calories (and therefore portion size) in check. Table 19-6 illustrates selected foods high in saturated fat. Table 19-7 provides examples of monounsaturated and polyunsaturated fat food sources and appropriate substitutions.

Patients also should be encouraged to read food labels and choose foods low in saturated fat. The Food and Drug Administration (FDA) provides guidelines for the following nutrient content claims regarding saturated fat[52]:

- "Low in saturated fat" means 1 g or less of saturated fat is provided per labeled serving. For main entrees, the food should contain no more than 1 g of saturated fat per 100 g.

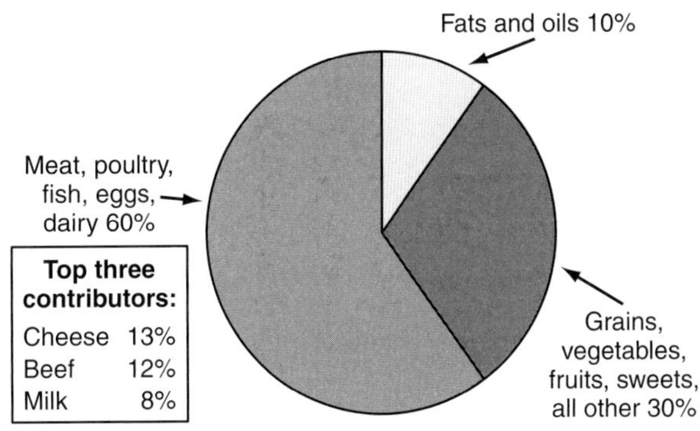

FIGURE 19-2 Major sources of saturated fatty acids.

TABLE 19-5 Saturated Fat Allowance Based on Varying Caloric Ranges at 7% of Calories (Rounded to Nearest 1/100).

Calorie Level	Saturated Fat (g)
2600	20.0
2400	18.5
2200	17.0
2000	15.5
1800	14.0
1600	12.5
1400	11.0
1200	9.0

TABLE 19-6 Major Foods Sources of Saturated Fat

High-fat meats like ground beef, spareribs, hot dogs, sausage, bologna and other processed meats
Poultry or game with skin (chicken, turkey, duck)
High-fat dairy such as whole or 2% milk, whole-milk yogurt, ice cream, cottage cheese, cheeses, cream, and half-and-half
Butter, lard
Sauces and gravies made from meat drippings
Fatback and salt pork
Palm oil and palm kernel oil
Coconut and coconut oil

TABLE 19-7 Food Sources Rich in Monounsaturated and Polyunsaturated Fats

Monounsaturated fats	Polyunsaturated fats
Olive oil and olives	Corn, cottonseed, safflower, soybean, and sunflower oils
Canola oil	Walnuts
Peanuts, peanut butter, peanut oil	Pumpkin seeds, sunflower seeds
Nuts and their butters, like almonds, cashews, and pecans	Salad dressings and mayonnaise
Avocados	Soft (tub) margarines

- "Saturated fat free" means that less than 0.5 g of saturated fat and less than 0.5 g of *trans* fat is provided per labeled serving.
- "Reduced/less saturated fat" means that the food contains at least 25% less saturated fat than an appropriate reference food.

Patients should be encouraged to look for foods bearing these claims. When nutrient content claims are not provided, an easy rule of thumb is to choose foods that contain no more than 1 g of saturated fat per 100 calories.

Once saturated fat food sources and appropriate substitutions have been provided to the patient (examples in Table 19-8), the focus should be on reducing *trans* fatty acid consumption. Although many strides have been made to reduce or eliminate *trans* fats from commercially available foods, *trans* fat consumption is still a concern. *Trans* fats, primarily derived from *partially hydrogenated oils*, can be found in a variety of foods. Table 19-9 and Figure 19-3 show examples.

A patient's best defense against consuming *trans* fats is to read food labels carefully, starting with the ingredients list. The words *hydrogenated* or *partially hydrogenated*, when referring to fats (e.g., safflower, sunflower, corn oils), indicates that a food contains *trans* fat. As a result of the January 2006 mandate established by the FDA that food labels must list *trans* fats, manufacturers have reduced and/or eliminated *trans* fats from many products. Consequently, the claim "0 grams trans fat" can be found on a number of previously *trans fat*-laden food products. Patients must be aware that the term *trans fat free,* similarly to *saturated fat free,* allows a food to contain up to but less than 0.5 g of *trans* fat per *serving.* Once the serving size has been exceeded, the food is no longer free of *trans* fat. In addition, as the list of *trans*-fat-free foods grows, so does the list of saturated fat–rich foods. This is because partially hydrogenated oils are commonly replaced with palm, palm kernel, or coconut oils, sources of saturated fat. Patients need to be aware of this and be vigilant when reading food labels to seek out foods free of *trans* fats *and* low in saturated fat. One way to do this is to choose foods that use liquid vegetable oil such as corn, safflower, sunflower, soy or canola in the ingredients.

TABLE 19-8 Saturated Fat Substitutions

Instead of...	Try...
Sautéing in butter	Sautéing in olive oil
Spreading toast with butter	Spreading toast with *trans*-fat-free tub margarine or peanut butter
Melting full-fat cheese on casserole	Melting low-fat or nonfat cheese on casserole
Pouring half-and-half in coffee	Using nonfat creamer in coffee
Drinking whole or 2% milk	Drinking 1% or nonfat (skim) milk
Spreading cream cheese over bagels	Spreading light or nonfat cream cheese over bagel
Enjoying a sundae made with full-fat ice cream	Trying low-fat yogurt or reduced-fat ice cream
Topping a baked potato with 2% to 4% milk fat cottage cheese	Topping a baked potato with 1% or nonfat cottage cheese
Ordering fettuccini alfredo	Ordering pasta with marinara sauce
Grilling spareribs	Grilling a tenderloin
Making burgers from ground beef	Making burgers from ground sirloin
Fried chicken with skin	Baked chicken with skin removed
2-egg omelet	Omelet made from 4 egg whites or ½ cup egg substitute
Tossing croutons on a salad	Tossing dry roasted nuts over salad

Step 2: Increase Intake of Omega-3 Fatty Acids

Essential long-chain polyunsaturated fats eicosapentaenoic acid (EPA) and docosahexaenoic acid (DHA), both derived from marine sources), and to a lesser extent α-linolenic acid (derived from plant sources) have

TABLE 19-9 Food Sources of *Trans* Fats

Fast foods, including fried chicken, French fries, home fries, biscuits, pies
Shortening
Stick margarine
Some tub margarines (although most have reduced or eliminated the *trans* fats)
Fried tortilla chips, corn chips, potato chips
Cookies, crackers, graham crackers, granola bars
Many commercial and local bakery baked goods and desserts
Powdered coffee creamers
Bread, tortillas
Some cheese dips, salad dressings, whipped toppings, sauces, gravies
Candy bars, energy bars

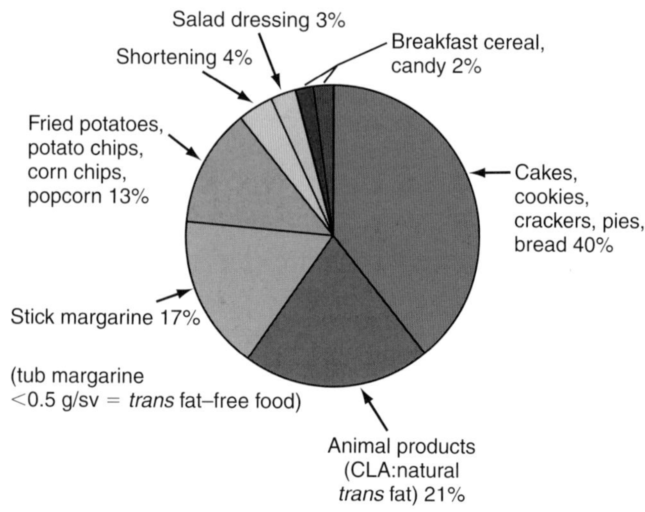

FIGURE 19-3 Major sources of *trans* fatty acids. CLA, conjugated linolenic acids.

increasingly been shown to confer protection from CVD and its related risk factors. As a result, patients should be encouraged to increase consumption. The American Heart Association in its latest scientific statement regarding omega-3 fatty acids recommends the following[53]:

- Patients without documented coronary disease should consume a variety of oily fish at least twice a week and include oils and foods rich in α-linolenic acid. This equates to approximately 500 mg of EPA and DHA daily.
- Patients with documented coronary disease should consume 1000 mg EPA and DHA per day, preferably from oily fish. Fish oil supplements could be considered.
- Patients with hypertriglyceridemia should consume 2 to 4 g of EPA and DHA per day provided as fish oil capsules under physician's care. Physicians need to review use of anticoagulants because supplementation at this level may interfere with blood clotting.

Cold water varieties of fish like mackerel, tuna, salmon, sardines, and herring are good sources of EPA and DHA (Table 19-10).

Although the conversion rate of α-linolenic acid to EPA and DHA is negligible, up to 1.2% of energy (approximately 2.7 g/day for a 2000-calorie diet) should be derived from α-linolenic acid–rich food sources according to the Institute of Medicine's Dietary Reference Intakes for Energy and Macronutrients.[54] As well as being a good source of polyunsaturated fat, α-linolenic acid–rich plant foods and their oils contain other heart-protective nutrients (e.g., ground flaxseed is a good source of fiber) and should be encouraged. Table 19-11 lists the α-linolenic acid content of selected foods.

TABLE 19-10 Omega-3 Fatty Acid Content of Selected SeaFood

Foods	Serving Size	Amount of Omega-3 (g)
Anchovies, canned	3 ounces drained	1.75
Atlantic herring	3 ounces cooked	1.71
Atlantic salmon, wild	3 ounces cooked	1.57
Sardines, canned	3 ounces in mustard sauce	1.37
Atlantic mackerel	3 ounces cooked	1.02
Salmon (chum), canned	3 ounces drained	1.0
Rainbow trout	3 ounces cooked	0.8
Sea bass (mixed species)	3 ounces cooked	0.65
Tuna, white meat canned	3 ounces drained	0.5
Catfish	3 ounces cooked	0.3
Yellowfin tuna	3 ounces cooked	0.24
Sole	3 ounces cooked	0.21
Prawns	6 pieces	0.15

Nutrient information gathered from ESHA Food Processor for Windows, version 8.6.0, ESHA Research, Salem, Oregon.

TABLE 19-11 Alpha-Linolenic Content of Selected Foods

Food Source	Serving Size	Amount of ALA (g)
Flaxseed oil	2 tsp	4.83
Ground flaxseed	2 Tbsp	3.71
Walnuts, raw	1 ounce	2.57
Walnut oil	2 tsp	0.94
Canola oil	2 tsp	0.87
Soybean oil	2 tsp	0.64

Nutrient information gathered from ESHA Food Processor for Windows, version 8.6.0, ESHA Research, Salem, Oregon.
ALA, α-linolenic acid.

The growth of omega-3–fortified foods available in the marketplace has skyrocketed in recent years. Foods like eggs, milk, soy milk, margarine, waffles, cereal, breads, pasta, juice, peanut butter, and chocolate can be included in the omega-3 fatty acid–fortified list. In most cases, the form of omega-3 contained in these foods is α-linolenic acid, although a growing number do contain marine omega-3 sources. Patients should be on the lookout for these foods and weigh health benefits against the number of calories and the amount of saturated fat and *trans* fat the food contains.

Step 3: Focus On Whole Grains And Dietary Fiber

Dietary fiber plays a key role in cardiovascular risk factor management. The NCEP ATP III guidelines suggest a minimum of 20 g of total dietary fiber daily, with at least 10 to 25 g derived from soluble fiber food sources. Patients with elevated LDL cholesterol should emphasize on foods rich in soluble fiber (Table 19-12).

To encourage an increase in whole grains, emphasis should be placed on substituting whole grain foods for their refined counterparts, such as substituting brown rice for white, whole wheat pasta for enriched pasta, whole grain cereals for refined sugary cereals, and 100% whole grain breads for white enriched versions. The following guidelines can help patients determine what foods are considered to be a whole grain:

- Look for foods that list 100% whole grain (e.g., corn, wheat, oat, barley) as the first ingredient. Terms like *enriched, bleached,* or *refined* are telltale signs that a food is not whole grain.
- Seek out foods that contain the voluntary food label called the Whole Grains Stamp, a special packaging symbol found on a growing list of packaged foods. The Whole Grain Stamp ensures that a food contains 100% whole grain. For more information on the stamp, visit http://www.wholegrainscouncil.org.
- Make sure foods contain as a minimum amount of dietary fiber level of:
  - Breads, crackers, rice, pasta: 2 to 3 g per serving
  - Ready-to-eat cereal: 5 g per serving
  - Hot cereal: 4 g per serving
  - Snack foods (e.g., pretzels, graham crackers, baked chips): 2 g per serving

TABLE 19-12 Soluble Fiber Content of Selected Foods

Food Source	Serving Size	Amount of Soluble Fiber (g)
Dried plums (prunes)	6 medium	3.1
Kidney beans, canned, drained	½ cup	2.7
Pear, fresh	1 medium	2.4
Pinto beans, canned, drained	½ cup	2.1
Garbanzo beans, canned, drained	½ cup	2.1
Orange, peeled	1 medium	2.1
Oat bran, dry	½ cup	2.0
Broccoli, cooked	1 cup	2.0
Old-fashioned oatmeal, dry	½ cup	1.9
Brussels sprouts, cooked	1 cup	1.9
Carrot, raw sticks	1 cup	1.5
Grapefruit	½ medium	1.4
Whole barley, cooked	½ cup	1.4
Flaxseed, ground or milled	2 Tbsp	1.1
Apple, with peel	1 medium	1.0
Eggplant, cooked with skin	1 cup	1.0

Nutrient information gathered from ESHA Food Processor for Windows, version 8.6.0, ESHA Research, Salem, Oregon.

Step 4: Build A Strong Foundation—increase Fruits, Vegetables, And Legumes

Fruits, vegetables, and legumes (beans, lentils, split peas) are not only excellent sources of dietary fiber, but they are also rich in antioxidant phytonutrients, vitamins, and minerals essential for optimal cardiovascular health. Few Americans are consuming the 5 to 9 servings of fruits and vegetables recommended by many groups. To help patients increase fruits and vegetables, consider the following tips:

- For breakfast: top cereal or yogurt with fresh fruit, add sautéed vegetables to omelets, add fresh fruit or 100% fruit juice to smoothies.
- For lunch: stuff sandwiches with vegetables, make tossed salads or vegetable or bean soups, finish lunch with fresh fruit.
- Snack ideas: dip fresh cubed fruit in yogurt, dip vegetables in hummus or low-fat dip, select fruit canned in its own juice or drink 100% fruit juice.
- For dinner: fill one half of the dinner plate with vegetables (cooked or raw), serve broth-based vegetable or bean soup with or before the meal, finish the meal with fresh fruit.

Step 5: Choose Protein Sources Wisely

Epidemiologic evidence, prospective cohorts, and the OmniHeart trial all show a strong argument for the need for patients to replace some or all of their animal-based meals with plant protein alternatives. Reducing animal protein–rich meals for plant sources can cut a considerable amount of saturated fat, while increasing levels of cardioprotective components like dietary fiber, potassium, B vitamins, antioxidants, and phytonutrients. To help encourage patients to adopt a higher plant-protein intake, consider the following tips:

- Encourage at least one meatless meal per week.
- Substitute soy protein (e.g., tofu, edamame, tempeh, soy milk), canned or dried beans, lentils, and nuts for animal protein in family-favorite recipes. Examples: stir fry with tofu, black bean burrito, spaghetti with cannellini beans, three-bean chili, grilled tempeh, toasted nuts on salad.
- Cut back on portion size (3–4 ounces) of meat served at meals, and choose leanest cuts possible. Just the practice of cutting back can have considerable benefits.
- Experiment with new ingredients and recipes to expand meatless meal options.

Step 6: Add Other Cardioprotective Components

As previously discussed, the NCEP ATP III guidelines suggest the use of soluble fiber and plant sterols/stanols as therapeutic options for managing lipids. Tips on increasing soluble fiber are listed in step 3. The use of plant sterols or their hydrogenated counterpart (stanols) in cholesterol management has been widely studied. The NCEP ATP III guidelines recommend that 2 g or more of plant sterols/stanols be consumed daily, generally via two servings of the sterol/stanol-fortified food. A growing list of foods marketed in the United States is fortified with plant sterols/stanols. These include tub margarine spreads, yogurt flavored drinks, juice, chocolate, cheese, granola bars, and yogurt. Patients and physicians need to be aware that these fortified foods, although effective at cholesterol lowering, must be skillfully added to a patient's dietary regimen in order to avoid caloric excess and corresponding weight gain. A sterol/stanol supplement is also on the market.

These first-line nutrition steps help patients make healthful food choices to decrease risk of CVD. With appropriate guidance and continued reinforcement, these dietary changes are a practical and cost-effective means of achieving optimal cardiovascular health.

The Role Of Registered Dietitians/nutrition Professionals In Nutrition Counseling

Individualized nutrition counseling is important for long-term adherence to a healthy dietary pattern. Registered dietitians (RDs) are uniquely qualified to tailor help for patients to effectively modify their diet to lower CVD risk factors. The limited number of eligible studies reviewed show that medical nutrition therapy (MNT) can be an effective approach to changing dietary intake and reducing total cholesterol, LDL cholesterol, and body weight.

As reviewed in a commentary (reference 55), studies on RD-delivered MNT for patients with hypercholesterolemia indicate that with two to six planned visits, patients reported dietary reductions in total fat from 32–36% to 25–28% of calories, and from 11–12% to 7–9% of calories for saturated fat. This was accompanied by reductions in total cholesterol of 6% to 13% and of 7% to 14% in LDL cholesterol. Decreases in TG and changes in HDL cholesterol were inconsistent. MNT included an initial scheduled visit ranging from 45 to 90 minutes and scheduled follow-up visits ranging from 30 to 60 minutes over 6 weeks to 6 months. Data on long-term adherence and sustained lipid response are unavailable. Thus, because of their expertise in nutrition and counseling, including behavior change, RDs are important for optimizing implementation of recommended dietary patterns that lower CVD risk.

The Role Of Physicians In Facilitating Healthful Lifestyle Behavior Change

Physician behavior can play an important role in promoting healthful lifestyle change. Two simple questions can provide both the patient and the physician with important insights as to whether behavior change is likely to be accomplished: (1) "On a scale of 1 to 10, tell me how likely you are to change" and (2) "On the same scale, tell me how prepared you are to change." This uses the Stages of Change model that can be adapted nicely to patients who need healthier lifestyles.[56] For those not ready to change, just encouraging patients to try not to gain weight may be an effective prevention message. For example, in CARDIA, for both men and women, simply not gaining weight (even if overweight to start) was an important way to reduce the chance of developing the metabolic syndrome.[57]

Behavioral experts recommend the use of multiple strategies including goal-setting, self-monitoring stimulus control, cognitive restructuring, stress management, relapse prevention, social support, and contracting.[58] Studies have shown that self-monitoring and regular physical activities are consistently associated with better weight control in the short and long term, respectively.[59]

Motivational interviewing is an intervention approach that also may be used by the clinician. For example, overweight diabetic women underwent motivational interviewing to promote weight loss, and significant changes were recorded at 6 months ($P = .01$) and 18 months ($P = .04$) compared to control subjects. Of note, this technique was not as effective in African American women.[60]

There are practical suggestions that can help as well. Having an office that has proper-sized blood pressure cuffs for those who are obese as well as appropriate chairs and gowns is important.[59]

Foster[59] suggested three simple guidelines:

1. Why? Be sure each patient knows the rationale for behavioral change.
2. What? Identify a goal and agree on a specific plan.
3. How? Identify facilitators and barriers to success.

One clinical practitioner summarizes these points to patients with metabolic risk factors at each visit by reminding them to "eat less, eat smart, and move more daily!" It's a brief and consistent message that patients are easily able to remember. There are considerable challenges ahead. A recent study found that most internal medicine residents fell short of the mark as adequate role models for promoting exercise adherence and recommended that they develop confidence in current guideline knowledge and personal physical activity enjoyment, and achieve self-efficacy in engaging in regular physical activity themselves.[61]

RESOURCES FOR CLINICAL PRACTICE

Resources from the American Heart Association:

- Fats 101. This website answers common questions about dietary fats. http://www.americanheart.org/presenter.jhtml?identifier=3045789
- My Fats Translator. This website presents a "fat calculator" for planning diets that contain healthy fats. http://www.myfatstranslator.com/
- Nutrition Facts. This website presents information about "Nutrition Facts." http://www.americanheart.org/presenter.jhtml?identifier=855
- Face the Fats. This website presents much information about dietary fat. http://www.americanheart.org/presenter.jhtml?identifier=3046074
- The Bad Fats Brothers Website. This website presents an informative podcast about saturated and *trans* fats. http://www.americanheart.org/presenter.jhtml?identifier=3048007
- Healthy Lifestyle. This website presents information about healthy lifestyle behaviors for decreasing risk of CVD. http://www.americanheart.org/presenter.jhtml?identifier=1200009

Resources from The National Heart, Lung, and Blood Institute:

- Portion Distortion Quiz. This website presents a PowerPoint file. http://hp2010.nhlbihin.net/portion/
- 10-year CVD Risk Calculator. This website can be used by individuals to calculate their 10-year risk of CVD. http://hp2010.nhlbihin.net/atpiii/calculator.asp?usertype=pub
- Body Mass Index Calculator. This website can be used by individuals to calculate their BMI. http://www.nhlbisupport.com/bmi/
- Menu Planner. This website can be used by individuals to plan healthy menus. http://hp2010.nhlbihin.net/menuplanner/menu.cgi
- Heart Health and Nutrition. This website presents a great deal of information for the public about heart health and nutrition. http://www.nhlbi.nih.gov/health/indexpro.htm#info

Other Resources:

Resources from International Food Information Council (IFIC):

Kidnetic. This website is for children and teaches principles of good nutrition and physical activity. http://www.kidnetic.com

Nutrition Information. This website provides multiple links to information about good nutrition. http://www.ific.org/index.cfm

The American Dietetic Association

Food and Nutrition Information—Consumer Resources. This website provides useful information for consumers about food and nutrition information. Also, if anyone is looking for a registered dietitian, this is the site to visit. http://www.eatright.org/cps/rde/xchg/ada/hs.xsl/nutrition.html

United States Department of Agriculture and The Department of Health and Human Services

MyPyramid.Gov. This website presents the Dietary Guidelines for Americans 2005, along with information for adults and children for planning diets http://www.mypyramid.gov/

Food Labeling and Nutrition.

Food and Drug Administration

This website provides food label education tools and information to help consumers understand the Nutrition Facts panel and nutrient content claims on food labels. http://www.cfsan.fda.gov/label.html

Shaping America's Health (An initiative of the American Diabetes Association). This website provides information about implementing healthy lifestyle practices. http://www.obesityprevention.org/

Shaping America's Youth. This website provides information about programs for lifestyle behaviors to promote health of America's youth. http://www.shapingamericasyouth.org/Default.aspx

SUMMARY

Major clinical trials and studies have defined dietary patterns that have very potent LDL cholesterol– and blood pressure–lowering effects. Dietary patterns also have been identified that favorably alter lipids and lipoproteins that characterize dyslipidemia. These dietary patterns that elicit marked effects involve substantive changes in single nutrients, as well as implementation of multiple dietary strategies to dramatically alter risk factor status. If healthy dietary change can be sustained long term, the evidence base is clear that CVD risk can be markedly reduced. Importantly, even small dietary modifications can have a benefit that is clinically significant. Many studies have shown that significant dietary changes can be achieved in the short term. However, over the long term, behavior changes are difficult to sustain entirely or even in part. This is associated with a diminution in CVD risk reduction. Thus, there is a pressing need to identify behavior change strategies that help patients maintain dietary changes that sustain an optimal reduction in CVD risk long term.

The rate-limiting step in achieving optimal reductions in CVD risk that are sustained long term is not related to our understanding of dietary patterns that potently reduce risk but, rather, is facilitating major dietary behavior changes that can be sustained over a lifetime. Thus, there is a key role for physicians and dietitians to serve as critically important resources for providing useful information and ongoing support to individuals to achieve and maintain a healthy dietary pattern.

REFERENCES

1. American Heart Association Nutrition Committee, Lichtenstein AH, Appel LJ, Brands M, et al: Diet and lifestyle recommendations revision 2006. A scientific statement from the American Heart Association Nutrition Committee. *Circulation* 2006;114:82-96.
2. Reddy KS, Katan MB: Diet, nutrition and the prevention of hypertension and cardiovascular diseases. *Public Health Nutr* 2004;7:167-186.
3. Van Horn L, McCoin M, Kris-Etherton P, et al: The evidence for dietary prevention and treatment of cardiovascular disease. *J Am Diet Assoc* 2008;108:287–331.
4. Ford ES, Ajani UA, Croft JB, et al: Explaining the decrease in U.S. deaths from coronary disease, 1980-2000. *N Engl J Med* 2007;356:2388-2398.
5. Appel LJ, Moore TJ, Obarzanek E, et al: A clinical trial of the effects of dietary patterns on blood pressure. DASH Collaborative Research Group. *N Engl J Med* 1997;336:1117-1124.
6. Sacks FM, Svetkey LP, Vollmer WM, et al: Effects on blood pressure of reduced dietary sodium and the Dietary Approaches to Stop Hypertension (DASH) diet. DASH-Sodium Collaborative Research Group. *N Engl J Med* 2001;344:3-10.
7. Appel LJ, Sacks FM, Carey VJ, et al: Effects of protein, monounsaturated fat, and carbohydrate intake on blood pressure and serum lipids: Results of the OmniHeart randomized trial. *JAMA* 2005;294:2455-2464.
8. Jenkins DJ, Kendall CW, Marchie A, et al: Effects of a dietary portfolio of cholesterol-lowering foods vs. lovastatin on serum lipids and C-reactive protein. *JAMA* 2003;290:502-510.
9. de Lorgeril M, Salen P, Martin JL, et al: Mediterranean diet, traditional risk factors, and the rate of cardiovascular complications after myocardial infarction: Final report of the Lyon Diet Heart Study. *Circulation* 1999;99:779-785.
10. Vincent-Baudry S, Defoort C, Gerber M, et al: The Medi-RIVAGE study: Reduction of cardiovascular disease risk factors after a 3-mo intervention with a Mediterranean-type diet or a low-fat diet. *Am J Clin Nutr* 2005;82:964-971.
11. Estruch R, Martinez-Gonzalez MA, Corella D, et al: Effects of a Mediterranean-style diet on cardiovascular risk factors: A randomized trial. *Ann Intern Med* 2006;145:1-11.
12. Grundy SM, Cleeman, JI, Merz CN, et al: Implications of recent clinical trials for the National Cholesterol Education Program Adult Treatment Panel III guidelines. *Circulation* 2004;110:227-239.
13. National Cholesterol Education Program (NCEP) Expert Panel on Detection, Evaluation, and Treatment of High Blood Cholesterol in Adults (Adult Treatment Panel III): Third report of the National Cholesterol Education Program (NCEP) Expert Panel on Detection, Evaluation, and Treatment of High Blood Cholesterol in Adults (Adult Treatment Panel III) final report. *Circulation.* 2002;106:3143-3421.
14. Jenkins DJ, Kendall CW, Faulkner DA, et al: Assessment of the longer-term effects of a dietary portfolio of cholesterol-lowering foods in hypercholesterolemia. *Am J Clin Nutr* 2006;83:582-591.
15. Ornish D, Brown SE, Scherwitz LW, et al: Can lifestyle changes reverse coronary heart disease? The Lifestyle Heart Trial. *Lancet* 1990;336:129-133.
16. Ornish D, Scherwitz LW, Billings JH, et al: Intensive lifestyle changes for reversal of coronary heart disease. *JAMA* 1998;280:2001-2007.
17. Daubenmier JJ, Weidner G, Sumner MD, et al: The contribution of changes in diet, exercise, and stress management to changes in coronary risk in women and men in the Multisite Cardiac Lifestyle Intervention Program. *Ann Behav Med* 2007;33:57-68.
18. Appel LJ, Champagne CM, Harsha DW, et al: Effects of comprehensive lifestyle modification on blood pressure control: Main results of the PREMIER clinical trial. *JAMA* 2003;289:2083-2093.

19. Elmer PJ, Obarzanek E, Vollmer WM, et al: Effects of comprehensive lifestyle modification on diet, weight, physical fitness, and blood pressure control: 18-month results of a randomized trial. *Ann Intern Med* 2006;144:485-495.
20. Ginsberg HN, Kris-Etherton P, Dennis B, et al: Effects of reducing dietary saturated fatty acids on plasma lipids and lipoproteins in healthy subjects: The DELTA Study protocol. *Arterioscler Thromb Vasc Biol* 1998;18:441-449.
21. Obarzanek E, Sacks FM, Vollmer WM, et al: Effects on blood lipids of a blood pressure-lowering diet: The Dietary Approaches to Stop Hypertension (DASH) Trial. *Am J Clin Nutr* 2001;74:80-89.
22. Griel AE, Ruder EH, Kris-Etherton PM: The changing roles of dietary carbohydrates: From simple to complex. *Arterioscler Thromb Vasc Biol* 2006;26:1958-1965.
23. Howard BV, Van Horn L, Hsia J, et al: Low-fat dietary pattern and risk of cardiovascular disease: the Women's Health Initiative Randomized Controlled Dietary Modification Trial. *JAMA* 2006;295:655-666.
24. Howard BV, Manson JE, Stefanick ML, et al: Low-fat dietary pattern and weight change over 7 years: The Women's Health Initiative Dietary Modification Trial. *JAMA* 2006;295:39-49.
25. Dayton S, Pearce ML, Hashimoto S, et al: A controlled clinical trial of a diet high in unsaturated fat in preventing complications of atherosclerosis. *Circulation* 1969;40:ii-1–ii-63.
26. Leren P: The Oslo Diet-Heart Study. Eleven-year report. *Circulation* 1970;42:935-942.
27. Research Committee. Controlled trial of soya-bean oil in myocardial infarction. *Lancet* 1968;ii:693-700.
28. Turpeinen O, Karvonen MJ, Pekkarinen M, et al: Dietary prevention of coronary heart disease: The Finnish Mental Hospital Study. *Int J Epidemiol* 1979;8:99-118.
29. National Institutes of Health. Clinical guidelines on the identification, evaluation, and treatment of overweight and obesity in adults—the evidence report. NIH Pub. No. 98-4083. Bethesda, MD: *National Heart, Lung and Blood Institute,* 1998;228 pages.
30. National Institutes of Health. Clinical guidelines on the identification, evaluation, and treatment of overweight and obesity in adults—the evidence report. Obesity Res, 1998; 6(suppl 2): 51S-209S.
31. United States Department of Health and Human Services. United States Department of Agriculture. Dietary Guidelines for Americans 2005. www.healthierus.gov/dietaryguidelines.
32. Mensink RP, Katan MB. Effect of monounsaturated fatty acids versus complex carbohydrates on high-density lipoproteins in healthy men and women. *Lancet* 1987;1:122-125.
33. Mensink RP, Zock PL, Kester ADM, et al: Effects of dietary fatty acids and carbohydrates on the ratio of serum total to HDL cholesterol and on serum lipids and apolipoproteins: a meta-analysis of 60 controlled trials. *Am J Clin Nutr* 2003;77:1146-1155.
34. Berglund L, Lefevre M, Ginsberg H, et al: Comparison of monounsaturated fat versus carbohydrates as replacement for saturated fat in subjects with a high metabolic risk profile: studies in the fasting and postprandial state. *Am J Clin Nutr* 2007;86:161–162.
35. The Seventh Report of the Joint National Committee on Prevention, Detection, Evaluation, and Treatment of High Blood Pressure. *National Heart, Lung, and Blood Institute.* 2004.
36. Svetkey LP, Simons-Morton D, Vollmer WM, et al: Effects of dietary patterns on blood pressure: Subgroup analysis of the Dietary Approaches to Stop Hypertension (DASH) randomized clinical trial. *Arch Intern Med* 1999;159:285–293
37. Vollmer WM, Sacks FM, Svetkey LP: New insights into the effects on blood pressure of diets low in salt and high in fruits and vegetables and low-fat dairy products. *Curr Control Trials Cardiovasc Med* 2001;2:71–74.
38. Vollmer WM, Sacks FM, Ard J, et al: Effects of diet and sodium intake on blood pressure: Subgroup analysis of the DASH-sodium trial. *Ann Intern Med* 2001;135:1019–1028.
39. Joshipura KJ, Hu FB, Manson JE, et al: The effect of fruit and vegetable intake on risk for coronary heart disease. *Ann Intern Med* 2001;134:1106–1114.
40. Liu S, Manson JE, Lee IM, et al: Fruit and vegetable intake and risk of cardiovascular disease: The Women's Health Study. *Am J Clin Nutr* 2000;72:922–1928.
41. Liu S, Lee IM, Ajani U, et al: Intake of vegetables rich in carotenoids and risk of coronary heart disease in men: The Physicians' Health Study. *Int J Epidemiol* 2001;30:130–135.
42. Bazzano LA, He J, Ogden LG, et al: Fruit and vegetable intake and risk of cardiovascular disease in US adults: The first National Health and Nutrition Examination Survey Epidemiologic Follow-up Study. *Am J Clin Nutr* 2002;76:93–99.
43. Mellen PB, Walsh TF, Herrington DM: Whole grain intake and cardiovascular disease: A meta-analysis. *Nutr Metab Cardiovasc Dis* 2008;18:283–290.
44. Mellen PB, Liese AD, Tooze JA, et al: Whole grain intake in carotid artery atherosclerosis in a multiethnic cohort: The Insulin Resistance Atherosclerosis Study. *Am J Clin Nutr* 2007;85: 1495-1502.
45. Psota TL, Gebauer SK, Kris-Etherton PM: Dietary omega-3 fatty acid intake and cardiovascular risk. *Am J Cardiol* 2006;98[suppl]: 3i-18i.
46. Pereira MA, Jacobs DR Jr, Van Horn L, et al: Dairy consumption, obesity and the insulin resistance syndrome in young adults: The CARDIA Study. *JAMA* 2002;287:2081-2089.
47. Elwood PC, Pickering JE, Fehily AM: Milk and dairy consumption, diabetes and the metabolic syndrome: The Caerphilly prospective study. *J Epidemiol Commun Health* 2007;61:695-698.
48. Kris-Etherton PM, Hu FB, Ros E, Sabaté J, et al: The role of tree nuts and peanuts in the prevention of coronary heart disease: Mutliple potential machanisms. *J Nutr* 2008; 138: 1746S–1751S.
49. Goldberg IJ, Mosca L, Piano MR, et al: Wine and your heart: A science advisory for healthcare professionals from the Nutrition Committee, Council on Epidemiology and Prevention, and Council on Cardiovascular Nursing of the American Heart Association. *Circulation* 2001;103:472-475.
50. Mukamal KJ, Chiuve SE, Rimm EB: Alcohol consumption and risk for coronary heart disease in men with healthy lifestyles. *Arch Intern Med* 2006;166:2145-2150.
51. Rimm EB, Stamfer EJ: Wine, beer, and spirits. Are they really horses of a different color? *Circulation* 2002;105:2806-2807.
52. Food and Drug Administration Guidelines on Nutrient-Content Claims for Food Labels. Available at www.cfsan.fda.gov/~dms/flg-6a.html.
53. Kris-Etherton PM, Harris WS, Appel LJ: Fish consumption, fish oil, omega-3 fatty acids, and cardiovascular disease. *Circulation* 2002;106;2747-2757.
54. Institute of Medicine (IOM): Dietary reference intakes for energy and macronutrients. Washington, DC: National Academy Press; 2002.
55. McColn M, Sikand G, Johnson EQ, et al: The effectiveness of medical nutrition therapy for disorders of lipid metabolism delivered by registered dietitians: A call for further research. *J Am Diet Assoc* 2008; 108:233–239.
56. Manson JE, Skerrett PJ, Greenland P, et al: The escalating pandemics of obesity and sedentary lifestyle. A call to action for clinicians. *Arch Intern Med* 2004;164:249-258.
57. Lloyd-Jones DM, Liu K, Colangelo LA, et al: Consistently stable or decreased body mass index in young adulthood and longitudinal changes in metabolic syndrome components: The Coronary Artery Risk Development in Young Adults study. *Circulation* 2007;115:1004-1011.
58. Foreyt JP: The role of lifestyle modification in dysmetabolic syndrome management. *Nestle Nutr Workshop Ser Clin Perform Programme* 2006;11:197-205.
59. Foster GD, Makris AP, Bailer BA: Behavioral treatment of obesity. *Am J Clin Nutr* 2005;82:230S-235S.
60. West DS, DiLillo V, Bursac Z, et al: Motivational interviewing improves weight loss in women with type 2 diabetes. *Diabetes Care* 2007;30:1081-1087.
61. Rogers LQ, Gutin B, Humphries MC, et al: Evaluation of internal medicine residents as exercise role models and associations with self-reported counseling behavior, confidence, and perceived success. *Teach Learn Med* 2006;18:215-221.

CHAPTER 20

Exercise and Lipids

Timothy S. Church and Carl J. Lavie

EXERCISE VERSUS PHYSICAL ACTIVITY

Before examining the relation between exercise and cholesterol, the working definitions of exercise and physical activity need to be examined. In general terms, aerobic exercise is defined as planned and structured bodily movement resulting in increased oxygen consumption and caloric expenditure. The specific goals of structured aerobic exercise may be improvements in fitness or general well-being, or aerobic exercise may be part of a weight loss (or maintenance) program. Examples include walking, jogging, swimming laps, and participating in an aerobics class. On the other hand, physical activity is any bodily movement produced by skeletal muscle that results in energy expenditure. Exercise is a type of physical activity, but most common forms of physical activity are activities of daily living, such as climbing stairs, gardening, and walking the dog. It is important to note that one can be very physically active yet never exercise. Because the research literature contains the use of both exercise and physical activity extensively, in this chapter we will use both terms throughout.

EXERCISE AND CORONARY HEART DISEASE

In examining the role of exercise in lipid therapy, one must keep in mind the overall role of exercise in the primary and secondary prevention of coronary heart disease (CHD) morbidity and mortality. The first modern epidemiologic studies looking at exercise and health were focused on work-related physical activity. Published in 1953, studies by Dr. Jeremy Morris compared the risk of having a myocardial infarction in bus drivers compared to bus conductors.[1] The buses were double-decker, and while the bus driver had essentially a sedentary work day, the conductors accumulated a substantial amount of physical activity each day as they climbed up and down the bus stairs to check tickets. The active conductors had about one-third the rate of CHD events compared with that of the sedentary bus drivers (Fig. 20-1A). Published in 1975, studies by Dr. Ralph Paffenbarger reported an inverse relation between risk of CHD death and work-related caloric expenditure in longshoremen (Fig. 20-1B).[2] As fewer individuals worked physically active jobs, the research shifted away from work-related physical activity toward total physical activity, with an emphasis on exercise. Dr. Steve Blair and colleagues published a series of manuscripts examining the risk of morbidity and mortality across levels of cardiorespiratory fitness as assessed by maximal treadmill test, which was taken as an excellent marker of physical activity habits in the weeks or months before the test.[3-6] The Aerobics Center Longitudinal Study (ACLS) is composed of men and women who came to the Cooper Clinic for a preventive medicine examination and underwent a maximal treadmill test. Based on the time on the treadmill, age, and gender, each individual's fitness was categorized as low, moderate, or high. For both men and women, there was an inverse relation between fitness level and risk of cardiovascular death. For both men and women, the risk of cardiovascular mortality in the moderate-fitness group was less than half the risk for the low-fitness group (Fig. 20-2). Thus it can be derived that substantial health benefit is associated with moving from being sedentary to being active. There have now been a large number of epidemiologic studies in a variety of populations that have confirmed benefits of regular physical activity on the primary and secondary prevention of CHD and other morbidities.[7-11]

Even though the goal of this chapter is to examine the role of exercise training in modifying lipids, it necessary to

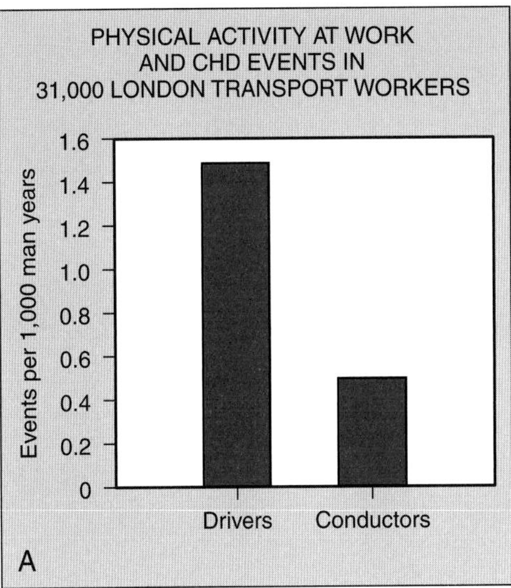

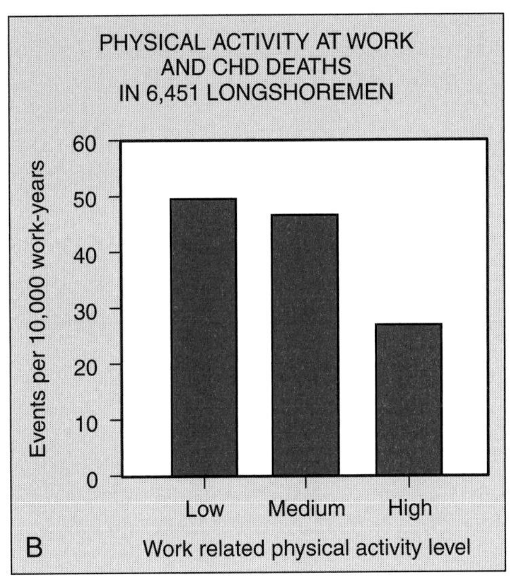

FIGURE 20-1 Work-related physical activity and risk for coronary heart disease. From Refs 1 and 2, with permission.

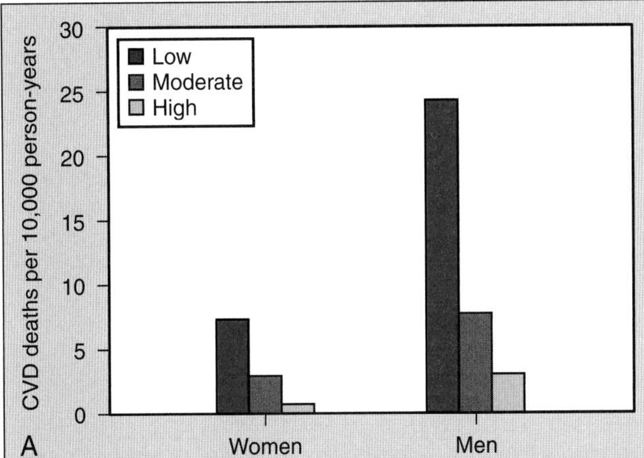

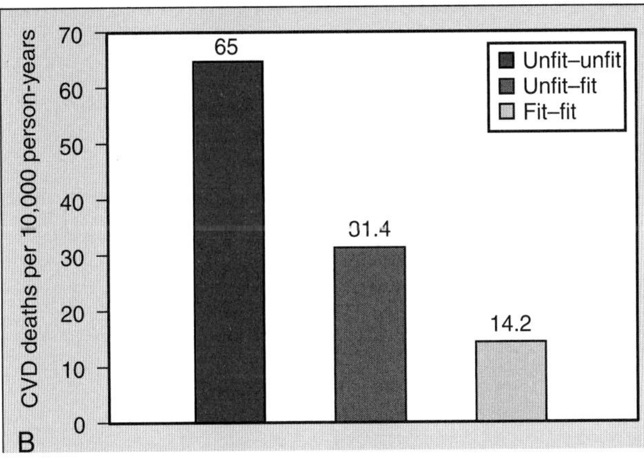

FIGURE 20-2 Baseline Cardiorespitatory fitness (A) and change in cardiorespitatory fitness (B) and risk for cardiovascular disease (CVD) death. From Refs. 5 and 6, with permission

TABLE 20-1	Benefits of Regular Exercise to Primary and Secondary Prevention of Coronary Heart Disease
Physiological Benefits	
Helps maintain healthy weight	Reduced abdominal adiposity
Improved heart rate variability	Reduced systemic inflammation
Reduced blood pressure	Improved insulin sensitivity
Improved endothelial function	Decreased myocardial oxygen demand
Increased myocardial function	Maintains lean mass
Decreased platelet aggregation	Increased fibrinolysis
Reduced blood and plasma viscosity	Increased capillary density
Increased mitochondrial density	
Reduced Risk of Developing Hypertension	
Metabolic syndrome	
Depression	
Type 2 diabetes	

at least review the numerous benefits of regular exercise that contribute to the reduced cardiovascular disease (CVD) risk associated with physical activity. As summarized in Table 20-1, the benefits associated with physical activity are diverse and include lower blood pressure, reduced sympathetic nervous system activity, prevention of insulin resistance, improved fibrinolytic activity, lower blood pressure, reduced visceral fat, lower markers of systemic inflammation, better cardiac function, healthier blood vessels, and lower resting heart rate. Furthermore, it is widely accepted that regular physical activity reduces the risk of developing hypertension, diabetes, and metabolic syndrome. Thus, in exploring the role of physical activity in modifying lipids, one needs to appreciate the many mechanisms, other than just lipids, whereby exercise confers health benefits.

Exercise and Cholesterol

Despite there being an abundance of data demonstrating the benefits of regular exercise on CHD incidence and mortality, the benefits of exercise training on blood lipids are relatively modest (Table 20-2).

TABLE 20-2 Effects of Exercise on Lipids and Lipoproteins

Lipid/Lipoprotein	Relationship to CHD	Effect of Regular Exercise	Comments
Total cholesterol	Positive	Little to no change	Exercise-induced improvements usually associated with weight loss
LDL	Positive	Little to no change	Exercise-induced improvements usually associated with weight loss
HDL	Negative	Increased but highly variable	Response greatest in those with elevated triglycerides
Triglyceride	Positive	Decrease	
Subfractions			
LDL particle size	Negative	Increases particle size and decreases percent of small LDL	
HDL particle size	Negative	Increases HDL particle size and increases percent of large HDL	

CHD, coronary heart disease; HDL, high-density lipoprotein; LDL, low-density lipoprotein.

Total Cholesterol

The data on exercise as a means to reduce total cholesterol are disappointing. Although some studies have demonstrated that exercise decreased total cholesterol, the vast majority of exercise training studies do not show that training lowers total cholesterol.[12-40] The exercise studies that have reported improvements in total cholesterol typically have significant exercise-induced weight loss.[13,41]

Low-Density Lipoprotein and Subfractions

Similar to total cholesterol, the majority of data suggest that exercise training does not substantially improve plasma low-density lipoprotein (LDL) concentrations in the absence of significant weight loss.[13-17,19,21,25-29] However, both cross-sectional and longitudinal data suggest that exercise training results in a shift away from smaller, more atherogenic LDL particles to larger, less atherogenic LDL particles. For example, Williams and colleagues and Halle and associates both reported that higher levels of activity are associated with lower concentrations of small dense LDL.[42,43] Kraus and colleagues reported that despite there being no change in LDL concentration, exercise training resulted in both an increase in the size of LDL particles and a reduction in the concentration of small LDL particles (Fig. 20-3).[44] The observation that even with no change in LDL concentration there was an increase in LDL particle size and a reduction in the concentration of LDL particles is an interesting and provocative finding, which may in part explain the apparent discrepancy between the benefit of regular exercise on reducing CHD risk and the lack of improvement in LDL concentration. This observation was groundbreaking and progressive given that it was initiated before the widespread acceptance of LDL particle size as an important CHD risk factor.

High-Density Lipoprotein and Subfractions, and Triglyclerides

Beginning with the pioneering work of Haskell and Wood in the 1980s, there have been numerous cross-sectional and prospective data demonstrating that exercise training leads to significant increases in high-density lipoprotein (HDL) cholesterol,[14,15,21,25-29,45,46] with the range of increases in HDL reported as a result of exercise training being quite large (3%–22%). Kraus and colleagues reported that exercise training increased HDL particle size and the concentration of large HDL particles (Fig. 20-4).[44] It has been noted that individuals with low HDL but normal triglycerides have much

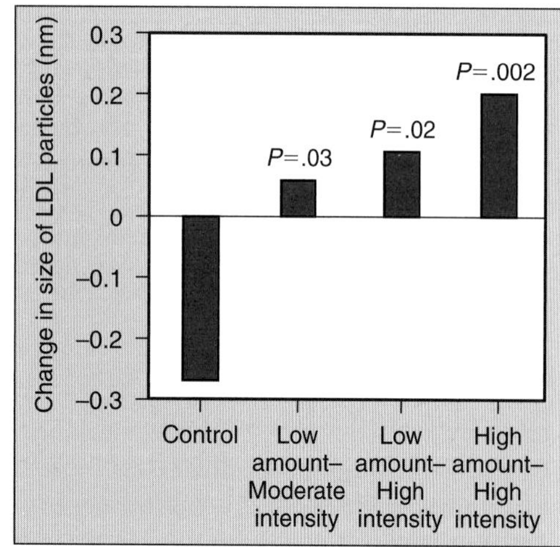

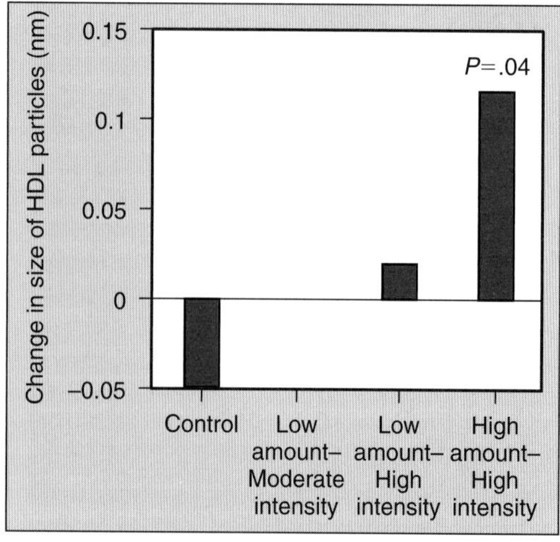

FIGURE 20-3 Exercise training and change in low-density lipoprotein (LDL) and high-density lipoprotein (HDL) particle size.

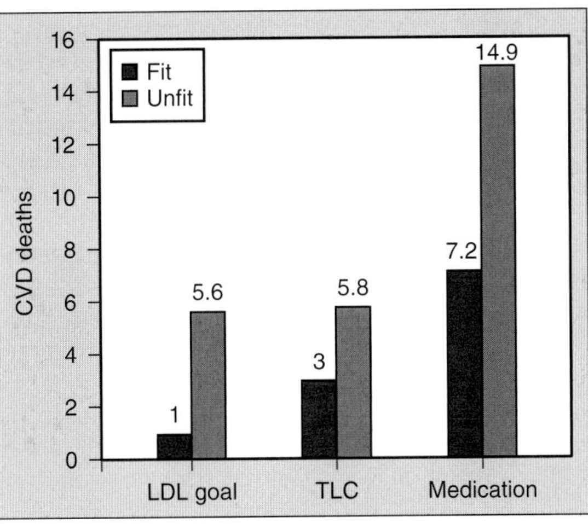

FIGURE 20-4 Relative risk for cardiovascular disease (CVD) mortality across updated adult treatment panel III treatment groups and fitness groups. LDL, low-density lipoprotein; TLC, therapeutic lifestyle changes. From Ref. 51, with permission.

smaller (if any) improvements in HDL in response to exercise training compared to individuals with low HDL and elevated triglycerides.[47]

Given the inverse relation between HDL cholesterol and triglycerides, it is not surprising that regular exercise is usually reported to result in a decrease in triglycerides.[14,15,21-23,25,27,28,48,49] In individuals without genetic abnormalities in triglyceride metabolism, typically the higher the initial triglyceride level, the greater the observed reductions in response to exercise training.

Potential Mechanisms for Improvements

Even though the mechanisms whereby regular exercise improves HDL and triglycerides are not fully understood, there are at least two potential physiologic pathways that likely play a role.[50] Lipoprotein lipase lowers very-low-density lipoprotein (VLDL) and chylomicron triglyceride levels, and exercise training increases lipoprotein lipase activity in adipose tissue and muscle. VLDL triglycerides are exchanged for cholesteryl esters in HDL and LDL, which are then hydrolyzed by lipases, causing a decrease in the size of particles. The exercise-induced decrease in VLDL triglycerides results in reduced availability of triglyceride for exchange and is probably a major mechanism underlying the increases in HDL cholesterol levels and the size of LDL particles.[50] In addition, hepatic lipase degrades HDL phospholipids, thus producing smaller HDL particles that are rapidly catabolized, and exercise has also been shown to decrease hepatic lipase activity.[47,50]

Interactions of Exercise and Cholesterol in Mortality

As noted in the beginning of this chapter, the modest improvements in lipid profiles associated with exercise training need to be kept in proper context. The reduction in CHD risk associated with regular exercise is well established, and the many mechanisms responsible for such benefit are detailed in Table 20-1. Thus, one should not lose enthusiasm toward exercise prescription because of the modest benefits to lipids. This concept is well demonstrated by the report by Arden and associates, which examined the benefit of fitness within levels of National Cholesterol Education Program Adult Treatment Panel III (NCEP ATP III) risk stratification.[51] As depicted in Figure 20-4, within each level of ATP III risk stratification, risk of CVD mortality was at least twofold higher for unfit individuals than for fit individuals. Restated, even in individuals whose LDL and risk factor profiles qualify them for cholesterol-lowering medications, living an active lifestyle and avoiding being unfit greatly reduced the risk of CVD mortality. Thus, despite the minimal benefit (if any) of regular exercise to reduce LDL cholesterol, those with elevated LDL, in a relative sense, stand to benefit the most from being physically active. Similar survival benefits associated with physical activity without reversal of the risk factor have been shown in individuals with hypertension, obesity, diabetes, and metabolic syndrome.[52-55] Whereas this may seem counterintuitive, it is not surprising given the broad range of physiologic benefits associated with physical activity.

EXERCISE PRESCRIPTION

Given the well-established health benefits, including improving plasma lipids, associated with regular physical activity, health care professionals should make physical activity counseling a regular component of health care encounters. For the purpose of general health, professionals should recommend 30 minutes or more of moderate-intensity physical activity such as brisk walking on most, preferably all, days of the week.[56] Participants starting a new activity program need to be reminded of the importance of starting slowly and increasing the amount and intensity conservatively.

The recommended amount of physical activity needed for weight loss or weight maintenance, although a topic of ongoing research, is suggested to be greater than 150 minutes per week for general health. For example, data from the National Weight Loss Registry noted that individuals who achieved and maintained considerable weight reduction over an extended period of time on average obtained more than 60 minutes per day of physical activity at least 6 days per week.[57] There is no consensus as to how much daily physical activity is necessary to promote weight loss. Whereas greater doses of exercise (200–300 min/week) have been shown to produce larger amounts of weight loss, the smaller doses of exercise (150 min/week), regardless of the prescribed exercise dose, are most effective in producing weight loss when combined with caloric restriction.[58,59]

CARDIAC REHABILITATION AND EXERCISE TRAINING

Given that cardiac rehabilitation and exercise training (CRET) has been shown to be beneficial to individuals with CHD and that exercise training plays an important role in CRET, the effect of therapy deserves mention.

Standard CRET programs involve not only exercise but also stress management, diet counseling, and smoking cessation. Thus it is hard to attribute the benefits of CRET to any single component of the program and necessitates that CRET be addressed separately from exercise only.

Numerous benefits of formal CRET programs have been established. In the early 1990s, before the routine use of statins, the effects of CRET programs on many of the cardiovascular risk factors, including plasma lipids, were assessed.[60] Following CRET, there were significant improvements in total cholesterol (−2%), triglycerides (−13%), HDL cholesterol (+7%), LDL cholesterol (−4%), and LDL cholesterol/HDL cholesterol ratio (−10%), which accompanied significant improvements in body mass index (−2%), percent body fat (−5%), and estimated exercise capacity (+26%).[60] Even though it is impossible to dissect out the benefits of exercise from the benefits of weight loss, it is clear that participation in CRET improves lipid profiles. Assessment of the predictors of improvements in lipids following CRET, using both univariable and multivariable analyses, found that the more abnormal the baseline values, the greater the improvement in LDL cholesterol, triglycerides, and HDL cholesterol following CRET.[60] In multivariable models, other independent predictors of improvements of LDL cholesterol following CRET were male gender, low change in exercise capacity, and low baseline triglycerides. Independent predictors for improving triglycerides with CRET were greater change in body mass index, older age, and greater increases in HDL cholesterol. Independent predictors of improving HDL cholesterol following CRET were greater changes in triglycerides, low baseline triglyceride, and female gender.

Because low levels of HDL cholesterol are extremely prevalent in patients with CHD and because low levels of HDL cholesterol may be the most potent lipid predictor of CHD, the effects of CRET on HDL cholesterol, especially in CHD patients with low levels of HDL cholesterol, is an important topic.[61,62] A substantial number of CHD patients have "isolated" low levels of HDL cholesterol, with relatively normal or only borderline-elevated levels of LDL cholesterol and triglycerides. In these patients, marked improvements occurred in HDL cholesterol (+17%; $P < .0001$) and LDL cholesterol/HDL cholesterol ratio (−11%; $P < .0001$) following CRET.[60]

Exercise and Markers of Inflammation

Measures of inflammation are increasingly being used in CHD risk stratification, and the most commonly used marker of inflammation is C-reactive protein (CRP). Although CRP is not a type of cholesterol, given the strong influence that weight and fitness have on CRP, the relation between exercise and CRP deserves mention. There is abundant cross-sectional evidence that physical activity (inversely) and weight (directly) are each independently associated with CRP (Fig. 20-5).[63-70] Cardiorespiratory fitness has also been shown to be inversely associated with CRP.[71] However, whereas a number of interventional trials have shown that weight loss reduced CRP, the available interventional trials that have examined the role of exercise in reducing CRP are both limited and conflicting.[72-79] One of the critical issues to be resolved is the question: "Does exercise reduce inflammation independent of exercise's benefits on body composition and weight?"

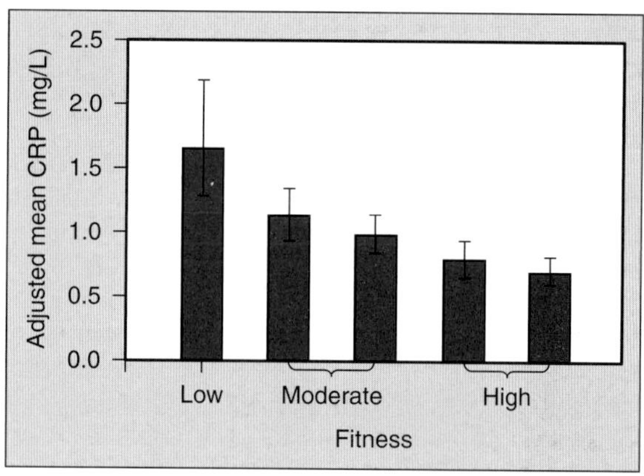

FIGURE 20-5 C-reactive protein (CRP) across fitness groups. From ref. 71, with permission.

CRET has been shown to reduce CRP by nearly 40%, and this reduction was independent of both changes in weight and the use of statins (Fig. 20-6).[80] In fact, even patients who gained weight with CRET had similar significant improvements in CRP levels. Once again it needs to be pointed out that standard CRET programs involve not only exercise but also stress management, diet counseling, and smoking cessation.

RISK AND SAFETY OF EXERCISE

Participation in physical activity or exercise is not without risk. However, these risks can be minimized with a few simple steps, and the risk for serious events is small when appropriate precautions are taken.[56] The most common risk of physical activity is musculoskeletal injury, with the risk increasing with obesity, sedentary lifestyle, amount of exercise, intensity of exercise, and participation in competitive sports. As a general principle, to minimize injury the amount or volume of daily activity should be increased gradually over time.

Risk for serious events such as sudden cardiac death or myocardial infarction acutely increases with participation in higher-intensity activities in individuals with either diagnosed or occult heart disease. For most individuals, it is not necessary to undergo

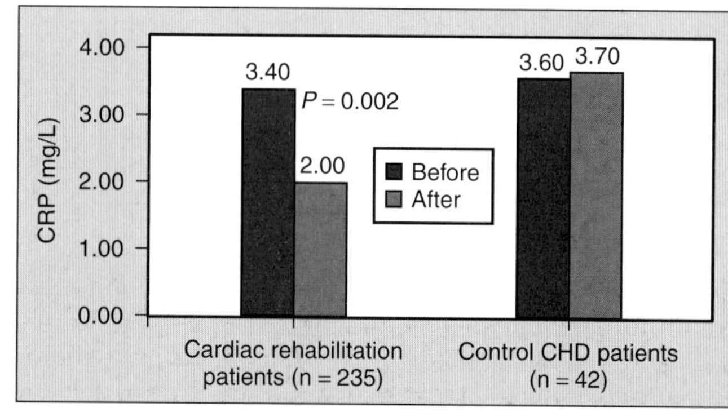

FIGURE 20-6 C-reactive protein (CRP) and cardiac rehabilitation. CHD, coronary heart disease. From Ref. 80, with permission.

exercise stress testing before starting a moderate-intensity exercise program that also includes a moderate rate of progression. However, individuals who wish to participate in higher-intensity activities, particularly those with major CVD risk factors, may need physician clearance before participating, and in some cases this should include an exercise stress test. The American College of Sports Medicine provides comprehensive screening algorithms for assessing the need for medical clearance and exercise stress testing before starting a new physical activity program.[81] As a general summary, for men younger than 45 years of age and women younger than 55 years with two or fewer CVD risk factors, exercise testing is not suggested before starting an exercise program of any intensity. Men 45 years of age and older and women 55 years of age and older, or those with two or more CVD risk factors should have a exercise stress test before initiating a high-intensity (vigorous) exercise program. Individuals with signs or symptoms of CVD or known cardiovascular, pulmonary, or metabolic disease should have a stress test before starting a moderate or intense (vigorous) exercise program. Thus, the higher the intensity of the proposed exercise program, the older the participant, and the more risk factors/disease present, the greater the need for an exercise stress test.

OTHER EXERCISE OPTIONS

Resistance training (weight lifting) has, in general, not been shown to substantially improve any lipid measures.[27] However, the amount of research focused on resistance training is much smaller than that focused on aerobic exercise, but it is an area deserving of further exploration.

SUMMARY

Despite the well-established benefits of regular exercise in the prevention of CHD, the benefits of exercise on plasma lipids are relatively modest and somewhat conflicting. It is generally accepted that exercise training results in an increase in HDL cholesterol and a reduction in triglycerides. Regular exercise has not consistently been shown to improve total cholesterol or LDL cholesterol but has been shown to decrease the percentage of smaller, more atherogenic LDL particles and increase the percentage of larger, less atherogenic LDL particles. Most importantly, it has been shown that in individuals with elevated LDL cholesterol (or diabetes, hypertension, or metabolic syndrome), leading a more physically active lifestyle is associated with a greatly reduced risk of CHD.

REFERENCES

1. Morris JN, Heady JA: Mortality in relation to the physical activity of work: A preliminary note on experience in middle age. *Br J Ind Med* 1953;10:245–254.
2. Paffenbarger RS Jr, Laughlin ME, Gima AS, et al: Work activity of longshoremen as related to death from coronary heart disease and stroke. *N Engl J Med* 1970;282:1109–1114.
3. Blair SN, Cooper KH, Gibbons LW, et al: Changes in coronary heart disease risk factors associated with increased treadmill time in 753 men. *Am J Epidemiol* 1983;118:352–359.
4. Blair SN, Goodyear NN, Gibbons LW, et al: Physical fitness and incidence of hypertension in healthy normotensive men and women. *JAMA* 1984;252:487–490.
5. Blair SN, Kohl HW III, Paffenbarger RS Jr, et al: Physical fitness and all-cause mortality: A prospective study of healthy men and women. *JAMA* 1989;262:2395–2401.
6. Blair SN, Kohl HW III, Barlow CE, et al: Changes in physical fitness and all-cause mortality: A prospective study of healthy and unhealthy men. *JAMA* 1995;273:1093–1098.
7. Manson JE, Hu FB, Rich-Edwards JW, et al: A prospective study of walking as compared with vigorous exercise in the prevention of coronary heart disease in women. *N Engl J Med* 1999;341:650–658.
8. Manson JE, Greenland P, LaCroix AZ, et al: Walking compared with vigorous exercise for the prevention of cardiovascular events in women. *N Engl J Med* 2002;347:716–725.
9. Paffenbarger RS Jr, Wing AL, Hyde RT: Physical activity as an index of heart attack risk in college alumni. *Am J Epidemiol* 1978;108:161–175.
10. Lee I-M, Hsieh C-C, Paffenbarger RS Jr: Exercise intensity and longevity in men: The Harvard Alumni Health Study. *JAMA* 1995;273:1179–1184.
11. Mora S, Redberg RF, Cui Y, et al: Ability of exercise testing to predict cardiovascular and all-cause death in asymptomatic women: A 20-year follow-up of the Lipid Research Clinics Prevalence Study. *JAMA* 2003;290:1600–1607.
12. Kiens B, Jorgensen I, Lewis S, et al: Increased plasma HDL-cholesterol and apo A-1 in sedentary middle-aged men after physical conditioning. *Eur J Clin Invest* 1980;10:203–209.
13. Després JP, Moorjani S, Trembly A: Heredity and changes in plasma lipids and lipoproteins after short-term exercise training in men. *Arteriosclerosis* 1988;8:402–409.
14. Belardinelli R, Paolini I, Cianci G, et al: Exercise training intervention after coronary angioplasty: The ETICA trial. *J Am Coll Cardiol* 2001;37:1891–1900.
15. LaRosa JC, Cleary P, Muesing RA, et al: Effect of long-term moderate physical exercise on plasma lipoproteins. The National Exercise and Heart Disease Project. *Arch Intern Med* 1982;142: 2269–2274.
16. Kokkinos PF, Holland JC, Narayan P, et al: Miles run per week and high-density lipoprotein cholesterol levels in healthy, middle-aged men. A dose-response relationship. *Arch Intern Med* 1995;155:415–420.
17. Thompson PD, Yurgalevitch SM, Flynn MM, et al: Effect of prolonged exercise training without weight loss on high-density lipoprotein metabolism in overweight men. *Metabolism* 1997;46:217–223.
18. Seip RL, Moulin P, Cocke T, et al: Exercise training decreases plasma cholesteryl ester transfer protein. *Arterioscler Thromb* 1993;13:1359–1367.
19. Wood PD, Haskell WL, Blair SN, et al: Increased exercise level and plasma lipoprotein concentrations: A one-year, randomized, controlled study in sedentary, middle-aged men. *Metabolism* 1983;32:31–39.
20. Marti B, Suter E, Riesen WF, et al: Effects of long-term, self-monitored exercise on the serum lipoprotein and apolipoprotein profile in middle-aged men. *Atherosclerosis* 1990;81:19–31.
21. Ballantyne FC, Clark RS, Simpson HS, et al: High-density and low-density lipoprotein subfractions in survivors of myocardial infarction and in control subjects. *Metabolism* 1982;31: 433–437.
22. Gelin J, Jivegard L, Taft C, et al: Treatment efficacy of intermittent claudication by surgical intervention, supervised physical exercise training compared to no treatment in unselected randomised patients I: One year results of functional and physiological improvements. *Eur J Vasc Endovasc Surg* 2001;22:107–113.
23. Plavsic C, Turkulin K, Perman Z, et al: The results of "exercise therapy in coronary prone individuals and coronary patients." *G Ital Cardiol* 1976;6:422–432.
24. Wilhelmsen L, Sanne H, Elmfeldt D, et al: A controlled trial of physical training after myocardial infarction: Effects on risk factors, nonfatal reinfarction, and death. *Prev Med* 1975;4: 491–508.
25. Yu CM, Li LS, Ho HH, et al: Long-term changes in exercise capacity, quality of life, body anthropometry, and lipid profiles after a cardiac rehabilitation program in obese patients with coronary heart disease. *Am J Cardiol* 2003;91:321–325.

26. Wosornu D, Bedford D, Ballantyne D: A comparison of the effects of strength and aerobic exercise training on exercise capacity and lipids after coronary artery bypass surgery. *Eur Heart J* 1996;17:854–863.
27. Durstine JL, Grandjean PW, Cox CA, et al: Lipids, lipoproteins, and exercise. *J Cardiopulm Rehabil* 2002;22:385–398.
28. Kelley GA, Kelley KS: Aerobic exercise and HDL_2-C: A meta-analysis of randomized controlled trials. *Atherosclerosis* 2006;184:207–215.
29. Leon AS, Sanchez OA: Response of blood lipids to exercise training alone or combined with dietary intervention. *Med Sci Sports Exerc* 2001;33:S502–S515.
30. Crouse SF, O'Brien BC, Grandjean PW, et al: Training intensity, blood lipids, and apolipoproteins in men with high cholesterol. *J Appl Physiol* 1997;82:270–277.
31. Duncan JJ, Gordon NF, Scott CB, et al: Women walking for health and fitness: How much is enough? *JAMA* 1991;266:3295–3299.
32. Huttunen JK, Lansimies E, Voutilainen E, et al: Effect of moderate physical exercise on serum lipoproteins. A controlled clinical trial with special reference to serum high-density lipoproteins. *Circulation* 1979;60:1220–1229.
33. King AC, Haskell WL, Young DR, et al: Long-term effects of varying intensities and formats of physical activity on participation rates, fitness, and lipoproteins in men and women aged 50 to 65 years. *Circulation* 1995;91:2596–2604.
34. Leaf DA, Parker DL, Schaad D: Changes in VO2max, physical activity, and body fat with chronic exercise: Effects on plasma lipids. *Med Sci Sports Exerc* 1997;29:1152–1159.
35. Leon AS, Rice T, Mandel S, et al: Blood lipid response to 20 weeks of supervised exercise in a large biracial population: The HERITAGE Family Study. *Metabolism* 2000;49:513–520.
36. Nicklas BJ, Katzel LI, Busby-Whitehead J, et al: Increases in high-density lipoprotein cholesterol with endurance exercise training are blunted in obese compared with lean men. *Metabolism* 1997;46:556–561.
37. Santiago MC, Leon AS, Serfass RC: Failure of 40 weeks of brisk walking to alter blood lipids in normolipemic women. *Can J Appl Physiol* 1995;20:417–428.
38. Stefanick ML, Mackey S, Sheehan M, et al: Effects of diet and exercise in men and postmenopausal women with low levels of HDL cholesterol and high levels of LDL cholesterol. *N Engl J Med* 1998;339:12–20.
39. Wood PD, Stefanick ML, Dreon DM, et al: Changes in plasma lipids and lipoproteins in overweight men during weight loss through dieting as compared with exercise. *N Engl J Med* 1988;319:1173–1179.
40. Wood PD, Stefanick ML, Williams PT, et al: The effects on plasma lipoproteins of a prudent weight-reducing diet with or without exercise in overweight men and women. *N Engl J Med* 1991;325:461–466.
41. Katzmarzyk PT, Leon AS, Rankinen T, et al: Changes in blood lipids consequent to aerobic exercise training related to changes in body fatness and aerobic fitness. *Metabolism* 2001;50:841–848.
42. Williams PT, Stefanick ML, Vranizan KM: The effects of weight loss by exercise or by dieting on plasma high-density lipoprotein levels in men with low, intermediate, and normal-to-high HDL at baseline. *Metabolism* 1994;43:917.
43. Halle M, Berg A, Konig D, et al: Differences in the concentration and composition of low-density lipoprotein subfraction particles between sedentary and trained hypercholesterolemic men. *Metabolism* 1997;46:186–191.
44. Kraus WE, Houmard JA, Duscha BD, et al: Effects of the amount and intensity of exercise on plasma lipoproteins. *N Engl J Med* 2002;347:1483–1492.
45. Kelley GA, Kelley KS, Franklin B: Aerobic exercise and lipids and lipoproteins in patients with cardiovascular disease: A meta-analysis of randomized controlled trials. *J Cardiopulm Rehabil* 2006;26:131–139.
46. Durstine JL, Grandjean PW, Davis PG, et al: Blood lipid and lipoprotein adaptations to exercise: A quantitative analysis. *Sports Med.* 2001;31:1033–1062.
47. Thompson PD, Rader DJ: Does exercise increase HDL cholesterol in those who need it the most? *Arterioscler Thromb Vasc Biol* 2001;21:1097-1098.
48. Kelley GA, Kelley KS, Vu TZ: Aerobic exercise, lipids and lipoproteins in overweight and obese adults: A meta-analysis of randomized controlled trials. *Int J Obes (Lond)* 2005;29:881–893.
49. Carson P, Phillips R, Lloyd M, et al: Exercise after myocardial infarction: a controlled trial. *J R Coll Physicians Lond* 1982;16:147–151.
50. Tall AR: Exercise to reduce cardiovascular risk—how much is enough? *N Engl J Med* 2002;347:1522–1524.
51. Ardern CI, Katzmarzyk PT, Janssen I, et al: Revised Adult Treatment Panel III guidelines and cardiovascular disease mortality in men attending a preventive medical clinic. *Circulation* 2005;112:1481–1488.
52. Church TS, LaMonte MJ, Barlow CE, et al: Cardiorespiratory fitness and body mass index as predictors of cardiovascular disease mortality among men with diabetes. *Arch Intern Med* 2005;165:2114–2120.
53. Church TS, Cheng YJ, Earnest CP, et al: Exercise capacity and body composition as predictors of mortality among men with diabetes. *Diabetes Care* 2004;27:83–88.
54. Church TS, Kampert JB, Gibbons LW, et al: Usefulness of cardiorespiratory fitness as a predictor of all-cause and cardiovascular disease mortality in men with systemic hypertension. *Am J Cardiol* 2001;88:651–656.
55. Katzmarzyk PT, Church TS, Blair SN: Cardiorespiratory fitness attenuates the effects of the metabolic syndrome on all-cause and cardiovascular disease mortality in men. *Arch Intern Med* 2004;164:1092–1097.
56. Pate RR, Pratt M, Blair SN, et al: Physical activity and public health: A recommendation from the Centers for Disease Control and Prevention and the American College of Sports Medicine. *JAMA* 1995;273:402–407.
57. Klem ML, Wing RR, McGuire MT, et al: A descriptive study of individuals successful at long-term maintenance of substantial weight loss. *Am J Clin Nutr* 1997;66:239–246.
58. Jakicic JM, Clark K, Coleman E, et al: American College of Sports Medicine position stand. Appropriate intervention strategies for weight loss and prevention of weight regain for adults. *Med Sci Sports Exerc* 2001;33:2145–2156.
59. Jakicic JM, Marcus BH, Gallagher KI, et al: Effect of exercise duration and intensity on weight loss in overweight, sedentary women: A randomized trial. *JAMA* 2003;290:1323–1330.
60. Lavie CJ, Milani RV: Factors predicting improvements in lipid values following cardiac rehabilitation and exercise training. *Arch Intern Med* 1993;153:982–988.
61. Milani RV, Lavie CJ: Prevalence and effects of nonpharmacologic treatment of "isolated" low-HDL cholesterol in patients with coronary artery disease. *J Cardiopulm Rehabil* 1995;15:439–444.
62. Lavie CJ, Milani RV: Effects of nonpharmacologic therapy with cardiac rehabilitation and exercise training in patients with low levels of high-density lipoprotein cholesterol. *Am J Cardiol* 1996;78:1286–1289.
63. Festa A, D'Agostino JR, Williams K, et al: The relation of body fat mass and distribution to markers of chronic inflammation. *Int J Obes Relat Metab Disord.* 2001;25:1407–1415.
64. Ford ES. Does exercise reduce inflammation? Physical activity and C-reactive protein among U.S. adults. *Epidemiology* 2002;13:561–568.
65. Geffken DF, Cushman M, Burke GL, et al: Association between physical activity and markers of inflammation in a healthy elderly population. *Am J Epidemiol* 2001;153:242–250.
66. LaMonte MJ, Durstine JL, Yanowitz FG, et al: Cardiorespiratory fitness and C-reactive protein among a tri-ethnic sample of women. *Circulation* 2002;106:403–406.
67. Manns PJ, Williams DP, Snow CM, et al: Physical activity, body fat, and serum C-reactive protein in postmenopausal women with and without hormone replacement. *Am J Hum Biol* 2003;15:91–100.
68. Visser M, Bouter LM, McQuillan GM, et al: Elevated C-reactive protein levels in overweight and obese adults. *JAMA* 1999;282:2131–2135.
69. Pischon T, Hankinson SE, Hotamisligil GS, et al: Leisure-time physical activity and reduced plasma levels of obesity-related inflammatory markers. *Obes Res* 2003;11:1055–1064.
70. Mora S, Lee IM, Buring JE, et al: Association of physical activity and body mass index with novel and traditional cardiovascular biomarkers in women. *JAMA* 2006;295:1412–1419.
71. Church TS, Barlow CE, Earnest CP, et al: Associations between cardiorespiratory fitness and C-reactive protein in men. *Arterioscler Thromb Vasc Biol* 2002;22:1869–1476.
72. Obisesan TO, Leeuwenburgh C, Phillips T, et al: C-reactive protein genotypes affect baseline, but not exercise training-induced

changes, in C-reactive protein levels. *Arterioscler Thromb Vasc Biol* 2004;24:1874–1879.

73. Kelley GA, Kelley KS: Effects of aerobic exercise on C-reactive protein, body composition, and maximum oxygen consumption in adults: A meta-analysis of randomized controlled trials. *Metabolism* 2006;55:1500–1507.
74. Selvin E, Paynter NP, Erlinger TP: The effect of weight loss on C-reactive protein: A systematic review. *Arch Intern Med* 2007;167:31–39.
75. Lakka TA, Lakka HM, Rankinen T, et al: Effect of exercise training on plasma levels of C-reactive protein in healthy adults: The HERITAGE Family Study. *Eur Heart J* 2005;26:2018–2025.
76. Okita K, Nishijima H, Murakami T, et al: Can exercise training with weight loss lower serum C-reactive protein levels? *Arterioscler Thromb Vasc Biol* 2004;24:1868–1873.
77. Huffman KM, Samsa GP, Slentz CA, et al: Response of high-sensitivity C-reactive protein to exercise training in an at-risk population. *Am Heart J* 2006;152:793–800.
78. Heilbronn LK, Noakes M, Clifton PM: Energy restriction and weight loss on very-low-fat diets reduce C-reactive protein concentrations in obese, healthy women. *Arterioscler Thromb Vasc Biol* 2001;21:968–970.
79. Mattusch F, Dufaux B, Heine O, et al: Reduction of the plasma concentration of C-reactive protein following nine months of endurance training. *Int J Sports Med* 2000;21:21–24.
80. Milani RV, Lavie CJ, Mehra MR: Reduction in C-reactive protein through cardiac rehabilitation and exercise training. *J Am Coll Cardiol* 2004;43:1056–1061.
81. Armstrong L, Balady GJ, Berry MJ, et al: ACSM's Guidelines for Exercise Testing and Prescription, 7th ed. Philadelphia: Lippincott Williams & Wilkins; 2006.

CHAPTER 21

Weight Loss

F. Xavier Pi-Sunyer

Obesity is highly prevalent in the United States and is growing throughout the world. The World Health Organization (WHO) has declared overweight as one of the top 10 risk conditions in the world and top 5 in developed nations. Its latest estimates indicate that globally in 2005 approximately 1.6 billion adults (age 15+) are overweight and at least 400 million are obese. The projection for 2015 is of approximately 2.3 billion adults overweight and more than 700 million obese. This also affects children, with at least 20 million children younger than 5 years who are overweight. Both the National Health and Nutrition Examination Survey (NHANES)[1] and the Behavioral Risk Factor Surveillance System (BRFSS)[2] indicate that the prevalence of obesity among adults continued to increase during the past decade. NHANES declared 66.3% of the adult population of the United States to be overweight and 32% to be obese.[2] This is a great unanticipated secular leap since the late 1980s.

The National Center for Health Statistics[3] has reported overweight in children and adolescents, tracking data acquired from 1963 to 2002. A significant increase in the prevalence of overweight has occurred in children aged 6 to 11 years, from 4% in 1963 to 1970, to 16% in 1999 to 2002, and in adolescents aged 12 to 19 years, from 5% in 1963 to 1970, to 16% in 2002 (Centers for Disease Control and Prevention [CDC] website: http://www.cdc.gov/).

The human organism seems unable to regulate energy intake appropriately, given the temptation of the modern food and beverage supply. The environment is so intrusive that only a consciously restrained eater can withstand the temptation to overeat in today's world. As a result, the average adult in the United States gains about 1.8 to 2.0 pounds per year between 20 and 60 years of age.[4]

The dramatic decrease in physical activity over the last few decades has also helped to fuel the obesity epidemic. Through mechanization and the creation of labor-saving devices, physical labor at work has all but disappeared. In addition, leisure-time activities have moved from active to passive, with the Internet, television, and spectator sports replacing active movement. Prentice and Jebb[5] have reported that the increase in weight in the United Kingdom in recent years is primarily due to a decrease in energy expenditure rather than to an increase in food intake.[5] As a result, people are expending less energy daily at a time when they are eating more calories, leading to inexorable weight gain.

Obesity brings with it a certain number of health risks. These include diabetes mellitus, dyslipidemia, hypertension, and cardiovascular disease. An increased risk for nonalcoholic steatohepatitis, gall stones, sleep apnea, osteoarthritis, and depression also exists. Dyslipidemia is a common problem in obese persons, particularly if the obesity is coupled with type 2 diabetes.

ASSESSMENT OF THE OBESE PATIENT WITH DYSLIPIDEMIA

It is important to know the total fat burden and the body fat distribution of a patient for the management of dyslipidemia. A simple and relatively accurate way to estimate total fat burden is to calculate the body mass index (BMI), which is weight in kg/height in m^2. The BMI correlates fairly well with the degree of obesity except in very muscular individuals.[6] According to the WHO, BMI of 18.5 to 24.9 kg/m^2 is defined as normal, 25 to 29.9 kg/m^2 as overweight, and more than 30 kg/m^2 as obese, with 30% to 34.9% defined as class 1 obesity, 35% to 39.9% as class 2, and more than 40% as class 3.

Central fat distribution is also correlated with dyslipidemia. Central obesity can be evaluated by measuring the waist circumference or the waist-to-hip ratio. Waist circumference should be measured at the uppermost border of the iliac crest. A waist circumference greater than 102 cm (40 inches) in men and 88 cm (35 inches) in women is considered abnormal and indicates increased risk for dyslipidemia, type 2 diabetes, hypertension, and cardiovascular disease. A waist-to-hip ratio greater than 1.0 in men and greater than 0.85 in women is considered abnormally high.[7]

Weight loss has been associated with an improvement in abnormal circulating lipids in a number of studies. Weight loss can be achieved with lifestyle interventions such as diet and exercise, with pharmacotherapy, or with surgery. The initial target of weight-loss therapy should be a reduction of body weight of about 10%. This weight-loss goal, which can reasonably be achieved with a combination of lifestyle modification and drug therapy, is associated with significant improvement in dyslipidemia.[7] With weight loss, patients with dyslipidemia may be able to discontinue antilipid medications.

OVERVIEW OF WEIGHT-LOSS THERAPY

Before starting a weight-loss program, a careful preliminary assessment has to be made. This should include the patient's usual diet, food preferences, and eating habits. Also, a history of previous weight-loss attempts and the reason why they failed should be taken. Losing weight is a difficult and time-consuming process, so the patient has to be appropriately motivated. Behavior modification is focused mainly on changing eating habits, increasing physical activity, altering attitudes, and developing support systems.

Patient motivation is a prerequisite for achieving the target of weight loss. Motivation can be increased by describing to the patient the health risks of obesity. Some things that have to be considered before starting the weight-loss procedure include the following:

1. How serious and determined to lose weight is the patient?
2. How well does the patient understand the dangers of being obese?
3. Can the patient's family and friends help him/her in the attempt to lose weight?
4. Is the patient prepared to start exercise together with diet therapy?
5. Does the patient have adequate time to spend on diet and exercise therapy?
6. Does the patient have adequate time to devote to the overall attempt to lose weight?

It is crucial for the patient to trust the physician or other healthcare workers involved in the weight-loss program and for the physician to show respect and concern for the patient. The patient–physician partnership is basic for the success of the weight-loss program.

Initially, the patient and the physician need to set an achievable goal. Patients usually have unrealistic and unachievable goals when they start a weight-loss program.[8] It is wise to begin with a modest goal of 8% to 10% because this can be met by a motivated person who is well managed. A number of recent guidelines have suggested a loss of about 10% from baseline weight.[7,9,10] This is realistic, attainable, and maintainable.[7,11] If the patient is successful at this, then maintenance at this lower weight for a time is wise. If the patient continues to follow the guidelines successfully, then further weight loss can be attempted. Setting more ambitious goals at the start can lead to disappointment, anger, and abandonment of the program.

BEHAVIOR THERAPY

The original premise of behavior therapy was that for obese patients, eating is maladaptive and that this can be changed for the better. More recently, as the cause of obesity has been recognized as being affected by much more than maladaptive eating, especially genetic, environmental, and social factors, the attempt at behavior change has broadened to include changes in physical activity, the environment, and the social setting of an individual attempting to lose weight.[12,13] Over the years, refinements of behavioral therapy techniques have been proposed.[14,15]

The aim of behavioral therapy is to change behavior by means of small, achievable steps. Because the behavior change will focus on diet and exercise, knowledge about this is a necessary step in therapy.

Specific behavioral strategies include self-monitoring, stress management, stimulus control, problem solving, contingency management, cognitive restructuring, and social support.[14] Self-monitoring has been found to be extremely important in weight control. It consists of observing and recording faithfully and as truthfully as possible various aspects of behavior, such as food intake, physical activity, and medication use.

Stimulus control is working at identifying what social or environmental cues lead to undesirable behavior. Once identified, a sustained effort is made to eliminate, change, or avoid these cues. This again requires self-examination by the patient with the help of the counselor. It requires honest confrontation with people and situations that cause excess eating. Stimulus control is closely tied to stress management. Stress may be free floating or brought on by special situations and circumstances. Learning to identify these causes and trying to change or avoid them is an important aim of behavior modification.

Contingency management involves the application of rewards for moving to appropriate behavior patterns for weight loss and maintenance. Behavior therapy stresses that a component of the therapy should be reward. This is based on the premise that weight control is difficult, and that reinforcement of constructive behavior can lead to patient satisfaction and continued motivation. This is done by exploring the kinds of rewards a patient would find positive and pleasurable (a movie, a new CD, some jewelry, a book, among others). This contingency management is often done with the use of contracts, whereby the patient agrees to modify a certain behavior (increase exercise bouts, decrease alcohol, decrease fried foods, and so forth) in return for which a reward is negotiated.

Problem solving is individually based. A patient needs to identify particular problems that affect eating and exercise, and formulate strategies for reversing them. This can be related to particular types of foods that are a problem, particular cooking techniques, portion sizes, snacking, caloric beverages, and so forth. Also, particular situations or people may be involved. Each must be confronted in turn and reversed. It is important not to try to change all identified problems at once, but to take them one at a time.

Cognitive restructuring is aimed at altering inappropriate cognition that affects eating and activity behavior. Because individuals develop behavior patterns primarily through cognitive processes, it is necessary to identify these and attempt to change maladaptive ones. These include coping skills strategies and problem-solving strategies.[16]

Social support can be helpful in achieving success. It is for this reason that group therapy has been the method of choice to deliver behavior therapy. Peers can help to establish appropriate and realistic intragroup norms for eating and exercise. They can help to counter the pressure of the outside world to see obese persons as unsuccessful if they do not reach ideal weight. Thinking patterns need to be diverted away from self-rejection and toward self-acceptance.[17]

Relapse prevention is an important component of behavior therapy. The major problem with all treatments for obesity is a slow return to baseline weight after the treatment intervention ends.[18] By 5 years after the start of a treatment program, most patients are back to baseline or beyond.[19] Relapse prevention training aims at teaching how to avoid or cope with slips and slides backward.[19] Continuing treatment beyond 6 months improves the maintenance of weight loss. Contact may be by actual group sessions, individual sessions, telephone calls, postcards, mailings, or Internet dialogue. These have been found to enhance weight maintenance.[20] Providing a locale for continued peer support group sessions has also proved helpful.[21]

A positive effect of behavior therapy is giving patients the major responsibility for the weight-loss strategy so that with success they can attribute increased power to themselves. This reinforces their motivation, increases their confidence, and is important in producing the will to maintain the effort over a long period.

It is important to individualize behavior change. The initial steps are to carefully identify present lifestyle habits and focus on what needs to be modified. This is greatly helped if a period of self-monitoring is used to detail dietary and activity habits. This includes time, quantity, and quality of meals and snacks, beverage intake, relationship to social and work situations, and mood changes. It is important to carefully evaluate macronutrient content of the diet, which can be done with food intake diaries and food frequency questionnaires. In addition, careful documentation of physical activity throughout the day should be done.

After a thorough account of present lifestyle habits has been documented, the next step is to begin to change habits to a more coherent and healthy way of eating. This deals with portion sizes, types of foods, kinds and amounts of beverages and snacks, macronutrient content of the diet, where and how food is eaten, and with whom. Stimuli that lead to eating need to be eliminated or controlled. For instance, stress-related eating, mood-related eating, and site-related eating need to be identified and changed. In addition, a beginning needs to be made in increasing physical activity, usually primarily by increased walking.

Stress management can often be important in helping a patient correct dysfunctional eating. Meditation, relaxation techniques, and social engagement all may help. Also, social support from family, friends, and work-site colleagues can be helpful in weight loss and weight maintenance.

A difficult issue is the maintenance of weight loss. It is common for persons to regain their weight in a period ranging from a few months to a few years. A weight-maintenance program is considered successful when weight regain is not more than 3 kg in 2 years.[7] Thus, the same effort at diet and physical activity needs to continue if maintenance is to be successful. The National Weight Loss Registry has shown that a continued effort in this regard is necessary to maintain weight.[22]

DIET

Diet is a key component of a weight-reduction effort. Obese persons consume a very high amount of calories,[23] and this must be reduced. A calorie-deficit diet can lead to significant weight loss and to improvement in an obese person with dyslipidemia. The typical American diet consists of about 15% protein, 35% fat, and 50% carbohydrates.[24] Fat should be decreased and total calories reduced. Sugar should be discouraged. High-fiber foods such as fruits and vegetables should be encouraged. Alcohol should be eliminated or drastically curtailed. One should aim at a deficit of about 1000 kcal/day; this would translate to about 1 kg of weight loss per week.

Many persons can benefit from a low-calorie formula diet for a period, usually 12 to 16 weeks.[25] Initially, this can be for all meals, and eventually it can be used for one or two meals a day. The advantage is that it gives good control of caloric intake. The disadvantage is that it can become extremely monotonous.

The aim of weight loss is to lose fat without losing too much lean body mass. The loss of some is inevitable, but it should be kept to a limit. This is done by eating enough protein and making it high-quality protein (e.g., egg whites, low-fat dairy products, lean meat, fish, poultry). The intake of protein should be at a level of 1.0 to 1.5 g/kg of ideal body weight. The ideal weight can be calculated using a BMI of 25 and finding the appropriate weight for height in a BMI table. A vegetarian diet can be used, but protein complementation is required to ensure appropriate essential amino acid intake.[26] Total fat should not exceed 30% of calories, with saturated fat not more than 8% to 10% of total calories. This is also true of polyunsaturated fats, whereas monounsaturates can be as high as 15%. The daily carbohydrate intake should include 20 to 30 g of fiber from fruits, vegetables, legumes, and grains. Fiber seems to help satiety at lower levels of caloric intake.[13] It is important also that adequate amounts of vitamins and minerals are taken daily.

There have been long-term trials (1 year or more) of both the low-fat balanced diet and the Mediterranean diet that have both shown their effectiveness and their safety.[27–29] One long-term trial of the high-carbohydrate/low-fat diet[30] also showed its effectiveness and safety over time. A number of randomized clinical trials comparing high-fat, low-carbohydrate diets with more balanced diets have been done, showing as good or better weight loss with the former as the latter.[31–35]

The effort to achieve a caloric deficit of between 500 and 1500 calories/day requires a careful dietary history. This can lead to a loss of between 1 and 2 lb/week.[13] A low-calorie diet includes 800 to 1500 calories/day. A diet of 1200 to 1500 calories/day for men and one of 1000 to 1200 calories/day for women is usually about right, but it needs to be individualized in relation to original intake and physical activity. These kinds of diets can cause a 10% weight loss in 6 months, with 75% being fat and 25% lean body mass.[36] Very-low-calorie diets of 300 to 800 calories/day have been used in the past but are not recommended. They require careful medical supervision because of potential electrolyte abnormalities, cardiac changes, and excess diuresis. They also have not been shown to produce greater weight loss.[37] Also, there tends to be a rapid regain once the very-low-calorie diet is abandoned.[38]

Generally, weight loss can continue for 4 to 6 months and then plateaus. This plateau is due to a new equilibrium in which energy intake once again is equivalent to energy expenditure. Maintenance of the weight loss requires continuing the same energy intake and a physical activity at least as great as a patient has been doing as his or her weight loss plateaus. Therefore, there can be no liberalization of food intake or reduction of physical activity, or else weight regain will occur.

PHYSICAL ACTIVITY

A number of studies have shown that increased physical activity will not particularly help in weight loss but can be effective in weight maintenance after weight is lost. Wing,[39] in a recent review of 13 randomized clinical trials of weight loss with and without an exercise component, found only two trials that demonstrated a significantly greater weight loss in the group that exercised. She also reviewed four studies that had a resistance exercise component and again found no statistically greater weight loss with exercise.[39] There has been less controversy as to whether exercise is helpful for weight maintenance. Pavlou and colleagues'[40] study showed a strong effect of exercise in the maintenance period on the ability to maintain weight loss. Those individuals who maintained an exercise regimen maintained their weight loss, whereas those who abandoned the exercise regained their weight. Also, a number of carefully conducted studies have reported the superiority for maintenance of adding exercise to diet.[39,41] For this reason, it is important to begin to modify behavior with regard to physical activity as one begins a program. In the absence of a contraindication such as a cardiac, orthopedic, or metabolic reason, exercise should always be encouraged. Initially, an effort is made simply to increase walking at a normal pace. The goal is to increase initially to 30 minutes per day and eventually to 60 minutes per day. The exercise does not need to be done all at once but can be done in bouts. The program needs to start slowly because many obese individuals are extremely sedentary. Eventually, depending on the age, weight, and fitness of the individual, jogging or biking can be done. Other activities, such as swimming, golf, and tennis, are encouraged.

The National Weight Loss Registry is a registry of persons who have lost at least 25 lb of their weight and kept it off for 5 years. To maintain their weight loss, these individuals expend at least 400 kcal/day in physical activity.[42] Other studies are available that also have documented that long-term weight loss is associated with increased physical activity.[43–45] For maintenance, therefore, good evidence exists that exercise will contribute to success. Exercise has been shown to improve lipid profiles.[46]

DRUG TREATMENT FOR WEIGHT LOSS

Because of the great difficulty of achieving weight loss and maintaining it over time, drug therapy is looked to for help. Because good data have been reported for the genetic underpinnings of obesity,[47,48] it is evident that obesity is a chronic disease that requires chronic treatment. Thus, if drug therapy is successful, it generally needs to be continued indefinitely. However, drug therapy should always be given in conjunction with diet and exercise. The inclusion of lifestyle modification in a program using drug therapy for weight loss leads to significantly greater weight loss and weight maintenance.[49]

Currently, only two drugs are approved for long-term use for weight loss in the United States (Table 21-1): orlistat and sibutramine. Another drug, phentermine, though approved only for short-term use, is actually used widely long term.

Orlistat

Orlistat is an inhibitor of pancreatic lipase.[50] The result of this inhibition is that about 30% of the daily ingested fat intake is not absorbed. This would lead to a 200-calorie deficit per day in an individual who consumed a diet of 2000 calories/day with 30% of calories as fat. The most common side effects of orlistat are gastrointestinal, such as fatty or oily stools, more frequent defecation, and fecal incontinence. Another side effect is a slight reduction in fat-soluble vitamins, generally not outside the reference range.

Several studies have confirmed the efficacy of orlistat in losing weight. The European Multicentre Orlistat Group conducted a double-blind study in which

TABLE 21-1 Drugs Approved by The Food and Drug Administration for Treating Obesity

Generic Name	Trade Name
Sibutramine	Meridia
Orlistat	Xenical, Alli
Phentermine	Adipex, Fastin, Lonamin

688 obese individuals (average BMI, 36 kg/m^2) were assigned to orlistat therapy or placebo for 1 year, in combination with a hypocaloric diet (minimum energy intake, 1000–1200 kcal/day). At the end of the first year, they were reassigned randomly to either orlistat or placebo for another year. At the end of the first year of the study, the mean weight loss was 10.2% for the orlistat group and 6.1% for the placebo group. During the second year of the study, the participants who were switched to placebo gained twice as much weight as those who continued on orlistat therapy. Participants who were switched from placebo to orlistat lost 0.9 kg more weight than in the first year of the trial.[51]

A U.S. study showed similar results.[52] In this trial, 892 obese individuals (BMI, 30–43 kg/m^2) who were previously on a 4-week controlled-energy diet plus placebo were randomized into either continuing placebo or starting orlistat 120 mg three times a day (tid). After 52 weeks, the participants started a weight-maintenance diet, and those in the orlistat group were rerandomized to continuing orlistat (60 or 120 mg tid) or placebo for another 52 weeks. Participants who were already taking placebo continued taking it. At the end of the first year, the participants taking orlistat had lost more weight than those taking placebo (8.76 ± 0.37 vs. 5.81 ± 0.67 kg). At the end of the second year, participants taking orlistat 120 mg tid regained less weight than those taking orlistat 60 mg tid or placebo (3.2 ± 0.45, 4.26 ± 0.57, and 5.63 ± 0.42 kg, respectively).

These studies showed that there is a significant weight loss with the use of orlistat in combination with diet during the first year, and that the tendency for weight regain that occurs during the second year is less with the use of orlistat. Weight loss with orlistat also helps in the treatment of comorbidities, including dyslipidemia.[52]

Sibutramine

The other drug that can be used for the treatment of obesity is sibutramine. Sibutramine is a serotonin and norepinephrine reuptake inhibitor that reduces appetite, thereby decreasing food intake and body weight.

The effect of sibutramine on weight loss was investigated in a multicenter dose-ranging study.[53] Participants (n = 1047) were randomly assigned to either sibutramine (1–30 mg) or placebo. After 6 months, dose-dependent weight loss was observed (1.2% weight loss with placebo compared with 2.7% with sibutramine 1 mg, 3.9% with 5 mg, 6.1% with 10 mg, 7.4% with 15 mg, 8.8% with 20 mg, and 9.4% with 30 mg).

Another study investigated the effect of sibutramine on weight loss, using very-low-calorie diet and sibutramine, compared with the same diet and placebo.[54] In the sibutramine group, 86% of the participants lost at least 5% of their initial body weight compared with 55% of the placebo group 6 months after study entry. At month 12, 75% of the sibutramine group maintained at least 100% of their weight loss, compared with 42% of the placebo group.

The Sibutramine Trial in Obesity Reduction and Maintenance (STORM) investigated the effect of sibutramine in maintaining weight that was lost on a hypocaloric formula diet.[55] In this trial, 605 obese patients, after losing weight, received 10 mg sibutramine daily for 6 months. After this period, participants who achieved at least 5% reduction in their body weight were randomly assigned either to continue with sibutramine for 18 more months or to receive placebo. Of the participants who completed the study, 43% of the sibutramine group maintained more than 80% of their original weight loss, whereas in the placebo group, only 16% maintained this level of weight loss.

The side effects of sibutramine include dry mouth, headache, insomnia, and constipation, but most importantly, it can increase heart rate by 4 to 6 beats/min and increase diastolic blood pressure by 2 to 3 mm Hg. Sibutramine should not be used in patients with a history of coronary heart disease, arrhythmias, or heart failure. Although some studies support sibutramine use in obese hypertensive patients,[56,57] it must be used with great caution or not at all in patients with uncontrolled hypertension. Patients taking sibutramine should regularly be monitored for their heart rate and blood pressure.

Phentermine

Other anorectic drugs have been approved for short-term use in the United States. They all act on the central nervous system, affecting either noradrenergic or serotoninergic systems. One of these drugs, phentermine, is being used extensively long term in the United States. It is an adrenergic drug. Two longer-term trials have been conducted with this drug.[58,59] One was conducted for 36 weeks as a randomized, controlled trial, with the drug arms being given the medication continually or intermittently every other week.[58] Weight loss was similar in the two drug arms. The drug reglmens yielded a 20.5% weight loss, whereas placebo gave a 6% loss. A second randomized trial of 6 months' duration reported a weight loss of 12.6% in the drug arm and 9.2% in the placebo arm.[59]

Phentermine was half of the phentermine–fenfluramine combination that was effective in eliciting weight loss but had severe adverse side effects of heart valve abnormalities and pulmonary fibrosis.[60–62] Although the Food and Drug Administration (FDA) banned fenfluramine, there was no evidence to implicate phentermine,[61] and it has remained in the market. No other long-term trials have been conducted, although no evidence of long-term toxicity has been reported.

SURGERY FOR WEIGHT LOSS

Not only is the prevalence of obesity increasing, but the size of individuals is getting larger and larger. Many of them have tried to lose weight numerous times and have failed repeatedly. As a result, they are turning to surgery to solve their predicament. A National Institutes of Health consensus conference[63] has produced guidelines suggesting a BMI of 40 or greater without comorbidities and BMI of 35 or greater with comorbid conditions as appropriate for referral to surgery.

The procedures being performed for obesity are gastric banding, vertical-banded gastroplasty, gastric bypass, and biliopancreatic bypass. Gastric banding and vertical-banded gastroplasty are restrictive procedures, reducing the ability to ingest food. The two others, gastric bypass and biliopancreatic bypass, are primarily malabsorptive. In general, the weight loss is least for banding, next for vertical-banded gastroplasty, next for gastric bypass, and most for biliopancreatic bypass. Biliopancreatic bypass is not commonly performed in the United States because it has significantly more adverse side effects. These include severe diarrhea and liver disease.[64,65]

The Swedish Obese Subjects (SOS) study has followed the outcomes of patients who had undergone surgery compared with a parallel group who had received medical therapy.[66] The weight loss was 23% ± 10% of excess weight in those undergoing vertical-banded gastroplasty and 33% ± 10% for those undergoing gastric bypass.[67] There was more improvement in glucose levels, lipids, and blood pressure in the surgical than the medical groups. In the 8-year follow-up report, although lipids improved and the development of type 2 diabetes was prevented, blood pressure had returned to its preoperative levels.[67] The SOS study showed that weight losses from baseline stabilized after 10 years at 25% for gastric bypass, 16% for vertical-banded gastroplasty, and 14% for banding (Figure 21-1).[68] Of 2010 volunteer subjects who underwent surgery and 2037 who received conventional medical treatment (matched control group), with a follow-up rate of 99.9% for an average of 10.9 years, there were 129 deaths in the control group and 101 deaths in the surgery group (Figure 21-2).[68]

Adams and colleagues'[69] recent retrospective study comparing patients who underwent gastric bypass with a baseline weight-matched control group showed a 40% decreased mortality rate in the surgery group over a mean follow-up of 7.1 years. A similar striking decrease occurred in cardiovascular mortality.

WEIGHT MAINTENANCE

Maintaining reduced weight after achieving weight loss is extremely difficult. The full reasons for this phenomenon are not known. A number of forces, however, seem relevant to this.

First, persons following hypocaloric diets decrease their basal metabolic rate and, therefore, require fewer calories to maintain weight.[70] Thus, as the weight loss proceeds, the caloric deficit becomes less than it originally was. At the end of the weight-loss phase, a patient will have a lower metabolic rate than at the start.

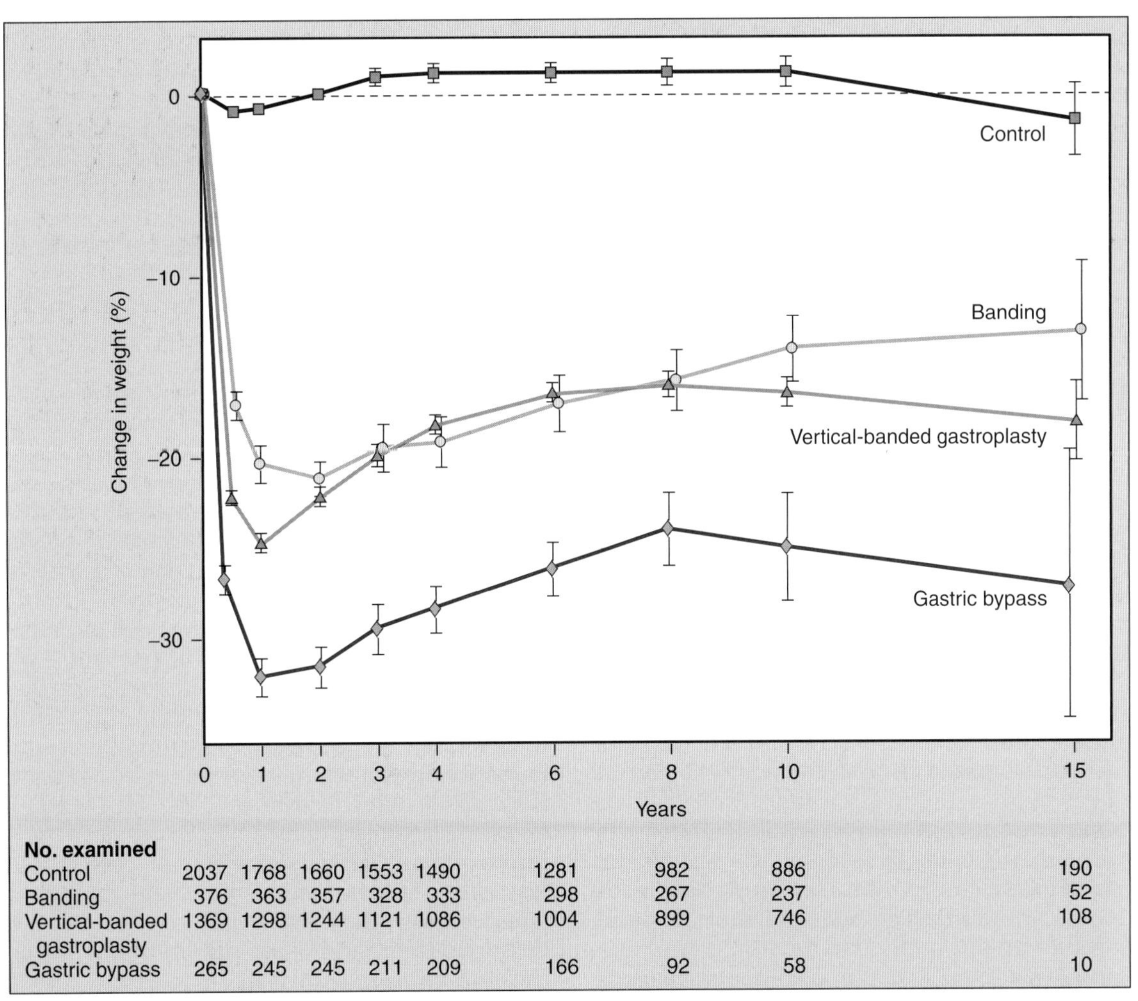

No. examined	0	1	2	3	4	6	8	10	15
Control	2037	1768	1660	1553	1490	1281	982	886	190
Banding	376	363	357	328	333	298	267	237	52
Vertical-banded gastroplasty	1369	1298	1244	1121	1086	1004	899	746	108
Gastric bypass	265	245	245	211	209	166	92	58	10

FIGURE 21-1 Mean percent weight change during a 15-year period in the control and the surgery group, according to the method of bariatric surgery. *(From Ref. 68, with permission.)*

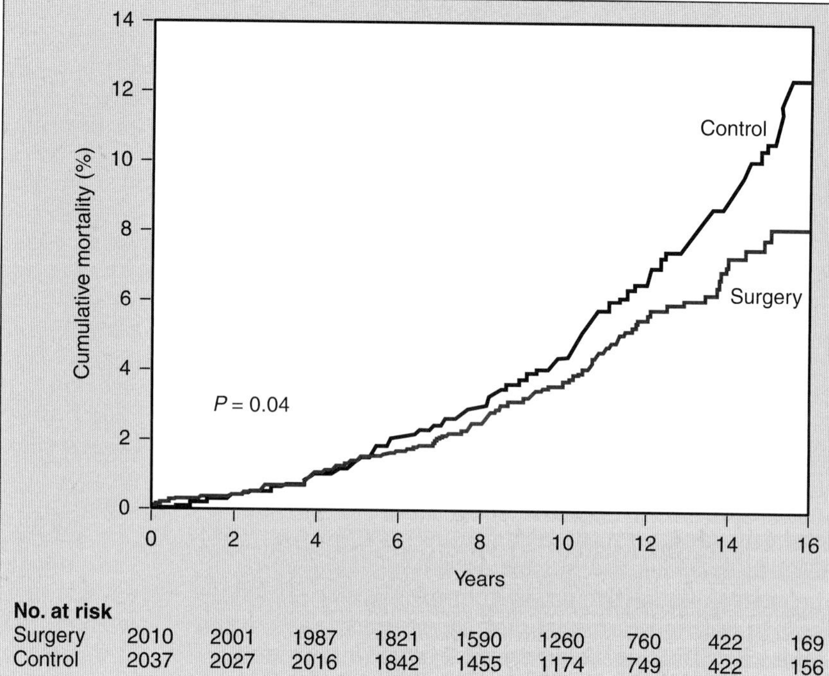

FIGURE 21-2 Unadjusted cumulative mortality in the Swedish Obese Subjects Study. The hazard ratio for mortality for subjects who underwent bariatric surgery (101 deaths) was 0.76 (95% CI, 0.59 to 0.99; P = 0.04) compared with control subjects (129 deaths). *(From Ref. 68, with permission.)*

This occurs because lean body mass is lost as well as fat, and the metabolic rate is directly related to the lean body mass.[71] Thus, the patient will require fewer calories at the end of a weight-loss period than he or she required before starting to lose weight.[72]

Second, as people lose weight, they become more efficient. That is, they require less energy to do the same physical task.[73] Thus, when a person who after a weight-loss phase returns to the total physical activity done previously, she/he will be in positive caloric balance because fewer calories are required to accomplish the same physical task. It is incumbent on every patient who has lost weight to increase his or her physical activity, and to increase it markedly (to some an extra 500–700 kcal/day).

Third, levels of lipoprotein lipase, an enzyme that breaks down circulating lipoprotein triglycerides and thus facilitates the entry of free fatty acids into cells, are increased in persons who are obese.[74] With weight reduction, the responsiveness of adipose tissue lipoprotein lipase to meals is increased,[74,75] suggesting a better ability to dispose of the triglyceride. This physiologic avidity of the adipose cells for the triglyceride makes the post–weight loss period a particularly difficult one in terms of regain.

Finally, there seems to be a heightened sensitivity to palatable foods.[76] Although this has not been adequately studied, there seems to be an enhanced taste threshold and an increased natural intake after a period of deprivation.[77]

A common psychological change with weight loss is actually overconfidence: the feeling that the weight has been lost and that the individual can now deal with maintenance without help. This is clearly not the case. Studies have shown repeatedly that the longer the relationship between patient and the therapeutic team is continued, the greater the likelihood of success.[78] As a result, caloric intake should be liberalized carefully and slowly after goal weight is reached, with daily weight monitoring. A permanent reduction in caloric intake is required because a patient's total energy expenditure will decline after weight loss. All the lifestyle changes learned during the weight-loss period must be continued, including the increased physical activity. If weight-loss drugs have been successful and without adverse effects, their chronic utilization can be recommended, with careful tracking for potential adverse effects.

EFFECT OF WEIGHT LOSS ON LIPIDS

The dyslipidemia of obesity is characterized by high triglycerides, reduced high-density lipoprotein (HDL) cholesterol, and small dense low-density lipoprotein (LDL) particles.[79,80] With weight loss, triglyceride concentrations decline, HDL cholesterol level increases, and small dense LDL particles become larger and less atherogenic.[81,82] Total and LDL cholesterol levels may be increased in some, but not all, persons with obesity.[83,84] On the other hand, HDL cholesterol levels and HDL cholesterol/LDL cholesterol ratios are typically decreased in obesity, whereas triglyceride levels are generally increased, leading to a greater atherogenic risk.[83,85] Short-term studies have confirmed the value of behavioral, low-calorie diet, and very-low-calorie diet interventions in decreasing total and LDL cholesterol levels, increasing HDL cholesterol levels and the HDL/LDL ratio, and reducing triglyceride level.[86–90] In most cases, short-term improvements have been observed, both in patients who lost substantial amounts of weight and in those who attained only moderate weight loss. The results of important long-term studies of the effects of weight loss on dyslipidemia are shown in Table 21-2.

In an early long-term study of the relationship between weight loss and dyslipidemia, Hall and

TABLE 21-2 Summary of Long-Term Studies of the Effects of Weight Loss on Dyslipidemia

Reference (Year): Study Name, Objective	No. and Characteristics of Patients	Study Duration and Intervention	Weight Change (kg, unless otherwise mentioned)	Changes in Lipid Levels
Hall et al. (1972)[91]: Evaluation of the cholesterol-lowering diet used in the Coronary Prevention Program in controlling hypertriglyceridemia	140 men, 90 with obesity and 50 with hypertriglyceridemia	1-year intervention with reduced-fat low-calorie diet	−10 lb	TC reduced by 12.1%* TG reduced by 17.3%* *$P = 0.01$
Mancini et al. (1981)[92]: Evaluation of the medical benefits of weight loss, including improved lipid levels	71 severely obese adults who maintained relatively stable weight losses	4- to 8-week intervention with very-low-calorie diet, followed by monitoring for 54 months	110.0 ± 2.8 (weight at start), 99.9 ± 2.6 (weight at 54 months) ($P < 0.005$)	Levels are given in mmol/L: TC: 4.8 ± 0.3 at start; 5.0 ± 0.2 at end (NS) TG: 2.0 ± 0.2 at start; 1.5 ± 0.1 at end ($P < 0.05$).
Wood et al. (1988)[93]: Randomized, controlled comparisons of the effect of decreased energy intake or increased exercise on fat weight	131 overweight sedentary men, 47 in the exercise group and 42 each in the diet and control groups	1-year intervention	Exercisers: −4.0 ± 3.9 Dieters: −7.2 ± 3.7 Control subjects: +0.6 ± 3.7	Levels are given in mmol/L: TC: −0.25 ± 0.64 in exercisers −0.36 ± 0.56 in dieters −0.23 ± 0.65 in control subjects (NS) LDL: −0.25 ± 0.61 in exercisers; −0.31 ± 0.64 in dieters; −0.21 ± 0.067 in control subjects (NS) HDL: +0.11 ± 0.15 in exercisers*; 0.12 ± 0.16 in dieters; −0.22 ± 0.11 in control subjects TC/HDL ratio: −0.62 ± 0.86 in exercisers*; 0.79 ± 0.69 in dieters†; −0.04 ± 0.84 in control subjects TG: −0.16 ± 0.53 in exercisers†; −0.27 ± 0.72 in dieters‡; + 0.08 ± 0.60 in control subjects *$P < 0.01$, †$P < 0.001$, ‡$P < 0.05$, versus control subjects
Brolin et al. (1990)[94]: Evaluation of the effect on dyslipidemia of weight loss after gastric bypass surgery	38 patients who underwent gastric bypass for severe obesity and had abnormal lipid levels at time of surgery	Mean follow-up period of 29 months	Weight of patients who lost <50% of excess weight: Group 1: 303 ± 53 at start; 251 ± 41 at 24 months; group 2: 303 ± 53 at start; 251 ± 41 at 24 months	Levels are given in mg/dL: TC: group 1: −263 ± 40 at start, 206 ± 36* at 24 months; group 2: −257 ± 37 at start, 240 ± 22 at 24 months HDL: group 1: −42 ± 3 at start, 55 ± 5* at 24 months; group 2: −36 ± 2 at start, 41 ± 5 at 24 months TG: group 1: −365 ± 275 at start, 150 ± 58* at 24 months; group 2: −341 ± 216 at start, 208 ± 107 at 24 months *$P < 0.05$, versus group 2
Weintraub et al. (1992)[95]: Determination of the efficacy of long-term drug therapy for promoting weight loss and the effect of weight loss on lipid values	121 obese adults	190 weeks of active treatment with low-calorie diets, exercise, and placebo or fenfluramine and phentermine: 20-week follow-up	Weight at start: 93.7 ± 1.3 Weight at week 554 (maximum mean weight loss): 79.6 ± 1.5 Weight at end: 91.4 ± 2.6	Levels are given mg/dl: TC: 198.6 ± 2.9 at start; 182.4 ± 3.1 at week 54*; 207.6 ± 6.0 at end (NS) LDL: 126.0 ± 2.5 at start; 113.9 ± 2.6 at week 54*; 133.6 ± 5.5 at end (NS) HDL: 45.5 ± 0.9 at start; 52.4 ± 1.2 at week 54*; 52.3 ± 2.4 at end* TC/HDL ratio: 4.56 ± 0.11 at start; 3.69 ± 0.12 at week 54 (NS); 4.20 ± 0.19 at end (NS) TG: 129.8 ± 8.5 at start; 89.6 ± 10.7 at week 54*; 109.0 ± 10.2 at end (NS) *$P < 0.01$, compared with corresponding baseline value

TABLE 21–2 Summary of Long-Term Studies of the Effects of Weight Loss on Dyslipidemia—cont'd

Reference (Year): Study Name, Objective	No. and Characteristics of Patients	Study Duration and Intervention	Weight Change (kg, unless otherwise mentioned)	Changes in Lipid Levels
Higgins et al. (1993)[96]: Longitudinal epidemiologic study of subset of Framingham Study population to determine the health effects of weight loss	2500 adults	10-year segment of a 20-year study	Weight changes are age-adjusted annual changes Men who lost weight: −0.52 ±1.14* Men with constant weight: +0.05 ± 1.14 Men who gained weight: 0.60 ± 1.33* Women who lost weight : −0.39 ± 0.86* Women with constant weight: +0.16 ± 0.36 (NS) Women who gained weight: +0.71 ± 1.58*	TC levels are given in mmol/L; changes in TC levels are age-adjusted means Men who lost weight: 6.1 at start; 5.9 at end† Men with constant weight: 6.1 at start; 6.1 at end (NS) Men who gained weight: 6.0 at start; 6.1 at end (NS) Women who lost weight: 6.1 at start; 6.4 at end (NS) Women with constant weight: 5.9 at start; 6.4 at end (NS) Women who gained weight: 5.8 at start; 6.4 at end (NS) *$P < 0.001$, †$P < 0.05$, both compared with no change

HDL, high-density lipoprotein; LDL, low-density lipoprotein; NS, not significant; TC, total cholesterol; TG, triglycerides.

coworkers[91] evaluated the efficacy of the cholesterol-lowering diet used in the Coronary Prevention Evaluation Program in controlling hypertriglyceridemia in 114 men, including 90 with obesity and 50 with hypertriglyceridemia. At the end of 1 year, patients lost a mean of 10 lb, whereas mean serum cholesterol levels decreased by 12.1% and mean serum triglyceride levels decreased by 17.3% ($P = 0.01$ for all changes). Maximum weight loss occurred at 7.4 months after the start of the study. Patients who had regained less than 4 lb by the end of the study at most had a 14.6% decrease in serum cholesterol and a 24.5% decrease in serum triglycerides at 1 year; patients who gained 4 lb or more had decreases of 8.4% and 10.0%, respectively.

In their long-term study of the health benefits of weight loss, Mancini and researchers[92] monitored lipid levels in 71 patients who were treated for severe obesity as hospital inpatients, receiving a very-low-calorie diet for 4 to 8 weeks, and then monitored for 54 months. Their mean body weights were 110.1 ± 2.8 kg at study entry, 97.7 ± 2.4 kg after 30 months, and 99.9 ± 2.6 kg after 54 months, indicating that these patients succeeded in sustaining marked weight loss over a long period. Triglyceride levels decreased significantly, although no significant change in cholesterol occurred.

Wood and coauthors[93] compared the effects on fat weight of decreasing energy intake without increasing exercise or of increasing energy expenditure without altering energy consumption in a 1-year randomized, controlled study including 121 men whose weight was 120% to 160% of ideal body weight. By the end of the study, mean decreases in fat weight for participants in the exercise, diet, and control groups were 4.1 ± 3.7 kg, 5.9 ± 4.1 kg, and 0.3 ± 3.3 kg, respectively ($P \leq 0.001$ for both treatment groups). Both exercisers and dieters lost significant amounts of total body weight when compared with control subjects ($P \leq 0.001$), whereas dieters lost significantly more weight than exercisers ($P \leq 0.01$). Weight loss had a beneficial effect on some lipid values, significantly increasing HDL cholesterol levels and significantly decreasing the ratio of total cholesterol to HDL cholesterol and the concentrations of total cholesterol and LDL cholesterol.

Brolin and colleagues[94] assessed the effect of weight loss in 38 patients who had dyslipidemia when they underwent gastric bypass surgery for severe obesity. At 24 months after surgery, patients were divided into those who had lost at least 50% of their excess weight (group 1) and those who had not (group 2). Group 1 included 26 patients who had lost between 51% and 88% of excess weight, with a mean loss of 64.5%. Group 2 consisted of 12 patients who had lost between 20% and 47% of their excess weight, with a mean loss of 35.2%. Although lipid levels improved in both groups, significant intergroup differences were noted. By the end of the study, hyperlipidemia had resolved in 32 patients, improved in 4 patients, and remained unchanged in 2 patients, although these results were not reported by treatment group. The authors observed that, as long as satisfactory weight loss was maintained, the greatest postoperative reductions in cholesterol and triglyceride levels were likely to occur in the patients with the greatest preoperative increases.

The long-term weight-control study undertaken by Weintraub and coworkers[95] is a particularly valuable contribution to our understanding of the association of lipid levels with obesity, weight loss, and weight regain because it reports weight and lipid levels at the start of the study, at several intermediate points, and at 210 weeks. Participants received 190 weeks of active treatment, including low-calorie diets, exercise, and either placebo or fenfluramine plus phentermine, followed by 20 weeks of follow-up. By week 54, the point of greatest mean weight loss, patients had lost 15% of their total body weight. Accompanying this significant decrease in weight were significant ($P < 0.01$) improvements in levels of total cholesterol, LDL cholesterol, HDL cholesterol, and triglycerides. The ratio of total cholesterol to HDL cholesterol also decreased, although this improvement did not reach statistical significance. By week 210, when patients had regained most of the weight they had lost earlier in the study, mean total cholesterol and LDL cholesterol levels had increased from baseline, whereas nonsignificant improvements in triglyceride levels and the ratio of total cholesterol to HDL cholesterol were sustained. Although the mean HDL cholesterol level decreased from its greatest level, 57.6 ± 1.6 mg/dL at week 139, it remained significantly improved over baseline ($P < 0.01$), suggesting that the maintenance of some degree of weight reduction is at least as important a factor in achieving improved HDL cholesterol levels as the magnitude of weight loss. Increased and sustained amounts of exercise may also have been a factor in improved HDL cholesterol levels.

As part of their 10-year study investigating the health effects of weight loss in 2500 members of the Framingham Study cohort, Higgins and coauthors[96] considered the relationship between weight loss and total cholesterol levels. Changes in cholesterol levels ranged from a decrease of 0.02 mmol/L per year for men who lost weight ($P < 0.05$ vs. men in the stable weight group) to increases of 0.01 to 0.02 mmol/L per year for those whose weight increased or remained unchanged. In women who lost weight, total cholesterol levels increased by 0.03 mmol/L per year, whereas other women had annual increases of 0.05 mmol/L. Because, as mentioned previously, this study did not distinguish between voluntary and disease-related involuntary weight loss, it was not possible to determine the health consequences of these changes in cholesterol levels. By the end of the study period, prevalence rates for both cardiovascular disease and coronary heart disease were greatest among men and women who lost weight.

In two studies of lifestyle intervention in subjects with impaired glucose tolerance, a modest weight loss of 6% from baseline showed an improvement of triglycerides, LDL cholesterol, and HDL cholesterol.[27,97] In the recent report of lifestyle intervention in subjects with type 2 diabetes, a weight loss of 9% was associated at 1 year with a similar improvement of triglycerides, LDL cholesterol and HDL cholesterol (Table 21-3).[98] Thus, the beneficial effect of weight loss on lipids occurs not only in individuals with normal glucose metabolism, but also in individuals with impaired glucose tolerance and type 2 diabetes.

Additional investigations of the type undertaken by Weintraub and coworkers[95] are likely to elucidate further the relationship between weight loss and lipid levels. In the meantime, however, the small size of the changes reported in some studies should not serve as a disincentive to embarking on a weight-loss program, because research indicates that even modest improvements in lipid levels are associated with a decreased risk for cardiovascular disease.[99,100]

TABLE 21–3 Lipid Outcomes in Look AHEAD (Action for Health in Diabetes) at 1 Year

Measure	Intensive Lifestyle Intervention	Diabetes Support and Education
Mean ± SE LDL-C level (mg/dL)		
Baseline	112.2 ± 0.4	112.4 ± 0.6
Year 1	107.0 ± 0.6	106.7 ± 0.7
Change	−5.2 ± 0.6	−5.7 ± 0.6
Mean ± SE HDL-C level (mg/dL)		
Baseline	43.5 ± 0.2	43.6 ± 0.2
Year 1	46.9 ± 0.3	44.9 ± 0.2
Change	3.4 ± 0.2	1.4 ± 0.1
Mean ± SE triglyceride level (mg/dL)		
Baseline	182.8 ± 2.3	180.0 ± 2.4
Year 1	152.5 ± 1.8	165.4 ± 1.9
Change	−30.3 ± 2.0	−14.6 ± 1.8
ADA LDL-C goal of <100 mg/dL (%) ± SE		
Baseline	37.1 ± 1.0	36.9 ± 1.0
Year 1	43.8 ± 1.0	44.9 ± 1.0
Change	6.7 ± 1.0	8.0 ± 1.0
Use of lipid-lowering medicines (%) ± SE		
Baseline	49.4 ± 1.0	48.4 ± 1.0
Year 1	53.0 ± 1.0	57.8 ± 1.0
Change	3.7 ± 0.8	9.4 ± 0.8

ADA, American Diabetes Association; HDL-C, high-density lipoprotein cholesterol; LDL-C, low-density lipoprotein cholesterol; SE, standard error.

From Ref. 98, with permission.

CONCLUSION

Weight loss is difficult to achieve and even more difficult to maintain. Lifestyle change is the method of choice, but it can often be aided by pharmacotherapy. Surgery is becoming significantly more popular for individuals with greater BMIs. Weight loss generally improves lipids in obese patients with dyslipidemia. The triad of low HDL cholesterol level, high triglyceride concentration, and small dense LDL particles is common and responds well to weight loss.

REFERENCES

1. Ogden CL, Carroll MD, Curtin LR, et al.: Prevalence of overweight and obesity in the United States, 1999-2004. *JAMA* 2006;295:1549–1555.
2. Mokdad AH, Serdula MK, Dietz WH, et al.: The spread of the obesity epidemic in the United States, 1991-1998. *JAMA* 1999;282:1519–1522.
3. National Center for Health Statistics: Obesity still a major problem, new data show. Hyattsville, MD: Centers for Disease Control and Prevention, 10-6-2006. 7-11-2007.
4. Hill JO, Wyatt HR, Reed GW, Peters JC: Obesity and the environment: Where do we go from here? *Science* 2003;299:853–855.
5. Prentice AM, Jebb SA: Obesity in Britain: Gluttony or sloth? *BMJ* 1995;311:437–439.
6. Gallagher D, Visser M, Sepulveda D, et al.: How useful is body mass index for comparison of body fatness across age, sex, and ethnic groups? *Am J Epidemiol* 1996;143:228–239.
7. National Heart Lung and Blood Institute: Clinical guidelines on the identification, evaluation, and treatment of overweight and obesity in adults—The evidence report. *Obes Res* 1998;6(suppl 2): 51S–210S.
8. Foster GD, Wadden TA, Vogt RA, Brewer G: What is a reasonable weight toss? Patients' expectations and evaluations of obesity treatment outcomes. *J Consult Clin Psychol* 1997;65:79–85.
9. Blackburn GL: Effect of degree of weight loss on health benefits. *Obes Res* 1995;3(suppl 2):211s–216s.
10. Thomas PR: Weighing the Options: Criteria for Evaluating Weight-Management Programs. Washington, DC, National Academy Press, 1995.
11. Pi-Sunyer FX: A review of long-term studies evaluating the efficacy of weight loss in ameliorating disorders associated with obesity. *Clin Ther* 1996;18:1006–1035.
12. Mahoney M: Cognition and Behavior Modification. Cambridge, MA: Ballinger, 1974.
13. Meichenbaum D: Cognitive Behavior Modification. New York: Plenum, 1977.
14. National Heart Lung and Blood Institute: The Practical Guide, Identification, Evaluation, and Treatment of Overweight and Obesity in Adults. 00-4084. Bethesda, MD: National Institutes of Health, 2000.
15. Wadden TA, Foster GD: Behavioral assessment and treatment of markedly obese patients. In Wadden TA, Van Itallie TB (eds): Treatment of the Severely Obese Patient. New York: Guilford, 1992, pp 290–330.
16. Wilson GT: Cognitive behavior therapy: Paradigm shift or passing phase? In Foreyt JP, Rathjen DP (eds): Cognitive Behavior Therapy. New York: Plenum Press, 2003, pp 7–32.
17. Perri MG, McAdoo WG, Spevak PA, et al.: Effect of a multicomponent maintenance program on long-term weight loss. *J Consult Clin Psychol* 1984;52:480–481.
18. Wadden TA, Sternberg JA, Letizia KA, et al.: Treatment of obesity by very low calorie diet, behavior therapy, and their combination: A five-year perspective. *Int J Obes* 1989;13(suppl 2):39–46.
19. Baum JG, Clark HB, Sandler J: Preventing relapse in obesity through posttreatment maintenance systems: Comparing the relative efficacy of two levels of therapist support. *J Behav Med* 1991;14:287–302.
20. Knowler WC, Barrett-Connor E, Fowler SE, et al.: Reduction in the incidence of type 2 diabetes with lifestyle intervention or metformin. *N Engl J Med* 2002;346:393–403.
21. Perri MG, McAdoo WG, McAllister DA, et al.: Effects of peer support and therapist contact on long-term weight loss. *J Consult Clin Psychol* 1987;55:615–617.
22. Hill JO, Wyatt HR, Phelan S, et al.: The National Weight Control Registry: Is it useful in helping deal with our obesity epidemic? *J Nutr Educ Behav* 2005;37:206–210.
23. Lichtman SW, Pisarska K, Berman ER, et al.: Discrepancy between self-reported and actual caloric intake and exercise in obese subjects. *N Engl J Med* 1992;327:1893–1898.
24. Centers for Disease Control and Prevention: Dietary Intake of Macronutrients, Micronutrients, and Other Dietary Constituents, USA, 1988-1994, series 11, no 245. Hyattsville, MD, National Center for Health Statistics, 2002.
25. Flechtner-Mors M, Ditschuneit HH, Johnson TD, et al.: Metabolic and weight loss effects of long-term dietary intervention in obese patients: Four-year results. *Obes Res* 2000;8:399–402.
26. Johnston PK: Vegetarian nutrition; proceedings of a symposium held in Arlington, VA. *Am J Clin Nutr* 1994;59:1099S–1262S.
27. Tuomilehto J, Lindstrom J, Eriksson JG, et al.: Prevention of type 2 diabetes mellitus by changes in lifestyle among subjects with impaired glucose tolerance. *N Engl J Med* 2001;344: 1343–1350.
28. Knowler WC, Barrett-Connor E, Fowler SE, et al.: Reduction in the incidence of type 2 diabetes with lifestyle intervention or metformin. *N Engl J Med* 2002;346:393–403.
29. de Lorgeril M, Salen P, Martin JL, et al.: Mediterranean diet, traditional risk factors, and the rate of cardiovascular complications after myocardial infarction: Final report of the Lyon Diet Heart Study. *Circulation* 1999;99:779–785.
30. Ornish D, Brown SE, Scherwitz LW, et al.: Can lifestyle changes reverse coronary heart disease? The Lifestyle Heart Trial. *Lancet* 1990;336:129–133.
31. Skov AR, Toubro S, Ronn B, et al.: Randomized trial on protein vs carbohydrate in ad libitum fat reduced diet for the treatment of obesity. *Int J Obes Relat Metab Disord* 1999;23:528–536.
32. Brehm BJ, Seeley RJ, Daniels SR, D'Alessio DA: A randomized trial comparing a very low carbohydrate diet and a calorie-restricted low fat diet on body weight and cardiovascular risk factors in healthy women. *J Clin Endocrinol Metab* 2003;88: 1617–1623.
33. Samaha FF, Iqbal N, Seshadri P, et al.: A low-carbohydrate as compared with a low-fat diet in severe obesity. *N Engl J Med* 2003;348:2074–2081.
34. Foster GD, Wyatt H, Hill JO, et al.: A randomized trial of a low-carbohydrate diet for obesity. *N Engl J Med* 2003;348:2082–2090.
35. Stern L, Iqbal N, Seshadri P, et al.: The effects of low-carbohydrate versus conventional weight loss diets in severely obese adults: One-year follow-up of a randomized trial. *Ann Intern Med* 2004;140:778–785.
36. Yang MU, Van Itallie TB: Reducing primary risk factors by therapeutic weight loss. In Wadden TA, Van Itallie TB (eds): Treatment of the Seriously Obese Patient. New York: Guilford Press, 1992:83–106.
37. Wadden TA, Foster GD, Letizia KA: One year behavioral treatment of obesity: Comparison of moderate and severe caloric restriction and the effects of weight maintenance therapy. *N Engl J Med* 1994;62:165–171.
38. Pi-Sunyer FX: The role of very-low-calorie diets in obesity. *Am J Clin Nutr* 1992;56:240S–243S.
39. Wing RR: Physical activity in the treatment of the adulthood overweight and obesity: Current evidence and research issues. *Med Sci Sports Exerc* 1999;31:S547–S552.
40. Pavlou KN, Krey S, Steffee WP: Exercise as an adjunct to weight loss and maintenance in moderately obese subjects. *Am J Clin Nutr* 1989;49:1115–1123.
41. Wadden TA, Vogt R, Andersen R, et al.: Exercise in the treatment of obesity: Effects of four interventions on body composition, resting energy expenditure, and mood. *J Consult Clin Psychol* 1997;65:269–277.
42. Klem ML, Wing RR, McGuire MT, et al.: A descriptive study of individuals successful at long-term maintenance of substantial weight loss. *Am J Clin Nutr* 1997;66:239–246.
43. Harris JK, French SA, Jeffrey RW, et al.: Dietary and physical activity correlates of long-term weight loss. *Obes Res* 1994;2: 307–313.

44. Kayman S, Bruvold W, Stern JS: Maintenance and relapse after weight loss in women: Behavioral aspects. *Am J Clin Nutr* 1990;52:800–807.
45. McGuire MT, Wing RR, Klem ML, et al.: What predicts weight regain in a group of successful weight losers? *J Consult Clin Psychol* 1999;67:177–185.
46. Stefanick ML, Mackey S, Sheehan M, et al.: Effects on diet and exercise in men and postmenopausal women with low levels of HDL cholesterol and high levels of low density lipoprotein (LDL) cholesterol. *N Engl J Med* 1998;339:12–20.
47. Bouchard C, Perusse L, Leblanc C, et al.: Inheritance of the amount and distribution of human body fat. *Int J Obes* 1988;12:205–215.
48. Bouchard C, Tremblay A, Despres JP, et al.: The response to long-term overfeeding in identical twins. *N Engl J Med* 1990;24:1477–1482.
49. Wadden TA, Berkowitz R, Sarwer D, et al.: Benefits of lifestyle modification in the pharmacologic treatment of obesity: A randomized trial. *Arch Intern Med* 2001;161:218–227.
50. Heck A, Yanovski J, Calis J: Orlistat, a new lipase inhibitor for the management of obesity. *Pharmacotherapy* 2000;20: 270–279.
51. Sjöström L, Rissanen A, Andersen T, et al.: Randomised placebo-controlled trial of orlistat for weight loss and prevention of weight regain in obese patients. European Multicentre Orlistat Study Group. *Lancet* 1998;352:167–172.
52. Davidson MH, Hauptman J, DiGirolamo M, et al.: Weight control and risk factor reduction in obese subjects treated for 2 years with orlistat: A randomized controlled trial. *JAMA* 1999;281: 235–242.
53. Bray GA, Blackburn GL, Ferguson JM, et al.: Sibutramine produces dose-related weight loss. *Obes Res* 1999;7:189–198.
54. Apfelbaum M, Vague P, Ziegler O, et al.: Long-term maintenance of weight loss after a very-low-calorie diet: A randomized blinded trial of the efficacy and tolerability of sibutramine. *Am J Med* 1999;106:179–184.
55. Hansen D, Astrup A, Toubro S, et al.: Predictors of weight loss and maintenance during 2 years of treatment by sibutramine in obesity. Results from the European multi-centre STORM trial. Sibutramine Trial of Obesity Reduction and Maintenance. *Int J Obes Relat Metab Disord* 2001;25:496–501.
56. McMahon FG, Weinstein SP, Rowe E, et al.: Sibutramine is safe and effective for weight loss in obese patients whose hypertension is well controlled with angiotensin-converting enzyme inhibitors. *J Hum Hypertens* 2002;16:5–11.
57. Sramek JJ, Leibowitz MT, Weinstein SP, et al.: Efficacy and safety of sibutramine for weight loss in obese patients with hypertension well controlled by beta-adrenergic blocking agents: A placebo-controlled, double-blind, randomised trial. *J Hum Hypertens* 2002;16:13–19.
58. Munro J, MacCuish A, Wilson E, et al.: Comparison of continuous and intermittent anoretic therapy in obesity. *Br Med J* 1968;1:352–356.
59. Williams RA, Foulsham BM: Weight reduction in osteoarthritis using phentermine. *Practitioner* 1981;225:231–232.
60. Connolly HM, Crary JL, McGoon MD, et al.: Valvular heart disease associated with fenfluramine-phentermine. *N Engl J Med* 1997;28:581–588.
61. Connolly H, McGoon M: Obesity drugs and the heart. *Curr Probl Cardiol* 1999;24:745–792.
62. Abenhaim L, Moride Y, Brenot F, et al.: Appetite-suppressant drugs and the risk of primary pulmonary hypertension. International Primary Pulmonary Hypertension Study Group. *N Engl J Med* 1996;335:609–616.
63. Gastrointestinal surgery for severe obesity: National Institutes of Health Consensus Development Conference Statement. *Am J Clin Nutr* 1992;55:615S–619S.
64. Scopinaro N, Gianetta E, Adami GF, et al.: Biliopancreatic diversion for obesity at eighteen years. *Surgery* 1996;119:261–268.
65. Sugerman HJ, Kellum JM, Engle KM, et al.: Gastric bypass for treating severe obesity. *Am J Clin Nutr* 1992;55:560S–566S.
66. Sjöström L, Larsson B, Backman L, et al.: Swedish Obese Subjects (SOS). Recruitment for an intervention study and a selected description of the obese state. *Int J Obes* 1992;16:465–479.
67. Sjöström C, Peltonen M, Wedel H, et al.: Differentiated long-term effects of intentional weight loss on diabetes and hypertension. *Hypertension* 2000;36:20–25.
68. Sjöström L, Narbro K, Sjostrom CD, et al.: Effects of bariatric surgery on mortality in Swedish obese subjects. *N Engl J Med* 2007;357:741–752.
69. Adams T, Gress R, Smith S, et al.: Long-term mortality after gastric bypass surgery. *N Engl J Med* 2007;357:753–761.
70. Bray GA: Effect of caloric restriction on energy expenditure in obese patients. *Lancet* 1969;2:397–398.
71. Nelson KM, Weinsier RL, Long CL, et al.: Prediction of resting energy expenditure from fat-free mass and fat mass. *Am J Clin Nutr* 1992;56:848–856.
72. Heshka S, Yang MU, Wang J, et al.: Weight loss and change in resting metabolic rate. *Am J Clin Nutr* 1990;52:981–986.
73. Weigle DS, Sande KJ, Iverius PH, et al.: Weight loss leads to a marked decrease in nonresting energy expenditure in ambulatory human subjects. *Metabolism* 2002;37:930–936.
74. Després JP: Lipoprotein metabolism in visceral obesity. *Int J Obes* 1991;15(suppl 2):45–52.
75. Ong JM, Simsolo RB, Saghizadeh M, et al.: Effects of exercise training and feeding on lipoprotein lipase gene expression in adipose tissue, heart, and skeletal muscle of the rat. *Metabolism* 1995;44:1596–1605.
76. Rodin J, Schank D, Striegel-Moore R: Psychological features of obesity. *Med Clin North Am* 1989;73:47–66.
77. Van Itallie TB, Kissileff HR: Physiology of energy intake: An inventory control model. *Am J Clin Nutr* 1985;42:914–923.
78. Perri MG, Nezu AM, Patti ET, et al.: Effect of length of treatment on weight loss. *J Consult Clin Psychol* 1989;57:450–452.
79. Despres JP, Moorjani S, Lupien PJ, et al.: Regional distribution of body fat, plasma lipoproteins, and cardiovascular disease. *Arteriosclerosis* 1990;10:497–511.
80. Krauss RM: Triglycerides and atherogenic lipoproteins: Rationale for lipid management. *Am J Med* 1998;105:58S–62S.
81. Dattilo AM: Effects of weight reduction on blood lipids and lipoproteins: A meta-analysis. *Am J Clin Nutr* 1992;56:320–328.
82. Eckel RH, Yost TJ: HDL subfractions and adipose tissue metabolism the reduced-obese state. *Am J Physiol* 1989;256(6 pt 1): E740–E746.
83. Kanders BS, Blackburn GL: Reducing primary risk factors by therapeutic weight loss. In Wadden TA, Van Itallie TB (eds): Treatment of the Seriously Obese Patient. New York: Guilford Press, 1992, pp 213–230.
84. Pi-Sunyer FX: Short-term medical benefits and adverse effects of weight loss. *Ann Intern Med* 1993;119:722–726.
85. Pi-Sunyer FX: Health implications of obesity. *Am J Clin Nutr* 1991;1595S–1603S.
86. Follick M, Abrams D, Smith T, et al.: Contrasting short- and long-term effects of weight loss on lipoprotein levels. *Arch Intern Med* 1984;144:1571–1574.
87. Carmena R, Ascaso J, Tebar J, et al.: Changes in plasma high-density lipoproteins after body weight reduction in obese women. *Int J Obes* 1984;8:135–140.
88. Fachnie JD, Foreback CC: Effects of weight reduction, exercise, and diet modification on lipids and apolipoproteins A-1 and B in severely obese persons. *Henry Ford Hosp Med J* 1987;35:216–220.
89. Schieffer B, Moore D, Funke E, et al.: Reduction of atherogenic risk factors by short-term weight reduction. Evidence of the efficacy of National Cholesterol Education Program guidelines for the obese. *Klin Wochenschr* 1991;69:163–167.
90. Wylie-Rosett J, Swencionis C, Peters MH, et al.: A weight reduction intervention that optimizes use of practitioner's time, lowers glucose level, and raises HDL cholesterol level in older adults. *J Am Diet Assoc* 1994;94:37–42.
91. Hall Y, Stamler J, Cohen DB, et al.: Effectiveness of a low saturated fat, low cholesterol, weight-reducing diet for the control of hypertriglyceridemia. *Atherosclerosis* 1972;16:389–403.
92. Mancini M, Di Biase G, Contaldo F, et al.: Medical complications of severe obesity: Importance of treatment by very-low-calorie diets: Intermediate and long-term effects. *Int J Obes* 1981;5: 341–352.
93. Wood PD, Stefanick ML, Dreon DM, et al.: Changes in plasma lipids and lipoproteins in overweight men during weight loss through dieting as compared with exercise. *N Engl J Med* 1988;319:1173–1179.
94. Brolin RE, Kenler HA, Wilson AC, et al.: Serum lipids after gastric bypass surgery for morbid obesity. *Int J Obes* 1990;14: 939–950.

95. Weintraub M, Sundaresan P, Schuster B: Long-term weight control study VII (weeks 0–210). *Clin Pharmacol Ther* 1992;51:634–641.
96. Higgins M, D'Agostino RB, Kannel W, et al.: Benefits and adverse effects of weight loss: Observations from the Framingham Study. *Ann Intern Med* 1993;119:758–763.
97. Knowler WC, Barrett-Connor E, Fowler SE, et al.: Reduction in the incidence of type 2 diabetes with lifestyle intervention or metformin. *N Engl J Med* 2002;346:393–403.
98. Pi-Sunyer FX, Blackburn GL, Brancati, et al.: Reduction in weight and cardiovascular disease risk factors in individuals with type 2 diabetes: One-year results of the Look AHEAD Trial. *Diabetes Care* 2007;30:1374–1383.
99. Goldstein DJ: Beneficial health effects of modest weight loss. *Int J Obes* 1992;16:397–415.
100. National Cholesterol Education Program: Second Report of the Expert Panel on Detection, Evaluation, and Treatment of High Blood Cholesterol in Adults (Adult Treatment Panel II). *Circulation* 1994;89:1333–1445.

CHAPTER 22

Statins

James M. McKenney, Peter Ganz, Barbara S. Wiggins, and Joseph S. Saseen

INTRODUCTION

The identification of inhibitors of the enzyme 3-hydroxy-3-methylglutaryl–coenzyme A (HMG-CoA) reductase led to the class of drugs known as *statins.* These agents have become arguably the most important discovery ever made in mankind's effort to reduce the burden of the number one killer of people throughout the world, atherosclerotic vascular disease. This discovery culminated in the labs of Dr. Akira Endo at Sankyo in Japan in the early 1970s, when the first statin, called *ML-236B* (later called *mevastatin* and *compactin*), was extracted from the fungus *Penicillium citrinum.*[1] Because of undefined "toxic effects" observed in dogs, mevastatin was not developed. However, another statin, pravastatin, was subsequently developed in this laboratory a decade later and marketed.

Building on Dr. Endo's discovery, scientists at Merck & Company isolated their first statin (initially called *mevinolin, monacolin K,* and *MK803*) from *Aspergillus terreus* in 1976. After completing clinical trials demonstrating low-density lipoprotein (LDL) cholesterol–lowering efficacy and safety, Merck & Company launched the first statin made available to the public, lovastatin (Mevacor), in 1987. Lovastatin and the other statins that followed have resulted in a substantial reduction in virtually all clinical manifestations of atherosclerotic vascular disease, including coronary events, strokes, and revascularization procedures, and have prolonged the lives of millions of people. As Paul Harvey, a radio personality in Chicago, would say, "and now we know the rest of the story"—the story of statins that will be reviewed briefly in this chapter.

CHEMISTRY

Six statins are currently on the U.S. market; three are derived from fungi (lovastatin, simvastatin, and pravastatin), and three are synthetic (fluvastatin, atorvastatin, and rosuvastatin) (Fig. 22-1). All statins share an HMG-CoA–like moiety, a dihydroxy heptanoic acid, which competes with HMG-CoA for binding with HMG-CoA reductase. The fungal statins have in common a naphthalenyl ester base structure and differ from each other only by a methyl or hydroxyl side group. The synthetic statins have in common a flurinated phenyl group, a methylethyl side chain, and a base structure made up of a five- or six-member ring with 1 or 2 carbon atoms substituted with a nitrogen atom (i.e., indole [fluvastatin], pyrrol [atorvastatin], and pyrimidine [rosuvastatin] rings) and side groups. Each of these structural elements participates in the interaction with the reductase enzyme, as will be explained later in the chapter.[2–7]

Fluvastatin exists as a racemic mixture with an active *3R,5S* enantiomer that contributes to LDL cholesterol lowering and an inactive *3S,5R* enantiomer that does not.[3]

MECHANISM OF ACTION

All isoprenoids and sterols in the body, including cholesterol, are derived from mevalonate. Mevalonate is derived from a 4-electron reduction of HMG-CoA, an early step in the biosynthesis of cholesterol catalyzed by the enzyme HMG-CoA reductase. All statins inhibit this step by competing for the catalytic binding domain for HMG-CoA in the HMG-CoA reductase molecule (Fig. 22-2). The HMG-CoA–like moiety of each statin (the dihydroxy heptanoic acid group) (see Fig. 22-1) occupies the HMG-CoA–binding pocket in the HMG-CoA reductase molecule and links via its O5 hydroxy group.[8] Statins are competitive inhibitors of HMG-CoA and have a several-fold higher affinity for binding sites in the reductase molecule than does HMG-CoA. Inhibitory constants for statins (K_i) are in the range of 5 to 44 nM, whereas the Michaelis constant (K_m) for HMG-CoA is 4 μM. Once the HMG-CoA moiety is in the binding

HMG-CoA

Simvastatin

Lovastatin

Pravastatin

Fluvastatin

Atorvastatin

Rosuvastatin

FIGURE 22-1 The chemical structure of statins.

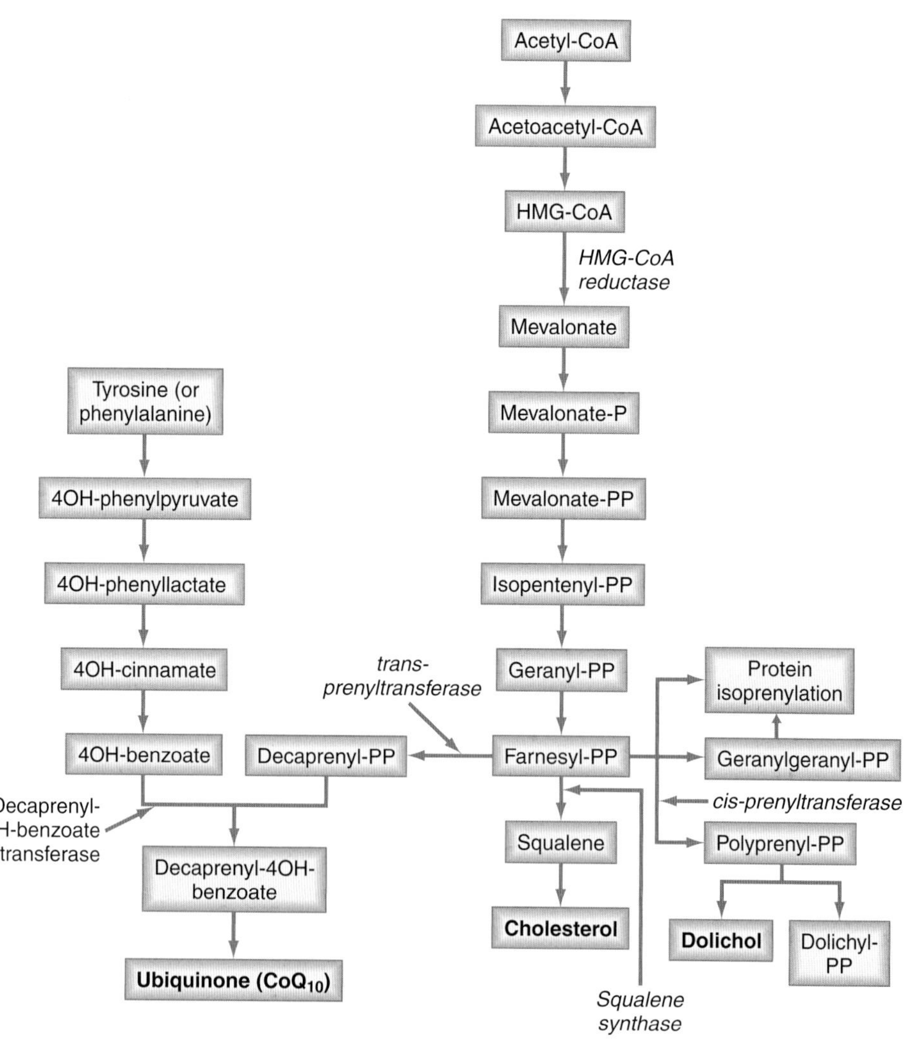

FIGURE 22-2 The cholesterol biosynthesis pathway. P, Phosphate; PP, pyrophosphate.

pocket, the remainder of the statin structure undergoes a conformational change in order to maximize contact with, and binding to, amino acid residues of the reductase. A variety of bonds are in play, including van der Walls contacts, hydrogen bonds, and polar interactions. The number and strength of these bonds vary among statins, and this in part dictates the length and degree of inhibition, which, in turn, results in the varying levels of LDL cholesterol–lowering efficacy. For example, rosuvastatin forms nine bonding interactions with the reductase and is the most potent LDL cholesterol–lowering statin. Atorvastatin forms eight bonding interactions with the enzyme and is the next most potent. The fungal statins have six bonding interactions with the enzyme.[8] By using a purified catalytic fragment of human HMG-CoA reductase in a cell-free system, the absolute potency of the statins has been determined. In these experiments, the statin concentrations required to inhibit 50% of the HMG-CoA reductase activity (IC_{50}) for pravastatin, fluvastatin, simvastatin, atorvastatin, and rosuvastatin were 44, 28, 11, 8.2, and 3.5 to 5.4 nM, respectively.[9,10]

Inhibition of HMG-CoA reductase leads to a reduction of cholesterol synthesis in the hepatocyte, a reduction in the cholesterol pool, and subsequent up-regulation of nuclear transcription factors, specifically sterol regulatory element–binding proteins (SREBPs), which increase the transcription of LDL receptors (also called B/E receptors) on the hepatic cell surface. The LDL receptors link with apolipoprotein (apo) B and apoE on the surface of circulating LDL and very-low-density lipoprotein (VLDL) particles and integrate them as well as their lipid content into the hepatocyte[11] (Fig. 22-3). The LDL receptors are also up-regulated when hepatic cholesterol is converted to bile acids through the action of CYP7A1, 7α-hydroxylase, to aid with the absorption of food from the gastrointestinal tract.

The reduction of circulating cholesterol with statin therapy has not been found to cause adverse systemic effects in nonhepatic cells that use cholesterol to manufacture sterol and other important biologic products. For example, andrology studies in statin-taking patients have shown that the quantity, quality, and functioning of sperm are not affected, nor are adrenal gland hormones.

Every cell in the body has the ability to synthesize cholesterol to help maintain membrane integrity. It is conceivable that statins could enter these cells, disrupt cholesterol biosynthesis, and interfere with normal cell functioning. This is one of the hypotheses given to explain the myotoxicity associated with these agents. A reduction of cholesterol synthesis in the muscle cell could lead to instability of the cell membrane that could, in turn, lead to cell lysis or rupture and symptoms of myopathy. More on this issue will be addressed in our discussion of adverse effects later in the chapter.

In addition to lowering blood cholesterol levels by up-regulating LDL receptors and removing circulating LDL and VLDL particles from the circulation, statins also reduce assembly and secretion of VLDL particles from the liver.[12,13] The more potent the inhibiting effect of the statin, the more this mechanism contributes to LDL cholesterol–lowering efficacy. Because of this mechanism, statins can lower LDL cholesterol levels in patients with no functional LDL receptors, such as occurs in homozygous familial hypercholesterolemia patients.

In reducing the production of mevalonate, other downstream products, in addition to cholesterol, are also reduced (see Fig. 22-2). For example, dolichols, which have an essential role in lipoprotein synthesis; ubiquinones, which are involved in electron transport; and isoprenoids, which take part in the post-translational modification of many proteins, including cell wall proliferation, are affected. The degree to which a reduction in these products of mevalonate is clinically important is widely debated. Some specialists hold that these and other changes contribute to the pleiotropic (non–LDL cholesterol) effects that are part of the coronary risk reduction properties of statins, while others point out that such changes may mediate the toxic effects of statins, particularly in the muscle and other organs.

LIPID-INDEPENDENT ACTIONS

Although statins have demonstrated reductions in cardiovascular morbidity and mortality, they confer only partial salvage and fail to reduce clinical events in approximately two thirds of treated subjects.[14–16] At present, decisions about the use and dosing of statins are linked to blood lipid concentrations.[17] A more complete understanding of the biologic actions that are independent of the lipid-lowering effects may lead to better utilization and greater effectiveness.

Because of the strong statistical association between serum cholesterol levels and cardiovascular events, reduction of serum cholesterol levels by statins has been proposed as the principal, if not the sole, mechanism underlying the beneficial effects of statins.[18] Furthermore, therapies that lower cholesterol independently of HMG-CoA reductase inhibition, such as partial ileal bypass surgery and cholestyramine, also improve cardiovascular outcomes, suggesting that statins at least in part also exert their benefit by lowering cholesterol.[19,20]

Nevertheless, evidence from basic and clinical studies suggests that statins also have several actions that are independent of cholesterol lowering: (1) Statins can attenuate inflammation and improve features associated with plaque stability in atheroma of nonhuman primates[21]; (2) blood C-reactive protein (CRP), a marker

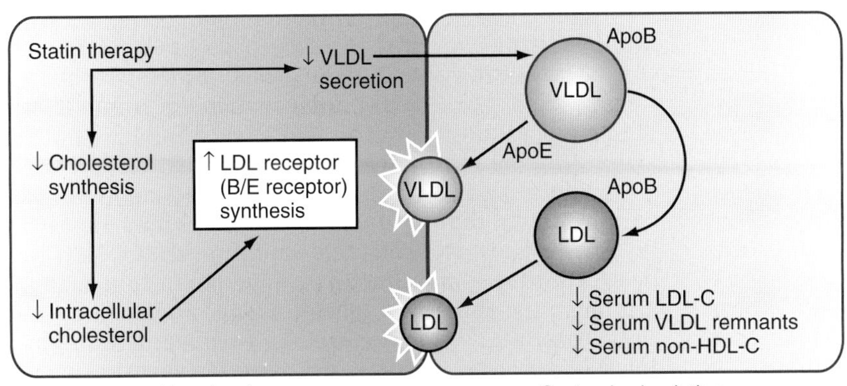

FIGURE 22-3 Statin mechanisms of action. Statins reduce hepatic cholesterol synthesis, lower intracellular cholesterol, stimulate up-regulation of low-density lipoprotein (LDL) receptors, reduce the secretion of very-low-density lipoprotein (VLDL) particles from the hepatocyte, and increase the uptake of non–high-density lipoprotein (non-HDL) particles (small dense LDL, VLDL remnants) from the systemic circulation. Apo, apolipoprotein; LDL-C, low-density lipoprotein cholesterol; HDL-C, high-density lipoprotein cholesterol.

of inflammation, is reduced by statins independently of the magnitude of cholesterol lowering[22,23] and probably too rapidly to be attributed to lipid lowering[24,25]; (3) consistent with these data, ezetimibe, which lowers cholesterol by reducing its absorption in the intestine without inhibiting HMG-CoA reductase,[26,27] fails to decrease CRP when used as the sole agent[28]; (4) in humans, statins improve endothelial function rapidly, before any appreciable reduction in serum cholesterol can be detected[29]; (5) in head-to-head comparisons, only statins, and not ezetimibe, improve endothelial function when identical reductions in LDL cholesterol are achieved by these agents[30,31]; (6) statins reverse endothelial dysfunction in young smokers with normal LDL cholesterol levels[32]; (7) regression of coronary atherosclerosis[22] and the improvement in clinical outcomes[33] with intensive statin therapy are also related equally and independently of CRP and LDL cholesterol reductions.

In sum, accumulating evidence suggests that statins exert an array of beneficial effects that are independent of LDL cholesterol lowering. Yet the concept of clinically relevant "lipid-independent" benefits of statins will most likely not be embraced until specific molecular pathways favorably altered by statins are convincingly identified in humans. Several molecular mechanisms have been proposed.[34] Among these, the inhibition of the Rho/Rho kinase (ROCK) signaling pathway by statins has the greatest support[35–37] and hence will be discussed in greater detail.

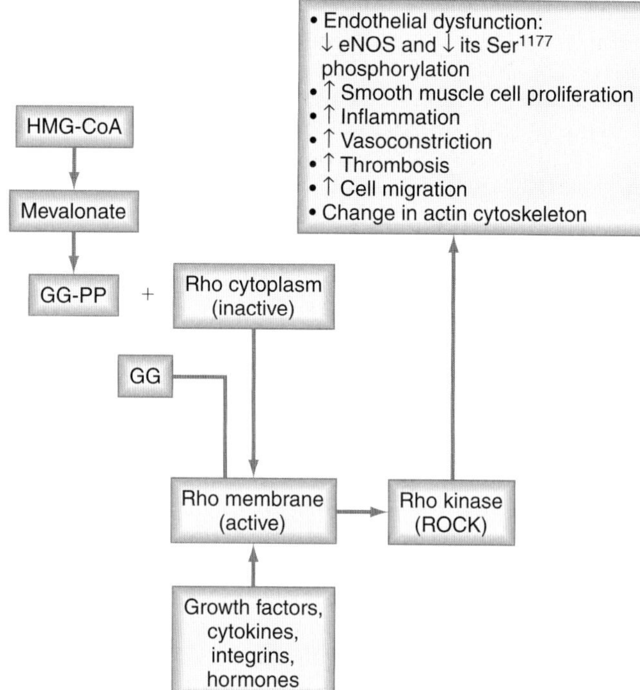

FIGURE 22-4 Rho/Rho kinase (Rho/ROCK) signaling pathway. Rho is present in the cytoplasm in an inactive state. Covalent modification of Rho by geranylgeranylation (isoprenylation) facilitates translocation of Rho to the cell membrane, where it can be activated (e.g., by growth factors, cytokines, integrins, and hormones). Rho in turn activates ROCK and leads to stimulation of characteristic cellular dysfunction associated with atherosclerosis (e.g., endothelial dysfunction, inflammation, cell migration, vascular smooth muscle contraction, and proliferation) eNOS, endothelial nitric oxide synthase; *GG*, geranylgeranyl; HMG-CoA, 3-hydroxy-3-methylglutaryl–coenzyme A; PP, pyrophoshate.

Rho/Rho kinase (Rho/ROCK) Signaling Pathway

Recent evidence has pointed to an important role for small GTP-binding proteins, such as Rho, in mediating diverse cellular functions.[38] Several classes of Rho described in mammals—RhoA, RhoB, and RhoC—have the same amino-acid sequence in their effector sequence, appear to have similar intracellular targets,[38,39] and are collectively referred to here as *Rho.* ROCK, a serine/threonine kinase, is the principal downstream effector of Rho.[40–42] Two isoforms of ROCK have overlapping functions but different cellular distributions.[40–43] The substrates of ROCK-mediated phosphorylation include components of the cytoskeleton and contractile apparatus.[39,43]

The Role of Rho/ROCK in Atherosclerosis

Through the control of the cytoskeleton, ROCK is a pivotal regulator of cell attachment, shape, contraction, movement, proliferation, and gene expression.[35,37,44] These functions constitute critical steps in the initiation and progression of atherosclerosis. Among the activators of Rho/ROCK, many are overexpressed in atherosclerosis, including oxidized LDL, various growth factors, cytokines, integrins, hormones, and G protein–coupled receptor ligands.[37,44,45,46] Stimulation of Rho/ROCK has proatherogenic consequences (Fig. 22-4). These include reduced endothelial nitric oxide synthase (eNOS) expression and its Ser[1177] phosphorylation,[44,46–49] enhanced vascular smooth muscle contraction,[50,51] heightened vascular inflammation,[50,52–55] increased endothelin-1,[56] increased plasminogen activator inhibitor–1 (PAI-1) accompanied by a reduction in tissue plasminogen activator (t-PA),[57,58] increased endothelial tissue factor expression,[59] increased angiotensin type 1 receptor density,[60] and increased vascular smooth muscle proliferation.[61,62] Thus, Rho/ROCK activation induces many characteristic dysfunctions that underlie atherosclerosis.

Selective Inhibitors of Rho/ROCK Support a Key Role for This Pathway in Cardiovascular Diseases

Rho/ROCK inhibitors have served as useful probes to delve into the role of this pathway in cardiovascular diseases *in vivo.* In animals, selective inhibition of Rho or ROCK reduces vascular leukocyte adhesion,[63] suppresses coronary neointimal formation, and regresses coronary arteriosclerosis.[53,64–66] It suppresses neointima formation after stent implantation,[67] prevents coronary artery spasm,[68] suppresses cardiac allograft vasculopathy,[69] prevents hypertension in spontaneously hypertensive rats,[70] improves left ventricular remodeling after myocardial infarction (MI),[71] and reduces infarct size following middle cerebral artery ligation.[36]

In humans, fasudil hydrochloride (1-[5-isoquinolinesulfonyl]-2-methylpiperazine, also known as HA1077, AT877, or Eril), is a selective inhibitor of ROCK. It has been approved for clinical use in Japan since 1987, although its ability to inhibit ROCK was recognized only recently.[37,72–75] In patients with variant angina, intracoronary fasudil prevents coronary vasospasm.[76–78]

Intrabrachial infusion of fasudil reduces the forearm vascular resistance in hypertensive subjects and in smokers over that of healthy controls, suggesting that vascular Rho/ROCK is overactive in the presence of atherogenic risk factors.[79–81] Fasudil markedly reduces myocardial ischemia in patients with stable coronary disease,[82,83] likely by improving endothelial function.[84]

Evidence of Inhibition of Rho/ROCK Pathway by Statins

The cholesterol biosynthetic pathway produces metabolic intermediates called *isoprenoids,* including farnesyl pyrophosphate (FPP) and geranylgeranyl pyrophosphate (GGPP)[35,36,45,46] (Fig. 22-5). FPP and GGPP are intracellular signaling molecules that bind to proteins (isoprenylation) and in particular activate a group of GTP-binding proteins that includes Rho.[35,36,45,46] Rho is present in the cytoplasm in an inactive GDP-bound state, and isoprenylation targets Rho to the cell membrane, where it cycles between the active GTP-bound and the inactive GDP-bound states.

Experimental studies have shown that by decreasing intracellular GGPP concentrations, statins reduce Rho/ROCK activity.[35,36,45,46] This produces a decrease or even a complete reversal of most of the proatherogenic cellular dysfunctions listed earlier, including enhanced production of endothelium-derived nitric oxide through eNOS mRNA stabilization, increased eNOS protein expression,[35,36,46,48] and enhanced eNOS Ser[1177] phosphorylation.[47,49,85] Furthermore, inhibition of Rho/ROCK signaling by statins leads to other favorable effects, including reductions in endothelin-1 production,[56] vascular smooth muscle cell proliferation,[61] vascular inflammation,[52–55] and propensity for thrombosis.[57–59] While the ability of relatively high doses of statins to inhibit the Rho/ROCK pathway has been shown across several species *in vivo,*[47,86] no information regarding whether statins inhibit Rho/ROCK pathway in doses used in humans in clinical practice is available. Therefore it is also not known whether this contributes to statins' ability to reverse cellular dysfunctions characteristic of atherosclerosis. Knowledge of the biologic effects of statins should lead to a more optimal utilization of these agents and should pave the way for the development of more effective statins or statin–ROCK inhibitor combinations.

PHARMACOKINETIC CHARACTERISTICS

Statins possess different pharmacokinetic properties, which may result in clinically relevant differences in their efficacy and safety. A comparison of some of the pharmacokinetic properties of these agents is listed in Table 22-1.

Lactone Forms

Two of the statins, lovastatin and simvastatin, are administered as prodrugs, in that they exist as an inactive lactone and must be converted to the active, open acid form once administered (Fig. 22-1; see Table 22-1) The lactone bond is easily hydrolyzed by enzymatic action, probably in the liver and potentially also in the gut. *In vivo,* statin prodrugs, and possibly all statins, exist in equilibrium between the lactone and open acid form. Lactone forms are highly lipid soluble and easily diffuse across cell membranes.

Lipophilicity

Statins also differ in their degree of lipophilicity or lipid solubility. The most lipid soluble are the lactone statins, lovastatin and simvastatin. The logarithm of the partition coefficient (log *P*) of statins (see Table 22-1) reflects their lipophilicity. The open acid forms of lovastatin and simvastatin, as well as fluvastatin and atorvastatin, have high log *P* values, identifying their relatively high lipophilicity.[87] The more lipid soluble the statin, the more easily it crosses cell membranes and gains access to hepatic and nonhepatic cells by passive diffusion. The hydroxyl substitution in the

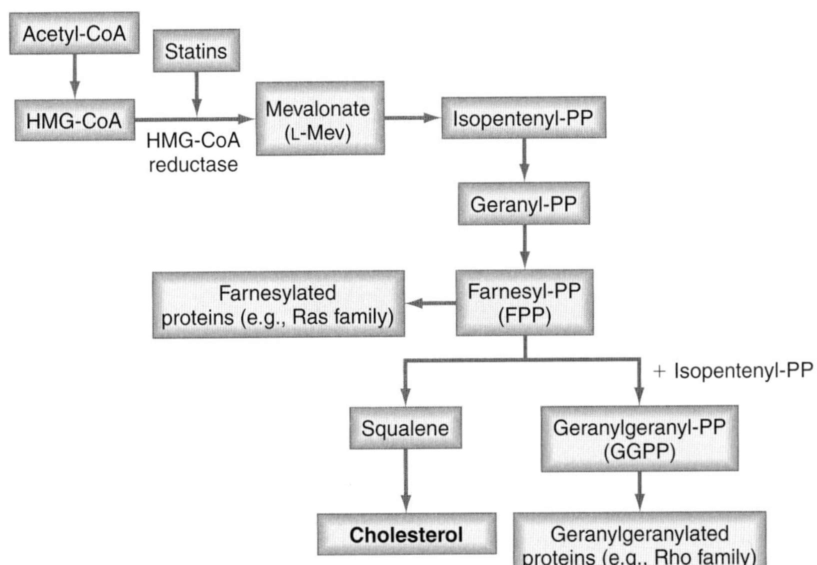

FIGURE 22-5 Cholesterol biosynthetic pathway. In addition to producing cholesterol, this pathway gives rise to intermediates with putative proatherogenic activities, such as geranylgeranyl and farnesyl pyrophosphate. These intermediates activate Rho and Ras signaling.

TABLE 22-1 Pharmacokinetic Variables of Marketed Statins

Variable	Atorvastatin	Fluvastatin	Lovastatin	Pravastatin	Rosuvastatin	Simvastatin
Prodrug	No	No	Yes	No	No	Yes
Lipophilicity (log *P*)	4.06	3.24	4.30	−0.23	0.13	4.68
T_{max} (h)	1.0–2.0	<1.0	2.0–4.0	1.0–1.5	3.0–5.0	4.0
Absorption (%)	30	98	30	34	40–60	60–80
Bioavailability (%)	14	24	<5	17	20	<5
Protein binding (%)	>98	98	>95	50	88	95
Major P450 metabolic enzyme	CYP3A4	CYP2C9 (minor)	CYP3A4	None	CYP2C (minor)	CYP3A4
Systemic active metabolites (n)	Yes (2)	No	Yes (4)	No	Minimal	Yes (3)
Renal excretion (%)	<2	<6	10	20	10	13
$T_{½}$ (h)	14	<3	2	2	19	1.4–3.0

pravastatin molecule and the methane sulfonamide group in the rosuvastatin molecule renders these statins relatively hydrophilic (see Table 22-1). The practical significance of this property is unknown, since even the hydrophilic statins, pravastatin and rosuvastatin, are transported across hepatic cell membranes by organic anion transporting polypeptides (OATP), most frequently OATP1B1.[88] Without the aid of a transport mechanism, these statins would have only limited access to nonhepatic cells, including the blood–brain barrier and the cells of the arterial wall.

Bioavailability

Relatively small amounts of administered drug (<25%) actually reach the systemic circulation (see Table 22-1). This is probably a desirable feature, as the statin's systemic concentration correlates with its propensity to cause adverse effects. The more bioavailable the statin, the higher the systemic concentration, and potentially the more risk for adverse effects. Fluvastatin, rosuvastatin, and pravastatin are the most bioavailable, possibly owing to their low lipid solubility. However, even the statins with low bioavailability may move across cell membranes more easily because of a high lipid solubility and be more prone to adverse effects. Conversely, a reduced bioavailability of statins in the systemic circulation could diminish desired pleiotropic effects by reducing their entry into vascular and other nonhepatic tissues.

Renal Elimination

Following oral administration, most of the statin dose (i.e., >80%) is eliminated via the liver and gastrointestinal tract, but some may be excreted through the kidneys. A greater portion of pravastatin and simvastatin is eliminated through the kidney, possibly owing to their low lipid solubility. However, only a small portion of atorvastatin and fluvastatin undergoes renal elimination (see Table 22-1). In patients with severe chronic kidney disease (i.e., estimated glomerular filtration rate [GFR] <30 mL/min), a statin with little renal elimination is preferred.

Elimination Half-Life

The elimination half-life of the statins varies from 1 to 3 hours for lovastatin, simvastatin, pravastatin, and fluvastatin, to 14 to 19 hours for atorvastatin and rosuvastatin (see Table 22-1). The longer the half-life of the statin, the longer the inhibition of reductase and thus a greater reduction in LDL cholesterol. However, the impact of inhibiting cholesterol synthesis persists even with statins that have a relatively short half-life. This is due to their ability to reduce blood levels of lipoproteins, which have a half-life of approximately 2 to 3 days. Because of this, all statins may be dosed once daily. The preferable time of administration is in the evening just before the peak in cholesterol synthesis. The LDL cholestrol–lowering efficacy has been shown to be slightly less when lovastatin is administered in the morning and slightly greater when the dose is administered twice daily, especially with doses of 40 to 80 mg/day.[5] These differences are modest and probably not clinically important. If a patient prefers to take his or her statin in the morning rather than at night, this is acceptable in order to encourage compliance with the therapy.

Metabolism

Lipid-soluble statins are converted to water-soluble salts and glucuronide conjugates for elimination from the body. Simvastatin and lovastatin are metabolized by cytochrome P450 3A4 (CYP3A4) enzymes (see Table 22-1). This is important because a large number of drugs are either inhibitors or substrates for this enzyme system and can result in drug–drug interactions, leading to increased blood levels. A list of select drug interactions with the statins is provided in Table 22-2. Atorvastatin also undergoes metabolism by the CYP3A4 enzymes, but to a lesser extent. Approximately 10% of fluvastatin and rosuvastatin are metabolized primarily by CYP2C9, and pravastatin undergoes no metabolism through the cytochrome P450 enzyme system.[9] Both fluvastatin and rosuvastatin are eliminated from the body largely unchanged as parent compounds by transporter-mediated excretion mechanisms in the liver into the feces via bile and into the urine.

TABLE 22-2 Selected and Significant Drug Interactions with Statins

Variable	Atorvastatin	Fluvastatin	Lovastatin	Pravastatin	Rosuvastatin	Simvastatin
Major P450 metabolic enzyme	CYP3A4	CYP2C9 CYP2C8	CYP3A4	None	CYP2C9 (minor)	CYP3A4
Azole antifungals (ketoconazole, itraconazole; not fluconazole)	Yes	No	Yes	No	No	Yes
Nondihydropyridine calcium-channel blockers (diltiazem, verapamil)	Rare cases	No	Yes (up to a fourfold increase in statin blood level)	No	No	Yes (up to a fourfold increase in statin blood level)
Amiodarone	NR	No	Yes	No	No	Yes
Cyclosporine	Yes	NR	Yes	Yes	Yes	Yes
Macrolide antibiotics (erythromycin, clarithromycin; not azithromycin)	No	No	Yes	No	No	Yes
Gemfibrozil	NR	No	Yes	Yes	Yes	Yes
Fenofibrate	NR	NR	NR	No	No	No
HIV protease inhibitors (indinavir, nelfinavir, ritonavir, saquinavir; indinavir less potent inhibitor)	Yes	No	Yes	No	No	Yes
Warfarin	No	No	Yes	No	Yes	Yes
Antidepressants (fluoxetine, fluoxamine, nefazodone, sertraline; not paroxetine or venalafaxine	Yes	No	Yes	No	No	Yes

HIV, human immunodeficiency virus; NR, not reported.

The open acid statins have been reported to undergo glucuronidation and subsequently lactonization.[89] Lactonized statins may be converted to the open acid form by an esterase enzyme and metabolized, excreted into the bile or urine, or directly metabolized by the cytochrome P450 system. Excretion of statins or their metabolites into the bile and feces is mediated by transport proteins, including OATP1B1 and multidrug resistance–associated protein–2 (MRP-2).

DRUG INTERACTIONS

CYP3A4 Interactions

Drugs that inhibit the CYP3A4 enzyme can interfere with the metabolism of atorvastatin, simvastatin, and lovastatin and result in an increase in the area under the statin concentration–time curve (AUC) and the C_{max} achieved. The principal agents that inhibit CYP3A4 are the azole antifungals (except fluconazole), macrolide antibiotics (except azithromycin), human immunodeficiency virus (HIV) protease inhibitors, antidepressants, and grapefruit juice (see Table 22-2).[90] Ritonavir, itraconazole, and ketoconazole are strong inhibitors of CYP3A4 and have been reported to raise the statin's AUC by as much as 20-fold. Conversely, the AUC increase for fluvastatin and pravastatin is negligible when either is given with itraconazole. The nondihydropyridine calcium-channel blockers (i.e., diltiazem and verapamil) are also inhibitors of the CYP3A4 system and are reported to raise the AUC of simvastatin and lovastatin (but not atorvastatin); dihydropyridine calcium-channel blockers (e.g., amlodipine, nifedipine) do not cause this effect. In most cases, the interacting drugs shown in Table 22-2 produce a twofold or greater increase in the affected statin's AUC and/or C_{max}, exposing the patient to a higher risk of concentration-related toxicity. Cases of rhabdomyolysis are encountered more commonly when a CYP3A4-metabolized statin is given with an inhibitor of this system.

As a general rule, atorvastatin is affected to a lesser extent by inhibitors of CYP3A4 than are lovastatin and simvastatin because it undergoes less metabolism.[88]

Selective inhibitors of CYP3A4 do not have a significant pharmacokinetic interaction with pravastatin, fluvastatin, or rosuvastatin because CYP3A4 has no appreciable role in the elimination of these statins.

Fresh or frozen grapefruit juice may increase the AUC and/or C_{max} of lovastatin, simvastatin, and atorvastatin because of an inhibitory effect on CYP3A4-mediated metabolism in the intestinal wall.[91–93] However, pravastatin and rosuvastatin pharmacokinetics are not affected. This inhibition is dose dependent and increases with the volume of grapefruit consumed. A glass of grapefruit juice (i.e., 200 mL) daily is reported to increase the AUC of simvastatin three- to fourfold, while larger doses (>1 quart per day) increase the AUC more than tenfold. When lovastatin or simvastatin is administered in the evening, a morning glass of grapefruit juice has no clinically relevant effect on the AUC.[94] The primary substance in grapefruit juice responsible for the inhibition is 6,7-dihydroxybergamuttin.[95] This substance is not found in orange juice, and no interactions of orange juice with CYP3A4 have been reported. Little is known about the potential for other citrus juices to cause potentiation of statin levels.

If a patient is taking a statin metabolized by CYP3A4 and requires therapy with a CYP3A4 inhibitor, there are several options. First, one could select a drug that does not inhibit CYP3A4. For example, use of the antifungal agent fluconazole or the antibiotic azithromycin may be good options. Alternatively, if a short course of a potentially interacting therapy is indicated, statin therapy can be safely suspended for this period as long as patients have no or stable cardiovascular disease.[96] Finally, one of the statins that is not affected by CYP3A4 inhibition, such as pravastatin, fluvastatin, or rosuvastatin, may replace the affected statin to allow concurrent use of the CYP3A4-inhibiting drug.

CYP2C9 Interactions

Among the drugs that inhibit CYP2C9 are omeprazole, tolbutamide, cimetidine, fluvoxamine, and azole antifungals (see Table 22-2). These drugs theoretically should affect the metabolism of fluvastatin, but few clinically important drug–drug interactions with fluvastatin have been reported. The most significant case is with fluconazole, with which the AUC of fluvastatin is modestly increased, but less than 100%.[97] Additionally, the AUC for rosuvastatin is increased only marginally when administered with fluconazole.

OATP1B1 Interactions

Drugs that interfere with OATP1B1 interfere with one of the most important mechanisms by which hydrophilic statins are transported into the liver. Some of the inhibitors of CYP3A4 also inhibit this transporter, including macrolide antibiotics (clarithromycin) and protease inhibitors (ritonavir, indinavir, and saquinavir). Another potent inhibitor of this and other transporters of statins is cyclosporine.[98] Cyclosporine also affects CYP3A4 and P-glycoprotein. Cyclosporine has been reported to raise the AUC of most statins by 2- to 25-fold (except fluvastatin).[88] Although these interactions are not completely understood, inhibition of OATP1B1 would be expected to decrease hepatic uptake of the statin, thus increasing its systemic concentration. Additionally, inhibition of transporters that mediate intestinal flux (e.g., multidrug resistance transporter–1 [MDR-1]) could decrease the statin's systemic clearance and increase the bioavailability of statins. Regardless of the mechanism, the interaction results in a significant increase in systemic statin concentration. However, it may also result in a reduction in lipid-lowering efficacy (because less of the drug is taken up in the liver to inhibit HMG-CoA reductase). Since most patients receiving cyclosporine will also require antiatherosclerosis treatment, the clinician will have to meet this challenge. Two solutions are available: small doses of a highly potent statin, such as 5 mg daily of rosuvastatin; or a maximal (80-mg) dose of fluvastatin, which does not adversely interact with cyclosporine. Long-term studies of fluvastatin in patients receiving cyclosporine after kidney transplantation did not report any cases of myopathy over a 5-year follow-up.[99]

Fibrate Interactions

Gemfibrozil, but not fenofibrate, adversely affects the pharmacokinetics of most statins. A summary of the effects of the fibrates on statin blood concentrations is listed in Table 22-3. Several mechanisms for this interaction appear to contribute.[100] Like cyclosporine, gemfibrozil interferes with OATP1B1-mediated transport of the statin into the hepatocyte, which could lead to an increased plasma concentration of the statin.[101] Gemfibrozil is also an inhibitor of CYP2C8, but this may only affect fluvastatin, and clinical studies reveal that the interaction is not clinically significant. It has been shown that statins undergo glucuronidation via UDP glucuronosyl transferase and subsequent lactonization.[89] Gemfibrozil interferes with these steps, thereby promoting a higher systemic concentration of the active, open acid form of statins. All statins (except atorvastatin and fluvastatin) are affected by this interaction (Table 22-3). Thus, if a statin–fibrate combination is to be used, fenofibrate should help avoid the adverse interaction or, if gemfibrozil is the fibrate selected for the combination, use of either atorvastatin or fluvastatin is advisable.

Warfarin Interactions

Small increases in prothrombin times and bleeding have been described with some statins when given to patients receiving warfarin therapy. The prescribing information for atorvastatin, fluvastatin, and pravastatin reports that no clinically significant effect on prothrombin time has been observed.[3,4,6] One explanation for this effect is the potential displacement of warfarin from plasma protein binding sites by the statin, although other mechanisms may contribute. While the increase in prothrombin time is modest and significant bleeding is uncommon, close monitoring of the international normalized ratio (INR) is advised when lovastatin, rosuvastatin, or simvastatin is added to or withdrawn from a regimen containing warfarin.[2,5,7]

TABLE 22-3 Effect of Fibric Acid Derivatives on Statin C_{max}

Statin	With Gemfibrozil	With Fenofibrate
Atorvastatin	Minor effect	No effect
Fluvastatin	No effect	No effect
Lovastatin	↑ in C_{max} by 2.8-fold	Not available
Pravastatin	↑ in C_{max} by 2-fold	No effect
Rosuvastatin	↑ in C_{max} by 2-fold	No effect
Simvastatin	↑ in C_{max} by 2-fold	No effect

Reprinted from Ref. 100, with permission.

LIPID-ALTERING EFFICACY

Effects on LDL Cholesterol

The evidence that lowering LDL cholesterol reduces cardiovascular risk is unequivocal. Thus, statins have become the preferred first-line treatment of choice in patients with coronary heart disease (CHD) risk sufficient to warrant pharmacologic therapy. Furthermore, the accumulated data support the "lower is better" paradigm and place additional emphasis on statin therapy because of the superior LDL cholesterol–lowering efficacy of statins compared with other therapies.

As suggested by experiments comparing the absolute potency of statins in inhibiting HMG-CoA reductase in a cell-free system (see the Mechanism of Action section earlier in the chapter), statins differ in their LDL cholesterol–lowering efficacy. The order of inhibiting potency reported in cell-free experiments correlates with the order of LDL cholesterol lowering with statins in humans. This was evaluated best in the Statin Therapies for Elevated Lipid Levels Compared Across Doses to Rosuvastatin (STELLAR) trial, a randomized, parallel-group, open-label, comparator-controlled trial in 2431 hypercholesterolemic adults that had sufficient statistical power to compare lipid and lipoprotein changes after 6 weeks for all of the statins and doses tested. The results of this trial demonstrated that on a milligram-to-milligram-basis, rosuvastatin was the most efficacious statin in lowering LDL cholesterol, followed by atorvastatin, simvastatin, and pravastatin. A comparison of the lipid-altering effects of selected statins is listed in Table 22-4.[103] Rosuvastatin lowered LDL cholesterol across its 10- to 40-mg dose range by 46% to 55%, compared with 37% to 51% for the atorvastatin 10- to 80-mg dose range, 28% to 46% for the simvastatin 10- to 80-mg dose range, and 20% to 30% for the pravastatin 10- to 40-mg dose range.

The LDL cholesterol–lowering efficacy of the statins is also reflected in their ability to attain National Cholesterol Education Program Adult Treatment Panel III (NCEP ATP III) LDL cholesterol treatment goals. Again using the STELLAR trial as a reference, the proportions of CHD or CHD risk-equivalent patients who achieved a treatment goal of less than 100 mg/dL with rosuvastatin 10 mg, atorvastatin 20 mg, simvastatin 40 mg, or pravastatin 40 mg (typical starting doses of these statins) were 55%, 43%, 31%, and 11%, respectively.[104] Furthermore, the proportions of patients with baseline triglycerides 200 mg/dL or greater who met both LDL cholesterol and non-HDL cholesterol treatment goals with rosuvastatin 10 mg, atorvastatin 20 mg, simvastatin 40 mg, or pravastatin 40 mg were 80%, 60%, 46%, and 37%, respectively.

The power of highly efficacious statins to achieve substantial LDL cholesterol lowering and to reach NCEP ATP III treatment goals is illustrated in an analysis of the response to rosuvastatin therapy in individual patients with very high baseline LDL cholesterol levels ranging from 190 to 240 mg/dL (Fig. 22-6). With rosuvastatin 10 mg, 37% of patients achieved a treatment goal of less than 100 mg/dL, greater than half the mean baseline LDL cholesterol level of the population, and 66% achieved the treatment goal of less than 100 mg/dL with rosuvastatin 20 mg. Most patients had a substantial LDL cholesterol reduction, especially with the 20-mg dose, even if the goal

TABLE 22-4 Comparison of the Lipid-Altering Effects with Statins from the STELLAR Trial[103]

Daily Statin Dose	Rosuvastatin	Atorvastatin	Simvastatin	Pravastatin
LDL Cholesterol (Baseline 187–194 mg/dL)				
10 mg	−46%	−37%	−28%	−20%
20 mg	−52%	−43%	−35%	−24%
40 mg	−55%	−48%	−39%	−30%
80 mg	NA	−51%	−46%	NA
HDL Cholesterol (Baseline 50–51 mg/dL)				
10 mg	8%	6%	5%	3%
20 mg	10%	5%	6%	4%
40 mg	10%	4%	5%	6%
80 mg	NA	2%	7%	NA
Triglycerides (Baseline 172–187 mg/dL)				
10 mg	−20%	−20%	−12%	−8%
20 mg	−24%	−23%	−18%	−8%
40 mg	−26%	−27%	−15%	−13%
80 mg	NA	−28%	−18%	NA
non-HDL Cholesterol (Baseline mean 222–230 mg/dL)				
10 mg	−42%	−34%	−26%	−19%
20 mg	−48%	−40%	−33%	−22%
40 mg	−51%	−45%	−35%	−27%
80 mg	NA	−48%	−42%	NA

HDL, high-density lipoprotein; LDL, low-density lipoprotein; NA, not available.

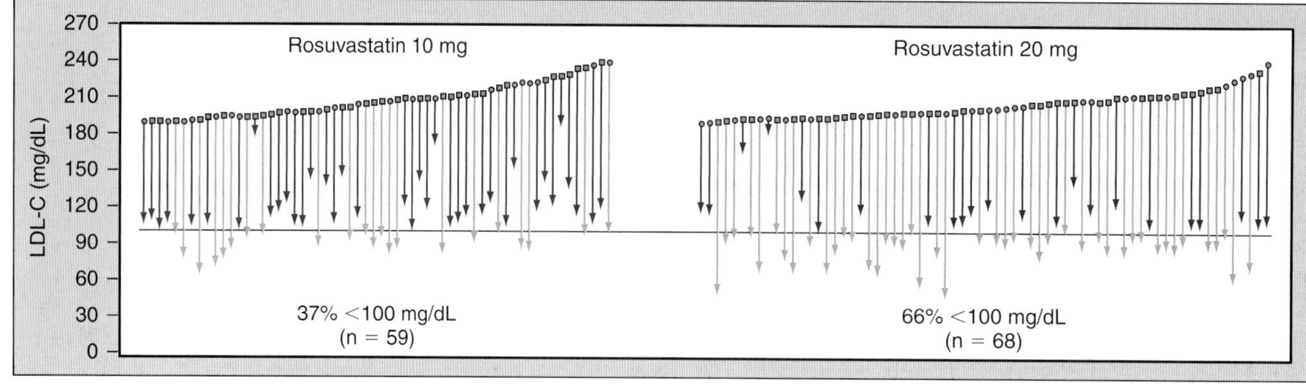

FIGURE 22-6 Reduction in low-density lipoprotein cholesterol (LDL-C) from a baseline of 190 to 240 mg/dL with rosuvastatin 10 mg (n = 59 subjects) and 20 mg (n = 68 subjects) in the STELLAR trial at 6 weeks.
Data on file, AstraZeneca.

of LDL cholesterol less than 100 mg/dL was not achieved. A few patients had minimal LDL cholesterol lowering (see Fig. 22-6), most commonly because of nonadherence with therapy. These data also demonstrate that even the most efficacious LDL cholesterol–lowering statin is not able to achieve treatment goals in all patients, illustrating the need for combination therapy in some patients.

Effects on Triglycerides

Statins also lower triglyceride levels, generally in the range of 15% to 30% (see Table 22-4). The efficacy of statins in lowering triglycerides mirrors their efficacy in lowering LDL cholesterol. The statins that are more efficacious in lowering LDL cholesterol are also more efficacious in lowering triglycerides. The lowering of triglycerides is also progressively greater with increasing baseline triglyceride levels and with escalating statin doses. For example, simvastatin at a starting dose of 20 mg daily has been shown to lower triglycerides by two times more in patients with triglycerides greater than 250 mg/dL than in patients with triglycerides less than 150 mg/dL. Furthermore, simvastatin has only modest and rather flat triglyceride-lowering effects across the 20- to 80-mg dose range in patients with triglycerides less than 150 mg/dL, but an escalating triglyceride-lowering effect in patients with triglycerides between 150 and 250 mg/dL or greater than 250 mg/dL. The effects of simvastatin on lowering triglycerides at various levels are depicted in Table 22-5.[105]

Atherogenic Dyslipidemia

Virtually all patients with a triglyceride level above 200 mg/dL have atherogenic dyslipidemia, a lipid disorder characterized by cholesterol-enriched VLDL remnant particles, small dense LDL, low high-density lipoprotein (HDL) cholesterol, and increased particle number. The key to reducing cardiovascular risk in these patients is not so much lowering their triglyceride levels as it is reducing the number and composition of cholesterol-carrying particles. Studies have shown that statins are highly efficacious in accomplishing this goal.

TABLE 22-5 Mean Percentage Lowering of Triglyceride with Simvastatin 20 to 80 mg Daily[105]

TG Levels (mg/dL)	20 mg Daily	40 mg Daily	80 mg Daily
<150	−12%	−7%	−11%
150–250	−30%	−22%	−25%
>250	−24%	−29%	−40%

TG, triglycende.

Studies in patients with atherogenic dyslipidemia have shown that particle concentration (number) is the best single predictor of atherosclerotic disease, and reducing this concentration is a key to risk reduction.[106] By their very mechanism of action, statins remove VLDL and LDL particles from the circulation, thus reducing particle concentration. All subfractions of VLDL, large and small, as well as VLDL particles containing apoC-III, are proportionately removed with statin therapy.[107,108] The cholesterol and triglyceride contents of these particles are also reduced. The same is true for LDL particles—particle number as well as cholesterol and triglyceride composition are reduced, but there is an important exception. In patients with atherogenic dyslipidemia, the concentration of small dense LDL particles makes up 50% to 70% of LDL particles prior to treatment, and these appear to be preferentially removed by statin therapy.[107–109] In one study, atorvastatin removed 44% of small dense LDL particles but only 10% of larger particles and 31% of all particles. By contrast, niacin, a drug commonly prescribed for patients with atherogenic dyslipidemia, shifted small LDL particles to larger ones and reduced particle number by only 14%.[107] The removal of small dense LDL particles and the reduction in the total number of particles with a statin would appear to be a more preferable treatment option.

Effects on non-HDL Cholesterol

The NCEP ATP III guidelines offer an easier way to address atherogenic dyslipidemia, with the recommendation that patients be treated first to their respective LDL cholesterol goal. If triglyceride levels remain 200 mg/dL or higher once this goal is reached, patients are to be treated to a second goal defined by non-HDL cholesterol. The rationale for the latter is that the presence of cholesterol-enriched VLDL remnant particles, one of the prime features of atherogenic dyslipidemia, would be reflected by an elevated non-HDL cholesterol and would prompt the clinician to manipulate the treatment regimen to address this second treatment goal. Since non-HDL cholesterol includes LDL cholesterol (and small dense LDL particles) as well as VLDL cholesterol (and remnant particles), it serves as a good surrogate for the multiple lipid disorders encountered in patients with this disorder.

Not surprisingly, statins are highly effective at reducing non-HDL cholesterol, as reflected in the STELLAR study data (see Table 22-4). In a similarly designed study in which statin doses were titrated to achieve NCEP ATP III LDL cholesterol goals, atorvastatin was reported to lower LDL cholesterol and non-HDL cholesterol by 42% and 38%, respectively, compared to 36% and 32% for simvastatin, 36% and 32% for lovastatin, 29% and 26% for fluvastatin, and 28% and 26% for pravastatin.[28]

Rather than reducing the cholesterol composition of lipoproteins, as is the case with non-HDL cholesterol, the clinician could choose to reduce the particle number by targeting apoB. Each VLDL and LDL particle has one apoB attached, so apoB can be used as a surrogate for particle number (concentration). Statins are highly effective at lowering apoB and do so in proportion to their lowering of LDL cholesterol. The alternative treatment goals using apoB would be less than 110 mg/dL for moderate-risk patients with 2 or more CHD risk factors and an LDL cholesterol goal of less than 130 mg/dL, and less than 90 mg/dL for high-risk patients with CHD or CHD risk equivalent and an LDL cholesterol goal of less than 100 mg/dL.[17]

Effects on HDL Cholesterol and ApoA-I

Statins generally produce modest increases in HDL cholesterol, but even these changes may be important (see Table 22-4). An analysis of the Scandinavian Simvastatin Survival Study (4S) data reported that the mean 6% increase in HDL cholesterol observed with simvastatin contributed a small but statistically significant effect to the positive outcome.[110] Most statins increase HDL cholesterol by 5% to 7%; rosuvastatin raises it by 8% to 10%. The increase is not strongly dose related. Atorvastatin raises HDL cholesterol at low doses but less so as the dose escalates[103] (see Table 22-4).

Statins may raise HDL cholesterol by up-regulating the transport protein ATP-binding cassette transporter A1 (ABCA1), which delivers free cholesterol to the cell surface in macrophages. A second potential mechanism is a reduction in transfer of cholesteryl esters from HDL to VLDL and LDL particles via inhibition of cholesteryl ester transfer protein (CETP).[111] Whether HDL cholesterol raising by CETP inhibition is beneficial remains to be demonstrated. Regardless of the mechanism, statins reduce the concentration of pre-β_1-HDL particles (nascent HDL), indicating that these particles are picking up cholesterol from macrophage cells. Additionally, α_1- and α_2-HDL particles (mature HDL) are increased in patients given statin therapy, indicating that cholesterol is being incorporated into these particles ostensibly for transport to the liver for elimination.[112]

While the effect of statins on HDL is small, it is still worthy of consideration when selecting a statin to treat patients who have an atherogenic dyslipidemia profile.

ADMINISTRATION

Patients should be started on therapeutic lifestyle changes, such as diet and exercise, prior to or concurrently with the initiation of statin therapy. Statins are best given once daily in the evening to coincide with the peak cholesterol biosynthesis at night, although the long-acting statins, atorvastatin and rosuvastatin, may be given at any time of day. From a practical point of view, the difference in LDL cholesterol lowering between morning and evening dosing is small, and therefore patients who prefer to take their statin dose in the morning can do so without significant loss of efficacy. It is recommended that lovastatin be administered with food to enhance its absorption, but the other statins may be taken with or without food. The LDL cholesterol–lowering effect may be seen within 2 weeks of initiating therapy, but the peak, steady-state lowering effects are usually seen after 4 weeks of therapy but may take as long as 6 weeks to be achieved with atorvastatin and rosuvastatin. Dosage changes should be made after these time periods.

Statin therapy should be initiated at recommended starting doses. A comparison of LDL cholesterol lowering at starting doses versus the maximum dose is presented in Table 22-6. Unless there are extenuating circumstances (e.g., drug interactions, prior statin intolerance), the starting dose should generally be one of the higher doses in keeping with the "lower is better" mantra. The exception is that atorvastatin 40 mg and rosuvastatin 20 mg should be reserved for patients with very high LDL cholesterol levels requiring substantial lowering (i.e., >40%–50%). At a minimum, the updated NCEP ATP III guidelines recommend an LDL cholesterol lowering of 30% to 40% to achieve even modest CHD risk reduction.[113] Every effort should be made to get patients to reach, if not exceed, the NCEP ATP III treatment goal. If LDL cholesterol lowering is insufficient with the initial dose, the statin dose may be doubled and will provide an additional 5% to 7% reduction in LDL cholesterol.

TABLE 22-6 LDL Cholesterol–Lowering Efficacy of Starting and Maximum Doses of Marketed Statins[2–7]

Statin	Starting Doses (Average LDL Cholesterol Reduction)	Maximum Dose (Average LDL Cholesterol Reduction)
Atorvastatin	10 mg (−39%) 20 mg (−43%) 40 mg* (−50%)	80 mg (−60%)
Fluvastatin	40 mg (−25%) 40 mg bid (−36%) 80 mg XL (−35%)	80 mg XL (−35%)
Lovastatin	20 mg (−27%)	40 mg bid (−40%)
Pravastatin	40 mg (−34%)	80 mg (−37%)
Rosuvastatin	5 mg (−45%) 10 mg (−52%) 20 mg† (−55%)	40 mg (−63%)
Simvastatin	20 mg (−38%) 40 mg (−41%)	80 mg (−47%)

*A 40-mg starting dose may be used when more than a 45% LDL cholesterol reduction is needed.

†A 20-mg starting dose may be used with marked hypercholesterolemia (i.e., LDL cholesterol >190 mg/dL) requiring aggressive lipid targets. LDL, low-density lipoprotein; XL, extended-release.

There are no clear guidelines defining the safety of low LDL cholesterol levels. Until such guidelines are established, it may be wise to back-titrate when levels fall below 50 mg/dL. Clinical trials have studied patients receiving statins with mean LDL cholesterol levels as low as 62 mg/dL (with a small number of patients below 40 mg/dL) for as long as 2 years without evidence of associated toxicity.[15] Dosing in geriatric, pediatric, renally impaired, and immunosuppressed patients is described later in this chapter. Asian patients may achieve higher blood levels of rosuvastatin than non-Asians and should be started at a dose of 5 mg and titrated upward as needed.

IMPACT ON MORBIDITY AND MORTALITY

Statins have been evaluated in more than 100,000 individuals participating in randomized, controlled clinical event endpoint trials. A summary of the key trials is shown in Tables 22-7 and 22-8. The conclusion from all of this evidence is that any adverse consequence of atherosclerotic vascular disease is reduced with statin therapy, including CHD death, nonfatal MI, coronary revascularization, acute coronary syndromes, unstable angina, stroke, peripheral artery disease (PAD), cardiac arrest, and heart failure. The statins not only help sustain the quality of life by reducing these events, but also help lengthen life by reducing total mortality. Reductions in total mortality have been specifically documented in 4S, the Long-Term Intervention with Pravastatin in Ischaemic Disease (LIPID), and Heart Protection Study (HPS).[114–116]

The extent of reduction in cardiovascular events is remarkably predictable and in accord with hypotheses derived from earlier population studies that estimated that for every 1% lowering in LDL cholesterol there could be a 1% lowering of CHD events. A glance at the LDL cholesterol change achieved in the randomized, placebo-controlled clinical trials and the change in CHD events (CHD death and nonfatal MI) in Table 22-7 confirms this relationship. Of course, the benefit is much more than 1% because statins reduce more than just CHD death, nonfatal MIs, and first cardiovascular events, which are often the outcome measures of these studies. An analysis of 14 of these trials and the 90,056 people who participated in them by the principal investigators for each trial has quantified this relationship even better: For every 1% lowering in LDL cholesterol with statins, first major CHD events are reduced by 0.88%.[117]

The statins are equally effective at reducing cardiovascular event rates in patients with existing vascular disease (secondary prevention) as in those with only risk factors (primary prevention). Of course, the absolute event reduction in secondary prevention trials is two- to threefold greater (because the event rate is higher) than in primary prevention trials, but the relative risk reduction is nearly the same. Statins are equally effective in reducing risk in men and women, irrespective of age. In fact, the Prospective Study of Pravastatin in the Elderly at Risk (PROSPER) specifically evaluated a population aged 70 to 82 years and reported a significant 19% reduction in CHD events with 5 years of pravastatin treatment.[118] The Cholesterol Treatment Trialists' Collaborators reported proportional 18% reductions in CHD events in patients older than 65 years as well as even in those older than 75 years.[117]

Statins have also shown effectiveness in reducing events in diabetic patients in many of the studies presented in Table 22-7. Given the growth in the number of patients with diabetes and the recognition of diabetes as a CHD risk equivalent by the NCEP ATP III, the fact that statins effectively reduce cardiovascular risk in these patients is important. Patients with diabetes often have an atherogenic dyslipidemic profile and only modestly elevated LDL cholesterol. In spite of this, statins are excellent treatment choices in these patients because statins effectively reduce small dense LDL particles, cholesterol-enriched remnant particles, and overall particle number as discussed above. Recently, the Collaborative Atorvastatin Diabetes Study (CARDS) specifically studied type 2 diabetic patients and reported a 37% relative event reduction, which was so robust that the trial was stopped prematurely. In fact, the eventual CHD event reduction of 37% at 3.9 years was actually achieved at 1 year of follow-up, and by 18 months of treatment with atorvastatin, this difference became statistically significant.[119] Post hoc analyses showed that elderly diabetic patients (65–75 years of age) in CARDS had a similar 38% relative risk reduction, but the absolute reduction was 3.9% compared to 2.7% for younger patients.[120]

The story of the treatment of dyslipidemia in a hypertensive population is similar to that of diabetes. In the Anglo-Scandinavian Cardiac Outcomes Trial–Lipid Lowering Arm (ASCOT-LLA), the CHD event reduction was so robust that the trial was discontinued at 3.3 years into the 5-year planned trial. Treatment with atorvastatin 10 mg resulted in a 36% CHD event reduction. Relative risk reduction in CHD events was apparent 30 days into the trial and statistically significant at 90 days.[121] Another statin study in hypertensive dyslipidemic patients reported a disappointing insignificant 9% reduction in CHD events.[122] The trial used a usual-care control group and was plagued by the drop-in of statin-treated patients in the usual care group and the drop-out of patients in the pravastatin treatment group. The result was only a net 16% reduction in LDL cholesterol, which the investigators argued was not sufficient to produce a significant CHD event reduction. The important lesson of this trial is that for any statin treatment to be successful in reducing risk, it must achieve a certain minimum cholesterol reduction. The NCEP ATP III has recommended that at least a 30% to 40% LDL cholesterol reduction should be achieved. This minimal reduction can and should be exceeded to maximize cardiovascular risk reduction.

Statins are as effective in reducing cardiovascular risk in patients with LDL cholesterol levels above 175 mg/dL as they are in those with levels below 135 mg/dL. In fact, the risk reduction is proportionately the same in individuals with LDL cholesterol less than 100 mg/dL prior to treatment. At one point, the NCEP ATP III guidelines recommended a LDL cholesterol treatment goal of less than 100 mg/dL, and so the fact that patients with baseline levels below this level could still demonstrate significant risk reduction was a surprise. This has important implications. In all of the

TABLE 22-7 Summary of Major Placebo-Controlled, Randomized, Double-Blind Clinical Event Endpoint Trials with Statins

Study	Follow-up (yr)	Patients	Treatment	LDL Cholesterol Beginning (End)	LDL Cholesterol Change	Change in CHD*	Comment
4S[114]	5.4	4444 adults with angina or prior MI	Simvastatin 40 mg/day	190 mg/dL (117 mg/dL)	−35%	−34%	Total mortality −30% ($P = 0.003$); CVA −30% ($P = 0.024$)
LIPID[115]	6.1	9014 adults with Hx prior MI or UA (smokers 10%, DM 9%, HTN 42%, obese 18%)	Pravastatin 40 mg/day	150 mg/dL (112 mg/dL)	−25%	−24%	Total mortality −22% ($P = 0.001$); CVA −19% ($P = 0.048$)
CARE[170]	5	4159 adults with prior MI	Pravastatin 40 mg/day	139 mg/dL (98 mg/dL)	−32%	−24%	
HPS[157]	5	20,536 adults with CHD, arterial disease, or diabetes (HTN 41%, no CHD 35%)	Simvastatin 40 mg/day	132 mg/dL (89 mg/dL)	−32%	−27%	All-cause mortality −13% ($P = 0.0003$); CVA −25% ($P = 0.001$)
ALERT[99]	5.1	2102 renal transplant patients, (smokers 19%, DM 19%, HTN 76%)	Fluvastatin 40 mg/day	159 mg/dL (108 mg/dL)	−32%	−35%	Primary endpoint: cardiac death, nonfatal MI, revascularization −17% ($P = 0.139$)
ALLHAT-LLT[122]	4.8	10,355 adults (smokers 23%, DM 35%, HTN 100%, CHD 14%)	Pravastatin 40 mg/day	146 mg/dL (105 mg/dL)	−17%	−9% (NS)	CVA −9% ($P = 0.31$)
PROSPER[118]	3.2	5804 adults, aged 70–82 (smokers 26%, DM 11%, PAD 7%, CHD 13%, TIA 11%, vascular disease 44%)	Pravastatin 40 mg/day	147 mg/dL (107 mg/dL)	−27%	−19%	Total mortality −3% ($P = 0.74$); CVA or TIA −4% ($P = 0.64$); vascular events −15% ($P = 0.014$)
ASCOT-LLA[14]	3.3	10,305 adults with HTN + ≥3 RF (DM 25%, smokers 32%, CVA/TIA 10%, PAD 5%)	Atorvastatin 10 mg/day	133 mg/dL (87 mg/dL)	−35%	−36%	CVA −27% ($P = 0.0236$); CV events −31% ($P = 0.0005$); total mortality −13% ($P = 0.1649$)
LIPS[190]	3.9	1677 adults post PCI (MI Hx 44%, smokers 25%, DM 14%, PAD 6%)	Fluvastatin 80 mg/day	132 mg/dL (96 mg/dL)	−27%	−31% ($P = 0.07$)	Primary endpoint: cardiac death, nonfatal MI, revascularization −22% ($P = 0.01$)
SPARCL[141]	4.9	4731 adults with prior CVA or TIA and no CHD (smokers 19%, HTN 62%, DM 17%)	Atorvastatin 80 mg/day	132 mg/dL (73 mg/dL)	−45%	−35%	First fatal or nonfatal CVA −16% ($P = 0.03$); CVA or TIA −23% ($P = 0.001$); hemorrhagic CVA +66%
CARDS[191]	3.9	2838 adults with DM + 1 RF, no CVD (smokers 23%, HTN 84%, obese 37%)	Atorvastatin 10 mg/day	118 mg/dL (78 mg/dL)	−31%	−35%	CVA −48% ($P = 0.001$); total mortality −27% ($P = 0.059$); CV events −37% ($P = 0.001$)
WOSCOPS[171]	4.9	6595 men with no CHD (HTN 15%, smoker 44%, DM 1%)	Pravastatin 40 mg/day	192 mg/dL (142 mg/dL)	−26%	−31%	Total mortality −22% ($P = 0.051$); CVA −11% ($P = 0.37$)
AFCAPS/TexCAPS[192]	5.2	6605 adults with no CHD, HDL cholesterol <35 mg/dL in men, <40 mg/dL in women (HTN 22%, smokers 13%)	Lovastatin 20–40 mg/day	150 mg/dL (115 mg/dL)	−25%	−40%	CHD events −37% ($P = 0.001$); CV events −25% ($P = 0.003$)

*CHD death and nonfatal myocardial infarction.

CHD, Coronary heart disease; CV, cardiovascular; CVA, cerebrovascular accident; CVD, cardiovascular disease; DM, diabetes mellitus; HDL, high-density lipoprotein; HTN, hypertension; Hx, history; LDL, low-density lipoprotein; MI, myocardial infarction; PAD, peripheral artery disease; PCI, percutaneaus coronary intervention; RF, risk factor; TIA, transient ischemic attack; UA, unstable angina.

TABLE 22-8 Summary of the Major Active-Controlled, Randomized, Double-Blind Clinical Event Endpoint Trials with Statins

Study	Follow-up	Patients	Treatment	LDL Cholesterol Beginning (End)	LDL Cholesterol Difference	Composite Endpoint	Comment
PROVE IT–TIMI 22[15]	24 month	4162 adults with ACS	Pravastatin 40 mg/day vs. atorvastatin 80 mg/day	106 mg/dL (95 mg/dL with pravastatin 40 mg/day) (62 mg/dL with atorvastatin 80 mg/day)	−35%	−16%* ($P = 0.005$) (emerged by 30 days, significant at 180 days)	Death or MI −18%; total mortality −28% (NS)
TNT[193]	4.9 yr	10,001 adults with stable CHD	Atorvastatin 10 mg/day vs. atorvastatin 80 mg/day	182 mg/dL (101 mg/dL with atorvastatin 10 mg/day) (77 mg/dL with atorvastatin 80 mg/day)	−24%	−22%† ($P < 0.001$)	Major CHD events −20% ($P = 0.002$); CVA −23% ($P = 0.007$); total mortality 1% (NS)
A to Z[172]	6–24 month	4497 adults with ACS	Simvastatin 20 mg/day vs. simvastatin 80 mg/day	111 mg/dL (77 mg/dL with simvastatin 20 mg/day) (63 mg/dL with simvastatin 80 mg/day)	−18%	−11%‡ ($P = 0.5$)	Total mortality −21% ($P = 0.08$); CV mortality −25% ($P = 0.05$)
IDEAL[194]	4.8 yr	8888 adults with stable CHD	Simvastatin 20 mg/day vs. atorvastatin 80 mg/day	121 mg/dL (104 mg/dL with simvastatin 20 mg/day) (81 mg/dL with atorvastatin 80 mg/day)	−22%	−16%§ ($P = 0.001$)	CV events (CHD events + CVA) −13% ($P = 0.02$); total mortality −2% ($P = 0.81$)

*Death, myocardial infarction (MI), unstable argina requiring hospitalization, revascularization, stroke.
†Coronary heart disease (CHD) death, nonfatal MI, resuscitation arrest, fatal or nonfatal stroke.
‡Cardiovascular (CV) death, nonfatal MI, readmission for acute coronary syndrome (ACS), stroke.
§CHD event = CHD death, nonfatal MI, cardiac arrest with resuscitation.
CVA, cerebrovascular accident; LDL, low-density lipoprotein; NS, nonsignificant

studies listed in Table 22-7, statin therapy was evaluated in patients who had a sufficient level of cardiovascular event risk to warrant treatment (and not a certain level of LDL cholesterol). The lesson is to select patients with sufficient cardiovascular risk for treatment and then to initiate statin (or other) therapy to achieve a rigorous LDL cholesterol reduction, regardless of baseline LDL cholesterol. The principal investigators of the trials listed in Table 22-7 concluded their extensive review of these studies with the following statement: " … treatment goals for statin treatment should aim chiefly to achieve substantial absolute reduction in LDL cholesterol (rather than to achieve particular target levels of LDL cholesterol), since the risk reductions are proportional to the absolute LDL cholesterol reductions."[117]

The active control studies have sought to determine whether there is added benefit from reducing LDL cholesterol to lower levels (see Table 22-8). In all cases, when a more efficacious LDL cholesterol–lowering statin or dose was compared with a less efficacious statin or dose, the more efficacious regimen produced a significant reduction in cardiovascular events. There was no evidence that the more aggressive treatment produced a higher margin of safety concerns. The most aggressive of these studies, the Pravastatin or Atorvastatin Evaluation and Infection Therapy (PROVE IT), compared patients with mean LDL cholesterol 95 mg/dL while receiving pravastatin 40 mg to patients with mean LDL cholesterol 62 mg/dL while receiving atorvastatin 80 mg and reported an additional 16% relative reduction in cardiovascular events with atorvastatin in just 2 years of treatment.[15] These data prompted the NCEP ATP III to recommend that clinicians consider a goal of <70 mg/dL in very-high-risk patients.[113]

SPECIAL POPULATIONS

Elderly

An important concern with the use of any medication in the elderly population is the greater potential for adverse effects compared with younger patients. There is valid reason for this concern, because the elderly may have reduced renal and hepatic function and altered body composition and are typically prescribed multiple pharmacologic therapies. As for the statins, there are limited data on whether there are important pharmacokinetic differences in the elderly, and if so, whether they matter. Data with atorvastatin have shown that the C_{max} is 43% higher and the elimination half-life is 36% longer in this patient population.[123] Yet, in randomized clinical trials, the clinical benefit of statin therapy in elderly subjects is the same as that demonstrated in younger subjects. While the relative benefit with statins may be somewhat smaller in elderly subjects, the absolute risk reduction may be larger because of the high prevalence of cardiovascular events in this population. Likewise, there were no differences in the adverse-event profiles among the elderly population shown in these trials. This evidence supports the proposition that statins are safe and effective in elderly patients at least to the same extent as in younger patients. Some lipid experts argue that age itself is one of the most important risk factors for cardiovascular events. Simply living long enough with any level of cholesterol may be sufficient to become a candidate for statin therapy. For example, a 70-year-old man with no risk factors has a Framingham-estimated 10-year CHD risk of 10%, which is at the threshold for therapeutic lifestyle change and possibly statin therapy. Just one or two additional risk factors propel the same person to a

10-year risk of more than 20%, which would qualify the patient as a CHD risk equivalent and warrant aggressive LDL cholesterol lowering. However, clinical judgment does come into play with elderly patients. If the patient's quality of life and prognosis are sufficient to support preventive therapy and if statin therapy is compatible with the concurrent drug regimen, there is certainly sufficient evidence to support initiation of statin therapy in practically any man older than 70 years of age and any woman older than 70 years of age with hypertension and either hypercholesterolemia or low HDL cholesterol as risk factors.

Pediatrics

The NCEP recommends screening children and adolescents over the age of 2 years if a parent has a known genetic lipid disorder or if there is a documented family history of premature cardiovascular disease in a parent or grandparent. Documented LDL cholesterol levels of 190 mg/dL or greater in children with no risk factors, or 160 mg/dL or greater with a family history of premature CHD events and two or more risk factors, warrants treatment with a minimal LDL cholesterol treatment goal of less than 130 mg/dL, but ideally less than 110 mg/dL.[124] Lifestyle modification is the cornerstone of therapy in this population, but high-risk pediatric patients may warrant treatment of lipid abnormalities with pharmacologic agents. Most of the statins have been evaluated in children and adolescents (beginning at 8–10 years of age) who have very high cholesterol levels, usually associated with familial hypercholesterolemia. These studies did not detect adverse effects on growth or sexual maturation in adolescent boys or on menstrual-cycle length in girls. However, the American Heart Association recommends that statin therapy be withheld until 10 years of age in boys and until after the onset of menses in girls.[124] Currently, all statins except rosuvastatin have pediatric-use labeling in their Food and Drug Administration (FDA)–approved prescribing information, based on clinical trials in children with familial hypercholesterolemia. Studies with rosuvastatin are currently under way. The choice of the statin is a matter of preference. The lowest effective doses of a statin should be used in these patients. The maximum daily dose studied is 40 mg for lovastatin, pravastatin, and simvastatin; 20 mg for atorvastatin; and 80 mg for fluvastatin. Girls given a statin should be advised about concerns with pregnancy, and all children and parents should be advised about potential drug interactions and symptoms of adverse effects. In addition to monitoring for liver- and muscle-related adverse effects while receiving statin therapy, children should be monitored for growth (height, weight, and body mass index).[2–7]

Renal Impairment

The presence of renal impairment is a risk factor for the development of statin-associated myopathy, especially for those statins that undergo significant renal elimination (see Table 22-1). The National Kidney Foundation has offered general guidance on the use of statins with varying degrees of GFR reduction.[125] Generally, atorvastatin is the preferred statin in patients with severely reduced GFR (<15 mL/min) because very little of the parent drug or active metabolites depend on renal mechanisms for elimination. Fluvastatin, the next least renally excreted statin, may be an alternative, although doses greater than 40 mg daily have not been studied in patients with severe renal impairment. Prescribing information for the remaining statins generally advises caution and close monitoring for potential adverse events (particularly myotoxicity) in patients with moderate to severe renal impairment, and advises the following dose parameters be employed: 5- to 10-mg maximum for rosuvastatin, 20-mg maximum for lovastatin, and a 5-mg starting dose for simvastatin.[2–7]

It should be noted that treatment with atorvastatin 20 mg daily versus placebo for 4 years in a population of diabetic subjects who were receiving maintenance hemodialysis did not demonstrate cardiovascular risk reduction.[126] Studies of statin therapy in other patient groups with renal impairment are ongoing.

Liver Dysfunction

Patients with nonalcoholic fatty liver disease (NAFLD) and nonalcoholic steatohepatitis (NASH) have a significantly increased cardiovascular risk and are candidates for lipid-lowering therapy. According to the National Lipid Association's (NLA) Liver Expert Panel, statins can be used safely in these patients.[127] This recommendation is based on the expert opinion of experienced authorities in the field and a forming evidence base. This evidence includes case–control studies showing that patients with presumed NAFLD and elevated liver transaminases are not at higher risk of statin hepatoxicity than those with normal baseline liver enzymes.[128,129] For example, a cohort study reported that 4.7% of patients with elevated baseline liver enzymes had elevated enzymes during a subsequent 6-month treatment with a statin compared with 1.9% of patients with normal enzymes at baseline followed by 6 months of a statin, and 6.4% of patients with elevated enzymes at baseline and no statin for 6 months. The evidence also includes descriptive studies reporting that statins may actually improve liver histology in patients with NASH.[130,131] Statin treatment was seen as improving liver densities (probably as a result of diminishing fat content), reducing transaminase levels, and improving the extent of inflammation. However, no change in the extent of fibrosis was seen. Larger studies are needed to confirm and extend these results. The NLA Liver Expert Panel advises that clinicians be alert to patient reports of jaundice, malaise, fatigue, lethargy, and related symptoms while undergoing statin therapy. Evidence for hepatotoxicity includes jaundice, hepatomegaly, increased indirect bilirubin level, and elevated prothrombin time.

NONTRADITIONAL USES

Chronic Renal Disease and Renoprotection

Are statins renoprotective? The answer to the question is unknown and will have to await results of ongoing randomized clinical trials powered to address this issue. However, the evidence to date is supportive of a positive answer. Post hoc analysis of the Greek Atorvastatin and Coronary Heart Disease Evaluation (GREACE) study reported that the estimated creatinine clearance (CrCl) improved 12% in those receiving atorvastatin therapy for 3 years but deteriorated 5% in usual-care patients not receiving statin therapy. The increase in CrCl with atorvastatin was greatest in those with the lowest baseline CrCl and with the highest doses of atorvastatin.[132] In a similar manner, a post hoc analysis of the Cholesterol and Recurrent Events (CARE) trial revealed that the rate of renal function loss slowed with pravastatin compared with placebo over 5 years of follow-up, with most of the benefit occurring in patients with the greatest renal impairment at baseline.[133] Finally, observation of more than 10,000 patients receiving open-label rosuvastatin 5 mg to 40 mg daily for up to 3.8 years revealed that estimated GFR either did not change or improved.[134] These results are consistent with a slowing or a halt in the progression of atherosclerosis that has been shown elsewhere to accompany statin therapy and suggest that statins may help preserve renal function in patients with increased risk of atherosclerotic vascular disease.

Many lipid specialists believe that chronic kidney disease (CKD) should be considered a CHD risk equivalent, given the strong association with atherosclerotic vascular disease and the increased risk of vascular events. However, it is not known whether targeting patients with CKD for lipid-altering therapy will reduce cardiovascular risk. A recent case–control analysis of 1574 adult kidney allograft recipients found that patients treated with statins had a statistically significant 24% lower mortality compared with untreated patients after controlling for baseline serum cholesterol levels, age, and transplant year.[135] A randomized, unblinded trial comparing statin therapy with no statin therapy reported a significant 32% reduction in total mortality and a 37% reduction in cardiovascular mortality with statin therapy in patients with end-stage renal disease.[136] Compared with placebo, fluvastatin 40 mg daily has been found to reduce CHD death and nonfatal MI (but not revascularization procedures or total mortality) in a 5-year randomized trial involving 2102 renal transplant patients.[99] A recent study in patients with type 2 diabetes receiving maintenance hemodialysis and either placebo or atorvastatin 20 mg daily for 4 years produced equivocal results. The primary endpoint, death from cardiac causes, nonfatal MI, and fatal and nonfatal stroke, was not significantly different from placebo ($P = 0.08$), but the composite of death from cardiac causes, nonfatal MI, and revascularization was reduced significantly ($P = 0.03$).[126] These results are encouraging but will require confirmation in larger trials before CKD becomes a CHD risk equivalent for determining need for and intensity of statin therapy. Until then, it is probably not appropriate to stratify patients with CKD as having a CHD risk equivalent. However, if these patients have dyslipidemia, as they often do, it is appropriate to risk stratify and provide lipid-altering treatment as indicated.

Cerebrovascular Accident

Statins have been shown to have neuroprotective effects, including an improvement of endothelial function, modulation of brain eNOS, inhibition of inflammatory processes associated with brain injury, and stabilization of cerebrovascular atherosclerotic plaques.[137] Statins have also been shown to reduce significantly the risk of ischemic stroke in CHD patients and are recommended by the American Stroke Association for use in the prevention of first stroke in patients with prior MI and average cholesterol levels as well as in patients with known CHD.[138,139] The NCEP ATP III guidelines recommend that patients with a history of stroke or transient ischemic attack (TIA) should be considered CHD risk equivalents and treated aggressively to reduce CHD events.[140]

The recent release of the Stroke Prevention by Aggressive Reduction in Cholesterol Levels (SPARCL) results has provided evidence for the first time that treatment of patients with a stroke or TIA but no known CHD with atorvastatin for 4.9 years to mean LDL cholesterol as low as 61 mg/dL resulted in a significant 16% relative reduction in rate of nonfatal and fatal strokes compared with placebo.[141] Major coronary events (i.e., cardiac death, nonfatal MI, and resuscitation after cardiac arrest) were reduced by 35% ($P = 0.003$) in the statin-treated group. However, the occurrence of hemorrhagic strokes was greater among statin-treated than placebo-treated patients (55 vs. 33 cases). A subsequent exploratory post hoc multivariable regression analysis of these 88 patients revealed that 86% of the increased risk of hemorrhagic stroke was accounted for by having a prior hemorrhagic stroke at study entry, being male, advancing in age, and being randomized to statin therapy.[141a] Notwithstanding prior epidemiologic trials reporting an association between low LDL cholesterol and hemorrhagic strokes,[158,159] the SPARCL investigators report that neither total cholesterol nor LDL cholesterol at baseline or at the visit prior to the hemorrhagic stroke was associated with an increased risk of hemorrhagic stroke, even in those patients with on-treatment LDL cholesterol levels below 40 mg/dL.

Other large statin clinical event endpoint trials in CHD patients have found little or no evidence of statin-associated hemorrhagic strokes. HPS, which involved 20,536 CHD patients assigned to simvastatin 40 mg/day or placebo for 5 treatment years, reported a 24% reduction in major CHD events (and a similar reduction in the 1820 patients with cerebrovascular disease but no CHD at study entry), a 30% reduction in ischemic stroke, and no difference in hemorrhagic strokes.[141b] However, among 3280 subjects in this study who had cerebrovascular disease at study entry, there were 21 (1.3%) who had a hemorrhagic stroke while receiving simvastatin, compared with 11 (0.7%) who received placebo. Analysis of more than 90,000 CHD patients participating in 14 randomized, placebo-controlled clinical trials (including HPS) involving treatment with various statins for 5 years revealed a 27% reduction in major CHD events for each 39-mg/dL reduction in LDL cholesterol, a 22% reduction in ishemic strokes for each 39-mg/dL reduction in LDL cholesterol, and no difference in rate of hemorrhagic stroke.[117]

According to current treatment guidelines, patients with a history of a stroke or TIA are indentified as CHD risk–equivalent patients and are targeted for aggressive treatment, usually with a statin in addition to lifestyle modification, to an LDL cholesterol below 100 mg/dL.[138,139] SPARCL data in patients with ischemic stroke history confirmed that cardiovascular risk reduction is substantial as is the reduction in the risk of recurrent strokes. As for patients with a hemorrhagic stroke history, while cardiovascular risk was reduced, in SPARCL more hemorrhagic strokes occurred than ischemic strokes were prevented. Based on this, and until new clarifying data emerge, clinicians should carefully weigh the factors contributing to the risk of cardiovascular events against those that increase the risk of hemorrhagic strokes prior to starting statin therapy in patients with a history of a hemorrhagic stroke. The patient's baseline cholesterol level, or that while receiving a statin, does not appear to be a factor raising the risk of a hemorrhagic stroke.

Peripheral Artery Disease

PAD is a CHD risk equivalent and, as such, patients with PAD are targeted for aggressive LDL cholesterol–lowering therapy to reduce coronary risk. However, there is growing evidence that statin therapy might also alter the natural history of PAD and improve claudication symptoms. A subanalysis of 4S reported that simvastatin treatment led to a 38% reduction in the risk of development or progression of intermittent claudication.[142] The Treatment of Peripheral Atherosclerotic Disease with Moderate or Intensive Lipid Lowering (TREADMILL) study was a randomized, double-blind, placebo-controlled, 12-month trial of the effects of atorvastatin on exercise performance in PAD patients with intermittent claudication. The study reported significant improvements in pain-free walking time, time to onset of claudication pain, and activity level, but not absolute walking time (i.e., from the beginning up to the time the patient was forced to stop walking because of claudication pain) in atorvastatin-treated patients.[143] These data suggest that selecting statin therapy in PAD patients for cardiovascular risk reduction may also improve daily claudication symptoms and impede the onset of PAD in some statin-treated patients.

Osteoporosis

The proposition that statins may increase bone mineral density and reduce fracture rates is contentious. *In vitro* studies have described an increase in the activity of bone morphogenetic proteins (BMPs), especially BMP-2, which controls osteoblast differentiation and enhances the expression of structural proteins of the bone matrix, such as type 1 collagen, osteopontin, osteocalcin, and bone sialoprotein.[144] In these experiments, lovastatin, simvastatin, fluvastatin, and atorvastatin have all been found to increase osteoblast cell numbers and new bone formation by approximately two- to threefold through induction of BMP-2.

The concept that statins may improve osteoporosis is supported by several large case–control observational studies reporting that populations of statin-taking patients have as many as 50% fewer hip fractures than non-statin-taking patients.[145,146] Some of these observational studies report that treatment with other lipid-altering therapies (e.g., fibrates) is not associated with a reduction in fracture risk. However, other observational studies have found no differences in fracture rates with statin therapy.[147] Part of the explanation for this may be that patients taking statins have "health-seeking" attributes that lower their risk of fractures, or that they are more likely to be overweight which could increase their bone mineral density and reduce fracture risk.

Randomized clinical trials offer less support for a positive statin effect on osteoporosis. Post hoc analyses of two placebo-controlled, outcome statin trials—4S with the lipophilic statin simvastatin and LIPID with the hydrophilic statin pravastatin—found no difference in fracture rates.[144,148] In the only randomized, placebo-controlled trial testing atorvastatin 10- to 80-mg daily doses in 626 postmenopausal women with high LDL cholesterol and lumbar spine bone mineral density T-score between 0.0 and −2.5, no significant changes in spine or hip bone mineral density or biomarkers were found.[149] These data offer little support for the use of statins to improve bone mineral density or reduce fracture rates. Until a well-designed, randomized trial has confirmed a beneficial effect, statins cannot be recommended in the treatment or prevention of osteoporosis.

Alzheimer's Disease

Alzheimer's disease (AD) is a neurodegenerative disorder manifested by cognitive decline, neuropsychiatric symptoms, and diffuse structural abnormalities in the brain. It is characterized by the deposition of amyloid-β in the form of neuritic plaques and by accumulation of intracellular neurofibrillary tangles, which are insoluble depositions resulting from altered metabolism of the cytoskeletal tau protein. Some have speculated that the synthesis of cholesterol and isoprenoid lipids is needed to provide amyloid peptides, which may provide the substrate for development of AD.

Most of the evidence that links cholesterol and AD has come from observational studies. It has been observed that an elevated cholesterol level in midlife increases the risk of AD by two- to threefold later in life.[150,151] Conversely, it has been observed that people who take statins and other lipid-lowering agents have a 60% to 75% reduction in the future risk of AD.[152,153] In animal studies, cholesterol feeding increased brain amyloid-β levels, and removing cholesterol from the feed was associated with a significant reduction in brain amyloid-β levels.[154,155]

One small, proof-of-concept, randomized, double-blind, placebo-controlled clinical trial has been conducted in 71 patients with a Mini-Mental State Examination (MMSE) score of 12 to 28 who randomly received atorvastatin 80 mg daily or placebo for 1 year.[156] A significant improvement in the primary efficacy measure for AD, the Alzheimer's Disease Assessment Scale–Cognitive Subscale (ADAS-COG), was reported. Based on the evidence to date, AD specialists believe that statin therapy may well be helpful in patients with mild disease (higher MMSE scores) who have cholesterol levels greater than 200 mg/dL and an $apoE_4$ allele. However, most specialists are waiting for the results of two large clinical trials testing statins in AD patients before routinely recommending them. One trial is the Cholesterol Lowering Agent to Slow Progression of Alzheimer's Disease (CLASP) with simvastatin 20 mg versus placebo, and the second is Lipitor's Effect in Alzheimer's Dementia (LEADe) with atorvastatin 80 mg versus placebo. It is appropriate to wait for the results of these important trials before recommending statin therapy in patients at risk for AD.

SAFETY

Very Low LDL Cholesterol

With the emphasis on aggressive LDL cholesterol lowering, the question becomes how low is too low? Unfortunately, the answer is not clear. However, comfort can be taken in the observation that the efficacy of a statin to lower LDL cholesterol is generally not related to an increased risk of liver or muscle adverse effects or other potential adverse effects. Said another way, the strength of the statin's interference with cholesterol biosynthesis and the resultant reduction in LDL cholesterol do not forecast adverse systemic effects, which appear more related to the concentration of the statin in the blood. So the key question is, is there an LDL cholesterol level at which those body functions and processes that depend on cholesterol begin to malfunction?

The clinical trials in Table 22-7 with the lowest on-treatment LDL cholesterol level achieved (e.g., ASCOT-LLA, SPARCL, and CARDS) and all of the studies in Table 22-8 did not report aberrant adverse effects. The one exception may be the SPARCL trial, which reported an adjusted hazard ratio of 1.66 for hemorrhagic stroke patients receiving statin[141] (see discussion earlier under "Cerebrovascular Accident").

A post hoc analysis of the PROVE IT trial, which achieved the lowest on-treatment LDL cholesterol level (a mean of 62 mg/dL), evaluated the occurrence of adverse events across on-treatment LDL cholesterol levels during treatment with either pravastatin 40 mg daily or atorvastatin 80 mg daily for 2 years. These are summarized in Table 22-9.[160] No adverse effect signal was noted in any safety measure, even in patients who achieved an LDL cholesterol below 40 mg/dL for 2 years. Safety measures included changes in hemorrhagic stroke, muscle toxicity, and discontinuation of statin therapy due to adverse effects.

Another way to try to answer the question of whether low LDL cholesterol is safe is to look at genetic dyslipidemias. Familial hypobetalipoproteinemia may be one such condition. Hypobetalipoproteinemia is a rare disorder (1:500 for heterozygotes and 1:1,000,000 for homozygotes) of apoB metabolism characterized by levels of plasma LDL cholesterol that are less than one-quarter to one-third normal. In heterozygotes, LDL cholesterol levels are mostly less than 70 mg/dL and much lower than this in homozygotes (i.e., approximately <40 mg/dL).[161] Homozygotes present with fat malabsorption, hepatic steatosis, and low plasma cholesterol levels at a young age and develop progressive neurologic degenerative disease, retinitis pigmentosa, and acanthocytosis over the first three decades of life before their demise. Heterozygotes are usually asymptomatic but have decreased LDL cholesterol and apoB levels, possibly a decreased risk of atherosclerosis, and normal longevity. This disorder is also associated with decreasing levels of hemostatic risk factors that may decrease clinical cardiac events through a reduction in thrombotic tendency.[162] While mechanistically not a perfect match for low LDL cholesterol with statin therapy, hypobetalipoproteinemia suggests that the current optional NCEP ATP III goal of LDL cholesterol less than 70 mg/dL for very-high-risk individuals is appropriate, but that achieving very low levels (e.g., <40 mg/dL) may be associated with unwanted adverse consequences. More research is needed to better characterize risks associated with very low LDL cholesterol.

Liver

Elevations of alanine aminotransferase (ALT) or aspartate aminotransferase (AST) to greater than three times the upper limit of normal (ULN) with statin therapy are rare, often just slightly more than observed in placebo-treated patients. In one survey of 35 randomized trials involving 74,102 patients, elevations in transaminase levels were reported in 1.4% of statin-treated patients compared with 1.1% of control patients.[163] In another review of 21 randomized trials involving 180,000 person-years, ALT elevation of three or more times the ULN was reported in only 300 statin-allocated patients per 100,000 person-years.[164]

TABLE 22-9 Percent of Patients with Safety Outcomes Receiving Either Pravastatin 40 mg/day or Atorvastatin 80 mg/day in the PROVE IT Trial Stratified by On-Treatment LDL Cholesterol[160]

	LDL Cholesterol (mg/dL)				
Safety Measures	80–100	60–80	40–60	<40	*P* trend
Myositis	0.4	0.6	0.6	0	0.75
CK >10 times ULN	0	0	0.3	0	0.45
Rhabdomyolysis	0	0	0	0	1.0
ALT >3 times ULN	3.2	3.0	3.2	2.6	0.98
Hemorrhagic stroke	0.4	0.2	0	0	0.12
Statin discontinued because of an adverse event	10.2	9.4	9.7	9.7	0.99
Death	1.1	1.4	1.3	0.5	0.59
Stroke	0.8	0.9	0.6	1.6	0.32

ALT, Alanine aminotransferase; CK, creatine kinase; LDL, low-density lipoprotein; ULN, upper limit of normal.

Transaminase elevations with statins appear related to the dose and not their LDL cholesterol–lowering efficacy. Transaminase elevations three times the ULN are observed in less than 1% of patients receiving low and intermediate statin doses and in 2% to 3% of patients receiving 80-mg doses.[127] However, analysis of prescribing information for each statin reveals that there is no relationship between the LDL cholesterol–lowering efficacy of the statin and elevations in ALT or AST (Fig. 22-7). In fact, in this analysis the most efficacious statins, atorvastatin and rosuvastatin, caused no more, and perhaps even fewer, elevations than the least efficacious statin, fluvastatin.

Transaminase elevations with statins are also transient. In the analysis of 180,000 individuals that reported 300 patients out of approximately 90,000 treated with a statin had a transaminase level greater than three times the ULN, only 110 had consecutive elevations. These data are summarized in Table 22-10.[164] This suggests that elevations resolve spontaneously in 70% of patients. It further suggests that clinicians should repeat liver function testing when faced with an isolated elevation in patients taking statins.

The more clinically relevant issue is whether statins cause serious liver dysfunction or failure.[127] Data for the oldest marketed statin, lovastatin, reveals that 22 cases of liver failure have been reported to the Merck Worldwide Adverse Event Database and/or the FDA Adverse Event Reporting System (AERS), representing a rate of 1 case per 1.14 million patient-treatment-years.[164] The 30 cases of liver failure in individuals taking any statin reported to the AERS database through 1999 represent a reporting rate of 1 case per 1 million person-years of statin prescription use.[165] The reporting rate of liver failure in the population *not* taking a statin is the same: about 1 case per million people.[166] This suggests one of two conclusions: (1) There is no relation between statin therapy and liver failure, or (2) cases of liver failure represent idiosyncratic reactions that very rarely occur in patients receiving statins.

The conclusion of the NLA Statin Safety Assessment Task Force is that the FDA should rescind the recommendation for routine monitoring of liver function tests for two reasons: (1) Monitoring is not likely to detect such a rare event, and (2) the identification of patients with isolated increased aminotransferase levels may prompt health professionals to discontinue therapy. While attempting to avoid a very remote risk of liver failure the patient will be exposed to a disproportionately high risk for cardiovascular events.[167]

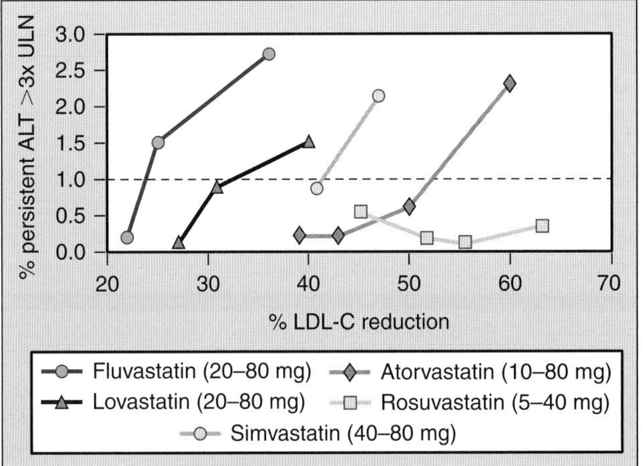

FIGURE 22-7 Increases in alanine aminotransferase (ALT) > 3 times the upper limit of normal (ULN) versus low-density lipoprotein cholesterol (LDL-C) reduction with statins across their dose range.

To deal with this issue, the NLA Statin Safety Assessment Task Force recommends that patients be routinely monitored for symptoms of hepatic dysfunction, including jaundice, malaise, lethargy, anorexia, and fatigue.[167] These recommendations are listed in Table 22-11. The liver experts consulting with the task force recommend that fractionated bilirubin be evaluated in patients with symptoms that, in the absence of biliary obstruction, is a more accurate prognosticator of liver injury than isolated transaminase elevations. If an aminotransferase level is found to be greater than three times the ULN on consecutive occasions, or if the fractionated bilirubin is elevated in a symptomatic patient, the statin should be withdrawn. However, if liver function tests are one to three times the ULN, there is no need to discontinue the statin. Furthermore, if ALT or AST are greater than three times the ULN in an asymptomatic patient, the test should be repeated, other etiologies ruled out, and consideration given to continuing statin therapy, reducing statin dose, or discontinuing statin therapy (see Table 22-11).

Muscle

In 2001, cerivastatin was withdrawn from the market because of a high incidence of rhabdomyolysis and associated deaths. Today, we know that serious muscle-related adverse effects with the statins remaining on the market are rare. On the basis of findings from 21 randomized clinical trials providing 180,000 person-years of follow-up on statin therapy or placebo, myopathy (muscle symptoms plus an increase in creative kinase [CK] of ≥10 times ULN) occurred in 5 patients per 100,000 person-years, and rhabdomyolysis in 1.6 patients per 100,000 person-years (placebo-corrected).[164] The AERS database yielded a reporting rate of 0.3 to 2.2 cases of myopathy and 0.3 to 13.5 cases of rhabdomyolysis per 1 million statin prescriptions.[168] According to an analysis of a large administrative managed-care claims database, which may come closest to reflecting a real-world estimate of the extent of this problem, 0.6 to 1.2 cases of hospitalized rhabdomyolysis occurred per 10,000 person-years of therapy with a statin. This information is summarized in Table 22-12. In this analysis, cerivastatin was associated with a reporting rate of 8.4 hospitalized rhabdomyolysis cases per 10,000 person-years.[169]

Muscle toxicity with statins is a class effect, but there may be differences in the rates of serious muscle toxicity for different statins. Considering only large randomized clinical outcome trials, pravastatin therapy has not been associated with a case of rhabdomyolysis in the 19,768 patients studied for 5 years.[115,170,171] Conversely, simvastatin produced rhabdomyolysis in 0.1% of the 2265 patients receiving 80 mg of simvastatin for 2 years in the A to Z trial.[172] The prescribing information for simvastatin reports a 0.5% rate of myopathy/rhabdomyolysis with 80 mg daily.[7]

TABLE 22-10 Number of Subjects with ALT >3 Times ULN out of 280,000 Patients Randomized to Statin Therapy or Placebo for an Average of 3 Years[164]

	Statin	Placebo	Net Risk
Single ALT measure	300	200	100
Consecutive ALT measures	110	40	70

ALT, Alanine aminotransferase; ULN, upper limit of normal.

TABLE 22-11 Recommendations to Health Professionals Regarding the Liver and Statin Safety[167]

1. During the routine general evaluation of patients being considered for statin and other lipid-lowering therapy, it is advisable to measure liver transaminase levels. If these levels are found to be abnormal, further investigation should be performed to determine the etiology of the abnormal test results.
2. Until there is a change in FDA-approved prescribing information for statins, it is appropriate to continue to measure transaminase levels according to prescribing information and clinical judgment.
3. The clinician should be alert to patient reports of jaundice, malaise, fatigue, lethargy, and related symptoms in patients taking statin therapy, as a signal of potential hepatotoxicity. Evidence for hepatotoxicity includes jaundice, hepatomegaly, increased indirect bilirubin level, and elevated prothrombin time (rather than simple elevations in liver transaminase levels).
4. The preferred biochemical test to ascertain significant liver injury is fractionated bilirubin, which, in the absence of biliary obstruction, is a more accurate prognosticator of liver injury than isolated aminotransferase levels.
5. Should the clinician identify objective evidence of significant liver injury in a patient receiving a statin, the statin should be discontinued. The etiology should be sought and, if indicated, the patient referred to a gastroenterologist or hepatologist.
6. If an isolated asymptomatic transaminase level is found to be elevated 1–3 times the ULN, there is no need to discontinue the statin.
7. If an isolated asymptomatic transaminase level is found to be >3 times the ULN during a routine evaluation of a patient receiving a statin, the test should be repeated and, if still elevated, other etiologies should be ruled out. Consideration should be given to continuing the statin, reducing its dose, or discontinuing it, based on clinical judgment.

TABLE 22-12 Incident Rates of Rhabdomyolysis from a Managed-Care Claims Database of 875,000 Statin-Taking Individuals in Which 42 Cases Were Confirmed with Chart Review

Drug	Patient-Years	Incident Rates per 10,000 Person-Years (95% CI)
Atorvastatin	261,567	0.6 (0.3–0.9)
Fluvastatin	12,635	1.6 (0.2–5.7)
Lovastatin	26,122	0.3 (0.1–2.1)
Pravastatin	64,254	1.1 (0.4–2.2)
Rosuvastatin	8,213	1.2 (0.03–6.7)
Simvastatin	54,394	0.6 (0.1–1.6)
Cerivastatin	4,719	8.4 (2.3–21.7)

CI, confidence interval.

The more common muscle-related adverse event with statins is myalgias, generally taken to mean muscle pain, soreness, or weakness. In clinical trials, myalgias, with or without a CK elevation, have been reported in approximately 3% to 15% of patients receiving statin therapy. Often, reports of myalgias with statins in clinical trials are the same as, or only slightly more than, those reported in patients receiving placebo.[163,164] In spite of the lack of a strong association with statin therapy, the occurrence of myalgias is the most common reason for patients (or health professionals) to discontinue therapy.

The exact mechanism of skeletal muscle toxicity associated with statins is unknown but appears to relate to an interruption of muscle function by statins, likely related to statins' inhibition of HMG-CoA reductase. Statins affect mostly type 2 (mitochondrial poor) muscle fibers. This suggests that statins may express their muscle toxicity through an action on these cells. One hypothesis is that statins reduce the cholesterol content of the sarcolemma (plasma membrane) of skeletal muscle cells, which may lead to instability or even rupture of some muscle cells.[88] A microarray of 14,500 well-characterized genes in normal volunteers receiving statin therapy and undergoing eccentric (muscle damaging) exercise has shown an up-regulation of genes of the ubiquitin proteasome pathway, which is active in protein degradation.[173] Recently, a genomewide scan of 85 subjects with definite or incipient myopathy and 90 controls, all of whom were receiving 80 mg of simvastatin daily, identified the rs4363657 single-nucleotide polymorphism located within *SLCO1B1* on chromosome 12 as a likely culprit of myopathy. *SLCO1B1* encodes for OATP1B1, the transport protein that regulates hepatic uptake of statins.[173a]

This rs4363657 polymorphism occurs in 15% of the population. In those affected, statins would not be taken up as freely into hepatic tissues, thus raising statin blood levels. In patients with this polymorphism, other factors that raise statin blood levels, such as use of a high statin dose and drug interactions that interfere with normal metabolic degradation of a statin, would increase the risk of myotoxicity. In the future, we may have genotyping to detect this SLCO1B1 polymorphism and thereby be alerted to an increased risk of myopathy in our statin-taking patients. Until then, it is important that we recognize and limit the factors that increase the risk of muscle toxicity (see Table 22-13).

Some investigators have speculated that a drop in ubiquinone levels may cause myotoxicity. Statins interfere with the formation of ubiquinone (also called *coenzyme Q10* [CoQ10]), a byproduct of cholesterol synthesis (see Fig. 22-2). Ubiquinone plays an important role in the cellular energy transduction of the mitochondrial electron transport system, supports ATP synthesis in the mitochondrial inner membrane, and stabilizes cell membranes, thus preserving cellular integrity and function.

Since ubiquinone is carried in LDL particles, serum levels drop with statin therapy along with LDL cholesterol, thus making this measure a poor indicator of the effects of statins on muscle energy metabolism. A better measure is the concentration of CoQ10 in the skeletal muscle cell. A recent study reported a reduction in muscle cell ubiquinone levels with simvastatin 80 mg but not with atorvastatin 40 mg, in spite of similar reductions in cholesterol levels, suggesting that this effect may be drug and dose dependent.[174] In subjects with the greatest reductions in muscle ubiquinone levels, a reduction in mitochondrial respiratory chain enzyme and citrate synthase activity was also reported. Many other studies in humans administered starting doses of statins have been unable to demonstrate a reduction in skeletal muscle CoQ10 levels. Studies in animals have also had inconsistent findings.

There have been conflicting results on the utility of administering ubiquinone to patients either to prevent or to treat muscle-related symptoms. In one study involving the use of very high experimental doses of lovastatin as a cancer treatment for 2.5 years, supplementation with CoQ10 240 mg daily did not reduce the frequency of myopathy compared with subjects not receiving this supplement.[175] In another small but well-designed study, statin-taking patients who had myalgia were randomized to CoQ10 100 mg/day or vitamin E 400 IU/day. Pain scores on a 10-point visual analogue scale were reduced from a mean of 5.0 to 3.0 with the CoQ10 supplementation, and most patients had some reduction in their pain score.[176] Given the equivocal nature of these data, CoQ10 deficiency cannot be attributed as the cause of statin-associated myopathy, nor does the evidence support the use of CoQ10 to prevent myopathic symptoms. Nevertheless, there are no known risks associated with CoQ10 supplementation, and thus supplementation with 200 mg daily may be tried in patients who develop myalgia and cannot otherwise tolerate statin therapy. Some patients may benefit from a placebo effect.[177]

Like liver transaminase elevations, muscle toxicity appears to relate to blood concentration of the statin and not to LDL cholesterol–lowering efficacy (Fig. 22-8). Thus, risk factors for the occurrence of muscle toxicity include those factors that can raise blood levels of statins, such as increasing dose, advanced age and frailty, female gender, renal insufficiency, hepatic dysfunction, hypothyroidism, and concurrent use of agents with pharmacokinetic interactions with statins, including gemfibrozil and agents that inhibit CYP3A4[164,178] (Table 22-13). Pravastatin is not subject to cytochrome P450 metabolism and therefore may be less likely than other statins to have pharmacokinetic interactions with cytochrome P450 inhibitors (e.g., verapamil, azole antifungals).[179] On the other hand, pravastatin, like other statins, is a substrate for OATP that mediates transport across cell walls and is susceptible to interference by cyclosporine, and other drugs that inhibit CYP3A4.[180]

Myotoxicity lies on a continuum of severity from mild myalgias to potentially fatal rhabdomyolysis. The NLA Statin Safety Assessment Task Force does not

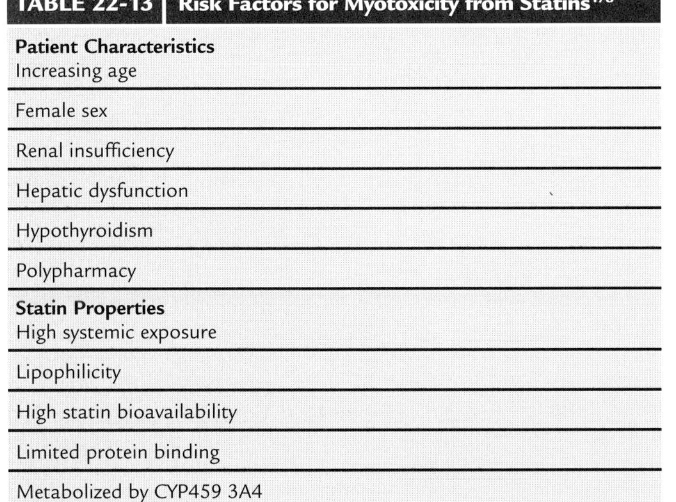

TABLE 22-13 Risk Factors for Myotoxicity from Statins[178]
Patient Characteristics
Increasing age
Female sex
Renal insufficiency
Hepatic dysfunction
Hypothyroidism
Polypharmacy
Statin Properties
High systemic exposure
Lipophilicity
High statin bioavailability
Limited protein binding
Metabolized by CYP459 3A4

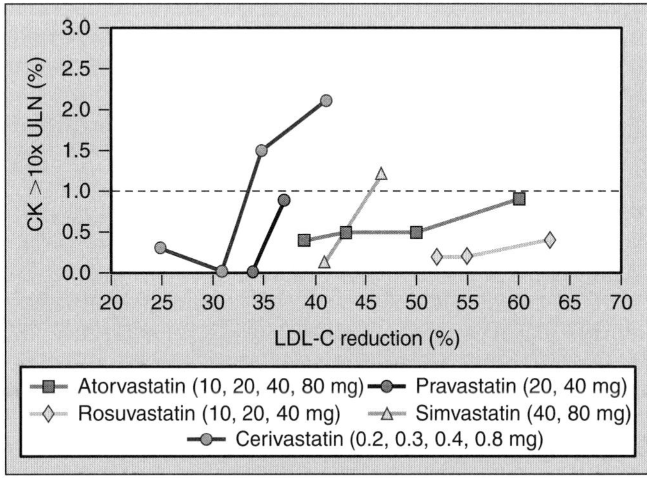

FIGURE 22-8 Incidence of increases in creatine kinase (CK) levels >10 times the upper limit of normal (ULN) versus low-density lipoprotein cholesterol (LDL-C) reduction with statins across their dose range.
Reprinted from Brewer HB Jr, Benefit-risk assessment of rosurastatin 10 to 40 milligrams. *Am J Cardiol* 2003;92:23K–29K.

recommend routine monitoring of CK levels. Instead, CK levels may be used to evaluate patients who report muscle symptoms. Statins should be discontinued in patients who develop intolerable muscle symptoms, with or without a CK elevation and in whom other etiologies have been ruled out. Statin therapy (with the same or a different agent) may be restarted at the same or a lower dose once the patient is asymptomatic, to test the reproducibility of the symptoms. These recommendations are summarized in Table 22-14.

Renal

During the premarket development for rosuvastatin, cases of 2+ or greater proteinuria in patients previously with negative or trace dipstick proteinuria were reported. This raised concerns that rosuvastatin and possibly other statins may impair renal function. In fact, this same phenomenon was found to occur with all statins but no more frequently than in a placebo-treated population (Fig. 22-9).

Today, we have a clearer understanding why this occurred. Low-molecular-weight proteins are filtered by the glomerulas and reabsorbed in the renal tubules. An *in vitro* experiment in opossum kidney proximal tubule cells demonstrated that inhibition of cholesterol synthesis with high concentrations of statins reduced renal tubular uptake of albumin (Fig. 22-10).[181] Further, addition of mevalonate restored the normal tubular reabsorption processes (Fig. 22-11). This experiment establishes the principle that the inhibition of HMG-CoA reductase in renal proximal tubule cells can reduce the rate of tubular protein uptake *in vivo,* providing a mechanistic explanation of statin-associated proteinuria. An analysis of proteinuria in 50 patients indicated the majority was tubular in origin, based on the presence of low-molecular-weight proteins.[179]

However, cases of acute renal failure have also been reported in patients treated with statins. The reporting rate for renal failure from the AERS database in statin-treated patients is low: 0.3 to 0.6 case per 1 million statin prescriptions.[168] This reporting rate is similar to that in a population not consuming statins. Further, examination of clinical trial data does not support the premise that statins cause renal failure. For example, data from three randomized clinical outcome trials with pravastatin—CARE, LIPID, and WOSCOPS—revealed that renal failure or other renal disease occurred more often in placebo controls (0.8%) than in pravastatin-treated patients (0.5%).[182] In 2005, the FDA conducted a case-by-case review of 38 reports of renal failure/insufficiency in patients receiving rosuvastatin and concluded that "no consistent pattern of clinical presentation or of renal injury (i.e., pathology) is evident among the cases of renal failure reported to date that clearly indicates causation by rosuvastatin or other statins."[183]

In contrast, several lines of evidence actually suggest a potential reno*protective* effect of long-term statin therapy, which is reviewed under Nontraditional Uses earlier in this chapter.

The consensus recommendations of the NLA Task Force to health professionals regarding the kidney and statins are that routine serum creatinine and proteinuria monitoring during therapy is not necessary for the purposes of identifying an adverse effect, and that if serum creatinine becomes elevated in the absence of rhabdomyolysis during statin therapy, statin therapy does not need to be discontinued. A dose adjustment may be required in some cases, based on prescribing information.

Neurologic

The potential risk of peripheral neuropathy with statin therapy is very small, if it exists at all.[167] This issue has been raised by case reports suggesting an association between peripheral neuropathy and statin use.[184] Symptoms of peripheral neuropathy appeared in 1 day

TABLE 22-14 Recommendations to Healthcare Professionals Regarding the Muscle and Statin Safety[167]
1. Whenever muscular symptoms or an increased CK level is encountered in a patient receiving statin therapy, health professionals should attempt to rule out other etiologies, because these are most likely to explain the findings. Other common etiologies include increased physical activity, trauma, falls, accidents, seizure, shaking chills, hypothyroidism, infections, carbon monoxide poisoning, polymyositis, dermatomyositis, alcohol abuse, and drug abuse (cocaine, amphetamines, heroin, or PCP).
2. Obtaining a pretreatment, baseline CK level may be considered in patients who are at high risk of muscle toxicity (e.g., older individuals or when combining a statin with an agent known to increase myotoxicity), but this is not routinely necessary in other patients.
3. It is not necessary to measure CK levels in asymptomatic patients during the course of statin therapy, because marked, clinically important CK elevations are rare and are usually related to physical exertion or other causes.
4. Patients receiving statin therapy should be counseled about the increased risk of muscle complaints, particularly if the initiation of vigorous, sustained endurance exercise or a surgical operation is being contemplated; they should be advised to report such muscle symptoms to a health professional.
5. CK measurements should be obtained in symptomatic patients to help gauge the severity of muscle damage and facilitate a decision of whether to continue therapy or alter doses.
6. In patients who develop intolerable muscle symptoms with or without a CK elevation and in whom other etiologies have been ruled out, the statin should be discontinued. Once the patient is asymptomatic, the same or a different statin at the same or a lower dose can be restarted to test the reproducibility of symptoms. Recurrence of symptoms with multiple statins and doses requires initiation of other lipid-altering therapy.
7. In patients who develop tolerable muscle complaints or are asymptomatic with a CK <10 times the ULN, statin therapy may be continued at the same or reduced doses and symptoms may be used as the clinical guide to stopping or continuing therapy.
8. In patients who develop rhabdomyolysis (CK >10,000 IU/L or CK >10 times the ULN with an elevation in serum creatinine or requiring IV hydration therapy), statin therapy should be stopped. IV hydration therapy in a hospital setting should be instituted if indicated for patients with rhabdomyolysis. Once the patient has recovered, the risk versus benefit of statin therapy should be carefully reconsidered.

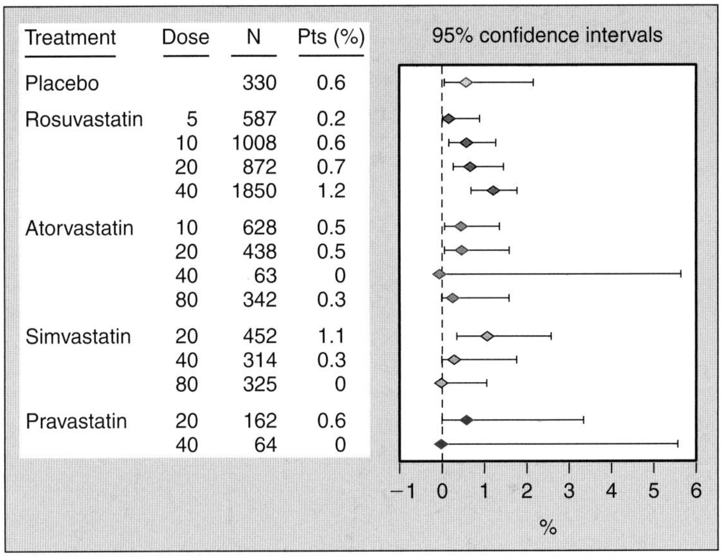

Treatment Dose N Pts (%)
Placebo 330 0.6
Rosuvastatin 5 587 0.2
10 1008 0.6
20 872 0.7
40 1850 1.2
Atorvastatin 10 628 0.5
20 438 0.5
40 63 0
80 342 0.3
Simvastatin 20 452 1.1
40 314 0.3
80 325 0
Pravastatin 20 162 0.6
40 64 0
95% confidence intervals
−1 0 1 2 3 4 5 6
%

FIGURE 22-9 Percentage of patients with negative to trace urine protein dipstick measurements at baseline and 2+ or greater measurements at the final study visit during treatment with statins at specified doses.

Simvastatin
Rosuvastatin
Pravastatin
Inhibition of albumin uptake (%)
100
80
60
40
20
0
0 10 20 30 40 50 60 70 80 90 100
Inhibition of cholesterol synthesis (%)

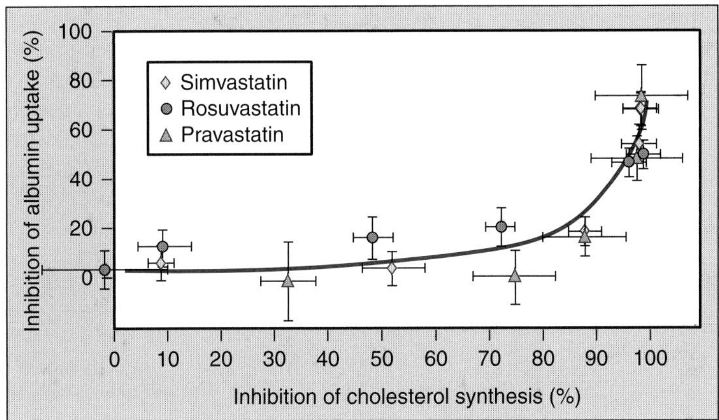

FIGURE 22-10 Comparison of percentage inhibition of cholesterol synthesis versus percentage inhibition of albumin uptake in a proximal tubule–derived opossum cell line.

Statin only
Statin + mevalonate
% interference with albumin uptake
120
100
80
60
40
20
0
Control
Simva 10 µm
Simva 100 µm
Rosuva 10 µm
Rosuva 100 µm
− + − + − + − + − +
Mevalonate 100 µm
Combined results of 2 experiments, mean ± SE

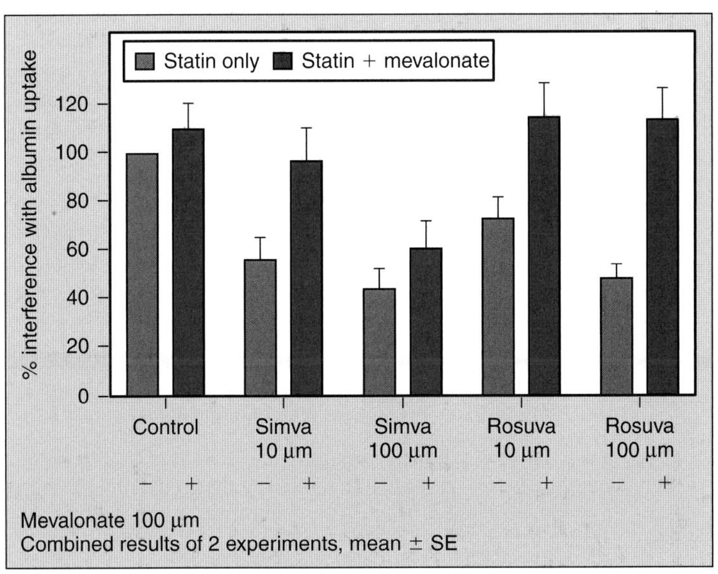

FIGURE 22-11 Impact of adding mevalonate on the percentage inhibition of albumin uptake by statins in a proximal tubule–derived opossum cell line.

to 7 years (average 6 months) and were confirmed by nerve conduction tests, and all patients improved—some completely within 1 to 9 months of discontinuing the statin. A meta-analysis of four cohort studies yielded a summary odds ratio of 1.8 (95% confidence interval, 1.1–3.0; $P < 0.001$), consistent with an increased risk of peripheral neuropathy with statin treatment.[164] However, these data alone are insufficient to prove causality, and they have not been confirmed by large, randomized clinical outcome trials. For example, during an average of 5 years of therapy in 20,536 patients randomized in HPS, no significant excess of peripheral neuropathy occurred in simvastatin-treated patients (11 cases) compared with controls (8 cases).[116] Similarly, PROSPER investigators found no evidence of statin-related peripheral neuropathy in the 5804 elderly patients (ages 70–82 years) receiving pravastatin 40 mg/day or placebo.[185]

The NLA Statin Safety Assessment Task Force concluded that although routine neurologic monitoring of patients for changes indicative of peripheral neuropathy are not recommended, systematic evaluation of patients who develop peripheral neuropathy while taking a statin is a reasonable approach to rule out secondary causes (e.g., diabetes mellitus, renal insufficiency, alcohol abuse, vitamin B_{12} deficiency).[167] If another etiology is not identified, statin therapy should be withdrawn for 3 to 6 months to establish whether an association with the statin exists. Although a presumptive diagnosis of statin-induced peripheral neuropathy can be made if the symptoms improve while off statin therapy, rechallenge (with a different statin and dose) should be considered so as not to forfeit the proven benefits of statin therapy.

Case reports also suggest that memory or cognitive impairment may occur rarely with statin therapy, but this most likely represents an idiosyncratic effect.[186] Most case reports involve memory loss. Symptoms began approximately 6 months after starting the statin. No memory tests were performed. Forty-two percent of cases reported improvement on withdrawing the statin. In four out of the four cases in which statin therapy was rechallenged, recurrent memory loss was reported. In order for a statin to alter cognition, it must gain access to the brain. The more lipophilic the statin, the greater the potential for permeability across the blood–brain barrier and thus the greater potential for central nervous system (CNS) effects.[187] Animal studies have demonstrated that the lipophilic statins, lovastatin and simvastatin, cross the blood–brain barrier, whereas hydrophilic statins (e.g., pravastatin) do so minimally.[188] The actual exposure of brain tissue to statins is a balance between the blood–brain barrier diffusion into the CNS and the movement out of the CNS by transporters. Any impact of the lipophilicity of statins on their clinical efficacy or safety has yet to be definitively proven.[187]

Large, randomized clinical trials do not support a relationship between statins and cognition changes. In HPS, cognitive impairment was detected in similar proportions of simvastatin-treated patients (23.7%) and controls (24.2%) after 5 years of therapy.[116,157] Likewise, cognitive function declined at the same rate in elderly pravastatin-treated patients and controls in PROSPER.[185]

Some clinical data suggest that statins may have a beneficial effect on CNS disorders such as Alzheimer's disease and other forms of dementia.[189] These data were discussed under Nontraditional Uses earlier in this chapter.

According to the NLA Statin Safety Assessment Task Force, if a patient has impaired cognition while receiving statin therapy, other etiologies should be ruled out, and if none are found, statin therapy should be withdrawn for 1 to 3 months. If improvement is not observed, statin therapy should be restarted based on a benefit–risk analysis.[167]

REFERENCES

1. Endo A: The discovery and development of HMG-CoA reductase inhibitors. *J Lipid Res* 1992;33:1569–1582.
2. Crestor Prescribing Information. AstraZeneca Pharmaceuticals, Wilmingon, DE. January, 2007.
3. Lescol Prescribing Information. Novartis Pharmaceuticals Corporation. East Hanover, NJ. April 2006.
4. Lipitor Prescribing Information. Pfizer, NY, NY. March 2007.
5. Mevacor Prescribing Information. Merck & Co, Whitehouse Station, NJ. November, 2005.
6. Pravachol Prescribing Information. Bristol-Myers Squibb, Princeton, NJ. August, 2005.
7. Zocor Prescribing Information. Merck & Co, Whitehouse Station, NJ. August, 2005.
8. Istvan ES, Deisenhofer J: Structural mechanism for statin inhibition of HMG-CoA reductase. *Science* 2001;292:1160–1164.
9. McTaggart F, Buckett L, Davidson R, et al: Preclinical and clinical pharmacology of rosuvastatin, a new 3-hydroxy-3-methylglutaryl coenzyme A reductase inhibitor. *Am J Cardiol* 2001;87 (suppl):28B–32B.
10. Holdgate GA, Ward WH, McTaggart F: Molecular mechanisms for inhibition of 3-hydroxy-3-methylglutaryl CoA (HMG-CoA) reductase by rosuvastatin. *Biochem Soc Trans* 2003;31:528–531.
11. Brown MS, Goldstein JL: A receptor-mediated pathway for cholesterol homeostasis. *Science* 1986;232:34–47.
12. Ginsberg HN, Le NA, Short MP, Ramakrishnan R, Desnick RJ: Suppression of apolipoprotein B production during treatment of cholesteryl ester storage disease with lovastatin: implications for regulation of apolipoprotein B synthesis. *J Clin Invest* 1987;80:1692–1697.
13. Arad Y, Ramakrishnan R, Ginsberg HN: Lovastatin therapy reduces low-density lipoprotein apoB levels in subjects with combined hyperlipidemia by reducing the production of apoB-containing lipoproteins: implications for the pathophysiology of apoB production. *J Lipid Res* 1990;31:567–582.
14. Sever PS, Dahlof B, Poulter NR, et al: Prevention of coronary and stroke events with atorvastatin in hypertensive patients who have average or lower-than-average cholesterol concentrations, in the Anglo-Scandinavian Cardiac Outcomes Trial–Lipid Lowering Arm (ASCOT-LLA): A multicentre randomised controlled trial. *Lancet* 2003;361:1149–1158.
15. Cannon CP, Braunwald E, McCabe CH, et al: Intensive versus moderate lipid lowering with statins after acute coronary syndromes. *N Engl J Med* 2004;350:1495–1504.
16. Collins R, Armitage J, Parish S, et al: MRC/BHF Heart Protection Study of cholesterol-lowering with simvastatin in 5963 people with diabetes: A randomised placebo-controlled trial. *Lancet* 2003;361:2005–2016.
17. Grundy SM: Approach to lipoprotein management in 2001 National Cholesterol Guidelines. *Am J Cardiol* 2002;90 (suppl): 11i–21i.
18. Baigent C, Keech A, Kearney PM, et al: Efficacy and safety of cholesterol-lowering treatment: Prospective meta-analysis of data from 90 056 participants in 14 randomised trials of statins. *Lancet* 2005;366:1267–1278.
19. Buchwald H, Varco RL, Matts JP, et al: Effect of partial ileal bypass surgery on mortality and morbidity from coronary heart disease in patients with hypercholesterolemia. Report of the Program on the Surgical Control of the Hyperlipidemias (POSCH). *N Engl J Med* 1990;323:946–955.

20. Lipid Research Clinics Program: The Lipid Research Clinics Coronary Primary Prevention Trial results. II. The relationship of reduction in incidence of coronary heart disease to cholesterol lowering. *JAMA* 1984;251:365–374.
21. Sukhova GK, Williams JK, Libby P: Statins reduce inflammation in atheroma of nonhuman primates independent of effects on serum cholesterol. *Arterioscler Thromb Vasc Biol* 2002;22:1452–1458.
22. Plenge JK, Hernandez TL, Weil KM, et al: Simvastatin lowers C-reactive protein within 14 days: An effect independent of low-density lipoprotein cholesterol reduction. *Circulation* 2002;106:1447–1452.
23. Nissen SE, Tuzcu EM, Schoenhagen P, et al: Statin therapy, LDL cholesterol, C-reactive protein, and coronary artery disease. *N Engl J Med* 2005;352:29–38.
24. Correia LC, Sposito AC, Lima JC, et al: Anti-inflammatory effect of atorvastatin (80 mg) in unstable angina pectoris and non–Q-wave acute myocardial infarction. *Am J Cardiol* 2003;92:298–301.
25. Laufs U, Wassmann S, Hilgers S, et al: Rapid effects on vascular function after initiation and withdrawal of atorvastatin in healthy, normocholesterolemic men. *Am J Cardiol* 2001;88:1306–1307.
26. Ballantyne CM, Houri J, Notarbartolo A, et al: Effect of ezetimibe coadministered with atorvastatin in 628 patients with primary hypercholesterolemia: A prospective, randomized, double-blind trial. *Circulation* 2003;107:2409–2415.
27. van Heek M, Farley C, Compton DS, et al: Ezetimibe potently inhibits cholesterol absorption but does not affect acute hepatic or intestinal cholesterol synthesis in rats. *Br J Pharmacol* 2003;138:1459–1464.
28. Ballantyne CM, Andrews TC, Hsia JA, et al: Correlation of non–high-density lipoprotein cholesterol with apolipoprotein B: Effect of 5 hydroxymethylglutaryl coenzyme A reductase inhibitors on non–high-density lipoprotein cholesterol levels. *Am J Cardiol* 2001;88:265–269.
29. Tsunekawa T, Hayashi T, Kano H, et al: Cerivastatin, a hydroxymethylglutaryl coenzyme A reductase inhibitor, improves endothelial function in elderly diabetic patients within 3 days. *Circulation* 2001;104:376–379.
30. Landmesser U, Bahlmann F, Mueller M, et al: Simvastatin versus ezetimibe: Pleiotropic and lipid-lowering effects on endothelial function in humans. *Circulation* 2005;111:2356–2363.
31. Fichtlscherer S, Schmidt-Lucke C, Bojunga S, et al: Differential effects of short-term lipid lowering with ezetimibe and statins on endothelial function in patients with CAD: Clinical evidence for 'pleiotropic' functions of statin therapy. *Eur Heart J* 2006;27:1182–1190.
32. Beckman JA, Liao JK, Hurley S, et al: Atorvastatin restores endothelial function in normocholesterolemic smokers independent of changes in low-density lipoprotein. *Circ Res* 2004;95:217–223.
33. Ridker PM, Cannon CP, Morrow D, et al: C-reactive protein levels and outcomes after statin therapy. *N Engl J Med* 2005;352:20–28.
34. Davignon J: The cardioprotective effects of statins. *Curr Atheroscler Rep* 2004;6:27–35.
35. Rikitake Y, Liao JK: Rho GTPases, statins, and nitric oxide. *Circ Res* 2005;97:1232–1235.
36. Laufs U, Liao JK: Targeting Rho in cardiovascular disease. *Circ Res* 2000;87:526–528.
37. Shimokawa H, Takeshita A: Rho-kinase is an important therapeutic target in cardiovascular medicine. *Arterioscler Thromb Vasc Biol* 2005;25:1767–1775.
38. Takai Y, Sasaki T, Matozaki T: Small GTP-binding proteins. *Physiol Rev* 2001;81:153–208.
39. Fukata Y, Amano M, Kaibuchi K: Rho–Rho-kinase pathway in smooth muscle contraction and cytoskeletal reorganization of non-muscle cells. *Trends Pharmacol Sci* 2001;22:32–39.
40. Ishizaki T, Maekawa M, Fujisawa K, et al: The small GTP-binding protein Rho binds to and activates a 160 kDa Ser/Thr protein kinase homologous to myotonic dystrophy kinase. *EMBO J* 1996;15:1885–1893.
41. Leung T, Manser E, Tan L, Lim L: A novel serine/threonine kinase binding the Ras-related RhoA GTPase which translocates the kinase to peripheral membranes. *J Biol Chem* 1995;270:29051–29054.
42. Matsui T, Amano M, Yamamoto T, et al: Rho-associated kinase, a novel serine/threonine kinase, as a putative target for small GTP binding protein Rho. *EMBO J* 1996;15:2208–2216.
43. Riento K, Ridley AJ: ROCKS: Multifunctional kinases in cell behaviour. *Nat Rev Mol Cell Biol* 2003;4:446–456.
44. Laufs U, Endres M, Stagliano N, et al: Neuroprotection mediated by changes in the endothelial actin cytoskeleton. *J Clin Invest* 2000;106:15–24.
45. Takemoto M, Liao JK: Pleiotropic effects of 3-hydroxy-3-methylglutaryl coenzyme A reductase inhibitors. *Arterioscler Thromb Vasc Biol* 2001;21:1712–1719.
46. Wolfrum S, Jensen KS, Liao JK: Endothelium-dependent effects of statins. *Arterioscler Thromb Vasc Biol* 2003;23:729–736.
47. Ming XF, Viswambharan H, Barandier C, et al: Rho GTPase/Rho kinase negatively regulates endothelial nitric oxide synthase phosphorylation through the inhibition of protein kinase B/Akt in human endothelial cells. *Mol Cell Biol* 2002;22:8467–8477.
48. Takemoto M, Sun J, Hiroki J, et al: Rho-kinase mediates hypoxia-induced downregulation of endothelial nitric oxide synthase. *Circulation* 2002;106:57–62.
49. Wolfrum S, Dendorfer A, Rikitake Y, et al: Inhibition of Rho-kinase leads to rapid activation of phosphatidylinositol 3-kinase/protein kinase Akt and cardiovascular protection. *Arterioscler Thromb Vasc Biol* 2004;24:1842–1847.
50. Kataoka C, Egashira K, Inoue S, et al: Important role of Rho-kinase in the pathogenesis of cardiovascular inflammation and remodeling induced by long-term blockade of nitric oxide synthesis in rats. *Hypertension* 2002;39:245–350.
51. Kandabashi T, Shimokawa H, Mukai Y, et al: Involvement of Rho-kinase in agonists-induced contractions of arteriosclerotic human arteries. *Arterioscler Thromb Vasc Biol* 2002;22:243–248.
52. Funakoshi Y, Ichiki T, Shimokawa H, et al: Rho-kinase mediates angiotensin II-induced monocyte chemoattractant protein-1 expression in rat vascular smooth muscle cells. *Hypertension* 2001;38:100–104.
53. Miyata K, Shimokawa H, Kandabashi T, et al: Rho-kinase is involved in macrophage-mediated formation of coronary vascular lesions in pigs *in vivo*. *Arterioscler Thromb Vasc Biol* 2000;20:2351–2358.
54. Lefer DJ, Scalia R, Jones SP, et al: HMG-CoA reductase inhibition protects the diabetic myocardium from ischemia-reperfusion injury. *FASEB J* 2001;15:1454–1456.
55. Endres M, Laufs U, Huang Z, et al: Stroke protection by 3-hydroxy-3-methylglutaryl (HMG)-CoA reductase inhibitors mediated by endothelial nitric oxide synthase. *Proc Natl Acad Sci U S A* 1998;95:8880–8885.
56. Hernandez-Perera O, Perez-Sala D, Navarro-Antolin J, et al: Effects of the 3-hydroxy-3-methylglutaryl-CoA reductase inhibitors, atorvastatin and simvastatin, on the expression of endothelin-1 and endothelial nitric oxide synthase in vascular endothelial cells. *J Clin Invest* 1998;101:2711–2719.
57. Bourcier T, Libby P: HMG-CoA reductase inhibitors reduce plasminogen activator inhibitor-1 expression by human vascular smooth muscle and endothelial cells. *Arterioscler Thromb Vasc Biol* 2000;20:556–562.
58. Essig M, Nguyen G, Prie D, et al: 3-Hydroxy-3-methylglutaryl coenzyme A reductase inhibitors increase fibrinolytic activity in rat aortic endothelial cells. Role of geranylgeranylation and Rho proteins. *Circ Res* 1998;83:683–690.
59. Eto M, Kozai T, Cosentino F, et al: Statin prevents tissue factor expression in human endothelial cells: role of Rho/Rho-kinase and Akt pathways. *Circulation* 2002;105:1756–1759.
60. Ichiki T, Takeda K, Tokunou T, et al: Downregulation of angiotensin II type 1 receptor by hydrophobic 3-hydroxy-3-methylglutaryl coenzyme A reductase inhibitors in vascular smooth muscle cells. *Arterioscler Thromb Vasc Biol* 2001;21:1896–1901
61. Lefer AM, Scalia R, Lefer DJ: Vascular effects of HMG-CoA-reductase inhibitors (statins) unrelated to cholesterol lowering: New concepts for cardiovascular disease. *Cardiovasc Res* 2001;49:281–287.
62. Laufs U, Marra D, Node K, Liao JK: 3-Hydroxy-3-methylglutaryl-CoA reductase inhibitors attenuate vascular smooth muscle proliferation by preventing rho GTPase-induced down-regulation of p27(Kip1). *J Biol Chem* 1999;274:21926–21931.
63. Slotta JE, Braun OO, Menger MD, Thorlacius H: Fasudil, a Rho-kinase inhibitor, inhibits leukocyte adhesion in inflamed large blood vessels *in vivo*. *Inflamm Res* 2006;55:364–367.
64. Morishige K, Shimokawa H, Eto Y, et al: Adenovirus-mediated transfer of dominant-negative Rho-kinase induces a regression of coronary arteriosclerosis in pigs *in vivo*. *Arterioscler Thromb Vasc Biol* 2001;21:548–554.

65. Eto Y, Shimokawa H, Hiroki J, et al: Gene transfer of dominant negative Rho kinase suppresses neointimal formation after balloon injury in pigs. *Am J Physiol Heart Circ Physiol* 2000;278: H1744–H1750.
66. Shimokawa H, Morishige K, Miyata K, et al: Long-term inhibition of Rho-kinase induces a regression of arteriosclerotic coronary lesions in a porcine model *in vivo*. *Cardiovasc Res* 2001;51: 169–177.
67. Matsumoto Y, Uwatoku T, Oi K, et al: Long-term inhibition of Rho-kinase suppresses neointimal formation after stent implantation in porcine coronary arteries: involvement of multiple mechanisms. *Arterioscler Thromb Vasc Biol* 2004;24:181–186.
68. Kandabashi T, Shimokawa H, Miyata K, et al: Evidence for protein kinase C-mediated activation of Rho-kinase in a porcine model of coronary artery spasm. *Arterioscler Thromb Vasc Biol* 2003;23:2209–2214.
69. Hattori T, Shimokawa H, Higashi M, et al: Long-term treatment with a specific Rho-kinase inhibitor suppresses cardiac allograft vasculopathy in mice. *Circ Res* 2004;94:46–52.
70. Mukai Y, Shimokawa H, Matoba T, et al: Involvement of Rho-kinase in hypertensive vascular disease: a novel therapeutic target in hypertension. *FASEB J* 2001;15:1062–1064.
71. Hattori T, Shimokawa H, Higashi M, et al: Long-term inhibition of Rho-kinase suppresses left ventricular remodeling after myocardial infarction in mice. *Circulation* 2004;109: 2234–2239.
72. Shibuya M, Asano T, Sasaki Y: Effect of Fasudil HCl, a protein kinase inhibitor, on cerebral vasospasm. *Acta Neurochir Suppl* 2001;77:201–204.
73. Nagata K, Kondoh Y, Satoh Y, et al: Effects of fasudil hydrochloride on cerebral blood flow in patients with chronic cerebral infarction. *Clin Neuropharmacol* 1993;16:501–510.
74. Masaoka H, Takasato Y, Nojiri T, et al: Clinical effect of Fasudil hydrochloride for cerebral vasospasm following subarachnoid hemorrhage. *Acta Neurochir Suppl* 2001;77:209–211.
75. Tanaka Y, Masuzawa T, Saito M, et al: Combined administration of Fasudil hydrochloride and nitroglycerin for treatment of cerebral vasospasm. *Acta Neurochir Suppl* 2001;77:205–207.
76. Masumoto A, Mohri M, Shimokawa H, et al: Suppression of coronary artery spasm by the Rho-kinase inhibitor fasudil in patients with vasospastic angina. *Circulation* 2002;105:1545–1547.
77. Inokuchi K, Ito A, Fukumoto Y, et al: Usefulness of fasudil, a Rho-kinase inhibitor, to treat intractable severe coronary spasm after coronary artery bypass surgery. *J Cardiovasc Pharmacol* 2004;44:275–277.
78. Mohri M, Shimokawa H, Hirakawa Y, et al: Rho-kinase inhibition with intracoronary fasudil prevents myocardial ischemia in patients with coronary microvascular spasm. *J Am Coll Cardiol* 2003;41:15–19.
79. Masumoto A, Hirooka Y, Shimokawa H, et al: Possible involvement of Rho-kinase in the pathogenesis of hypertension in humans. *Hypertension* 2001;38:1307–1310.
80. Noma K, Higashi Y, Jitsuiki D, et al: Smoking activates rho-kinase in smooth muscle cells of forearm vasculature in humans. *Hypertension* 2003;41:1102–1105.
81. Noma K, Goto C, Nishioka K, et al: Smoking, endothelial function, and Rho-kinase in humans. *Arterioscler Thromb Vasc Biol* 2005;25:2630–2635.
82. Shimokawa H, Hiramori K, Iinuma H, et al: Anti-anginal effect of fasudil, a Rho-kinase inhibitor, in patients with stable effort angina: A multicenter study. *J Cardiovasc Pharmacol* 2002;40:751–761.
83. Vicari RM, Chaitman B, Keefe D, et al: Efficacy and safety of fasudil in patients with stable angina: A double-blind, placebo-controlled, phase 2 trial. *J Am Coll Cardiol* 2005;46:1803–1811.
84. Nohria A, Grunert ME, Rikitake Y, et al: Rho kinase inhibition improves endothelial function in human subjects with coronary artery disease. *Circ Res* 2006;99:1426–1432.
85. Kureishi Y, Luo Z, Shiojima I, et al: The HMG-CoA reductase inhibitor simvastatin activates the protein kinase Akt and promotes angiogenesis in normocholesterolemic animals. *Nat Med* 2000;6:1004–1010.
86. Rikitake Y, Kim HH, Huang Z, et al: Inhibition of Rho kinase (ROCK) leads to increased cerebral blood flow and stroke protection. *Stroke* 2005b;36:2251–2257.
87. Davidson MH, Robinson JG: Lipid-lowering effects of statins: A comparative review. *Expert Opin Pharmacother* 2006;7:1701–1714.
88. Shitara Y, Sugiyama Y: Pharmacokinetic and pharmacodynamic alterations of 3-hydroxy-3-methylglutryl coenzyme A (HMG-CoA) reductase inhibitor: Drug-drug interactions and interindividual differences in transporter and metabolic enzyme functions. *Pharmacol Ther* 2006;112:71–105.
89. Prueksaritanont T, Zhao JJ, Ma B, et al: Mechanistic studies on metabolic interactions between gemfibrozil and statins. *J Pharmacol Exp Ther* 2002;301:1042–1051.
90. Neuvonen PJ, Niemi M, Backman JT: Drug interactions with lipid-lowering drugs: Mechanism and clinical relevance. *Clin Pharmacol Ther* 2006;80:565–581.
91. Lilja JJ, Neuvonen M, Neuvonen PJ: Effects of regular consumption of grapefruit juice on the pharmacokinetics of simvastatin. *Br J Clin Pharmacol* 2004;58:56–60.
92. Kantola T, Kivisto KT, Neuonen PJ: Grapefruit juice greatly increases serum concentrations of lovastatin and lovastatin acid. *Clin Pharmacol Ther* 1998;63:397–402.
93. Lilja JJ, Kivisto KT, Neuvonen PJ: Grapefruit juice increases serum concentrations of atorvastatin and has no effect on pravastatin. *Clin Pharmacol Ther* 1999;66:118–127.
94. Lilja JJ, Kivisto KT, Neuvonen PJ: Duration of effect of grapefruit juice on the pharmacokinetics of the CYP 3A4 substrate simvastatin. *Clin Pharmacol Ther* 2000;68:384–390.
95. Fuhr U, Frummert AL: The fate of naringin in humans: A key to grapefruit juice–drug interactions. *Clin Pharmacol Ther* 1995;58:365–373.
96. Stone NJ: Stopping statins. *Circulation* 2004;110:2280–2282.
97. Kantola T, Backman JT, Niemi M, et al: Effect of fluconazole on plasma fluvastatin and pravastatin concentrations. *Eur J Clin Pharmacol* 2000;56:225–229.
98. Shitara Y, Itoh T, Sato H, et al: Inhibition of transporter-mediated hepatic uptake as a mechanism for drug-drug interaction between cerivastatin and cyclosporine A. *J Pharmacol Exp Ther* 2003;304:610–616.
99. Holdaas H, Fellstrom B, Jardine AG, et al: Effect of fluvastatin on cardiac outcomes in renal transplant recipients: A multicentre, randomised, placebo-controlled trial. *Lancet* 2003;361:2024–2031.
100. Bellosta S, Paoletti R, Corsini A: Safety of statins: Focus on clinical pharmacokinetics and drug interactions. *Circulation* 2004;109 (suppl III):50–57.
101. Shitara Y, Hirano M, Santo H, Sugiyama Y: Gemfibrozil and its glucuronide inhibit the organic anion transporting polypeptide 2 (ASTP2/OATP1B1:SLC21A6)-mediated hepatic uptake and CYP2C8-mediated metabolism of cerivastatin: Analysis of the mechanism of the clinically relevant drug-drug interaction between cerivastatin and gemfibrozil. *J Pharmacol Exp Ther* 2004;311:228–236.
102. The FIELD Investigators: Effects of long-term fenofibrate therapy on cardiovascular events in 9795 people with type 2 diabetes mellitus (the FIELD study): Randomised controlled trial. *Lancet* 2006;366:1849–1861.
103. Jones PH, Davidson MH, Stein EA, et al: Comparison of the efficacy and safety of rosuvastatin versus atorvastatin, simvastatin, and pravastatin across doses (STELLAR Trial). *Am J Cardiol* 2003;92:152–160.
104. McKenney JM, Jones PH, Adamczyk MA, et al: Comparison of the efficacy of rosuvastatin versus atorvastatin, simvastatin and pravastatin in achieving lipid goals: Results from the STELLAR trial. *Curr Med Res Opin* 2003;19:689–698.
105. Stein EA, Lane M, Laskarzewski P: Comparison of statins in hypertriglyceridemia. *Am J Cardiol* 1998;81 (suppl 4A):66B–69B.
106. Rosenson R, Otvos JD, Freedman DS: Relations of lipoprotein subclass levels and low-density lipoprotein size to progression of coronary artery disease in the Pravastatin Limitation of Atherosclerosis in the Coronary Arteries (PLAC-I) Trial. *Am J Cardiol* 2002;90:89–94.
107. McKenney JM, McCormick LS, Schaefer EJ, et al: Effect of niacin and atorvastatin on lipoprotein subclasses in patients with atherogenic dyslipidemia. *Am J Cardiol* 2001;88:270–274.
108. Sacks FM, Alaupovic P, Moye LA: Effect of pravastatin on apolipoprotein B and C-III in very low-density lipoproteins and low-density lipoproteins. *Am J Cardiol* 2002;90:165–167.
109. Sasaki S, Kuwahara N, Kunitomo K, et al: Effects of atorvastatin on oxidized low-density lipoprotein, low-density lipoprotein subfraction distribution, and remnant lipoprotein in patients with mixed hyperlipidemia. *Am J Cardiol* 2002;89:386–389.
110. Pedersen TR, Anders GO, Ole F, et al: Lipoprotein changes and reduction in the incidence of major coronary heart disease

events in the Scandinavian Simvastatin Survival Study (4S) *Circulation* 1998;97:1453–1460.

111. Geurin M, Egger P, Le Goff W, et al: Atorvastatin reduces postprandial accumulation and cholesteryl ester transfer protein-mediated remodeling of triglyceride-rich lipoprotein subspecies in type IIb hyperlipidemia. *J Clin Endocrinol Metab* 2002;87:4991–5000.

112. Asztalos BF, Maulf FL, Dallal GE, et al: Comparison of the effects of high doses of rosuvastatin versus atorvastatin on the subpopulation of high-density lipoprotein. *Am J Cardiol* 2007;99:681–685.

113. Grundy SM, Cleeman JI, Meraz CNB, et al: Implications of recent clinical trials for the National Cholesterol Program Adult Treatment Panel III guidelines. *Circulation* 2004;110:227–239.

114. Scandinavian Simvastatin Survival Study Group: Randomised trial of cholesterol lowering in 4444 patients with coronary heart disease: The Scandinavian Simvastatin Survival Study (4S). *Lancet* 1994;344:1383–1389.

115. The Long-term Intervention with Pravastatin in Ischaemic Disease (LIPID) Study Group: Prevention of cardiovascular events and death with pravastatin in patients with coronary heart disease and a broad range of initial cholesterol levels. *N Engl J Med* 1998;339:1349–1357.

116. Heart Protection Study Collaborative Group: Effects of cholesterol-lowering with simvastatin on stroke and other major vascular events in 20 536 people with cerebrovascular disease or other high-risk conditions. *Lancet* 2004;363:757–767.

117. Cholesterol Treatment Trialists' (CTT) Collaborators: Efficacy and safety of cholesterol-lowering treatment: Prospective meta-analysis of data from 90 056 participants in 14 randomised trials of statins. *Lancet* 2005;366:1267–1278.

118. Shepherd J, Blauw GJ, Murphy MB, et al: Pravastatin in elderly individuals at risk of vascular disease (PROSPER); A randomised controlled trial. *Lancet* 2002;360:1623–1630.

119. Colhoun HM, Betteridge DJ, Durrington PN, et al: Rapid emergence of effect of atorvastatin on cardiovascular outcomes in the Collaborative Atorvastatin Diabetes Study (CARDS). *Diabetologia* 2005;48:2482–2485.

120. Neil HA, DeMicco DA, Luo DJ, et al: Analysis of efficacy and safety in patients aged 65-75 years at randomization. Collaborative Atorvastatin Diabetes Study (CARDS). *Diabetes Care* 2006;29: 2378–2384.

121. Sever PS, Poulter NR, Dahlof B, et al: Different time course for prevention of coronary and stroke events by atorvastatin in the Anglo-Scandinavian Cardiac Outcomes Trial–Lipid Lowering Arm (ASCOT-LLA). *Am J Cardiol* 2005;96 (suppl):39F–44F.

122. ALLHAT officers and coordinators for the ALLHAT collaborative research group: Major outcomes in moderately hypercholesterolemic, hypertensive patients randomized to pravastatin vs. usual care. The Antihypertensive and Lipid-Lowering Treatment to Prevent Heart Attack Trial (ALLHAT-LLT). *JAMA* 2002;288:2998–3007.

123. Gibson DM, Bron NJ, Richens A, et al: Effect of age and gender on pharmacokinetics of atorvastatin in humans. *J Clin Pharmacol* 1996;36:242–246.

124. McCrindle BW, Urbina EM, Dennison BA, et al: Drug therapy of high-risk lipid abnormalities in children and adolescents: A scientific statement from the American Heart Association Atherosclerosis, Hypertension, and Obesity in Youth Committee, Council of Cardiovascular Disease in the Young, with the Council on Cardiovascular Nursing. *Circulation* 2007;115:1948–1967.

125. Kasiske BL, Wanner C, O'Neill WC: An assessment of statin safety by nephrologists. *Am J Cardiol* 2006;97 (suppl):82C–85C.

126. Wanner C, Krane V, März W, et al: Atorvastatin in patients with type 2 diabetes mellitus undergoing hemodialysis. *N Engl J Med* 2005;353:238–248.

127. Cohen DE, Anania FA, Chalasani N: An assessment of statin safety by hepatologists. *Am J Cardiol* 2006;97:77C–81C.

128. Chalasani N, Aljadhey H, Kesterson J, et al: Patients with elevated liver enzymes are not at higher risk for statin hepatotoxicity. *Gastroenterology* 2004;126:1287–1292.

129. Vuppalanchi R, Teal E, Chalasani N: Patients with elevated baseline liver enzymes do not have a higher frequency of hepatoxicity from lovastatin than those with normal baseline liver enzymes. *Am J Med Sci* 2005;329:62–65.

130. Kiyici M, Gulten M, Gurel M, et al: Ursodeoxycholic acid and atorvastatin in the treatment of nonalcoholic steatohepatitis. *Can J Gastroenterol* 2003;17:713–718.

131. Rallidis LS, Drakoulis CK, Parasi AS: Pravastatin in patients with nonalcoholic steatohepatitis: Results of a pilot study. *Atherosclerosis* 2004;174:193–196.

132. Athyros VG, Mikhailidis DP, Papageorgiou AA, et al: The effect of statins versus untreated dyslipidemia on renal function in patients with coronary heart disease. A subgroup analysis of the Greek Atorvastatin and Coronary Heart Disease Evaluation (GREACE) study. *J Clin Pathol* 2004;57:728–734.

133. Tonelli M, Moyé L, Sacks FM, et al: Effect of pravastatin on loss of renal function in people with moderate chronic renal insufficiency and cardiovascular disease. *J Am Soc Nephrol* 2003;14:1605–1613.

134. Vidt DG, Cressman MD, Harris S, et al: Rosuvastatin-induced arrest in progression of renal disease. *Cardiology* 2004;102: 52–60.

135. Cosio FG, Pesavento TE, Pelletier RP, et al: Patient survival after renal transplantation III: The effects of statins. *Am J Kidney Dis* 2002;40:638–643.

136. Seliger SL, Weiss NS, Gillen DL, et al: HMG-CoA reductase inhibitors are associated with reduced mortality in ESRD patients. *Kidney Int* 2002;61:297–304.

137. Vaughan CJ, Delanty N: Neuroprotective properties of statins in cerebral ischemia and stroke. *Stroke* 1999;30:1969–1673.

138. Goldstein LB, Adams R, Alberts MJ, et al: Primary prevention of ischemic stroke: A guideline from the American Heart Association/American Stroke Association Stroke Council. *Circulation* 2006;113:e873–e923.

139. Sacco RL, Adams R, Albers G, et al: Guidelines for prevention of stroke in patients with ischemic stroke or transient ischemic attack: A statement for healthcare professionals from the American Heart Association/American Stroke Association Council on Stroke. *Circulation.* 2006;113:409–449.

140. National Cholesterol Education Program: Third Report of the Expert Panel on Detection, Evaluation, and Treatment of High Blood Cholesterol in Adults (Adult Treatment Panel III). Final Report. *Circulation* 2002;106:3143–3421.

141. Stroke Prevention by Aggressive Reduction in Cholesterol Levels (SPARCL) Investigators: High-dose atorvastatin after stroke or transient ischemic attack. *N Engl J Med.* 2006;355: 549–559.

141a. Goldstein LB, Amarenco P, Szarek M, et al: Hemorrhagic stroke in the Stroke Prevention by Aggressive Reduction in Cholesterol Levels study. *Neurology* 2008;70:2364–2370.

141b. Heart Protection Study Collaborative Group: Effects of cholesterol-lowering with simvastatin on stroke and other major vascular events in 20 536 people with cerebrovascular disease or other high-risk conditions. *Lancet* 2004;363:757–767.

142. Pedersen TR, Kjekshus J, Pyörälä K, et al: Effect of simvastatin on ischemic signs and symptoms in the Scandinavian Simvastatin Survival Study (4S). *Am J Cardiol* 1998a;81:333–335.

143. Mohler ER, Hiatt WR, Creager MA, et al: Cholesterol reduction with atorvastatin improves walking distance in patients with peripheral arterial disease. *Circulation* 2003;108:1481–1486.

144. Jadhav SB, Jain GK: Statins and osteoporosis: New role for old drugs. *J Pharm Pharmacol* 2006;58:3–18.

145. Wang PS, Solomon DH, Mogun H, Avorn J: HMG-CoA reductase inhibitors and the risk of hip fractures in elderly patients. *JAMA* 2000;283:3211–3216.

146. Meier CR, Schlienger RG, Kraenzlin ME, et al: HMG-CoA reductase inhibitors and the risk of fractures. *JAMA* 2000;283: 3205–3210.

147. Van Staa TP, Wegman S, de Vries F, et al: Use of statins and risk of fractures. *JAMA* 2001;285:1850–1855.

148. Reid IR, Hague W, Emberson J, et al: Effect of pravastatin on frequency of fracture in the LIPID study; secondary analysis of a randomized controlled trial. *Lancet* 2001;357:509–512.

149. McClung MR, Kiel DP, Lindsay RS, et al: A 12-month, dose response study of atorvastatin effects on bone in postmenopausal women. Poster presented to the American Society of Nephrology, November 17, 2006.

150. Kivipelto M, Helkala EL, Laakso MP, et al: Midlife vascular risk factors and Alzheimer's disease in later life: Longitudinal, population based study. *BMJ* 2001;322:1447–1451.

151. Notkola IL, Sulkava R, Pekkanen J, et al: Serum total cholesterol, apolipoprotein E epsilon 4 allele, and Alzheimer's disease. *Neuroepidemiology* 1998;17:14–20.

152. Rockwood K, Kirkland S, Hogan DB, et al: Use of lipid-lowering agents, indication bias, and the risk of dementia

in community-dwelling elderly people. *Arch Neurol* 2002;59: 223–227.
153. Wolozin B, Kellman W, Rousseau P, et al: Decreased prevalence of Alzheimer disease associated with 3-hydroxy-3-methylglutaryl coenzyme A reductase inhibitors. *Arch Neurol* 2000;57: 1439–1443.
154. Sparks DL, Scheff SW, Hunsaker JC III, et al: Induction of Alzheimer-like β amyloid immunoreactivity in the brains of rabbits with dietary cholesterol. *Exp Neurol* 1994;126:88–94.
155. Sparks DL: Intraneuronal β-amyloid immunoreactivity in the CNS. *Neurobiol Aging* 1996;17:291–299.
156. Sparks DL, Sabbagh MN, Connor DJ, et al: Atorvastatin for the treatment of mild to moderate Alzheimer disease: Preliminary results. *Arch Neurol* 2005;62:753–757.
157. Heart Protection Study Collaborative Group: MRC/BHF Heart Protection Study of cholesterol lowering with simvastatin in 20 536 high-risk individuals: A randomised placebo-controlled trial. *Lancet* 2002;360:7–22.
158. Iso H, Jacobs DR Jr: Serum cholesterol levels and six-year mortality from stroke in 350,977 men screened for the Multiple Risk Factor Intervention Trial. *N Engl J Med* 1989;320:904–910.
159. Yano K, Reed DM, MacLean DJ: Serum cholesterol and hemorrhagic stroke in the Honolulu Heart Program. *Stroke* 1989;20:1460–1465.
160. Wiviott SD, Cannon CP, Morrow DA, et al: Can low-density lipoprotein be too low? The safety and efficacy of achieving very low, low-density lipoprotein with intense statin therapy. A PROVE IT-TIMI 22 substudy. *J Am Coll Cardiol* 2005;46:1411–1416.
161. Schonfeld G: Familial hypobetalipoproteinemia: A review. *J Lipid Res* 2003;44:878–883.
162. Welty FK, Mittleman MA, Wilson PWF, et al: Hypobetalipoproteinemia is associated with low levels of hemostatic risk factors in the Framingham offspring population. *Circulation* 1997;95:825–830.
163. Kashani A, Phillips CO, Foody JM, et al: Risks associated with statin therapy. A systematic overview of randomized clinical trials. *Circulation* 2006;114:2788–2797.
164. Law M, Rudnicka AR: Statin safety: A systemic review. *Am J Cardiol* 2006;97(suppl):52C–60C.
165. US Food and Drug Administration, Center for Drug Evaluation and Research: Statins and hepatotoxicity. (US Food and Drug Administration Web site) Available at: http://www.fda.gov/ohrms/dockets/ac/00/backgrd/3622b2b_safety_review.pdf. Accessed August 15, 2005.
166. Tolman KG: The liver and lovastatin. *Am J Cardiol* 2002;89:1374–1380.
167. McKenney JM, Davidson MH, Jacobson TA, Guyton JR: Final conclusions and recommendations of the National Lipid Association Statin Safety Assessment Task Force. *Am J Cardiol* 2006 (suppl);97:89C–94C.
168. Davidson MH, Clark JA, Glass LM, Kanumalla A: Statin safety: an appraisal from the Adverse Event Reporting System. *Am J Cardiol* 2006;97(suppl):32C–43C.
169. Cziraky MJ, Willey VJ, McKenney JM, et al: Statin safety: an assessment using an administrative claims database. *Am J Cardiol* 2006;97(suppl):61C–68C.
170. Sacks FM, Pfeffer MA, Moye LA, et al: The effect of pravastatin on coronary events after myocardial infarction in patients with average cholesterol levels. *N Engl J Med* 1996;335:1001–1009.
171. Shepherd J, Cobbe SM, Ford I, et al: Prevention of coronary heart disease with pravastatin in men with hypercholesterolemia. *N Engl J Med* 1995;333:1301–1307.
172. de Lemos JA, Blazing MA, Wiviott SD, et al: Early intensive vs a delayed conservative simvastatin strategy in patients with acute coronary syndromes. Phase Z of the A to Z trial. *JAMA* 2004;292:1307–1316.
173. Urso ML, Clarkson PM, Hittel D, et al: Changes in ubiquitin proteasome pathway gene expression in skeletal muscle with exercise and statins. *Arterioscler Thromb Vasc Biol* 2005;25:2560–2566.
173a. The SEARCH Collaborative Group. *SLCO1B1* variants and statin-induced myopathy—A genomewide study. *N Engl J Med* 2008;359:789–799.
174. Paiva H, Thelen KM, Coster V, et al: High dose statins and skeletal muscle metabolism in humans: a randomized, controlled trial. *Clin Pharmacol Ther* 2005;78:60–68.
175. Thibault A, Samid D, Tompkins AC, et al: Phase I study of lovastatin, an inhibitor of the mevalonate pathway, in patients with cancer. *Clin Cancer Res* 1996;2:483–491.
176. Caso G, Kelly P, McNurlan MA, Lawson WE: Effect of coenzyme Q10 on myopathic symptoms in patients treated with statin. *Am J Cardiol* 2007;99:1409–1412.
177. Marcoff L, Thompson PD: The role of coenzyme Q10 in statin-associated myopathy: a systematic review. *J Am Coll Cardiol* 2007;49:2231–2237.
178. Rosenson RS: Current overview of statin-induced myopathy. *Am J Med* 2004;116:408–416.
179. Jacobson TA. Statin safety: Lessons from New Drug Applications for marketed statins. *Am J Cardiol* 2006;97(suppl):44C–51C.
180. Bottorff M, Hansten P: Long-term safety of hepatic hydroxymethyl glutaryl coenzyme A reductase inhibitors. *Arch Intern Med* 2000;160:2273–2280.
181. Sidaway JE, Davidson RG, McTaggart F: Inhibitors of 3-hydroxy-3-methylglutaryl-CoA reductase reduce receptor-mediated endocytosis in opossum kidney cells. *J Am Soc Nephrol* 2004;15:2258–2265.
182. Pfeffer MA, Keech A, Sacks FM, et al: Safety and tolerability of pravastatin in long-term clinical trials. *Circulation* 2002;105: 2341–2346.
183. US Food and Drug Administration: FDA Public Health Advisory on Crestor (rosuvastatin). Center for Drug Evaluation and Research. (FDA Web site) Available at: http://www.fda.gov/cder/drug/advisory/crestor_3_2005.htm. Accessed February 6, 2006.
184. Chong PH, Boskovich A, Stevkovic N, Bartt RE: Statin-associated peripheral neuropathy: Review of the literature. *Pharmacotherapy* 2004;24:1194–1203.
185. PROspective Study of Pravastatin in the Elderly at Risk (PROSPER) Study Group: Pravastatin in elderly individuals at risk of vascular disease (PROSPER): A randomised controlled trial. *Lancet* 2002;360:1623–1630.
186. Wagstaff LR, Mitton MW, Arvik BM, Doraiswamy PM: Statin-associated memory loss: Analysis of 60 case reports and review of the literature. *Pharmacotherapy* 2003;23:871–880.
187. Bays H: Statin safety: An overview and assessment of the data—2005. *Am J Cardiol* 2006;97(suppl):6C–26C.
188. Saheki A, Terasaki T, Tamai I, Tsuji A: *In vivo* and *in vitro* blood-brain barrier transport of 3-hydroxy-3-methylglutaryl coenzyme A (HMG-CoA) reductase inhibitors. *Pharm Res* 1994;11:305–311.
189. Brass LM, Alberts MJ, Sparks L: An assessment of statin safety by neurologists. *Am J Cardiol* 2006;97(suppl):86C–88C.
190. Serruys PWJ, de Feyter P, Macaya C, et al: Fluvastatin for prevention of cardiac events following successful first percutaneous coronary intervention. A randomized controlled trial. *JAMA* 2002;287:3215–3222.
191. Colhoun HM, Betteridge DJ, Durrington PN, et al: Primary prevention of cardiovascular disease with atorvastatin in type 2 diabetes in the Collaborative Atorvastatin Diabetes Study (CARDS): Multicentre randomised placebo-controlled trial. *Lancet* 2004;364:685–696.
192. Downs JR, Clearfield M, Weis S, et al: Primary prevention of acute coronary events with lovastatin in men and women with average cholesterol levels: Results of AFCAPS/TexCAPS. *JAMA* 1998;279:1615–1622.
193. LaRosa JC, Grundy SM, Waters DD, et al: Intensive lipid lowering with atorvastatin in patients with stable coronary disease. *N Engl J Med* 2005;352:1425–1435.
194. Pedersen TR, Faergeman O, Kastelein JJ, et al: High-dose atorvastatin vs usual-dose simvastatin for secondary prevention after myocardial infarction. The IDEAL study: A randomized controlled trial. *JAMA* 2005;294:2437–2445.

CHAPTER 23

Bile Acid Sequestrants

John R. Guyton and Anne Carol Goldberg

INTRODUCTION

Bile acid sequestrants (BAS) effectively reduce plasma low-density lipoprotein (LDL) cholesterol by interrupting the enterohepatic circulation of bile acids, with consequent diversion of hepatic cholesterol toward the synthesis of new bile acids. BAS have been shown to inhibit atherogenesis and reduce cardiovascular events in multiple randomized trials, including one large monotherapy trial. Pharmaceutical BAS are large polymers that lack systemic absorption and thus avoid systemic side effects. However, their adsorptive mechanism of action requires bulk administration, leading to inconvenience and sometimes to gastrointestinal side effects. Because of these drawbacks, BAS are generally regarded as second-line or additive agents for treating hypercholesterolemia. They can be drugs of choice in situations in which patient safety is the key consideration, such as in children or in women of childbearing potential.

HISTORY

Cholestyramine, the first BAS, was developed at Merck in the late 1950s (MK-135). It is an insoluble styrene-divinyl benzene copolymer bearing quaternary ammonium ions–an anion exchange resin. In 1959, Bergen et al. reported that cholestyramine reduced serum total cholesterol in humans by an average of 20%.[1] This marked the discovery of a second effective agent for hypercholesterolemia, following niacin earlier in the decade. Besides hypercholesterolemia, another early successful therapeutic target for cholestyramine was the pruritus of primary biliary cirrhosis caused by excessive circulating bile acids.[2]

An upper limit to the dosing of cholestyramine was established in an early study in which a dose of 30 g daily was shown to induce steatorrhea by impairing intestinal lipase activity in normal subjects.[3] Subsequently, cholestyramine was used in large clinical trials with a target of 24 g daily in three divided doses.[4,5]

Colestipol was introduced at the beginning of the 1970s. It is a high–molecular weight, insoluble copolymer of diethylenetriamine and 1-chloro-2, 3-epoxypropane. Like cholestyramine, colestipol is an insoluble anion exchange compound with a slightly lower binding capacity for bile salts. Thus, the highest dose of colestipol recommended clinically is slightly higher, at 30 g daily.[6] In clinical use, the effects on lipoproteins and the side effects of colestipol have been indistinguishable from those of cholestyramine.[7]

Colesevelam is a polyallylamine cross-linked with epichlorohydrin and alkylated with 1-bromodecane and 6-bromohexyltrimethylammonium bromide. The presence of alkylated amines in this compound enhances the binding capacity and affinity for bile salts. Colesevelam gained marketing approval in the United States in 2000. Major advantages are its lack of drug interactions and low rates of gastrointestinal side effects.

Colestimide, a 2-methylimidazole-epichlorohydrin polymer, is a new BAS administered in tablet form and currently marketed (2007) in Japan. It has been shown to be effective in combination therapy for familial hypercholesterolemia.[8] Current clinical trials with this compound are focused on lowering phosphate in patients undergoing kidney dialysis and on combined lipid and glucose amelioration in diabetes.[9]

MECHANISM OF ACTION

Bile acids are synthesized by the liver from cholesterol. They exist mostly as glycine or taurine conjugates and as secondary dehydroxylated products of gut bacterial action.[10] Their function is to solubilize dietary fats and other nonpolar nutrients through the formation of mixed micelles in the intestinal lumen, facilitating intestinal absorption of these substances. Solubilization and absorption of cholesterol, for example, is completely dependent on the presence of bile acids. Bile acid micelles deliver fatty substances to mucosal absorptive cells throughout the small intestine, but the bile acids themselves undergo limited absorption until they reach the terminal ileum. The apical sodium bile acid transporter (ASBT, *SLC10A2*), a 348–amino acid protein with seven transmembrane-spanning domains, is expressed in the terminal ileum and is responsible for efficient uptake of bile acids. More than 95% of intestinal bile acids are absorbed in the small intestine, and less than 5% are excreted in feces (Fig. 23-1). The absorbed bile acids are carried by portal blood flow to the liver, where a transport protein (termed the Na^+-taurocholate cotransporting polypeptide, or NTCP) mediates their uptake into hepatocytes. ASBT and NTCP are homologous, sharing 35% amino acid identity.[11]

The pK_a of bile acids is approximately 5, indicating that more than 95% exist in the ionized form at physiologic pH. Cholestyramine binds conjugated and unconjugated bile salt anions with apparent dissociation constants of 20 to 100 $\times$ 10^{-6} M. The capacity of the polymers for binding bile salt anions is high. A typical 24 g daily dose of cholestyramine can bind as much as 10 g of cholate under simulated physiologic conditions *in vitro*. However, the adsorption of organic anions to the older BAS, cholestyramine and colestipol, is quite nonspecific. For example, fatty acid anions bind with equal or greater affinity compared with bile salt anions.[12]

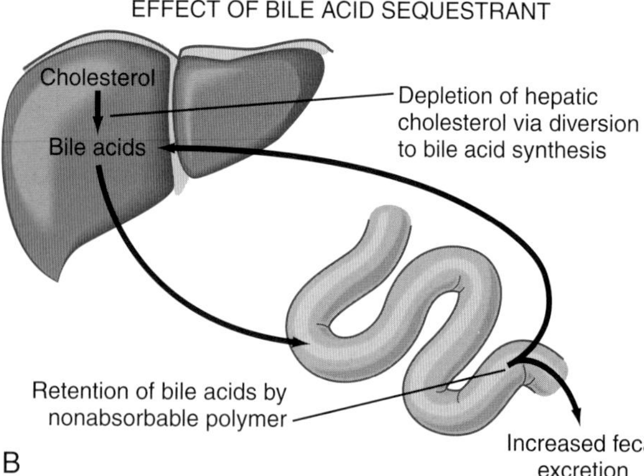

FIGURE 23-1 Effect of bile acid sequestrants on the enterohepatic circulation of bile acids. **A,** Bile acids are synthesized in the liver from cholesterol. In the terminal ileum, more than 95% of bile acids are absorbed and return to the liver. **B,** Binding of bile acids to nonabsorbable polymer leads to 3- to 10-fold increases in fecal excretion. Hepatic synthesis from cholesterol increases to a similar degree in response to bile acid depletion. Consequently, hepatic cholesterol levels fall, leading to increased synthesis of cholesterol and increased expression of hepatic low-density lipoprotein (LDL) receptors. Plasma LDL levels fall because of increased uptake in the liver.

Daily Synthesis and Excretion

The daily synthetic rate of bile acids in humans, approximately 300 to 500 mg, is essentially equal to fecal bile acid excretion, because no other elimination pathway exists.[10,13,14] Utilization of hepatic cholesterol for bile acid synthesis represents a substantial fraction of the total body turnover of cholesterol, which is approximately 1000 mg per day, of which 800 mg is derived from *de novo* synthesis and 200 mg from dietary sources (only half of the usual 400 mg dietary cholesterol intake is absorbed).[14,15]

With administration of BAS, fecal bile acid excretion can increase to 1000 to 3000 mg daily (see Fig. 23-1).[16] Bile acid synthesis from cholesterol may increase 5- to 10-fold.[10] In addition, the intestinal absorption of cholesterol decreases modestly because of intestinal bile acid depletion, thus increasing the fecal elimination of biliary cholesterol. These effects establish a substantial drain from the total body cholesterol pool, but the decrease is partially compensated by augmentation of cholesterol synthesis. By kinetic analysis of injected radioisotopically labeled cholesterol, whole body cholesterol production rates were estimated to increase an average of 86% in humans during long-term treatment with colestipol 15 g daily.[17] Cholesterol synthesis in the liver can increase markedly following bile acid depletion, based on animal studies.[18,19]

In 1999, the key transcriptional regulator of bile acid pathways in the intestine and liver was discovered to be the farnesoid X receptor (FXR, see Fig. 23-2).[20,21] FXR is also called FXR-α to distinguish it from the FXR-β found in some species, but FXR-β is a pseudogene in humans and primates. Activation of FXR by bile acids is strong and occurs at biologically appropriate concentrations, unlike the weak and unphysiologic activation by the isoprenoid farnesol. Therefore, despite the name *farnesoid* X receptor, bile acids are the natural activators of FXR. FXR forms a heterodimer with its obligate partner 9-*cis* retinoic acid receptor–α (RXR-α), and the FXR/RXR-α heterodimer binds DNA. The hormone response element to which FXR/RXR-α binds is termed a bile acid response element (BARE). Many target genes for FXR/RXR-α have been identified in the liver, intestine, kidney, and adrenal gland.[22,23]

Bile acids down-regulate the rate-limiting enzyme of bile acid synthesis, cholesterol 7α-hydroxylase (CYP7A1) by two major mechanisms (see Fig. 23-2). In ileal absorptive cells, ligation of FXR increases transcription of fibroblast growth factor–19 (FGF-19, or FGF-15 in mice), which is secreted into the portal vein. Subsequently, FGF-19 binds the cell surface receptor FGFR-4 on hepatocytes, activating the c-Jun N-terminal kinase (JNK) pathway, which inhibits CYP7A1. In

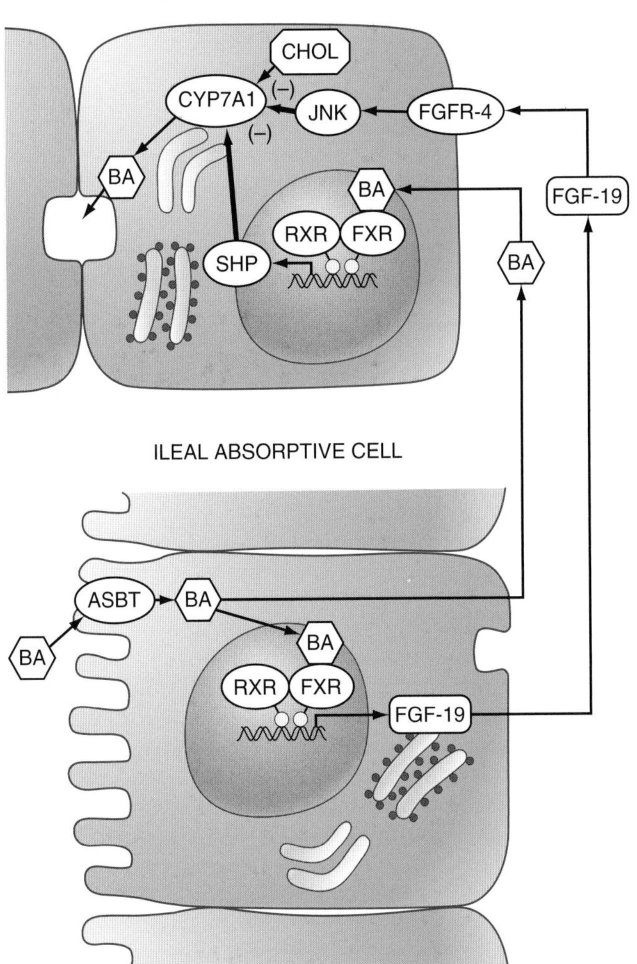

FIGURE 23-2 Regulatory mechanisms of bile acid metabolism. Cytochrome P450 isoenzyme 7A1 (CYP7A1) mediates 7α-hydroxylation of cholesterol, the rate-limiting step in bile acid (BA) synthesis from cholesterol (CHOL). CYP7A1 is under negative regulation via the c-Jun N-terminal kinase (JNK) cascade and is also subject to transcriptional down-regulation via small heterodimer partner (SHP). Ileal absorptive cells express the apical sodium bile acid transporter (ASBT), which mediates uptake of bile acids from the intestinal lumen. Bile acids activate the farnesoid X receptor (FXR), a transcription factor that binds DNA as a heterodimer with the 9-*cis* retinoic acid receptor–α (RXR). One target gene up-regulated by FXR/RXR in ileal cells encodes fibroblast growth factor–19 (FGF-19). FGF-19 travels by the portal circulation to the liver, where it interacts with the transmembrane tyrosine kinase receptor, FGF receptor–4 (FGFR-4), on the surface of hepatocytes, negatively regulating bile acid synthesis via JNK. In hepatocytes, bile acid–activated FXR/RXR promotes transcription of SHP. SHP dimerizes with and inactivates the transcription factors—liver X receptor (LXR, not shown) and liver receptor homolog–1 (LRH-1, not shown)—leading to down-regulation of CYP7A1 expression and decreased bile synthesis. See references in text.

hepatocytes, bile acid activation of FXR increases expression of small heterodimer partner (SHP), a member of the nuclear receptor superfamily that lacks a DNA-binding domain. SHP then dimerizes with and inactivates liver X receptor (LXR) and liver receptor homology–1 (LRH-1), leading to decreased CYP7A1 expression.[13,22,23]

The diversion of hepatic cholesterol to bile acid synthesis by BAS ultimately results in the lowering of plasma LDL. Depletion of hepatic cholesterol is sensed by endoplasmic reticulum proteins that escort sterol regulatory element–binding proteins (SREBPs) to the Golgi complex, where they are cleaved. SREBPs then translocate to the nucleus where they increase the expression of HMG-CoA reductase and the LDL receptor.[24] Plasma LDL lowering is a result of increased expression of hepatic LDL receptors. Using radiolabeled LDL and cyclohexanedione-modified LDL, plasma LDL lowering by cholestyramine was shown to be associated with a doubling of the fractional catabolic rate by the receptor-mediated route, but no change in fractional catabolic rate by receptor-independent clearance was found.[25]

Elucidation of the transport and signaling systems for bile acids and cholesterol, as partially described above, has potential implications for the effects of BAS beyond LDL lowering. In addition, improved understanding may lead to new pharmacologic modulators. FXR in particular affects genes involved in triglyceride metabolism, mediating positive regulation of apolipoprotein (apo) C-II and apoA-V, very-low-density lipoprotein (VLDL) receptor, and phospholipid transfer protein and negative regulation of apoC-III and hepatic lipase. The net result in human clinical studies appears to be a transient lowering of plasma triglyceride by administration of bile acids, and conversely, a mild increase in plasma triglyceride by BAS.[13,23] In the intestinal enterocyte, FXR induces gene expression of angiogenin, carbonic anhydrase–XII, and inducible nitric oxide synthase. These effects may potentially protect cells from adverse effects of bile acids and/or may play a role in the response of the intestine to bacterial overgrowth.[26]

Pharmacologic inhibition of the ileal ASBT might accomplish LDL lowering as an alternative to the use of BAS.[27,28] The same goal is achieved by partial ileal resection to prevent reabsorption of bile acids.[29] However, ileal resection is often accompanied by increased frequency of stool and sometimes by watery diarrhea.[29,30] In clinical studies involving perfusions of the human colon by bile acid solutions, dihydroxy bile acids (chenodeoxycholic and deoxycholic acids) induced an inhibition of absorption or, at higher concentrations, the actual secretion of sodium, potassium, and water.[31] Both steatorrhea and diarrhea are features of a rare recessive disorder in which ASBT is nonfunctional. The disorder is treated with BAS.[32] It might be possible to combine BAS with an ASBT inhibitor to provide a greater perturbation of bile acid/cholesterol metabolism without the induction of diarrhea, but no definitive study has been done. On an empirical basis, the older BAS, cholestyramine and colestipol, are widely used for the treatment of diarrhea in various clinical settings.

Links between glucose and bile acid metabolism have been described.[33] In small randomized clinical trials, cholestyramine 24 g daily given to nondiabetic subjects and colesevelam 3.75 g daily given to diabetic subjects were shown to reduce fasting plasma glucose levels.[34,35] Colesevelam also lowered hemoglobin A1c levels by 0.5% ($p = 0.007$) compared with placebo-treated subjects.[35] The mechanism of this effect is unexplained at present. Activation of FXR in mice has been shown to increase insulin sensitivity and lead to hypoglycemia.[23] Therefore, deactivation of FXR related to the use of BAS might be expected to raise glucose, not lower it. Nevertheless, decreased FXR activity might lead via decreased SHP to up-regulation of hepatic LXR, which can decrease gluconeogenesis.[36]

Moreover, transgenic expression of human FGF-19 in genetically obese mice was shown to prevent or reverse diabetes and ameliorate several aspects of the metabolic syndrome.[37]

EFFECTS ON PLASMA LIPOPROTEINS

The major effect of the BAS is the reduction of LDL cholesterol levels with a corresponding decrease of total cholesterol. The effect on high-density lipoprotein (HDL) cholesterol is typically a modest increase in the range of 0% to 5%.[38] As monotherapy, BAS lower LDL cholesterol by 5% to 30% in a dose-dependent manner.[39–45] The effect is seen within 2 to 4 weeks of the start of therapy and generally remains stable over time.[40,43,46,47] Colestipol tablets or granules lower LDL cholesterol by 12% at a dose of 4 g/day and 24% at 16 g/day.[46] The dose response seen in the Lipid Research Clinics Coronary Primary Prevention Trial (LRC-CPPT) for cholestyramine over the dose range of 4 to 24 g/day was a 6.6% to 28.3% decrease in LDL cholesterol.[5,48]

Because colesevelam has greater bile acid–binding efficacy than cholestyramine or colestipol, it can be used at doses lower than those used for the older BAS.[38,40] The decrease seen in LDL cholesterol is usually about 15% at 3.8 g/day and 18% at 4.3 g/day (seven 625-mg tablets).[1,39,43]

The BAS can increase cholesterol synthesis by affecting HMG-CoA reductase. Use of an HMG-CoA reductase inhibitor, or statin, ameliorates this effect, leading to substantial LDL cholesterol reductions when BAS are combined with statins. The combination of BAS and HMG-CoA reductase inhibitor can lower LDL cholesterol levels by up to 60%.[38,39,49–52] The statin decreases the rise of triglyceride levels that can occur with BAS, but the BAS may also decrease the amount of triglyceride reduction that can be seen with the more-potent statins.

All three of the available BAS have been studied in combination with different HMG-CoA reductase inhibitors. The decreases in LDL cholesterol range from 24% to 60% depending on the dose of BAS and of the statin.[49–51,53]

Because BAS can provide 10% to 25% further reduction of LDL when added to statins,[54] their use can make it possible to reach LDL cholesterol goals in patients who cannot tolerate high statin doses. For example, colesevelam 3.8 g/daily, plus atorvastatin 10 mg daily lowered LDL by 48%, compared with 53% reduction with atorvastatin 80 mg daily.[50] Thus, the use of a BAS can make it possible for LDL cholesterol goals to be reached with less than maximum doses of statins in patients who have side effects from high statin doses. However, cholestyramine and colestipol can interfere with absorption of statins if taken at the same time, leading to a decrease in efficacy.[52] Colesevelam does not affect statin absorption.

The combination of statin, BAS, and niacin has been used in patients with heterozygous familial hypercholesterolemia where even greater LDL cholesterol reductions are required.[55] A typical approach would use the maximum statin doses, BAS at maximally tolerated doses, and up to 2 g/day of niacin.

Before the availability of HMG-CoA reductase inhibitors, the combination of BAS and niacin was a typical drug regimen for patients with high LDL cholesterol levels. This combination was used in the Cholesterol Lowering Atherosclerosis Study (CLAS) and the Familial Atherosclerosis Treatment Study (FATS) with reductions of LDL cholesterol by 30% to 40% with 30 g/day of colestipol plus 3 g/day or more of niacin. HDL cholesterol increased by more than 35% with this approach.[56,57] However, tolerance problems are significant with both the high dose of BAS as well as the high dose of niacin.

Some patients are unwilling to take statins or are intolerant of all statins even when given in very low doses. High doses of BAS and niacin can treat patients with very high LDL cholesterol levels. Combining colesevelam and extended-release niacin can produce good effects with fewer side effects than older resins and high-dose crystalline niacin. Another possible combination is the addition of ezetimibe to colesevelam, which can lower LDL cholesterol by 32%.[58]

Patients with high triglycerides who have elevated LDL cholesterol levels after treatment with a fibric acid derivative may be candidates for the addition of a BAS. BAS have been combined with clofibrate, bezafibrate, gemfibrozil, or fenofibrate.[38,41,42,59] The combination of colesevelam and fenofibrate in patients with mean baseline LDL cholesterol levels of 159 mg/dL and median triglyceride levels of 230 mg/dL resulted in a 17% reduction of LDL cholesterol, 32% reduction of triglycerides, and 11.5% increase of HDL cholesterol.[59]

NONLIPID EFFECTS

In addition to the effect of BAS on glucose,[34,35] there are reports of reduction of CRP.[60,61] Devaraj et al. found a reduction of high-sensitivity C-reactive protein (hs-CRP) of 18.7% compared with placebo. There was no correlation between LDL cholesterol lowering and hs-CRP lowering. No significant changes were seen in levels of interleukin-6 and tumor necrosis factor–α.[61] Bays et al. pooled data from three combination trials with colesevelam and statin and found a 23% reduction of hs-CRP in patients on statin plus colesevelam compared with that seen in patients on statin alone.[60]

PREVENTION OF ATHEROSCLEROSIS AND CARDIOVASCULAR EVENTS

BAS have been shown in randomized trials to inhibit atherogenesis and reduce cardiovascular events. The most significant monotherapy outcome trial was the LRC-CPPT in which 3806 men aged 35 to 59 with elevated total cholesterol and without evident coronary heart disease were randomized to therapy with cholestyramine 24 g daily or placebo. The primary outcome of combined coronary heart disease death and nonfatal myocardial infarction was significantly reduced by 19%.[5,48] In other trials involving resins alone or in combination with other agents, cholestyramine and colestipol have shown beneficial effects on coronary disease. The National Heart, Lung, and Blood Institute (NHLBI) Type II Coronary Intervention Study used cholestyramine

24 g/day versus placebo and showed decreased progression of coronary artery lesions with greater than 50% stenosis at baseline in the cholestyramine group.[4] The St. Thomas' Atherosclerosis Regression Study (STARS) was an angiographic study comparing the effects of an intensive diet or intensive diet plus cholestyramine 8 g twice a day with usual care in men with coronary artery disease. Angiographic evidence of progression of coronary artery disease was less, and there was more evidence of improvement in luminal diameter in patients treated with diet and cholestyramine compared with the group on a usual diet.[62]

Angiographic studies with colestipol include CLAS, in which the combination of colestipol 30 g/day and niacin 4.3 g/day was associated with decreased progression and increased regression of coronary artery atherosclerosis compared with placebo.[56] In FATS, the combinations of lovastatin 40 mg daily with colestipol 30 g daily and niacin 4 g daily plus colestipol 30 g daily produced greater regression and less progression of atherosclerosis as well as fewer clinical events compared with conventional therapy.[57] Kane et al. used a combination of lovastatin, niacin, and colestipol compared with diet alone in patients with familial hypercholesterolemia and very high LDL cholesterol levels, studied in the University of California, San Francisco, Specialized Center of Research (UCSF-SCOR) study. Angiographic evidence of regression of atherosclerotic lesions occurred in the drug combination group compared with evidence of progression in the diet-only group.[63]

TABLE 23-1 Adverse Effects Associated with Bile Acid Sequestrants

Nonselective Polymers—Cholestyramine and Colestipol	
Common Adverse Events	
Constipation	Bloating
Flatulence	Abdominal pain
Aggravation of hemorrhoids	Indigestion and heartburn
Increase of plasma triglycerides (usually mild)	
Infrequent Adverse Events	
Nausea and vomiting	Diarrhea
Dysphagia, esophageal obstruction (colestipol tablets)	Rash
Urticaria	Dermatitis
Hepatic transaminase elevations	Alkaline phosphatase elevation
Musculoskeletal pain	Headache
Impaired absorption of vitamins	Swelling of hands or feet
Hypoprothrombinemic bleeding (rare)	Fatigue, weakness
Hyperchloremic acidosis (at high doses)	Steatorrhea (at very high drug doses)
Selective Polymer—Colesevelam	
Infrequent Adverse Events	
Potentially the same as those with nonselective polymers, but less frequently observed	

From Refs 13,16,49,62,70,72-74, with permission.

SAFETY AND TOLERABILITY

BAS are regarded as extraordinarily safe LDL-lowering agents because systemic exposure to the administered drugs is essentially nil.[6,64] By inhibiting the presentation of bile acids to the intestinal mucosa and to the liver, they exert systemic effects including the target effect of LDL cholesterol lowering. Nevertheless, the polymers themselves remain in the gastrointestinal tract, and they deserve to be called nonsystemic. The safety of BAS is emphasized by the fact that patients with prior statin-induced myotoxicity tolerate colesevelam well, despite aggravation of myalgia or weakness by most or all other cholesterol-lowering therapies.[65] BAS are the only cholesterol-lowering agents that should be used by premenopausal women without contraception.[66]

Adverse Effects

Adverse effects associated with BAS are largely gastrointestinal (Table 23-1). Constipation is the most common side effect, and it can be severe. A large fraction, 10% to 30%, of people treated with the older nonselective BAS—cholestyramine and colestipol—experience constipation, bloating, abdominal discomfort, and/or aggravation of hemorrhoids. Cholestyramine and colestipol are essentially equivalent in side-effect profiles.[6] Colesevelam appears to be better tolerated than the nonselective, older BAS, although no direct comparison has been done. In an integrated analysis of placebo-controlled trials, constipation was reported by 11% of colesevelam-treated subjects compared with 7% of placebo-treated subjects.[64] The selectivity of colesevelam for bile acid anions compared with fatty acid and other organic anions may partly explain the improved side-effect profile.

Recommendations for minimizing constipation and bloating associated with BAS include increased fluid intake, increased fiber intake, and the provision of stool softeners such as docusate sodium. These measures are more important in elderly or debilitated patients. Colesevelam may not require such ancillary measures.[64] For the older, nonselective BAS, a slow increase of dosage has been recommended, perhaps over a period of months.[67]

Patients tend to prefer colesevelam or colestipol tablets over cholestyramine or colestipol granules. One should advise patients to be sure that tablets placed in the mouth are entirely wet before swallowing to avoid the discomfort of a tablet sticking in the back of the throat. When more than 18% to 20% LDL cholesterol lowering is needed, granular formulations find greater acceptance. Patients should be informed that the granules do not dissolve but can be suspended in a variety of liquids, including water and fruit juice, or mixed with applesauce.

Experimentation to find a palatable vehicle should be encouraged. Mixing the granules with psyllium powder and ample liquid may help to counter constipation and hardness of stools while potentially gaining further LDL-lowering from psyllium.[68] With either tablets or granules, it is helpful to advise swallowing carefully, without gulping, to minimize concomitant air swallowing, a major source of intestinal gas.[69]

BAS can worsen hypertriglyceridemia. They are contraindicated as monotherapy in persons with high triglyceride levels (>400 mg/dL) and in type III hyperlipoproteinemia (dysbetalipoproteinemia).[70] Patients with normal baseline triglyceride levels have minimal triglyceride increase, but those with baseline triglyceride levels greater than 200 mg/dL may get substantial further elevation.[5,71,72]

Interference with Absorption of Drugs and Vitamins

Only the nonselective BAS are known to interfere substantially with absorption of concomitantly administered drugs; colesevelam avoids this problem. Colesevelam has been shown not to affect the bioavailability of digoxin, lovastatin, metoprolol, quinidine, valproic acid, and warfarin. Small decreases in plasma levels of sustained-release verapamil were seen, but the clinical significance is unclear.[64]

The nonselective BAS, cholestyramine and colestipol, bind and inhibit the absorption of a wide range of drugs. These include, but are not limited to, thiazide diuretics, furosemide, penicillin, tetracycline, and gemfibrozil. In general, other drugs should be taken 1 hour before nonselective BAS or 4 hours after.[67] Particular care is necessary when drugs with narrow toxic-to-therapeutic ratios are prescribed, such as digoxin, thyroxine, or warfarin. The guideline for scheduling nonselective BAS around other drugs, however, can make adherence difficult. Scheduling can be relaxed if a measurable target such as lipoprotein levels, blood pressure, or blood glucose is attained as other drugs are taken closer to or even simultaneously with nonselective BAS.

The possibility of malabsorption of the fat-soluble vitamins A, D, E, and K and the anionic vitamin folate has been investigated in BAS-treated subjects. Decreased folic acid was identified among children treated with cholestyramine; the deficiency could be overcome by supplementing folic acid 5 mg daily.[73] Among children treated with colestipol, vitamin A and vitamin E were reduced in a subgroup with high drug adherence, but all vitamin concentrations remained within normal limits.[74] Neither 25-hydroxyvitamin D nor parathyroid hormone levels were altered in cholestyramine-treated patients, suggesting that BAS should not induce osteomalacia.[74,75] Rarely, vitamin K deficiency has occurred after treatment with cholestyramine or colestipol, and bleeding with hypoprothrombinemia has been reported.[76]

REFERENCES

1. Bergen SS Jr, Van Itallie TB, Tennent DM, Sebrell WH: Effect of an anion exchange resin on serum cholesterol in man. *Proc Soc Exp Biol Med* 1959;102:676–679.
2. Effects of cholestyramine, a bile acid sequestering exchange resin: *Nutr Rev* 1961;19:292–293.
3. Hashim SA, Bergen SS Jr, Van Itallie TB: Experimental steatorrhea induced in man by bile acid sequestrant. *Proc Soc Exp Biol Med* 1961;106:173–175.
4. Levy RI, Brensike JF, Epstein SE, et al: The influence of changes in lipid values induced by cholestyramine and diet on progression of coronary artery disease: Results of the NHLBI Type II Coronary Intervention Study. *Circulation* 1984;69:325–337.
5. Lipid Research Clinics Program: The Lipid Research Clinics Coronary Primary Prevention Trial results. I. Reduction in incidence of coronary heart disease. *JAMA* 1984;251:351–374.
6. Heel RC, Brogden RN, Pakes GE, et al: Colestipol: a review of its pharmacological properties and therapeutic efficacy in patients with hypercholesterolaemia. *Drugs* 1980;19:161–180.
7. Glueck CJ, Ford S Jr, Scheel D, Steiner P: Colestipol and cholestyramine resin. Comparative effects in familial type II hyperlipoproteinemia. *JAMA* 1972;222:676–681.
8. Kawashiri MA, Higashikata T, Nohara A, et al: Efficacy of colestimide coadministered with atorvastatin in Japanese patients with heterozygous familial hypercholesterolemia (FH). *Circ J* 2005;69:515–520.
9. Colestimide. ClinicalTrials.gov. Accessed 11-17-2007.
10. Hofmann AF: The enterohepatic circulation of bile acids in health and disease. In Sleisinger MH, Fordtran JS, (eds): Gastrointestinal Disease: Pathophysiology, Diagnosis, and Management, 3rd ed. Philadelphia, Saunders, 1983, pp 115–131.
11. Love MW, Dawson PA: New insights into bile acid transport. *Curr Opin Lipidol* 1998;9:225–229.
12. Johns WH, Bates TR: Quantification of the binding tendencies of cholestyramine. II. Mechanism of interaction with bile salt and fatty acid salt anions. *J Pharm Sci* 1970;59:329–333.
13. Claudel T, Staels B, Kuipers F: The farnesoid X receptor: a molecular link between bile acid and lipid and glucose metabolism. *Arterioscler Thromb Vasc Biol* 2005;25:2020–2030.
14. Grundy SM: Cholesterol metabolism in man. *West J Med* 1978;128:13–25.
15. Grundy SM, Ahrens EH Jr: Measurements of cholesterol turnover, synthesis, and absorption in man, carried out by isotope kinetic and sterol balance methods. *J Lipid Res* 1969;10:91–107.
16. Grundy SM: Treatment of hypercholesterolemia by interference with bile acid metabolism. *Arch Intern Med* 1972;130:638–648.
17. Goodman DS, Noble RP, Dell RB: The effects of colestipol resin and of colestipol plus clofibrate on the turnover of plasma cholesterol in man. *J Clin Invest* 1973;52:2646–2655.
18. Schneider DL, Gallo DG, Sarett HP: Effect of cholestyramine on cholesterol metabolism in young adult swine. *Proc Soc Exp Biol Med* 1966;121:1244–1248.
19. Moutafis CD, Myant NB: Increased hepatic synthesis of cholesterol after ileal by-pass in monkeys. *Clin Sci* 1968;34:541–548.
20. Makishima M, Okamoto AY, Repa JJ, et al: Identification of a nuclear receptor for bile acids. *Science* 1999;284:1362–1365.
21. Parks DJ, Blanchard SG, Bledsoe RK, et al: Bile acids: natural ligands for an orphan nuclear receptor. *Science* 1999;284:1365–1368.
22. Edwards PA, Kast HR, Anisfeld AM: BAREing it all: the adoption of LXR and FXR and their roles in lipid homeostasis. *J Lipid Res* 2002;43:2–12.
23. Lee FY, Lee H, Hubbert ML, et al: FXR, a multipurpose nuclear receptor. *Trends Biochem Sci* 2006;31:572–580.
24. Yabe D, Brown MS, Goldstein JL: Insig-2, a second endoplasmic reticulum protein that binds SCAP and blocks export of sterol regulatory element-binding proteins. *Proc Natl Acad Sci USA* 2002;99:12753–12758.
25. Shepherd J, Packard CJ, Bicker S, et al: Effect of cholestyramine on low-density lipoproteins. *N Engl J Med* 1980;303:943–944.
26. Inagaki T, Moschetta A, Lee YK, et al: Regulation of antibacterial defense in the small intestine by the nuclear bile acid receptor. *Proc Natl Acad Sci USA* 2006;103:3920–3925.
27. Booker ML: S-8921 (Shionogi). *Curr Opin Investig Drugs* 2001;2:393–395.
28. Telford DE, Edwards JY, Lipson SM, et al: Inhibition of both the apical sodium-dependent bile acid transporter and HMG-CoA reductase markedly enhances the clearance of LDL apoB. *J Lipid Res* 2003;44:943–952.
29. Buchwald H, Varco RL, Matts JP, et al: Effect of partial ileal bypass surgery on mortality and morbidity from coronary heart disease in patients with hypercholesterolemia. *N Engl J Med* 1990;323:946–955.
30. Hofmann AF: The continuing importance of bile acids in liver and intestinal disease. *Arch Intern Med* 1999;159:2647–2658.

31. Mekjian HS, Phillips SF, Hofmann AF: Colonic secretion of water and electrolytes induced by bile acids: perfusion studies in man. *J Clin Invest* 1971;50:1569–1577.
32. Oelkers P, Kirby LC, Heubi JE, Dawson PA: Primary bile acid malabsorption caused by mutations in the ileal sodium-dependent bile acid transporter gene *(SLC10A2)*. *J Clin Invest* 1997;99: 1880–1887.
33. Staels B, Kuipers F: Bile acid sequestrants and the treatment of type 2 diabetes mellitus. *Drugs* 2007;67:1383–1392.
34. Garg A, Grundy SM: Cholestyramine therapy for dyslipidemia in non-insulin-dependent diabetes mellitus. A short-term, double-blind, crossover trial. *Ann Intern Med* 1994;121:416–422.
35. Zieve FJ, Kalin MF, Schwartz SL, et al: Results of the glucose-lowering effect of WelChol study (GLOWS): A randomized, double-blind, placebo-controlled pilot study evaluating the effect of colesevelam hydrochloride on glycemic control in subjects with type 2 diabetes. *Clin Ther* 2007;29:74–83.
36. Commerford SR, Vargas L, Dorfman SE, et al: Dissection of the insulin-sensitizing effect of liver X receptor ligands. *Mol Endocrinol* 2007;21:3002–3012.
37. Tomlinson E, Fu L, John L, et al: Transgenic mice expressing human fibroblast growth factor-19 display increased metabolic rate and decreased adiposity. *Endocrinology* 2002;143: 1741–1747.
38. Insull W: Clinical utility of bile acid sequestrants in the treatment of dyslipidemia: a scientific review. *South Med J* 2006;99:257–273.
39. Adridge MA, Ito MK: Colesevelam hydrochloride: A novel bile acid-binding resin. *Ann Pharmacother* 2001;35:898–907.
40. Davidson MH, Dillon MA, Gordon B, et al: Colesevelam hydrochloride (Cholestagel). A new, potent bile acid sequestrant associated with a low incidence of gastrointestinal side effects. *Arch Intern Med* 1999;159:1893–1900.
41. Hunninghake DB, Bell C, Olson L: Effect of colestipol and clofibrate, singly and in combination, on plasma lipid and lipoproteins in type IIb hyperlipoproteinemia. *Metabolism* 1981;30:610–615.
42. Hunninghake DB, Probstfield JL, Crow LO, et al: Effect of colestipol and clofibrate on plasma lipid and lipoproteins in type IIa hyperlipoproteinemia. *Metabolism* 1981;30:605–609.
43. Insull W, Toth P, Mullican W, et al: Effectiveness of colesevelam hydrochloride in decreasing LDL cholesterol in patients with primary hypercholesterolemia: A 24-week randomized controlled trial. *Mayo Clin Proc* 2001;76:971–982.
44. Lipid Research Clinics Program. The Lipid Research Clinics Coronary Primary Prevention Trial results. II. The relationship of reduction in incidence of coronary heart disease to cholesterol lowering. *JAMA* 1984;251:365–374.
45. Lyons D, Webster J, Fowler G, et al: Colestipol at varying dosage intervals in the treatment of moderate hypercholesterolemia. *Br J Clin Pharmac* 1994;37:59–62.
46. Insull W, Davidson MH, Demke DM, et al: The effects of colestipol tablets compared with colestipol granules on plasma cholesterol and other lipids in moderately hypercholesterolemic patients. *Atherosclerosis* 1995;112:223–235.
47. Vecchio TJ, Linden CV, O'Connell JMJ, et al: Comparative efficacy of colestipol and clofibrate in type IIa hyperlipoproteinemia. *Arch Intern Med* 1982;142:721–723.
48. Lipid Research Clinics Program. The Lipid Research Clinics Coronary Primary Prevention Trial results. II. The relationship of reduction in incidence of coronary heart disease to cholesterol lowering. *JAMA* 1984;251:365–374.
49. Davidson MH, Toth P, Weiss S, et al: Low-dose combination therapy with colesevelam hydrochloride and lovastatin effectively decreases low-density lipoprotein cholesterol in patients with primary hypercholesterolemia. *Clin Cardiol* 2001;24:467–474.
50. Hunninghake D, Insull W, Toth P, et al: Coadministration of colesevelam hydrochloride with atorvastatin lowers LDL cholesterol additively. *Atherosclerosis* 2001;158:407–416.
51. Knapp HH, Schrott H, Ma P, et al: Efficacy and safety of combination simvastatin and colesevelam in patients with primary hypercholesterolemia. *Am J Med* 2001;110:352–360.
52. Pan HY, DeVault AR, Swites BJ, et al: Pharmacokinetics and pharmacodynamics of pravastatin alone and with cholestyramine in hypercholesterolemia. *Clin Pharmacol Ther* 1990;48:201–207.
53. Denke MA, Grundy SM: Efficacy of low-dose cholesterol-lowering drug therapy in men with moderate hypercholesterolemia. *Arch Intern Med* 1995;155:393–399.
54. Davidson MH, Dicklin MR, Maki KC, Kleinpell RM: Colesevelam hydrochloride: a non-absorbed, polymeric cholesterol-lowering agent. *Exp Opin Invest Drugs* 2000;9:2663–2671.
55. Malloy MJ, Kane JP, Kunitake ST: Complementarity of colestipol, niacin, and lovastatin in treatment of severe familial hypercholesterolemia. *Ann Intern Med* 1987;107:616–623.
56. Blankenhorn DH, Nessim SA, Johnson RL, et al: Beneficial effects of combined colestipol-niacin therapy on coronary atherosclerosis and coronary venous bypass grafts. *JAMA* 1987;257:3233–3240.
57. Brown G, Albers JJ, Fisher LD, et al: Regression of coronary artery disease as a result of intensive lipid-lowering therapy in men with high levels of apolipoprotein B. *N Engl J Med* 1990;323:1289–1298.
58. Bays H, Rhyne J, Abby S, et al: Lipid-lowering effects of colesevelam HCl in combination with ezetimibe. *Curr Med Res Opin* 2006;22:2191–2200.
59. McKenny J, Jones M, Abby S: Safety and efficacy of colesevelam hydrochloride in combination with fenofibrate for the treatment of mixed hyperlipidemia. *Curr Med Res Opin* 2005;21:1403–1412.
60. Bays HE, Davidson M, Jones MR, Abby SL: Effects of colesevelam hydrochloride on low-density lipoprotein cholesterol and high-sensitivity C-reactive protein when added to statins in patients with hypercholesterolemia. *Am J Cardiol* 2006;97:1198–1205.
61. Devaraj S, Autret B, Jialal I: Effects of colesevelam hydrochloride (WelChol) on biomarkers of inflammation in patients with mild hypercholesterolemia. *Am J Cardiol* 2006;98:641–643.
62. Watts GF, Lewis B, Brunt JN, et al: Effects on coronary artery disease of lipid-lowering diet, or diet plus cholestyramine, in the St. Thomas' Atherosclerosis Regression Study (STARS) *Lancet* 1992;339:563–569.
63. Kane JP, Malloy MJ, Ports TA, et al: Regression of coronary atherosclerosis during treatment of familial hypercholesterolemia with combined drug regimens. *JAMA* 1990;264:3007–3012.
64. WelChol (colesevelam) product information. Physicians Desk Reference. Montvale, NJ, Thomson PDR, 2005, pp 2978–2979.
65. Antons KA, Williams CD, Baker SK, Phillips PS: Clinical perspectives of statin-induced rhabdomyolysis. *Am J Med* 2006;119: 400–409.
66. Stone NJ, Blum CB: Management of Lipids in Clinical Practice, 5th ed. Caddo, OK, Professional Communications, 2005, pp 284–289.
67. Colestid (colestipol) product information. Physicians Desk Reference. Montvale, NJ, Thomson PDR, 2004, pp 2740–2742.
68. Spence JD, Huff MW, Heidenheim P, et al: Combination therapy with colestipol and psyllium mucilloid in patients with hyperlipidemia. *Ann Intern Med* 1995;123:493–499.
69. Abraczinskas D, Goldfinger SE: Intestinal gas and bloating. In Rose BD (ed): UpToDate. Waltham, MA, UpToDate, 2007.
70. Adult Treatment Panel III: Third Report of the National Cholesterol Education Program (NCEP) Expert Panel on Detection, Evaluation, and Treatment of High Blood Cholesterol in Adults. Bethesda, MD, NIH Publication No. 02-5215, National Institutes of Health, 2002, pp. VI-9–VI-10.
71. Crouse JR III: Hypertriglyceridemia: A contraindication to the use of bile acid binding resins. *Am J Med* 1987;83:243–248.
72. Witztum JL, Schonfeld G, Weidman SW, et al: Bile sequestrant therapy alters the compositions of low-density and high-density lipoproteins. *Metabolism* 1979;28:221–229.
73. West RJ, Lloyd JK: The effect of cholestyramine on intestinal absorption. *Gut* 1975;16:93–98.
74. Schwarz KB, Goldstein PD, Witztum JL, Schonfeld G: Fat-soluble vitamin concentrations in hypercholesterolemic children treated with colestipol. *Pediatrics* 1980;65:243–250.
75. Hoogwerf BJ, Hibbard DM, Hunninghake DB: Effects of long-term cholestyramine administration on vitamin D and parathormone levels in middle-aged men with hypercholesterolemia. *J Lab Clin Med* 1992;119:407–411.
76. Vroonhof K, van Rijn HJ, van Hattum J: Vitamin K deficiency and bleeding after long-term use of cholestyramine. *Neth J Med* 2003;61:19–21.

CHAPTER 24

Cholesterol Absorption Inhibitors

G. D. Norata and A. L. Catapano

INTRODUCTION

In humans, sterols are required for a number of physiologic processes, but excess sterol production or absorption can be detrimental because it may contribute to the development of atherosclerosis. The net effects of dietary cholesterol absorption, endogenous cholesterol synthesis, and biliary cholesterol excretion regulate whole-body cholesterol balance, either by transformation into bile acids or through direct cholesterol excretion.[1–3] Recent studies have significantly advanced our understanding of intestinal sterol absorption at the molecular level.[4] Nuclear hormone receptors (e.g., liver X receptor [LXR], farnesoid X receptor [FXR], and retinoid X receptor [RXR]) regulate the absorption of dietary sterols by modulating the transcription of several genes involved in cholesterol metabolism.[4] One of these genes encodes a molecule (ATP-binding cassette [ABC] transporter) that transports dietary cholesterol from enterocytes to the intestinal lumen, thereby limiting the amount of cholesterol absorbed.[4] By the same mechanism, ABC transporters also provide an efficient barrier against the absorption of plant sterols. Another key process that affects intestinal sterol absorption is the synthesis of cholesteryl esters. Mice lacking the enzyme for cholesterol esterification in the small intestine have a reduced capacity to absorb dietary cholesterol and are protected against diet-induced hypercholesterolemia, gallstone formation, and atherosclerosis.[4] Furthermore, a key protein involved in cholesterol transport, named Niemann–Pick C1–like 1 protein (NPC1L1), has been characterized recently. NPC1L1-deficient mice have impaired cholesterol absorption, and the lack of responsiveness to ezetimibe in these mice suggests that NPC1L1 is likely to be the main target of this new cholesterol-lowering drug.

The pharmacologic treatment of elevated blood cholesterol levels has been dramatically modified over the past 15 years by the introduction of statins as the main approach to therapy; that is, the focus has switched from reducing the intake of fat to modulating cholesterol in the body. However, many patients cannot reach the target for low-density lipoprotein (LDL) cholesterol level through the use of statins or fibrates or ion-exchange resins alone. As a consequence, the need for coadministering drugs with different mechanisms of action emerges. New molecules are under intensive investigation, and ezetimibe, a specific inhibitor of cholesterol absorption, is available and appears to complement the efficacy of the major classes of hypolipidemic drugs available.

In this chapter, we first focus on the molecular mechanisms involved in cholesterol absorption and then describe the different approaches available, which directly or indirectly interfere with cholesterol absorption.

INTESTINAL CHOLESTEROL ABSORPTION

Within the intestinal lumen, dietary cholesterol is presented to the brush border of mucosal enterocytes as a micelle formed by the action of bile salts, cholesterol, and fatty acids.[4,5] The initial point of contact between these micelles and the intestinal cells that absorb cholesterol occurs at the surface of the enterocyte brush border in the intestine.[4,5] Cholesterol appears to be specifically removed from the micelles as part of the absorption process: it is absorbed mainly in the duodenum and jejunum, but bile acids are not absorbed to an appreciable degree at these sites. Rather, specific bile acid transporters located in the ileum subsequently absorb bile acids, delivering them back to the liver and thus giving rise to an enterohepatic circulation.[5] A key protein involved in cholesterol absorption in the intestine, NPC1L1, has a

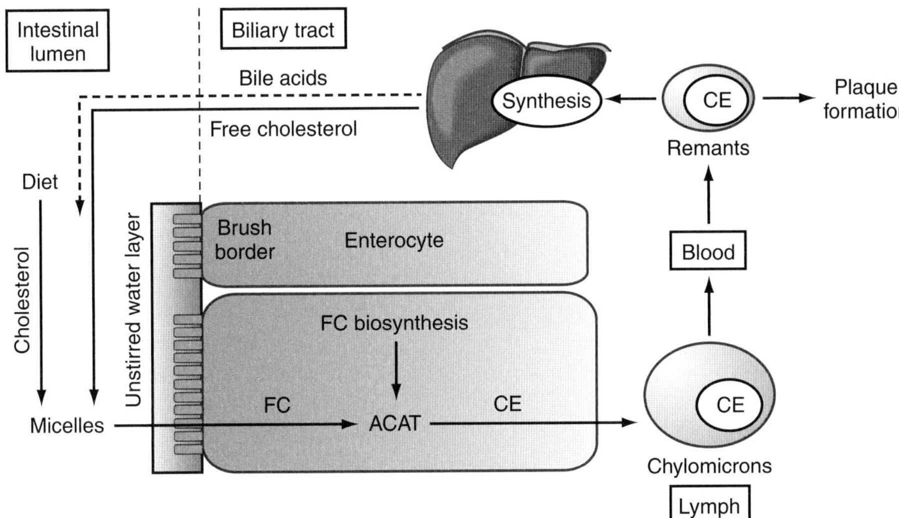

FIGURE 24-1 Pathway of exogenous cholesterol metabolism. Exogenous cholesterol is hydrolyzed to free cholesterol (FC) by pancreatic lipases secreted into the intestine. It is then transferred by micelles to the brush border of enterocytes, where it diffuses through the epithelial membrane to the interior of the cell. In the smooth endoplasmic reticulum, exogenous cholesterol is converted to cholesteryl ester (CE) by acyl–coenzyme A: cholesterol acyltransferase (ACAT), then packaged into chylomicrons. These chylomicrons are pumped through the thoracic lymph duct into the blood, where lipoprotein lipase hydrolyzes them into chylomicron remnants. These particles are then transported to the liver for further processing, or if they are small enough (≤45 nm), they may penetrate arterial cells via transcytotic vesicles.

fundamental role in promoting cholesterol transport through the enterocyte brush border membrane.[6] This critical protein is abundantly expressed in animal small intestine, and mice deficient in NPC1L1 have a markedly reduced sterol absorption.[6] A specific inhibitor of this transporter, ezetimibe, is now available for lowering plasma cholesterol by an additional 15% to 25%. A few years ago, noncholesterol sterols did not appear to be absorbed; however, more recently, new insights into sitosterolemia or phytosterolemia depicted a different situation. Phytosterolemia is a rare autosomal recessive disorder caused by hyperabsorption and impaired biliary secretion of cholesterol and plant sterols, which subsequently accumulate in tissues, causing tendon xanthoma and premature coronary artery disease. The disease appears to be caused by mutations in two ABC transporters, ABCG5 and ABCG8, which are localized at the apical membrane of the enterocyte and at the canalicular membrane in the liver. When functional, these proteins together form a full, active transporter and limit the net absorption of both plant sterols and cholesterol by actively pumping them from enterocytes back into the intestinal lumen. These transporters may also promote the elimination of sterols in the liver by enhancing their excretion into bile. Mice lacking *abcg5*/*abcg8* genes mimic the major phenotypes of human sitosterolemia.[6,7] After absorption, free cholesterol and fatty acids are re-esterified in the enterocyte by the action of acyl–coenzyme A: cholesterol acyltransferase (ACAT), packaged with triglycerides, phospholipids, and apolipoprotein (apo) B-48 into chylomicrons, and they are finally secreted from the basolateral site of the enterocytes, from where they enter the lymphatic channels and eventually are transported into the peripheral circulation[4,5] (see Fig. 24-1). Recent studies have significantly advanced our understanding of intestinal sterol absorption at the molecular level. Two nuclear hormone receptors are believed to be involved in the regulation of cholesterol homeostasis: LXR and FXR. The natural ligands for LXR and FXR are oxysterols (oxidized derivatives of cholesterol) and bile acids, respectively.[8,9] To modulate transcriptional activity, ligand-activated LXR or FXR form a heterodimer with one additional nuclear hormone receptor, RXR. These heterodimers control the transcription of several important genes that participate in cholesterol metabolism, sometimes appearing to antagonize the effects of each other. Two mechanisms are involved in the reduction of cholesterol following FXR–RXR and LXR–RXR activation.[10,11] The FXR–RXR heterodimer suppresses CYP7A1 expression and decreases bile acid synthesis. Because nonpolar lipids such as cholesterol have limited solubility in the aqueous environment of the intestinal lumen, bile acids are required to solubilize these nonpolar compounds and allow their absorption. By suppressing bile acid production, the activated FXR–RXR heterodimer decreases the solubilization and absorption of dietary cholesterol. Even though activation of the LXR–RXR heterodimer could not counterbalance the FXR–RXR–mediated suppression of CYP7A1 expression, the activated LXR–RXR heterodimer has a powerful effect on cholesterol homeostasis by inducing the expression of ABC transporters (specifically, ABCA1) in enterocytes. This increase in ABCA1 expression represents the second mechanism by which the administration of the RXR ligand decreases cholesterol absorption. ABCA1 normally pumps cholesterol from enterocytes back out to the intestinal lumen, thereby limiting the amount of cholesterol absorbed.[12] Mice treated with the RXR ligand present an increased intestinal expression of ABCA1, mediated by the activation of the LXR–RXR heterodimer. As a consequence, pharmacologic activation of the nuclear hormone receptors RXR, LXR, and FXR, including peroxisome proliferator–activated receptor (PPAR) agonists, positively affects ABCA1 expression and activity[13,14] and may represent a pharmacologic target for controlling hypercholesterolemia. In addition to transporting cholesterol, ABC transporters appear to be involved in the metabolism of plant sterols. Normally, the human intestine provides an efficient barrier against the absorption of plant sterols; that is, less than 5% of dietary plant sterols are absorbed, compared with 40% to 60% of dietary cholesterol.[15,16] Because plant sterols are also preferentially removed by the liver and excreted into bile, plasma concentrations of plant sterols in humans are usually low.[17] This defense against the absorption of plant sterols is disrupted in β-sitosterolemia, a rare autosomal recessive disorder characterized by the accumulation of large amounts of plant sterols in most tissues.[18] As a result, almost all affected patients develop coronary artery disease at an early age. The genetic defect was localized to chromosome 2p21 in 1998,[19] and recently two groups independently identified the genes as members of the ABC transporter family[20,21]: ABCG5 and ABCG8, two half-transporters that associate to form a fully active transporter. After absorption into the enterocyte, ABCG5 and ABCG8 mediate the transport of plant and shellfish sterols as well as cholesterol from the enterocyte back into the lumen, thereby decreasing their absorption; thus, a mutation in ABCG5 or ABCG8 results in a dysfunctional transporter that fails to eliminate plant and shellfish sterols from the body.[12] Another molecule that plays a key role in the absorption of sterols is ACAT, the enzyme that catalyzes the synthesis of cholesteryl esters.[22–24] The esterification of free cholesterol within cells allows the cholesterol to be stored as a neutral lipid in cytosolic droplets. Cholesteryl ester synthesis also participates in the packaging of cholesterol into lipoprotein particles for export. The precise role of cholesterol esterification in intestinal cholesterol absorption is not fully understood. However, because enterocytes take up only free cholesterol but secrete mostly cholesteryl esters onto lipoprotein particles (chylomicrons), cholesteryl ester synthesis is important in enhancing cholesterol absorption, perhaps by creating an intracellular diffusion gradient for free cholesterol.[4]

AGENTS AFFECTING CHOLESTEROL ABSORPTION

Different therapeutic approaches that could interfere with cholesterol absorption are currently available. (Fig. 24-2) These include molecules such as phytosterols and bile acid sequestrants that interfere with cholesterol dispersion into the micelles and that bind and impair the reabsorption of bile acids. More recently, new selective molecules for specific targets have emerged. These include ezetimibe, which inhibits NPC1L1; ACAT inhibitors, which inhibit cholesterol esterification; and microsomal triglyceride transfer protein (MTP) inhibitors, which indirectly affect cholesterol absorption.

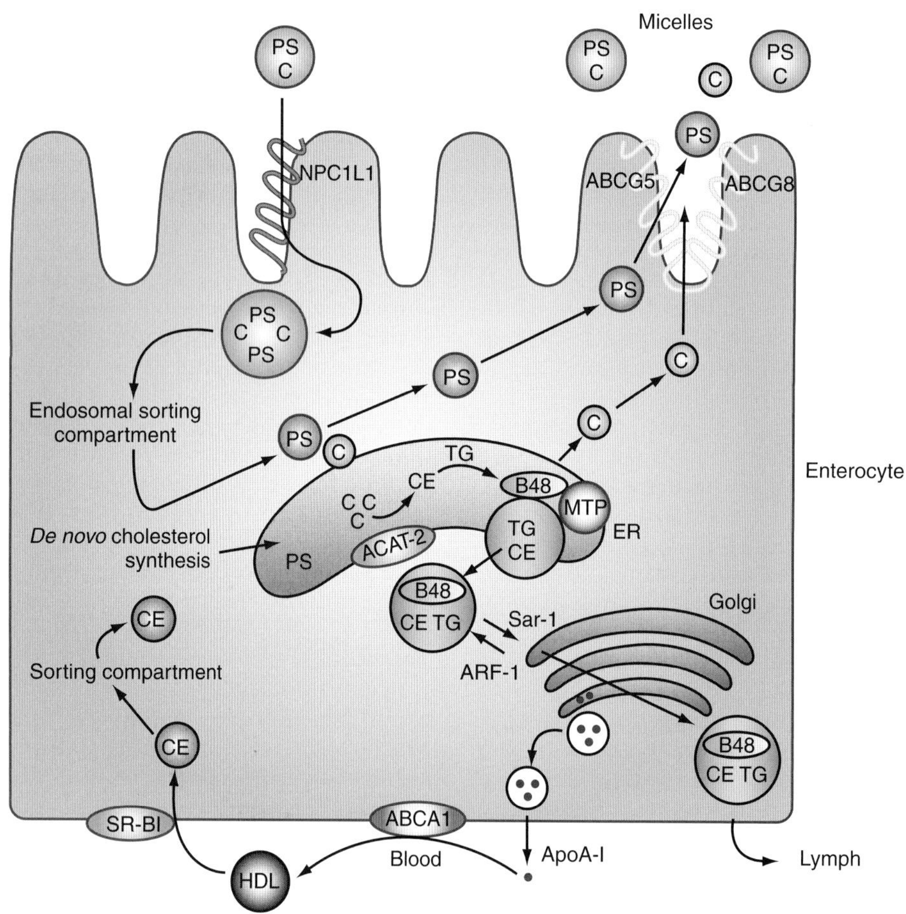

FIGURE 24-2 Inhibition of cholesterol absorption. Most of the cholesterol (C) entering the intestinal lumen is biliary cholesterol; the remainder is obtained from the diet. The luminal cholesterol is initially packaged into micelles, then taken up by microvilli in the brush border membrane of enterocytes. Bile acid sequestrants (e.g., cholestyramine) reduce the efficiency of cholesterol absorption by reducing the size of the bile acid pool and by reducing micelle formation. Plant sterols (PS) limit cholesterol absorption by either competing with cholesterol for solubilization into micelles or competing with cholesterol for proteins that facilitate sterol uptake into the small intestine. Uptake of micellar cholesterol is driven by the concentration of cholesterol in the micelle and the permeability coefficient and involves the Niemann–Pick C1–like 1 (NPC1L1) protein. Once in the epithelial cell, cholesterol is either esterified by acyl–coenzyme A:cholesterol acyltransferase–(ACAT-2), incorporated into chylomicrons (CM) and absorbed, or returned to the lumen by the ATP-binding cassette A1 (ABCA1) transporter. If ACAT-2 activity is inhibited or if ABCA1 gene activity is up-regulated, cholesterol absorption will be inhibited. New approaches to lipid management include the selective inhibition of intestinal cholesterol absorption via the exogenous cholesterol pathway. Apo, apolipoprotein; B48, apoB-48; CE, cholesteryl ester; ER, endoplasmic reticulum; HDL, high-density lipoprotein; MTP, microsomal triglyceride transfer protein; SR-BI, scavenger receptor class B type I; TG, triglyceride.

Phytosterols

Phytosterols are cholesterol-like molecules found in all plant foods, with the highest concentrations occurring in vegetable oils.[25] They are absorbed only in trace amounts but inhibit the absorption of intestinal cholesterol, including recirculating endogenous biliary cholesterol, a key step in cholesterol elimination. Natural dietary intake varies from about 167 to 437 mg/day. Attempts to measure biologic effects in feeding studies have been impeded by limited solubility in both water and fat. Esterification of phytosterols with long-chain fatty acids increases fat solubility by 10-fold and allows delivery of several grams daily in fatty foods such as margarine.[25] A dosage of 2 g/day as the ester reduces LDL cholesterol by 10%, and little difference is observed in the hypercholesterolemic activity between Δ^5-sterols and 5α-reduced sterols (stanols). Phytosterols can also be dispersed in water after emulsification with lecithin and reduce cholesterol absorption when added to foods. In contrast to these supplementation studies, much less is known about the effect of low phytosterol levels in the diet.[25] However, reduction of cholesterol absorption can be measured at a dose as low as 150 mg during otherwise sterol-free test meals, suggesting that natural food phytosterols may be clinically important. Current literature suggests that phytosterols are safe when added to the diet, and that measured absorption and plasma levels are very small.[26] However, the effects of large doses on plant phytosterol levels require careful evaluation. Increasing the aggregate amount of phytosterols consumed in a variety of foods may be an important way of reducing population cholesterol levels and preventing coronary heart disease on a population basis.

COLESTYRAMINE

—CH—CH2—CH—CH2—

—CH2—CH— CH2N+(CH3)3Cl− n

COLESTIPOL

HNCH2CH2NCH2CH2NCH2CH2NCH2CH2NH

CH2 CH2 CH2 CH2 CH2

HCOH HCOH HCOH HCOH HCOH

CH2 CH2 CH2 CH2 CH2

—CH2CH2NCH2CH2N HNCH2CH2N HNCH2CH2— n

COLESEVELAM

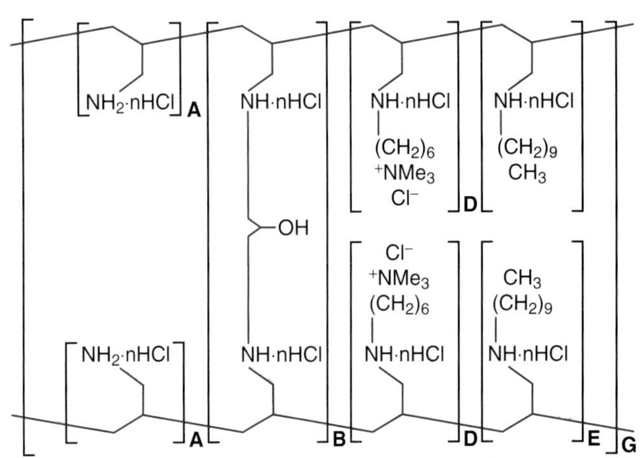

FIGURE 24-3 Molecular structure of bile acid sequestrants.

Bile Acid Sequestrant Resins

Drugs that interfere with cholesterol absorption have been used since it was discovered in the 1960s that ileal exclusion, designed to reduce dietary cholesterol intake, also reduced bile acids.[27] The two original resins, cholestyramine and colestipol, are both bile acid (anion)–binding exchange resins (Fig. 24-3). Neither is systemically absorbed or altered by digestive enzymes. The beneficial clinical effects are indirect. The binding of bile acids, and the subsequent elimination into the feces, reduces bile acid reabsorption in the ileum. The liver synthesizes cholesterol to cope with the increased demand for bile acids. The efficacy of these drugs, however, is limited by the need to mix the powders in liquid. The inconvenience, combined with the taste and the gastrointestinal side effects, limits the top dose to 24 g/day of cholestyramine or 30 g/day of colestipol—enough to result in a mean reduction in serum cholesterol of 15% to 17% or a reduction in serum LDL cholesterol of 18% to 25%, respectively.[28] Association of cholestyramine or colestipol with statins increases the lipid-lowering effects of statins.[28] Gastrointestinal adverse effects (most commonly flatulence and constipation) are often present with low dosages, as low as 2 g/day, and increase with increasing dosage. Most patients will stop taking bile acid sequestrant resins within a few weeks, although some patients adjust to the therapy. Patients should have levels of fat-soluble vitamins checked whenever they experience a severe response, such as steatorrhea, for a prolonged period.

A persistent concern with early lipid-lowering agents was the potential for reduced steroid hormone levels, because, like bile, steroid hormones are produced from cholesterol stores. Many trials examined the effects of various markers in normal and dyslipidemic populations as an indication of adequate steroid hormone production. In all of these trials, growth has not been limited; sexual maturation, sperm production, and fertility have not been affected; and all other similar endpoints, such as steroid production following stimulation with cortisone of the adrenal glands, have been normal. Early studies with resins indicated that the levels of steroid hormones did decrease, but rarely below the lower limits of normal; in addition, patients who were stimulated often responded as rapidly as patients who were not taking lipid-altering drugs.[29]

Colesevelam represents a new formulation of the bile acid–binding resins.[29] It is essentially a more "tailored" compound that offers more bile acid–binding sites for a given length of polymer backbone. The amount of colesevelam required to achieve significant results in reducing LDL cholesterol is less than that needed with colestipol or cholestyramine.[29] In combination with statins, colesevelam provided a significant incremental additive effect. The combination of 20 mg of simvastatin with 2.3 g of colesevelam reduced LDL cholesterol by 42%, as did 10 mg of simvastatin with 3.8 g of colesevelam. In combination with 10 mg of atorvastatin, 3.8 g of colesevelam decreased LDL cholesterol by 48%, which is similar to the effects expected with 40 mg of atorvastatin alone.[30] Although colesevelam will bind avidly with bile acids and cholesterol, it does not have a significant interaction with digoxin, lovastatin, metoprolol, quinidine, valproic acid, or warfarin.[31] Colesevelam should be used with appropriate caution following major gastrointestinal surgery and in patients with dysphagia, patients with marked hypertriglyceridemia, and patients suspected of having or being susceptible to fat-soluble vitamin deficiencies.

The bile acid–binding resins are widely used for lowering cholesterol in children. Multiple studies have reported the experience of chronic treatment, although most of these studies are of small size. Significant efficacy in children is usually achieved with doses proportional to their body size, or about half the dose needed in adults. As with adults, the use of resins does not decrease fat-soluble vitamins in the blood unless the patient develops significant gastrointestinal problems. Still, multivitamins are often used in pediatric practice with patients who are taking these drugs. Children often tolerate the resins better than adults and have significantly fewer adverse events, although they are more prone to discontinue therapy. Although bile acid sequestrants have not undergone placebo-controlled testing in children, they have been effectively and safely used in at least two generations of patients. It has been shown that triple therapy (using a combination of stanol ester with moderate dose of statin and resin) makes it possible to control LDL cholesterol levels effectively in hypercholesterolemic subjects[32]; future studies should investigate this issue.

Ezetimibe

Ezetimibe (SCH 58235) (Fig. 24-4) is a highly potent and selective cholesterol absorption inhibitor that reduces absorption of cholesterol from dietary and biliary sources by preventing transport of cholesterol through the intestinal wall.[33,34]

A major advance in the understanding of ezetimibe's mechanism of action occurred in 2004, when Altmann, Davis, and colleagues evaluated sequence data from human, rat, and mouse gastrointestinal cDNA libraries to identify proteins with features such as transmembrane domains and known cholesterol-sensing motifs that would be expected to be seen in a putative cholesterol transporter.[35] A candidate emerged from this search, namely NPC1L1 protein, whose gene is designated as *Npc1l1* in mouse and *NPC1L1* in human. NPC1L1 was first described in 2000[36]; its name was derived from the fact that it shared 42% amino acid identity with Niemann–Pick type C1 protein (NPC1), which encodes a protein involved in intracellular cholesterol transport and is also the causative gene for Niemann–Pick disease type C1.[37] In mouse, rat, and human, the small intestine showed high level of NPC1L1 mRNA expression.[35] With the exception of human liver, which showed similar levels of expression as the intestine, NPC1L1 expression in all other tissues was less than 10% of intestinal expression and was barely detectable in many tissues, in contrast with the fairly ubiquitous tissue expression of NPC1. Further analysis of the duodenal–ileal axis of rat small intestine demonstrated that peak expression of Npc1L1 mRNA and Npc1L1 protein occurred in the proximal jejunum, which was also the predominant site for sterol absorption.[35]

Interestingly, ezetimibe has also been shown to block the uptake of oxidized LDL by human macrophages through inhibition of both NPC1L1 and ANX2/CAV1,[38] which suggests that the actions of this agent may extend beyond the intestinal epithelium. Aminopeptidase N (CD13) in the brush border membrane may represent an additional molecular target for ezetimibe. Ezetimibe has been shown to bind to aminopeptidase N, thereby blocking the endocytosis of cholesterol from micelles in the intestinal lumen.[39] Additional evidence has come from *in vitro* binding assays that tested directly the interaction between the drug and NPC1L1. Garcia-Calvo and colleagues[40] developed a binding assay and showed that labeled ezetimibe glucuronide bound specifically to a single site in intestinal epithelial brush border membranes and in embryonic kidney cells engineered to express NPC1L1. Furthermore, the binding affinities of ezetimibe and its analogues to recombinant NPC1L1 were indistinguishable from those observed for native enterocyte membranes. Values for the dissociation constant of ezetimibe glucuronide for NPC1L1 were evaluated in intestinal enterocyte membranes and human embryonic kidney cells engineered to express NPC1L1 from various species. Binding affinities were highest for rhesus monkey, compared with more moderate values for rat and human; the lowest values reported were for mouse, which also correlates well with the *in vivo* potency observed for ezetimibe across species. Also, ezetimibe failed to affect cholesterol absorption in Npc1L1−/− mice compared with wild-type mice. These results established NPC1L1 as ezetimibe's target. More recently it has been shown that NPC1L1 is expressed in the membrane of primate hepatocytes and that NPC1L1 facilitates cholesterol uptake in hepatoma cells.[41] Transgenic mice expressing human NPC1L1 in hepatocytes (L1-TG mice) show a 10- to 20-fold decrease in biliary cholesterol concentration but not in phospholipid and bile acid

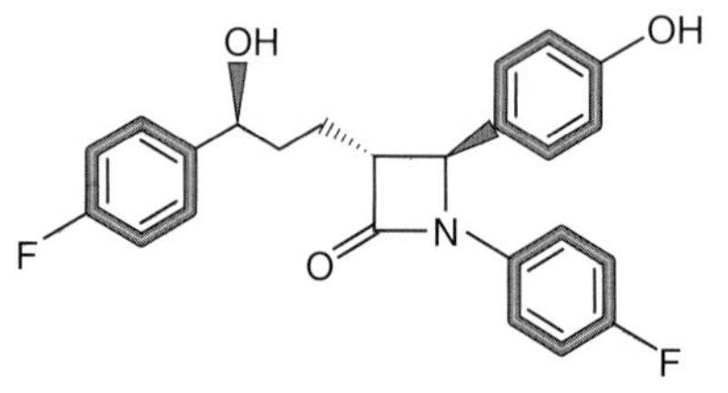

FIGURE 24-4 Molecular structure of ezetimibe (SCH 58325).

concentrations. This decrease is associated with a 30% to 60% increase in plasma cholesterol, mainly because of the accumulation of apoE-rich high-density lipoprotein (HDL). Biliary and plasma cholesterol concentrations in these animals virtually returned to normal with ezetimibe treatment. These findings suggest that in humans, ezetimibe may reduce plasma cholesterol by inhibiting NPC1L1 function in both intestine and liver; furthermore, hepatic NPC1L1 may have evolved to protect the body from excessive biliary loss of cholesterol.[41]

Ezetimibe interferes with intestinal absorption of cholesterol without affecting absorption of triglycerides, fatty acids, bile acids, or fat-soluble vitamins,[34] unlike pancreatic lipase inhibitors (e.g., orlistat), which affect the absorption of triglycerides and may decrease the absorption of fat-soluble vitamins.[42] Furthermore, ezetimibe also differs from the bile acid sequestrants (e.g., cholestyramine), which interfere with absorption of vitamins A, D, E, and K; taurocholate; and bile acids.[43] Ezetimibe undergoes phase II metabolism,[33] yielding a glucuronide that is pharmacodynamically active. Following intraduodenal delivery to rodents, ezetimibe is rapidly and extensively glucuronidated in the intestinal wall, is absorbed into the portal plasma, and passes through the liver into the bile within minutes.[33] Once glucuronidated, ezetimibe circulates enterohepatically, repeatedly returning to the primary site of action (the intestine), thus limiting peripheral exposure. This recirculation may explain the long duration of action of ezetimibe. Ezetimibe localizes in the intestinal wall, mainly as the phenolic glucuronide (SCH 60663).[33] Comparative studies suggest that the glucuronide is a more potent inhibitor of cholesterol absorption than ezetimibe,[33] and the localization of the glucuronide at the intestinal villi may explain its apparent increase in potency compared with ezetimibe. Specific localization of radiolabeled ezetimibe to the intestinal villi, its site of action, has been demonstrated in bile-cannulated rats intravenously injected with ^{3}H-ezetimibe.[33] Autoradiographic analysis of cross sections of the intestines of these rats shows that ezetimibe is located throughout the intestinal villi and is concentrated in the tips of the intestinal villi. Results from preclinical studies in various animal models have demonstrated the lipid-lowering and antiatherosclerotic properties of ezetimibe as a single agent, as well as a synergistic effect when combined with a statin. In cholesterol-fed rhesus monkeys, ezetimibe reduced both plasma cholesterol (ED_{50} = 0.0005 mg/kg/day) and LDL cholesterol in a dose-dependent manner.[44] In apoE-knockout mice, ezetimibe reduced serum cholesterol by more than 50% and decreased carotid (97%) and aortic (47% to 87%) atherosclerosis.[45] Ezetimibe inhibited the rise of plasma cholesterol in cholesterol-fed dogs (ED_{50} = 0.007 mg/kg/day).[46] In animals fed cholesterol-free diets, ezetimibe caused only modest reductions in plasma cholesterol levels, likely the result of an up-regulation of hepatic cholesterol synthesis.[47] Ezetimibe reduces the delivery of dietary and biliary cholesterol to the liver from the intestine, resulting in a decrease of hepatic cholesterol stores and an up-regulation of hepatic 3-hydroxy-3-methylglutaryl–coenzyme A (HMG-CoA) reductase activity. The drug therefore has a mode of action complementary to that of the statins in lowering plasma cholesterol concentrations, as ezetimibe inhibits the absorption of cholesterol, whereas statins decrease synthesis of cholesterol. The synergistic reduction in plasma total cholesterol concentration in dogs treated with ezetimibe (0.007 mg/kg/day) and lovastatin (5 mg/kg/day) has also been demonstrated with ezetimibe and pravastatin (2.5 mg/kg/day) or fluvastatin (2.5 mg/kg/day).[46]

In humans, the efficacy and safety of ezetimibe in monotherapy in phase II studies were evaluated in patients with mild to moderate primary hypercholesterolemia (LDL cholesterol = 130–250 mg/dL and TG ≤350 mg/dL), who were given 10 mg of ezetimibe for 12 weeks. Depending on the study,[47,48] compared with placebo, directly measured LDL cholesterol was 17.3% to 18.5% lower with ezetimibe. This effect occurred within 2 weeks and persisted throughout the 12-week treatment period. The response to ezetimibe was generally consistent across all subgroups, regardless of risk factor status, gender, age, race, or baseline lipid profile.[47,48] In addition, a modest increase in HDL cholesterol (2.3% to 2.9%) was observed. The adverse event profiles for the ezetimibe and placebo groups were similar. Overall, the nature, number, and pattern of occurrence of adverse events that led to study discontinuation suggested no differential risk with ezetimibe treatment relative to placebo (3% of placebo and 4% of ezetimibe recipients discontinued because of adverse events). The incidence of elevated liver function test values (alanine aminotransferase [ALT] or aspartate aminotransferase [AST] ≥3× the upper limit of normal [ULN] at two consecutive visits >1 week apart) was less than 1% in both placebo and ezetimibe treatment groups. Elevated muscle enzyme values (creatine kinase [CK] ≥10× ULN) were reported in less than 1% of both placebo and ezetimibe treatment groups. All the observed increases were asymptomatic and either transient with continued treatment or reversible following treatment discontinuation (Table 24-1).

The effect of ezetimibe (10 mg/day) on cholesterol absorption and synthesis, sterol excretion, and plasma concentrations of cholesterol and noncholesterol sterols was investigated in individuals with mild to moderate hypercholesterolemia.[49] Ezetimibe reduced cholesterol absorption by 54% ($P < 0.001$) while increasing cholesterol synthesis by 89%; furthermore, bile acid synthesis was slightly but not significantly increased. These results suggest that ezetimibe inhibits cholesterol absorption and promotes a compensatory increase in cholesterol synthesis, followed by clinically relevant reductions in LDL and total cholesterol concentrations. Ezetimibe also reduces plasma concentrations of the noncholesterol sterols sitosterol and campesterol, suggesting an effect on the absorption of these compounds as well.

Despite the established efficacy of statins, many patients taking statins do not achieve the lipid goals of the U.S. National Cholesterol Education Program Adult Treatment Panel III (NCEP ATP III). Combining lipid-modifying agents that act through complementary pathways may provide more effective LDL cholesterol–lowering.[50] Ezetimibe plus statin (80 mg) is almost four times more effective in reducing LDL cholesterol than is doubling the statin dose from 40 mg to 80 mg, the maximum recommended dose, in patients with homozygous

TABLE 24-1 Ezetimibe in Monotherapy: Treatment-Emergent Clinical and Laboratory Adverse Events

	Placebo (n = 226)	Ezetimibe (n = 666)
Clinical Adverse Events*		
Upper respiratory infection	25 (11%)	57 (9%)
Headache	18 (8%)	53 (8%)
Back pain	11 (5%)	33 (5%)
Musculoskeletal pain	9 (4%)	31 (5%)
Arthralgia	12 (5%)	28 (4%)
Laboratory Adverse Events		
ALT ≥3× ULN, consecutive	0	1 (<1%)
AST ≥3× ULN, consecutive	1 (<1%)	2 (<1%)
CK ≥10× ULN	1 (<1%)	3 (<1%)

*Occurring in more than 4% of patients in any group.
ALT, alanine aminotransferase; AST, aspartate aminotransferase; CK, creatine kinase; ULN, upper unit of normal

familial hypercholesterolemia.[51] LDL cholesterol reductions were seen within 2 weeks, were sustained throughout the study, and were obtained in patients receiving dietary therapy and, in half of the patients, concomitant LDL apheresis.[51] The relevance of these findings is highlighted by the limitations of pharmacologic therapy (including high-dose statin therapy) in reducing LDL cholesterol in patients with homozygous familial hypercholesterolemia as compared with other types of hypercholesterolemia. Ezetimibe exerts comparable actions in other forms of severe hypercholesterolemia. The effect of statins in homozygous familial hypercholesterolemia seems to be significantly limited by the inability of these patients to effectively up-regulate the LDL receptor, whereas the primary mechanism responsible for ezetimibe-induced LDL cholesterol lowering, inhibition of cholesterol absorption at the intestinal brush border, seems to be largely unaffected by the pathophysiologic milieu of homozygous familial hypercholesterolemia. As for safety, ezetimibe and statin have shown an overall tolerability and safety profile similar to statin alone; no excess of myopathy or myositis associated with ezetimibe compared with statin or placebo was observed.[51]

Moreover, when administered with statins, ezetimibe had no effect on the pharmacokinetics profile of statins, digoxin, oral contraceptives (ethinyl estradiol and levonorgestrel), glipizide, tolbutamide, midazolam, or warfarin,[51] because ezetimibe is not metabolized via cytochrome P450. The efficacy of ezetimibe coadministered with statins has been proved for lovastatin,[52] simvastatin,[53] pravastatin,[54] and atorvastatin[55] (Fig. 24-5). A broader lipid control is achieved when ezetimibe is coadministered with low doses of statins than when the dose of the statin alone is increased.[52–55] Pooled efficacy results show an additional reduction of LDL cholesterol of 14% to 18%, an additional reduction of triglycerides of 10%, and an additional increase of HDL cholesterol of up to 5%. Of note, a recent trial has shown that the association of ezetimibe with atorvastatin provided a significant additional 10% reduction in high-sensitivity C-reactive protein versus atorvastatin alone.[55] This finding suggests an added anti-inflammatory effect of the combination, possibly resulting from the overall complex effect of ezetimibe on the lipid profile.

In clinical practice, ezetimibe coadministered with a statin may enable more patients to achieve recommended

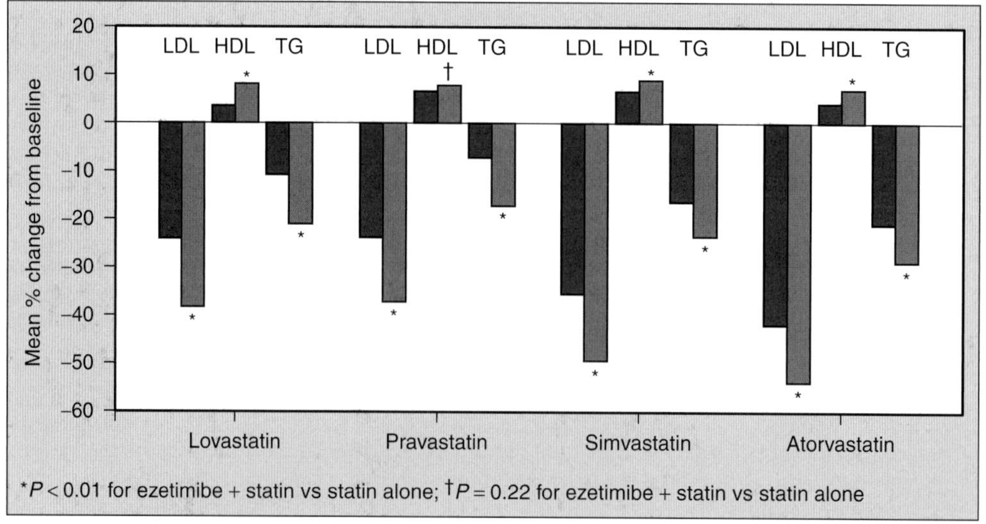

FIGURE 24-5 Effects of the association of ezetimibe and statins on plasma lipids. The red bars represent the mean percent changes of statin treatment versus placebo; the gray bars represent the mean percent change of statin plus ezetimibe treatment versus placebo. *$P < 0.01$ for ezetimibe + statin versus statin alone; ‡$P = 0.22$ for ezetimibe + statin versus statin alone. HDL, high-density lipoprotein cholesterol; LDL, low-density lipoprotein cholesterol; TG, triglycerides.

target LDL cholesterol levels by offering greater lowering with few dosage titrations and may also be a well-tolerated alternative for patients in whom maximum-dose statin monotherapy is inadequate.

The efficacy of ezetimibe was also studied in patients with β-sitosterolemia.[56] Thirty-seven patients were randomized to receive either ezetimibe 10 mg/day or placebo for 8 weeks in a randomized double-blind trial. Ezetimibe induced a 21% and 24% decrease in sitosterol and campesterol concentrations, respectively, versus a placebo-induced 4% and 3% increase, respectively.

Acyl–Coenzyme A: Cholesterol Acyl–Transferase Inhibitors

Enterocytes take up only free cholesterol but secrete mostly cholesteryl esters onto lipoprotein particles (chylomicrons); thus, cholesteryl ester synthesis may be important in enhancing cholesterol absorption, perhaps by creating an intracellular diffusion gradient for free cholesterol.[4] Mice lacking ACAT-2, the main enzyme responsible for cholesterol esterification in the mouse small intestine, that were fed a high-fat, high-cholesterol diet showed a twofold decrease in plasma cholesterol as compared with wild-type mice.[57] Avasimibe is a novel orally bioavailable ACAT inhibitor that has been tested in phase III human trials (Fig. 24-6). It is safe when administered to rats, dogs, and humans. *In vitro* studies in human macrophages demonstrated that avasimibe reduces foam cell formation not only by enhancing free cholesterol efflux but also by inhibiting the uptake of modified LDL.[58] Avasimibe induces cholesterol 7α-hydroxylase and increases bile acid synthesis in cultured rat hepatocytes; its administration to rats does not produce an increase of the bile in the lithogenicity index. The hypolipidemic efficacy of the compound was demonstrated in cholesterol-fed as well as in non-cholesterol-fed animals. In these models, plasma cholesterol levels were reduced, mainly because of the decrease in the non-HDL cholesterol fraction.[58] In a study performed in 130 men and women with combined hyperlipidemia and hypoalphalipoproteinemia, avasimibe 50 to 500 mg/day significantly reduced plasma total triglyceride and very-low-density lipoprotein (VLDL) cholesterol.[59] Although total cholesterol, LDL cholesterol, and HDL cholesterol were unchanged, it must be stressed that animal data suggest that avasimibe may possess direct antiatherosclerotic activity in addition to its cholesterol-lowering effect. Avasimibe treatment may also contribute to increased plaque stability and prevent the progression of atherosclerosis.[60] Moreover, avasimibe and statins have been shown to have synergistic effects, and the combination may not only inhibit atherosclerotic lesion progression but also induce lesion regression, independently of changes in plasma cholesterol.[61] In humans the effects of avasimibe at dosages of 50, 250, and 750 mg/day on the progression of coronary atherosclerosis was assessed by intravascular ultrasound (IVUS).[62] Surprisingly, the percentage of atheroma volume increased by 0.7%, 0.8%, and 1.0% in the respective avasimibe groups and by 0.4% with placebo (P = NS). Furthermore, LDL cholesterol increased during the study by 1.7% with placebo but by 7.8%, 9.1%, and 10.9% in the respective avasimibe groups ($P < 0.05$ in all groups). These data suggest that in humans, avasimibe did not favorably alter coronary atherosclerosis as assessed by IVUS; however, further studies in humans are warranted to clarify this issue.

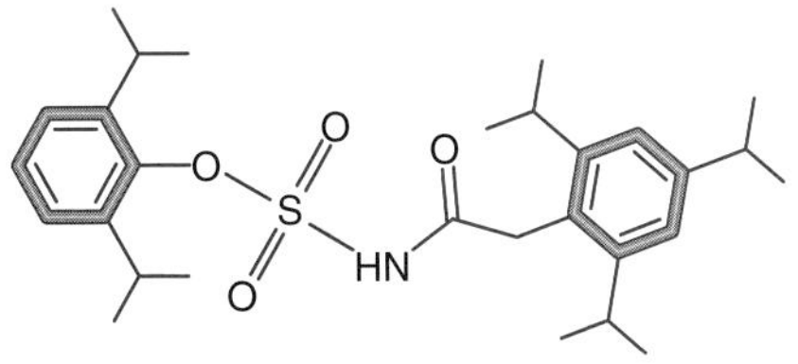

FIGURE 24-6 Molecular structure of avasimibe (CI-1011).

Microsomal Triglyceride Transfer Protein Inhibitors

Different proteins and enzymes involved in lipid metabolism are currently under investigation to develop new therapeutic approaches to limit cholesterol and lipid absorption. Among these, many studies are currently focused on the role of MTP. MTP is a heterodimeric protein consisting of a unique 97-kD subunit and a 58-kD ubiquitous multifunctional protein disulfide isomerase that possess both an apoB-binding domain and a lipid transfer domain. The protein is believed to act as a chaperone, stabilizing nascent apoB polypeptide within the endoplasmic reticulum, and is also known to facilitate lipid transfer from the endoplasmic reticulum membrane to nascent apoB by a shuttle mechanism. Although the binding and transfer activities of MTP function independently, both activities are essential for the assembly and secretion of apoB-containing lipoproteins. MTP transfers lipids by transiently interacting with a membrane, extracting the lipids, dissociating from the membrane, and then binding to another membrane to deliver the lipids. Inhibitors of MTP have exhibited potential as lipid-lowering agents; however, any process that decreases the export of triglyceride-rich lipoproteins may alter fat absorption and promote the development of fatty liver and excess fat in the intestines.[63] The MTP inhibitor implitapide has demonstrated lipid-lowering effects and an ability to suppress atherosclerosis in apoE-knockout mice. The antiatherosclerotic effects of the compound were also associated with inhibition of the postprandial triglyceride response. However, the development of this drug has been discontinued for undisclosed reasons. CP-346086 is another potent inhibitor of MTP. The compound lowered plasma concentrations of apoB-containing lipoproteins in experimental animals and in humans, with no effect on HDL levels. However, CP-346086 exhibited a potential for adverse events related to hepatic lipid accumulation. The compound JTT-130 is an orally active inhibitor of MTP. The compound is currently undergoing phase II clinical trials to assess its potential for the treatment of hyperlipidemia. This compound has been claimed to lack hepatic MTP activity because of a rapid metabolism in the portal blood and liver. The lack of such activity of this compound may thus result in an avoidance of the liver toxicity issues that have occurred with systemically active MTP inhibitors.[63] The publication of the results of clinical trials with JTT-130 will help clarify its potential in inhibiting lipoprotein synthesis and lipid absorption in the intestine.

CONCLUSIONS

Serum cholesterol levels are regulated primarily by two organs: the liver, which produces cholesterol for use in digestion, and the intestine, which absorbs cholesterol from food and from bile. Recent studies show the involvement of NPC1L1, ABCG5, ABCG8, LXR, and FXR in cholesterol metabolism in the enterocyte, suggesting possible new targets to inhibit cholesterol absorption and control homozygous sitosterolemia. Moreover, new drugs that control cholesterol absorption in the intestine are current available or are under clinical development. Statins inhibit cholesterol biosynthesis in the liver, so agents that inhibit cholesterol absorption in the intestine might be expected to have additive effects when used in combination with statins. These drugs will be useful in patients at high risk of coronary artery disease, in whom an aggressive lipid-lowering therapy is required for an optimal management of dyslipidemia.

REFERENCES

1. Gould RG, Jones RJ, LeRoy GV, et al: Absorbability of beta-sitosterol in humans. *Metabolism* 1969;18:652–662
2. Dietschy JM, Turley SD, Spady DK: Role of liver in the maintenance of cholesterol and low-density lipoprotein homeostasis in different animal species, including humans. *J Lipid Res* 1993;34:1637–1659.
3. Jolley CD, Woollett LA, Turley SD, et al: Centripetal cholesterol flux to the liver is dictated by events in the peripheral organs and not by the plasma high-density lipoprotein or apolipoprotein A-I concentration. *J Lipid Res* 1998;39:2143–2149.
4. Chen HC: Molecular mechanisms of sterol absorption. *J Nutr* 2001;131:2603–2605.
5. Love MW, Dawson PA: New insights into bile acid transport. *Curr Opin Lipidol* 1998;9:225–229.
6. Levy E, Spahis S, Sinnett D, et al: Intestinal cholesterol transport proteins: an update and beyond. *Curr Opin Lipidol* 2007;18:310–318.
7. Salen G, Tint GS, Shefer S, et al: Increased sitosterol absorption is offset by rapid elimination to prevent accumulation in heterozygotes with sitosterolemia. *Arterioscler Thromb* 1992;12:563–568.
8. Repa JJ, Mangelsdorf DJ: Nuclear receptor regulation of cholesterol and bile acid metabolism. *Curr Opin Biotechnol* 1999;10:557–563.
9. Russell DW: Nuclear orphan receptors control cholesterol catabolism. *Cell* 1999;97:539–542.
10. Repa JJ, Mangelsdorf DJ: The liver X receptor gene team: potential new players in atherosclerosis. *Nat Med* 2002;8:1243–1248.
11. Repa JJ, Turley SD, Lobaccaro JMA, et al: Regulation of absorption and ABC1-mediated efflux of cholesterol by RXR heterodimers. *Science* 2000;289:1524–1529.
12. Brewer HB Jr, Santamarina-Fojo S: New insights into the role of the adenosine triphosphate-binding cassette transporters in high-density lipoprotein metabolism and reverse cholesterol transport. *Am J Cardiol* 2003;91:3E–11E.
13. Chinetti G, Lestavel S, Bocher V, et al: PPAR-alpha and PPAR-gamma activators induce cholesterol removal from human macrophage foam cells through stimulation of the ABCA1 pathway. *Nat Med* 2001;7:53–58.
14. Norata GD, Pellegatta F, Catapano AL: Peroxisome proliferator activated receptors and cardiovascular disorders. *Ital Heart J* 2003;4(1 Suppl.):8–18.
15. Wilson MD, Rudel LL: Review of cholesterol absorption with emphasis on dietary and biliary cholesterol. *J Lipid Res* 1994;35:943–955.
16. Dawson PA, Rudel LL: Intestinal cholesterol absorption. *Curr Opin Lipidol* 1999;10:315–320.
17. Salen G, Ahrens EH, Grundy SM: Metabolism of β-sitosterol in man. *J Clin Invest* 1970;49:952–967.
18. Bhattacharyya AK, Connor WE: Beta-sitosterolemia and xanthomatosis. A newly described lipid storage disease in two sisters. *J Clin Invest* 1974;53:1033–1043.
19. Patel SB, Salen G, Hidaka H, et al: Mapping a gene involved in regulating dietary cholesterol absorption. The sitosterolemia locus is found at chromosome 2p21. *J Clin Invest* 1998;102:1041–1044.
20. Berge KE, Tian H, Graf GA, et al: Accumulation of dietary cholesterol in sitosterolemia caused by mutations in adjacent ABC transporters. *Science* 2000;290:1771–1775.
21. Lee MH, Lu K, Hazard S, et al: Identification of a gene, ABCG5, important in the regulation of dietary cholesterol absorption. *Nat Genet* 2001;27:79–83.
22. Chang TY, Chang CCY, Cheng D: Acyl-coenzyme A:cholesterol acyltransferase. *Annu Rev Biochem* 1997;66:613–638.
23. Meiner V, Tam C, Gunn MD, et al: Tissue expression studies of mouse acyl CoA:cholesterol acyltransferase gene *(Acact)*: findings supporting the existence of multiple cholesterol esterification enzymes in mice. *J Lipid Res* 1997;38:1928–1933.
24. Cases S, Novak S, Zheng YW, et al: ACAT-2, a second mammalian acyl-coA:cholesterol acyltransferase. Its cloning, expression, and characterization. *J Biol Chem* 1998;273:26755–26764.
25. Ostlund RE Jr: Phytosterols in human nutrition. *Annu Rev Nutr* 2002;22:533–549.
26. Plat J, Mensink RP: Effects of plant sterols and stanols on lipid metabolism and cardiovascular risk. *Nutr Metab Cardiovasc Dis* 2001;11:31–40.
27. Grundy SM, Ahrens EH, Salen G: Interruption of the enterohepatic circulation of bile acids in man: comparative effects of cholestyramine and ileal exclusion on cholesterol metabolism. *J Lab Clin Med* 1971;78:94–121.
28. Black DM: Gut-acting drugs for lowering cholesterol. *Curr Atheroscler Rep* 2002;4:71–75.
29. Davidson MH, Dillon MA, Gordon B, et al: Colesevelam hydrochloride (Cholestagel): a new potent bile acid sequestrant associated with a low incidence of gastrointestinal side effects. *Arch Intern Med* 1999;159:1893–1900.
30. Hunninghake D, Insull W Jr, Toth P, et al: Coadministration of colesevelam hydrochloride with atorvastatin lowers LDL cholesterol additively. *Atherosclerosis* 2001;158:407–416.
31. Donovan JM, Stypinski D, Stiles MR, et al: Drug interactions with colesevelam hydrochloride, a novel, potent lipid-lowering agent. *Cardiovasc Drugs Ther* 2000;14:681–690.
32. Gylling H, Mettinen TA: LDL cholesterol lowering by bile acid malabsorption during inhibited synthesis and absorption of cholesterol in hypercholesterolemic coronary subjects. *Nutr Metab Cardiovasc Dis* 2002;12:19–23.
33. van Heek M, Farley C, Compton DS, et al: Comparison of the activity and disposition of the novel cholesterol absorption inhibitor, SCH58235, and its glucuronide, SCH60663. *Br J Pharmacol* 2000;129:1748–1754.
34. van Heek M, Farley C, Compton D, et al: The novel cholesterol absorption inhibitor, ezetimibe, selectively inhibits the intestinal absorption of free cholesterol in the presence and absence of exocrine pancreatic function [abstract]. *Atherosclerosis* 2000;151:155.
35. Altmann SW, Davis HR Jr, Zhu LJ, et al: Niemann-Pick C1 like 1 protein is critical for intestinal cholesterol absorption. *Science* 2004;303:1201–1204.
36. Davies JP, Ioannou YA: Topological analysis of Niemann-Pick C1 protein reveals that the membrane orientation of the putative sterol-sensing domain is identical to those of 3-hydroxy-3-methylglutaryl-CoA reductase and sterol regulatory element binding protein cleavage-activating protein. *J Biol Chem* 2000;275:24367–24374.
37. Carstea ED, Morris JA, Coleman KG, et al: Niemann-Pick C1 disease gene: homology to mediators of cholesterol homeostasis. *Science* 1997;277:228–231.
38. Seedorf U, Engel T, Lueken A, et al: Cholesterol absorption inhibitor ezetimibe blocks uptake of oxidized LDL in human

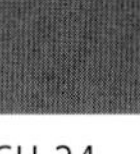

macrophages. *Biochem Biophys Res Commun* 2004;320:1337–1341.

39. Kramer W, Girbig F, Corsiero D, et al: Aminopeptidase N (CD13) is a molecular target of the cholesterol absorption inhibitor ezetimibe in the enterocyte brush border membrane. *J Biol Chem* 2005;280:1306–1320.
40. Garcia-Calvo M, Lisnock J, Bull HG, et al: The target of ezetimibe is Niemann-Pick C1-like 1 (NPC1L1). *Proc Natl Acad Sci U S A* 2005;102:8132–8137.
41. Temel RE, Tang W, Ma Y, et al: Hepatic Niemann-Pick C1-like 1 regulates biliary cholesterol concentration and is a target of ezetimibe. *J Clin Invest* 2007;117:1968–1978.
42. Heck AM, Yanovski JA, Calis KA: Orlistat, a new lipase inhibitor for the management of obesity. *Pharmacotherapy* 2000;20:270–279.
43. West RJ, Lloyd JK: The effect of cholestyramine on intestinal absorption. *Gut* 1975;16:93–98.
44. van Heek M, Compton DS, Davis HR: The cholesterol absorption inhibitor, ezetimibe, decreases diet-induced hypercholesterolemia in monkeys. *Eur J Pharmacol* 2001;415:79–84.
45. Davis HR Jr, Compton DS, Hoos L, et al: Ezetimibe, a potent cholesterol inhibitor, inhibits the development of atherosclerosis in apo E knockout mice. *Arterioscler Thromb Vasc Biol* 2001;21:2032–2038
46. Davis HR Jr, Pula KK, Alton KB, et al: The synergistic hypocholesterolemic activity of the potent cholesterol absorption inhibitor, ezetimibe, in combination with 3-hydroxyl-3-methylglutaryl coenzyme A reductase inhibitors in dogs. *Metabolism* 2001;50:1234–1241.
47. Dujovne CA, Ettinger MP, McNeer JF, et al: Efficacy and safety of a potent new selective cholesterol absorption inhibitor, ezetimibe, in patients with primary hypercholesterolemia. *Am J Cardiol* 2002;90:1092–1097.
48. Knopp RH, Gitter H, Truitt T, et al: Effects of ezetimibe, a new cholesterol absorption inhibitor, on plasma lipids in patients with primary hypercholesterolemia. *Eur Heart J* 2003;24:729–741.
49. Sudhop T, Lutjohann D, Kodal A, et al: Inhibition of intestinal cholesterol absorption by ezetimibe in humans. *Circulation* 2002;106:1943–1948.
50. Farmer JA, Gotto AM Jr: Antihyperlipidaemic agents: drugs interaction of clinical significance. *Drug Saf* 1994;11:301–309.
51. Gagne C, Gaudet D, Bruckert E: Efficacy and safety of ezetimibe coadministered with atorvastatin or simvastatin in patients with homozygous familial hypercholesterolemia. *Circulation* 2002;105:2469–2475.
52. Kerzner B, Corbelli J, Sharp S, et al: Efficacy and safety of ezetimibe coadministered with lovastatin in primary hypercholesterolemia. *Am J Cardiol* 2003;91:418–424.
53. Davidson MH, McGarry T, Bettis R, et al: Ezetimibe coadministered with simvastatin in patients with primary hypercholesterolemia. *J Am Coll Cardiol* 2002;40:2125–2134.
54. Melani L, Mills R, Hassman D, et al: Efficacy and safety of ezetimibe coadministered with pravastatin in patients with primary hypercholesterolemia: a prospective, randomized, double-blind trial. *Eur Heart J* 2003;24:717–728.
55. Ballantyne CM, Houri J, Notarbartolo A, et al: Effect of ezetimibe coadministered with atorvastatin in 628 patients with primary hypercholesterolemia. A prospective, randomized, double-blind trial. *Circulation* 2003;107:2409–2415.
56. von Bergamann K, Salen G, Lutjohann D, et al: Ezetimibe effectively reduces serum plant sterols in patients with sitosterolemia [abstract]. Presented at 73rd European Atherosclerosis Society Congress, 2002.
57. Buhman KK, Accad M, Novak S, et al: Resistance to diet-induced hypercholesterolemia and gallstone formation in ACAT2-deficient mice. *Nat Med* 2000;6:1341–1347.
58. Llaverias G, Laguna JC, Alegret M: Pharmacology of the ACAT inhibitor avasimibe (CI-1011). *Cardiovasc Drug Rev* 2003;21:33–50.
59. Insull W Jr, Koren M, Davignon J, et al: Efficacy and short-term safety of a new ACAT inhibitor, avasimibe, on lipids, lipoproteins, and apolipoproteins, in patients with combined hyperlipidemia. *Atherosclerosis* 2001;157:137–144.
60. Tardif JC, Gregoire J, Lesperance J, et al: Design features of the Avasimibe and Progression of Coronary Lesions assessed by intravascular UltraSound (A-PLUS) clinical trial. *Am Heart J* 2002;144:589–596.
61. Bocan TM, Krause BR, Rosebury WS, et al: The combined effect of inhibiting both ACAT and HMG-CoA reductase may directly induce atherosclerotic lesion regression. *Atherosclerosis* 2001;157:97–105.
62. Tardif JC, Grégoire J, L'Allier PL, et al: Effects of the acyl coenzyme A:cholesterol acyltransferase inhibitor avasimibe on human atherosclerotic lesions. *Circulation* 2004;110:3372–3377.
63. Burnett JR, Watts GF: MTP inhibition as a treatment for dyslipidaemias: time to deliver or empty promises? *Expert Opin Ther Targets* 2007;11:181–189.

CHAPTER 25

Nicotinic Acid

B. Greg Brown, Paul L. Canner, Mark E. McGovern, John R. Guyton, and Lars A. Carlson

INTRODUCTION

Nicotinic acid, or niacin, has been a child of the 20th century, but its most important roles may lie ahead. Designated in the mid-1930s as a B-complex vitamin, the deficiency of which causes pellagra, it was found in 1955 to reduce plasma cholesterol in humans and atherosclerosis in the rabbit. It was subsequently shown to have major dose-dependent effects on a broad spectrum of plasma lipoproteins—effects that are predictably favorable in terms of atherosclerosis risk. An evolving understanding of the metabolic mechanisms of niacin's effects, and of its side effects, has put us in a position to engineer its gastrointestinal release profile and to combine it with adjunctive treatments to minimize its side effects. Specifically, identification of the so-called "niacin receptor," a G_i-coupled membrane protein on the adipocyte and the cutaneous Langerhans cell, holds promise for the development of more effective and tolerable pharmaceuticals. Because lipid therapies focused on raising high-density lipoprotein (HDL) cholesterol and lowering low-density lipoprotein (LDL) cholesterol are comparably beneficial and are additive in their impact on vascular disease, niacin's most predictable future is its use in combination with LDL cholesterol–lowering agents such as the statins. As the current most effective HDL cholesterol–raising agent, niacin in various combinations appears to hold great promise for improved prevention of cardiovascular disease.

EARLY HISTORY OF NICOTINIC ACID

Dr Lars Carlson and his colleagues forged a pioneering understanding of the diverse effects of nicotinic acid and helped open the door to its use for atherosclerosis prevention.[1]

Early Discoveries

Nicotinic acid from liver extract was found, circa 1937, to prevent and cure pellagra. The active vitamin ingredient was *nicotinamide,* an amide metabolite of nicotinic acid, now a member, B_3, of the B-complex vitamin group. In 1955, Altschul and colleagues showed that niacin, but not nicotinamide, lowered cholesterol in humans and that it reduced lipid accumulation in aortas of cholesterol-fed rabbits.[2,3] Parsons and colleagues found that niacin 3 to 6 g daily lowered total cholesterol by 16%, but reduced the β/α cholesterol ratio (~LDL/HDL) from 5.0 to 2.8 (44%) in humans, first suggesting niacin's increase of HDL cholesterol.[4]

Early Pharmacologic, Metabolic, and Lipid Studies

Initially, Carlson and colleagues focused on niacin's suppression of lipolytic fatty acid release from adipose and on plasma free fatty acid (FFA) metabolism and its relation to catechol-induced energy production.[5–9] Briefly summarized, these metabolic studies, conducted almost entirely in human volunteers, found that FFAs originated from adipose tissue,[10] were rapidly esterified,[11] and were rapidly converted to hepatic triglycerides and then to plasma triglycerides (very-low-density lipoprotein [VLDL]).[12,13] Niacin given intravenously was shown to reduce strikingly plasma levels of FFA (although there was a large compensatory rebound in levels at 1–2 hours). Furthermore, niacin greatly suppressed the release of FFA and glycerol (an index of rate of lipolysis) stimulated by norepinephrine.[5] As a harbinger of the discovery of the "niacin receptor,"[14–16] and of β-hydroxybutyrate as its endogenous ligand,[17] they demonstrated that, following radiolabeled nicotinic acid infusion into mice, virtually all of the label was present in adipose tissue,[18] a tissue distribution that experts in the field had never seen before but that is now well explained by the adipocyte location of the nicotinic acid receptor. Furthermore, niacin suppressed the production of β-hydroxylated fatty acids and splanchnic ketone bodies. The niacin flush is associated with an abrupt fourfold rise in forearm blood flow (but rarely a fall in blood pressure) that is nearly completely prevented by 1-hour pretreatment with indomethacin 100 mg.[19] The flow increase is followed by an abrupt 500-fold rise in the prostaglandin PGD_2 metabolite 9α,11β-PGF2 suggesting that the flush is driven by the release of PGD_2.[20] Subsequent studies examined the effects of niacin on energy metabolism and interactions with catecholamines.[21–23] Because daily fatty acid release and transport is equivalent to roughly 1000 calories of daily energy production by oxidative metabolism, the question arose whether niacin's effect on FFA release would alter total body or myocardial metabolism. After intravenous niacin in healthy volunteers, and despite a striking fall in plasma fatty acids, total body oxygen consumption and temperature remained constant, as did myocardial oxygen use. Total body and transcardiac extraction and utilization of fatty acids decreased, and that of glucose increased, such that oxidative metabolism shifted isocalorically from fat to carbohydrate.[9,24]

Niacin: A Potential Therapy for Lipid Disorders and Associated Atherosclerosis

As the understanding of cholesterol's association with atherosclerosis emerged[1,25–28] along with the classification of different types of hyperlipidemia,[29–31] the focus turned to the effects of niacin on serum lipoprotein levels and therapeutic reduction of heart disease risk.[32] In studies of niacin in men displaying lipoprotein profiles commonly associated with coronary disease (types IIa, IIb, and IV), total cholesterol fell on average by 8% to 21%, and triglycerides fell by 29% to 55%.[33] Corresponding figures for women were 25% to 26% and 36% to 59%.[33] Subsequent studies showed the effect of niacin 4.0 g/day, for 6 weeks, on plasma lipoproteins in dyslipidemic subjects: On average, total cholesterol decreased by 14%, triglycerides by 26%, VLDL cholesterol by 47%, LDL cholesterol by 16%, and Lp(a) by 40%. In these subjects, HDL cholesterol, HDL_2 cholesterol, and HDL_3 cholesterol increased by 40%, 90%, and 8%, respectively.[34] Of note, niacin is the only lipid drug that has a substantial effect on Lp(a). Another unique effect of niacin is the powerful reduction of the extremely high triglyceride levels in the rare type V hyperlipoproteinemia, from 20 to 100 mmol/L to below 5 mmol/L. This reduction is associated with a disappearance of the life-threatening recurrent attacks of pancreatitis characteristic of this genetic disorder.[35]

The Stockholm Ischaemic Heart Disease Secondary Prevention Study

Given the convergence of this evidence predicting clinical benefit from combined LDL cholesterol lowering and HDL cholesterol raising, the Stockholm Ischaemic Heart Disease Secondary Prevention Study[36,37] randomized survivors of myocardial infarction (MI) in a single Stockholm hospital to niacin 3.0 g daily plus clofibrate 2.0 g daily, or to no lipid therapy (not placebo). On average, the therapy combination reduced total cholesterol by 13% and triglycerides by 19% relative to control. Total mortality and coronary heart disease (CHD) mortality were reduced in the niacin/clofibrate treatment group by 26% ($P < 0.05$) and 36% ($P < 0.01$), respectively. Of note, this therapy benefit was seen in the subgroup above age 60. Benefit was seen only in the 215 of 276 treated patients with baseline triglycerides greater than 1.5 mmol/L (143 mg/dL) and was most pronounced in the 44% of patients achieving at least a 30% triglyceride reduction with therapy. HDL cholesterol was not measured, but in a somewhat comparable study,[38] HDL cholesterol rose by 42%.

THE CORONARY DRUG PROJECT: A PIONEERING LANDMARK PREVENTION TRIAL

Design and Methods of the Coronary Drug Project

Much of the impetus for the current use of nicotinic acid (or niacin) in the treatment of hyperlipidemia originates from the Coronary Drug Project (CDP). The CDP, conducted during 1966 to 1974 in 53 clinical centers, was a randomized, double-blind, placebo-controlled trial of five lipid-modifying agents in 8341 men with previous ECG-documented MI.[39] All patients at entry were at least three months post-MI, in NYHA functional class I or II with clinically stable coronary disease and no other major illnesses, and free from specified diseases or conditions incompatible with any of the study medications.[39]

The study included five drug treatment regimens—conjugated estrogens at two dosage levels (2.5 and 5.0 mg/day), clofibrate (1.8 g/day), dextrothyroxine sodium (6.0 mg/day), and immediate-release niacin (3.0 g/day)—and a lactose placebo (3.8 g/day). Approximately five patients were allocated to the placebo group for every two patients in any of the active treatment groups. The primary outcome variable was designated as all-cause mortality for the entire study period.[39] Patient enrollment took place over a 3.6-year period; patient follow-up ranged from 4.5 to 8.5 years. While the mean follow-up was 6.2 years, the initial report was based on follow-up data at 5 years.[40]

Baseline Findings

A total of 1119 and 2789 patients were enrolled in the niacin and placebo groups, respectively. At entry, the mean age of the participants was 52.4 years; 93% were white, and 37% were current cigarette smokers. Mean serum cholesterol and triglyceride levels at entry were 251 mg/dL and 183 mg/dL, respectively. Mean fasting and 1-hour plasma glucose levels were 102 mg/dL and 173 mg/dL, respectively. Oral hypoglycemic agents were being taken by 5.2% of the study population at entry;

patients taking insulin or any cholesterol-lowering agents at screening were excluded.[39]

Treatment Effects with Respect to Mortality and Cardiovascular Morbidity

Both of the estrogen regimens and dextrothyroxine were discontinued before the scheduled end of the trial because of adverse effects.[41–43] For this report, all data have now been analyzed to completion of the full treatment trial (mean 6.2 years of follow-up). These new results, presented here for the first time, are little changed in magnitude but provide greater statistical confidence in the treatment comparisons.[44] Niacin gave no evidence of benefit over placebo with respect to all-cause mortality at the end of patient follow-up on study treatment (24.8% vs. 25.9%; P = NS). However, niacin significantly reduced the risk of definite nonfatal MI (10.7% for niacin vs. 14.8% for placebo; $P = 0.001$). Also, only 3.3% of niacin patients, compared with 7.2% of placebo patients, had any cardiovascular surgery during the study ($P < 0.0001$) (Fig. 25-1). By comparison, these percentages for clofibrate versus placebo were 13.8% versus 14.8%, and 6.3% versus 7.2%, despite the similar effects of niacin and clofibrate on total cholesterol and triglycerides. Higher percentages of patients in the niacin group than in the placebo group had atrial fibrillation (5.3% vs. 3.4%; $P = 0.009$) or other cardiac arrhythmias (37.0% vs. 32.6%; $P = 0.011$) (Table 25-1).

Other Effects of Niacin

Niacin reduced serum cholesterol and triglycerides by 10% and 26%, respectively, compared with placebo over the course of the study. Comparable figures for clofibrate were 6% and 22%.[40] In addition, niacin significantly affected many other biochemical measures as well as some hematologic measures (Table 25-2). Greater percentages of niacin-treated than placebo patients experienced gastrointestinal problems, acute gouty arthritis, decreased appetite, or unexpected loss of weight. As expected, 91% of niacin patients ever described flushing; 49%, itching; 7%, urticaria; and 20%, other types of rash. Clinical findings of ichthyosis, acanthosis nigricans, and hyperpigmentation of the skin were reported in 3%, 4%, and 5%, respectively. As a result of these unpleasant side effects, significantly more niacin patients had reduced adherence to study medication over the course of the study ($P < 0.0001$) (see Table 25-2).[40] On the other hand, there were no significant differences between niacin and placebo at year 5 in serum direct bilirubin, presence of glycosuria, urine protein, hematocrit, systolic and diastolic blood pressures, and body weight.

Conclusions from the Main Study

The CDP Research Group reasoned that although crystalline niacin at the recommended 3.0 g daily dose may be beneficial with respect to nonfatal MI, 1) this was not the primary study outcome, 2) niacin showed no significant benefit at 5 years' follow-up with respect to either all-cause or coronary mortality, and 3) excess incidence of arrhythmias, gastrointestinal problems, and abnormal chemistry levels occurred in the niacin group. Therefore, they concluded that "great care and caution must be exercised if this drug is to be used for treatment of persons with CHD."[40]

Design and Methods of the Mortality Follow-Up

Owing to these rather guarded conclusions of the CDP Research Group, there was only limited interest in niacin as a lipid-modifying medication for the next several years. In 1981, the CDP Coordinating Center was awarded a contract by the National Heart, Lung, and Blood Institute for mortality follow-up of CDP patients who were alive at the end of the trial. The primary objectives were to update vital status and obtain death certificates as appropriate for the 6008 CDP patients known to be alive in February 1975 and to relate the findings to the CDP treatment group.[45] There was a

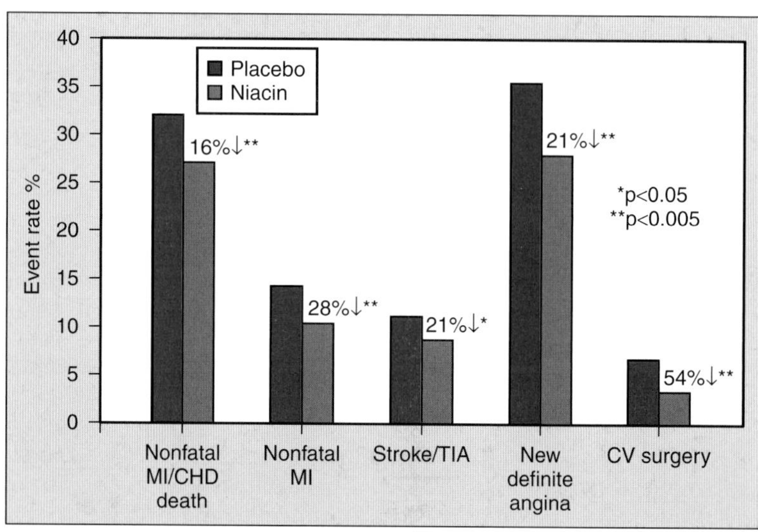

FIGURE 25-1 Clinical cardiovascular (CV) outcomes for complete Coronary Drug Project (CDP) treatment follow-up (mean 6.2 years) were all significantly reduced with nicotinic acid. The predefined primary event was total mortality, which was reduced by 4.3% (NS). CHD, coronary heart disease; MI, myocardial infarction; TIA, transient ischemic attack.

TABLE 25-1 Coronary Drug Project: Percentages of Patients with Selected Clinical Findings, Niacin and Placebo Groups, Total Follow-up Experience, Mean 6.2 Years

Finding	Niacin	Placebo	z	P
All-cause mortality	24.8%	25.9%	−0.75	NS
Cardiovascular Findings				
Definite nonfatal MI	10.7%	14.8%	−3.30	0.001
Coronary death or definite nonfatal MI	27.0%	32.0%	−3.08	0.002
Cardiovascular surgery	3.2%	7.2%	−4.55	<0.0001
Fatal or nonfatal stroke or TIA	8.8%	11.1%	−2.19	0.029
New definite angina pectoris	28.6%	36.2%	−2.81	0.005
Atrial fibrillation	5.3%	3.4%	2.62	0.009
Other cardiac arrhythmias	37.0%	32.6%	2.55	0.011
Other Clinical Findings				
Gastrointestinal problems	27.5%	21.8%	3.66	0.0003
Acute gouty arthritis	8.3%	4.7%	4.08	<0.0001
Acanthosis nigricans	3.7%	0.7%	6.72	<0.0001
Patient Complaints				
Flushing	90.7%	4.3%	53.77	<0.0001
Itching of the skin	48.8%	6.4%	30.84	<0.0001
Urticaria	7.2%	1.5%	9.37	<0.0001
Other types of rash	19.8%	5.8%	13.36	<0.0001
Decreased appetite	4.0%	1.5%	4.72	<0.0001
Unexpected loss of weight	2.7%	0.9%	4.28	<0.0001

[a]The values in this table have been recomputed by the author (PLC), updating those originally published, most of which were for the first 5 years of follow-up rather than the total follow-up period. Only variables with z-value for niacin-placebo exceeding ± 2.00 ($P < 0.05$) are presented in this table (with one exception); see the original publication for results for other findings. MI, myocardial infarction; NS, non-significanse; TIA, transient ischemic attack. From Ref. 40.

TABLE 25-2 Coronary Drug Project: Mean Levels of Selected Variables at Year 5, Niacin and Placebo Groups

Variable	Niacin	Placebo*	z	P
Serum cholesterol, mg/dL	228	250	−13.28	<0.0001
Serum triglycerides, mg/dL	149	207	−9.40	<0.0001
Serum total bilirubin, mg/dL	0.596	0.639	−3.88	0.0001
Serum glutamic oxaloacetic transaminase, Henry units	32.0	29.8	3.18	0.001
Serum alkaline phosphatase, King-Armstrong units	8.32	7.57	8.49	<0.0001
Serum creatine phosphokinase, IU	94.2	80.9	4.22	<0.0001
Plasma fasting glucose, mg/dL	110	107	2.41	0.016
Plasma 1-hour glucose, mg/dL	186	175	5.02	<0.0001
Plasma urea nitrogen, mg/dL	14.9	16.5	−9.69	<0.0001
Serum uric acid, mg/dL	6.77	6.25	8.86	<0.0001
Serum potassium, mEq/L	4.15	4.24	−5.73	<0.0001
Serum sodium, mEq/L	140.3	140.0	3.06	0.002
White blood cell count, cells/mm^3	6660	7061	−4.77	<0.0001
Absolute neutrophil count, cells/mm^3	4006	4331	−4.56	<0.0001
< 20% adherence to study prescription, %	14.3	4.2	8.54	<0.0001
< 80% adherence to study prescription, %	21.8	9.4	7.86	<0.0001

The values in this table have been recomputed by the author (PLC), updating those originally published which did not include all of the year 5 data. Ns for the data in this table range from 616 to 771 for the niacin group and from 1587 to 1972 for the placebo group. There were no baseline determinations of serum creatine phosphokinase, serum potassium, and serum sodium. Serum creatine phosphokinase was performed at only the nonannual follow-up visits; thus the values in the table are for month 56 rather than year 5. From Ref. 40.

*The year 5 (Y5) means for the placebo group were adjusted for the niacin-placebo differences at baseline (BL); that is, placebo(Y5 adjusted) = placebo(Y5) + niacin(BL) − placebo(BL).

particular interest in learning whether the trend for excess cancer mortality in the low-dose estrogen group[120] persisted and extended to the high-dose estrogen group with the passage of time.

For this follow-up study, vital status was ascertained from: 1) CDP investigators, 2) regular and certified mail and telephone calls to the patients, 3) telephone calls to the patients' known contacts, 4) a National Death Index search for years 1979 to 1981, 5) Social Security and Veterans Administration file searches, and 6) a national search agency. Death certificates were obtained to determine cause of death. Information on vital status as of June 1983 was obtained on all but 24 of the 6008 patients still alive at the end of the trial in 1975, and death certificates were obtained for 91% of the deaths reported.[45]

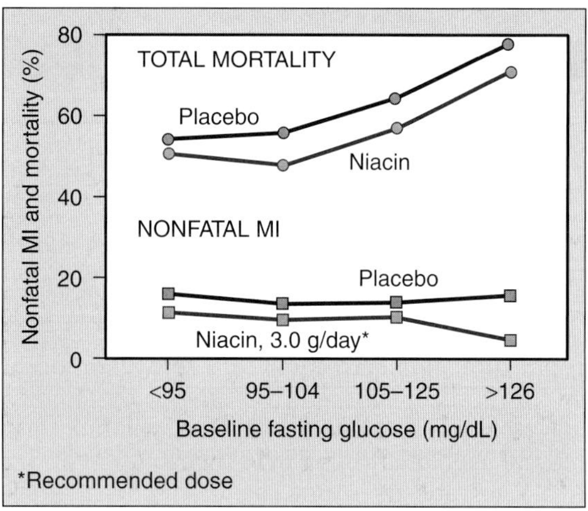

FIGURE 25-2 Total mortality at 15 years (a mean 6.2 years on trial and 8.8 years after trial completion) was significantly reduced by 11%, overall ($P < 0.0005$). Nonfatal myocardial infarction (MI), overall, was reduced by 28% at 6.2 years ($P < 0.005$). When event rates were compared within various ranges of pretreatment fasting glucose, tests for heterogeneity were nonsignificant, supporting the position that niacin's generally small effect on insulin resistance does not detract from its clinical benefits by these measures, even among those with baseline diabetes mellitus. *(Based on data from Ref. 48.)*

Results of the Mortality Follow-Up

Quite unexpectedly, the niacin treatment group was the only one that showed results of interest in this follow-up study. For a mean follow-up period of 15 years (6.2 years during the study and 8.8 years post-study), all-cause mortality was 52.0% for niacin compared with 58.2% for placebo ($P = 0.0004$). Most of this difference was in CHD mortality (36.5% vs. 41.3%; $P = 0.005$). For all of the other major categories of cause of death (cerebrovascular, other cardiovascular, cancer, other causes, unknown cause) the percentage of niacin patients was slightly lower than that of placebo patients.[45]

Mortality and Cardiovascular Morbidity by Levels of Baseline Plasma Glucose

In spite of the renewed interest in prescribing niacin for lipid modification resulting from the CDP mortality follow-up, caution has been urged in the use of niacin among patients with elevated fasting glucose levels or overt diabetes.[46,47] This caution was largely based on the finding shown in Table 25-2 that niacin at a 3.0 g dose elevates fasting and 1-hour glucose levels.

In 2002, Kos Pharmaceuticals, Inc., provided funding to the CDP Coordinating Center in order to carry out additional analyses of the niacin and placebo group data on all-cause mortality and definite nonfatal MI according to different levels of baseline and follow-up plasma glucose. These analyses revealed that niacin's beneficial effect with respect to 6-year definite nonfatal MI (Fig. 25-2), to coronary death or definite nonfatal MI, or to 15-year all-cause mortality (see Fig. 25-2) was homogeneous across the different levels of baseline fasting and 1-hour plasma glucose as well as across different levels of change (decrease, small increase, large increase) in fasting and 1-hour glucose from baseline to year 1.[48] For example, 15-year all-cause mortality in the niacin and placebo groups was 49.4% versus 55.0% in patients whose fasting glucose decreased, 45.4% versus 51.9% in those whose fasting glucose increased by 0 to 9 mg/dL, and 49.8% versus 64.1% in those whose fasting glucose increased by 10 mg/dL or more between baseline and year 1.[48] In this example, the most beneficial effect of niacin was observed in patients who experienced the largest *increase* in plasma glucose levels during the first year of the original study. These analyses showed that elevated baseline glucose levels, a rapid increase in levels during the first year of treatment, or glucose intolerance at baseline, did not translate into any disadvantage with respect to cardiovascular events or mortality risk.[48] Thus, the use of niacin in patients with abnormal glucose metabolism or overt diabetes mellitus does not increase (it in fact decreases) the rate of macrovascular complications of atherosclerosis in these long-term cardiovascular analyses of the CDP. Nevertheless, caution is appropriate when starting niacin in the patient with poor glycemic control.

Mortality and Cardiovascular Morbidity by Presence or Absence of the Metabolic Syndrome

Similarly, CDP patients were grouped according to the presence or absence of the metabolic syndrome using criteria similar to those defined in the guidelines of the National Cholesterol Education Program Adult Treatment Panel III.[46] The Adult Treatment Panel III defines the metabolic syndrome by the presence of three or more of the following criteria: abdominal obesity (waist circumferences >40 mg/dL for men), serum triglyceride levels ≥150 mg/dL, HDL cholesterol levels <40 mg/dL for men, systolic blood pressure ≥130 mm Hg or diastolic blood pressure ≥85 mm Hg, and fasting glucose levels ≥110 mg/dL. A body mass index of 28 kg/m^2 or more was used as a substitute for waist circumference. Baseline HDL cholesterol data were available for only 492 patients in the niacin and placebo groups in the CDP, and in this subpopulation the metabolic syndrome was defined as the presence of three or more of the five criteria. Without HDL cholesterol measures, it was defined by the presence of three or more of four criteria.[49]

As with the analyses by baseline glucose, the niacin–placebo differences in 6-year definite nonfatal MI and 15-year total mortality were homogeneous with respect to presence or absence of the metabolic syndrome at baseline, for both the three or more of five criteria and the three or more of four criteria definitions of the metabolic syndrome. For example, for the total group of patients (three or more of four criteria definition), 15-year total mortality for patients without the metabolic syndrome was 50.4% versus 56.9% for 933 niacin and 2314 placebo patients, respectively; for patients with the metabolic syndrome at baseline, it was 59.7% versus 63.8% for 186 and 473 patients, respectively. Hazard ratios for niacin versus placebo obtained using the Cox proportional hazards model[45,50] were both 0.86 at 15 years for patients with or without the metabolic syndrome.[49]

In conclusion, this analysis shows that the elevation of plasma glucose level by niacin does not adversely affect its clinical benefits in patients presenting with the metabolic syndrome.

NICOTINIC ACID IN ATHEROSCLEROSIS IMAGING TRIALS

Therapies to prevent or reverse atherosclerosis or its complications can be tested in terms of their effects on risk factor levels; on plaque size, composition, or severity of arterial obstruction; or on the frequency of clinical events. Nicotinic acid therapy has been extensively examined in trials using coronary arteriography and also carotid ultrasound. These trials, briefly described here, were among the first to pioneer the use of atherosclerosis imaging methods. Each trial and its results are detailed in Table 25-3; results from several trials are illustrated in Fig. 25-3 through 25-6.

CLAS

The Cholesterol Lowering Atherosclerosis Study (CLAS),[51] one of the original coronary arteriographic trials, compared immediate-release niacin (3–12 g/day) plus colestipol (30 g/day) with placebo over 2 years. Patients with previous coronary bypass surgery underwent baseline coronary arteriography, were randomized to either of these 2 regimens, and were followed clinically for 2 years with a final arteriogram. Change, per patient, in arterial obstruction was estimated by visual comparison of individual coronary segments using a consensus panel of three expert arteriographers. Patients were classified in terms of the number of "visually progressing" native lesions per patient and the percent of subjects with visual graft progression. The principal finding of this landmark study was that, relative to placebo, the active drug combination reduced the frequency of native artery lesion progression and increased that of regression ($P < 0.03$). This trial was the first to demonstrate clinically that regression of stenosis could be induced by lipid therapy. There was no significant reduction in cardiovascular event rate, in part because these patients were protected from major events by their bypass surgery.

CLAS-II

In a subgroup of the CLAS patients, the study was extended for 2 years on the same randomized therapy. This study further confirmed the observations of the original CLAS (Table 25-3).[52] Later, a serial ultrasound analysis of the progression of carotid artery intima–media thickness (CIMT) in these patients confirmed that the combination of niacin and colestipol also slowed the atherosclerotic process in the carotid vascular bed; the improvements were related to the in-treatment plasma levels of triglyceride-rich lipoproteins, as indicated by apolipoprotein (apo)-CIII concentrations.[53]

TABLE 25-3 Arterial Imaging Trials with Nicotinic Acid Combinations: In-trial Lipid Responses Relative to Placebo, and Reduction in Coronary Stenosis Progression and Clinical Events

					Angiographic Endpoint		Clinical Endpoint Frequency	
Trial	No	%↓ LDL Cholesterol*	%↓ TG *	%↑ HDL Cholesterol*	Δ%S Placebo	Δ%S Rx	Placebo Primary Event, %	Rx, % Reduction
CLAS[51]	188	−39	−17	+35	NA	NA	NA	NA
CLAS II[52]	138	−34	−13	+35	NA	NA	NA	NA
FATS N+C[56]	100	−25	−44	+35	+2.1	−0.9	23%	−78
FATS L+C[56]	98	−39	−10	+10	+2.1	−0.7	23%	−66
UC-SCOR[54]	97	−27	−22	+24	+0.8	−1.5	NA	NA
HARP[65]	91	−41	−26	+13	+2.4	+1.5	21%	−33†
SCRIP[62]	300	−19	−26	+7	+0.9	+0.3	22%	−43
FATS-TRx[66]	176	−36	−42	+18	NA	NA	19%	−69
HATS[69]	160	−36	−35	+26	+3.9	−0.4	23%	−60
AFREGS[38]	148	−26	−50	+36	+1.5	−0.8	26%	−53

* Lipid changes during active treatment (Rx) are placebo-adjusted.† not significant.⁺
Δ % S, change in percent sterosis; HDL, high-density lipoprotein; LDL, low-density lipoprotein; † NA, not available; TG, triglycerides.

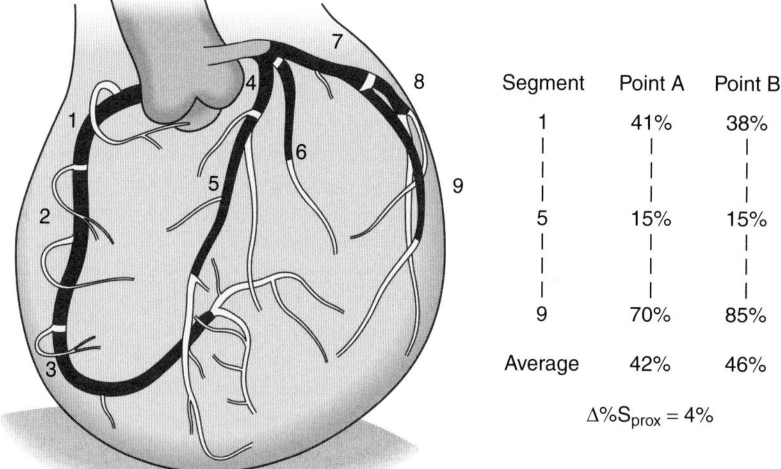

FIGURE 25-3 Method for estimation of mean per-patient change in the worst percent stenosis in each of nine proximal coronary segments. A computer-assisted, fully blinded analysis was used. Approaches similar to this were used in all quantitative arteriographic studies described. *(Reproduced from Ref. 56, with permission.)*

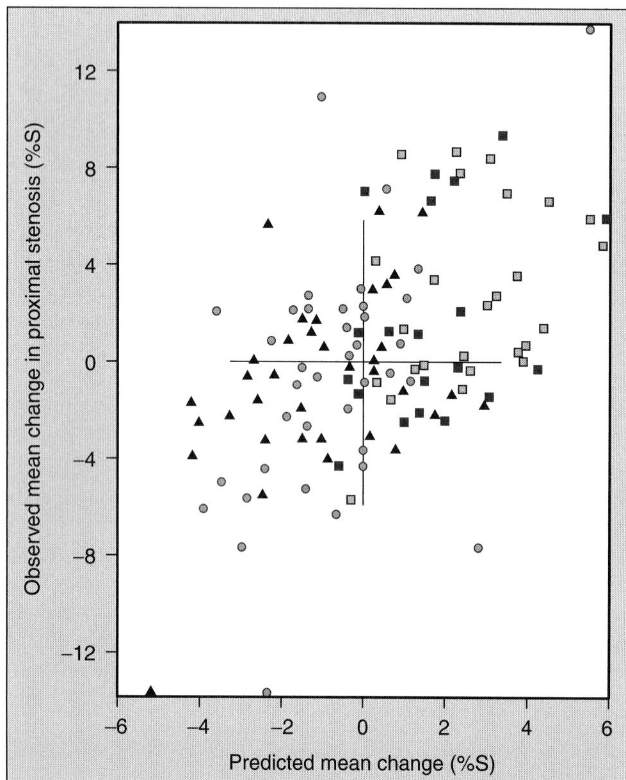

FIGURE 25-4 A multivariate linear regression analysis produced an expression containing variables significantly and independently predictive of mean proximal percent stenosis change: [$\Delta\%S_{prox}$ = 0.035 %ΔLDL cholesterol − 0.045 %ΔHDL cholesterol + 0.14 %ΔSBP − 0.8ΔST + 1.2]. The predicted change computed for each patient correlated highly with the measured change ($r = 0.47$, $p < 0.0001$). *(Reproduced from Ref. 56, with permission.)*

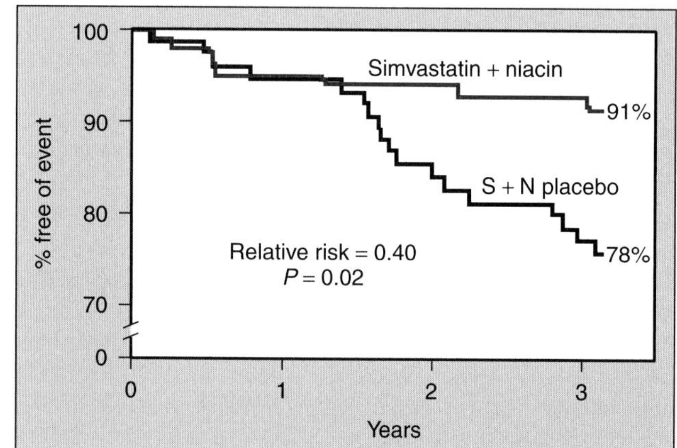

FIGURE 25-5 Kaplan–Meier curves with Cox proportional hazards comparison of predefined primary event composite in HATS intention-to-treat comparison of patients randomized to simvastatin plus niacin or to their placebos. Clinical event rate was reduced by 60% with this drug combination. *(Reproduced from Ref. 69, with permission.)*

UC-SCOR

In the University of California Specialized Center of Research in Atherosclerosis Intervention Trial (UC-SCOR),[54] Kane et al. compared combination therapy with niacin (1.5– 7.5 g/day), colestipol (up to 30 g/day), and, when available in 1987, lovastatin (40–60 mg/day) versus their placebos for their effects on atherosclerosis progression by using a computer-assisted quantitative arteriographic technique (quantitative coronary angiography [QCA]) in their laboratories. These asymptomatic subjects were selected for familial hypercholesterolemia, with mean pretreatment LDL cholesterol of 278 mg/dL, and for at least some degree of atherosclerotic obstruction on the protocol baseline coronary arteriogram. A follow-up arteriogram at 2 years showed that the combination therapies induced, on average over the entire active treatment group, a small *regression* of atherosclerosis, while the placebo group showed continued significant progression (see Table 25-3). The simultaneous publications of UC-SCOR and the Familial Atherosclerosis Treatment Study (FATS) study confirmed with similar QCA techniques[55] that it was possible to completely halt the average progression of obstructive disease in an entire group of patients at high risk for atherogenesis. There were virtually no cardiovascular events in this short primary prevention study.

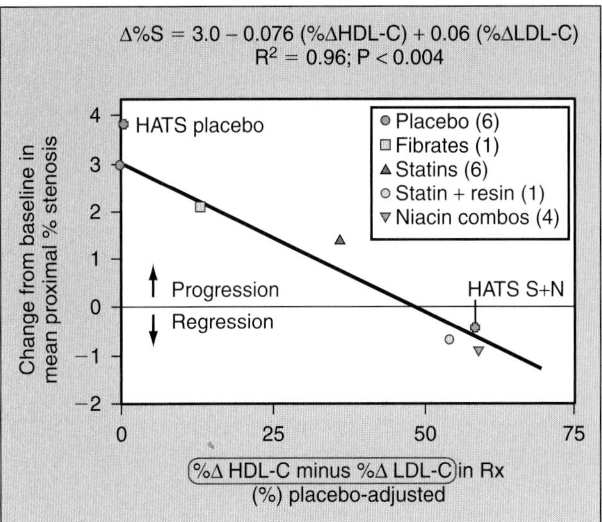

FIGURE 25-6 Plot of average change in proximal percent diameter coronary stenosis during treatment in 12 studies reported with 4 drug treatment classes and the placebo control groups for the 6 statin studies. The mean changes in percent stenosis for the drug classes are almost completely explained ($R^2 = 0.96$) by the sum of in-trial percent increase in HDL cholesterol (HDL-C) and the percent reduction in LDL cholesterol (LDL-C), averaged over the trials in each drug class and adjusted for the placebo arm effects on lipids. *(Reproduced from Ref. 73, with permission.)*

FATS

In FATS,[56] among 145 patients with clinically established coronary disease, a strong family history of CHD, and high levels of apoB, two active treatment combinations (niacin 4 g/day plus colestipol 30 g/day; or lovastatin 40 mg/day plus colestipol 30 g/day) were compared with the then-conventional treatment regimen (diet counseling and placebo, or in about half, colestipol 30 g/day for LDL cholesterol ≥90th population percentile). In arteriograms taken at baseline and at 2.5-year follow-up, the most severe stenoses found in each of nine standard proximal coronary segments were systematically measured; the average severity of these nine stenoses was computed at these two time-points; their difference (+4% stenosis in Fig. 25-3) was the primary arteriographic endpoint. A secondary endpoint, *patient progression only*, was defined as a worsening by +10% stenosis (3 standard deviations [SD] of the method's variance) of at least one of these nine stenoses without any stenosis improving by that amount. *Patient regression only* was similarly defined. While the conventional therapy group had significant mean proximal stenosis progression, and its patients displayed a high prevalence (46%) of progression only and rare (11%) regression only, the two intensive therapy groups had net regression of proximal stenosis (see Table 25-3), significantly lower prevalence (23%) of progression only, and more frequent (36%) regression only. A subgroup of previously asymptomatic FATS patients showed comparable arteriographic benefits.[57] FATS, taken together with CLAS and UC-SCOR, suggested the striking arteriographic benefits of therapies that raised HDL cholesterol while lowering LDL cholesterol. Indeed, a stepwise multivariate FATS analysis selected percent change from baseline (%Δ) HDL cholesterol, %ΔLDL cholesterol, and %Δ systolic blood pressure during therapy as significant independent variables predicting change in mean proximal percent stenosis (see Fig. 25-4).[58,59]

Of interest, the two groups given the intensive combination regimens had a 73% lower frequency ($P < 0.03$) than the control group of the primary event composite end point—cardiovascular death, MI, or revascularization for worsening ischemia. Thus, FATS suggested that the observed arterial benefits could translate to striking clinical benefits among patients at risk of progressive native coronary disease. In a subsequent analysis,[60] the mechanism of benefit from intensive lipid therapy in FATS was best explained by prevention of abrupt progression of mild and moderate stenoses to severe obstructive atherothrombotic lesions. That is, lipid therapy appeared to stabilize the vulnerable plaques against rupture.

In a subsequent FATS analysis, Maher et al. determined that, in the high-risk setting with elevation of both LDL cholesterol and Lp(a), LDL cholesterol should be aggressively lowered by 40% or more and that treatment should probably include added niacin, the only lipid drug that effectively reduces Lp(a).[61]

SCRIP

The Stanford Coronary Risk Intervention Program (SCRIP) compared the effects of an intensive combination of several risk factor interventions (including lipid-lowering and antihypertensive therapy, and weight, antismoking, and exercise programs) with usual care on coronary disease progression over 4 years among 300 patients with established coronary disease.[62,63] The lipid therapy, when used, included colestipol, niacin, and lovastatin targeting certain lipid abnormalities, if present. Not all intensive risk reduction patients received all three drugs. Compared with usual care, the patients assigned to intensive treatment had significant slowing of measured stenosis progression and a trend toward reduced clinical events (see Table 25-3). Of interest, patients with small dense LDL particle size distribution at baseline showed substantially greater arteriographic benefit from the intensive therapy than those with large buoyant particles.[64]

HARP

The Harvard Atherosclerosis Reversal Project (HARP) reported the effects of a combination of niacin, gemfibrozil, and pravastatin compared with the effects of their placebos on measured progression of coronary obstruction among 91 patients with established coronary disease.[65] In this relatively small study, there was a trend toward slowed stenosis progression, but not reduced clinical events, in the intensively treated group (see Table 25-3).

FATS-TRx10

The FATS–10-year triple therapy observational follow-up (FATS-TRx10) was initiated after exactly half of the 176 FATS patients had completed that study and returned to the usual care of their physicians.[66] Surprisingly, less than 30% of these very-high-risk patients were given any lipid drugs by their physicians, circa 1988. As a consequence, all patients completing FATS from then on were offered a triple therapy combination similar to that used in the UC-SCOR trial (niacin 2–4 g/day as tolerated, lovastatin 40 mg/day, and colestipol 20 g/day). Seventy-five of 88 accepted. These two groups of patients—101 patients continuing under the care of their physicians on usual care and 75 on triple therapy (TRx)—have since been followed closely. Indeed, the TRx/UC usual care follow-up continues to this point at a mean *TRx* duration of 18 years. The comparison of both groups has been reported to a mean of 10 years.[66] The intention-to-treat Cox proportional hazards analysis of freedom from cardiac death or nonfatal MI demonstrated a first event rate of 22% among the usual care group and of 7% among the TRx group, with an odds ratio of 0.33 ($P < 0.025$).

A random subgroup of eight TRx patients was selected to undergo bilateral carotid bifurcation magnetic resonance imaging (MRI) studies; another group of eight patients was selected from the catheterization laboratory, who matched the TRx subgroup for age, gender, coronary disease severity, and untreated lipoprotein profile levels, and who had never received any lipid therapy.[67] In both groups, all 16 of the carotid bifurcations contained MRI-demonstrated atherosclerotic plaque. For each bifurcation, the section with the largest plaque was chosen for plaque size and composition analysis. The only difference between these two groups of plaques was the percent lipid content; 17% of plaque area was lipid in the untreated patients, and 1% in the patients receiving TRx for 10 years ($P < 0.01$). There was no between-group difference in plaque area (58 mm^2 with TRx versus 64 mm^2 with no treatment), fibrous connective tissue percent area (84% vs. 77%), and calcium and calcified lipid percent area (15% vs. 6%). This substantial difference in carotid plaque lipid content between these intensively treated and untreated patients with coronary disease and hyperlipidemia implies that plaque lipid depletion is the principal effect of intensive therapy. Based on coronary histopathology studies in fatal MI,[68] lipid depletion would have the effect of stabilizing the vulnerable plaque against rupture of its fibrous cap with resulting thrombotic occlusion. The hypothesis[11] that lipid therapy reduces atherothrombotic event risk by depletion of lipid and lipid-rich inflammatory macrophages from the plaques' lipid-rich core and from macrophage foam cells is supported by this evidence[46,67] and is widely accepted.

HATS

The HDL Atherosclerosis Treatment Study (HATS) randomized 160 patients with established coronary disease, HDL cholesterol of 35 mg/dL or more (men) or 50 mg/dL or more (women), and LDL cholesterol of 140 mg/dL or more to simvastatin (13 mg/day, taken) plus niacin (2.4 g/day taken) or to their placebos and, in a 2×2 factoril design, to antioxidant vitamins (E, C, β-carotene, and selenium) or to their placebos.[69] Atherosclerosis progression was measured by QCA. Patients given simvastatin and niacin had, on average, a virtual halting of the progression of proximal coronary stenosis. Those given placebos for simvastatin, niacin, and antioxidants had on average a 3.9% worsening of proximal stenosis severity (see Table 25-3). Again, a regimen (simvastatin plus niacin) that reduced LDL cholesterol by 42% from baseline and increased HDL cholesterol by 26% reduced the atherothrombotic event composite, endpoint (cardiovascular death, MI, stroke, and revascularization for progressive ischemia) by 60% ($P < 0.02$) (see Fig. 25-5). Antioxidant vitamins significantly blunted the HDL cholesterol and HDL$_2$ response to simvastatin and niacin and did not protect against progression of proximal stenosis or reduce the frequency of atherothrombotic events.

AFREGS

The Air Force Regression Study (AFREGS) has made an important contribution to our appreciation of the role of HDL cholesterol–raising therapy in prevention of atherothrombotic disease.[38] It compared a triple-drug combination (niacin 3 g/day plus gemfibrozil 1200 mg/day plus cholestyramine 16 g/day) with their placebos in a group of patients with established coronary disease who all underwent an intensive diet and exercise program. Progression of obstructive coronary disease was measured by QCA with methods similar to those of FATS, HATS, and UC-SCOR. Patients receiving only lifestyle counseling had moderate disease progression, whereas those randomized to the intensive drug regimen experienced modest regression ($P < 0.05$) (see Table 25-3). The incidence of the prespecified cardiovascular event composite endpoint was reduced by 54% among those receiving the intensive regimen. Of note, these benefits were achieved without statins and with only 18% LDL cholesterol lowering (placebo-adjusted), but with 42% HDL cholesterol raising—the dominant lipid change.

ARBITER 2 and 3

In the two carotid ultrasound studies, Arterial Biology for the Investigation of the Treatment Effects of Reducing Cholesterol (ARBITER) 2 and 3,[70,71] a group of 160 patients with established coronary disease and on chronic statin therapy with a mean LDL cholesterol of 87 mg/dL were initially randomized to either continued statin therapy plus extended-release niacin (1 g/day) or to statin plus niacin placebo. Far wall common CIMT was measured at baseline and 1 year. At 1 year, 130 of the 149 patients who completed the study agreed to continue on open-label extended-release niacin for another year at the same dose, with CIMT measured at 2 years. During the first year, using paired data from completers, those on placebo increased their mean CIMT by +0.042 mm ($P < 0.001$ versus baseline). In those 125 treated with extended-release niacin for just 1 year in the combined randomized and open-label studied, CIMT regressed by −0.027 ($P < 0.001$ vs. pre–extended-release, niacin baseline). In those 57 treated for 24 months in the combined studies, CIMT regressed by −0.041 mm ($P < 0.001$ vs. baseline). Although there are concerns about the lack of an intention-to-treat analysis in a setting of moderate dropout, and about the open-label treatment phase, these trials, taken together, are the first to demonstrate an atherosclerosis treatment benefit with the addition of niacin to an established statin regimen. Of note, statin monotherapy in the 1-year blinded phase of extended-release niacin placebo was associated with continued significant CIMT progression despite a group mean LDL cholesterol level in the mid-80-mg/dL range. This finding of continued progression with statins is similar to that seen for change in coronary stenosis during statin monotherapy. And as with the coronary stenosis findings, regression occurred when niacin was combined with statin.

A Meta-Analysis of Quantitative Coronary Imaging Trials

A number of prospective, randomized, blinded, placebo-controlled trials of lipid therapy have used QCA in patients with clinically established native coronary disease. In a published meta-analysis of eleven of these trials, results from all studies using a given drug class (e.g., placebo, fibrate, statin, combined statin–resin, or niacin/LDL cholesterol–lowering combinations) were averaged together and presented as a drug class effect in terms of the average mean treatment-induced patient changes in LDL cholesterol, HDL cholesterol, percent diameter coronary stenosis, or the prespecified primary cardiovascular event composite.[72] In this meta-analysis of arteriographic effects (see Fig. 25-6), monotherapy with statins or fenofibrate moderately slowed stenosis progression, while combinations of statin with resin and combinations of niacin with LDL cholesterol–lowering therapies consistently produced small, but highly significant, regression of stenosis. The sum of the percent increase in HDL cholesterol and the percent reduction in LDL cholesterol averaged over the given drug class was highly predictive of that class's effect on stenosis change ($R^2 = 0.96$; $P < 0.001$) and, as well, of the percent reduction in the predefined primary clinical event rate.[72,73]

NICOTINIC ACID PREPARATIONS

Both the efficacy and the side effect profile of nicotinic acid are governed by its rate of absorption from the gastrointestinal tract, and nicotinic acid formulations with varying release rates may have very different therapeutic effects and adverse side effects.[74,75] It is important that clinicians understand this unique feature of nicotinic acid in order to select the appropriate formulation to prescribe for patients. Immediate-release formulations of nicotinic acid, also known as "crystalline" nicotinic acid, cause intense cutaneous vasodilation ("flushing"), thus limiting their use and patient acceptability. Sustained-release formulations of nicotinic acid (also sometimes called slow-release, controlled-release, time-release, long-acting, etc.) were developed to reduce the frequency and intensity of flushing by slowing the rate of absorption and decreasing peak plasma drug concentrations. However, this slower rate of absorption can result in loss of effectiveness (particularly for HDL cholesterol) and an increase in the risk of liver toxicity.[76,77] To understand why this is so, it is necessary to understand the unique metabolic profile and nonlinear pharmacokinetics of nicotinic acid. Nicotinic acid is metabolized along two distinct pathways in the liver.[74,75] One, which is associated with flushing, is a conjugative pathway with relatively low affinity but high capacity leading to the formation of nicotinuric acid (Fig. 25-7). The other, a nonconjugative pathway with relatively high affinity but low capacity, leads to the formation of nicotinamide and nicotinamide adenine dinucleotide (NAD); this pathway is associated with liver toxicity. Immediate-release formulations of nicotinic acid rapidly saturate the high-affinity but low-capacity nonconjugative pathway (pathway 2), resulting in a greater percentage of the drug being eliminated by conjugation (pathway 1, with lower affinity but higher capacity). The result is a high incidence of cutaneous flushing. On the other hand, sustained-release formulations, by delaying absorption, increase the proportion of drug that can be eliminated by nonconjugative metabolism (pathway 2) and thereby decrease flushing. However, they may increase the risk of hepatic toxicity, particularly in the case of the ultra-long-acting formulations (Fig. 25-8).[75,78,79] Sustained-release formulations may also lack the efficacy of immediate-release formulations (Figure 25-9), possibly because more drug is diverted into nicotinamide, which has no effect on the plasma lipids. A once-daily extended-release formulation of nicotinic acid with an intermediate-release rate is available by prescription. By optimizing the release rate (and the ratio of pathway 1 to pathway 2 metabolites) and by virtue of once-daily dosing, extended-release nicotinic acid reduces the incidence of flushing compared with immediate-release nicotinic acid (Fig. 25-10) and avoids the hepatic toxicity associated with older, longer-acting,

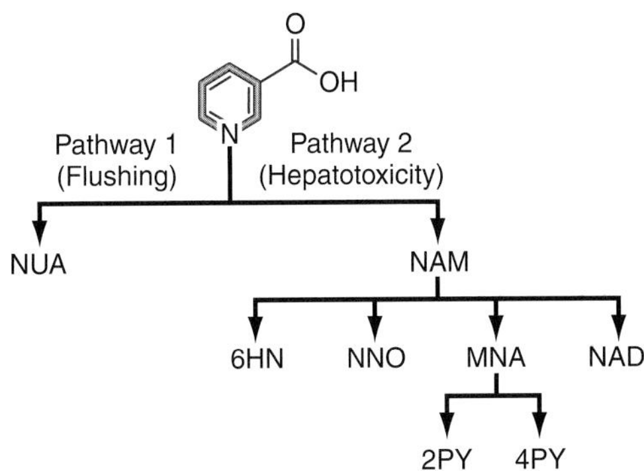

FIGURE 25-7 Metabolic pathways of nicotinic acid in the liver. Pathway 1, conjugation with glycine to form nicotinuric acid (NUA), is a low-affinity but high-capacity pathway associated with flushing. Pathway 2 is a nonconjugative pathway with high affinity but low capacity, leading to formation of nicotinamide (NAM) and nicotinamide adenine dinucleotide (NAD); it is associated with increased risk for hepatotoxicity. *6HN, 6-hydroxy NAM, MNA, N-methyl NAM; MNO, NAM-N-oxide; 2PY, N-methyl-2-pyridone-s-carboxomide; 4 PY, N-methyl-4-pyridone-5-carboxamide. (Reproduced from Ref. 75, with permission.)*

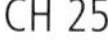

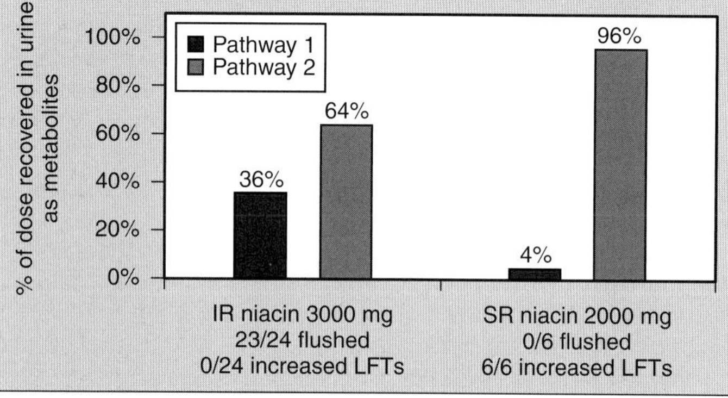

FIGURE 25-8 The metabolic profile of nicotinic acid changes depending on the rate of absorption, thus influencing the clinical effects observed. The left side shows results from a single-dose study of immediate-release nicotinic acid (IR niacin) administered to healthy subjects as a 3 g dose. Nearly all patients flushed, and no elevations in liver tests were observed. Thirty-six percent of the parent drug was recovered as pathway 1 metabolites. The right side shows results from a separate single-dose study of an ultra-long-acting nicotinic acid formulation (SR niacin). No patients flushed, but all six had elevations in liver function tests (LFTs) (approximately ninefold mean change), prompting discontinuation of the study. Ninety-six percent (96%) of the parent drug was recovered as pathway 2 metabolites. *(Based on data from Refs. 78 and 79.)*

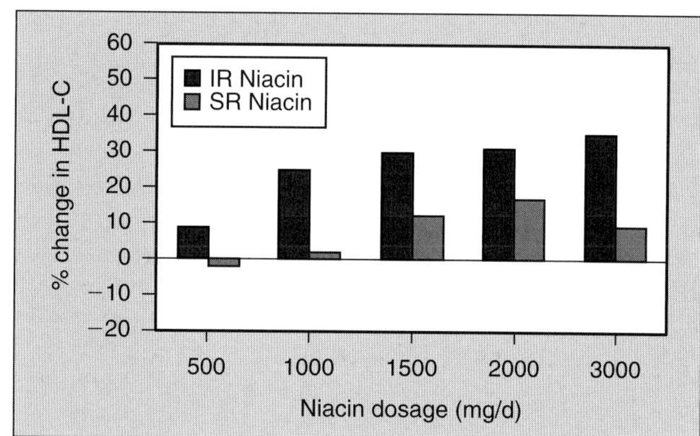

FIGURE 25-9 Results of a head-to-head dose-escalation comparison of immediate-release nicotinic acid (IR niacin) and an ultra-slow-release nicotinic acid (SR niacin) formulation (the same formulation shown in the right side of Figure 25-8). At all doses studied, immediate-release nicotinic acid had a greater effect on HDL cholesterol (HDL-C) than the slow-release formulation. *(Based on data from Ref. 77.)*

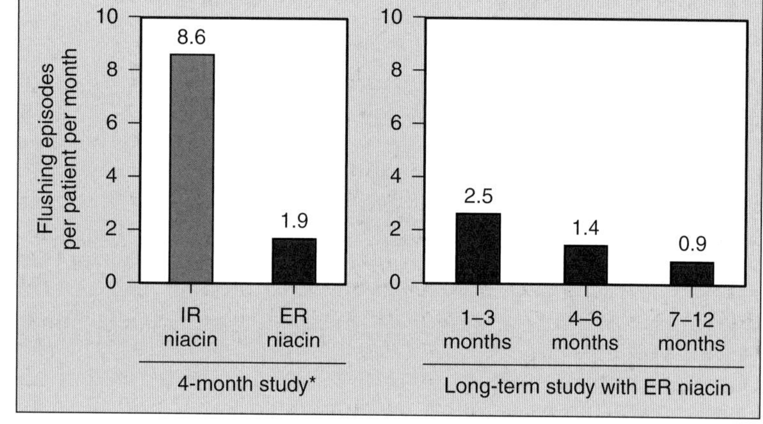

FIGURE 25-10 Decrease in flushing incidence with once-daily extended-release nicotinic acid (ER niacin) is shown in the left panel in a head-to-head comparison against immediate-release nicotinic acid (IR niacin). The right panel shows how flushing decreases during long-term therapy as patients develop tolerance. Results are for flushing episodes per patient per 4-week period, obtained from diary cards. *(Reproduced from Ref. 81, with permission.)*

twice-daily sustained-release preparations.[80,81] Extended-release nicotinic acid also retains the efficacy of immediate-release nicotinic acid (Fig. 25-11).[82,83] Because of these nuances in the efficacy and safety of nicotinic acid preparations related to their release rates, administration of nicotinic acid is best managed by a physician or other healthcare practitioner familiar with its use. Furthermore, because of variations in the deliverable dose, composition, and quality,[84] and lack of physician oversight with nonprescription preparations, the prescription forms of niacin are recommended.[85] Prescription forms of niacin currently available in the United States include Niacor (immediate-release) and Niaspan (extended-release).

While nicotinic acid broadly affects the lipoprotein profile (see Fig. 25-11), its effects on LDL cholesterol are considerably less than those of the statins. For this reason, combination therapy involving a statin and nicotinic acid is a rational choice.[86] The effects of nicotinic acid and a statin taken together appear to be directly additive for major lipoprotein classes.[87] Once-daily fixed-dose combinations of extended-release nicotinic acid with lovastatin (Advicor) (Fig. 25-12)[88] or with simvastatin, (Simcor)[89a] are currently available or investigational.

NICOTINIC ACID—SAFETY ISSUES

Hyperglycemia

Niacin causes insulin resistance and increases fasting glucose levels by approximately 5%.[40,90,91] An average 20% to 28% decline in insulin sensitivity was shown after 2 weeks' administration of immediate-release niacin

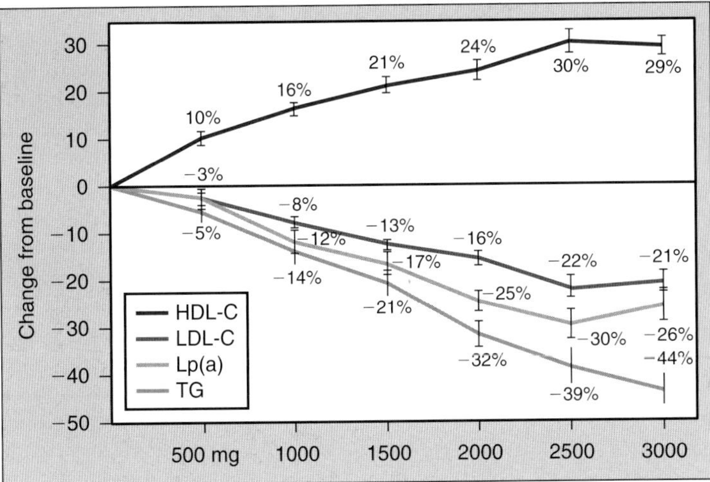

FIGURE 25-11 Dose–response effects of once-daily extended-release nicotinic acid across the dosing range of 1000 mg to 2000 mg. Exposure to each dose level was 4 weeks. Nicotinic acid favorably affects all major lipoprotein classes that are independently associated with risk for atherosclerosis and coronary heart disease. HDL-C, high-density lipoprotein cholesterol; LDL-C, low-density lipoprotein cholesterol; Lp(a), lipoprotein(a); TG, triglycerides. *(Reproduced Ref. 82, with permission.)*

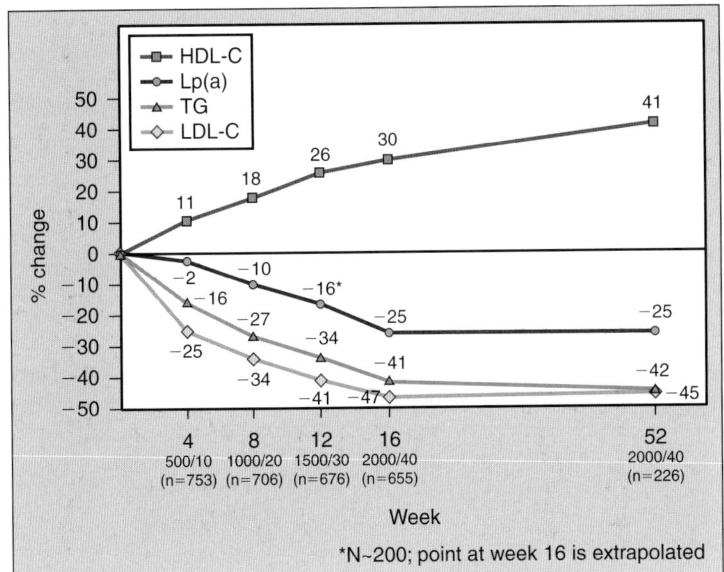

FIGURE 25-12 Dose response effects of a fixed-dose combination of nicotinic acid with lovastatin. Additivity in the lovastatin and niacin effects on lipoproteins is evident compared with Figure 25-11. Note the progressive increase in HDL cholesterol between 16 weeks and 52 weeks, an established phenomenon with niacin called "niacin HDL creep." HDL-C, high-density lipoprotein cholesterol; LDL-C, low-density lipoprotein cholesterol; Lp(a), lipoprotein(a); TG, triglycerides. *(Reproduced from Ref. 130, with permission.)*

at 1000 mg twice daily.[92,93] The mechanism of insulin resistance may relate to a rebound increase in plasma nonesterified fatty acids following their initial drop.[94] Long-term administration of niacin might have a lesser effect on glucose–insulin homeostasis. Before and after 4 months' treatment with extended-release niacin 2 g at bedtime, glucose and insulin responses to an oral glucose challenge were indistinguishable.[95] Theoretically, niacin might promote new-onset diabetes mellitus in persons at risk. However, in the CDP, niacin did not increase new prescriptions for insulin, new prescriptions for oral hypoglycemics, or instances of dipstick-positive glycosuria.[40]

Recent data suggest that niacin can be used safely in diabetes, although such use historically has been discouraged.[47] Hemoglobin A1c levels were 0.3% higher in each of two randomized studies using niacin doses of 2.6 and 1.5 g/day compared with placebo. In both studies, increases in antidiabetic medication were modestly more common in the niacin-treated patients, but the overall hyperglycemic effect of niacin was minor[96,97] and diminished after 4 to 8 months.[91]

Liver Function

Sustained-release niacin, which is generally prescribed twice daily in the morning and evening, has a much greater propensity for hepatic toxicity than immediate-release or extended-release niacin. While some preparations of sustained-release niacin may be used safely in doses up to 1 g twice daily, other formulations have given significant hepatic transaminase elevations in up to 25% of patients at this dose.[76,77,98,99] Patients who had liver toxicity with sustained-release niacin have subsequently used immediate-release niacin without liver dysfunction.[99] Extended-release niacin given once daily at bedtime has modest adverse effects on the liver, as less than 1% of patients had transaminase elevations greater than 3 times the upper limit of normal in a large clinical trial,[100] and no case reports of liver failure have been published.

Myopathy

Myopathy has not been described as an adverse effect of niacin in clinical trials involving immediate-release or extended-release formulations.[40,74] The few case reports associated with niacin in clinical practice generally do not meet current criteria for myopathy.[101,102] A more persistent issue has been whether the addition of niacin may potentiate the myopathic risk of statin therapy, but recent data point toward a lack of such risk. A handful of case reports that associated niacin–statin combination therapy with rhabdomyolysis were published soon after the introduction of lovastatin to clinical practice.[103–105] However, at least half of these cases allowed alternative explanations. Moreover, since that time no new evidence has appeared to confirm a niacin–statin interaction. No case of myopathy has been reported among more than 6000 patients who have taken niacin–statin combination therapy in clinical trials (the formulation was largely extended-release niacin).[106–108] The rate of reports to the U.S. Food and Drug Administration of rhabdomyolysis associated with niacin–statin combination therapy, indexed for prescriptions from market data, was no higher than rates with statin or niacin monotherapy.[109] Thus, the risk of potentiating myopathy by using immediate-release or extended-release niacin with a statin appears to be very small. However, niacin-induced hepatic toxicity in a statin-treated patient, perhaps resulting from administration of sustained-release niacin, could lead to decreased first-pass hepatic extraction of the statin, increased peripheral blood levels, and the potential for myopathy.

Other Safety Issues with Niacin

Uncommon adverse clinical events with niacin may occur in the skin, eye, gastrointestinal tract, and joints. Flushing is almost universal, but infrequently a skin rash may persist between doses. The rash generally should not be regarded as allergic or urticarial, but may be an eczematoid reaction related to skin dryness. Acanthosis nigricans is an idiosyncratic reaction in a few patients, generally manageable by reducing the dose. Psoriasis is not known to be affected by niacin.[110] Blurring of vision may occur with high doses of niacin, generally 3 g daily or higher.[111] Fundoscopic examination can show cystoid macular edema.[112,113] In the past, peptic ulcer, nausea, and vomiting were associated with high niacin doses,[114] but these adverse effects are rare today. Niacin can raise uric acid levels about 10% through competitive inhibition of the tubular secretion of uric acid, leading to gout in susceptible persons.[40,90,115]

Although atrial fibrillation was reported with increased frequency in niacin-treated patients in the CDP,[40] it has not emerged as a significant adverse experience in subsequent smaller randomized trials with niacin. Clinical trials have revealed small laboratory variations of uncertain significance, including reductions in serum potassium (~2%) and increases in serum alkaline phosphatase (~10%) and prothrombin time (mean 4%) (see Table 25-2).[40,90]

THE FUTURE OF NICOTINIC ACID

Why Bother with this Old Drug?

First, we believe the next advances in cardiovascular disease prevention will be based on evidence of benefit from treatment of dyslipidemia, and specifically from raising HDL cholesterol. HDL cholesterol–raising drugs will most likely be given in combination with the well-proven statins.[116,117] Niacin is the most effective currently-available agent for raising HDL cholesterol[113] and for increasing LDL particle size,[118] is the only lipid drug that lowers Lp(a),[61] is as effective as fibrates in lowering triglycerides,[83] and has, in numerous trials cited in this chapter, demonstrated significant arterial and clinical benefit. Because of these facts, niacin is experiencing renewed interest. Second, we believe that modified niacin preparations will improve its dose tolerability and thus its efficacy. Niacin's best days may lie ahead.

Niacin's Resurgence

As long-time users and investigators of niacin, we can offer the following thoughts. First, as detailed in this chapter, we have great enthusiasm for combination LDL cholesterol– and HDL cholesterol–targeted therapies. An important question is whether niacin will become the dominant HDL cholesterol–raising ingredient of such therapy. For this to happen, (1) niacin must prove clinically more effective, or more cost-effective, than other existing or emerging HDL cholesterol–active agents,[119] and (2) its principal limiting side effects, flushing and itching, must be reduced to minor issues. Regarding possible competing agents, the failure of torcetrapib was a great disappointment but does not necessarily doom the cholesteryl ester transfer protein (CETP) inhibitor drug class. Ongoing analyses should resolve this question. Regarding flushing, extended-release niacin preparations have reduced the frequency of severe or moderately severe flushing by greater than 80% in comparison with immediate-release niacin.[120] Despite this development, flushing remains a complaint in the subgroup of flush-sensitive patients, a common reason for some physicians to reject niacin use out-of-hand, and the basis for a rate of 6% to 10% for early drug discontinuation by patients. A recent advance is a modified version of extended-release niacin that yields even lower peak niacin plasma levels and reduced flushing, particularly when combined with aspirin.[121,122]

The overarching reason for niacin's underuse is the relative complexity of its initiation.[76,110] Key "nuisance" aspects are flushing, dose up-titration over 1 to 4 months, aspirin coadministration, timed snacks before bedtime, and the need for more than the usual amount of counseling and patient (and physician) education. However, the effort to promote sustained compliance with the regimen is usually rewarded in 1 or 2 months with the development of a surprising degree of tolerance of the flushing response. Patients committed to stay with the drug for at least 2 months and who have supportive medical care providers are, in our experience, almost always successful with its chronic use.

The "Niacin Receptor"

Direct pharmacologic suppression of niacin-induced flushing may become possible. As illustrated in Fig. 25-13, flushing has been shown to result from subcutaneous release of PGD_2 mediated by niacin's action as a ligand for the dermal Langerhans cell G_i-coupled receptor, GRP109A,[14,15 123,124] also known as HM74 in humans.[16] Activation by niacin of this same receptor in adipocytes (see Fig. 25-13) results in at least some of niacin's desired pharmacologic effects (decreased hormone-sensitive triglyceride lipase activity with diminished lipolysis and reduced plasma FFA, VLDL-triglyceride, and LDL levels). Other putative mechanisms of niacin's lipid effects have been described that are probably not GRP109A mediated.[125–127] The endogenous ligand for GRP109A is β-hydroxybutyrate,[17] implicating its evolutionary role in metabolic adaptations to starvation ketosis. Understanding the role of GRP109A-mediated release of PGD_2 in dermal cells as the mediator of the flushing side effect has led to the development and investigation of an agent (MK0524, laropiprant) that blocks the PGD_2-mediated activation of a vascular smooth muscle cell receptor,

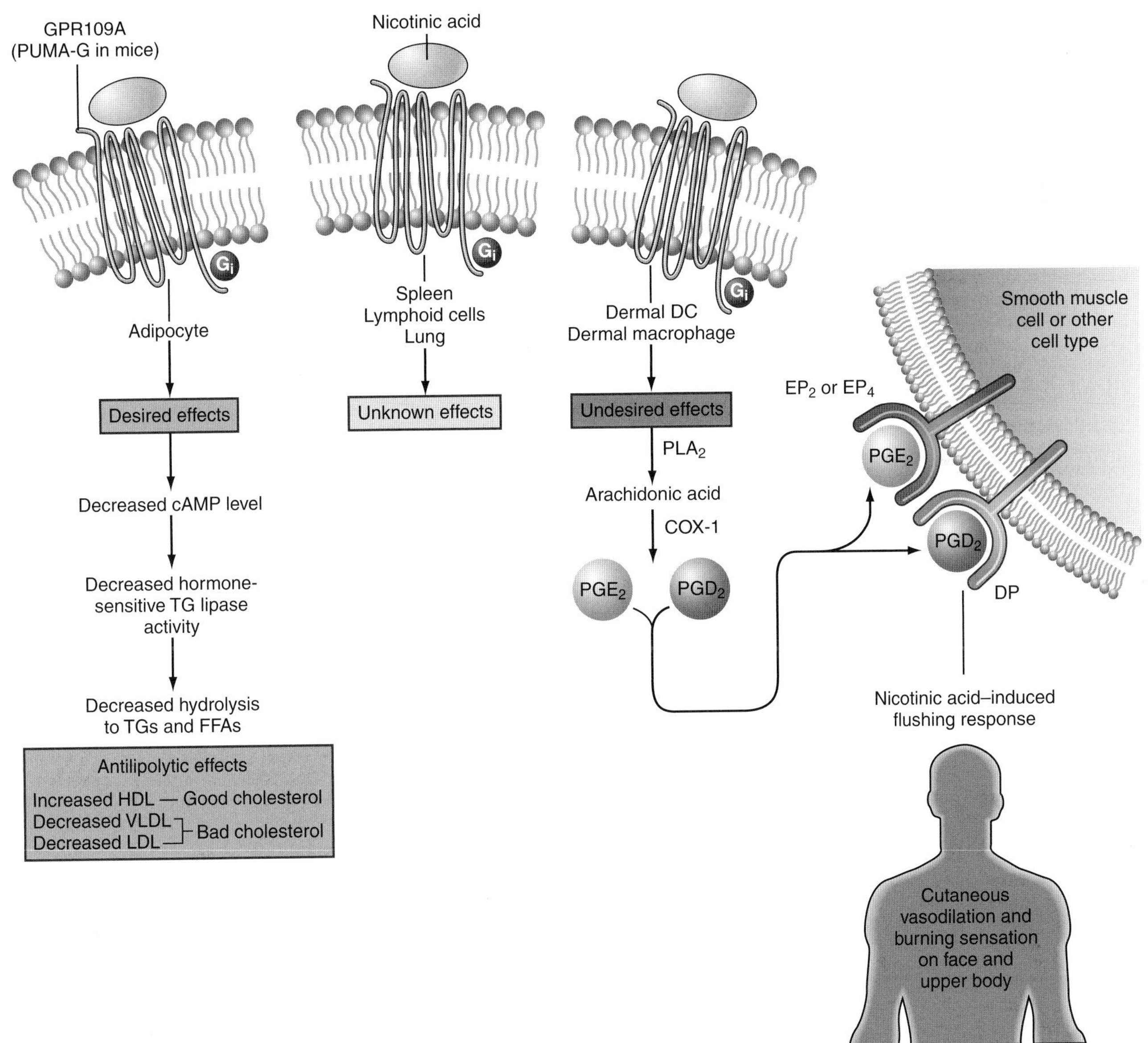

FIGURE 25-13 Activation of the G_i protein–coupled receptor GPR109A can produce differential responses depending on the location of the receptor. Lipid effects are mediated through the receptors located on the adipocytes, and flushing is mediated through the receptors located on the cutaneous Langerhans cells. cox-1, cyclo-oxygenase-1; DC, dendritic cell; DP, PGD_2 receptor; EP, PGE_2 receptor; FFA, free fatty acid; PGD_2, prostaglandin D_2; PGE_2, prostaglandin E_2; PLA_2, phospholipase A_2; TG, triglyceride. *(Reproduced from Ref. 15, with permission.)*

D1P, that triggers vasodilation and thus flushing, but does not alter the adipocyte metabolic effects of niacin. In preliminary studies, MK0524 reduced the intensity and duration of flushing significantly in both human and mouse models and continues under active development.[128,129]

CONCLUSION

As documented in this chapter, nicotinic acid has a long track record of significant clinical benefit in prevention of cardiovascular complications of atherosclerosis, whether as monotherapy or in combinations. These benefits are statistically associated with its effects on both HDL cholesterol and LDL cholesterol, and possibly on LDL particle size, triglycerides, and Lp(a). Its greatest promise would seem to be in its combinations with LDL cholesterol–lowering agents. Whether it fully realizes this promise depends on rapidly emerging developments related to the niacin and PGD_2 receptors and to modified drug release profiles, and also on the absence of a superior alternative to niacin.

REFERENCES

1. Carlson LA: Nicotinic acid: The broad spectrum drug. A 50th anniversary review. *J Intern Med* 2005;258:94–114.
2. Altschul R, Hoffer A, Stephen JD: Influence of nicotinic acid on serum cholesterol in man. *Arch Biochem* 1955;54:558–559.
3. Anitschokov N: Experimental arteriosclerosis in animals. In Cowdry EV (ed): Arteriosclerosis: A Survey of the Problem. New York, Macmillan, 1933, pp 271–322.
4. Parsons WB, Flinn JH: Reduction of serum cholesterol levels and beta-lipoprotein cholesterol levels by nicotinic acid. *Arch Intern Med* 1959;103:783–790.
5. Carlson LA, Oro L: The effect of nicotinic acid on the plasma free fatty acids. *Acta Med Scand* 1962;172:641–645.
6. Carlson LA: Studies on the effect of nicotinic acid on catecholamine stimulated lipolysis in adipose tissue *in vitro*. *Acta Med Scand* 1963;173:719–722.
7. Carlson LA, Havel RJ, Ekelund LG, Holmgren A: Effect of nicotinic acid on the turnover rate and oxidation of the free fatty acids in man during exercise. *Metabolism* 1963;12:837–845.
8. Carlson LA, Lassers BW, Wahlqvist ML, Kaijser L: The relationship in man between plasma free fatty acids and myocardial metabolism of carbohydrate substrate. *Cardiology* 1972;57:51–54.
9. Havel RJ, Carlson LA, Eckelund LG, Holmgren A: Studies on the relation between mobilization of free fatty acids and energy metabolism in man: Effects of norepinepherine and nicotinic acid. *Metabolism* 1964;13:1402–1412.
10. Gordon RS Jr, Cherkes A: Unesterified fatty acids in human blood plasma. *J Clin Invest* 1956;35:206–212.
11. Laurell S: Recycling of intravenously injected palmitic acid-1-C^{14} as esterified fatty acid in the plasma of rats, and turnover rate of plasma triglycerides. *Acta Physiol Scand* 1959;47:218–223.
12. Carlson LA: Studies on the incorporation of injected palmitic acid-1-C14 into liver and plasma lipids in man. *Acta Soc Med Ups* 1960;65:85–89.
13. Havel RJ: Conversion of plasma free fatty acids into triglycerides of plasma lipoprotein fractions in man. *Metab Clin Exp* 1961;10:1031–1036.
14. Benyo Z, Gille A, Kero J, et al.: GPR109A (PUMA-G/HM74A) mediates nicotinic acid-induced flushing. *J Clin Invest* 2005;115: 3634–3640.
15. Pike NB: Flushing out the role of GPR109A (HM74A) in the clinical efficacy of nicotinic acid. *J Clin Invest* 2005;115:3400–3403.
16. Tunaru S, Kero J, Schaub A, et al.: PUMA-G and HM74 are receptors for nicotinic acid and mediate its antilipolytic effect. *Nat Med* 2003;9:352–355.
17. Taggart AK, Kero J, Gan X, et al.: (D)-beta-Hydroxybutyrate inhibits adipocyte lipolysis via the nicotinic acid receptor PUMA-G. *J Biol Chem* 2005;280:26649–26652.
18. Carlson LA, Hanngren A: Initial distribution in mice of ^{3}H-labelled nicotinic acid studied by autoradiography. *Life Sci* 1964;3:867–871.
19. Kaijser L, Eklund B, Olsson AG et al.: Dissociation of the effects of nicotinic acid on vasodilatation and lipolysis by a prostaglandin synthesis inhibitor, indomethacin, in man. *Med Biol* 1979;57:114–117, 773–782.
20. Morrow JD, Parsons WG III, Roberts LJ, et al.: Release of markedly increased quantities of prostaglandin D2 *in vivo* in humans following the administration of nicotinic acid. *Prostaglandins* 1989;38:263–274.
21. Carlson LA, Ostman J: Plasma beta-hydroxybutyric acid response to nicotinic acid-induced plasma free fatty acid decrease in man. *Diabetologia* 1966;2:127–129.
22. Carlson LA, Freyschuss U, Kjellberg J, Ostman J: Suppression of splanchnic ketone body production in man by nicotinic acid. *Diabetologia* 1967;3:494–499.
23. Carlson LA, Levi L, Oro L: Plasma lipids and urinary excretion of catecholamines in man during experimentally induced emotional stress, and their modification by nicotinic acid. *J Clin Invest* 1968;47:1795–1805.
24. Lassers BW, Wahlqvist ML, Kaijser L, Carlson LA: Effect of nicotinic acid on myocardial metabolism in man at rest and during exercise. *J Appl Physiol* 1972;33:72–80.
25. Carlson LA: Serum lipids in men with myocardial infarction. *Acta Med Scand* 1960;167:399–413.
26. Castelli W: Epidemiology of triglycerides: A view from Framingham. *Am J Cardiol* 1992;70:3H–9H.
27. Gordon T, Castelli WP, Hjortland MC, et al.: High-density lipoprotein as a protective factor against coronary heart disease. The Framingham Study. *Am J Med* 1977;62:707–714.
28. Miller GJ, Miller NE: Plasma high-density lipoprotein concentration and development of ischaemic heart disease. *Lancet* 1975;I:16–19.
29. Beaumont JL, Carlson LA, Cooper GR, et al.: Classification of hyperlipidemias and hyperlipoproteinemias. *Bull World Health Organization* 1970;43:891–915.
30. Fredrickson DA, Levy RI, Lees RS: Fat transport in lipoproteins: an integrated approach to mechanisms and disorders. *N Engl J Med* 1967;276:34–44, 94–103, 148–156, 215–225, 273–281.
31. Havel RJ, Eder HA, Bragdon JH: The distribution and chemical composition of ultracentrifugally separated lipoproteins in human serum. *J Clin Invest* 1955;34:1345–1353.
32. Johansson JO, Egberg N, Asplund-Carlson A, et al.: Nicotinic acid treatment shifts the fibrinolytic balance favourably and decreases plasma fibrinogen in hypertriglyceridaemic men. *J Cardiovasc Risk* 1997;4:165–171.
33. Carlson LA, Oro L: Effect of treatment with nicotinic acid for one month on serum lipids in patients with different types of hyperlipidemia. *Atherosclerosis* 1973;18:1–9.
34. Carlson LA, Hamsten A, Asplund A: Pronounced lowering of serum levels of lipoprotein Lp(a) in hyperlipidaemic subjects treated with nicotinic acid. *J Intern Med* 1989;226:271–276.
35. Lithell H, Vessby B, Walldius G, Carlson LA: Hypertriglyceridemia, acute pancreatitis and ischemic heart disease in a pair of monozygotic twins. *Acta Med Scand* 1987;221:311–316.
36. Carlson LA, Danielson M, Eckberg I, et al.: Reduction of myocardial reinfarction by the combined treatment with clofibrate and nicotinic acid. *Atherosclerosis* 1977;28:81–86.
37. Carlson LA, Rosenhamer G: Reduction of mortality in the Stockholm Ischaemic Heart Disease Secondary Prevention Study by combined treatment with clofibrate and nicotinic acid. *Acta Med Scand* 1988;223:405–418.
38. Whitney EJ, Krasuski RA, Personius BE, et al.: A randomized trial of a strategy for increasing high-density lipoprotein cholesterol levels: Effects on progression of coronary heart disease and clinical events. *Ann Intern Med* 2005;142:95–104.
39. The Coronary Drug Project Research Group: The Coronary Drug Project. Design, methods, and baseline results. *Circulation* 1973;47(Suppl I):I1–I50.
40. The Coronary Drug Project Research Group: Clofibrate and niacin in coronary heart disease. *JAMA* 1975;231:360–381.
41. The Coronary Drug Project Research Group: The Coronary Drug Project: Initial findings leading to modifications of its research protocol. *JAMA* 1970;214:1303–1313.

42. The Coronary Drug Project Research Group: The Coronary Drug Project: findings leading to further modifications of its protocol with respect to dextrothyroxine. *JAMA* 1972;220:996–1008.
43. The Coronary Drug Project Research Group: The Coronary Drug Project: findings leading to discontinuation of the 2.5 mg/day estrogen group. *JAMA* 1973;226:652–657.
44. Cox DR: Regression models and life-tables. *J R Statist Soc B* 1972;34:187–202.
45. Canner PL, Berge KG, Wenger NK, et al., for the Coronary Drug Project Research Group: fifteen-year mortality in Coronary Drug Project patients: long-term benefit with niacin. *J Am Coll Cardiol* 1986;81:1245–1255.
46. Expert Panel on Detection, Evaluation, and Treatment of High Blood Cholesterol in Adults (Adult Treatment Panel III): Third Report of the National Cholesterol Education Program (NCEP) Expert Panel on Detection, Evaluation, and Treatment of High Blood Cholesterol in Adults (Adult Treatment Panel III) final report. *Circulation* 2002;106:3143–3421.
47. Garg A, Grundy SM: Nicotinic acid as therapy for dyslipidemia in non-insulin-dependent diabetes mellitus. *J Am Med Assoc* 1990;264:723–726.
48. Canner PL, Furberg CD, Terrin ML, McGovern ME: Benefits of niacin by glycemic status in patients with healed myocardial infarction (from the Coronary Drug Project). *Am J Cardiol* 2005;95:254–257.
49. Canner PL, Furberg CD, McGovern ME: Benefits of niacin in patients with versus without the metabolic syndrome and healed myocardial infarction (from the Coronary Drug Project). *Am J Cardiol* 2006;97:477–479.
50. SAS Language: Reference, 1st ed, 8.2 version. Cary, NC: SAS Institute, Inc, 2002.
51. Blankenhorn DH, Nessim SA, Johnson RL, et al.: Beneficial effects of combined colestipol-niacin therapy on coronary atherosclerosis and coronary venous bypass grafts. *JAMA* 1987;257:3233–3240.
52. Cashin-Hemphill L, Mack WJ, Pogoda JM, et al.: Beneficial effects of colestipol-niacin on coronary atherosclerosis. A 4-year follow-up. *JAMA* 1990;264:3013–3017.
53. Hodis HN, Mack WJ: Triglyceride-rich lipoproteins and progression of atherosclerosis. *Eur Heart J* 1998;19(Suppl A):A40–44.
54. Kane JP, Malloy MJ, Ports TA, et al.: Regression of coronary atherosclerosis during treatment of familial hypercholesterolemia with combined drug regimens. *JAMA* 1990;264:3007–3012.
55. Brown BG, Hillger LA, Lewis C, et al.: A maximum confidence approach for measuring progression and regression of coronary artery disease in clinical trials. *Circulation* 1993;87(Suppl II):II66–II73.
56. Brown G, Albers JJ, Fisher LD, et al.: Regression of coronary artery disease as a result of intensive lipid-lowering therapy in men with high levels of apolipoprotein B. *N Engl J Med* 1990;323:1289–1298.
57. Zhao XQ, Brown BG, Hillger L, et al.: Effects of intensive lipid-lowering therapy on the coronary arteries of asymptomatic subjects with elevated apolipoprotein B. *Circulation* 1993;88:2744–2753.
58. Assman G, Schulte H, von Eckardstein A, et al.: High-density lipoprotein cholesterol as a predictor of coronary heart disease risk. The PROCAM experience and pathophysiological implications for reverse cholesterol transport. *Atherosclerosis* 1996;124(Suppl):S11–S20.
59. Gordon DJ, Probstfield JL, Garrison LJ, et al.: High-density lipoprotein cholesterol and cardiovascular disease. Four prospective American studies. *Circulation* 1989;79:8–15.
60. Brown BG, Zhao XQ, Sacco DE, Albers JJ: Lipid lowering and plaque regression. New insights into prevention of plaque disruption and clinical events in coronary disease. *Circulation* 1993;87:1781–1791.
61. Maher VM, Brown BG, Marcovina SM, et al.: Effects of lowering elevated LDL cholesterol on the cardiovascular risk of lipoprotein(a). *JAMA* 1995;274:1771–1774.
62. Haskell WL, Alderman EL, Fair JM, et al.: Effects of intensive multiple risk factor reduction on coronary atherosclerosis and cardiac events in men and women with coronary artery disease. The Stanford Coronary Risk Intervention Project (SCRIP). *Circulation* 1994;89:975–990.
63. Quinn TG, Alderman EL, McMillan A, et al.: Development of new coronary atherosclerotic lesions during a 4-year multiple risk factor reduction program: the Stanford Coronary Risk Intervention Project (SCRIP). *J Am Coll Cardiol* 1994;24:900–908.
64. Miller BD, Alderman EL, Haskell WL, et al.: Predominance of dense low-density lipoprotein particles predicts angiographic benefit or therapy in the Stanford Coronary Risk Intervention Project. *Circulation* 1996;94:2146–2153.
65. Sacks FM, Pasternac RC, Gibson CM, et al.: Effects on coronary atherosclerosis of decrease in plasma cholesterol concentrations in normocholesterolemic patients. *Lancet* 1994;344:1182–1186.
66. Brown BG, Brockenbrough A, Zhao XQ, et al.: Very intensive lipid therapy with lovastatin, niacin, and colestipol for prevention of death and myocardial infarction: a 10-year Familial Atherosclerosis Treatment Study (FATS) follow up. *Circulation* 1998;98(Suppl 1):I–635.
67. Zhao XQ, Yuan C, Hatsukami TS, et al.: Effects of prolonged intensive lipid-lowering therapy on the characteristics of carotid atherosclerotic plaques *in vivo* by MRI: a case–control study. *Arterioscler Thromb Vasc Biol* 2001;21(10):1623–1629.
68. Davies MJ, Richardson PD, Woolf N, et al.: Risk of thrombosis in human atherosclerotic plaques. Role of extracellular lipid, macrophages, and smooth muscle cell content. *Brit Heart J* 1993;69:377–381.
69. Brown BG, Zhao XQ, Chait A, et al.: Simvastatin and niacin, antioxidant vitamins, or the combination for the prevention of coronary disease. *N Engl J Med* 2001;345:1583–1592.
70. Taylor AJ, Sullenberger LE, Lee HJ, et al.: Arterial Biology for the Investigation of the Treatment Effects of Reducing cholesterol (ARBITER) 2. A double-blind, placebo-controlled study of extended release niacin on atherosclerosis progression in secondary prevention patients treated with statins. *Circulation* 2004:110:3512–3517.
71. Taylor AJ, Lee HJ, Sullenberger LE: The effect of 24 months of combination statin and extended release niacin on carotid intima–media thickness. ARBITER 3. *Curr Med Res Opin* 2006:22;2243–2250.
72. Brown BG, Stukovsky KH, Zhao XQ: Simultaneous low-density lipoprotein-C lowering and high-density lipoprotein-C elevation for optimum cardiovascular disease prevention with various drug classes, and their combinations: a meta-analysis of 23 randomized lipid trials. *Curr Opin Lipidol* 2006;17:631–636.
73. Brown BG, Zhao XQ, Cheung MC: Should both HDL cholesterol and LDL cholesterol be targets for lipid therapy? A review of current evidence. *J Clin Lipidology* 2007;1:88–94.
74. Guyton JR: Extended-release niacin for modifying the lipoprotein profile. *Expert Opin Pharmacother* 2004;5:1385–1398.
75. Piepho RW: The pharmacokinetics and pharmacodynamics of agents proven to raise high-density lipoprotein cholesterol. *Am J Cardiol* 2000;86(Suppl):35L–40L.
76. Knopp RH, Ginsberg J, Albers JJ, et al.: Contrasting effects of unmodified and time-release forms of niacin on lipoproteins in hyperlipidemic subjects: clues to mechanism of action of niacin. *Metabolism* 1985;34:642–650.
77. McKenney JM, Proctor JD, Harris S, Chinchili VM: A comparison of the efficacy and toxic effects of sustained- vs immediate-release niacin in hypercholesterolemic patients. *J Am Med Assoc* 1994;271:672–677.
78. Cefali EA, Adams MH: Extended-release niacin pharmacokinetics following multiple-dose administration. *Pharmacotherapy* 2003;23:125.
79. Cefali EA: Effect of over-the-counter sustained-release niacin on serum transaminases. *Pharmacotherapy* 2003;23:126.
80. McCormack PL, Keating GM: Prolonged-release nicotinic acid. A review of its use in the treatment of dyslipidaemia. *Drugs* 2005;65:2719–2740.
81. McGovern M: Niaspan: Creating a new concept for raising HDL cholesterol. *Eur Heart J* 2005;7(Suppl F);F41–F47.
82. Sprecher DL: Raising high-density lipoprotein cholesterol with niacin and fibrates: a comparative review. *Am J Cardiol* 2000;86(Suppl):46L–50L.
83. Stroes ES, Birjmohum RS, Hutten BA, Kastelein JJ: Efficacy and safety of high-density lipoprotein cholesterol-increasing compounds: a meta-analysis of randomized controlled trials. *J Am Coll Cardiol* 2005;45:185–197.
84. Myers CD, Carr MC, Park S, Brunzell JD: Varying cost and free nicotinic acid content in over-the-counter niacin preparations for dyslipidemia. *Ann Inter Med* 2003;139:996–1002.
85. Mosca L, Appel LJ, Benjamin EJ, et al.: American Heart Association: evidence-based guidelines for cardiovascular disease prevention in women. *Circulation* 2004;109:672–692.

86. Levy DR, Pearson TA: Combination niacin and statin therapy in primary and secondary prevention of cardiovascular disease. *Clin Cardiol* 2005;28:317–320.
87. Hunninghake DB, McGovern ME, Koren M, et al.: A dose-ranging study of a new, once-daily, dual-component drug product containing niacin extended-release and lovastatin. *Clin Cardiol* 2003;26:112–118.
88. Kashyap ML, McGovern ME, Berra K, et al.: Long-term safety and efficacy of a once-daily niacin/lovastatin formulation for patients with dyslipidemia. *Am J Cardiol* 2002;89:672–678.
89. Ballantyne CM, Davidson MH, McKenney J, et al.: Comparison of the safety and efficacy of a combination tablet of niacin extended release and simvastatin vs simvastatin monotherapy in patients with increased non-HDL cholesterol (from the SEACOAST I Study). *Am J Cardiol* 2008;101:1428–1436.
89a. Ballantyne CM, Davidson MH, McKenney JM, et al.: Comparison of thet efficacy and safety of a combination tablet of niacin extended-release and simvastatin with simvastatin 80 mg monotherapy: the SEACOAST II (high-dose) study. *J Clin Lipidol* 2008;2:79–90.
90. Guyton JR, Goldberg AC, Kreisberg RA, et al.: Effectiveness of once nightly dosing of extended-release niacin alone and in combination for hypercholesterolemia. *Am J Cardiol* 1998;82:737–743.
91. Zhao XQ, Morse JS, Dowdy AA, et al.: Safety and tolerability of simvastatin plus niacin in patients with coronary artery disease and low high-density lipoprotein cholesterol (The HDL Atherosclerosis Treatment Study). *Am J Cardiol* 2004;93:307–312.
92. Kelly JJ, Lawson JA, Campbell LV, et al.: Effects of nicotinic acid on insulin sensitivity and blood pressure in healthy subjects. *J Hum Hypertens* 2000;14:567–572.
93. Rasouli N, Hale T, Kahn SE, et al.: Effects of short-term experimental insulin resistance and family history of diabetes on pancreatic beta-cell function in nondiabetic individuals. *J Clin Endocrinol Metab* 2005;90:5825–5833.
94. Poynten AM, Gan SK, Kriketos AD, et al.: Nicotinic acid-induced insulin resistance is related to increased circulating fatty acids and fat oxidation but not muscle lipid content. *Metabolism* 2003;52:699–704.
95. Vega GL, Cater NB, Meguro S, et al.: Influence of extended-release nicotinic acid on nonesterified fatty acid flux in the metabolic syndrome with atherogenic dyslipidemia. *Am J Cardiol* 2005;95:1309–1313.
96. Elam MB, Hunninghake DB, Davis KE, et al.: Effect of niacin on lipid and lipoprotein levels and glycemic control in patients with diabetes and peripheral arterial disease. The ADMIT study: A randomized trial. *JAMA* 2000;284:1263–1270.
97. Grundy SM, Vega GL, McGovern ME, et al.: Efficacy, safety, and tolerability of once-daily niacin for the treatment of dyslipidemia associated with type 2 diabetes. *Arch Intern Med* 2002;162:1568–1576.
98. Christensen NA, Achor RWP, Berge KG, et al.: Nicotinic acid treatment of hypercholesterolemia. *J Am Med Assoc* 1961;177:76–80.
99. Henkin Y, Johnson KC, Segrest JP: Rechallenge with crystalline niacin after drug-induced hepatitis from sustained-release niacin. *J Am Med Assoc* 1990;264:241–243.
100. Capuzzi DM, Guyton JR, Morgan JM, et al.: Efficacy and safety of an extended-release niacin (Niaspan): A long-term study. *Am J Cardiol* 1999;82:74U–81U.
101. Gharavi AG, Diamond JA, Smith DA, et al.: Niacin-induced myopathy. *Am J Cardiol* 1994;74:841–842.
102. Litin SC, Anderson CF: Nicotinic acid-associated myopathy: A report of three cases. *Am J Med* 1989;86:481–483.
103. Cooke HM: Lovastatin- and niacin-induced rhabdomyolysis. *Hosp Pharm* 1994;29:33–34.
104. Norman DJ, Illingworth DR, Munson J, et al.: Myolysis and acute renal failure in a heart-transplant recipient receiving lovastatin [letter]. *N Engl J Med* 1988;318:46–47.
105. Reaven P, Witztum JL: Lovastatin, nicotinic acid, and rhabdomyolysis. *Ann Intern Med* 1988;109:597–598.
106. Duvall WL, Blazing MA, Saxena S, et al.: Targeting cardiovascular risk associated with both low-density and high-density lipoprotein using statin-niacin combination therapy. *J Cardiovasc Risk* 2002;9:339–347.
107. Advicor Prescribing Information. Abbott Laboratories, North Chicago, IL. August 2007.
108. Rubenfire M: Safety and compliance with once-daily niacin extended-release/lovastatin as initial therapy in the Impact of Medical Subspecialty on Patient Compliance to Treatment (IMPACT) study. *Am J Cardiol* 2004;94:306–311.
109. Sheikh-Ali AA, Karas RH: Safety of lovastatin/extended release niacin compared with lovastatin alone, atorvastatin alone, pravastatin alone, and simvastatin alone (from the United States Food and Drug Administration adverse event reporting system). *Am J Cardiol* 2007;99:379–381.
110. Guyton JR, Bays HE: Safety considerations with niacin therapy. *Am J Cardiol* 2007;99(Suppl C):22C–31C.
111. Fraunfelder FW, Fraunfelder FT, Illingworth DR: Adverse ocular effects associated with niacin therapy. *Brit J Opthalmol* 1995;79:54–56.
112. Bressler NM: Cystoid macular edema from niacin typically is not accompanied by fluorescein leakage on angiography. *Am J Ophthalmol* 2005;139:951.
113. Gass JD: Nicotinic acid maculopathy. *Am J Ophthalmol* 1973;76:500–510.
114. Mosher LR: Nicotinic acid side effects and toxicity: A review. *Am J Psychiatry* 1970;126:1290–1296.
115. Gershon SL, Fox IH: Pharmacologic effects of nicotinic acid on human purine metabolism. *J Lab Clin Med* 1974;84:179–186.
116. Heart Protection Study Collaborative Group: MRC/BHF Heart Protection Study of cholesterol lowering with simvastatin in 20 536 high-risk individuals: A randomized placebo-controlled trial. *Lancet* 2002;360:7–22.
117. LaRosa JC, He J, Vupputuri S: Effect of statins on risk of coronary disease: A meta-analysis of randomized controlled trials. *JAMA* 1999;282:2340–2346.
118. Brown BG, Zambon A, Lanman RB, et al.: Frequency and importance of conversion to large buoyant LDL with simvastatin and niacin therapy: Comparison of four methods. *Circulation* 2003;108(Suppl IV):IV–197.
119. Clark RW, Sutfin TA, Ruggeri RB, et al.: Raising high-density lipoprotein in humans through inhibition of cholesteryl ester transfer protein: An initial multidose study of torcetrapib. *Arterioscler Thromb Vasc Biol* 2004;24:490–497.
120. Knopp RH, Alagona P, Davidson M, et al.: Equivalent efficacy of a time-release form of niacin (Niaspan) given once-a-night versus plain niacin in the management of hyperlipidemia. *Metabolism* 1998;47:1097–1104.
121. Cefali EA, Simmons PD, Stanek EJ, Shamp TR: Improved control of niacin-induced flushing using an optimized once-daily, extended-release niacin formulation. *Int J Clin Pharmacol Ther* 2006;44:633–640.
122. Cefali EA, Simmons PD, Stanek EJ: Aspirin reduces cutaneous flushing after administration of an optimized extended-release niacin formulation. *Int J Clin Pharmacol Ther* 2007;45:78–88.
123. Benyo Z, Gille A, Bennett CL, et al.: Nicotinic acid-induced flushing is mediated by activation of epidermal Langerhans cells. *Mol Pharmacol* 2006;70:1844–1849.
124. Lorenzen A, Stannek C, Lang H, et al.: Characterization of a G protein-coupled receptor for nicotinic acid. *Mol Pharmacol* 2001;59:349–357.
125. Jin FY, Kamanna VS, Kashyap ML: Niacin accelerates intracellular ApoB degradation by inhibiting triacylglycerol synthesis in human hepatoblastoma (HepG2) cells. *Arterioscler Thromb Vasc Biol* 1999;19:1051–1059.
126. Jin FY, Kamanna VS, Kashyap ML: Niacin decreases the removal of high-density lipoprotein apolipoprotein A-I but not cholesterol ester by HepG2 cells. Implications for reverse cholesterol transport. *Arterioscler Thromb Vasc Biol* 1997;17:2020–2028.
127. Rubic T, Trottman M, Lorenz RL: Stimulation of CD 36 and the key effector of reverse cholesterol transport ATP-binding cassette A1 in monocytoid cells by niacin. *Biochem Pharmacol* 2004;67:411–419.
128. Paolini JF, Mitchel YB, Reyes R, et al.: Effects of laropiprant on nicotinic acid-induced flushing in patients with dyslipidemia. *Am J Cardiol* 2008;101:625–630.
129. Lai E, De Lepeleire I, Crumley TM, et al.: Suppression of niacin-induced vasodilation with an antagonist to prostaglandin D2 receptor subtype 1. *Clin Pharmacol Ther* 2007;81:849–857.
130. Xydakis AM, Ballantyne CM: Combination therapy for combined dyslipidemia. *AM J Cardiol* 2002;90(Suppl):21K-29K.

CHAPTER 26

Fibrates

Peter H. Jones

The fibrate drug class has been in clinical use since the late 1960s, with clofibrate as the first member followed by the approval of fenofibrate, bezafibrate, gemfibrozil, and ciprofibrate over the next several decades. Early clinical investigations with clofibrate in the World Health Organization (WHO) primary prevention trial[1,2] and in secondary prevention trials (Coronary Drug Project, Newcastle, and Edinburgh)[3–5] suggested that this class had benefit in coronary heart disease (CHD) risk reduction but raised some questions about noncardiovascular disease adverse outcomes. Although it was known that clofibrate and gemfibrozil primarily reduced serum triglycerides along with modest reductions in total cholesterol, the newer-generation fibrates (fenofibrate, bezafibrate, ciprofibrate) had greater total cholesterol and low-density lipoprotein (LDL) cholesterol reductions. Despite this, the mechanism of action of fibrates was not known before the early 1990s. More recent clinical trials with both angiographic outcomes and hard CHD outcomes confirm the benefits of fibrates and have alleviated most of the safety concerns. This chapter will review the mechanism of action of fibrates on lipid and lipoprotein metabolism, the demonstrated clinical officacy and safety in monotherapy and in combination with other lipid-modifying drugs, and the clinical trials with surrogate and clinical cardiovascular disease event outcomes.

MECHANISM OF ACTION ON LIPID METABOLISM AND CELLULAR FUNCTION

The fibrates are synthetic ligands that bind to peroxisome proliferator–activated receptor (PPAR)–α. PPARs belong to a family of nuclear hormone receptors, and they can bind to natural ligands such as fatty acids and fatty acid–derived eicosonoids, resulting in a conformational change in the PPAR protein such that it forms a heterodimer partnership with another nuclear hormone receptor, retinoid X receptor (RXR).[6] This heterodimer complex can then bind to certain PPAR response elements (PPREs) in the promoter region of selected target genes. This binding to PPREs will affect gene transcription by either activation or, infrequently, repression (Fig. 26-1).[7] The recruitment of coactivators and/or release of corepressors are also an important component of proper gene transcription. There are two other types of PPARs, PPAR-γ and -β (or -δ). PPAR-α is expressed in metabolically active tissues such as the liver, kidney, heart, skeletal muscle, and brown fat, as well as in monocytes and vascular endothelial and smooth muscle cells. Fibrates are known to clinically reduce serum triglyceride levels, and this depends on PPAR-α–mediated mechanisms, which include 1) increased fatty acid uptake (by inducing fatty acid transport protein) and increased fatty acid β-oxidation, which reduces the substrate needed for the formation of very-low-density lipoproteins (VLDL); and 2) increased transcription of lipoprotein lipase (LPL) and repressed transcription of apolipoprotein (CPU) C-III, which inhibits LPL activity.[8,9] These two actions result in enhanced triglyceride-rich lipoprotein lipolysis, which results in lower chylomicron and VLDL levels and allows the released free fatty acids to be stored in adipose tissue or used for energy in skeletal muscle. Fibrates also increase high-density lipoprotein (HDL) cholesterol levels, and this depends on PPAR-α activation of hepatic apoA-I and A-II production.[10] The process of reverse cholesterol transport, which is thought to be one of the main beneficial actions of HDL particles, may be enhanced by PPAR-α activation in macrophages, which increases the expression of the ATP-binding cassette (ABC) A1 transporter, possibly through a modest effect on the liver X receptor (LXR).[11]

In addition to the PPAR-α–mediated effects of fibrates that result in lower serum triglycerides and increased HDL cholesterol, there are other PPAR-α

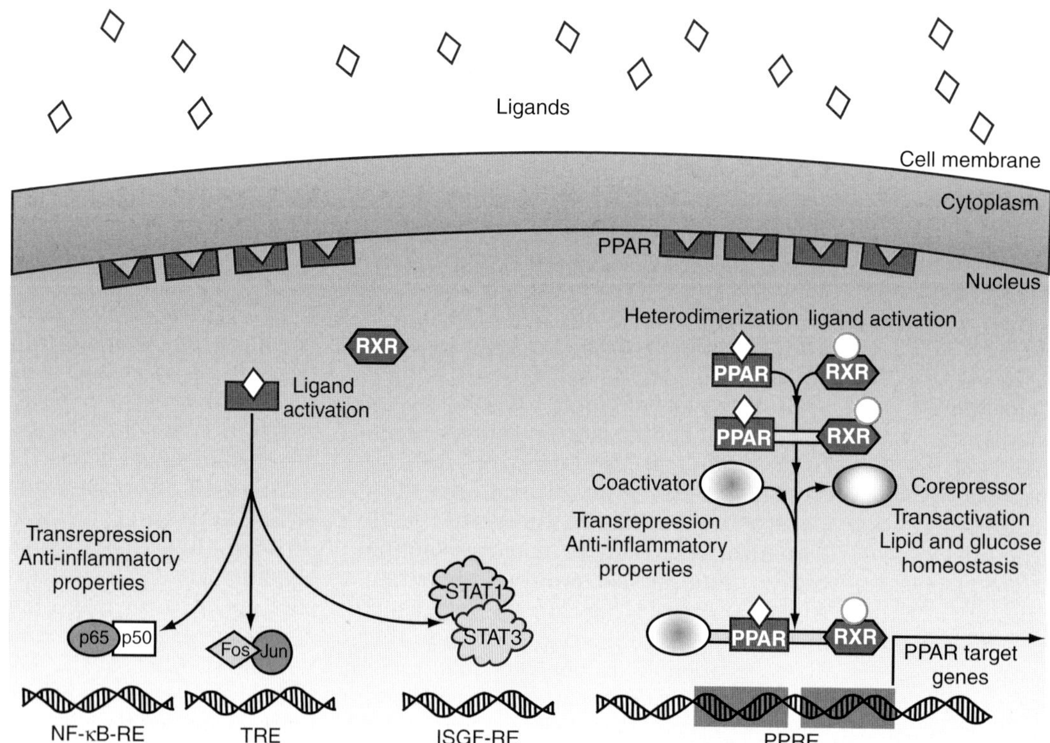

FIGURE 26-1 Mechanisms by which peroxisome proliferator–activated receptors (PPARs) affect gene transcription. *ISGF-RE, interferon-stimulated gene factor responsive element; NF-κB-RE–κB nuclear factor B response element; PPRE, PPAR response element; RXR, retinoid X receptor; STAT, signal transducer and activator of transcription; TRE, O-tetradecanoylphorbol 13-acetate–responsive element. (Reprinted from Ref. 7, with permission.)*

mechanisms that could be considered anti-inflammatory and antiatherosclerotic (Table 26-1). *In vitro* experiments have demonstrated that fibrates reduce the expression of vascular cell adhesion molecule–1 (VCAM) on cytokine-stimulated endothelial cells, as well as reduce the release of monocyte chemoattractant protein–1 (MCP-1), both of which should reduce the attachment and transmigration of monocytes into the arterial wall.[12] PPAR-α agonists have also been shown to reduce the expression of tissue factor and the release of matrix metalloproteinases by monocytes and macrophages, actions that could reduce the vulnerability of plaques to rupture and subsequent thrombosis.[13,14] Many proinflammatory genes depend on nuclear factor–κB (NF-κB), and it has been suggested that PPAR-α agonists may reduce the expression of these genes.[15] As a result, PPAR-α agonists such as fibrates have been shown to reduce inflammatory markers such as interleukin-6, fibrinogen, serum amyloid A, C-reactive protein (CRP), and tumor necrosis factor–α.

As mentioned previously, there are other PPARs, such as PPAR-γ and -δ, and synthetic ligands have been made that activate each. Some synthetic ligands have activity on more than one PPAR, such as dual PPAR-α and -γ, and pan-PPAR agonists. The fibrates most common in clinical use, gemfibrozil, bezafibrate, and fenofibrate, are mostly PPAR-α agonists; however, bezafibrate and fenofibrate may have weak PPAR-γ agonist activity. There is evidence that fenofibrate and bezafibrate improve insulin sensitivity, potentially through increased expression of adiponectin.[16,17]

TABLE 26-1	PPAR α Effect on Cellular Function and Inflammation
Decreases VCAM-1	
Decreases tissue factor expression	
Decreases matrix metalloproteinase release	
Decreases monocyte chemoattractant protein (MCP)-1	
Reduces inflammatory markers	
Fibrinogen	
IL-6	
C-reactive protein	
Serum amyloid A	
Tumor necrosis factor (TNF) α	

CLINICAL EFFICACY OF FIBRATES ON LIPIDS/LIPOPROTEINS/APOLIPOPROTEINS

Fibrates are prescribed as first-line agents for reducing elevated triglycerides because of their superior efficacy in decreasing triglyceride-rich lipoproteins (VLDL and intermediate-density lipoproteins [IDL]).[18] Fibrates also reduce the magnitude and duration of postprandial lipemia in patients with hypertriglyceridemia.[19] All of the clinically available fibrates reduce fasting triglyceride levels by 30% to 50% on average, and the higher the baseline triglyceride level, the greater the reduction can be.[20–26] In the rare genetic dyslipidemia resulting from homozygosity for apoE_2, termed type III dysbetalipoproteinemia, the fibrates produce very significant reductions in the cholesterol-enriched VLDL remnants, resulting in large decreases in total cholesterol (40%–50%) and triglycerides (50%–70%), and in regression of the xanthomas typically found in this disorder.[27]

Low levels of HDL cholesterol can occur in isolation from abnormalities in other lipoproteins but more frequently are associated with elevated triglycerides. Fibrates increase total HDL cholesterol levels most effectively in individuals with hypertriglyceridemia,[28] and this results from several mechanisms. First, reducing triglyceride-rich lipoproteins will decrease the neutral lipid exchange by cholesteryl ester transfer protein (CETP) between triglyceride-rich lipoproteins and HDL, which results in less triglyceride enrichment of HDL particles and less opportunity for hepatic lipase remodeling of them to a smaller size. Second, the enhanced LPL-induced lipolysis of triglyceride-rich lipoproteins by fibrates provides important surface coat constituents that facilitate HDL maturation, and the increase in hepatic apoA-I production will also contribute to increased HDL precursors. Although most patients will have an increase in HDL cholesterol with fibrates, there have been rare reports of a profound, paradoxical decrease in HDL cholesterol in patients with type 2 diabetes when fenofibrate or bezafibrate were added to a thiazolidinedione.[29–31] This was reversible when the fibrate was discontinued. The mechanism responsible for this rare occurrence is not known.

Fibrates are not considered first-line therapy for lowering LDL cholesterol because of their limited efficacy compared with statins. The newer-generation fibrates (fenofibrate, bezafibrate, ciprofibrate) have modest LDL cholesterol–lowering efficacy (−15% to −20%) in hypercholesterolemic patients with normal baseline triglycerides.[18,26] ApoB levels are also reduced by 10% to 20%. If baseline triglycerides are high, LDL cholesterol levels may increase, probably resulting from a shift in the predominant size of LDL particles from small and dense to a larger particle without a significant change in LDL particle number.[8,32] Total apoB levels may decline, however, because of reduced VLDL particle numbers. The effect of fibrates on levels of lipoprotein(a) [Lp(a)] are mixed. In some studies, bezafibrate and gemfibrozil have reduced Lp(a), but not in all. It appears that there is heterogeneity of response of Lp(a) to fibrates depending on baseline triglyceride levels. In normotriglyceridemic patients, gemfibrozil reduced Lp(a) by 17% and by 25% in those with baseline Lp(a) levels greater than 20 mg/dL. However, in hypertriglyceridemic patients, gemfibrozil had no significant effect on Lp(a). The reason for such a difference of response based on pretreatment triglyceride levels is not clear, but possible explanations are that reduced VLDL production by fibrates in subjects with hypertriglyceridemia permits more apoB availability for Lp(a) assembly, thereby increasing Lp(a) production, and/or that reduced VLDL levels decrease the interaction of Lp(a) with VLDL to form complexes, which would normally be cleared by the LDL receptor.[33]

Head-to-head comparative trials of the lipid efficacy of the fibrates are limited but generally show equivalent triglyceride lowering and increases in HDL cholesterol in their recommended doses.[23,25] The range of lipid/lipoprotein/apolipoprotein efficacy for the fibrates is in Table 26-2.

FIBRATES AND OTHER BIOCHEMICAL EFFECTS

As previously mentioned, fibrates can alter cellular processes through PPAR-α activation that can result in anti-inflammatory activities. High sensitivity CRP is primarily produced by the liver in response to cytokine mediators and has been shown to be an independent predictor of CHD in men and women. Many therapies that are known to be beneficial in reducing CHD risk, such as weight loss, exercise, aspirin, and statins, have been shown to reduce CRP. Similarly, fibrates have been shown to reduce CRP in subjects with dyslipidemia in most studies, but not all.[17,26,34–37] Lipoprotein-associated phospholipase A_2 (LpPLA_2) has also been suggested as a marker of increased vascular disease risk, particularly stroke. Statins have been shown to reduce Lp-PLA_2, probably because most Lp-PLA_2 mass is carried in LDL particles. Fenofibrate has recently been shown to lower Lp-PLA_2 to a similar degree as statins in type 2 diabetes and mixed dyslipidemia subjects.[35] Fibrinogen has been associated with increased vascular risk and is an

TABLE 26-2 Clinical Lipid Efficacy of Fibrates

Fibrate	TG	HDL	LDL	TC	apoB	apoA-I
Gemfibrozil 1200 mg/day	−30% to −50%	+5% to +20%	−10%	−10% to −15%	−10% to −20%	+5%
Bezafibrate 400–600 mg/day	−30% to −48%	+5% to +17%	−15% (Type II) +7% (Type IV)	−15%		
Ciprofibrate 100 mg/day	−37% to −73%	+18% to +39%	−18% to −29% (Type II) +36% (Type IV)	−15% to −25%	−15% to −20%	+8% to +10%
Fenofibrate 200–300 mg/day	−30% to −45%	+10% to +15%	−10% to −15%	−10% to −15%	−10% to −15%	+10%

apo, apolipoprotein; HDL, high-density lipoprotein cholesterol; LDL, low-density lipoprotein cholesterol; TC, total cholesterol; TG, triglycerides.

acute-phase reactant. The newer-generation fibrates have all been shown to lower fibrinogen levels in dyslipidemic subjects.[17,23,25,26,37,38]

Elevated uric acid levels are frequently seen in individuals with the metabolic characteristics of the metabolic syndrome,[39] and hyperuricemia has been suggested as an independent predictor of cardiovascular disease.[40,41] Fenofibrate has been shown to reduce uric acid levels, most likely by increasing renal excretion[42]; however, this has not been demonstrated for bezafibrate or gemfibrozil.[43] Homocysteine elevations appear to have an association with increased vascular disease risk, but randomized clinical trials of folate plus B_{12} and B_6 supplementation in high-risk subjects have failed to demonstrate any risk reduction by lowering homocysteine levels.[44] Fenofibrate has increased homocysteine levels in short-term efficacy studies[45–48] and in long-term cardiovascular disease outcome trials (Fenofibrate Intervention and Event Lowering in Diabetes [FIELD] and Diabetes Atherosclerosis Intervention Study [DAIS].[49,50] In the FIELD trial, the homocysteine increase was reversible when fenofibrate was discontinued, and the clinical impact of this elevation on the primary endpoint, which did not reach statistical significance, is not clear. In the quantitative angiographic analysis in DAIS, the increase in homocysteine by fenofibrate did not appear to alter the favorable fenofibrate effect of slowing atherosclerosis progression compared with placebo.[51]

Serum creatinine levels have increased in some patients treated with fenofibrate and ciprofibrate.[26,49] This increase was reversible after 5 years of fenofibrate therapy in the FIELD trial, and evidence suggests that this is not representative of a decline in glomerulor filtration rate (GFR), but rather the result of increased creatinine production.[52] In an analysis of patients in the Veterans Affairs High-density Lipoprotein Intervention Trial (VA-HIT) with baseline estimated GFR of 30 to 60 mL/min/1.73m², there was no change in the estimated GFR with gemfibrozil treatment compared with placebo over 5 years, regardless of whether the patients had type 2 diabetes or the metabolic syndrome. Also, a transient increase in serum creatinine was noted in 10% of the gemfibrozil group compared with 4% in the placebo group.[53] Fibrates have not been associated with acute renal deterioration; in fact, fenofibrate has been shown to reduce progression of microalbuminuria in subjects with type 2 diabetes.[49,54]

The National Kidney Foundation (NKF),[54a] the National Lipid Association, and others[54b] have provided practical advice about the use of fibrates in patients with stage 2 or greater chronic kidney disease, since fibrates require renal excretion for elimination. In general, fibrate monotherapy should be used with caution, the dose of fenofibrate should be reduced for GFR 30 to 60 mL/min/1.73 m², and fibrates should be avoided for end-stage renal disease. Gemfibrozil may be preferred, possibly at a lower dose, for patients with GFR less than 30 mL/min/1.73m². Caution should be used in combining fibrates with statins in stage 2 to 4 chronic kidney disease; while gemfibrozil monotherapy is preferred over fenofibrate by the NKF, fenofibrate may be safer if a statin is to be added. If gemfibrozil is to be used, the safest statin in combination is probably fluvastatin because there is no pharmacokinetic interaction.

The dyslipidemia of insulin resistance, which is characterized by elevated serum triglycerides and low HDL cholesterol, is uniquely suited for fibrates. The important question is whether fibrates have mechanisms of action that could also improve insulin sensitivity, such as by serving as weak agonists for PPAR-γ and/or increasing adiponectin levels. Bezafibrate does have weak agonist effects for PPAR-γ, and it was shown in the Bezafibrate Infarction Prevention (BIP) trial to reduce the progression to type 2 diabetes in a post hoc analysis of subjects with the metabolic syndrome.[55,56] The same authors showed in a post hoc subgroup that homeostasis model assessment of insulin resistance (HOMA-IR) progressed in the placebo group, while there was no significant change in the bezafibrate group over 2 years.[57] Gemfibrozil did not change the progression rate to diabetes in VA-HIT compared with placebo.[58] It is not clear if fenofibrate has an agonist effect on PPAR-γ, but there is evidence that measures of insulin resistance are improved with treatment of subjects with metabolic syndrome.[17] Fenofibrate has been shown to increase adiponectin levels,[17,38] which is an adipocyte-secreted protein that seems to improve glucose use and correlates inversely with insulin resistance. Whether this effect on adiponectin has clinical relevance for fenofibrate-treated patients awaits further investigation.

REVIEW OF FIBRATE RANDOMIZED CLINICAL TRIALS

The history of cardiovascular event outcome trials with fibrates started with clofibrate in the 1960s. Table 26-3 contains the important fibrate trials that evaluated either cardiovascular outcomes or the effect of therapy on a surrogate measure of atherosclerosis, such as quantitative angiography or B-mode ultrasound. All of these studies were placebo controlled.

The early clofibrate studies, Newcastle[4] and Edinburgh,[5] were small and performed in CHD subjects who had high total cholesterol levels. Both reported significant reductions in fatal and nonfatal CHD events, and one had a reduction in total mortality (Newcastle) over 5 to 6 years that accompanied a modest 10% to 20% reduction in total cholesterol. The Coronary Drug Project had a clofibrate arm for men with CHD and reported a nonsignificant 9% reduction in fatal and nonfatal CHD events over 5 years.[3] The WHO primary prevention trial evaluated 5000 individuals treated with clofibrate and found a significant 25% reduction in nonfatal myocardial infarction (MI) and no change in CHD death; this trial also raised concern, as previously mentioned, with the finding that total mortality was increased.[1,2] Importantly, the first post–acute coronary syndrome trial, the Stockholm Ischaemic Heart Disease Study, treated consecutive survivors of an MI with clofibrate plus niacin versus placebo and found that CHD death was reduced by 36% and total mortality was reduced by 26% over 5 years.[59]

Despite the success of most of these trials, the acceptance of clofibrate treatment for CHD prevention was limited by the adverse effect on mortality noted in the WHO study. Fibrate therapy received an important

TABLE 26-3 Summary of Clinical Trials with Fibrates

Trial	Population; Duration	Lipid/Nonlipid Effects	Outcome
Clofibrate			
Coronary Drug Project[3]	1103 men with CHD; 5 yr	TC −6.5% TG −22%	No effect on total mortality; −9% reduction in CHD death and nonfatal MI (NS).
WHO[1,2]	15,745 men without CHD; 5000 received clofibrate; 5.3 yr	TC −9%	Nonfatal MI reduced by 25%; no effect on CHD death. Increased total mortality with clofibrate.
Newcastle[4]	497 CHD subjects; PBO-controlled; 5 yr	TC −9% to −15%	Significant reduction in total mortality, particularly sudden death. Significant reduction in nonfatal MI.
Edinburgh[5]	717 CHD subjects; PBO-controlled; 6 yr	TC −15% to −20%	Significant reduction in fatal and nonfatal CHD events. No effect on total mortality.
Stockholm IHD [59]	556 consecutive MI survivors; clofibrate plus niacin vs. PBO; 5 yr		Clofibrate plus niacin reduced total mortality by 26% and CHD mortality by 36% compared with PBO.
Gemfibrozil			
HHS[60]	4081 men without CHD; PBO-controlled; 5 yr	TC −11% TG −43% HDL +10% LDL −10% Non-HDL−14%	Reduced CHD events by 34%. In subgroup with LDL/HDL ratio >5 and TG >200 mg/dL, CHD events reduced by 71%.
VA-HIT[58]	2531 men with CHD; PBO-controlled; 5yr	TC −4% LDL no change TG −31% HDL +6%	22% reduction in CHD death and nonfatal MI.
Angiographic			
LOCAT[85]	395 men post CABG with HDL <43 mg/dL; PBO-controlled; 2.5 yr	LDL −5% TG −36% HDL +21%	QCA at 32 months showed less progression in native coronaries and fewer new lesions.
Bezafibrate			
BIP[64]	3090 with CHD; PBO-controlled; 6.2 yr	TG −21% HDL +18% LDL −6.5% Fibrinogen −12%	10% reduction in CHD events (NS). 40% reduction in CHD events if TG >200 mg/dL (post hoc).
LEADER[86]	1568 men with PAD; PBO-controlled; 3 yr	TC −8% LDL −8% HDL +8% TG −23% Fibrinogen −13%	No effect on CHD or stroke. Benefit on nonfatal MI in men younger than 65 yr. Reduced severity of claudication.
Angiographic			
BECAIT[87]	92 post MI; PBO controlled; 5 yr	TC −9% TG −37% HDL +9% Fibrinogen −12%	QCA at 2 and 5 years showed less angiographic progression and fewer coronary events (NS).
B-mode Ultrasound			
SENDCAP[88]	164 type 2 DM without CVD; PBO-controlled; 3 yr	TC −7% TG −32% HDL +6% LDL −10% Fibrinogen −18%	No benefit on carotid or femoral B-mode ultrasound measurement of progression.
Fenofibrate			
FIELD[49]	9795 type 2 DM; PBO-controlled; 5 yr	TC −11% LDL −12% TG −29% HDL +2% apoB −7.5%	−11% (NS) reduction in fatal CHD and nonfatal MI. −24% reduction in nonfatal MI. Total CV events reduced significantly by 11%.
Angiographic			
DAIS[50]	418 type 2 DM PBO-controlled; 3 yr	TC −10% LDL −5% HDL +8% TG −28%	QCA showed significantly smaller increase in % diameter stenosis and decrease in MLD with fenofibrate. Fewer CHD events with fenofibrate (NS).

CABG, coronary artery bypass grafting; CHD, coronary heart disease; CV, cardiovascular; CVD, CV disease; DM, diabetes mellitus; HDL, high-density lipoprotein cholesterol; LDL, low-density lipoprotein cholesterol; MI, myocardiel infarction; MLD, minimum lumen diameter; NS, nonsignificant; PBO, placebo; QCA, quantitative coronary angiography; TC, total cholesterol; TG, triglycerides lift from the results of the Helsinki Heart Study in 1987.[60] This primary prevention trial of gemfibrozil or placebo in men without CHD who had a non-HDL cholesterol level greater than 200 mg/dL demonstrated a significant 34% reduction in the primary endpoint of fatal and nonfatal MI, and most importantly, found that gemfibrozil had no adverse effect on total or noncardiovascular disease mortality. Post hoc analysis revealed that the greatest CHD benefit occurred in the subgroup with a LDL cholesterol/HDL cholesterol ratio greater than 5 plus a triglyceride level greater than 204 mg/dL who were treated with gemfibrozil.[61] An analysis of 18 years of follow-up, comparing the original placebo group with the gemfibrozil group, showed that CHD death was significantly lower in the original gemfibrozil cohort and that total mortality was also lower in the gemfibrozil subgroup with a body mass index of 27.5 or greater and triglycerides greater than or equal to 184 mg/dL, which are components suggestive of the metabolic syndrome.[62] The other pivotal gemfibrozil trial was VA-HIT, which randomized men with CHD and low HDL cholesterol to gemfibrozil or placebo for 5 years.[58] Nearly half of the population had either type 2 diabetes or the metabolic syndrome, and mean baseline lipids included LDL cholesterol levels of 111 mg/dL, HDL cholesterol levels of 32 mg/dL, and triglyceride levels of 160 mg/dL. Gemfibrozil increased HDL cholesterol by 6% and reduced triglycerides by 31%, and this resulted in a 22% lower incidence of a composite endpoint of nonfatal MI, CHD death, and stroke. There was a nonsignificant reduction in total mortality. Further subgroup analysis of those with type 2 diabetes has provided evidence of gemfibrozil's significant reduction of stroke risk and has shown that gemfibrozil had the greatest benefit on CHD events in nondiabetic individuals who were in the highest quartile of fasting plasma insulin levels.[63]

These trials with gemfibrozil provide important information about the target population most likely to benefit from fibrate treatment. This would include primary prevention patients with either high non-HDL cholesterol or LDL cholesterol/HDL cholesterol ratios greater than 5 with triglycerides greater than 200 mg/dL, and secondary prevention patients with predominantly low HDL cholesterol and either type 2 diabetes or evidence of insulin resistance. The studies with bezafibrate further elucidate the role of fibrates in patients with the metabolic syndrome and dyslipidemia. In the BIP trial, CHD subjects with low HDL cholesterol had a nonsignificant 9% reduction in CHD events over 6 years with bezafibrate compared with placebo.[64] Post hoc analysis showed a significant 39% reduction in CHD events in the subgroup with baseline triglycerides 200 mg/dL or greater, and in subjects with the metabolic syndrome, the primary endpoint (fatal and nonfatal MI and sudden death) was significantly reduced by 23% (Fig. 26-2).[55] In addition, on-treatment HDL cholesterol significantly affected subsequent cardiac mortality, such that a 5-mg/dL increase in HDL cholesterol resulted in a 27% decrease in cardiac death.[65]

The quantitative angiographic trials with gemfibrozil, fenofibrate, and bezafibrate have all shown a slowing of atherosclerosis progression, which is similar to

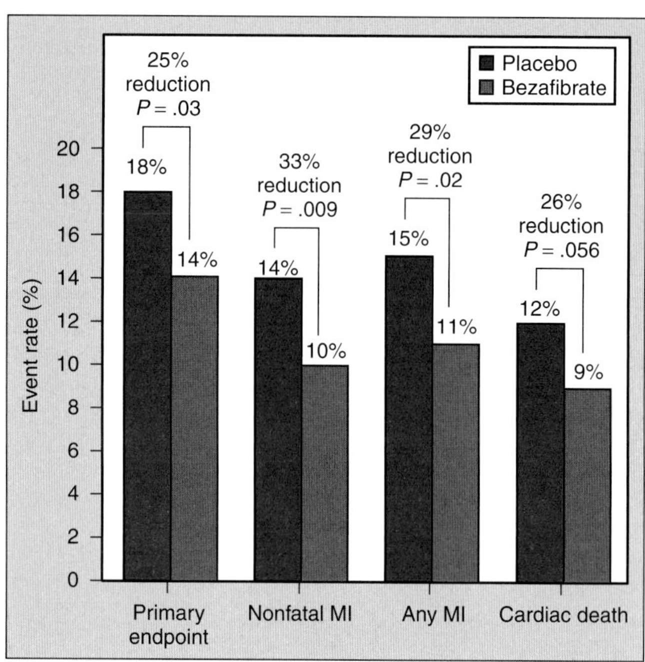

FIGURE 26-2 Event rate reduction in patients with the metabolic syndrome in the Bezafibrate Infarction Prevention (BIP) Study. In BIP patients with the metabolic syndrome, risk for the primary endpoint (composite of fatal and nonfatal myocardial infarction [MI] and sudden death) was significantly reduced by 25% with bezafibrate. *(From Ref. 55.)*

the placebo-controlled studies of statins.[50,85–87] The most recent large fibrate trial was the FIELD study.[49] This study randomized 9795 subjects with type 2 diabetes and total cholesterol greater than 250 mg/dL, triglycerides greater than or equal to 89 mg/dL, a total cholesterol/HDL cholesterol ratio of 4 or greater, and no indication for lipid therapy to receive either placebo or fenofibrate (micronized, 200 mg) for 5 years. Most of the population (78%) had no clinical history or evidence of baseline cardiovascular disease. The primary endpoint of CHD death and nonfatal MI was reduced by a nonsignificant 11% (P = 0.16). The secondary endpoint of total cardiovascular disease events was significantly reduced by 11%, as was the incidence of nonfatal MI (−24%) and coronary revascularizations (−21%). In a prespecified analysis, the patients without baseline cardiovascular disease (N = 7664) had a significant 25% reduction in the primary endpoint (P = 0.014) and an 11% reduction in the secondary endpoint (P = 0.004; Fig. 26-3). The FIELD protocol did allow for other lipid-lowering agents to be prescribed by the subjects' healthcare provider if necessary, and at the end of the study 32% of the placebo group and 16% of the fenofibrate group were taking a statin. It appeared that this disproportionate use of statins in the placebo group had an effect on the primary outcome, because a prespecified adjustment for statin use showed that the original randomization to fenofibrate had a significant 19% reduction in the primary endpoint. Of interest, fenofibrate therapy significantly reduced the tertiary endpoints of need for laser treatment for retinopathy and of progression of microalbuminuria. These effects on the microvascular complications of diabetes need to be tested in future clinical trials.

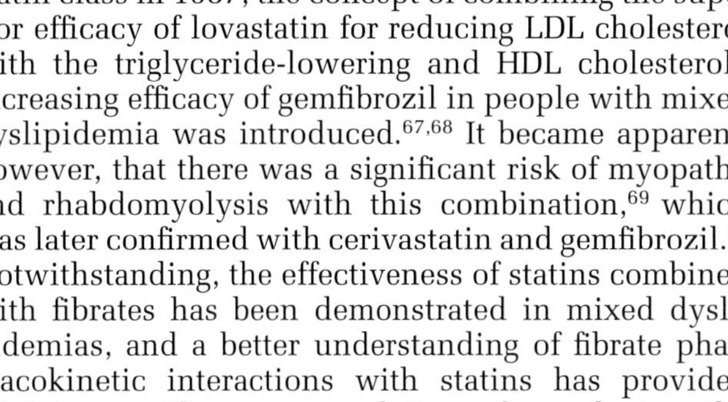

FIGURE 26-3 Effects on coronary heart disease (CHD) events and total cardiovascular disease (CVD) events in the Fenofibrate Intervention and Event Lowering in Diabetes (FIELD) Study. Fenofibrate treatment had a particularly beneficial effect in patients without prior cardiovascular disease (78% of the study population). *(From Ref. 49.)*

COMBINATION TREATMENT OF FIBRATES WITH OTHER LIPID-ALTERING AGENTS

For the vast majority of patients at significant risk for cardiovasular disease, statins will be the cornerstone of lipid treatment. Residual risk exists for some people with low HDL cholesterol and/or high triglycerides who are at their LDL cholesterol goal on statins, and the addition of fibrates could be useful. For a few selected individuals with severe hypertriglyceridemia, two or more drugs, such as fibrates, niacin, and omega-3 fatty acids, are needed to reduce triglycerides to below 500 mg/dL. In addition, a few individuals who are intolerant to statins because of muscle-related adverse symptoms may benefit from fibrates plus intestinally acting drugs such as bile acid resins and/or ezetimibe to control their dyslipidemia. The efficacy and safety studies discussed here were not designed to evaluate hard cardiovascular disease outcomes. As mentioned previously, the Stockholm Ischaemic Heart Disease Study with clofibrate plus niacin is the only clinical event outcome trial of fibrate combination therapy. Post hoc analysis of the FIELD trial may be able to assess the impact of adding a statin to fenofibrate in type 2 diabetes subjects compared with fenofibrate alone. The Action to Control Cardiovascular Risk in Diabetes (ACCORD) trial in patients with type 2 diabetes will evaluate cardiovascular disease events with simvastatin plus fenofibrate versus simvastatin alone in 5800 people, and the results are anticipated in 2009 or 2010.[66]

Fibrates and Statins

After the introduction of lovastatin as the first in the statin class in 1987, the concept of combining the superior efficacy of lovastatin for reducing LDL cholesterol with the triglyceride-lowering and HDL cholesterol–increasing efficacy of gemfibrozil in people with mixed dyslipidemia was introduced.[67,68] It became apparent, however, that there was a significant risk of myopathy and rhabdomyolysis with this combination,[69] which was later confirmed with cerivastatin and gemfibrozil.[70] Notwithstanding, the effectiveness of statins combined with fibrates has been demonstrated in mixed dyslipidemias, and a better understanding of fibrate pharmacokinetic interactions with statins has provided clinicians with recommendations for reducing the myopathy risk.

The majority of the recent statin–fibrate efficacy studies have evaluated fenofibrate or fenofibric acid, an investigational agent that is the active component of fenofibrate (Table 26-4).[71–77c] In general, the addition of fenofibrate or fenofibric acid to a statin provides greater reductions in triglycerides and increases in HDL cholesterol than statin monotherapy. In the study by Grundy et al. the combination of simvastatin and fenofibrate resulted in a shift of LDL particle size from predominantly small to intermediate and large, whereas there was no change in particle size in the simvastatin monotherapy group.[77] This was also shown with the use of fenofibric acid in combination with rosuvastatin 10 and 20 mg, LDL particle size increased significantly in subjects with baseline mixed dyslipidemia receiving combination therapy compared with rosuvastatin 10 and 20 mg monotherapy.[77d] In a few of these trials, fenofibrate was found to reduce uric acid levels and to result in a slight increase in serum creatinine. None of these studies reported a significant difference in the incidence of muscle adverse events between monotherapy and combination therapy.

The myositis risk of gemfibrozil coadministered with statins may be related to the pharmacokinetic interaction it has with all statins, except fluvastatin, resulting in significant increases in the serum concentration maximum (C_{max}) of each statin.[78,79] Gemfibrozil interferes with the glucuronidation of statins, which is an important process for statin elimination, while fenofibrate does not. Similar pharmacokinetic studies with fenofibrate coadministration with statins reveals no change in statin C_{max}.[80] Although the mechanism by which statins can cause myositis is not clear, higher than expected active statin blood concentrations do appear to be an important factor.

Fenofibrate and Ezetimibe

Recent clinical trials suggest that the combination of fenofibrate and ezetimibe in subjects with mixed dyslipidemia results in better lipid effects than either treatment alone. In one study, fenofibrate 160 mg/day and ezetimibe 10 mg/day reduced LDL cholesterol by 5% and 13%, respectively.[81] The combination reduced LDL cholesterol by 20% without additional triglyceride

TABLE 26-4 Combination Statin and Fenofibrate Efficacy Studies

	N	Percent Change in Lipids/Lipoproteins		
		LDL Cholesterol	TG	HDL Cholesterol
Ellen RL[71]				
Statin	39	−30	−9	+15
Fenofibrate	41	0	−41	+14
Statin plus fenofibrate	80	−28	−41	+22
Farnier M[72]				
Fenofibrate 200 mg	32	−21	−29	+4
Fenofibrate plus fluvastatin 20 mg	33	−32	−39	+14
Fenofibrate plus fluvastatin 40 mg	31	−41	−40	+3
Athynos VG[73]				
Atorvastatin 20 mg	40	−40	−30	+9
Fenofibrate 200 mg	40	−15	−41	+16
Atorvastatin plus fenofibrate	40	−46	−50	+22
Derosa G[74]				
Fluvastatin 80 mg	23	−25	−17	+14
Fluvastatin 80 mg plus fenofibrate 200 mg	25	−35	−32	+34
Durrington PN[75]				
Fenofibrate 201 mg	49	+1	−34	+9
Rosuvastatin 5 mg plus fenofibrate 201 mg	60	−34	−41	+11
Rosuvastatin 10 mg plus fenofibrate 201 mg	53	−42	−47	+12
Grundy SM[77]				
Simvastatin 20 mg	207	−26	−20	+10
Simvastatin 20 mg plus fenofibrate 160 mg	411	−31	−43	+19
Goldberg AC [77a]				
Atorva 20 mg	101	−37	−16	+6
Atorva 20 mg + fenofibric acid 135 mg	95	−34	−46	+14
Atorva 40 mg	95	−40	−23	+5
Atorva 40 mg + fenofibric acid 135 mg	96	−35	−42	+13
Mohiuddin SM[77b]				
Simva 20 mg	116	−22	−14	+7
Simva 20 mg + fenofibric acid 135 mg	109	−24	−37	+18
Simva 40 mg	106	−32	−22	+8
Simva 40 mg + fenofibric acid 135 mg	108	−25	−43	+19
Jones PH[77c]				
Rosuvastatin 10 mg	243	−38	−24	+8
Rosuvastatin 10 + fenofibric acid 135 mg	231	−45	−47	+20
Rosuvastatin 20 mg	238	−45	−26	+10
Rosuvastatin 20 + fenofibric acid 135 mg	230	−39	−43	+19

and HDL cholesterol effects beyond that of fenofibrate monotherapy. The combination was well tolerated without significant adverse events compared with the monotherapies. In a placebo-controlled trial of fenofibrate 160 mg/day (n = 160), ezetimibe/simvastatin 10/20 mg/day (n = 179), and the combination (n = 180) in subjects with mixed dyslipidemia, LDL cholesterol was reduced by 16%, 47%, and 46%, triglycerides were reduced by 41%, 29%, and 50%, and HDL cholesterol was increased by 18%, 9%, and 19%, respectively.[82] There were no significant differences in safety and tolerability among the three active treatment groups, particularly in muscle or liver adverse events. There were more subjects with slight creatinine elevations in the two fenofibrate arms but no discontinuations because of this finding.

Fibrates and Bile Acid Resins

A trial with fenofibrate 160 mg/day for 8 weeks was followed by randomization to coadministration of colesevelam 3.75 g/day or placebo for an additional 6 weeks.[83] The combination produced greater reductions in LDL cholesterol and apoB than fenofibrate monotherapy but did not change HDL cholesterol and triglycerides compared with fenofibrate monotherapy. There were no significant adverse event differences with the combination.

There is a substantial minority of patients, particularly at older ages, who have adverse events with statin treatment, mostly related to myalgias with normal creatine kinase levels. Many of these people will not persist with statins because of the symptoms. Bile acid resins and ezetimibe are alternatives to statins for lowering LDL cholesterol, and the trials discussed above which combined the intestinally active drugs with fibrates may be important options for such individuals. In a quantitative coronary angiography trial in men with CHD and low HDL cholesterol, the stepwise addition of gemfibrozil 1200 mg/day, niacin 3000 mg/day, and cholestyramine 16 g/day was compared with placebo in 71 and 72 subjects, respectively, for 30 months.[84] Compared with placebo, the combination therapy reduced LDL cholesterol by 26% and triglycerides by 50%, and increased HDL cholesterol by 36%. The triple therapy reduced the progression of atherosclerosis and had a nonsignificant trend toward reducing the composite cardiovascular disease endpoint.

SAFETY OF FIBRATES

As mentioned previously, the early trials with clofibrate raised concern about an increase in noncardiovascular disease mortality. Part of this was related to increases in cholelithiasis, in complications from cholecystectomy, and in pancreatitis; however, there was also some concern about an increase in gastrointestinal malignancies. Experience with the newer fibrates has not demonstrated a relationship with malignancy risk, but there are higher incidences of cholelithiasis and pancreatitis. A recent thorough review of the safety of fibrates has addressed these risks and other safety concerns such as increases in serum creatinine and homocysteine, changes in INR with concomitant coumarin administration, myopathy risk in monotherapy and in combination with statins, and a risk of thromboembolic events.[80] The authors made the following recommendations to healthcare professionals: 1) Obtain baseline serum creatinine before initiating fibrate therapy. If impaired renal function is present at baseline, such as estimated GFR less than 60 mL/min/1.73m^2, used when the lowest dose of fenofibrate or gemfibrozil. It is recommended the fenofibrate not be used with GFR less than 30 mL/min/1.73m^2. 2) There is no need to monitor creatinine levels, but if they are found to be increased without another cause, consider stopping the fibrate. 3) Obtain baseline creatine kinase level if adding fenofibrate to a statin, and monitor symptoms of muscle pain or weakness. It is suggested that gemfibrozil not be used with any statin other than fluvastatin. It is best to use as low a statin dose as possible. If the patient has renal insufficiency (GFR 30–60 mL/min), caution should be used when adding any fibrate to statin therapy. 4) Routine monitoring of homocysteine is not indicated at this time. 5) Monitor INR in patients on coumarin when a fibrate is added. 6) Even though fibrates may increase the risk for cholelithiasis, it is not recommended to screen for gallstones before fibrate therapy. The benefit versus the risk for giving a fibrate to patients with known cholelithiasis should be weighed.

CONCLUSION

The fibrate class of drugs is clinically indicated to lower serum triglycerides and increase HDL cholesterol. Fibrates also reduce postprandial lipemia and increase the size of LDL particles. The newer fibrates, fenofibrate and bezafibrate, can moderately reduce LDL cholesterol in hypercholesterolemic subjects, and they may improve insulin sensitivity in insulin-resistant individuals. The lipid-modifying effects of fibrates are mediated through activation of PPAR-α, and this effect may also have anti-inflammatory and antiatherosclerotic consequences. Preliminary data suggest that fibrates may delay progression of microalbuminuria in diabetes and may delay diabetic retinopathy; however, these results await longer, well-designed trials for confirmation. Randomized clinical trials show that fibrate monotherapy is most effective in reducing quantitative measures of coronary atherosclerosis progression and in reducing cardiovascular events in patients with high triglycerides and/or low HDL cholesterol, especially those who have the metabolic syndrome. However, the relative risk reduction in clinical outcomes is not as great as that with statin monotherapy in similar high-risk populations. The suggested clinical indications for fibrate monotherapy are listed in Table 26-5 and are derived from both clinical trial evidence and clinical practice experience. The substantial cardiovascular disease risk that remains in statin-treated high-risk patients may in part be related to persistent elevation in triglyceride-rich lipoproteins and low HDL cholesterol levels, and it would appear that concomitant fibrate and statin therapy is more effective in improving all lipoprotein levels than are statins or fibrates alone and is comparably safe. Whether this combination will provide incremental risk reduction over statin monotherapy awaits future trial evidence.

TABLE 26-5 Clinical Indications for Fibrate Therapy
1. Triglycerides >500 mg/dL
2. Primary prevention in men without CHD and non-HDL cholesterol >200 mg/dL, especially if LDL/HDL ratio >5 and triglycerides >200 mg/dL, and/or statin intolerance
3. Type 2 diabetes patients without CVD who are statin intolerant
4. Men with CHD and low HDL cholesterol and near goal LDL cholesterol, especially those who are statin intolerant
5. Combination therapy of fenofibrate and statin if triglycerides >200 mg/dL and non-HDL cholesterol is not at goal in high-risk patients
6. Combination therapy with niacin and/or omega-3 fatty acids for persistent severe hypertriglyceridemia

REFERENCES

1. Report of the Committee of Principal Investigators: WHO Cooperative Trial on primary prevention of ischemic heart disease using clofibrate to lower serum cholesterol: Mortality follow-up. *Lancet* 1980;ii:379–385.
2. Committee of Principal Investigators: A co-operative trial in the primary prevention of ischaemic heart disease using clofibrate. *Br Heart Journal* 1978;40:1069–1118.
3. The Coronary Drug Project Research Group: Clofibrate and niacin in coronary heart disease. *JAMA* 1975;231:360–381.

4. Trial of clofibrate in the treatment of ischaemic heart disease: Five year study by a group of physicians of the Newcastle upon Tyne region. *Br Med J* 1971;4:767–775.
5. Research Committee of the Scottish Society of Physicians: Ischaemic heart disease: A secondary prevention trial using clofibrate. *Br Med J* 1971;4:775–784.
6. Berger J, Moller DE: The mechanisms of action of PPARs. *Annu Rev Med* 2002;53:409–435.
7. Libby P, Plutzky J: Inflammation in diabetes mellitus: Role of peroxisome proliferator-activated receptor–α and peroxisome proliferator-activated receptor–γ agonists. *Am J Cardiol* 2007;99: 27B–40B.
8. Staels B, Dallongeville J, Auwerx J, et al.: Mechanism of action of fibrates on lipid and lipoprotein metabolism. *Circulation* 1998;98:2088–2093.
9. Watts GF, Dimmitt SB: Fibrates, dyslipoproteinemia and cardiovascular disease. *Curr Opin Lipidol* 1999;10:561–574.
10. Staels B, Auwerx J: Regulation of apo A-I gene expression by fibrates. *Atherosclerosis* 1998;137(Suppl.):S19–S23.
11. Chinetti G, Lestavel S, Bocker V, et al.: PPAR-alpha and PPAR-gamma activators induce cholesterol removal from human macrophages from cells through stimulation of the ABCA1 pathway. *Nat Med* 2001;7:53–58.
12. Marx N, Sukhova GK, Collins T, et al.: PPAR alpha activators inhibit cytokine-induced vascular cell adhesion molecule-1 expression in human endothelial cells. *Circulation* 1999;99:3125–3131.
13. Marx N, Mackman N, Schonbeck U, et al.: PPAR alpha agonists inhibit tissue factor expression in human monocytes and macrophages. *Circulation* 2001;103:213–219.
14. Shu H, Wong B, Zhou G, et al.: Activation of PPAR alpha or gamma reduces secretion of matrix metalloproteinase 9 but not interleukin 8 from human monocytic THP-1 cells. *Biochem Biophys Res Commun* 2000;267:345–349.
15. Delerive P, Fruchart JC, Staels B: Peroxisome proliferation-activated receptors in inflammation control. *J Endocrinol* 2001;169:453–459.
16. Wysocki J, Belowski D, Kalina M, et al.: Effects of micronized fenofibrate on insulin resistance in patients with metabolic syndrome. *Int J Clin Pharmacol Ther* 2004;42:212–217.
17. Koh KK, Han SH, Quon MF, et al.: Beneficial effects of fenofibrate to improve endothelial dysfunction and raise adiponectin levels in patients with primary hypertriglyceridemia. *Diabetes Care* 2005;28:1419–1424.
18. Zimetbaum P, Frishman WH, Kahn S: Effects of gemfibrozil and other fibric acid derivatives on blood lipids and lipoproteins. *J Clin Pharmacol* 1991;31:25–37.
19. Cavallero E, Piolot A, Jacotot B: Postprandial lipoprotein clearance in type 2 diabetes: Fenofibrate effects. *Diabetes Metab* 1995;21:118–120.
20. Mellies M, Stein E, Khoury P, et al.: Effects of fenofibrate on lipids, lipoproteins and apolipoproteins in 33 subjects with primary hypercholesterolaemia. *Atherosclerosis* 1987;63:57–64.
21. Cattin L, Da Col PG, Feruglio FS, et al.: Efficacy of ciprofibrate in primary type II and IV hyperlipidemia: The Italian multicenter study. *Clin Ther* 1990;12:482–488.
22. Bradford R, Goldberg A, Schonfeld G, et al.: Double-blind comparison of bezafibrate versus placebo in male volunteers with hyperlipoproteinemia. *Atherosclerosis* 1992;92:31–40.
23. Knipscheer H, Valois J, Ende B, et al.: Ciprofibrate versus gemfibrozil in the treatment of primary hyperlipidemia. *Atherosclerosis* 1996;124(Suppl.):S75–S81.
24. Gotto AM Jr, Breen WJ, Corder CN, et al.: Once-daily, extended-release gemfibrozil in patients with dyslipidemia. The Lopid SR Work Group I. *Am J Cardiol* 1993;71:1057–1063.
25. Aguilar-Salinas CA, Fanganel-Salmon G, Meza E, et al.: Ciprofibrate vs. gemfibrozil in the treatment of mixed hyperlipidemias: An open-label, multicenter study. *Metabolism* 2001;50:729–733.
26. Rizos E, Bairaktari E, Ganotakis E, et al.: Effect of ciprofibrate on lipoproteins, fibrinogen, renal function, and hepatic enzymes. *J Cardiovasc Pharmacol Ther* 2002;7:219–226.
27. Larsen M, Illingworth D, O'Malley J: Comparative effects of gemfibrozil and clofibrate in type III hyperlipoproteinemia. *Atherosclerosis* 1994;106:235–240.
28. Miller M, Bachorik PS, McCrindle BW, et al.: Effect of gemfibrozil in men with primary isolated low high-density lipoprotein cholesterol: A randomized, double-blind, placebo-controlled, crossover study. *Am J Med* 1993;94:7–12.
29. Ebcioglu Z, Morgan J, Carey C, Capuzzi D: Paradoxical lowering of high-density lipoprotein cholesterol level in 2 patients receiving fenofibrate and a thiazolidinedione [letter]. *Ann Intern Med* 2003;139:E-797–E-798.
30. Senba H, Kawano M, Kawakami M: Severe decrease in serum HDL cholesterol during combination therapy of bezafibrate and pioglitazone. *J Artheroscler Thromb* 2006;13:263–264.
31. Goldberg RB, Mendez AF: Severe, acquired (secondary) high-density lipoprotein deficiency. *J Clin Lipidol* 2007;1:41–56.
32. Lahdenpera S, Tilly-Kiesi M, Vuorinen-Markkola H, et al.: Effects of gemfibrozil on low-density lipoprotein particle size, density distribution, and composition in patients with Type II diabetes. *Diabetes Care* 1993;16:584–592.
33. Jones PH, Pownall HJ, Patsch W, et al.: Effect of gemfibrozil on levels of lipoprotein[a] in Type II hyperlipoproteinemic subjects. *J Lipid Res* 1996;37:1298–1308.
34. Despres JP, Lemieux I, Pascot A, et al.: Gemfibrozil reduces plasma C-reactive protein levels in abdominally obese men with the atherogenic dyslipidemia of the metabolic syndrome. *Arterioscler Thromb Vasc Biol* 2003;23:702–703.
35. Muhlestein J, May H, Jensen J, et al.: The reduction of inflammatory biomarkers by statin, fibrate, and combination therapy among diabetic patients with mixed dyslipidemia. The DIACOR (Diabetes and Combined Lipid Therapy Regimen) study. *J Am Coll Cardiol* 2006;48:396–401.
36. Jeong Kim C: Effects of fenofibrate on C-reactive protein levels in hypertriglyceridemic patients. *J Cardiovasc Pharmacol* 2006;74:758–763.
37. Jonkers IJ, Mohrschladt MF, Westendorp RG, et al.: Severe hypertriglyceridemia with insulin resistance is associated with systemic inflammation: Reversal with bezafibrate therapy in a randomized controlled trial. *Am J Med* 2002;112:275–280.
38. Koh KK, Quon MJ, Hon SH, et al.: Additive beneficial effects of fenofibrate combined with atorvastatin in the treatment of combined hyperlipidemia. *J Am Coll Cardiol* 2005;45: 1649–1653.
39. Onat A, Uyarel H, Hergenc G, et al.: Serum uric acid is a determinant of metabolic syndrome in a population-based study. *Am J Hypertens* 2006;19:1055–1062.
40. Bos MJ, Koudstaal PJ, Hofman A, et al.: Uric acid is a risk factor for myocardial infarction and stroke: The Rotterdam study. *Stroke* 2006;37:1503–1507.
41. Coutinho TDA A, Turner ST, Peyser PA, et al.: Associations of serum uric acid with markers of inflammation, metabolic syndrome, and subclinical coronary atherosclerosis. *Am J Hypertens* 2007;20:83–89.
42. Elisaf M, Tsimichodimos V, Bairaktari E, et al.: Effect of micronized fenofibrate and losartan combination on uric acid metabolism in hypertensive patients with hyperuricemia. *J Cardiovasc Pharmacol* 1999;34:60–63.
43. Bastow MD, Durrington PN, Ishola M: Hyper TG and hyperuricemia: effects of 2 fibric acid derivatives (bezafibrate and fenofibrate) in a double-blind placebo-controlled trial. *Metabolism* 1988;37:217–220.
44. Bazzaro LA, Reynolds K, Holder KN, He J: Effect of folic acid supplementation on risk of cardiovascular disease. A meta-analysis of randomized controlled trials. *JAMA* 2006;296:2720–2726.
45. Milionis HJ, Papakostas J, Kakafika A, et al.: Comparative effects of atorvastatin, simvastatin, and fenofibrate on serum homocysteine levels in patients with primary hyperlipidaemia. *J Clin Pharmacol* 2003;43:825–830.
46. Bissonnette R, Treacy E, Rozen R, et al.: Fenofibrate raises plasma homocysteine levels in the fasted and fed states. *Atherosclerosis* 2001;155:455–462.
47. Dierkes J, Westphal S, Luley C: Serum homocysteine increases after therapy with fenofibrate or bezafibrate [letter]. *Lancet* 1999;354:219–220.
48. Westphal S, Dierkes J, Luley C: Effects of fenofibrate and gemfibrozil on plasma homocysteine [letter]. *Lancet* 2001;358:39–40.
49. Keech A, Simes RJ, Barter P, et al.: Effects of long-term fenofibrate therapy on cardiovascular events in 9795 people with type 2 diabetes mellitus (the FIELD study): Randomized controlled trial. *Lancet* 2005;366:1849–1861.
50. Diabetes Atherosclerosis Intervention Study Investigators: Effect of fenofibrate on progression of coronary artery disease in type 2 diabetes: The Diabetes Atherosclerosis Intervention Study, a randomized trial. *Lancet* 2001;357:905–910.
51. Genest J, Frohlich J, Steiner G: Effect of fenofibrate-mediated increase in plasma homocysteine on the progression of coronary artery disease in type 2 diabetes mellitus. *Am J Cardiol* 2004;93:848–853.

52. Hottelart C, El Esper N, Rose F, et al.: Fenofibrate increased creatininemia by increasing metabolic production of creatinine. *Nephron* 2002;92:536–541.
53. Tonelli M, Collins D, Robins S, et al.: Effect of gemfibrozil or change in renal function in men with moderate chronic renal insufficiency and coronary disease. *Am J Kidney Dis* 2004;44:832–839.
54. Ansquen J-C, Foucher C, Rattier S, et al.: Fenofibrate reduces progression to microalbuminuria over 3 years in a placebo-controlled study in Type 2 diabetes: Results from the Diabetes Atherosclerosis Intervention Study (DAIS). *Am J Kidney Dis* 2005;45:485-493.
54a. K/DOQI clinical practice guidelines for managing dyslipidemia in chronic kidney disease. *Am J Kidney Dis* 2003;41:(Suppl: B):51–237.
54b. Harper CR, Jacobsen TA: Managing dyslipidemia in chronic kidney disease. *J Am Coll Cardiol* 2008;51:2375-2384.
55. Tenenbaum A, Motro M, Fisman EZ, et al.: Bezafibrate for the secondary prevention of myocardial infarction in patients with metabolic syndrome. *Arch Intern Med* 2005;165:1154–1160.
56. Tenenbaum A, Motro M, Fisman EZ, et al.: Peroxisome proliferator-activated receptor ligand bezafibrate for prevention of type 2 diabetes mellitus in patients with coronary artery disease. *Circulation* 2004;109:2197–2202.
57. Tenenbaum A, Fisman EZ, Boyko V, et al.: Attenuation of prevention of insulin resistance in patients with coronary artery disease by bezafibrate. *Arch Intern Med* 2006;166:737–741.
58. Rubins HB, Robins SJ, Collins D, et al.: Gemfibrozil for the secondary prevention of coronary heart disease in men with low levels of high-density lipoprotein cholesterol. *N Engl J Med* 1999;341:410–418.
59. Carlson LA, Rosenhaner G: Reduction of mortality in the Stockholm Ischaemic Heart Disease Secondary Prevention Study by combined treatment with clofibrate and nicotinic acid. *Acta Med Scand* 1988;223:405–418.
60. Frick MH, Elo O, Haapa K, et al.: Helsinki Heart Study: Primary prevention trial with gemfibrozil in middle-aged men with dyslipidemia. *N Engl J Med* 1987;317:1237–1245.
61. Manninen V, Tendanen L, Koskinen P, et al.: Joint effects of serum triglyceride and LDL cholesterol and HDL cholesterol concentrations on coronary heart disease risk in the Helsinki Heart Study. *Circulation* 1992;85:37–45.
62. Tenkanen L, Manttari M, Kovanen PT, et al.: Gemfibrozil in the treatment of dyslipidemia. An 18 year mortality follow-up of the Helsinki Heart Study. *Arch Intern Med* 2006;166:743–748.
63. Rubins HB, Robins SF, Collins D, et al.: Diabetes, plasma insulin, and cardiovascular disease: Subgroup analysis from the Department of Veterans Affairs High-Density Lipoprotein Intervention Trial (VA-HIT). *Arch Intern Med* 2002;162:2597–2604.
64. The BIP Study Group: Secondary prevention by raising HDL cholesterol and reducing triglycerides in patients with coronary artery disease: The Bezafibrate Infarction Prevention (BIP) Study. *Circulation* 2000;102:21–27.
65. Goldenberg I, Goldbourx U, Boyko V, et al.: Relation between on-treatment increments in serum high-density lipoprotein cholesterol levels and cardiac mortality in patients with coronary heart disease (from the Bezafibrate Infarction Prevention Trial). *Am J Cardiol* 2006;97:466–471.
66. ACCORD: Available at http://www.accordtrial.org. Accessed April 2, 2007.
67. Glueck CJ, Oakes N, Speirs J, et al.: Gemfibrozil-lovastatin therapy for primary hyperlipoproteinemias. *Am J Cardiol* 1992;70:1–9.
68. Garg A, Grundy SM: Gemfibrozil alone and in combination with lovastatin for treatment of hypertriglyceridemia in NIDDM. *Diabetes* 1998;38:364–372.
69. Pierce LR, Wysowski DK, Gross TP: Myopathy and rhabdomyolysis associated with lovastatin-gemfibrozil combination therapy. *JAMA* 1990;264:71–75.
70. Chang JT, Staffa JA, Parks M, Green L: Rhabdomyolysis with MHG-CoA reductase inhibitors and gemfibrozil combination therapy. *Pharmacoepidemiol Drug Saf* 2004;13:417–426.
71. Ellen RL, McPherson R: Long-term efficacy and safety of fenofibrate and a statin in the treatment of combined hyperlipidemia. *Am J Cardiol* 1998;81(Suppl.):60B–65B.
72. Farnier M, Dejager S: Effect of combined fluvastatin-fenofibrate therapy compared with fenofibrate monotherapy in severe primary hypercholesterolemia. French Fluvastatin Study Group. *Am J Cardiol* 2000;85:53–57.
73. Athyros VG, Papgeorgiou AA, Athyrou VV, et al.: Atorvastatin and micronized fenofibrate alone and in combination in type 2 diabetes with combined hyperlipidemia. *Diabetes Care* 2002;25:1198–1202.
74. Derosa G, Cicero AE, Bertone G, et al.: Comparison of fluvastatin + fenofibrate combination therapy and fluvastatin monotherapy in the treatment of combined hyperlipidemia, type 2 diabetes mellitus, and coronary heart disease: A 12-month, randomized, double-blind, controlled trial. *Clin Ther* 2004;26:1599–1607.
75. Durrington PN, Tuomilehto J, Hamann A, et al.: Rosuvastatin and fenofibrate alone and in combination in type 2 diabetes patients with combined hyperlipidaemia. *Diabetes Res Clin Pract* 2004;64:137–151.
76. Vega GL, Ma PT, Cater NP, et al.: Effects of adding fenofibrate (200 mg/day) to simvastatin (10 mg/day) in patients with combined hyperlipidemia and metabolic syndrome. *Am J Cardiol* 2003;91:956–960.
77. Grundy SM, Vega GL, Yuan Z, et al.: Effectiveness and tolerability of simvastatin plus fenofibrate for combined hyperlipidemia (the SAFARI trial). *Am J Cardiol* 2005;95:462–468.
77a. Goldberg AC, Bays HE, Ballantyne CM, et al.: Efficacy and safety of a novel fibrate, ABT-335, in combination with atorvastatin in patients with mixed dyslipidemia: a 12 week Phase 3 study [abstract]. *J Am Coll Cardiol* 2008; 51 (Suppl):A327.
77b. Mohiuddin SM, Pepine CJ, Kelly MT, et al.: Efficacy and safety of a novel fibrate, ABT-335, in combination with simvastatin in patients with mixed dyslipidemia: a Phase 3 study [abstract]. *J Am Coll Cardiol* 2008;51(Suppl):A327.
77c. Jones PH, Davidson MH, Kashyap ML, et al.: Efficacy and safety of ABT-335 (fenofibric acid) in combination with rosuvastatin in patients with mixed dyslipidemia: a Phase 3 study. *J Clin Lipidol* 2008:2:218–219.
77d. Jones PH, Dayspring T, Kelly MT, et al.: Effects of ABT-335 in combination with rosuvastatin on low-density lipoprotein particle size in patients in mixed dyslipidemia. *J Clin Lipidol* 2008;2:219–220.
78. Prueksaritanont T, Tang C, Qiu Y, et al.: Effects of fibrates on metabolism of statins in hepatocytes. *Drug Metab Dispos* 2002;30:1280–1287.
79. Preuksaritanont T, Zhao JJ, Ma B, et al.: Mechanistic studies on metabolism interactions between gemfibrozil and statins. *J Pharmacol Exp Ther* 2002;301:1042–1051.
80. Davidson MH, Armani A, McKenney JM, Jacobson TA: Safety considerations with fibrate therapy. *Am J Cardiol* 2007;99(Suppl.):3C–18C.
81. Farnier M, Freeman MW, Macdonell G, et al.: Efficacy and safety of the coadministration of ezetimibe with fenofibrate in patients with mixed hyperlipidaemia. *Eur Heart J* 2005;26:897–905.
82. Farnier M, Roth E, Gil-Extremera B, et al.: Efficacy and safety of the co-administration ezetimibe/simvastatin with fenofibrate in patients with mixed dyslipidemia. *Am Heart J* 2007;153:335.e1–335.e8.
83. McKenney J, Jones M, Abby S: Safety and efficacy of colesevelam hydrochloride in combination with fenofibrate for the treatment of mixed hyperlipidemia. *Curr Med Res Opin* 2005;21:1403–1412.
84. Whitney EJ, Krauski RA, Personius BE, et al.: A randomized trial of a strategy for increasing high-density lipoprotein cholesterol levels: Effects on progression of coronary heart disease and clinical events. *Ann Intern Med* 2005;142:95–104.
85. Frick MH, Syvanne M, Nieminen MS, et al.: Prevention of the angiographic progression of coronary and vein-graft atherosclerosis by gemfibrozil after coronary bypass surgery in men with low levels of HDL cholesterol. *Circulation* 1997;96:2137–2143.
86. Meade T, Zhuric R, Cook C, et al.: Bezafibrate in men with lower extremity arterial disease: Randomized controlled trial. *BMJ* 2005;325:1–5.
87. Ericsson C-G, Hamster A, Nilsson J, et al.: Angiographic assessment of effects of bezafibrate on progression of coronary artery disease in young male postinfarction patients. *Lancet* 1996;347:849–853.
88. Elkeles RS, Diamond JR, Poulter C, et al.: Cardiovascular outcomes in Type 2 diabetes. A double-blind placebo-controlled study of bezafibrate: The St. Mary's, Ealing, Northwick Park Diabetes Cardiovascular Disease Prevention (SENDCAP) Study. *Diabetes Care* 1998;21:641–648.

CHAPTER 27

Omega-3 Fatty Acids

William S. Harris and Terry A. Jacobson

INTRODUCTION

It was the pioneering observations made among Greenland Inuit in the 1970s by Bang and Dyerberg that were primarily responsible for the modern interest in marine oils and cardiovascular disease.[1,2] These Danish investigators reported that despite a diet high in saturated fat and cholesterol, serum lipids—particularly triglyand (TG)—were significantly lower in the Inuits compared with Danes.[3] It was hypothesized that the omega-3 fatty acids (FAs) found in abundance in marine oils may have been responsible for this hypolipidemic effect.[4]

But the Danes were not the first to observe the lipid-lowering effects of fish (marine) oils. Ahrens et al. reported in 1959 that a diet containing 40% of the energy as menhaden (fish) oil lowered serum TG by 50% in a patient whose TG levels were 486 mg/dL on a corn oil diet rich in linoleic acid (the primary omega-6 FA in the diet).[5] In 1981, the effect on TG concentrations was replicated by feeding purified eicosapentaenoic acid (EPA) and docosahexaenoic acid (DHA) in healthy subjects,[6] confirming that it was this particular class of polyunsaturated FAs (PUFAs) that had hypotriglyceridemic effects.

DEFINITIONS

There are two families of dietary PUFAs: omega-3 and omega-6 (or n-3 and n-6). These derive their names from the chemical structure of each family, with the final double bond being either three or six positions from the terminal methyl group (the omega, or nth, carbon in the molecule). These are depicted in Fig. 27-1. There are two subclasses of omega-3 FAs in the human diet, plant-derived and marine-derived. There is one omega 3 FA in the former group, α-linolenic acid (ALA, C18:3n-3), whereas there are threein the latter: EPA (C20:5n-3), docosapentaenoic acid (DPA, C22:5n-3) and DHA (C22:6n-3). (This FA nomenclature originated in 1963 with Mohrhauer and Holman[7] and gives the carbon number [C] followed by the number of double bonds and the family.) Dietary sources of the marine-based omega-3 FAs are given in Table 27-1.

EFFECTS ON LIPID CLASSES

Triglycerides

As noted above, the omega-3 FAs appeared to have unique TG-lowering properties not shared by the omega-6 FAs. Early studies documenting this effect used what are by today's standards exceedingly high doses of omega-3 FAs. For example, controlled-feeding studies used 20 to 25 g of EPA and DHA (the most abundant omega-3 FA in fish oils) in healthy volunteers[8] and in hyperlipidemic patients.[9] In the former, TG reductions of 33% (going from 76 to 50 mg/dL) were observed, whereas in the latter, 65% reductions were seen in patients with combined dyslipidemia whose average baseline TGs were 344 mg/dL. This intake reduced TG levels by 71% in patients with severe hypertriglyceridemia (HTG) (841 mg/dL on the control diet).[9] This dose was achieved by feeding a salmon steak twice every day and drinking about 100 mL of salmon oil. This is obviously impractical, so lower doses were subsequently investigated. Based on a meta-analysis of 72 placebo-controlled trials, 3 to 4 g of EPA and DHA produced TG reductions of 25% to 35%, with greater reductions in patients with higher TG levels (Fig. 27-2).[10] For example, patients with severe HTG (TG >500 mg/dL) treated with 3.4 g of omega-3 acid ethyl esters had a 45% reduction in TG levels (Fig. 27-3).[11] In this study, the time course of TG change was followed and was essentially complete within 1 month.

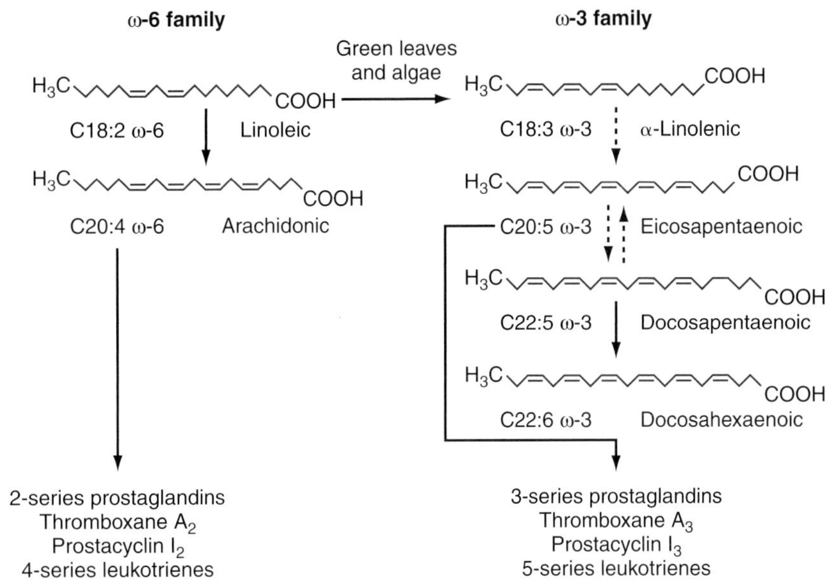

ω-6 family

H_3C — COOH
C18:2 ω-6 Linoleic

H_3C — COOH
C20:4 ω-6 Arachidonic

2-series prostaglandins
Thromboxane A_2
Prostacyclin I_2
4-series leukotrienes

Green leaves and algae

ω-3 family

H_3C — COOH
C18:3 ω-3 α-Linolenic

H_3C — COOH
C20:5 ω-3 Eicosapentaenoic

H_3C — COOH
C22:5 ω-3 Docosapentaenoic

H_3C — COOH
C22:6 ω-3 Docosahexaenoic

3-series prostaglandins
Thromboxane A_3
Prostacyclin I_3
5-series leukotrienes

FIGURE 27-1 The omega-6 and omega-3 families of polyunsaturated fatty acids. Of the omega-3 fatty acids, α-linolenic acid is found in plant oils, whereas eicosapentaenoic acid (EPA) and docosahexaenoic acid DHA are found in fish oils. There is minimal conversion of the former to the latter two. Both arachidonic acid and EPA are substrates for cyclo-oxygenases and lipoxygenases, each producing a different family of compounds with differing physiologic actions.

Cholesterol

The early high-dose studies also observed cholesterol-lowering effects (relative to a saturated fat diet) that were similar to those seen with vegetable oils.[8,9] This effect was later shown to be largely caused by the removal of saturated fat, not the addition of omega-3 FA per se. Fish oils, when given as supplements to a stable background diet, do not typically affect the total cholesterol level.[10] The only exception to this would be when the total cholesterol is elevated because of an excessive number of chylomicrons (Fredrickson types I or V-hyperlipoproteinemia) or of very-low-density lipoproteins (VLDL, type IV hypertipoproteinemia) that are causing the hypercholesterolemia. In these cases, omega-3 FAs will, in reducing the concentrations of these two classes of TG-rich particles that also carry some cholesterol, reduce the total serum cholesterol levels (see Fig. 27-3). Omega-3 FAs do not typically lower the low-density lipoprotein (LDL) cholesterol concentration, and as described later, they can actually increase LDL cholesterol levels in some patients.

EFFECTS ON LIPOPROTEIN CLASSES

Chylomicrons

Chylomicrons are the largest and most TG-rich lipoproteins in the blood. Chylomicrons are usually present only in the postprandial state, because they carry dietary fat from the intestines to other tissues (see Chapter 1). Because omega-3 FAs are known to significantly reduce fasting TG concentrations, their effects on postprandial TG metabolism have been examined in some detail. As expected, treatment with omega-3 FAs markedly reduced the rise in serum TG after a fatty meal.[12,13] The effect was not a result of malabsorption of omega-3 FAs, because fish oil–rich test meals produced similar Postprandial triglyceridemic curves as control fats.[12,14] Their effect on the postmeal excursion of serum TGs appeared only after weeks of prefeeding with omega-3 FAs, and the blunting of postprandial triglyceridemia occurred regardless of the type of fat in the test meal (Fig. 27-4). The dose of omega-3 FAs necessary to effect a reduction in postprandial lipemia has been shown to be as low as 1 g/day.[15,16] The extent to which the diminution of postmeal lipemia contributes to cardiovascular risk reduction is currently unknown, but this may be one mechanism by which these FAs mitigate against the development of coronary heart disease (CHD).

VLDL

Very-low-density lipoproteins (VLDL) carry 90% of the serum TGs in the fasting state. VLDL TGs are made in the liver from FAs that are either synthesized *de novo*, extracted from the circulation as nonesterified FAs, or recycled from lipoprotein remnants cleared by hepatic receptors. Like chylomicron TG, VLDL TG is cleared from the circulation by the action of lipoprotein lipase (LPL), the lipolytic enzyme found on capillary endothelial cells. As noted earlier, at doses of 3 to 4 g of EPA and DHA per day, omega-3 FAs can lower serum VLDL cholesterol and total TG by 30% to 50% depending on baseline TG levels (see Fig. 27-3).

LDL

Diets rich in the omega-6 fatty acid linoleic acid can actively reduce LDL cholesterol levels beyond the reduction seen from simply removing saturated FAs (see Chapter 19). The long-chain omega-3 FA, however, can paradoxically have the opposite effect. Indeed, when concentrated omega-3 FA products became available in the mid-1980s, supplementation trials (instead of whole food substitution trials) revealed that not only did omega-3 FAs not lower cholesterol, but also they actually could raise LDL cholesterol and apolipoprotein (apo) B-100 levels when given in doses of about 6 g/day to hypertriglyceridemic patients.[17] In one study, in which TG levels decreased from 407 to 252 mg/dL

TABLE 27-1 Dietary, Supplemental, and Pharmaceutical Sources of Long-Chain Omega-3 Fatty Acids

Fish	EPA and DHA g/3 oz Serving (Edible Portion)	Ounces per Day Required to Provide ≈1 g of EPA and DHA per Day
Tuna		
Light, canned in water	0.26	12
White, canned in water	0.73	4
Fresh	0.24–1.28	2.5–12
Sardines	0.98–1.70	2–3
Salmon		
Sockeye or Pink	1.05	3
Chinook	1.48	2
Atlantic, farmed	1.09–1.83	1.5–2.5
Atlantic, wild	0.9–1.56	2–3.5
Mackerel	0.34–1.57	2–8.5
Herring		
Pacific	1.81	1.5
Atlantic	1.71	2
Trout, rainbow		
Farmed	0.98	3
Wild	0.84	3.5
Cod		
Atlantic	0.13	23
Pacific	0.24	12.5
Catfish		
Farmed	0.15	20
Wild	0.2	15
Flounder/Sole	0.42	7
Oyster		
Pacific	1.17	2.5
Eastern	0.47	6.5
Lobster	0.07–0.41	7.5–42.5
Crab, Alaskan King	0.35	8.5
Shrimp, mixed species	0.27	11
Clam	0.24	12.5
Scallop	0.17	17.5
Supplements	**Omega-3 Fatty Acids g/g of Oil**	**g of Oil/Day**
Cod liver oil*	0.19	5
Standard fish oil	0.30	3
Omega-3 FA concentrates	0.50	2
Drugs		
Omega-3 acid ethyl esters	0.84	1

*This amount of cod liver oil would provide the Recommended Dietary Allowance of vitamin A and twice that of vitamin D.

Fish intakes are only estimates because eicosapentaenoic acid (EPA) and docosahexaenoic acid (DHA) content can vary markedly with season, diet, age, and storage/preparation methods.

Data from references 90, 91, and 94.

FA, fatty acid.

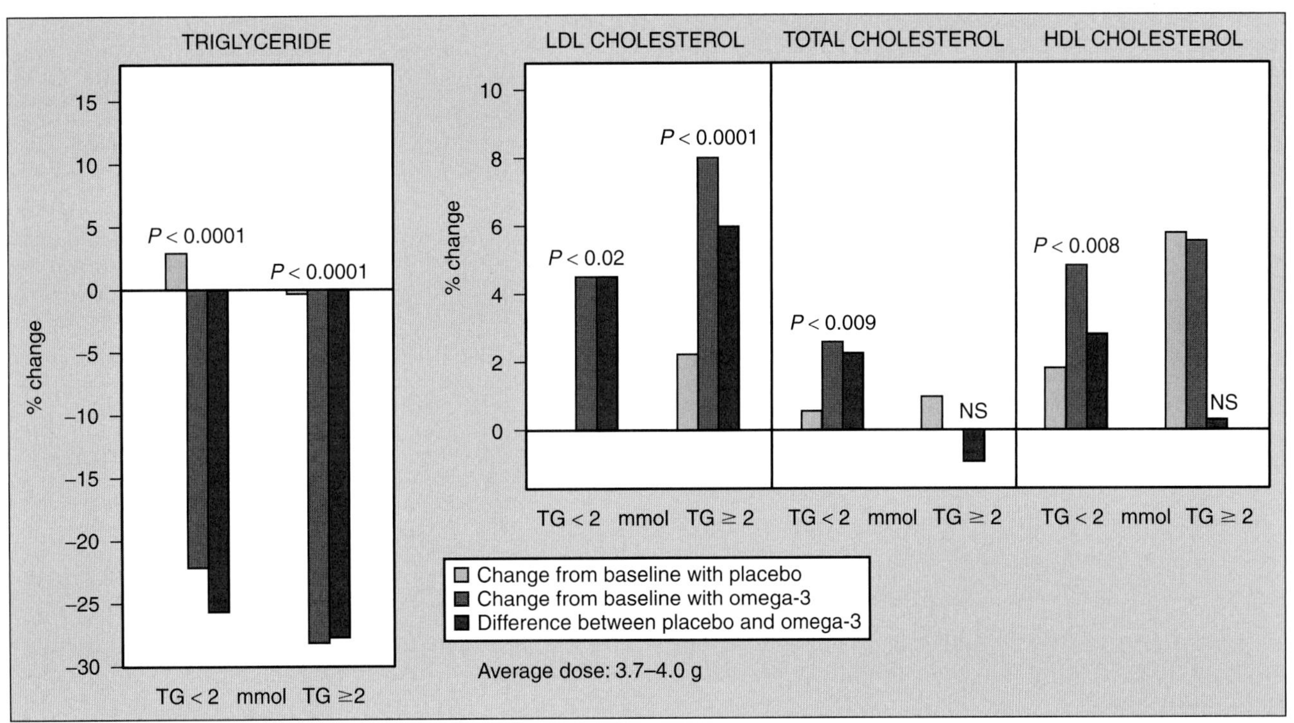

FIGURE 27-2 Meta-analysis of 72 placebo-controlled studies examining the effects of omega-3 Fatty acid supplementation on serum lipids and lipoproteins. To convert mmol/L to mg/dL, multiply by 0.1129. LDL, low-density lipoprotein; HDL, high-density lipoprotein; TG, triglyceride. *(Adapted from Ref. 10.)*

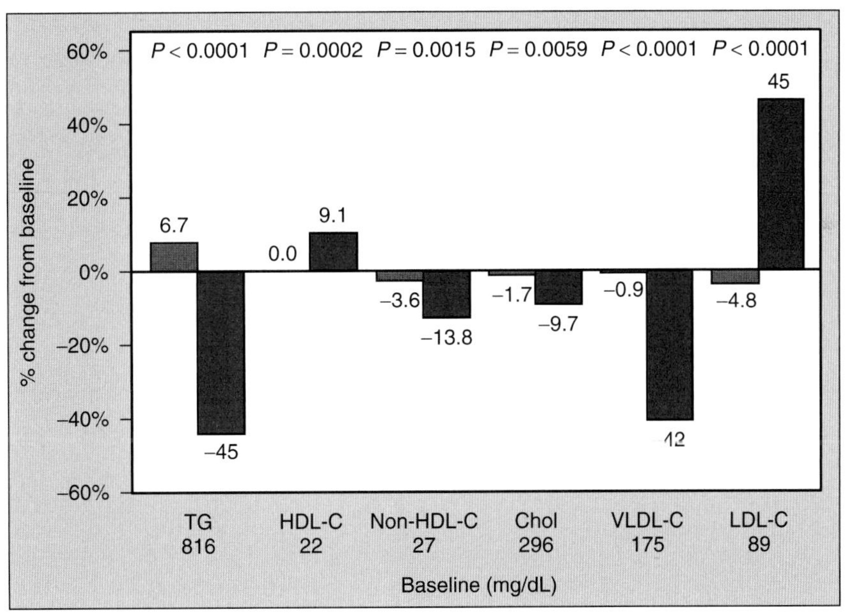

FIGURE 27-3 Effects of omega-3 acid ethyl esters (four1-g capsules/day; n = 41) and placebo (corn oil; n = 41) on serum lipid and lipoprotein concentrations in patients with severe hypertriglyceridemia. Combined data from two studies differing only in duration of treatment: 6 weeks (Ref. 90) and 16 weeks (Ref. 11). P-values compare the change in the placebo group (gray bars) with that in the omega-3 group (red bars). Chol, cholesterol; LDL-C, low-density lipoprotein cholesterol; HDL-C, high-density lipoprotein cholesterol; TG, triglycerides; VLDL-C, very-low-density lipoprotein cholesterol.

(38%) in patients with isolated HTG, and from 261 to 177 mg/dL (32%) in those with combined dyslipidemia, LDL cholesterol rose from 129 to 152 mg/dL (18%) in the former group and from 162 to 181 mg/dL (12%) in the latter (both changes $p < 0.05$). An even larger percent increase can occur in patients with severe (TG >500 mg/dL; see Fig. 27-3), partly because baseline LDL cholesterol is abnormally depressed in these patients (mean 89 mg/dL[11]), and thus a modest absolute increase in LDL cholesterol (in this study, 40 mg/dL) produced a 45% rise in LDL cholesterol.

When it became clear in the late 1980s that fish oil could increase LDL cholesterol levels in some settings, there was a marked drop-off in the interest in these oils, based on the reasonable assumption at the time that LDL cholesterol levels were the primary determinants of risk for CHD. This increase in LDL cholesterol (which also occurs in patients with severe HTG treated

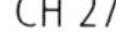

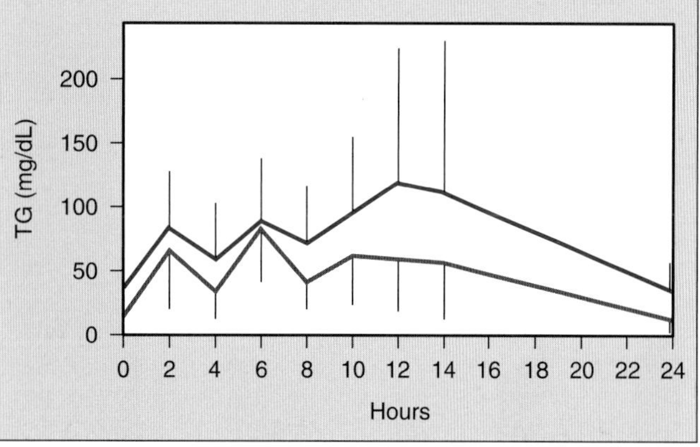

FIGURE 27-4 Effects on the 24-hour time course of serum triglycendes (TG) in eight healthy subjects studied after 4 weeks of treatment with 4.5 g of omega-3 fatty acids (FA)/day *(gray line)* and after 4 weeks of placebo *(red line)*. Three standardized meals of solid food (containing no omega-3 FAs) providing the indicated percent of total kilocalories (shown in parentheses) were given at 8 AM (20%), noon (30%), 5 PM (40%), and 10 PM (10%). The area under the curve was 31% lower after chronic treatment with omega-3 FAs ($P < 0.01$). *From Ref. 93, with permission.*

with gemfibrozil[18] or fenofibrate[19]) is not, however, believed to increase risk for CHD, although this has never been directly tested (as discussed later). Despite the rise in LDL cholesterol observed in these patients at this dose, research continued with omega-3 FAs in an effort to characterize the mechanisms by which they reduced serum TG levels, and to understand why, in some situations, they raised LDL cholesterol.

The rise in LDL cholesterol could result from increases in the number of LDL particles or an increase in LDL particle size (i.e., with each particle carrying more cholesterol). Larger LDL particles are believed to be less atherogenic than the smaller, denser particles characteristic of the HTG state (see Chapter 9).[20] It appears that in some patients with HTG, omega-3 FA treatment will increases both LDL subclasses,[21] whereas in others it increases the larger subclass only,[22] and in yet other situations, it actually decreases the levels of the small dense fraction (Table 27-2).[23] The primary determinant of whether a decrease in TG levels will result in a shift in LDL particle size is related to the ultimate TG concentration reached, not the percent or absolute decrease achieved. Accordingly, LDL size distributions shift away from a preponderance of small dense particles to large buoyant particles when the TG levels fall below about 150 mg/dL.

HDL

Omega-3 FAs typically have a minor high-density lipoprotein (HDL)–raising effect. In the meta-analysis noted above, HDL cholesterol concentrations increased

TABLE 27-2 Effects of Omega-3 Fatty Acids on Low-Density Lipoprotein Size are Related to the TG Level Achieved

Change in TG (mg/dL)	Change in LDL cholesterol (mg/dL)	Change in LDL Size	Reference
558 to 363	102 to 125	None	[21]
232 to 183	162 to 203	↑ larger/mid LDL	[22]
221 to 144	173 to 185	↓ small LDL	[23]

LDL, low-density lipoprotein; TG, triglycende.

(relative to baseline) by 3% to 5% in both normolipidemic ($P < 0.008$) and HTG patients but was not statistically significant in the latter group.[10] In patients with very high TGs (>500 mg/dL), 4 g of omega-3 acid ethyl esters per day produced a 9% increase in HDL cholesterol.[11] Kinetic studies examining the mechanism of this effect in patients with the metabolic syndrome who were treated with 4 g/day of omega-3 acid ethyl esters revealed a combination of slowed production and slowed clearance of apoA-I.[24] These effects essentially cancelled each other, resulting in no net change in HDL cholesterol in this study. HDL_2 cholesterol was, however, increased.

EFFECTS OF OMEGA-3 FATTY ACIDS IN DYSLIPIDEMIC PATIENTS

Primary Hypertriglyceridemia

Omega-3 FAs have been used to treat HTG in virtually all primary disorders. These include familial HTG (type IV hyperlipoproteinemia),[17,25,26] familial hyperchylomicronemia (type V hyperlipoproteinemia),[27–29] dysbetalipoproteinemia (type III hyperlipoproteinemia),[25,30,31] and combined dyslipidemia (type IIb hyperlipoproteinemia).[17,22,32] Serum TG is also reduced in patients with atherogenic dyslipidemia.[33,34] This lipoprotein phenotype (elevated TG and depressed HDL, not one of the original Fredrickson phenotypes) is part of the definition of the metabolic syndrome.[35] There is evidence (from one patient) that omega-3 FA therapy can reduce TG levels even in lipoprotein lipase deficiency (type I hyperlipoproteinemia),[36] although this obviously needs further study. Omega-3 FAs have a minimal impact on the lipid profile in patients with isolated hypercholesterolemia (type IIa hyperlipoproteinemia).[37] In summary, for patients with primary HTG, doses of 3 to 4 g of EPA and DHA will lower serum TG by 25% to 50%, depending on starting levels.

Mixed Hyperlipidemia (Elevated Low-Density Lipoprotein, Triglycerides)

Statins are the cornerstone of therapy for patients with elevated LDL, and omega-3 FAs can also be used safely in patients on statins who continue to have elevations in triglycerides or non-HDL cholesterol. Many patients on statin therapy who have LDL cholesterol levels at goal still have large residual CHD risk because of either uncontrolled triglycerides, elevated non-HDL cholesterol, or low HDL cholesterol. Omega-3 FAs can lower triglycerides by about 25% to 30% and non-HDL cholesterol by 7% to 9% in patients with TGs of 200 to 499 mg/dL on concurrent statin therapy (Fig. 27-5).[38] In this setting, there was a net 4.6% rise in HDL cholesterol and a 3.5% rise in LDL cholesterol.

Secondary Hypertriglyceridemias

Patients with hemodialysis-induced HTG respond to omega-3 FA treatment,[39] but few randomized, controlled trials of more than 1 month's duration are available in this patient population. Similarly, fish oil

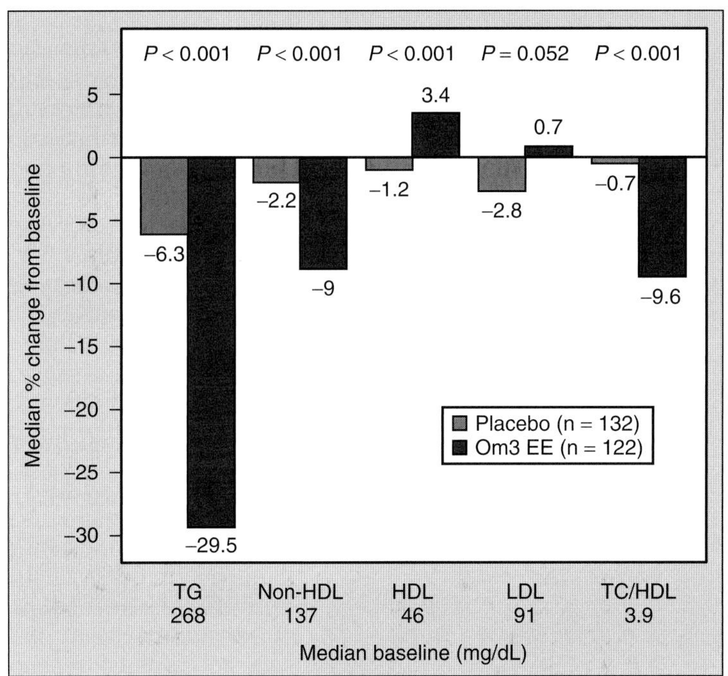

FIGURE 27-5 Effects of 8 weeks of treatment with omega-3 acid ethyl esters (Om3 EE, four 1-g capsules/day; $n = 123$) and placebo (corn oil; $n = 133$) on serum lipid and lipoprotein concentrations in patients with triglyceride levels of 200 to 499 mg/dL while on stable treatment with simvastatin (40 mg/day) (Ref 38). *P*-values compare the change in the placebo group with that in the omega-3 group. LDL, low-density lipoprotein; HDL, high-density lipoprotein; TC, Total serum cholesterol; TG, triglycerides.

treatment in nephrotic syndrome appears to be effective,[40] but placebo-controlled trials are rare. Patients with type 2 diabetes mellitus consistently respond to fish oil supplementation, with a decrease in triglycerides but with no effect on glycemia.[41] There is less experience with patients with type 1 diabetes (likely because HTG is far less common in this form), but it appears that they respond similarly to patients with type 2 diabetes.[42] The effects of omega-3 FAs in other forms of secondary HTG or in other disease or physiologic states (e.g., pregnancy) are less well studied.

Drug-Induced

HTG (or more typically, exacerbation of pre-existing HTG) is a side effect of a variety of drugs. These include estrogen, corticosteroids, β-blockers, thiazide diuretics, retinoids, antiretrovirals, bile acid–binding resins, and some immunosuppressants. Alcohol, whether considered a drug or a food, can also raise serum TG levels. There have been no systematic, well-controlled studies of the ability of omega-3 FAs to ameliorate the TG-raising effects of any of these drugs, with the exception of the antiretrovirals and retinoids. HTG associated with the former can be reduced by 25% to 30% with 1.8 to 2.9 g/day of omega-3 FA,[43] and similar effects have been seen with retinoid-induced (e.g., isotretoinin and etrentinate) HTG with 3 g/day of EPA and DHA.[44]

MECHANISMS UNDERLYING THE LIPID-ALTERING EFFECTS OF OMEGA-3 FATTY ACIDS

Reduced Hepatic Lipogenesis

Lipoprotein kinetic studies in HTG patients given omega-3 FAs have consistently reported reduced appearance (hepatic production/secretion) of VLDL TG.[45] A review of mechanistic studies conducted in fish oil–fed rats demonstrated that omega-3 FAs inhibit hepatic FA synthesis (lipogenesis) and stimulate FA β-oxidation.[45] These effects are summarized in Fig. 27-6. Omega-3 FAs accomplish this by altering levels of a group of nuclear transcription factors (e.g., sterol receptor element–binding protein [SREBP]–1c and peroxisome proliferator–activated receptor [PPAR]–α) that together result in diminished hepatic TG production, reduced VLDL assembly and secretion, and enhanced VLDL TG clearance from the circulation (Fig. 27-7).[46,47] Evidence in humans that omega-3 FA can reduce lipogenesis was obtained in a study in which carbohydrate-induced HTG (which is caused by enhanced TG synthesis in response to increased carbohydrate intake) was completely blocked by omega-3 FAs.[48]

Enhanced Plasma Lipolytic Activity and Endothelial Binding

Studies of LPL activity in postheparin plasma have typically shown no effect of omega-3 FA supplementation,[12,49] although there are exceptions.[50] However, the lipolytic activity of normal (non-heparin-stimulated) plasma is enhanced by omega-3 FA treatment.[51,52] In addition to, but perhaps independent of, enhanced LPL activity, the binding of chylomicron-like particles to the endothelium appears to be enhanced by omega-3 FA treatment.[53] Together these findings suggest that omega-3 FAs stimulate plasma TG clearance. However, numerous studies tracing lipoprotein kinetics have consistently failed to document enhanced VLDL particle (i.e., VLDL apoB) clearance,[45,54] suggesting that although the TG component of these particles may be removed more quickly, the particles themselves are not.

The LDL-raising effect of omega-3 FAs appears to result from the removal of the blockade in VLDL catabolism (which is partly responsible for both the HTG and an unusually low baseline LDL cholesterol

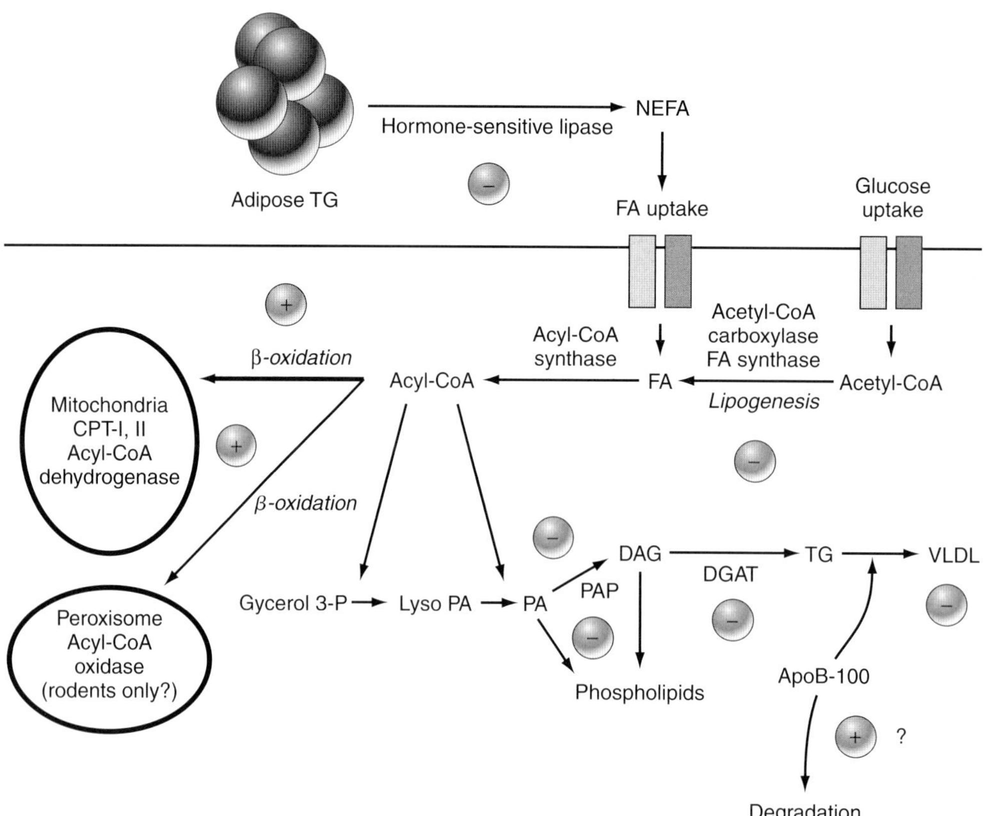

FIGURE 27-6 Potential mechanisms by which omega-3 fatty acids (FAs) influence hepatic triglyceride (TG) metabolism. Feeding omega-3 FA to rats has been shown to inhibit (−) lipogenesis and the activities of diacylglycerol acyl transferase (DGAT), phosphatidic acid phosphohydrolase (PA), and hormone-sensitive lipase; and to stimulate (+) β-oxidation, phospholipid synthesis, and apolipoprotein (apo) B degradation. The end result is a reduced rate of secretion of very-low-density lipoprotein (VLDL) TG. Serum nonesterified fatty acids (NEFA) also provide FAs for TG synthesis, but the extent to which decreases in NEFAs are responsible for the reduction in TG levels is not known. *(From Ref. 45.)*

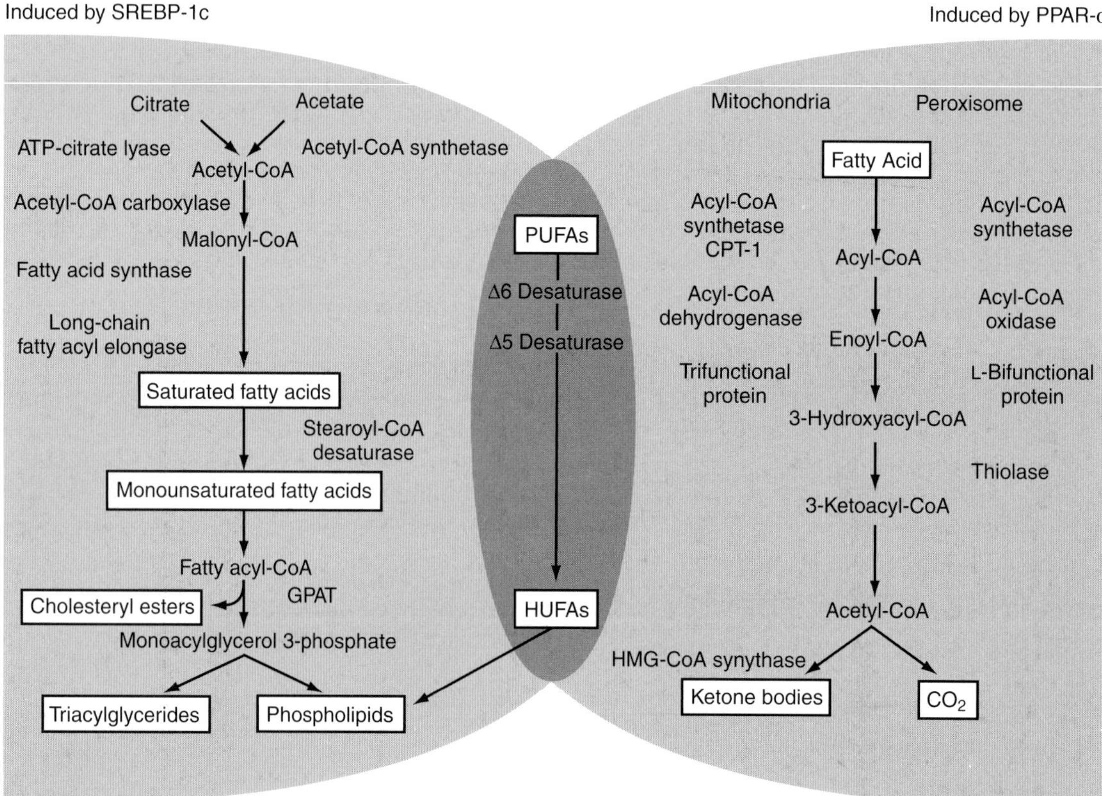

FIGURE 27-7 Regulation of lipogenic and fatty acid oxidative enzyme pathways by omega-3 fatty acids (FAs). Omega-3 FAs can lower expression of sterol regulatory element–binding protein (SREBP)–1c, which reduces triglyceride (TG) synthesis, and simultaneously can increase the expression of peroxisome proliferator-activated receptor (PPAR)–α which increases FA β-oxidation. *(From Ref. 47.)*

seen in these patients). Kinetic studies have shown that treatment with 4 g of omega-3 acid ethyl esters reduces the hepatic production (secretion) of VLDL and enhances the conversion of VLDL to LDL.[54] With the improvement in VLDL clearance (by stimulation of lipolysis), LDL levels rise. There appear to be factors intrinsic to omega-3–enriched VLDL at play as well, because VLDL particles derived from patients taking omega-3 FAs are more susceptible to *in vitro* lipolytic degradation and conversion to LDL than particles taken from the same patients taking placebos.[55] The molecular events underlying this effect are not known.

EFFECTS ON CARDIOVASCULAR EVENTS

There are a wealth of data from population,[56] case–control,[57] prospective cohort,[58,59] and randomized controlled trials[60–62a] supporting a cardioprotective effect of omega-3 FAs that is independent of lipid lowering. The three major randomized controlled trials are summarized below. The Gruppo Italiano per lo Studio della Sopravvivenza nell'Infarto Miocardico (GISSI)–Prevenzione study enrolled 11,234 Italian patients with recent myocardial infarction (MI) (<3 months) and randomized them to 0.85 g/day of EPA and DHA for 3.5 years. There was a significant reduction of 21% in total mortality and 44% in sudden death by the end of the study. The former result was achieved after only 3 months of treatment, and the latter after 4 months (Fig. 27-8).[60] The primary endpoint (death, nonfatal MI, and nonfatal stroke) was significantly reduced by 15% (95% confidence interval [CI], 2% to 26%) with omega-3 FA treatment. Of note, there was a nonsignificant change in the relative risk of nonfatal MI (0.86; 95% CI, 0.70 to 1.18) and nonfatal stroke (1.22; 95% CI, 0.75 to 1.97). During the trial, there were no clinically meaningful changes in lipids, as expected with this low dose of omega-3 FAs. Because of the rapid time course in the reduction of sudden death and total mortality, it was hypothesized that at these doses, the primary mechanism of benefit was antiarrhythmic. Although the GISSI study was a landmark trial because of its sheer size and at-risk population, it did have a few methodological weaknesses, including the use of a usual-care control group instead of a placebo group (i.e., an open-label design).

An other major omega-3 FA trial was the Japan EPA Lipid Intervention Study (JELIS). JELIS tested the hypothesis that the addition of 1.8 g/day of highly purified EPA to statin therapy can reduce the incidence of major cardiovascular events in Japanese patients with hypercholesterolemia.[62] JELIS randomized 14,981 primary prevention patients and 3664 secondary prevention patients in a prospective open-label, blinded endpoint study with a 4.6-year follow-up. Most notable in this study, in addition to the large sample size, was that all patients were given low-dose statin therapy and continued to consume the typical Japanese diet, one rich in omega-3 FAs. At the end of 54 months, the incidence of major coronary events was reduced by 19% (95% CI, 5% to 31%, $P = 0.011$), including the composite endpoint of nonfatal MI, CHD death, unstable angina, and revascularization procedures (Fig. 27-9). The incidence of unstable angina and nonfatal coronary events was significantly reduced by 14% ($P = 0.014$) and 19% ($P = 0.015$), respectively, but the incidence of sudden death and coronary death was unchanged. In JELIS, the trends toward reduction of the incidence of unstable angina and nonfatal coronary events suggest that important plaque-stabilizing properties may also be involved with omega-3 FA therapy. Although risk reduction was 19% for the whole cohort, this remained significant only for the secondary prevention subgroup; it was not significant for the primary prevention cohort ($P = 0.13$). In interpreting JELIS, one must realize that the benefit seen was with combined statin therapy in a population already consuming high amounts of omega-3 FAs. The very low rate of cardiac death in both the intervention and the control groups (8 times lower than in the

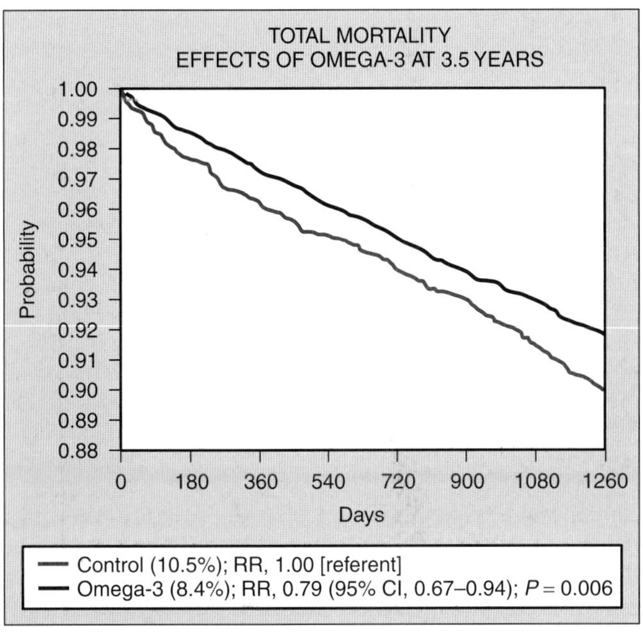

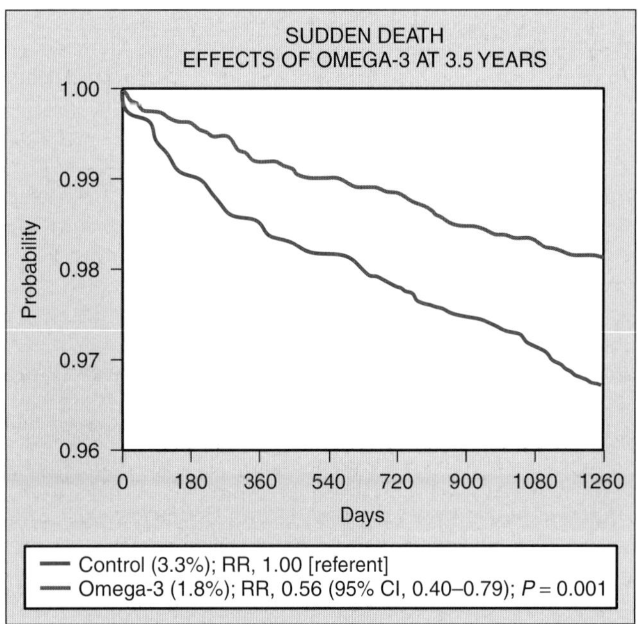

FIGURE 27-8 GISSI Prevenzione Study. Effects of omega-3 acid ethyl esters (1 g, providing 850 mg EPA and DHA) versus usual care on total mortality *(left)* and sudden death *(right)*. *From Ref. 60, with permission.*
CI, confidence interval; RR, relative risk.

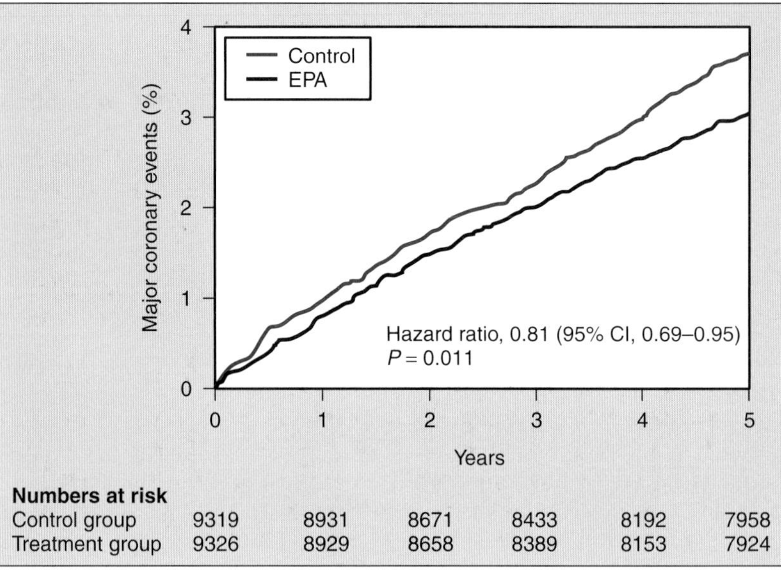

FIGURE 27-9 Major coronary event rates in the Japan EPA Lipid Intervention Study (JELIS). Hypercholesterolemic patients on statin therapy were randomized to usual care with or without 1.8 g of EPA and followed for a mean of 4.6 years. Kaplan–Meier estimates for the control and EPA groups are shown for all 18,645 patients. *From Ref. 62, with permission.*

GISSI-Prevenzione study), supports the view that intakes of around 800 to 1000 mg/day of EPA and DHA (typical of this Japanese population[59]) provide significant protection against fatal CHD.

The GISSI–Heart Failure (GISSI-HF) trial randomized 6,975 patients with stage II-IV congestive heart failure (CHF) of any etiology to either 1 g/day omega-3 FA (0.85 g EPA and DHA) or placebo for a median of 3.9 years.[62a] The primary endpoints were time to death, and time to death or hospitalization for cardiovascular reasons. Total mortality was reduced by 9% (adjusted hazard ratio [HR], 0.91; 95.5% CI, 0.833 to 0.998; $P = 0.041$), and the combined endpoint of total mortality and hospitalizations for cardiovascular reasons was reduced by 8% (adjusted HR, 0.92; 99% CI, 0.849 to 0.999; $P = 0.009$). The Kaplan–Meier curves began to diverge around 2 years. Although there was a significant reduction in cardiovascular mortality from any cause (adjusted HR, 0.90; 95% CI, 0.81 to 0.99; $P = 0.045$), the reduction in sudden death (adjusted HR, 0.93; 95% CI, 0.79 to 1.08) did not reach statistical significance ($P = 0.333$). Most of the cardiovascular deaths in the study were due to either worsening heart failure or presumed arrhythmic deaths. Similar to the results of GISSI-Prevenzione in post-MI patients, there was no significant reduction in MI or stroke in GISSI-HF. Interstingly, a nested study within the GISSI-HF trial using rosuvastatin showed no benefit on clinical outcomes. The mechanisms by which EPA and DHA may slow the progression of HF are unclear but may include improved oxygen utilization, reduced cardiac fibrosis, and improved left ventricular function.[62b]

It is beyond the scope of this review to cover in detail the proposed non-lipoprotein-related mechanisms of action for omega-3 FAs. Briefly, however, these include reductions in risk for fatal arrhythmias,[63] enhanced plaque stability,[64] reductions in heart rate,[65] improved endothelial function,[66] and a variety of antiatherosclerotic and antithrombotic processes.[67] The intakes associated with these benefits are typically below 1 g/day, a dose with minimal[15,68] to no[69] TG-lowering effects. These doses are, however, 2 to 4 times higher than current U.S. dietary intakes.[70] The interested reader is referred to recent reviews.[71,72]

SPECIAL POPULATIONS—IMPLANTABLE CARDIAC DEFIBRILLATORS

Although much evidence has accumulated on the role of omega-3 FAs in the prevention of sudden death, ventricular fibrillation (VF), ventricular tachycardia (VT), and atrial fibrillation, their use at this time in these conditions requires further evaluation. Of special note have been three studies in which the efficacy of omega-3 FAs in suppressing VT/VF in patients with implantable cardioverter defibrillators (ICDs) was tested.[73–75] The primary outcomes of these studies were consistent: there was no effect of omega-3 FA supplementation on the time of first ICD discharge. There were, however, differences in secondary outcomes, with Leaf et al.[73] and Brouwer et al.[75] reporting benefits in some groups, and Raitt et al.[74] reporting some adverse effects in a subgroup of patients with a history of VT. The somewhat confused outcomes of these trials have been critically reviewed.[63] Available data to date do not suggest an important therapeutic effect of omega-3 FAs in the ICD patient population.

AVAILABLE OMEGA-3 FATTY ACID PRODUCTS

Although there are a myriad of omega-3 FA dietary supplements on the market, as of 2008 there was only one omega-3 FA product approved by the Food and Drug Administration (FDA) for the treatment of HTG (Lovaza, BlaxaSmithKline, Research Triangle Park, NC; formerly Omacor, Reliant Pharmaceuticals, Liberty Corner, NJ). Referred to generically as omega-3 acid ethyl esters, this product is indicated as adjunct therapy along with diet and exercise for the treatment of severe HTG (TG >500 mg/dL). It has also been found to be effective and safe in reducing TG and non-HDL cholesterol in patients with TG or greater than 200 mg/dL despite ongoing statin therapy,[38] but it is not currently indicated in this population. The approved dose of omega-3 acid ethyl esters is four 1-g capsules per day, which provides 3.4 g of EPA and DHA. To obtain this dose of EPA and DHA from dietary supplements (which range from 65% to 20% EPA and DHA per 1-g capsule) would require 5 to 17 capsules per day, respectively. It should be noted, however, that as an FDA-approved drug, omega-3 acid ethyl esters have been tested for purity, potency, safety, and efficacy, and its manufacturing processes are subject to FDA investigation. The same cannot be said about dietary supplements, which are not subject to the same level of regulatory oversight and are not intended to treat disease. That said, a Consumers' Union evaluation of 16 fish oil supplements reported that label potencies for EPA and DHA were generally achieved, and that the capsules were free of pollutants.[76] Consequently, supplements are likely to be safe and may be effective in TG lowering, but the large number of capsules required to achieve TG-lowering doses of EPA and DHA may hinder compliance. The additional non–omega-3 FAs contained in supplements also provide extra, unneeded calories. Ultimately, direct evidence for the efficacy of most specific supplements is generally lacking.

As noted earlier, ALA is the plant-derived, shorter chain omega-3 FA. Since it can be grown in essentially unlimited amounts (flaxseed oil is 55% ALA), there has been much interest in whether it can substitute for EPA and DHA as a TG-lowering agent. The short answer is that it cannot. In a 2006 meta-analysis of 14 studies, ALA was found to be ineffective at lowering serum TG levels or altering other cardiovascular risk factors.[77] In one study there was a reported TG-lowering effect,[78] but it required 38 g/day of ALA (normal intakes are about 1.5 g/day). Using doses of ALA generally recommended as safe (3 to 4 g) consistently demonstrates no effects on triglycerides.

SAFETY AND TOLERABILITY OF OMEGA-3 FATTY ACIDS

The safety of EPA and DHA was assumed from the outset, given that Inuit populations have been consuming gram quantities of these fatty acids from seal, whale, and fish for millennia and that the Japanese traditionally consume 800 to 1000 mg/day, or about eight times the typical Western intake.[59] Neither of these populations suffers any obvious harm from this intake; indeed, the latter are remarkably free of cardiovascular disease.

Because omega-3 FAs can inhibit platelet function through competition with arachidonic acid for incorporation into membrane phospholipids and for conversion to eicosanoids by cyclo-oxygenase,[79] concerns regarding bleeding exist, but these concerns have been more theoretical than real. A review of several studies in which lipid-lowering doses of EPA and DHA had been given to patients undergoing major vascular surgery revealed no evidence for clinically significant bleeding, even when combined with other antiplatelet drugs.[80] The combined effects of omega-3 FAs and clopidogrel have not been evaluated.

Only omega-3 acid ethyl esters have been formally evaluated by the FDA for safety. The package insert lists no contraindications (other than hypersensitivity to the agent) and no warnings, and the only precautions of note are recommendations to periodically monitor alanine aminotransferase and LDL, and to watch for signs of bleeding in patients also taking omega-3 acid ethyl esters and anticoagulants. The only minor clinical side effects include occasional eructation (<5%) or fish aftertaste (<3%).

There are several advantages in choosing to use omega-3 FAs with statins versus combining statins with niacin or fibrates in patients. A particular advantage is that there are no drug–drug interactions between statins and omega-3 acid ethyl esters,[81] and they do not worsen blood glucose control (as can occur with niacin[82]) or creatinine and homocysteine levels (as can occur with fibrates[83]). Omega-3 FAs may thus have particular advantages in HTG patients with diabetes or renal insufficiency, or who are taking multiple medications known to interact with the cytochrome P450 system, including statins. Disadvantages include the need for four capsules, which can be given either once a day or twice a day. Although data exist for the benefits of using omega-3 FA ethyl esters with simvastatin in JELTS,[62] the dose used in that study was only 1.8 g/day of pure EPA, and it produced negligible effects on serum lipids. It remains to be determined whether the doses of omega-3 fatty acid ethyl esters necessary for TG reduction (4 g/day) can result in cardiovascular risk reduction when used with statin therapy.

BLOOD OMEGA-3 FATTY ACID LEVELS AS A RISK FACTOR

Target blood levels of EPA and DHA have also been suggested as markers of cardioprotection.[84] For example, red blood cell membrane levels EPA and DHA of greater than 8% appear to be associated with the lowest risk for CHD death[84] and are associated with reduced risk for acute coronary syndromes. In contrast, patients with red blood cell membrane EPA and DHA levels less than 4% are considered to have higher risk for cardiovascular events.[85] Low blood omega-3 FA levels are associated with an increased risk of sudden cardiac death.[58] Optimal membrane levels of omega-3 FA usually are achieved with the consumption of 1 to 1.5 g of EPA and DHA daily,[84] an intake not dissimilar from that in Japan.

CLINICAL APPLICATIONS

As noted previously, the only FDA-approved use for omega-3 FAs is for the treatment of very high TG levels (>500 mg/dL) for which the indicated dose is 4 g/day EPA and DHA ethyl esters. Although they have been shown to be effective in reducing TG and non-HDL cholesterol in patients taking statins whose TG levels are between 200 to 400 mg/dL, they are currently not indicated for this purpose. It is important to note that clinically significant reductions in TGs would not be expected from lower doses of omega-3 acid ethyl esters because although a dose–response relationship exists, most of it occurs above the 3- to 4-g/day level.[86] In the United States, these agents are also not indicated for the secondary prevention of CHD, although this is the case in Europe.

The American Heart Association (AHA) currently recommends that patients with CHD consume about 1 g/day of a combination of EPA and DHA per day.[87,88] This is based largely on the results of the GISSI-Prevenzione study in which 850 mg was used. For individuals without known CHD or HTG, the AHA recommends the consumption of about two (preferably oily) fish meals per week. This would translate into 450 to 500 mg/day EPA and DHA and would raise red blood cell EPA and DHA levels by at least 50%.[89] Even half of this intake has been suggested as a cardioprotective target in the general population.[71] Given the modest reductions in total mortality and cardiovascular hospitalizations in the GISSI-HF trial, 1 g of EPA and DHA should also be considered for most CHF patients.

CONCLUSIONS

Evidence continues to accumulate for a beneficial effect of omega-3 FA in forestalling CHD. Future large-scale, placebo-controlled clinical event endpoint trials are needed to confidently establish the utility of these nutrients in cardiovascular protection and to determine whether TG-lowering doses of omega-3 FAs (3–4 g/day) are equally or even more effective at reducing CHD risk than lower doses.

REFERENCES

1. Dyerberg J, Bang HO, Stoffersen E, et al: Eicosapentaenoic acid and prevention of thrombosis and atherosclerosis? *Lancet* 1978;i:117–119.
2. Dyerberg J: Linolenate-derived polyunsaturated fatty acids and prevention of atherosclerosis. *Nutr Rev* 1986;44:125–134.
3. Bang HO, Dyerberg J: Lipid metabolism and ischemic heart disease in Greenland Eskimos. *Adv Nutr Res* 1980;3:1–22.
4. Dyerberg J, Bang HO, Hjorne N: Fatty acid composition of the plasma lipids in Greenland Eskimos. *Am J Clin Nutr* 1975;28: 958–966.
5. Ahrens EH Jr, Insull W Jr, Hirsch J, et al: The effect on human serum-lipids of a dietary fat, highly unsaturated, but poor in essential fatty acids. *Lancet* 1959;i:115–119.
6. Bronsgeest-Schoute HC, van Gent CM, Luten JB, Ruiter A: The effect of various intakes of omega-3 fatty acids on the blood lipid composition in healthy human subjects. *Am J Clin Nutr* 1981;34:1752–1757.
7. Mohrhauer H, Holman RT: The effect of dose level of essential fatty acids upon fatty acid composition of rat liver. *J Lipid Res* 1963;58:151–159.
8. Harris WS, Connor WE, McMurry MP: The comparative reductions of the plasma lipids and lipoproteins by dietary polyunsaturated fats: Salmon oil versus vegetable oils. *Metabolism* 1983;32:179–184.
9. Phillipson BE, Rothrock DW, Connor WE, et al: Reduction of plasma lipids, lipoproteins and apoproteins by dietary fish oils in patients with hypertriglyceridemia. *N Engl J Med* 1985;312: 1210–1216.
10. Harris WS: n-3 Fatty acids and serum lipoproteins: Human studies. *Am J Clin Nutr* 1997;65 (Suppl):1645S–1654S.
11. Harris WS, Ginsberg HN, Arunakul N, et al: Safety and efficacy of Omacor in severe hypertriglyceridemia. *J Cardiovasc Risk* 1997;4:385–392.
12. Harris WS, Connor WE, Alam N, Illingworth DR: Reduction of postprandial triglyceridemia in humans by dietary omega-3 fatty acids. *J Lipid Res* 1988;29:1451–1460.
13. Westphal S, Orth M, Ambrosch A, et al: Postprandial chylomicrons and VLDLs in severe hypertriacylglycerolemia are lowered more effectively than are chylomicron remnants after treatment with n-3 fatty acids. *Am J Clin Nutr* 2000;71:914–920.
14. Weintraub MS, Zechner R, Brown A, et al: Dietary polyunsaturated fats of the w-6 and w-3 series reduce postprandial lipoprotein levels. *J Clin Invest* 1988;82:1884–1893.
15. Roche HM, Gibney MJ: Postprandial triacylglycerolaemia: The effect of low-fat dietary treatment with and without fish oil supplementation. *Eur J Clin Nutr* 1996;50:617–624.
16. Agren JJ, Hanninen O, Julkunen A, et al: Fish diet, fish oil and docosahexaenoic acid rich oil lower fasting and postprandial plasma lipid levels. *Eur J Clin Nutr* 1996;50:765–771.
17. Harris WS, Dujovne CA, Zucker M, Johnson B: Effects of a low saturated fat, low cholesterol fish oil supplement in hypertriglyceridemic patients: A placebo-controlled trial. *Ann Intern Med* 1988;109:465–470.
18. Leaf DA, Connor WE, Illingworth DR, et al: The hypolipidemic effects of gemfibrozil in type V hyperlipidemia. *JAMA* 1989;262: 3154–3160.
19. Goldberg AC, Schonfeld G, Feldman EB, et al: Fenofibrate for the treatment of type IV and V hyperlipoproteinemias: a double-blind, placebo-controlled multicenter US study. *Clin Ther* 1989;11:69–83.
20. Austin MA, Breslow JL, Hennekens CH, et al: Low-density lipoprotein subclass patterns and risk of myocardial infarction. *JAMA* 1988;260:1917–1921.
21. Lu G, Windsor SL, Harris WS: Omega-3 fatty acids alter lipoprotein subfraction distributions and the *in vitro* conversion of very-low-density lipoproteins to low-density lipoproteins. *J Nutr Biochem* 1999;10:151–158.
22. Calabresi L, Donati D, Pazzucconi F, et al: Omacor in familial combined hyperlipidemia: Effects on lipids and low-density lipoprotein subclasses. *Atherosclerosis* 2000;148:387–396.
23. Minihane AM, Khan S, Leigh-Firbank EC, et al: ApoE polymorphism and fish oil supplementation in subjects with an atherogenic lipoprotein phenotype. *Arterioscler Thromb Vasc Biol* 2000;20:1990–1997.
24. Chan DC, Watts GF, Nguyen MN, Barrett PH: Factorial study of the effect of n-3 fatty acid supplementation and atorvastatin on the kinetics of HDL apolipoproteins A-I and A-II in men with abdominal obesity. *Am J Clin Nutr* 2006;84:37–43.
25. Otto C, Ritter MM, Soennichsen AC, et al: Effects of n-3 fatty acids and fenofibrate on lipid and hemorrheological parameters in familial dysbetalipoproteinemia and familial hypertriglyceridemia. *Metabolism* 1996;45:1305–1311.
26. Harris WS, Windsor SL, Dujovne CA: Effects of four doses of n-3 fatty acids given to hyperlipidemic patients for six months. *J Am Coll Nutr* 1991;10:220–227.
27. Singer P, Wirth M, Berger I, et al: Influence on serum lipids, lipoproteins and blood pressure of mackerel and herring diet in patients with type IV and V hyperlipoproteinemia. *Atherosclerosis* 1985;56:111–118.
28. Pschierer V, Richter WO, Schwandt P: Primary chylomicronemia in patients with severe familial hypertriglyceridemia responds to long-term treatment with (n-3) fatty acids. *J Nutr* 1995;125:1490–1494.
29. Richter WO, Jacob BG, Ritter MM, Schwandt P: Treatment of primary chylomicronemia due to familial hypertriglyceridemia by ω-3 fatty acids. *Metabolism* 1992;41:1100–1105.
30. Dallongeville J, Boulet L, Davignon J, Lussier-Cacan S: Fish oil supplementation reduces β-very-low-density lipoprotein in type III dysbetalipoproteinemia. *Arterioscler Thromb* 1991;11:864–871.
31. Molgaard J, von Schenck H, Lassvik C, et al: Effect of fish oil treatment on plasma lipoproteins in type III hyperlipoproteinaemia. *Atherosclerosis* 1990;81:1–9.
32. Grundt H, Nilsen DW, Hetland O, et al: Improvement of serum lipids and blood pressure during intervention with n-3 fatty acids was not associated with changes in insulin levels in subjects with combined hyperlipidaemia. *J Intern Med* 1995;237:249–259.
33. Leigh-Firbank EC, Minihane AM, Leake DS, et al: Eicosapentaenoic acid and docosahexaenoic acid from fish oils: Differential associations with lipid responses. *Br J Nutr* 2002;87:435–445.
34. Chan DC, Watts GF, Mori TA, et al: Randomized controlled trial of the effect of n-3 fatty acid supplementation on the metabolism of apolipoprotein B-100 and chylomicron remnants in men with visceral obesity. *Am J Clin Nutr* 2003;77:300–307.
35. Grundy SM: Metabolic syndrome: A multiplex cardiovascular risk factor. *J Clin Endocrinol Metab* 2007;92:399–404.
36. Rouis M, Dugi KA, Previato L, et al: Therapeutic response to medium-chain triglycerides and omega-3 fatty acids in a patient with the familial chylomicronemia syndrome. *Arterioscler Thromb Vasc Biol* 1997;17:1400–1406.
37. Demke DM, Peters GR, Linet OI, et al: Effects of a fish oil concentrate in patients with hypercholesterolemia. *Atherosclerosis* 1988;70:73–80.
38. Davidson MH, Stein EA, Bays HE, et al: Efficacy and tolerability of adding prescription omega-3 fatty acids 4 g/d to simvastatin

40 mg/d in hypertriglyceridemic patients: An 8-week, randomized, double-blind, placebo-controlled study. *Clin Ther* 2007;29: 1354–1367.

39. Turpeinen O, Karvonen MJ, Pekkarinen M, et al: Dietary prevention of coronary heart disease: The Finnish Mental Hospital Study. *Int. J Epidemiol* 1979;8:99–118.
40. Hall AV, Parbtani A, Clark WF, et al: Omega-3 fatty acid supplementation in primary nephrotic syndrome: Effects on plasma lipids and coagulopathy. *J Am Soc Nephrol* 1992;3:1321–1329.
41. Montori VM, Farmer A, Wollan PC, Dinneen SF: Fish oil supplementation in type 2 diabetes. A quantitative systematic review. *Diabetes Care* 2000;23:1407–1415.
42. Mori TA, Vandongen R, Masarei JR, et al: Comparison of diets supplemented with fish oil or olive oil on plasma lipoproteins in insulin-dependent diabetics. *Metabolism* 1991;40:241–246.
43. De Truchis P, Kirstetter M, Perier A, et al: Reduction in triglyceride level with N-3 polyunsaturated fatty acids in HIV-infected patients taking potent antiretroviral therapy: A randomized prospective study. *J Acquir Immune Defic Syndr* 2007;44: 278–285.
44. Ashley JM, Lowe NJ, Borok ME, Alfin-Slater RB: Fish oil supplementation results in decreased hypertriglyceridemia in patients with psoriasis undergoing etretinate or acitretin therapy. *J Am Acad Dermatol* 1988;19:76–82.
45. Harris WS, Bulchandani D: Why do omega-3 fatty acids lower serum triglycerides? *Curr Opin Lipidol* 2006;17:387–393.
46. Davidson MH: Mechanisms for the hypotriglyceridemic effect of marine omega-3 fatty acids. *Am J Cardiol* 2006;98:27i–33i.
47. Nakamura MT, Cheon Y, Li Y, Nara TY: Mechanisms of regulation of gene expression by fatty acids. *Lipids* 2004;39:1077–1083.
48. Harris WS, Connor WE, Inkeles SB, Illingworth DR: Dietary omega-3 fatty acids prevent carbohydrate-induced hypertriglyceridemia. *Metabolism* 1984;33:1016–1019.
49. Nozaki S, Garg A, Vega GL, Grundy SM: Postheparin lipolytic activity and plasma lipoprotein response to ω-3 polyunsaturated fatty acids in patients with primary hypertriglyceridemia. *Am J Clin Nutr* 1991;53:638–642.
50. Khan S, Minihane AM, Talmud PJ, et al: Dietary long-chain n-3 PUFAs increase LPL gene expression in adipose tissue of subjects with an atherogenic lipoprotein phenotype. *J Lipid Res* 2002;43:979–985.
51. Park Y, Harris WS: Omega-3 fatty acid supplementation accelerates chylomicron triglyceride clearance. *J Lipid Res* 2002;44: 455–463.
52. Harris WS, Lu G, Rambjor GS, et al: Influence of n-3 fatty acid supplementation on the endogenous activities of plasma lipases. *Am J Clin Nutr* 1997;66:254–260.
53. Park Y, Jones PG, Harris WS: Triacylglycerol-rich lipoprotein margination: A potential surrogate for whole-body lipoprotein lipase activity and effects of eicosapentaenoic and docosahexaenoic acids. *Am J Clin Nutr* 2004;80:45–50.
54. Chan DC, Watts GF, Barrett PHR, et al: Regulatory effects of HMG CoA reductase inhibitor and fish oils on apolipoprotein B-100 kinetics in insulin-resistant obese male subjects with dyslipidemia. *Diabetes* 2002;51:2377–2386.
55. Harris WS, Lu G, Windsor SL: Fish oil accelerates the conversion of VLDL to LDL *in vitro* [abstract]. *J Invest Med* 1995;43:302A.
56. He K, Song Y, Daviglus ML, et al: Accumulated evidence on fish consumption and coronary heart disease mortality: A meta-analysis of cohort studies. *Circulation* 2004;109:2705–2711.
57. Siscovick DS, Raghunathan TE, King I, et al: Dietary intake and cell membrane levels of long-chain n-3 polyunsaturated fatty acids and the risk of primary cardiac arrest. *JAMA* 1995;274:1363–1367.
58. Albert CM, Campos H, Stampfer MJ, et al: Blood levels of long-chain n-3 fatty acids and the risk of sudden death. *N Engl J Med* 2002;346:1113–1118.
59. Iso H, Kobayashi M, Ishihara J, et al: Intake of fish and n3 fatty acids and risk of coronary heart disease among Japanese: The Japan Public Health Center-Based (JPHC) Study Cohort I. *Circulation* 2006;113:195–202.
60. Marchioli R, Barzi F, Bomba E, et al: Early protection against sudden death by n-3 polyunsaturated fatty acids after myocardial infarction: Time-course analysis of the results of the Gruppo Italiano per lo Studio della Sopravvivenza nell'Infarto Miocardico (GISSI)-Prevenzione. *Circulation* 2002;105:1897–1903.
61. Burr ML, Fehily AM, Gilbert JF, et al: Effects of changes in fat, fish, and fibre intakes on death and myocardial reinfarction: Diet and Reinfarction Trial (DART). *Lancet* 1989;2:757–761.
62. Yokoyama M, Origasa H, Matsuzaki M, et al: Effects of eicosapentaenoic acid on major coronary events in hypercholesterolaemic patients (JELIS): A randomised open-label, blinded endpoint analysis. *Lancet* 2007;369:1090–1098.

62a. GISSI-HF Investigators: Effect of n-3 polyunsaturated fatty acids in patients with chronic heart failure (the GISSI-HF trial): a randomised, double-blind, placebo-controlled trial. *Lancet.* In press.

62b. Stanley WC, Recchia FA, Okere IC: Metabolic therapies for heart disease: Fish for prevention and treatment of cardiac failure? *Cardiovasc Res* 2005;68:175–177.

63. Reiffel JA, McDonald A: Antiarrhythmic effects of omega-3 fatty acids. *Am J Cardiol* 2006;98:50i–60i.
64. Thies F, Garry JM, Yaqoob P, et al: Association of n-3 polyunsaturated fatty acids with stability of atherosclerotic plaques: A randomised controlled trial. *Lancet* 2003;361:477–485.
65. Mozaffarian D, Geelen A, Brouwer IA, et al: Effect of fish oil on heart rate in humans: A meta-analysis of randomized controlled trials. *Circulation* 2005;112:1945–1952.
66. Nestel P, Shige H, Pomeroy S, et al: The n-3 fatty acids eicosapentaenoic acid and docosahexaenoic acid increase systemic arterial compliance in humans. *Am J Clin Nutr* 2002;76: 326–330.
67. Robinson JG, Stone NJ: Antiatherosclerotic and antithrombotic effects of omega-3 fatty acids. *Am J Cardiol* 2006;98:39i–49i.
68. Schwellenbach LJ, Olson KL, McConnell KJ, et al: The triglyceride-lowering effects of a modest dose of docosahexaenoic acid alone versus in combination with low dose eicosapentaenoic acid in patients with coronary artery disease and elevated triglycerides. *J Am Coll Nutr* 2006;25:480–485.
69. Radack KL, Deck CC, Huster GA: n-3 fatty acid effects on lipids, lipoproteins, and apolipoproteins at very low doses: Results of a randomized controlled trial in hypertriglyceridemic subjects. *Am J Clin Nutr* 1990;51:599–605.
70. Psota TL, Gebauer SK, Kris-Etherton P: Dietary omega-3 fatty acid intake and cardiovascular risk. *Am J Cardiol* 2006;98: 3i–18i.
71. Mozaffarian D, Rimm EB: Fish intake, contaminants, and human health: Evaluating the risks and the benefits. *JAMA* 2006;296:1885–1899.
72. Jacobson TA: Secondary prevention of coronary artery disease with omega-3 fatty acids. *Am J Cardiol* 2006;98:61i–70i.
73. Leaf A, Albert CM, Josephson M, et al: Prevention of fatal arrhythmias in high-risk subjects by fish oil n-3 fatty acid intake. *Circulation* 2005;112:2762–2768.
74. Raitt MH, Connor WE, Morris C, et al: Fish oil supplementation and risk of ventricular tachycardia and ventricular fibrillation in patients with implantable defibrillators: A randomized controlled trial. *JAMA* 2005;293:2884–2891.
75. Brouwer IA, Zock PL, Camm AJ, et al: Effect of fish oil on ventricular tachyarrhythmia and death in patients with implantable cardioverter defibrillators: The Study on Omega-3 Fatty Acids and Ventricular Arrhythmia (SOFA) randomized trial. *JAMA* 2006;295:2613–2619.
76. Omega-3 oil: Fish or pills? Consumer Reports 2003;30–32.
77. Wendland E, Farmer A, Glasziou P, Neil A: Effect of alpha linolenic acid on cardiovascular risk markers: A systematic review. *Heart* 2006;92:166–169.
78. Singer P, Berger I, Wirth M, et al: Slow desaturation and elongation of linoleic and α-linolenic acids as a rationale of eicosapentaenoic acid-rich diet to lower blood pressure and serum lipids in normal, hypertensive and hyperlipemic subjects. *Prostaglandins Leukot Med* 1986;24:173–193.
79. Calder PC: n-3 polyunsaturated fatty acids, inflammation, and inflammatory diseases. *Am J Clin Nutr* 2006;83:1505S–1519S.
80. Harris WS: Expert opinion: Omega-3 fatty acids and bleeding—cause for concern? *Am J Cardiol* 2007;99:S44–S46.
81. McKenney JM, Swearingen D, Di Spirito M, et al: Study of the pharmacokinetic interaction between simvastatin and prescription omega-3-acid ethyl esters. *J Clin Pharmacol* 2006;46: 785–791.
82. Elam MB, Hunninghake DB, Davis KB, et al: Effect of niacin on lipid and lipoprotein levels and glycemic control in patients with diabetes and peripheral arterial disease. The ADMIT study: A randomized trial. *JAMA* 2000;284:1263–1270.
83. Keech A, Simes RJ, Barter P, et al: Effects of long-term fenofibrate therapy on cardiovascular events in 9795 people with type 2 diabetes mellitus (the FIELD study): Randomised controlled trial. *Lancet* 2005;366:1849–1861.

84. Harris WS, von Schacky C: The Omega-3 Index: A new risk factor for death from coronary heart disease? *Prev Med* 2004;39: 212–220.
85. Block RC, Harris WS, Reid KJ, et al: EPA and DHA in blood cell membranes from acute coronary syndrome patients and controls. *Atherosclerosis* 2007;197:821–828.
86. Harris WS: n-3 fatty acids and lipoproteins: Comparison of results from human and animal studies. *Lipids* 1996;31: 243–252.
87. Kris-Etherton PM, Harris WS, Appel LJ: Fish consumption, fish oil, omega-3 fatty acids, and cardiovascular disease. *Circulation* 2002;106:2747–2757.
88. Smith SC Jr, Allen J, Blair SN, et al: AHA/ACC guidelines for secondary prevention for patients with coronary and other atherosclerotic vascular disease: 2006 update. *Circulation* 2006;113:2363–2372.
89. Harris WS, Pottala JV, Sands SA, Jones PG: Comparison of the effects of fish and fish-oil capsules on the n 3 fatty acid content of blood cells and plasma phospholipids. *Am J Clin Nutr* 2007;86:1621–1625.
90. Ackman RG: Nutritional composition of fats in seafoods. *Prog Food Nutr Sci* 1989;13:161–289.
91. Hepburn FN, Exler J, Weihrauch JL: Provisional tables on the content of omega-3 fatty acids and other fat components of selected foods. *J Am Diet Assoc* 1986;86:788–793.
92. Harris WS, Poston WC, Haddock CK: Tissue n-3 and n-6 fatty acids and risk for coronary heart disease events. *Atherosclerosis* 2007;193:1–10.
93. Harris WS, Muzio F: Fish oil reduces postprandial triglyceride concentrations without accelerating lipid emulsion removal rates. *Am J Clin Nutr* 1993;58:68–74.
94. The USDA Nutrient Data Laboratory: Available at http://www.nal.usda.gov/fnic/foodcomp/.

CHAPTER 28

Endocannabinoid Receptor Blockers

Jean-Pierre Després

OBESITY AND THE ATHEROGENIC DYSLIPIDEMIA OF INSULIN RESISTANCE: IMPORTANCE OF BODY FAT DISTRIBUTION AND VISCERAL ADIPOSITY

Although obesity is recognized as a health hazard,[1,2] physicians have been challenged by the absence of complications in some patients despite their very significant obesity. On the other hand, some moderately overweight individuals are characterized by a whole cluster of atherogenic and diabetogenic metabolic abnormalities including type 2 diabetes and/or clinical signs of cardiovascular disease (CVD). In this regard, numerous imaging and metabolic studies conducted over the last two decades have revealed that, in both men and women, the amount of visceral (intra-abdominal) adipose tissue, which can be reliably assessed by imaging techniques such as computed tomography, is a critical correlate of the presence of a constellation of atherogenic and diabetogenic metabolic abnormalities.[3–8] Thus, although excess fatness per se increases the risk of chronic complications, there is compelling evidence that viscerally obese patients represent the subgroup of obese patients characterized by the most severe metabolic abnormalities (Fig. 28-1).

ATHEROGENIC DYSLIPIDEMIA OF VISCERAL OBESITY: THE "PORTAL" THEORY

Numerous studies have been conducted to shed some light on the factors explaining the link between abdominal obesity (particularly excess visceral adiposity) and insulin resistance/atherogenic dyslipidemia (Fig. 28-2). First, there is ample evidence showing that increased adipose tissue mass is associated with impaired *in vivo* insulin action. However, Reaven and colleagues[9–13] have documented on numerous occasions that some obese patients are insulin sensitive, whereas some apparently normal-weight individuals nevertheless show significant insulin resistance. In this regard, studies that have used imaging techniques to measure subcutaneous versus visceral adipose tissue accumulation have shown that among individuals with the same amount of total body fat or with similar levels of obesity, those with a selective excess of intra-abdominal, or visceral, adipose tissue had the most severe insulin-resistant state.[4,7,14,15] Because of the specific metabolic properties of adipose cells from the visceral depot and their strategic anatomic location (some of this fat depot is drained by the portal vein), an increased accumulation of hyperlipolytic visceral adipose tissue could be associated with impaired free fatty acid (FFA) metabolism, hypertrophied visceral adipocytes have been shown to be resistant to the antilipolytic effect of insulin and also are characterized by impaired FFA esterification.[16,17] Such flux of FFA toward the liver favors an increased secretion of triglyceride-rich lipoproteins, reduced hepatic degradation of apolipoprotein B (as there is a need to increase hepatic triglyceride output to limit liver fat infiltration leading to steatosis) and of insulin leading to hyperapolipoprotein B and hyperinsulinemia, and increased hepatic glucose production contributing to glucose intolerance.[18,19]

Obese patients with an excess accumulation of visceral (intra-abdominal) adipose tissue are also characterized by an exaggerated postprandial triglyceride response,[3] as the increased number of very-low-density lipoprotein (VLDL) particles found in patients with fasting hypertriglyceridemia compete with dietary chylomicrons

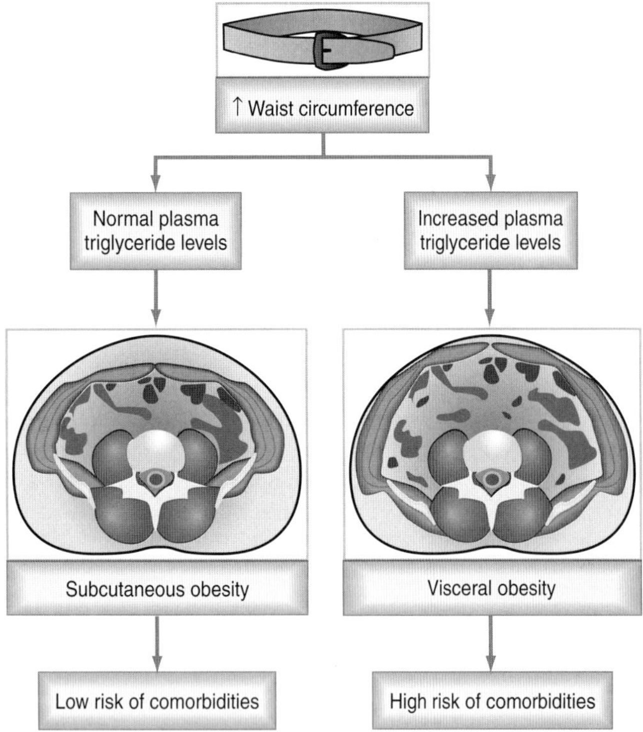

FIGURE 28-1 Importance of measuring waist circumference and fasting plasma triglyceride levels to identify in clinical practice individuals with high levels of visceral (intra-abdominal) adipose tissue. Under this approach, measuring waist circumference is a critical first step to find individuals with high levels of abdominal fat. As a second step to distinguish between subcutaneous versus visceral abdominal obesity, the clinician should pay attention to fasting triglyceride concentrations. If fasting triglyceride levels are normal, the expanded waistline may be the result of excess subcutaneous fat deposition, and such an obesity phenotype is less likely to be associated with the constellation of abnormalities of the metabolic syndrome. However, in the presence of fasting hypertriglyceridemia, there is a high probability that the patient may be characterized by excess visceral adiposity and by the related features of the metabolic syndrome. Thus, "hypertriglyceridemic waist" as a marker of excess visceral adiposity is predictive of an increased risk of comorbidities.

for lipolysis by the enzyme lipoprotein lipase, which becomes saturated in the postprandial state. Such an elevated concentration of triglyceride-rich lipoproteins (VLDL, chylomicrons, and their remnants) found in viscerally obese patients contributes to an increased transfer of triglyceride molecules from these triglyceride-rich lipoproteins to low-density lipoprotein (LDL) and high-density lipoprotein (HDL) in exchange for cholesteryl esters located in LDL and HDL. This process, which is mediated by the enzyme cholesteryl ester transfer protein (CETP), leads to the triglyceride enrichment of LDL and HDL particles, which are then subjected to lipolysis by the enzyme hepatic lipase. There is some evidence suggesting that hepatic lipase activity is elevated in viscerally obese patients,[20,21] and increased activity of this enzyme promotes the formation of small LDL particles. Thus, the increased bi-directional exchange of triglyceride–cholesteryl ester molecules in hypertriglyceridemic patients with visceral obesity leads to the formation of cholesteryl ester–depleted, small LDL and HDL particles. Such a process explains the increased proportion of small LDL particles in visceral obesity and contributes to the reduced HDL cholesterol concentration found in this condition. This is why the small dense LDL and HDL phenotype is a component of the high-triglyceride, reduced–HDL cholesterol dyslipidemic state of viscerally obese, insulin-resistant patients. In this regard, it is also very important to point out that plasma LDL cholesterol concentrations are generally not increased in viscerally obese patients. It has been reported that plasma LDL cholesterol concentrations show no correlation with LDL and HDL particle sizes.[6,8,22] Thus, clinicians should not rely on LDL cholesterol levels to identify patients likely to have small LDL or HDL particles.

In summary, there is therefore a metabolic rationale explaining why an expanded abdominal visceral adipose tissue mass and altered lipolytic activity are related to the high-triglyceride, low–HDL cholesterol, small-LDL dyslipidemia generally found in insulin-resistant abdominally obese patients.

STRESS AND STEROIDS

It is, however, relevant to mention that this "portal theory" has been at times questioned.[23,24] For instance, it has been shown that the expanded visceral adipose depot does not represent a large proportion of the total adipose tissue mass. In addition, it has been shown by Jensen[25] that although visceral adipocytes have a hyperlipolytic state, a large percentage of adipose tissue–derived fatty acids originate from subcutaneous fat. In this regard, the possibility has been raised that excess visceral fat deposition may also be a marker of the relative inability of subcutaneous adipose tissue to store the excess energy induced by a positive energy balance resulting from the overconsumption of an energy-dense diet and/or a lack of physical activity/exercise (see later section).[26] Another hypothesis has been promoted by Björntorp,[27,28] who put forward the notion that visceral obesity is also a marker of a more primary neuro endocrine abnormality partitioning the energy surplus preferentially in visceral rather than in subcutaneous adipose tissue (see Fig. 28-2). In this model, the higher glucocorticoid receptor density found in visceral rather than subcutaneous fat cells could make the visceral fat depot exquisitely sensitive to the activation of the hypothalamo-pituitary–adrenal axis leading to preferential lipid accumulation in the visceral (intra-abdominal) fat depots.[27,29] Steroid hormones have also been involved in the control of body fat distribution. Estrogens in women increase peripheral fat accumulation, whereas androgen levels in men appear to limit visceral fat deposition.[30] Trans-sexuals receiving hormone replacement therapy change their regional body fat patterning, a finding which clearly shows the remarkable effects of sex steroids on body fat distribution and cardiometabolic risk profile.[31,32] Thus, visceral obesity is associated with a specific neuroendocrine profile. Once the visceral depot is expanded, the peculiar metabolic profile of the hypertrophied visceral adipocytes could contribute to further deteriorate the patient's condition. Thus, the viscerally obese patient may enter a vicious cycle exacerbating his or her risk of diabetes and coronary heart disease (CHD).

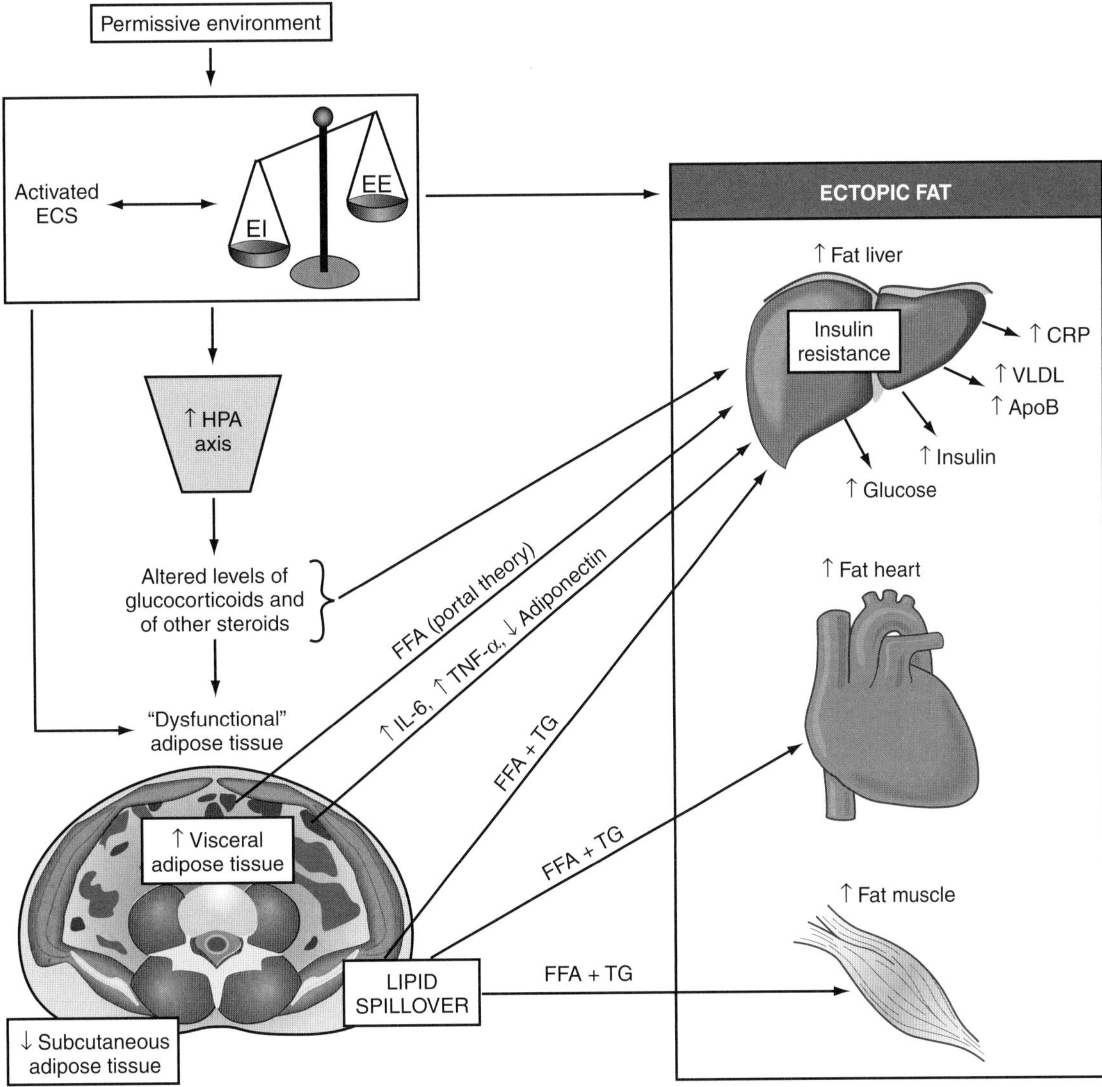

FIGURE 28-2 Overview of theories proposed to explain the link between excess visceral adiposity and insulin resistance as well as features of the metabolic syndrome. First, the combination of an energy-dense diet and a sedentary lifestyle both contribute to the development of a positive energy balance. Among genetically susceptible individuals, such a positive energy balance may contribute to activate the hypothalamic–pituitary–adrenal (HPA) axis. It has been suggested that this activated HPA axis may lead to altered glucocorticoid and other steroid levels. Such an altered neurohormonal milieu may promote visceral fat and ectopic fat deposition and the development of related metabolic abnormalities. Another recently proposed hypothesis is that the activation of the endocannabinoid system (ECS) may be a cause or a consequence of a positive energy balance. Again, among genetically susceptible individuals, an activated ECS may promote visceral fat deposition and ectopic fat deposition through the interaction of overproduced endocannabinoids, with specific CB_1 receptors located not only in key areas of the brain involved in the regulation of energy balance but also in important metabolic tissues such as the adipose tissue, the liver, the skeletal muscle, the heart, the gut (not shown), and the pancreas (not shown). Under the popular "portal" theory, the resulting excess of hyperlipolytic visceral adipose tissue generates an increased flux of free fatty acids (FFA) that, through the portal circulation, impair liver metabolism, contributing to liver fat deposition and steatosis. However, the portal theory has been challenged. The recently discovered endocrine properties of adipose tissue is another possible explanation for the health hazards of visceral obesity. Under this theory, the cytokines produced by the large visceral adipose depot could expose the liver to altered concentrations of various cytokines (adipokines such as interleukin-6 [IL-6, which is increased], tumor necrosis factor–α [TNF-α, which is increased], and adiponectin [which is decreased]) in visceral obesity. Finally, it has also been proposed that excess visceral adiposity is only a marker of ectopic fat deposition. Under this model, excess visceral fat deposition may be a marker of the relative inability of subcutaneous fat to clear and store excess calories from the diet, leading to fat accumulation at undesired sites (ectopic fat) such as the liver, the heart, the skeletal muscle, and other tissues (not shown). It is likely that all the above theories are involved in the development of the constellation of metabolic abnormalities associated with excess visceral adiposity. ApoB, apolipoprotein B; CRP, C-reactive protein; EE, energy expenditure; EI, energy intake; TG, triglycerides; VLDL, very-low-density lipoprotein.

ADIPOSE TISSUE AS AN ENDOCRINE ORGAN

Studies conducted over the last decade have emphasized the notion that adipose tissue is also an "endocrine organ" that produces numerous prothrombotic and inflammatory molecules.[33] Such "adipokines" could exacerbate the patient's risk of diabetes and CHD (see Fig. 28-2). For instance, viscerally obese patients have been shown to have impaired fibrinolysis and increased susceptibility to thrombosis.[34–36] Furthermore, patients with excess visceral adiposity are characterized by a chronic inflammatory state.[5,37] Increased plasma C-reactive protein (CRP) concentrations have been reported in abdominally obese patients, the highest levels being found in obese patients with a selective excess of visceral adipose tissue.[5] Such elevated CRP levels may be the consequence of altered cytokine levels such as interleukin-6 (IL-6) and tumor necrosis factor–α (TNF-α) originating from the expanded abdominal adipose tissue mass[38,39] and promoting a chronic inflammatory state that could also contribute to the etiology of insulin resistance and CVD. As opposed to IL-6 or TNF-α, another adipose tissue–derived cytokine, adiponectin, has been reported to be reduced in concentration in the blood of abdominally obese patients.[40,41] Such a low adiponectin concentration has been suggested to contribute to the development of insulin resistance and CHD in abdominally obese patients with the features of the metabolic syndrome.[40,42,43] Cross-sectional studies have reported that plasma adiponectin levels were reduced in type 2 diabetic patients as well as in patients with documented CHD.[44,45] A recent prospective study has shown that a low adiponectin concentration could predict an increased CHD risk beyond the contribution of classical CHD risk factors,[46] although other studies have generally failed to reach similar conclusions.[47] Nevertheless, it is now clear that patients with type 2 diabetes or CHD with visceral obesity have markedly reduced plasma adiponectin levels.

VISCERAL ADIPOSE TISSUE: A MARKER OF "DYSFUNCTIONAL" ADIPOSE TISSUE?

Even though the hyperlipolytic state and endocrine properties of visceral adipose tissue could, along with a given neuroendocrine profile, explain the constellation of metabolic abnormalities of patients with visceral adiposity, it has been proposed that excess visceral adiposity may not be causally related to features of the metabolic syndrome.[48] Indeed, it has been suggested that excess visceral adiposity may instead represent one feature of ectopic fat deposition (see Fig. 28-2).[26] Under such a theory, individuals who could not store the excess energy that results from their affluent/sedentary lifestyle in subcutaneous adipose tissue would then store lipids at undesired sites such as the liver, the heart, the skeletal muscle, and the intra-abdominal cavity. Thus, the amount of visceral fat would be correlated with the metabolic syndrome only because it is an excellent marker of ectopic fat deposition. However, as shown in Fig. 28-2, it is more likely that all the above theories contribute, at least to a certain extent, to the dysmetabolic profile of viscerally obese patients.

Therefore, viscerally obese patients, even in the absence of classical CVD risk factors such as hypertension, smoking, hyperglycemia, and elevated LDL cholesterol concentrations, could be at high risk for an acute coronary event not only because of the presence of an atherogenic metabolic profile that includes the high-triglyceride, low–HDL cholesterol, small-LDL, elevated–apolipoprotein B dyslipidemic state, but also because of a prothrombotic and inflammatory profile (Fig. 28-3).[22,49] However, although several features of this constellation of abnormalities, often called the metabolic syndrome, have been shown to predict an increased CHD risk, we presently do not know which of these variables to assess in order to improve our ability to predict CHD events once traditional risk factors have been taken into account.[26] Additional studies are clearly warranted on this issue, and this question will likely become a very fertile area of investigation.

VISCERAL OBESITY AND CHD RISK: THE ATHEROGENIC DYSLIPIDEMIA AND BEYOND

Over the years, several groups have attempted to quantify the CHD risk associated with the features of the metabolic syndrome found in abdominal obesity. Several prospective

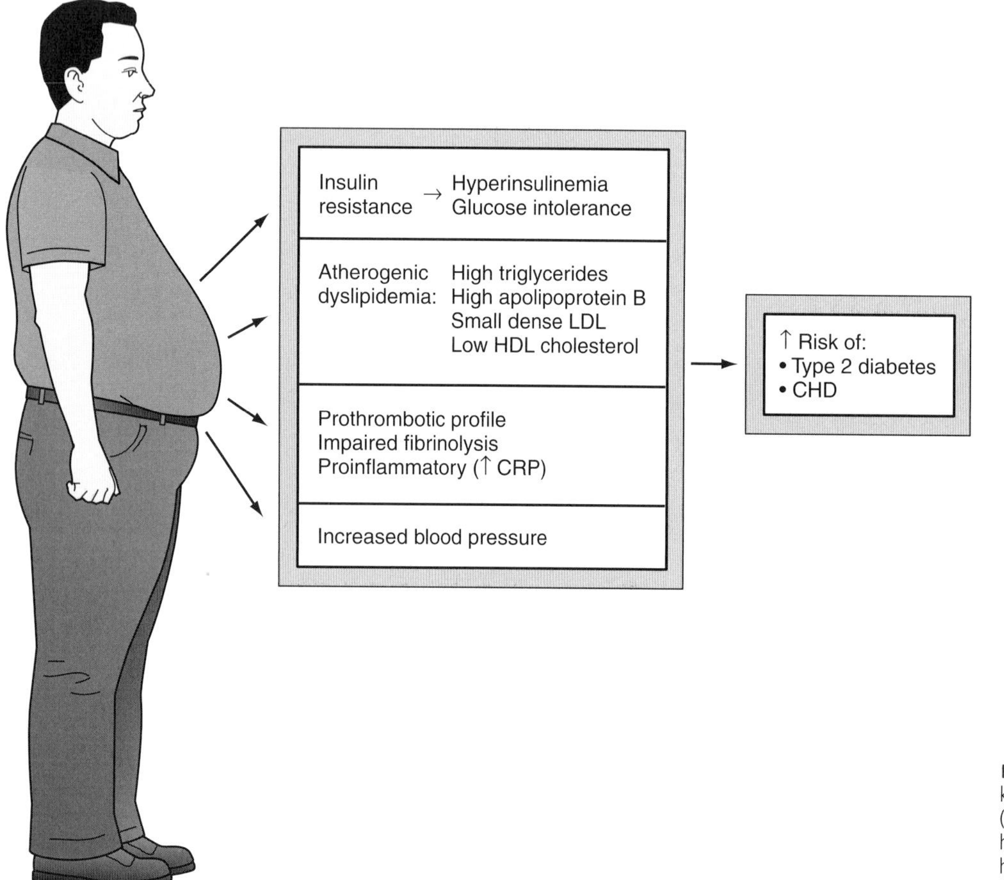

FIGURE 28-3 Simplified overview of the key metabolic abnormalities found in visceral (intra-abdominal) obesity. CHD, coronary heart disease; CRP, C-reactive protein; HDL, high-density lipoprotein; LDL, Low-density lipoprotein.

studies have suggested that fasting hyperinsulinemia, which is often used as a crude marker of insulin resistance in nondiabetic individuals, was predictive of an increased CHD risk.[50–54] In the sample of 2103 asymptomatic middle-aged men of the Québec Cardiovascular Study followed for incidence of a first CHD event over 5 years, we found that some of the metabolic features of abdominal obesity, namely fasting hyperinsulinemia, an elevated apolipoprotein B concentration, small LDL particles, an elevated cholesterol/HDL cholesterol ratio, and an elevated CRP concentration, were all predictive of an increased risk of CHD.[50,55–58] We also found that the simultaneous presence of these features of the metabolic syndrome were predictive of a markedly elevated risk of CHD.[59] As these markers are not well accepted CHD risk factors in current medical practice and in national guidelines, we have compared the ability of some of these features of the insulin resistance syndrome (what we have referred to as the atherogenic metabolic triad of elevated insulin and apolipoprotein B levels and small LDL particles) to predict CHD risk with commonly used algorithms such as the Framingham Risk Score.[60] Not surprisingly, we found that a high Framingham Risk Score was predictive of an increased risk of CHD in the men of the Québec Cardiovascular Study.[60] However, even in the absence of classical risk factors (and therefore among men with a low Framingham score), we found the features of the metabolic syndrome also to be predictive of an equally increased risk of CHD.[60] Therefore, these results provide evidence that our current risk assessment algorithms based on traditional risk factors do not always identify high-risk subjects with the features of the metabolic syndrome if these individuals do not have traditional risk factors such as hypertension, smoking, elevated cholesterol, or type 2 diabetes. There is therefore a need to further refine current CHD risk assessment algorithms by potentially considering relevant markers of the metabolic syndrome. However, identifying the combination of markers that will provide the optimal discrimination of high-risk individuals while being manageable in the context of primary care medicine will require further work.

It is with this last objective in mind that we have proposed to use "hypertriglyceridemic waist"[61] as a phenotype providing physicians with a simple screening test to identify at very low cost the subgroup of abdominally obese patients with the atherogenic features of the metabolic syndrome (see Fig. 28-1). The National Cholesterol Education Program Adult Treatment Panel III (NCEP ATP III) guidelines[62] had also previously acknowledged the importance of considering both waist girth and fasting triglycerides as two key clinical variables to identify individuals with the metabolic syndrome, although different cut-off values were proposed. Additional work is under way to validate the screening tools proposed by various organizations, because the selection of variables and cut-off values by most of these working groups was not based on their ability to predict hard clinical events.[49]

MANAGING THE ATHEROGENIC DYSLIPIDEMIA OF ABDOMINAL OBESITY

Thus, the typical atherogenic dyslipidemia of abdominal obesity does not consist of an elevated concentration of LDL cholesterol.[8,63] Rather, numerous studies have shown that abdominal obesity is associated with increased plasma triglyceride levels, an increased apolipoprotein B concentration, an increased proportion of small dense LDL, and reduced HDL cholesterol concentrations.[4,7,8] This typical dyslipidemic state has often been referred to as the atherogenic dyslipidemia of insulin resistance and of the metabolic syndrome. Prospective studies have shown that the presence of this profile increases CHD risk at any given LDL cholesterol concentration.[59,64–66]

In this regard, one of the key markers of increased CHD risk at any given LDL cholesterol level is the HDL cholesterol concentration. Several prospective studies that have stratified individuals (men and women) on the basis of LDL cholesterol and HDL cholesterol concentrations have shown that reduced HDL cholesterol levels are predictive of an increased risk of CHD.[67–70] Numerous mechanisms have been proposed to explain the cardioprotective effect of high HDL. For instance, it has been well documented that HDL is involved in reverse cholesterol transport, a process mediated by receptors and enzymes, including CETP. In addition, we now also understand that HDL has important anti-inflammatory, antioxidant, and antithrombotic properties.[71] Thus, such properties of HDL could explain why numerous epidemiological studies have reached the conclusion that a low HDL cholesterol concentration is predictive of an increased CHD risk.[70,72,73] However, with the current epidemic of obesity and type 2 diabetes, we also need to keep in mind that a low HDL cholesterol concentration is often a marker of the presence of abdominal obesity, insulin resistance, and a whole cluster of atherothrombotic and inflammatory abnormalities that we often refer to as the metabolic syndrome.[22,49] Thus, it should be kept in mind that in clinical practice, a low HDL cholesterol concentration is rarely seen in the absence of the above risk factors and metabolic abnormalities resulting from a sedentary lifestyle and unhealthy dietary habits.

If the anti-inflammatory, antioxidant, and antithrombotic properties of HDL play a role in cardioprotection, any pharmacologic approach that increases HDL levels should theoretically reduce CHD risk. However, recently published negative results on the powerful "HDL raiser" torcetrapib have failed to provide evidence that increasing HDL concentration alone is a valid therapeutic target.[74,75] Of course, whether this specific modality to raise HDL is characterized by an overall "negative class effect" or whether some specific properties of torcetrapib (such as its blood pressure–raising effect) have offset the potential cardiovascular benefits of raising HDL by this specific CETP inhibitor is currently unknown. In addition, it is also possible that the magnitude of CETP inhibition produced an unphysiologic lipoprotein transport system leading to very high HDL concentrations with little or no cardiovascular benefits. Further studies will be needed to explore whether a more subtle CETP inhibition or other CETP inhibitors would still represent a clinically relevant approach to treating patients with low HDL.

On the other hand, studies using fibrates to increase HDL have shown some benefits, especially among patients with abdominal obesity, insulin resistance, and the metabolic syndrome, but the positive results published with gemfibrozil (Veterans Affairs HDL Intervention Trial [VA-HIT])[76] and bezafibrate (Bezafilorate Infarction

Prevention [BIP])[64] have not been reproduced with fenofibrate in the Fenofibrate Intervention and Event Lowering Diabetes (FIELD) trial.[77]

There is very likely a possibility that a treatment that would target the core features of the most prevalent form of low HDL cholesterol in clinical practice (abdominal obesity and insulin resistance) could have a significant impact on CHD events. However, before we review the evidence that losing weight and abdominal fat by targeting the endocannabinoid system could substantially improve the lipoprotein profile of patients with visceral obesity, it is important to acknowledge at this stage that we do not have adequate global cardiometabolic risk assessment algorithms to translate improvements in the cardiometabolic risk profile (including changes in the lipid profile described below) produced by losing abdominal fat (in response to a lifestyle modification program and/or by pharmacotherapic aimed at loss of visceral fat) into estimates of CHD risk reduction. Comprehensive metabolic epidemiologic studies with full cardiometabolic risk profiling along with proper measurements of total and visceral adiposity will be necessary to answer this clinically important question.

THE ENDOCANNABINOID SYSTEM

It is now well established that the endocannabinoid system has significant effects on energy as well as on carbohydrate and lipid metabolism[78–80] Not only is the endocannabinoid system involved in the central regulation of appetite and satiety, but this system has a major impact on hepatic lipid metabolism as well as on insulin sensitivity and plasma glucose–insulin homeostasis through effects on peripheral tissues such as the liver, the adipose tissue, the gut, the skeletal muscle, and the pancreas.[79] Endocannabinoids are endogeneous phospholipid derivatives (the two most studied with reported effects on energy metabolism being anandamide and 2-arachidonoylglycerol [2-AG]) that bind to type 1 and 2 cannabinoid receptors (CB_1 and CB_2 receptors, respectively).[81,82] The CB_1 receptor is a G-protein–coupled receptor that is involved in the regulation of the central effects of endocannabinoids on appetite.[83] Under normal circumstances, key physiologic functions of the endocannabinoid system are, when activated on demand, to reduce anxiety and pain, to modulate body temperature and blood pressure, and to sedate and reduce motor behavior while increasing food intake.[84] In the presence of chronic conditions of activation such as chronic overeating and obesity, the activated endocannabinoid system has numerous potentially deleterious effects not only on food intake but also on carbohydrate and lipid metabolism.[83] Administration of endocannabinoids in animals has been shown to increase food intake, even in satiated animals, and this effect is not found in CB_1 receptor–knockout animals, suggesting that the effects of anandamide and 2-AG on energy balance and metabolism are mediated by CB_1 receptors.[78,85,86] CB_1-knockout mice have a lean phenotype and are also resistant to diet-induced obesity compared with wild-type animals.[78]

Until recently, evidence of an activated endocannabinoid system in human abdominal obesity was lacking. However, two independent groups have now reported evidence of elevated plasma endocannabinoid levels (2-AG) in the specific subgroup of viscerally obese patients.[87,88] Furthermore, such elevated 2-AG levels were found to be correlated with several alterations in the cardiometabolic risk profile of viscerally obese patients, including insulin resistance, hypertriglyceridemia, low HDL cholesterol, and reduced adiponectin levels. In this regard, the reduced plasma adiponectin concentration found in patients with visceral obesity is a finding that is fully compatible with the presence of CB_1 receptors on fat cells and with the effects of endocannabinoids on adiponectin production by fat cells.[89] The latter finding supports the notion that the elevated endocannabinoid levels found in viscerally obese patients could explain their reduced plasma adiponectin concentrations. Another question that has not been adequately addressed in humans is whether the activated endocannabinoid system is a consequence or a cause of overeating and visceral obesity. Because obesity per se (in the absence of excess visceral fat) did not appear to be associated with elevated concentrations of the abundant endocannabinoid 2-AG,[87,88] these findings suggest that the endocannabinoid system may indeed play a role in the regulation of body fat distribution and ectopic fat deposition.

On the basis of these findings, it would be relevant to propose the hypothesis that CB_1 antagonism could represent a relevant approach to specifically treat overweight or obese patients with visceral obesity, excess liver fat, and related metabolic abnormalities. The next sections will review the published evidence on the effect of rimonabant, the first CB_1 antagonist developed and available in clinical practice in several countries but not yet in North America.

PUBLISHED CLINICAL TRIALS WITH THE CANNABINOID RECEPTOR TYPE 1 ANTAGONIST RIMONABANT: IMPACT ON THE LIPID AND CARDIOMETABOLIC RISK PROFILE

The four phase III studies (Rimonabant In Obesity [RIO] program) conducted and published with the first CB_1 antagonist developed (rimonabant) have shown that antagonism of the endocannabinoid system could reduce body weight, but more importantly induce a significant loss of abdominal fat (as estimated by the reduction in waist circumference), improve insulin sensitivity (indices of plasma glucose–insulin homeostasis), decrease plasma triglyceride and increase HDL cholesterol levels, decrease the proportion of small LDL particles, reduce inflammation (CRP), and increase plasma adiponectin concentrations (Figs. 28-4 and 28-5 and Table 28-1).[90–93]

Furthermore, subgroup analyses revealed that when subjects were stratified as a function of the magnitude of weight loss, the greater the weight loss achieved, the more substantial were the improvements in the lipid profile. However, for any given weight loss, there was a further reduction in triglyceride levels

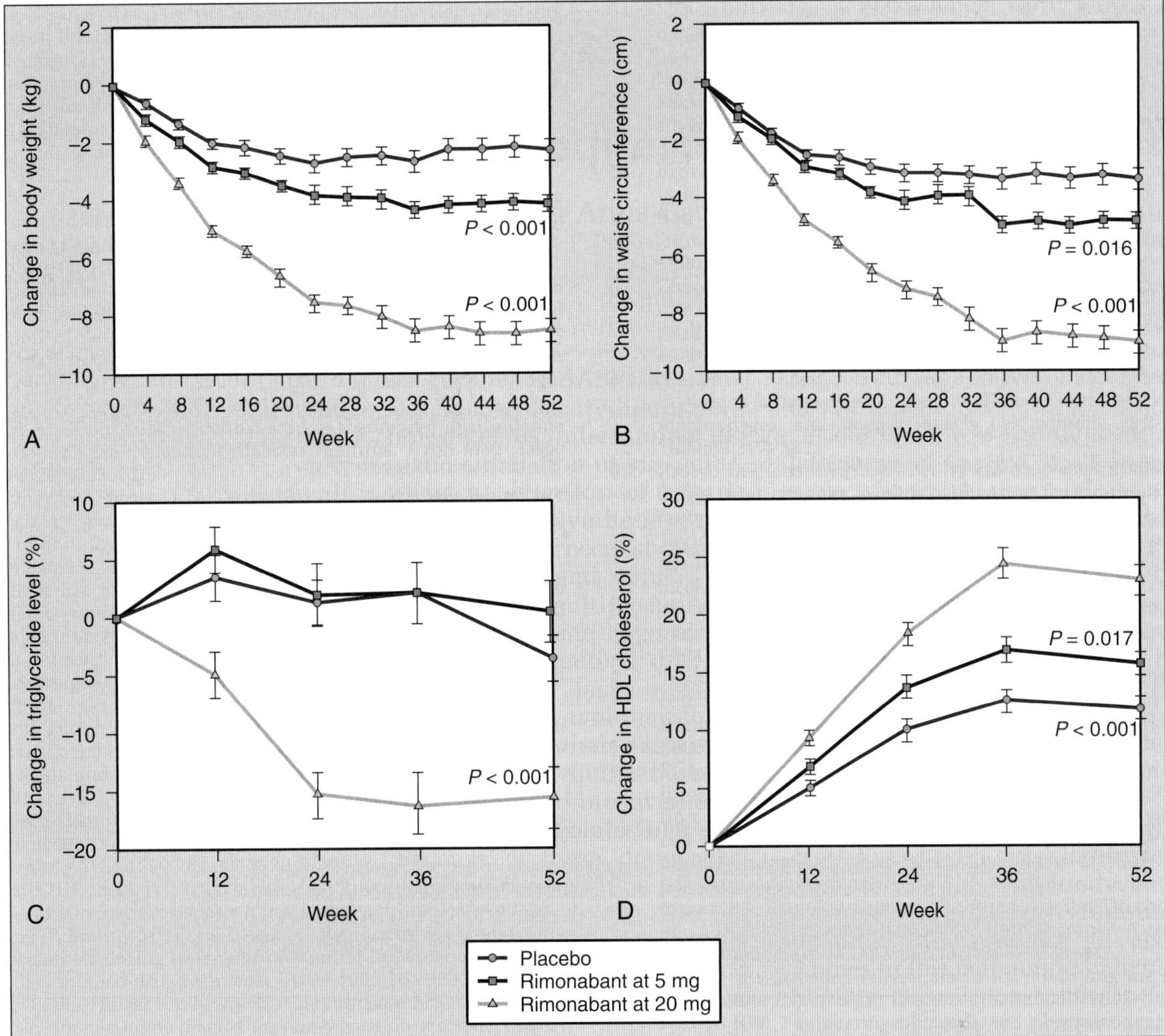

FIGURE 28-4 Effect of a 1-year treatment with the CB_1 antagonist rimonabant on body weight, waist circumference, plasma triglycerides, and HDL cholesterol in overweight or obese dyslipidemic patients of the RIO-Lipids trial. *(From Ref. 90. Copyright © 2005 Massachusetts Medical Society. All rights reserved.)*

and a further increase in plasma HDL cholesterol concentrations.[91–93] Overall, about half of the effect of rimonabant on triglycerides, HDL cholesterol, indices of insulin sensitivity, and adiponectin could not be explained by the magnitude of weight loss alone.[90–93] Two trials in which liver fat and visceral fat will be measured by computed tomography (An International Study of Rimonabant in Dyslipidemia with Atherogenic Risk in Abdominally Obese Patients ([ADAGIO]-Lipids and Visceral Fat Reduction Assessed by CT-Scan on Rimonabant [VICTORIA]) currently underway to test the hypothesis that such a weight loss–independent effect on metabolic risk markers is partly the consequence of a selective loss of visceral fat that is expected to be greater than what could be predicted by weight loss. For instance, intervention studies have shown that weight loss in viscerally obese patients is generally associated with a selective loss of visceral adipose tissue.[94–98] As a rule of thumb, the greater the initial level of visceral adiposity, the more substantial will be the relative loss of visceral fat with interventions aiming at weight loss.

Effect of Cannabinoid Receptor Type 1 Antagonism on Low-Density Lipoprotein Particle Size

Rimonabant has been reported to have little or no effect on LDL cholesterol concentration (Fig 28-6).[90,92,93] This lack of effect is not surprising because abdominal obesity is not associated with increased LDL cholesterol levels but rather with an increased proportion of small LDL particles.[8] As weight loss and exercise training have been shown to induce a shift in LDL particle size in the absence of major changes in LDL cholesterol concentrations,[99–101] the shift in LDL particle size observed in the RIO-Lipids trial supports the notion that the assessment of LDL cholesterol concentration does not allow the clinician to appreciate the impact of weight loss or of rimonabant therapy on LDL quality in abdominally obese patients. Prospective studies have shown that an increased proportion of small LDL is predictive of an increased CHD risk.[56,102–104] However, whether the presence of an increased proportion of small LDL particles predicts an elevated CHD risk beyond traditional risk

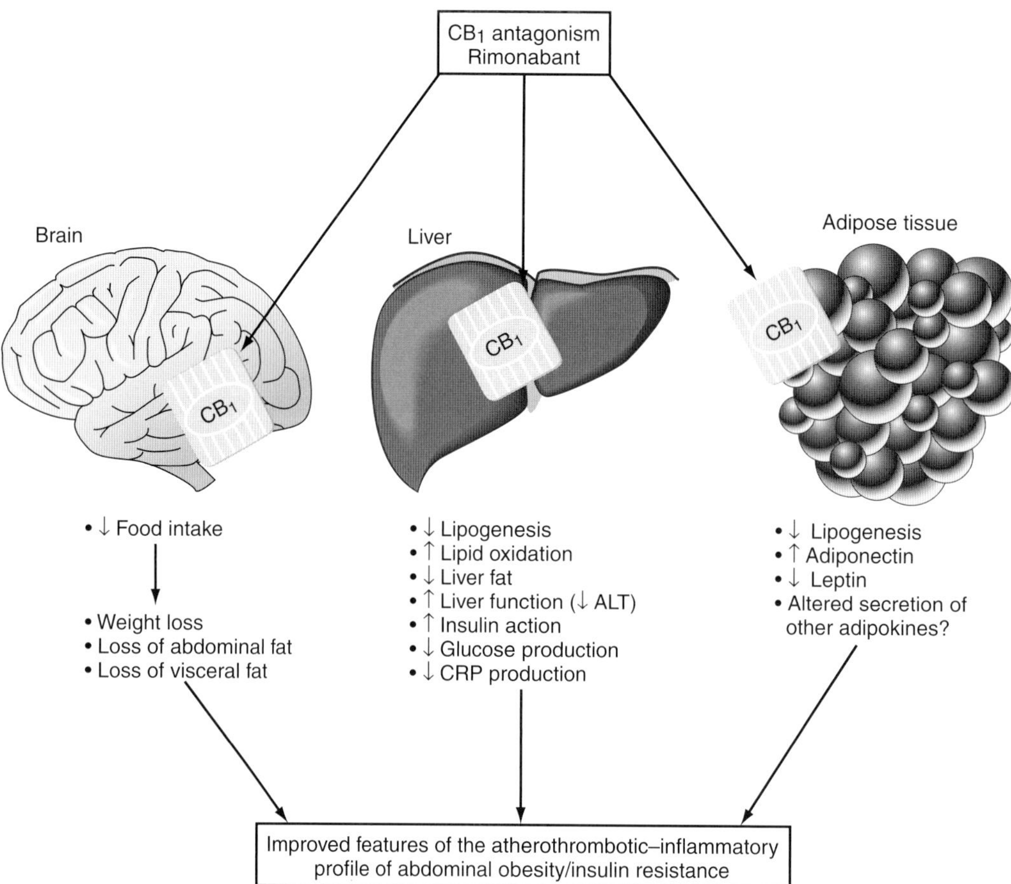

FIGURE 28-5 Overview of the known mechanisms by which antagonism of an overactivated endocannabinoid system could lead to improvements in numerous features of the insulin resistant–atherothrombotic–inflammatory profile of the viscerally obese patient with an atherogenic dyslipidemia and/or type 2 diabetes. CB_1, cannabinoid recepter type 1; CRP, C-reactive protein; ALT, alanine aminotransferase.

factors, including triglycerides and HDL cholesterol, is doubtful. Furthermore, no intervention study has been conducted to test the impact of increasing LDL particle size as a target for primary or secondary CHD prevention. However, the finding that LDL particle size is not an independent predictor of CHD after control for triglycerides and HDL cholesterol does not imply that small LDL particles do not promote atherosclerosis. For instance, several *in vitro* studies have provided mechanistic insights as to why small LDL particles could contribute to atherosclerosis (reduced affinity for LDL receptor, increased susceptibility to oxidation, etc.).[105] Finally, despite the fact that rimonabant has no impact on LDL cholesterol levels, it has been found that statin-treated patients in the RIO program responded equally well to this CB_1 antagonist in terms of decreases in triglycerides and increases in HDL cholesterol compared with non-statin-treated patients.[106] Therefore, the added value of rimonabant therapy for abdominal obesity and for metabolic risk markers that cannot be managed by statin therapy is worth considering.

Effect of Cannabinoid Receptor Type 1 Antagonism on Triglyceride Levels

Plasma triglyceride levels are increased in abdominally obese patients.[4,7] Triglyceride molecules do not appear to be atherogenic per se, and whether an elevated triglyceride concentration is an independent predictor of CHD risk remains a matter of debate.[107–109] However, hypertriglyceridemia accompanied by abdominal obesity is predictive of a high probability of finding patients with the whole cluster of atherothrombotic and inflammatory abnormalities linked to insulin resistance that is often referred to as the metabolic syndrome (see Fig. 28-1).[61] Therefore, the reduction in triglyceride levels and of waist circumference observed in the RIO studies suggests that CB_1 antagonism with drugs like rimonabant could have a significant impact on the cluster of metabolic abnormalities of the metabolic syndrome by treating the core cause of the metabolic syndrome (see Fig. 28-4). This is probably the most important consequence of targeting the endocannabinoid system for emphasis rather than focusing on the response of only a single marker such as HDL cholesterol, for which change cannot be translated, for the time being, into clinical benefits when considered as an isolated target.

Effect of Cannabinoid Receptor Type 1 Antagonism on Inflammation

Rimonabant does more to CHD risk markers than simply improve the high-triglyceride, low–HDL cholesterol dyslipidemic state. Because abdominal obesity is probably the most important correlate of elevated CRP concentration (a marker of inflammation),[5,38] weight loss and loss of abdominal fat with rimonabant should theoretically reduce plasma CRP levels.[37,110] This is exactly what was

TABLE 28-1 Effects of the Cannabinoid-1 Receptor Blocker Rimonabant on Anthropometric and Cardiometabolic Risk Variables
Anthropometric Variables:
↓ Body weight
↓ Waist circumference
Lipoprotein and Lipid Variables:
↑ HDL cholesterol
↓ Cholesterol/HDL cholesterol ratio
↓ Triglycerides
↓ Apolipoprotein B/apolipoprotein A-I ratio
↑ LDL peak particle size
↓ % small LDL particles
Glucose and Insulin Variables:
↑ Insulin sensitivity (HOMA index)
↓ Fasting insulin
↓ Fasting glucose
↓ HbA_{1c}
Inflammatory Variables:
↑ Adiponectin
↓ Leptin
↓ C-reactive protein
Hemodynamic Variables:
↓ Systolic blood pressure
↓ Diastolic blood pressure

found with rimonabant therapy in RIO-Lipids.[90] The effect of CB_1 blockade on CRP was also confirmed in the RIO-Diabetes trial.[92] For the time being, the results available suggest that this effect is probably entirely explained by weight loss and loss of abdominal fat.

Effect of Cannabinoid Receptor Type 1 Antagonism on Adiponectin

It is now well accepted that adipose tissue does much more than store and mobilize lipids. It is also a remarkable endocrine organ. An expanded abdominal adipose tissue mass shows signs of macrophage infiltration leading to an increased production of inflammatory cytokines. Some of these cytokines (such as TNF-α) have a significant effect on the production of an important adipose tissue–derived cytokine, adiponectin.[111] Adiponectin is the most important cytokine produced by adipose tissue, and its plasma levels are markedly reduced in patients with visceral obesity, type 2 diabetes, and CHD.[40,46,112] In RIO-Lipids, we found that rimonabant treatment increased plasma adiponectin levels.[90] Part of this increase in adiponectin levels with therapy was explained by the magnitude of weight loss. However, more than half of the increase in adiponectin levels could not be explained by weight loss, a finding compatible with data showing the presence of CB_1 receptors on fat cells.[113] Animal data had previously shown that agonists for the CB_1 receptor decreased adiponectin gene expression and protein secretion in adipose tissue and that rimonabant could stimulate adiponectin production by fat cells.[89] Because adiponectin has numerous potentially important metabolic effects (probably affecting liver metabolism, affecting the insulin signaling pathway, improving insulin sensitivity, and affecting processes involved in the regulation of plasma HDL cholesterol levels),[42,44] the effect of rimonabant on adiponectin levels could be one of the mechanisms explaining the weight loss–independent effect of the drug on metabolic risk factors. This hypothesis is under investigation.

Effects of Cannabinoid Receptor Type 1 Antagonism on Blood Pressure

Despite the fact that no phase III trial with rimonabant was specifically designed to examine the effect of this CB_1 antagonist on blood pressure as a primary endpoint, rimonabant was found to lower blood pressure.[90,92] Because the patients as a group were not hypertensive, the average reduction in blood pressure has been reported to be modest. However, a subgroup analysis of patients with moderate hypertension in RIO-Lipids revealed a robust blood pressure–lowering effect of rimonabant on systolic and diastolic blood pressure.[90] As for CRP, such a reduction in blood pressure with rimonabant therapy appeared to be entirely explained by the magnitude of weight loss.

Effects of Cannabinoid Receptor Type 1 Antagonism on Liver Fat and Function

Liver enzyme levels are raised in abdominally overweight/obese patients with dyslipidemia because of hepatic fat deposition resulting from excess visceral adiposity.[114,115] In RIO-Lipids, the effects of rimonabant on liver enzymes were examined.[116]

Concentrations of five liver enzymes were assayed at baseline, every 3 months, and after 1 year of treatment. At 1 year, the mean reductions in alanine aminotransferase (ALT), aspartate aminotransferase (AST), and alkaline phosphatase levels were significantly greater for rimonabant 20 mg/day than for placebo. The proportion of patients with ALT levels above the upper normal range decreased from 12.5% at baseline to 10.2% at 1 year with placebo and from 10.2% to 3.1% with rimonabant 20 mg/day (between-group difference: $P < 0.001$).[116] Regression analyses showed a relationship between change in body weight and change in ALT levels in the placebo and rimonabant 20 mg/day groups. There was also a correlation between reduction in waist circumference and ALT levels in the rimonabant 20 mg/day group, but not in the placebo group. Therefore, in abdominally obese/overweight patients with untreated dyslipidemia, treatment with rimonabant 20 mg/day was associated with reduced ALT, AST, and alkaline phosphatase levels. For rimonabant 20 mg/day, reductions in ALT, a crude but clinically relevant marker of fatty liver disease,[117] were correlated with changes in body weight and waist circumference. Another recently completed trial (ADAGIO-Lipids) has not only confirmed that rimonabant could improve liver function, but also a computed tomography substudy revealed that antagonism of CB_1, receptors could induce

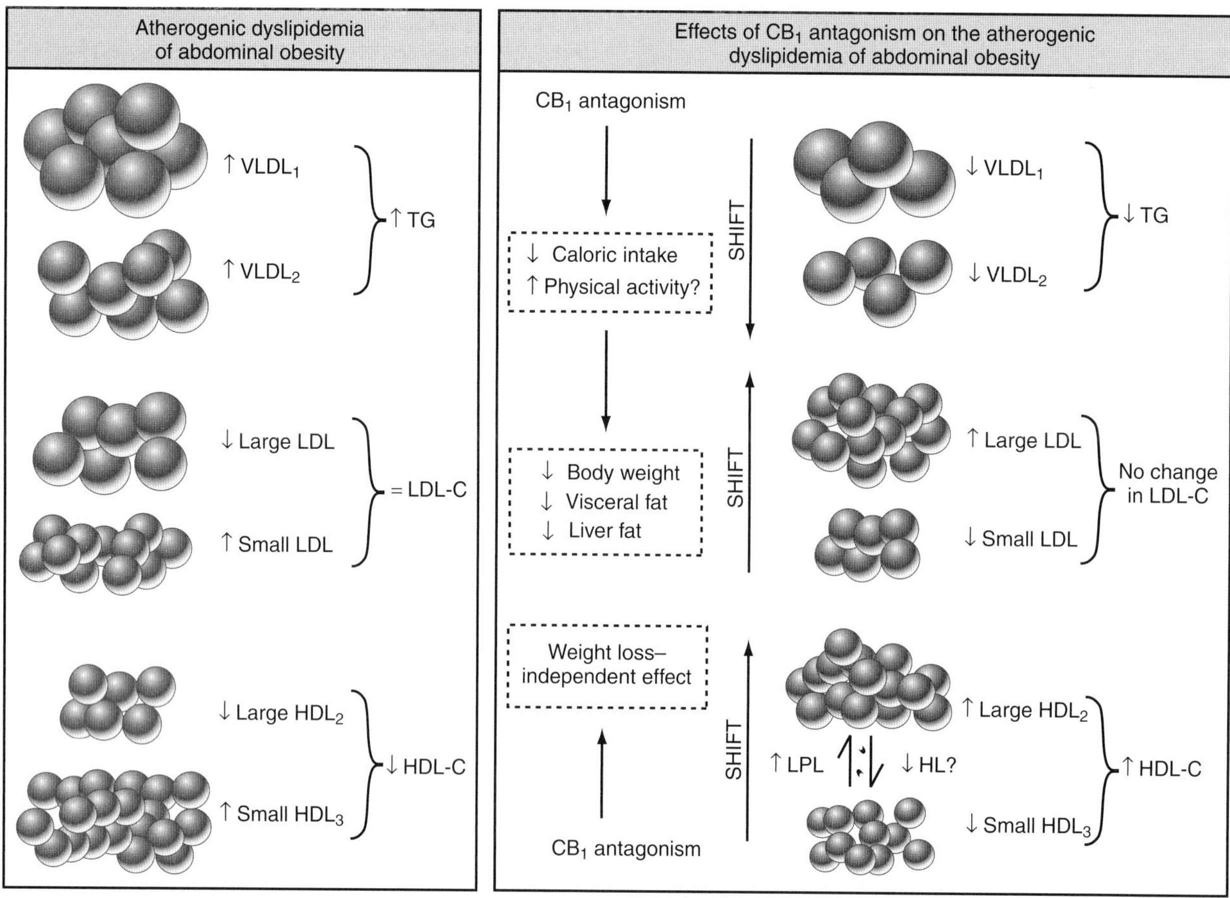

FIGURE 28-6 Schematic representation of the atherogenic lipoprotein profile of patients with visceral (intra-abdominal) obesity *(left panel)*. Viscerally obese, insulin resistant patients have increased fasting triglyceride (TG) levels because of an overproduction of large, TG-rich very-low-density lipoprotein$_1$ (VLDL$_1$) particles. Plasma low-density lipoprotein cholesterol (LDL-C) levels are generally in the normal range in viscerally obese patients, which is potentially misleading information to the clinician because these individuals are often characterized by an increased proportion of small, cholesteryl ester–depleted low-density lipoprotein (LDL) particles. Plasma high-density lipoprotein (HDL) cholesterol levels are also reduced in viscerally obese patients, particularly the concentration of the large, cholesteryl ester–rich HDL$_2$ subfraction, leading to a reduced HDL particle size. Two mechanisms have been proposed to explain the improvements in the plasma lipoprotein profile produced by CB$_1$ antagonism with rimonabant: (1) weight loss and loss of abdominal fat; (2) improvements in the lipoprotein profile that are weight loss–independent through the specific effects of rimonabant on target tissues such as adipose tissue and the liver. For instance, CB$_1$ antagonism has been shown to "boost" adiponectin production by adipose tissue as well as to reduce lipogenesis in the liver, contributing to the documented effect of rimonabant on liver function (reduced alanine aminotransferase [ALT]). Rimonabant treatment induces changes not only in lipoprotein concentration but also in particle size. Finally, it is important to point out that the shift in LDL particle size (increase) reported with rimonabant cannot be appreciated by the measurement of LDL cholesterol concentrations, which show no change. (Note: Differences in particle size between VLDL [very large], LDL [intermediate], and HDL [small] could not be appropriately scaled in this simplified illustration.)

a significant loss of visceral adipose tissue and mobilization of liver fat.[118]

Are the Effects of Rimonabant on Lipoproteins and Lipids Underestimated?

When the effects of rimonabant on plasma lipoproteins/lipids is examined, a critically important point to highlight is the design of the four phase III studies.[90–93] Indeed, in those studies, it is important to point out that baseline measurements were performed after a 1-month placebo run-in period during which patients were instructed to reduce their daily caloric intake by 600 kcal. Therefore, the baseline measurements in the RIO studies were performed after an initial weight loss of about 2 kg induced by the run-in period, and this negative energy balance had already produced some reductions in plasma triglyceride and HDL cholesterol levels. For instance, it is well known that HDL cholesterol levels tend to go down when subjects are actively losing weight and that HDL cholesterol levels increase once patients are weight stable.[119] Thus, the absolute effects of rimonabant on triglyceride levels are likely to be underestimated, whereas the absolute increase in HDL cholesterol levels with rimonabant therapy (about 20% to 25%) are probably overestimated. However, irrespective of the baseline levels, the effect of rimonabant on HDL cholesterol levels compared with placebo has been shown to be robust and very consistent. Irrespective of baseline HDL cholesterol levels, rimonabant at 20 mg/day has been shown to increase HDL cholesterol levels by about 8% over the placebo response. However, as many metabolic parameters are rapidly improved when patients follow a hypocaloric diet (which was the case during the 1-month run-in period preceding the four RIO phase III trials), there is a need to properly quantify the effects of rimonabant on metabolic risk parameters. Another trial without a hypocaloric diet run-in period (ADAGIO-Lipids) has been specifically designed to properly quantify the effects of rimonabant on metabolic risk variables. Results of ADAGIO-Lipids confirmed the effects of rimonabant on the comprehensive set of cardiometabolic risk markers presented in Table 28-1. Furthermore, the computed tomography imaging substudy of ADAGIO-Lipids provided for the first time evidence that rimonabant therapy could induce significant losses of visceral and liver fat.[118]

Metabolic Effects of Cannabinoid Receptor Type 1 Antagonist with Rimonabant: More Than a High-Density Lipoprotein–Raising Drug

All phase III studies with rimonabant have shown that this CB_1 antagonist raise HDL cholesterol levels (see Fig. 28-4), with the increase being greater than what could be attributed to weight loss. Despite the robust effect of rimonabant on abdominal obesity and related metabolic abnormalities, it would be an error to focus only on the HDL-raising properties of the drug to explain its potential benefits for CHD risk (under investigation in imaging and CVD morbidity/mortality trials). Other therapeutic approaches (CETP inhibitors, nicotinic acid) can also increase HDL levels to a much greater extent than rimonabant.[75,120,121] However, none of these drugs have been shown to have a favorable impact on most metabolic consequences of abdominal obesity (including insulin sensitivity, plasma glucose–insulin homeostasis, and blood pressure). Furthermore, raising HDL levels by the CETP inhibitor torcetrapib has not been found to reduce CHD morbidity and mortality,[75] suggesting that raising HDL alone, depending on the mechanism used, may not necessarily represent a legitimate therapeutic target. Unfortunately, clinicians are presently ill equipped to quantify the impact of improving all these markers on the risk of hard CHD events. Trials are under way to address this important question. However, it is likely that the impact of CB_1 antagonism on CHD risk will be at least as important (without considering the metabolic improvements not explained by weight loss) as the impact of weight loss and loss of abdominal fat produced by a lifestyle modification program. Whether the additional metabolic properties of CB_1 antagonists such as rimonabant could translate into further CHD risk reduction beyond body weight loss is for the time being a speculation that should be tested in cardiometabolic trials with hard CHD endpoints. However, from the known mechanisms of action of this new class of drugs, it is proposed that insulin-resistant or type 2 diabetic patients with visceral obesity, ectopic fat deposition, and high-triglyceride, low–HDL cholesterol atherogenic dyslipidemia would particularly benefit from the antagonism of their overactivated endocannabinoid system.

ACKNOWLEDGMENTS

The work of Dr. Jean-Pierre Després has been supported by research grants from the Canadian Institutes of Health Research, the Canadian Diabetes Association, the Heart and Stroke Foundation, and the Foundation of the Québec Heart Institute. Dr. Després is the Scientific Director of the International Chair on Cardiometabolic Risk, which is supported by an unrestricted grant from Sanofi Aventis awarded to Université Laval.

REFERENCES

1. Kissebah AH, Freedman DS, Peiris AN: Health risk of obesity. *Med Clin North Am* 1989;73:111–138.
2. Bray GA: Complications of obesity. *Ann Intern Med* 1985;103: 1052–1062.
3. Couillard C, Bergeron N, Prud'homme D, et al: Postprandial triglyceride response in visceral obesity in men. *Diabetes* 1998;47:953–960.
4. Després JP, Moorjani S, Lupien PJ, et al: Regional distribution of body fat, plasma lipoproteins, and cardiovascular disease. *Arteriosclerosis* 1990;10:497–511.
5. Lemieux I, Pascot A, Prud'homme D, et al: Elevated C-reactive protein: another component of the atherothrombotic profile of abdominal obesity. *Arterioscler Thromb Vasc Biol* 2001;21:961–967.
6. Pascot A, Lemieux I, Prud'homme D, et al: Reduced HDL particle size as an additional feature of the atherogenic dyslipidemia of abdominal obesity. *J Lipid Res* 2001;42:2007–2014.
7. Pouliot MC, Després JP, Nadeau A, et al: Visceral obesity in men. Associations with glucose tolerance, plasma insulin, and lipoprotein levels. *Diabetes* 1992;41:826–834.
8. Tchernof A, Lamarche B, Prud'homme D, et al: The dense LDL phenotype. Association with plasma lipoprotein levels, visceral obesity, and hyperinsulinemia in men. *Diabetes Care* 1996;19: 629–637.
9. Reaven GM: Banting lecture 1988. Role of insulin resistance in human disease. *Diabetes* 1988;37:1595–1607.
10. Reaven GM: Pathophysiology of insulin resistance in human disease. *Physiol Rev* 1995;75:473–486.
11. Abbasi F, Brown BW Jr, Lamendola C, et al: Relationship between obesity, insulin resistance, and coronary heart disease risk. *J Am Coll Cardiol* 2002;40:937–943.
12. McLaughlin T, Abbasi F, Cheal K, et al: Use of metabolic markers to identify overweight individuals who are insulin resistant. *Ann Intern Med* 2003;139:802–809.
13. Reaven GM: The metabolic syndrome: is this diagnosis necessary? *Am J Clin Nutr* 2006;83:1237–1247.
14. Ross R, Aru J, Freeman J, et al: Abdominal adiposity and insulin resistance in obese men. *Am J Physiol Endocrinol Metab* 2002;282:E657–E663.
15. Ross R, Freeman J, Hudson R, et al: Abdominal obesity, muscle composition, and insulin resistance in premenopausal women. *J Clin Endocrinol Metab* 2002;87:5044–5051.
16. Marette A, Mauriège P, Marcotte B, et al: Regional variation in adipose tissue insulin action and GLUT4 glucose transporter expression in severely obese premenopausal women. *Diabetologia* 1997;40:590–598.
17. Zierath JR, Livingston JN, Thorne A, et al: Regional difference in insulin inhibition of non-esterified fatty acid release from human adipocytes: relation to insulin receptor phosphorylation and intracellular signalling through the insulin receptor substrate-1 pathway. *Diabetologia* 1998;41:1343–1354.
18. Adeli K, Taghibiglou C, Van Iderstine SC, et al: Mechanisms of hepatic very low-density lipoprotein overproduction in insulin resistance. *Trends Cardiovasc Med* 2001;11:170–176.
19. Arner P: Free fatty acids—do they play a central role in type 2 diabetes? *Diabetes Obes Metab* 2001;3(Suppl 1):S11–S19.
20. Després JP, Ferland M, Moorjani S, et al: Role of hepatic-triglyceride lipase activity in the association between intra-abdominal fat and plasma HDL cholesterol in obese women. *Arteriosclerosis* 1989;9:485–492.
21. Carr MC, Hokanson JE, Zambon A, et al: The contribution of intraabdominal fat to gender differences in hepatic lipase activity and low/high-density lipoprotein heterogeneity. *J Clin Endocrinol Metab* 2001;86:2831–2837.
22. Després JP: Health consequences of visceral obesity. *Ann Med* 2001;33:534–541.
23. Frayn KN: Visceral fat and insulin resistance—causative or correlative? *Br J Nutr* 2000;83(Suppl 1):S71–S77.
24. Miles JM, Jensen MD: Counterpoint: visceral adiposity is not causally related to insulin resistance. *Diabetes Care* 2005;28: 2326–2328.
25. Jensen MD: Lipolysis: contribution from regional fat. *Annu Rev Nutr* 1997;17:127–139.
26. Després JP, Lemieux I: Abdominal obesity and metabolic syndrome. *Nature* 2006;444:881–887.
27. Björntorp P: Do stress reactions cause abdominal obesity and comorbidities? *Obes Rev* 2001;2:73–86.
28. Björntorp P: Metabolic implications of body fat distribution. *Diabetes Care* 1991;14:1132–1143.
29. Rebuffe-Scrive M, Walsh UA, McEwen B, et al: Effect of chronic stress and exogenous glucocorticoids on regional fat distribution and metabolism. *Physiol Behav* 1992;52:583–590.
30. Bélanger C, Luu-The V, Dupont P, et al: Adipose tissue intracrinology: potential importance of local androgen/estrogen metabolism in the regulation of adiposity. *Horm Metab Res* 2002;34:737–745.

31. Elbers JM, Asscheman H, Seidell JC, et al: Effects of sex steroid hormones on regional fat depots as assessed by magnetic resonance imaging in transsexuals. *Am J Physiol* 1999;276: E317–E325.
32. Elbers JM, Giltay EJ, Teerlink T, et al: Effects of sex steroids on components of the insulin resistance syndrome in transsexual subjects. *Clin Endocrinol (Oxf)* 2003;58:562–571.
33. Flier JS: The adipocyte: storage depot or node on the energy information superhighway? *Cell* 1995;80:15–18.
34. Juhan-Vague I, Alessi MC: Plasminogen activator inhibitor 1 and atherothrombosis. *Thromb Haemost* 1993;70:138–143.
35. Juhan-Vague I, Alessi MC: Regulation of fibrinolysis in the development of atherothrombosis: role of adipose tissue. *Thromb Haemost* 1999;82:832–836.
36. Juhan-Vague I, Morange P, Renucci JF, et al: Fibrinogen, obesity and insulin resistance. *Blood Coagul Fibrinolysis* 1999;10: S25–S28.
37. Tchernof A, Nolan A, Sites CK, et al: Weight loss reduces C-reactive protein levels in obese postmenopausal women. *Circulation* 2002;105:564–569.
38. Hak AE, Stehouwer CD, Bots ML, et al: Associations of C-reactive protein with measures of obesity, insulin resistance, and subclinical atherosclerosis in healthy, middle-aged women. *Arterioscler Thromb Vasc Biol* 1999;19:1986–1991.
39. Yudkin JS, Stehouwer CD, Emeis JJ, et al: C-reactive protein in healthy subjects: associations with obesity, insulin resistance, and endothelial dysfunction: a potential role for cytokines originating from adipose tissue? *Arterioscler Thromb Vasc Biol* 1999;19:972–978.
40. Côté M, Mauriège P, Bergeron J, et al: Adiponectinemia in visceral obesity: impact on glucose tolerance and plasma lipoprotein and lipid levels in men. *J Clin Endocrinol Metab* 2005;90:1434–1439.
41. Motoshima H, Wu X, Mahadev K, et al: Adiponectin suppresses proliferation and superoxide generation and enhances eNOS activity in endothelial cells treated with oxidized LDL. *Biochem Biophys Res Commun* 2004;315:264–271.
42. Ukkola O, Santaniemi M: Adiponectin: a link between excess adiposity and associated comorbidities? *J Mol Med* 2002;80:696–702.
43. Yamamoto Y, Hirose H, Saito I, et al: Correlation of the adipocyte-derived protein adiponectin with insulin resistance index and serum high-density lipoprotein-cholesterol, independent of body mass index, in the Japanese population. *Clin Sci (Lond)* 2002;103:137–142.
44. Hotta K, Funahashi T, Arita Y, et al: Plasma concentrations of a novel, adipose-specific protein, adiponectin, in type 2 diabetic patients. *Arterioscler Thromb Vasc Biol* 2000;20:1595–1599.
45. Kumada M, Kihara S, Sumitsuji S, et al: Association of hypoadiponectinemia with coronary artery disease in men. *Arterioscler Thromb Vasc Biol* 2003;23:85–89.
46. Pischon T, Girman CJ, Hotamisligil GS, et al: Plasma adiponectin levels and risk of myocardial infarction in men. *JAMA* 2004;291:1730–1737.
47. Sattar N, Wannamethee G, Sarwar N, et al: Adiponectin and coronary heart disease: a prospective study and meta-analysis. *Circulation* 2006;114:623–629.
48. Lemieux I: Energy partitioning in gluteal-femoral fat: does the metabolic fate of triglycerides affect coronary heart disease risk? *Arterioscler Thromb Vasc Biol* 2004;24:795–797.
49. Després JP: Is visceral obesity the cause of the metabolic syndrome? *Ann Med* 2006;38:52–63.
50. Després JP, Lamarche B, Mauriège P, et al: Hyperinsulinemia as an independent risk factor for ischemic heart disease. *N Engl J Med* 1996;334:952–957.
51. Eschwège E, Richard JL, Thibult N, et al: Coronary heart disease mortality in relation with diabetes, blood glucose and plasma insulin levels: the Paris prospective study, ten years later. *Horm Metab Res* 1985;15:41–46.
52. Pyörälä K: Relationship of glucose tolerance and plasma insulin to the incidence of coronary heart disease: results from two population studies in Finland. *Diabetes Care* 2: 1979;131–141.
53. Welborn TA, Wearne K: Coronary heart disease incidence and cardiovascular mortality in Busselton with reference to glucose and insulin concentrations. *Diabetes Care* 1979;2:154–160.
54. Yarnell JWG, Sweetnam PM, Marks V, et al: Insulin in ischaemic heart disease: are associations explained by triglyceride concentrations? The Caerphilly prospective study. *Br Heart J* 1994;71:293–296.
55. Lamarche B, Moorjani S, Lupien PJ, et al: Apolipoprotein A-I and B levels and the risk of ischemic heart disease during a five-year follow-up of men in the Québec cardiovascular study. *Circulation* 1996;94:273–278.
56. Lamarche B, Tchernof A, Moorjani S, et al: Small dense low-density lipoprotein particles as a predictor of the risk of ischemic heart disease in men. Prospective results from the Québec Cardiovascular Study. *Circulation* 1997;95:69–75.
57. Lemieux I, Lamarche B, Couillard C, et al: Total cholesterol/HDL cholesterol ratio vs LDL cholesterol/HDL cholesterol ratio as indices of ischemic heart disease risk in men. The Quebec Cardiovascular Study. *Arch Intern Med* 2001;161:2685–2692.
58. Pirro M, Bergeron J, Dagenais GR, et al: Age and duration of follow-up as modulators of the risk for ischemic heart disease associated with high plasma C-reactive protein levels in men. *Arch Intern Med* 2001;161:2474–2480.
59. Lamarche B, Tchernof A, Mauriège P, et al: Fasting insulin and apolipoprotein B levels and low-density lipoprotein particle size as risk factors for ischemic heart disease. *JAMA* 1998;279: 1955–1961.
60. Lemieux I, Poirier P, Bergeron J, et al: Hypertriglyceridemic waist: A useful screening phenotype in preventive cardiology? *Can J Ccardiol* 2007;23(suppl. B):23B–31B.
61. Lemieux I, Pascot A, Couillard C, et al: Hypertriglyceridemic waist. A marker of the atherogenic metabolic triad (hyperinsulinemia, hyperapolipoprotein B, small dense LDL) in men? *Circulation* 2000;102:179–184.
62. Executive Summary of The Third Report of The National Cholesterol Education Program (NCEP) Expert Panel on Detection, Evaluation, and Treatment of High Blood Cholesterol In Adults (Adult Treatment Panel III). *JAMA* 2001;285:2486–2497.
63. Després JP, Moorjani S, Ferland M, et al: Adipose tissue distribution and plasma lipoprotein levels in obese women. Importance of intra-abdominal fat. *Arteriosclerosis* 1989;9:203–210.
64. Secondary prevention by raising HDL cholesterol and reducing triglycerides in patients with coronary artery disease: the Bezafibrate Infarction Prevention (BIP) study. *Circulation* 2000;102:21–27.
65. Jeppesen J, Hein HO, Suadicani P, et al: Relation of high TG-low HDL cholesterol and LDL cholesterol to the incidence of ischemic heart disease. An 8-year follow-up in the Copenhagen Male Study. *Arterioscler Thromb Vasc Biol* 1997;17:1114–1120.
66. Manninen V, Tenkanen L, Koshinen P, et al: Joint effects of serum triglyceride and LDL cholesterol and HDL cholesterol concentrations on coronary heart disease risk in the Helsinki Heart Study: implications for treatment. *Circulation* 1992;85:37–45.
67. Castelli WP: Cholesterol and lipids in the risk of coronary artery disease—the Framingham Heart Study. *Can J Cardiol* 1988;4:5A–10A.
68. Assmann G, Schulte H, von Eckardstein A, et al: High-density lipoprotein cholesterol as a predictor of coronary heart disease risk. The PROCAM experience and pathophysiological implications for reverse cholesterol transport. *Atherosclerosis* 1996;124(Suppl):S11–S20.
69. Sharrett AR, Ballantyne CM, Coady SA, et al: Coronary heart disease prediction from lipoprotein cholesterol levels, triglycerides, lipoprotein(a), apolipoproteins A-I and B, and HDL density subfractions: The Atherosclerosis Risk in Communities (ARIC) Study. *Circulation* 2001;104:1108–1113.
70. Després JP, Lemieux I, Dagenais GR, et al: HDL cholesterol as a marker of coronary heart disease risk: the Quebec cardiovascular study. *Atherosclerosis* 2000;153:263–272.
71. Barter PJ, Nicholls S, Rye KA, et al: Antiinflammatory properties of HDL. *Circ Res* 2004;95:764–772.
72. Gordon T, Castelli WP, Hjortland MC, et al: High-density lipoprotein as a protective factor against coronary heart disease: the Framingham study. *Am J Med* 1977;62:707–714.
73. Castelli WP, Garrison RJ, Wilson PWF, et al: Incidence of coronary heart disease and lipoprotein cholesterol levels: the Framingham Study. *JAMA* 1986;256:2835–2838.
74. Kastelein JJ, van Leuven SI, Burgess L, et al: Effect of torcetrapib on carotid atherosclerosis in familial hypercholesterolemia. *N Engl J Med* 2007;356:1620–1630.
75. Nissen SE, Tardif JC, Nicholls SJ, et al: Effect of torcetrapib on the progression of coronary atherosclerosis. *N Engl J Med* 2007;356:1304–1316.
76. Rubins HB, Robins SJ, Collins D, et al: Gemfibrozil for the secondary prevention of coronary heart disease in men with low levels of high-density lipoprotein cholesterol. Veterans Affairs High-Density Lipoprotein Cholesterol Intervention Trial Study Group. *N Engl J Med* 1999;341:410–418.

77. Keech A, Simes RJ, Barter P, et al: Effects of long-term fenofibrate therapy on cardiovascular events in 9795 people with type 2 diabetes mellitus (the FIELD study): randomised controlled trial. *Lancet* 2005;366:1849–1861.
78. Cota D, Marsicano G, Tschop M, et al: The endogenous cannabinoid system affects energy balance via central orexigenic drive and peripheral lipogenesis. *J Clin Invest* 2003;112:423–431.
79. Di Marzo V, Bifulco M, De Petrocellis L: The endocannabinoid system and its therapeutic exploitation. *Nat Rev Drug Discov* 2004;3:771–784.
80. Horvath TL: Endocannabinoids and the regulation of body fat: the smoke is clearing. *J Clin Invest* 2003;112:323–326.
81. Devane WA, Hanus L, Breuer A, et al: Isolation and structure of a brain constituent that binds to the cannabinoid receptor. *Science* 1992;258:1946–1949.
82. Sugiura T, Kondo S, Sukagawa A, et al: 2-Arachidonoylglycerol: a possible endogenous cannabinoid receptor ligand in brain. *Biochem Biophys Res Commun* 1995;215:89–97.
83. Howlett AC, Barth F, Bonner TI, et al: International Union of Pharmacology. XXVII. Classification of cannabinoid receptors. *Pharmacol Rev* 2002;54:161–202.
84. Di Marzo V, Petrosino S: Endocannabinoids and the regulation of their levels in health and disease. *Curr Opin Lipidol* 2007;18:129–140.
85. Di Marzo V, Goparaju SK, Wang L, et al: Leptin-regulated endocannabinoids are involved in maintaining food intake. *Nature* 2001;410:822–825.
86. Kirkham TC, Williams CM, Fezza F, et al: Endocannabinoid levels in rat limbic forebrain and hypothalamus in relation to fasting, feeding and satiation: stimulation of eating by 2-arachidonoyl glycerol. *Br J Pharmacol* 2002;136:550–557.
87. Bluher M, Engeli S, Kloting N, et al: Dysregulation of the peripheral and adipose tissue endocannabinoid system in human abdominal obesity. *Diabetes* 2006;55:3053–3060.
88. Côté M, Matias I, Lemieux I, et al: Circulating endocannabinoid levels, abdominal adiposity and related cardiometabolic risk factors in obese men. *Int J Obes Lond* 2007;31:692–699.
89. Bensaid M, Gary-Bobo M, Esclangon A, et al: The cannabinoid CB1 receptor antagonist SR141716 increases Acrp30 mRNA expression in adipose tissue of obese fa/fa rats and in cultured adipocyte cells. *Mol Pharmacol* 2003;63:908–914.
90. Després JP, Golay A, Sjöström L: Effects of rimonabant on metabolic risk factors in overweight patients with dyslipidemia. *N Engl J Med* 2005;353:2121–2134.
91. Pi-Sunyer FX, Aronne LJ, Heshmati HM, et al: Effect of rimonabant, a cannabinoid-1 receptor blocker, on weight and cardiometabolic risk factors in overweight or obese patients: RIO-North America: a randomized controlled trial. *JAMA* 2006;295:761–775.
92. Scheen AJ, Finer N, Hollander P, et al: Efficacy and tolerability of rimonabant in overweight or obese patients with type 2 diabetes: a randomised controlled study. *Lancet* 2006;368:1660–1672.
93. Van Gaal LF, Rissanen AM, Scheen AJ, et al: Effects of the cannabinoid-1 receptor blocker rimonabant on weight reduction and cardiovascular risk factors in overweight patients: 1-year experience from the RIO-Europe study. *Lancet* 2005;365: 1389–1397.
94. Paré A, Dumont M, Lemieux I, et al: Is the relationship between adipose tissue and waist girth altered by weight loss in obese men? *Obes Res* 2001;9:526–534.
95. Goodpaster BH, Kelley DE, Wing RR, et al: Effects of weight loss on regional fat distribution and insulin sensitivity in obesity. *Diabetes* 1999;48:839–847.
96. Després JP, Lamarche B: Effects of diet and physical activity on adiposity and body fat distribution: implications for the prevention of cardiovascular disease. *Nutr Res Rev* 1993;6:137–159.
97. Zamboni M, Armellini F, Turcato E, et al: Effect of weight loss on regional body fat distribution in premenopausal women. *Am J Clin Nutr* 1993;58:29–34.
98. Leenen R, van der Kooy K, Deurenberg P, et al: Visceral fat accumulation in obese subjects: relation to energy expenditure and response to weight loss. *Am J Physiol* 1992;263: E913–E919.
99. Baumstark MW, Frey I, Berg A: Acute and delayed effects of prolonged exercise on serum lipoproteins. II. Concentration and composition of low-density lipoprotein subfractions and very low-density lipoproteins. *Eur J Appl Physiol Occup Physiol* 1993;66:526–530.
100. Houmard JA, Bruno NJ, Bruner RK, et al: Effects of exercise training on the chemical composition of plasma LDL. *Arterioscler Thromb Vasc Biol* 1994;14:325–330.
101. Williams PT, Krauss RM, Vranizan KM, et al: Effects of exercise-induced weight loss on low-density lipoprotein subfractions in healthy men. *Arterioscler Thromb Vasc Biol* 1989;9:623–632.
102. St-Pierre AC, Ruel IL, Cantin B, et al: Comparison of various electrophoretic characteristics of LDL particles and their relationship to the risk of ischemic heart disease. *Circulation* 2001;104:2295–2299.
103. Stampfer MJ, Krauss RM, Ma J, et al: A prospective study of triglyceride level, low-density lipoprotein particle diameter, and risk of myocardial infarction. *JAMA* 1996;276:882–888.
104. Gardner CD, Fortmann SP, Krauss RM: Association of small low-density lipoprotein particles with the incidence of coronary artery disease in men and women. *JAMA* 1996;276:875–881.
105. Lamarche B, Lemieux I, Després JP: The small dense LDL phenotype and the risk of coronary heart disease: Epidemiology, patho-physiology and therapeutic aspects. *Diabetes Metab* 1999;25:199–211.
106. Després JP, Van Gaal L, Scheen AJ, et al: Rimonabant improves cardiometabolic risk factors in overweight/obese patients irrespective of treatment with statins: pooled data from the RIO program. *Atheroscler* 2006;7:*suppl*:329.
107. Austin MA, McKnight B, Edwards KL, et al: Cardiovascular disease mortality in familial forms of hypertriglyceridemia: a 20-year prospective study. *Circulation* 2000;101:2777–2782.
108. Nordestgaard BG, Benn M, Schnohr P, et al: Nonfasting triglycerides and risk of myocardial infarction, ischemic heart disease, and death in men and women. *JAMA* 2007;298: 299–308.
109. Bansal S, Buring JE, Rifai N, et al: Fasting compared with nonfasting triglycerides and risk of cardiovascular events in women. *JAMA* 2007;298:309–316.
110. Heilbronn LK, Noakes M, Clifton PM: Energy restriction and weight loss on very-low-fat diets reduce C-reactive protein concentrations in obese, healthy women. *Arterioscler Thromb Vasc Biol* 2001;21:968–970.
111. Weisberg SP, McCann D, Desai M, et al: Obesity is associated with macrophage accumulation in adipose tissue. *J Clin Invest* 2003;112:1796–1808.
112. Spranger J, Kroke A, Mohlig M, et al: Adiponectin and protection against type 2 diabetes mellitus. *Lancet* 2003;361: 226–228.
113. Roche R, Hoareau L, Bes-Houtmann S, et al: Presence of the cannabinoid receptors, CB1 and CB2, in human omental and subcutaneous adipocytes. *Histochem Cell Biol* 2006;126:177–187.
114. Church TS, Kuk JL, Ross R, et al: Association of cardiorespiratory fitness, body mass index, and waist circumference to nonalcoholic fatty liver disease. *Gastroenterology* 2006;130: 2023–2030.
115. Yamada J, Tomiyama H, Yambe M, et al: Elevated serum levels of alanine aminotransferase and gamma glutamyltransferase are markers of inflammation and oxidative stress independent of the metabolic syndrome. *Atherosclerosis* 2006;189:198–205.
116. Després JP, Golay A, Sjöström L: Evidence that rimonabant has beneficial effects on liver enzymes in overweight/obese patients with dyslipidemia—RIO-Lipids Trial (abstract). *Circulation* 2006;114:II–223.
117. Marchesini G, Forlani G: NASH: from liver diseases to metabolic disorders and back to clinical hepatology. *Hepatology* 2002;35:497–499.
118. Després JP, Ross R, Boka G, et al: Rimonabant reduces both intra-abdominal adiposity and liver fat and improves cardiometabolic risk factors: The ADAGIO-Lipids trial. Presented at the 77th European Atherosclerosis Society Congress, Istanbul, 29 April 2008.
119. Dattilo AM, Kris-Etherton PM: Effects of weight reduction on blood lipids and lipoproteins: a meta-analysis. *Am J Clin Nutr* 1992;56:320–328.
120. Brown BG, Zhao XQ, Chait A, et al: Simvastatin and niacin, antioxidant vitamins, or the combination for the prevention of coronary disease. *N Engl J Med* 2001;345:1583–1592.
121. Brown G, Albers JJ, Fisher LD, et al: Regression of coronary artery disease as a result of intensive lipid-lowering therapy in men with high levels of apolipoprotein B. *N Engl J Med* 1990;323:1289–1298.

CHAPTER 29

Combination Therapy for Dyslipidemia

Michael H. Davidson

Coronary heart disease (CHD) is responsible for 52% of the 870,000 deaths that occur annually from cardiovascular disease in the United States.[1] Aggressive risk-reduction therapies are indicated for patients with CHD to improve survival, reduce recurrent events, and improve quality of life for these patients. 3-Hydroxy-3-methylglutaryl–coenzyme A reductase inhibitors (statins) are used in CHD prevention to target the reduction of increased low-density lipoprotein (LDL) level and to improve the lipid-level profile. Yet, statin therapy is often insufficient in achieving sufficient risk reduction for many patients with CHD, who often require the use of combination therapy to achieve target goals. This chapter reviews the use of combination therapy for dyslipidemia, highlighting the options available for maximizing risk reduction in CHD.

RATIONALE FOR COMBINATION THERAPY

Currently, only a small percentage of patients, including those with CHD, are reaching lipid goals. Early aggressive use of effective lipid-lowering agents is critical to achieve target lipid levels in the growing number of individuals at risk for CHD. It is now well established that cardiovascular benefit for lipid lowering to less than current cholesterol goal levels (LDL cholesterol level <70 mg/dL) for those with chronic CHD is beneficial (Table 29-1). Combination therapy increases the likelihood of achieving target lipid levels, especially in those patients with residual risk. Several reasons exist for combining therapeutic modalities to target both the endogenous and exogenous pathways of cholesterol synthesis. These include lack of achievement of LDL goals, lack of achievement of non–high-density lipoprotein (non-HDL) cholesterol goals, safety of high-dose statins, and residual risk despite statin therapy in many patients with CHD.

Lack of Achievement of Low-Density Lipoprotein Cholesterol Goals

Lipid-lowering drugs are among the most prescribed medications in the world, with more than 20 million people prescribed this class of drugs. Statins have been the most widely used for the treatment of dyslipidemia to reduce the risk for CHD. Early aggressive use of the effective lipid-lowering agents currently available is critical to achieve target lipid levels in a greater number of patients, and the use of combination drug therapy further enhances the likelihood of achieving target lipid levels.

Statins are used to target the reduction of increased LDL level and to improve the lipid-level profile. Statins have other non-LDL lipid effects, including decreasing triglycerides (TGs) and increasing HDL cholesterol that could also contribute to the risk reduction.[5,6] Other therapies with significant non-LDL-lowering effects, such as fibrates and niacin, which reduce TGs and increase HDL, also have been shown to reduce CHD events despite less potent effects on reducing LDL.[7] Yet, despite these therapeutic options, a significant number of patients with CHD do not achieve LDL goals. The National Cholesterol Education Program Adult Treatment Panel III (NCEP ATP III) guidelines outline that in high-risk patients with a low HDL cholesterol level, consideration should be given to combination therapy with a fibrate or nicotinic acid in addition to an LDL-lowering drug.[8] Other widely used lipid-altering drugs include fibrates, niacin, and intestinally active drugs, such as ezetimibe and colesevelam.

TABLE 29-1 Summary of Adult Treatment Panel III Guidelines for Dyslipidemia

	LDL Cholesterol Goal, mg/dL	Non-HDL Cholesterol Goal, mg/dL (if TG ≥ 200 mg/dL)
Low risk: <2 risk factors*	<160	<190
Moderate risk: ≥2 risk factors,* 10-year risk <10%	<130	<160
Moderately high risk: ≥2 risk factors,* 10-year risk = 10–20%	<130 (optional: <100)	<160
High risk†: CHD or CHD risk equivalents PAD, AAA, carotid artery disease‡ Diabetes§ 10-year risk >20%	<100	<130
Very high risk: CHD + other risk factors Multiple major risk factors (especially diabetes§) Multiple components of metabolic syndrome (especially high TG + high non-HDL cholesterol + low HDL cholesterol) Severe or poorly controlled risk factors (especially cigarette smoking) Acute coronary syndrome	<70 (optional)	<100 (optional)

*Cigarette smoking, hypertension (≥140/90 mm Hg or taking antihypertensive medication), low high-density lipoprotein cholesterol (HDL cholesterol; <40 mg/dL), family history of premature coronary heart disease (CHD; male first-degree relative <55 years old, female first-degree relative <65 years old), age (men ≥45 years old, women ≥55 years old); high HDL cholesterol (≥60 mg/dL) is a negative risk factor and decreases by 1 the total number of risk factors.

†American Heart Association/Centers for Disease Control and Prevention guidelines also include individuals at intermediate risk who have C-reactive protein level >3 mg/L.[2] National Kidney Foundation Guidelines recommend treating all patients with stage 1 to 4 chronic kidney disease in accordance with the high-risk category of Adult Treatment Panel III (ATP III).[3]

‡Transient ischemic attack, stroke of carotid origin, or >50% obstruction of a carotid artery.

§American Diabetes Association guidelines recommend that all patients with type 2 diabetes 40 years or older reduce low-density lipoprotein cholesterol (LDL cholesterol) level by 30% to 40% regardless of baseline LDL cholesterol.[4]

From Expert Panel on Detection, Evaluation, and Treatment of High Blood Cholesterol in Adults: Executive summary of the Third Report of the National Cholesterol Education Program (NCEP) Expert Panel on Detection, Evaluation, and Treatment of High Blood Cholesterol in Adults (Adult Treatment Panel III). JAMA 2001;285:2486-2497; and Grundy SM, Cleeman JI, Merz CN, et al: Implications of recent clinical trials for the National Cholesterol Education Program Adult Treatment Panel III guidelines. Circulation 2004;110:227-239, by permission.

AAA, abdominal aortic aneurysm; *PAD*, peripheral artery disease; *TG*, triglycerides.

Lack of Achievement of Non–High-Density Lipoprotein Cholesterol Goals

Many patients with CHD have therapeutic needs that exceed simple reductions in LDL cholesterol using statins. The NCEP ATP III has acknowledged the increasing evidence of an independent association between hypertriglyceridemia and CHD by issuing guidelines that identify non-HDL cholesterol as a secondary target for therapy in patients with increased TG levels.[9] This association is likely related to the atherogenicity of some species of TG-rich lipoproteins, particularly small very-low-density lipoprotein (VLDL) and intermediate-density lipoprotein particles. Increase of these “remnant” lipoproteins has been shown to contribute to atherosclerosis in mice.[10] Evidence exists that genetic dyslipidemias characterized by increased concentrations of remnant lipoproteins are associated with the development of premature CHD, and remnant lipoprotein levels strongly predict the progression of atherosclerosis.[9] In addition, in both observational studies and during treatment in clinical trials, levels of apolipoprotein (apo) B, reflecting the total number of circulating atherogenic particles (LDL plus VLDL), have been found to be associated with CHD risk more than the LDL cholesterol concentration.[11]

It is recognized that more aggressive therapy is needed to achieve non-HDL cholesterol goals than LDL cholesterol goals. In the Atorvastatin Cholesterol Efficacy and Safety Study (ACCESS), fewer patients on statin therapy achieved non-HDL cholesterol targets than LDL cholesterol targets. For example, with atorvastatin therapy, 72% of patients achieved an LDL cholesterol level ≤100 mg/dL compared with 60% who reached a non-HDL cholesterol level of ≤125 mg/dL (the level corresponding to the population percentile for non-HDL cholesterol equivalent to that for an LDL cholesterol concentration of 100 mg/dL).[12] After achievement of LDL cholesterol goals, non-HDL cholesterol level can be managed more aggressively by reducing LDL cholesterol or by using strategies that target a reduction in VLDL cholesterol.[13] As the prevalence of hypertriglyceridemia is increasing, enhanced efforts to improve non-HDL cholesterol goal achievement have the potential to produce a substantial effect on CHD.

Safety of High-Dose Statins

Concerns about the safety of high-dose statins and associated adverse events has surfaced as a result of statin-associated myotoxicity, including skeletal muscle necrosis that may result in life-threatening rhabdomyolysis, and persistent liver enzyme elevation. The recent heightened awareness of rhabdomyolysis is related, in part, to the clinical experience with cerivastatin (Baycol; Bayer Corp., West Haven, CT), a statin that was associated with increased reporting rate of fatal rhabdomyolysis nearly 80 times greater than rates reported for other statins available at the time, specifically atorvastatin (Lipitor; Pfizer Inc., New York, NY), fluvastatin (Lescol and Lescol XL; Novartis, East

Hanover, NJ), lovastatin (Mevacor; Merck & Co., West Point, PA), pravastatin (Pravachol; Bristol-Myers Squibb, Princeton, NJ) and simvastatin (Zocor; Merck & Co).[14,15]

Although the reported occurrence of muscle-related adverse events in clinical trials of statins is low, few clinical trials are of sufficient size, duration, or design to detect rhabdomyolysis. In addition, differing definitions of adverse events are used. Nonfatal rhabdomyolysis is defined as muscle symptoms plus creatine kinase more than 40 times the upper limit of normal. In the Heart Protection Study,[16] the largest clinical trial of statin therapy to date, five cases (0.05%) of nonfatal rhabdomyolysis were reported in patients receiving simvastatin 40 mg compared with three cases (0.03%) in patients receiving placebo. Although the absolute event rate for rhabdomyolysis remains low at all doses for approved statins, the greatest approved dose of a statin does have an increased risk for muscle adverse effects. Therefore, an important clinical challenge remains to further reduce the residual CHD risk on optimal statin therapy without adversely affecting patient safety.

Residual Risk on Statin Therapy

With the recognition that additional event reduction can be obtained by more intensive LDL cholesterol reductions in some patients at very high risk for CHD events, the NCEP ATP III recommends the therapeutic optional goal of LDL level less than 70 mg/dL and non-HDL level less than 100 mg/dL.[17] Cholesterol-lowering therapy with statins has been established as an effective method of reducing death and myocardial infarction among patients with CHD. However, a significant amount of individuals who are receiving statin therapy continue to have high residual risk. An important clinical challenge exists in reducing residual CHD risk with optimal therapies without increasing adverse effects. Combination therapy appears most appropriate for patients with a high rate of events despite optimal statin therapy. In addition to lifestyle modification, the use of combination therapy in CHD is an acknowledged strategy in optimal management to prevent or delay the morbidity and mortality associated with CHD and its risk factors. Current recommendations for CHD prevention and treatment advise the use of combination drug therapy for high-risk patients including those with combined hyperlipidemia and diabetic dyslipidemia.[12,18]

In light of the residual risk for CHD events in statin trials within certain subgroups, combination therapy appears most appropriate in patients with a high rate of events despite optimal statin therapy. The updated NCEP ATP III guidelines recommend an optional LDL cholesterol goal of less than 70 mg/dL in patients at very high risk, including those with established cardiovascular disease in conjunction with multiple major risk factors, severe or poorly controlled risk factors, multiple metabolic syndrome components, or acute coronary syndromes.[8] In a national survey of compliance with the NCEP ATP III guidelines, 75% of patients with CHD met the definition of "very high risk," yet only 18% had an LDL cholesterol level less than 70 mg/dL, and only 4% had an LDL cholesterol level less than 70 mg/dL and a non-HDL cholesterol level less than 100 mg/dL when TG levels were greater than 200 mg/dL.[19] These data substantiate the use of more aggressive statin therapy and implementation of combination therapy to reduce residual risks of statins.

LOW-DENSITY LIPOPROTEIN CHOLESTEROL REDUCTION

Statin clinical event outcome trials have proved conclusively that reducing LDL cholesterol results in significant improvement in cardiovascular morbidity or mortality (Table 29-2). The relationship between LDL cholesterol and CHD events appears to be linear, with considerable evidence supporting the "lower is better" hypothesis. However, even with low LDL levels, the residual risk for subsets of high-risk patients continues to be increased. In the Treating to New Targets (TNT) trial, patients taking atorvastatin 80 mg (with a mean LDL cholesterol level of 77 mg/dL) had a cardiovascular event rate of 28%, compared with a 33% event rate for patients taking 10 mg atorvastatin (with mean LDL cholesterol level of 101 mg/dL), which represents a 22% relative risk reduction.[25]

Statin therapy generally reduces LDL cholesterol level by 25% to 35% with fluvastatin, lovastatin, or pravastatin, and 35% to 45% with atorvastatin, simvastatin, or rosuvastatin.[9,26,27] Each doubling of the dose usually produces an additional 5% to 7% reduction in LDL cholesterol level and a slightly smaller percentage decrease in non-HDL cholesterol.[9,27] Larger incremental reductions of 10% to 20% may be achieved by adding a second agent targeting enhanced LDL cholesterol reduction. The second agent may be a nonpharmacologic product such as viscous fiber or plant sterol/stanols,[9,28,29] or another pharmacological agent such as a cholesterol absorption inhibitor or bile acid sequestrant.[30,31]

Compared with adding an agent to target LDL cholesterol, the addition of a fibrate or niacin usually has a lesser impact on LDL cholesterol; however, it reduces non-HDL cholesterol because of the decrease of VLDL cholesterol.[32]

Several combination therapies can be used to target LDL cholesterol reduction. These include combination therapy with a statin plus ezetimibe or a statin plus a bile acid sequestrant.

Statins Plus Ezetimibe

LDL cholesterol reduction can be enhanced by combining a statin, which reduces hepatic cholesterol synthesis and increases hepatic LDL receptor activity, with ezetimibe, a selective cholesterol absorption inhibitor that blocks cholesterol absorption at the intestinal brush border to reduce LDL cholesterol. Combination therapy with ezetimibe plus statins has been evaluated in several randomized clinical trials of patients with primary hypercholesterolemia. Ezetimibe 10 mg coadministered with simvastatin 10 mg resulted in 44% LDL cholesterol level reductions similar to those obtained with simvastatin 80 mg alone, and coadministration of ezetimibe 10 mg with simvastatin doses of 10 to 80 mg resulted in TG reductions of 26% to 31% and HDL cholesterol increases of

TABLE 29-2 **Risk for Cardiovascular Events by Diabetes Status or Baseline High-Density Lipoprotein Cholesterol Level in Major Statin Trials**

	Without Diabetes		With Diabetes	
Trial	**Statin**	**Placebo/Control**	**Statin**	**Placebo/Control**
HPS*[16]	19.8%	25.7%	33.4%	37.8%
CARE†[20]	19.6%	24.6%	28.7%	36.8%
LIPID*[21]	11.7%	15.2%	19.7%	22.8%
PROSPER*[22]	13.1%	16%	23.1%	18.4%
ASCOT*[23]	4.9%	8.7%	9.6%	11.4%
TNT‡[24]	7.8%§	9.7%¶	13.8%§	17.9%¶
	High HDL Cholesterol on Statin	***High HDL Cholesterol on Placebo***	***Low HDL Cholesterol on Statin***	***Low HDL Cholesterol on Placebo***
HPS*[16]	17%	20.9%	22.0%	29.9%
CARE/LIPID*†[20,21]	18.5%	22.4%	25%	30.8%
PROSPER*[22]	12.8%	11.6%	13%	19.3%

*Coronary artery disease (CAD) death, nonfatal myocardial infarction, coronary or noncoronary revascularization, or stroke.

†CAD death and nonfatal myocardial infarction

‡CAD death, nonfatal myocardial infarction, resuscitated cardiac arrest, or fatal or nonfatal stroke.

§80 mg/day atorvastatin.

¶10 mg/day atorvastatin.

ASCOT, Anglo-Scandinavian Cardiac Outcomes Trial[23]; CARE, Cholesterol and Recurrent Events[20]; HDL, high-density lipoprotein; HPS, Heart Protection Study[16]; LIPID, Long-Term Prevention with Pravastatin in Ischaemic Disease[21]; PROSPER, Prospective Study of Pravastatin in the Elderly at Risk[22]; TNT, Treating to New Targets.[24]

8% to 11%.[33] Similarly, compared with monotherapy, coadministration of ezetimibe 10 mg and atorvastatin 10, 20, 40, or 80 mg resulted in significant improvements in LDL cholesterol (12% reduction), HDL cholesterol (3% increase), TGs (8% reduction), and high-sensitivity C-reactive protein (10% reduction) levels.[34]

In a study comparing lovastatin monotherapy at 10, 20, or 40 mg or ezetimibe 10 mg with combination therapy of ezetimibe 10 mg plus lovastatin 10, 20, or 40 mg, the coadministration of ezetimibe provided an incremental 14% LDL cholesterol decrease, a 5% HDL cholesterol increase, and a 10% decrease in TGs compared with pooled lovastatin alone. Ezetimibe plus lovastatin provided mean LDL cholesterol level decreases of 33% to 45%, median TG concentration decreases of 19% to 27%, and mean HDL cholesterol level increases of 8% to 9%, depending on the statin dose.[35]

Similarly, compared with monotherapy, combination therapy with ezetimibe 10 mg and pravastatin 10, 20, or 40 mg resulted in significant incremental reductions in LDL cholesterol and TG levels compared with pooled pravastatin alone ($P < 0.01$). Coadministration therapy reduced LDL cholesterol level by 34% to 41% and TG level by 21% to 23%, and increased HDL cholesterol level by 7.8% to 8.4%, depending on the dose of pravastatin.[36]

Statins Plus Bile Acid Sequestrants

Bile acid sequestrants are a class of antihyperlipidemic drugs developed to reduce LDL cholesterol levels. Two of the most commonly prescribed bile acid sequestrants, cholestyramine and colestipol, have been used since the 1980s and have been proved effective and safe as nonsystemic approaches to cholesterol reduction. The clinical benefit of bile acid sequestrants has been demonstrated in several clinical trials, including the Lipid Research Clinics Coronary Primary Prevention Trial[37] and the Familial Atherosclerosis Treatment Study.[38] The use of bile acid sequestrants in clinical practice is difficult, due in part to adherence issues related to poor palatability of the drug and to the occurrence of adverse gastrointestinal effects, particularly constipation. As a result, colesevelam hydrochloride has become the preferred drug of this class.

Colesevelam hydrochloride (Welchol; Sankyo Pharma Inc., Parsippany, NJ) is a nonabsorbed lipid-lowering agent that can be used in monotherapy or in combination therapy to reduce LDL cholesterol level in patients with hypercholesterolemia. Combination therapy with colesevelam hydrochloride and lovastatin,[39] simvastatin,[40] or atorvastatin[41] can significantly reduce LDL cholesterol levels in patients with hypercholesterolemia.

Low-dose combination therapy with colesevelam hydrochloride (2.3 g) and lovastatin (10 mg) resulted in LDL cholesterol level decreases of 34% (60 mg/dL; $P < 0.0001$) when administered together and 32% (53 mg/dL; $P < 0.0001$) when administered separately in patients with primary hypercholesterolemia.[39]

Similarly, combination therapy with simvastatin 10 and 20 mg and colesevelam hydrochloride 2.3 and 3.8 g resulted in mean LDL cholesterol level decreases in all active treatment groups ($P < 0.0001$). Groups treated with combination therapy had a mean reduction in LDL cholesterol levels of 42% (−80 mg/dL; $P < 0.0001$ compared with baseline), which exceeded reductions for simvastatin 10 mg (−26%, −48 mg/dL) or 20 mg (−34%, −61 mg/dL) alone or for colesevelam hydrochloride 2.3 g (−8%, −17 mg/dL) or 3.8 g (−16%, −31 mg/dL) alone ($P < 0.001$).[41]

In an additional study, coadministration of colesevelam hydrochloride 3.8 g and atorvastatin 10 mg or 80 mg/day resulted in LDL cholesterol level decreases of 12% to 53% in all active treatment groups ($P < 0.01$).

Combination therapy resulted in significant decreases in LDL cholesterol levels (48%) compared with colesevelam hydrochloride (12%) or low-dose atorvastatin (38%) alone ($P < 0.01$) but similar to those achieved with atorvastatin 80 mg/day (53%). In addition, total cholesterol level decreased by 6% to 39% in all active treatment groups and HDL cholesterol level increased significantly for all groups ($P < 0.05$).[41]

COMBINED DYSLIPIDEMIA

Non–High-Density Lipoprotein Cholesterol Reduction

The NCEP ATP III identified non-HDL cholesterol as a secondary therapeutic target for individuals with increased TG levels (≥200 mg/dL). Non-HDL cholesterol goals are set 30 mg/dL greater than the LDL cholesterol goal for the patient's risk category (see Table 29-1), a level based on the Friedewald formula,[42] in which VLDL cholesterol levels are estimated to be one fifth of the TG concentration. Because TG concentrations less than 150 mg/dL are considered normal, a VLDL concentration less than 30 mg/dL represents the reference range. As TG levels increase, the fraction of non-HDL cholesterol accounted for by LDL cholesterol declines.

Non-HDL cholesterol correlates well with apoB concentration and is, therefore, a good proxy for the total number of circulating atherogenic particles.[12] Consistent with this relationship, population studies have shown non-HDL cholesterol to be a somewhat stronger predictor of cardiovascular disease[43,44] and mortality[45] risk than LDL cholesterol.

Statin Plus Fibrates

Fibrates are an important class of drugs for the management of dyslipidemia. This class of drugs is generally well tolerated but is infrequently associated with several safety issues. Fibrates, most likely by an effect mediated by peroxisome proliferator–activated receptor–α (PPAR-α), may reversibly increase creatinine and homocysteine but are not associated with an increased risk for renal failure in clinical trials. In patients with combined dyslipidemia, fibrate–statin combination therapy can be used to promote reductions in LDL cholesterol and TGs and simultaneous increases in HDL cholesterol level.

Fibrates are associated with a slightly increased risk (<1.0%) for myopathy, cholelithiasis, and venous thrombosis. In clinical trials, in patients without increased TG and/or low HDL cholesterol levels, fibrates are associated with an increase in noncardiovascular mortality. Gemfibrozil generally should be avoided in combination with statins. The preferred option is fenofibrate, which is not associated with an inhibition of statin metabolism. Clinicians are advised to measure serum creatinine before fibrate use and adjust the dose accordingly for renal impairment. Routine monitoring of creatinine is not required, but if a patient has a clinically important increase in creatinine and other potential causes of creatinine increase have been excluded, consideration should be given to discontinuing fibrate therapy or reducing the dose.[46]

The additive effects of simvastatin and fenofibrate on lipid parameters have been documented in the Simvastatin Plus Fenofibrate for Combined Hyperlipidemia (SAFARI) trial.[47] Monotherapy with simvastatin 20 mg/day was compared with combination therapy of simvastatin 20 mg/day plus fenofibrate 160 mg/day in patients with combined hyperlipidemia (fasting TG levels ≥150 and ≤500 mg/dL and LDL cholesterol level >130 mg/dL). When compared with monotherapy, mean LDL cholesterol levels significantly decreased with combination therapy (by 25.8% and 31.2%, respectively; $P < 0.001$). In addition, when compared with monotherapy, mean HDL cholesterol levels significantly increased with combination therapy (by 9.7% and 18.6%, respectively; $P < 0.001$), without the occurrence of any drug-related serious adverse events.[47]

Statin Plus Niacin

Statin–niacin combination therapy has been used to reduce residual cardiovascular risk. Niacin is often added to a statin in patients with combined hyperlipidemia, especially if the HDL level is low or lipoprotein(a) level is high. Although statins have demonstrated an approximate reduction in CHD events by 30%, combination therapy with statins and niacin has resulted in reductions of 75%. This significant reduction in CHD events suggests that other effects of niacin, such as TG reduction, lipoprotein(a) reduction, and HDL cholesterol increase may also contribute to the benefits.

Adding niacin to a statin is a likely combination because niacin has the most significant effects on increasing HDL level. There have also been a number of trials that have demonstrated the safety of this combination and efficacy in inhibiting the progression of atherosclerosis. Most trials have used either immediate-release niacin or extended-release niacin (Niaspan; Abbott Laboratories, North Chicago, IL). Because of the safety data on extended-release niacin in combination with a statin, there has been increased interest in the use of combination therapy to maximize risk reduction in patients with dyslipidemia.

As demonstrated by the Arterial Biology for the Investigation of the Treatment Effects of Reducing Cholesterol (ARBITER) 2 trial, the addition of extended-release niacin to statin therapy was demonstrated to increase HDL cholesterol level by 21% and slow the progression of atherosclerosis measured by change in carotid intima–media thickness compared with statin therapy alone in patients with known CHD and low HDL cholesterol levels.[48]

In the HDL-Atherosclerosis Treatment Study (HATS), simvastatin (10–20 mg/day) plus niacin (2–4 g/day) therapy resulted in significant risk reduction for composite cardiovascular endpoints (death from coronary causes, confirmed myocardial infarction or stroke, or revascularization) by 90% in the group treated with simvastatin plus niacin compared with placebo ($P = 0.03$).[49] In addition, simvastatin–niacin combination therapy resulted in a 0.4% regression in coronary stenosis but progression in other treatment groups receiving antioxidants alone, simvastatin plus niacin plus antioxidants, or placebo

($P < 0.001$).[50] Studies evaluating statin plus niacin combination therapy have consistently demonstrated the efficacy in increasing HDL cholesterol and reducing TG and LDL cholesterol.[51–54] Additional studies comparing statin monotherapy with statin–niacin combination therapy indicate that statins and niacin have additive effects on HDL cholesterol. Angiographic studies further support the effect of statin-niacin combination therapy in impeding the progression of CHD.[49]

Statin Plus Omega-3 Fatty Acids

Omega-3 fatty acids, or fish oils, are essential fatty acids that are thought to inhibit VLDL and TG synthesis in the liver, although the exact molecular mechanisms are not well understood. Omega-3 fatty acids have been demonstrated to significantly reduce TG levels and increase LDL cholesterol levels in patients with high TG concentration. Dietary supplementation with the n-3 polyunsaturated fatty acids (PUFAs) eicosapentaenoic acid (EPA) and docosahexaenoic acid (DHA) has also been shown to reduce the risk for death, nonfatal coronary events, and stroke after myocardial infarction.[55] PUFAs have been demonstrated to reduce TG levels by 20% to 30%, and up to 50% in patients with severe hypertriglyceridemia (TG >750 mg/dL [>8.47 mmol/L]).[56,57] In studies of combination therapy with statins and n-3 PUFAs, LDL cholesterol reductions of 13% to 24% and TG reductions of 27% to 30% have been demonstrated when n-3 PUFAs were added to pravastatin 40 mg/day[58] or simvastatin 20 mg/day.[59] Similarly, combination therapy with atorvastatin 10 mg resulted in significant reductions of the concentration of small dense LDL particles and increases in HDL cholesterol compared with monotherapy.[60]

A highly purified, pharmaceutical-grade, omega-3 fatty acid marine fish oil formulation contains high concentrations of EPA and DHA (440 and 260 mg, respectively, for a total of 800 mg EPA + DHA), together with 4 mg (6 IU) vitamin E in each 1-g capsule. Prescription omega-3 fatty acid marine oils are indicated for the treatment of hypertriglyceridemia and have been demonstrated to significantly reduce serum TGs by 19% to 55% at doses of 4 capsules per day when administered over periods ranging from 6 weeks to several years. When combined with therapy with gemfibrozil and simvastatin, marine oil reduces TG levels by an additional 37% and 46%, respectively. In a recent study assessing combination therapy with simvastatin 40 mg and omega-3 acid ethyl esters 4 g/day, median percentage decrease in non-HDL cholesterol was significantly greater with combination therapy compared with placebo plus simvastatin (9.0% vs. 2.2%, respectively; $P < 0.001$). In addition, combination therapy significantly reduced TG concentration (29.5%) and VLDL cholesterol (27.5%), increased HDL cholesterol (3.4%), and decreased total cholesterol/HDL cholesterol ratio (9.6%; $P \leq 0.001$ vs. placebo for all).[61]

SEVERE HYPERTRIGLYCERIDEMIA

Severe hypertriglyceridemia is usually due to impairment or deficiency of lipoprotein lipase, the vascular enzyme that degrades chylomicrons into remnant particles and liberates the TG into free fatty acids for energy use or for fat storage. In some cases, severe forms of familial dysbetalipoproteinemia (type III hyperlipidemia) or overproduction of VLDL (familial hypertriglyceridemia) may result in severe hypertriglyceridemia. If the total cholesterol is greater than 300 mg/dL and the TG concentration is between 500 and 1000 mg/dL, the patient may have a genetic cause of dyslipidemia (type III or familial combined hyperlipidemia).

Serum TGs are primarily carried in apoB-containing lipoproteins and have been demonstrated to be predictive of CHD risk.[62] High levels of fasting TG (≥200 mg/dL) often represent an increase in plasma concentration of VLDL particles, the cholesterol content of which is correlated with the number of atherogenic particles.[6] According to NCEP ATP III guidelines, a statin is recommended as initial therapy for reducing LDL cholesterol and non-HDL cholesterol in patients with hypertriglyceridemia (200–499 mg/dL). However, statin monotherapy is often insufficient to achieve non-HDL cholesterol targets. For patients with persistent hypertriglyceridemia (≥200 mg/dL) receiving statin therapy, adding a TG-lowering agent is recommended as a therapeutic option to reduce non-HDL cholesterol levels.[9]

Dietary fat and simple carbohydrate restriction are indicated to reduce chylomicrons and VLDL. If dietary therapy fails, the drug therapy options include niacin and fibrates. Fibrates are recommended therapy in patients whose primary abnormality is increased TG levels and low HDL cholesterol. Both fibrate plus niacin and fibrate plus omega-3 fatty acid combination therapy can also be used for the management of hypertriglyceridemia.

LOW HIGH-DENSITY LIPOPROTEIN

Low serum concentrations of HDL cholesterol have consistently emerged as an independent risk factor for CHD. In the Framingham Study[63] and the Quebec Cardiovascular Study,[64] there was a well-defined escalation in risk as HDL cholesterol levels decreased. Results from the Framingham Study demonstrated that with every 20-mg/dL reduction in HDL cholesterol, CHD risk increased by 50%. Other studies, including the Honolulu Heart Study,[65] Israeli Ischemic Heart Disease Study,[66] Belgian Interuniversity Research on Nutrition and Health Study,[67] and Poland and United States Collaborative Study on Cardiovascular Epidemiology,[68] demonstrated that low serum levels of HDL cholesterol predispose to the development of CHD.

Often, lifestyle modification can be used to target common causes of low HDL cholesterol level such as excess body weight and physical inactivity. The NCEP ATP III guidelines identify therapeutic lifestyle changes as the initial intervention for increasing HDL cholesterol levels and include targeting dietary intake of cholesterol, use of plant stanols/sterols and fiber to reduce LDL cholesterol level, and a focus on total calories and physical activity to maintain desirable weight. Additional components such as smoking cessation, weight loss, aerobic exercise, and moderate alcohol intake are also advocated.

Pharmacologic therapy is indicated in the management of low HDL cholesterol when therapeutic lifestyle changes are not adequate to achieve target goals. The

NCEP ATP III guidelines outline that in high-risk patients with a low HDL cholesterol level, consideration should be given to combination therapy in addition to an LDL-lowering drug.[9] Traditionally, the principal drug classes used for the management of low HDL cholesterol include statins, niacin, and fibrates.

Based on the results of the large statin endpoint trials (West of Scotland Coronary Prevention Study, Air Force/Texas Coronary Atherosclerosis Prevention Study), patients with high LDL and low HDL levels may have significant benefits from statin therapy. Statins should be used as first-line agents in patients with CHD or CHD risk equivalent, and in those who have isolated low HDL cholesterol or low HDL cholesterol levels combined with increased LDL cholesterol level.

Niacin is the most effective HDL cholesterol–increasing pharmacologic agent, and although the specific mechanism of action of niacin is not well understood, it appears that niacin reduces apoB secretion, thereby reducing both VLDL and LDL, increasing apoA-I, and reducing lipoprotein(a).

Fibrates are PPAR-α ligands and lead to increased lipoprotein lipase expression and decreased apoC-III expression, which results in enhanced catabolism of TG-rich particles. Fibrates also increase the expression of apoA-I and apoA-II, with a net result of decreasing hypertriglyceridemia and increasing HDL cholesterol level. As a result, fibrate combination therapy is used for patients with hypertriglyceridemia and low HDL level.

Combination therapy is often indicated for the management of low HDL cholesterol in CHD. Options include statin combination therapy with ezetimibe, fibrates, or niacin. Adding niacin to a statin is the most likely combination because niacin has the most significant effects on increasing HDL cholesterol level. Adding a fibrate is desirable when TG concentrations are increased.

A newer approach to increasing HDL cholesterol level is through the inhibition of cholesteryl ester transfer protein (CETP). CETP plays an important role in cholesterol metabolism because it is responsible for the transfer of cholesteryl esters from HDL to VLDL and LDL. Results from recent clinical trials question the therapeutic use of at least one CETP inhibitor, torcetrapib, which was demonstrated to increase blood pressure and have no effect on decreasing the progression of coronary atherosclerosis; however, other CETP inhibitors are in development.

Other emerging approaches to increasing HDL level include infusion of mutant forms of apoA-I such as apoA-I_{Milano}, delipidated HDL, oral apoA-I mimetics, and apoA-I_{Milano} gene transfer. Additional novel therapies that may prove beneficial in increasing HDL cholesterol levels include activators of nuclear receptors liver X and farnesoid X receptors, which may also stimulate reverse cholesterol transport, and PPAR agonists targeting one or more of the PPAR-α, -δ, or -γ receptors.

SAFETY OF COMBINATION THERAPY

Although combination therapy is widely used and often recommended by expert panels for the management of hypertension and diabetes, for the treatment of dyslipidemia, combination treatment is seldom applied clinically in practice. In the National Cholesterol Education Program Evaluation Project Utilizing Novel E-Technology (NEPTUNE) II Survey,[19] only 5% of patients receiving treatment were on combination therapies (Figs. 29-1 and 29-2). The perception of adverse events associated with combining a statin with niacin or a fibrate is one of the major reasons that combination therapy has not been widely utilized in practice. In the labeling for all statins are cautionary notes regarding the combination with niacin or a fibrate, stating that the potential benefits should outweigh the increased risk for myopathy. The concern regarding the combination of niacin with a statin is based on early case reports that documented myopathy with lovastatin in combination with high doses of niacin (≥2.5 g/day). Because niacin does not alter the pharmacokinetics of lovastatin and excessive doses of niacin monotherapy have documented hepatotoxicity, the most likely explanation for the cases of myopathy associated with combination statin–niacin therapy is that the liver impairment associated with niacin toxicity results in delayed clearance of the statin, leading to an increased risk for myopathy. Statin-induced myopathy is almost always associated with factors that increase the area under the curve, such as increased dosage, hypothyroidism, renal or hepatic impairment, or drugs that interfere with statin metabolism such as cytochrome P450 3A4 inhibitors. In the absence of hepatotoxicity, it is unlikely that niacin would increase the risk for

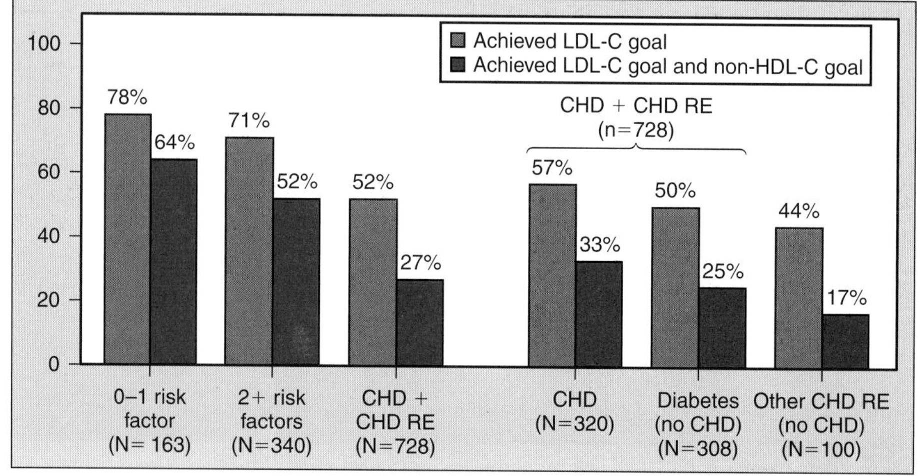

FIGURE 29-1 Percentage of patients with triglyceride concentrations ≥200 mg/dL having achieved low-density lipoprotein cholesterol (LDL-C) and non-high-density lipoprotein cholesterol (non-HDL-C) treatment goals according to risk category. *(Adapted from Ref. 19, with permission.) CHD, coronary heart disease; RE, risk equivalent.*

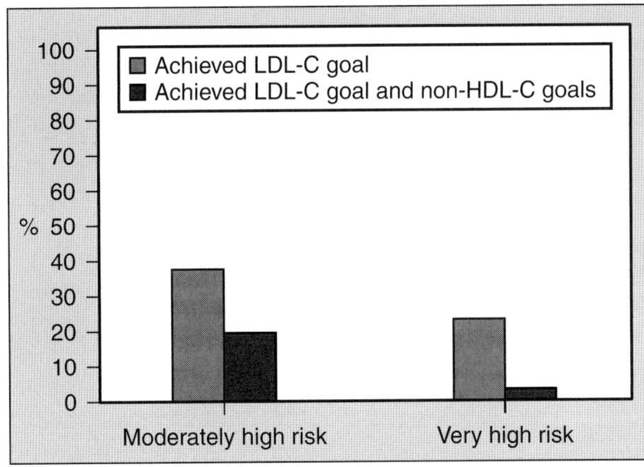

FIGURE 29-2 Achievement of optional low-density lipoprotein cholesterol (LDL-C) and combined LDL cholesterol and non-high-density lipoprotein cholesterol (non-HDL-C) goals among patients with triglyceride concentrations ≥200 mg/dL in the National Cholesterol Education Program Evaluation Project Utilizing Novel E-Technology II (NEPTUNE II) Survey. *(Adapted from Ref. 19, with permission.)*

statin myopathy, and since the first two reports of niacin and lovastatin myopathy, there have been no additional reports in the medical literature.

An appraisal of statin therapy from the U.S. Food and Drug Administration (FDA) Adverse Event Reporting System (AERS) demonstrated that a before-and-after cerivastatin withdrawal comparison showed a substantial increase in the reporting of adverse events of interest for the statin class overall. Report proportion analyses indicated that the burden of rosuvastatin-associated adverse events was similar to that for other statin agents. Analyses of monthly reporting rates showed that the reporting of rosuvastatin-associated rhabdomyolysis and renal failure increased after adverse event–specific mass media publicity. Adverse event reporting patterns after the introduction of rosuvastatin were comparable with those seen with other statins and did not resemble those of cerivastatin.[69]

Adverse event reports under the MedWatch program to the FDA have also documented a low incidence of myopathy associated with statin combined with niacin.[70] Extended-release niacin, which has a low rate of hepatotoxicity, especially when compared with sustained-release niacin, has few reports of myopathy in the AERS database despite several hundred thousand prescriptions written in combination with a statin. Therefore, the AERS data, although not conclusive, support the safety of doses of extended-release niacin up to 2 g/day in combination with a statin.

In regard to fibrate therapy, there appears to be a clinically significant difference in safety with the combination of statin with gemfibrozil compared with fenofibrate. There are at least 60 case reports of gemfibrozil–statin myopathy in the medical literature compared with two cases for fenofibrate in combination with a statin. Recent reviews of the FDA AERS database have documented that after correcting for prescription utilization, the rate of myopathy for gemfibrozil with a statin is 30 times more than for combination therapy with fenofibrate.[71,72] Cerivastatin, in combination with gemfibrozil, was associated with more than 4000 times the rate of rhabdomyolysis compared with statin therapy alone, and numerous fatalities were reported, resulting in the removal of cerivastatin from the worldwide market. An analysis of several managed-care prescription and hospitalization event databases have estimated that the rate of rhabdomyolysis requiring hospitalization from cerivastatin in combination with gemfibrozil was at least one in ten patients. The Lipid and Diabetes Study,[73] which had a 2 × 2 factorial design, utilized cerivastatin–fenofibrate combination therapy or placebo in more than 2000 patients with diabetes (more than 1000 for more than 12 weeks) before the study was discontinued when cerivastatin was withdrawn from the market. In the patients taking the combination of cerivastatin and fenofibrate, there were no case reports of myopathy. In a Veterans Administration database evaluation during a 2-year period (October 1, 2002, to September 30, 2003), there were 93,677 patients taking a combination of gemfibrozil and statin and 1830 patients taking fenofibrate with a statin during the evaluation period. During the 2 years evaluated, there were 149 cases of rhabdomyolysis or acute tubular necrosis in the 93,677 patients taking gemfibrozil with any statin for an overall rate of 0.16%. No cases of rhabdomyolysis or acute tubular necrosis were reported in the 1830 patients taking fenofibrate with any statin.[8] Therefore, the AERS data and the information from the Lipid and Diabetes Study support a much greater safety margin for combining a statin with fenofibrate than with gemfibrozil. The reason for the much greater propensity for gemfibrozil to increase the risk for myopathy with a statin is most likely due to the difference in the pharmacokinetic interactions between the two fibrates. Lipophilic statins are hydrolyzed by the cytochrome P450 enzymes to increase water solubility for renal excretion. Statins are also metabolized by another secondary pathway known as glucuronidation. Gemfibrozil utilizes the same family of glucuronidation enzymes as the statins, but fenofibrate utilizes a different enzyme family. This explains the marked increase in area under the curve for statins in conjunction with gemfibrozil, whereas fenofibrate has no significant effects on statin blood levels. Gemfibrozil is also a potent cytochrome P450 2C8 (CYP2C8) inhibitor, which is a metabolic pathway for cerivastatin. The more prominent increase in the area under the curve for gemfibrozil and cerivastatin may be because of the effect of both CYP2C8 and glucuronidation. Rosiglitazone and repaglinide are also metabolized by CYP2C8, and blood levels are increased in combination with gemfibrozil but not with fenofibrate. Therefore, gemfibrozil is problematic not only for combination therapy with statins but also for use with antidiabetes drugs that utilize the CYP2C8 pathway. In patients with diabetes, who have documented benefits from statin therapy but a high residual risk, combination therapy with fenofibrate appears to be the most appropriate add-on treatment to further improve the lipid profile, if necessary, and to avoid the significant safety problems associated with gemfibrozil therapy. The Action to Control Cardiovascular Risk in Diabetes (ACCORD) trial is under way to determine the enhanced clinical benefit of adding fenofibrate to the treatment of patients receiving simvastatin therapy, and the Atherothrombosis Intervention in Metabolic Syndrome with Low HDL/High Triglycerides and Impact on Global Health Outcomes (AIM-HIGH) trial will be evaluating the potential clinical benefits of increasing HDL cholesterol level with niacin in patients with CHD and the metabolic syndrome.[74]

CONCLUSION

Combination therapy that further improves the lipid profile appears to be frequently necessary for patients at very high risk who have not yet achieved the optional therapeutic target. A notable finding from NEPTUNE II[19] was that the prevalence of combination therapy was not different in 2003 (9.6%) compared with that observed among Lipid Treatment Assessment Project (L-TAP) participants (10.2%) in the 1990s.[75] Combination therapy is beneficial for patients who do not achieve recommended goals despite the use of statin therapy or if more aggressive lipid-modifying therapy is necessary to achieve the desired target goals. Bile acid sequestrants (cholestyramine, colestipol, and colesevelam hydrochloride), niacin (extended release), and ezetimibe reduce LDL cholesterol by 15% to 20%, depending on the dose. A 15% to 20% decrease in LDL cholesterol is approximately equivalent to tripling the dose of the statin. For every doubling the dose of the statin, there is a further decrease in LDL cholesterol of approximately 6%. Therefore, the use of combination therapy with the aforementioned nonstatin drugs results in LDL cholesterol reductions equivalent to or greater than the highest dose of the statin. Combination therapy can be successfully utilized to maximize safety of lipid-lowering therapy.

The use of combination therapy may have been impacted by the history of increased risk for myopathy with gemfibrozil in combination with a statin. However, other lipid-altering agents such as bile acid sequestrants, extended-release niacin, ezetimibe, and fenofibrate do not have a pharmacokinetic interaction with statins and appear to have a low risk for increasing statin-related side effects. The improved safety of these agents with a statin has stimulated a new era of clinical trials evaluating the potential clinical benefits of combination therapy for CHD risk reduction.

REFERENCES

1. Rosamond W, Flegal K, Friday G, et al: Heart Disease and Stroke Statistics—2007 Update: A Report from the American Heart Association Statistics Committee and Stroke Statistics Subcommittee. *Circulation* 2007;115:e69–e171.
2. Pearson TA, Mensah GA, Alexander RW, et al: Markers of inflammation and cardiovascular disease: application to clinical and public health practice: a statement for healthcare professionals from the Centers for Disease Control and Prevention and the American Heart Association. *Circulation* 2003;107:499–511.
3. National Kidney Foundation: Clinical practice guidelines for managing dyslipidemias in chronic kidney disease. *Am J Kidney Dis* 2003;41(suppl 3):S39–S58.
4. American Diabetes Association: Standards of medical care in diabetes—2007. *Diabetes Care* 2007;30:S4–S41.
5. Gotto AM JR, Whitney E, Stein EA, et al: Relation between baseline and on-treatment lipid parameters and first acute major coronary events in the Air Force/Texas Coronary Atherosclerosis Prevention Study (AFCAPS/TexCAPS). *Circulation* 2000;101: 477–484.
6. Stein EA, Lane M, Saskarzewski P: Comparison of statins in hypertriglyceridemia. *Am J Cardiol* 1998;81:66B–69B.
7. Birjmohun RS, Hutten BA, Kastelein JJP, Stroes ESG: Efficacy and safety of high-density lipoprotein cholesterol-increasing compounds: a meta-analysis of randomized controlled trials. *J Am Coll Cardiol* 2005;45:185–197.
8. Grundy SM, Cleeman JI, Merz CN, et al: Implications of recent clinical trials for the National Cholesterol Education Program Adult Treatment Panel III guidelines. *Circulation* 2004;110: 227–239.
9. Expert Panel on Detection, Evaluation, and Treatment of High Blood Cholesterol in Adults: executive summary of the Third Report of the National Cholesterol Education Program (NCEP) Expert Panel on Detection, Evaluation, and Treatment of High Blood Cholesterol in Adults (Adult Treatment Panel III). *JAMA* 2001;285:2486–2497.
10. Breslow JL: Mouse models of atherosclerosis. *Science* 1996;272:685–688.
11. Sniderman AD, Furberg CK, Keech A, et al: Apolipoproteins versus lipids as indicators of coronary risk and as targets for statin therapy. *Lancet* 2003;361:777–780.
12. Ballantyne CM, Andrews TC, Hsia JA, et al; for the ACCESS Study Group: correlation of non-high-density lipoprotein cholesterol with apolipoprotein B: Effect of 5-hydroxymethylglutaryl coenzyme A reductase inhibitors on non-high density lipoprotein cholesterol levels. *Am J Cardiol* 2001;88:265–269.
13. Maki CK, Galant R, Davidson MH: Non-high-density lipoprotein cholesterol: the forgotten therapeutic target. *Am J Cardiol* 2005;96(suppl):59K–64K.
14. Staffa JA, Chang J, Green L: Cerivastatin and reports of fatal rhabdomyolysis. *N Engl J Med* 2002;346:539–540.
15. Davidson MH: Controversy surrounding the safety of cerivastatin. *Expert Opin Drug Saf* 2002;1:207–212.
16. Heart Protection Study Collaborative Group: MRC/BHF Heart Protection Study of cholesterol lowering with simvastatin in 20,536 high-risk individuals: a randomized placebo-controlled trial. *Lancet* 2002;360:7–22.
17. Grundy SM, Cleeman JI, Merz CN, et al: National Heart, Lung, and Blood Institute. American College of Cardiology Foundation. American Heart Association. Implications of Recent Clinical Trials for the National Cholesterol Education Program Adult Treatment Panel III Guidelines. *Circulation* 2004;110:227–239.
18. American Diabetes Association: Management of dyslipidemia in adults with diabetes. *Diabetes Care* 2003;26(suppl):S83–S86.
19. Davidson MH, Maki KC, Pearson TA, et al: Results of the National Cholesterol Education Program (NCEP) Evaluation Project Utilizing Novel E-Technology (NEPTUNE) II Survey: implications for treatment under the recent NCEP Writing Group recommendations. *Am J Cardiol* 2005;96:556–563.
20. Sacks FM, Rouleau JL, Moye LA, et al: Baseline characteristics in the Cholesterol and Recurrent Events (CARE) Trail of secondary prevention in patients with average serum cholesterol levels. *Am J Cardiol* 1995;75:621–623.
21. Lipid Study Group: Prevention of cardiovascular events and death with pravastatin in patients with coronary heart disease and a broad range of initial cholesterol levels: the Long-Term Intervention with Pravastatin in Ischaemic Disease (LIPID) Study Group. *N Engl J Med* 1998;339:1349–1357.
22. Shepherd J, Blauw GJ, Murphy MB, et al: Pravastatin in elderly individuals at risk of vascular disease (PROSPER): a randomized controlled trial. *Lancet* 2002;360:1623–1630.
23. Sever PS, Dahlof B, Poulter NR, et al; for the ASCOT Investigators: Prevention of coronary and stroke events with atorvastatin in hypertensive patients who have average or lower-than-average cholesterol concentrations in the Anglo-Scandinavian Cardiac Outcomes Trial—Lipid Lowering Arm (ASCOT-LLA): a multicenter randomized controlled trial. *Lancet* 2003;361:1149–1158.
24. Shepherd J, Barter P, Cermena R, et al; for the Treating to New Targets Investigators: Effect of lowering LDL cholesterol substantially below currently recommended levels in patients with coronary heart disease and diabetes. *Diabetes Care* 2006;29:1220–1226.
25. LaRosa JC, Grundy SM, Waters DD, et al; Treating to New Targets (TNT) Investigators: intensive lipid lowering with atorvastatin in patients with stable coronary disease. *N Engl J Med* 2005;352:1425–1435.
26. Davidson M, Ma P, Stein EA, et al: Comparison of effects on low-density lipoprotein cholesterol and high-density lipoprotein cholesterol with rosuvastatin versus atorvastatin in patients with type IIa or IIb hypercholesterolemia. *Am J Cardiol* 2002;89:268–275.
27. Jones PH, Davidson MH, Stein EA, et al; for the STELLAR Study Group: Comparison of the efficacy and safety of rosuvastatin

versus atorvastatin, simvastatin, and pravastatin across doses (STELLAR trial). *Am J Cardiol* 2003;92:152–160.

28. Katan MB, Grundy SM, Jones P, et al; Stresa Workshop Participants: Efficacy and safety of plant stanols and sterols in the management of blood cholesterol levels. *Mayo Clin Proc* 2003;78:965–978.
29. Moreyra AE, Wilson AC, Koraym A: Effect of combining psyllium fiber with simvastatin in lowering cholesterol. *Arch Intern Med* 2005;165:1161–1166.
30. Davidson MH: The use of colesevelam hydrochloride in the treatment of dyslipidemia: a review. *Expert Opin Pharmacother* 2007;8:2569–2578.
31. Davidson MH, Toth PP: Combination therapy in the management of complex dyslipidemias. *Curr Opin Lipidol* 2004;15: 423–431.
32. Davidson MH: Combination therapy for dyslipidemia: safety and regulatory considerations. *Am J Cardiol* 2002;90(suppl): 50K–60K.
33. Davidson MH, McGarry T, Bettis R, et al: Ezetimibe coadministered with simvastatin in patients with primary hypercholesterolemia. *J Am Coll Cardiol* 2002;40:2125–2134.
34. Ballantyne CM, Houri J, Notarbartolo A, et al: Effect of ezetimibe coadministered with atorvastatin in 628 patients with primary hypercholesterolemia. *Circulation* 2003;107:2409–2415.
35. Kerzner B, Corbelli J, Sharp S, et al; Ezetimibe Study Group: Efficacy and safety of ezetimibe coadministered with lovastatin in primary hypercholesterolemia. *Am J Cardiol* 2003;91:418–424.
36. Melani L, Mills R, Hassman D, et al; Ezetimibe Study Group: Efficacy and safety of ezetimibe coadministered with pravastatin in patients with primary hypercholesterolemia: a prospective, randomized, double-blind trial. *Eur Heart J* 2003;24:717–728.
37. The Lipid Research Clinics Program: The Lipid Research Clinics Coronary Primary Prevention Trial results. I: reduction in incidence of coronary heart disease. *JAMA* 1984;251:351–364.
38. Brown G, Albers JJ, Fisher LD, et al: Regression of coronary artery disease as a result of intensive lipid lowering therapy in men with high levels of apolipoprotein B. *N Engl J Med* 1990;323:1289–1298.
39. Davidson MH, Toth P, Weiss S, et al: Low-dose combination therapy with colesevelam hydrochloride and lovastatin effectively decreases low-density lipoprotein cholesterol in patients with primary hypercholesterolemia. *Clin Cardiol* 2001;24:467–474.
40. Knapp HH, Schrott H, Ma P, et al: Efficacy and safety of combination simvastatin and colesevelam in patients with primary hypercholesterolemia. *Am J Med* 2001;110:352–360.
41. Hunninghake D, Insull W Jr, Toth P, et al: Coadministration of colesevelam hydrochloride with atorvastatin lowers LDL cholesterol additively. *Atherosclerosis* 2001;158:407–416.
42. Friedewald WT, Levy RI, Fredrickson DS: Estimation of the concentration of low-density lipoprotein cholesterol in plasma, without use of the preparative ultracentrifuge. *Clin Chem* 1972;18:499–502.
43. Lu W, Resnick HE, Jablonski KA, et al: Non HDL cholesterol as a predictor of cardiovascular disease in type 2 diabetes: the Strong Heart Study. *Diabetes Care* 2003;26:16–23.
44. Shai I, Rimm EB, Hankinson SE, et al: Multivariate assessment of lipid parameters as predictors of coronary heart disease among postmenopausal women: potential implications for clinical guidelines. *Circulation* 2004;110:2824–2830.
45. Cui Y, Blumenthal RS, Flaws JA, et al: Non-high-density lipoprotein cholesterol level as a predictor of cardiovascular disease mortality. *Arch Intern Med* 2001;161:1413–1419.
46. Davidson MH, Armani A, McKenney JM, Jacobson TA: Safety considerations with fibrate therapy. *Am J Cardiol* 2007;99: 3C–18C.
47. Grundy SM, Vega LG, Yuan Z, et al: Effectiveness and tolerability of simvastatin plus fenofibrate for combined hyperlipidemia (the SAFARI trial). *Am J Cardiol* 2005;95:462–468.
48. Taylor AJ, Sullenberger LE, Lee HJ, et al: Arterial Biology for Investigation of the Treatment Effects of Reducing Cholesterol (ARBITER) 2: a double-blind placebo-controlled study of extended-release niacin on atherosclerosis progression in secondary prevention patients treated with statins. *Circulation* 2004;110:3512–3517.
49. Brown B, Brockenbrough A, Zhao X-Q, et al: Very intensive lipid therapy with lovastatin, niacin, and colestipol for prevention of death and myocardial infarction: a 10-year Familial Atherosclerosis Treatment Study (FATS) follow-up [abstract 3341]. *Circulation* 1998;98:I-635.
50. Brown BG, Zhao XQ, Chait A, et al: Simvastatin and niacin, antioxidant vitamins, or the combination for the prevention of coronary disease. *N Engl J Med* 2001;345:1583–1592.
51. Yim BT, Chong PH: Niacin-ER and lovastatin treatment of hypercholesterolemia and mixed dyslipidemia. *Ann Pharmacother* 2003;37:106–115.
52. Kashyap ML, McGovern ME, Berra K, et al: Long-term safety and efficacy of a once-daily niacin/lovastatin formulation for patients with dyslipidemia. *Am J Cardiol* 2002;89:672–678.
53. Hunninghake DB, McGovern ME, Koren M, et al: A dose-ranging study of a new, once-daily, dual-component drug product containing niacin extended-release and lovastatin. *Clin Cardiol* 2003;26:112–118.
54. Bays HE, Dujovne CA, McGovern ME, et al: Comparison of once-daily, niacin extended-release/lovastatin with standard doses of atorvastatin and simvastatin (the Advicor Versus Other Cholesterol-modulating Agents Trial Evaluation [ADVOCATE]). *Am J Cardiol* 2003;91:667–672.
55. GISSI-Prevenzione Investigators: Dietary supplementation with n-3 polyunsaturated fatty acids and vitamin E after myocardial infarction: results of the GISSI-Prevenzione trial. *Lancet* 1999;354:447–455.
56. O'Keefe JH, Harria WS: From inuit to implementation: omega-3 fatty acids come of age. *Mayo Clin Proc* 2000;75:607–614.
57. Harris WS, Ginsberg HN, Arunakul N, et al: Safety and efficacy of omacor in severe hypertriglyceridemia. *J Cardiovasc Risk* 1997;4:385–391.
58. Contacos C, Barter PJ, Sullivan DR: Effect of pravastatin and omega-3 fatty acids on plasma lipids and lipoproteins in patients with combined hyperlipidemia. *Arterioscler Thromb* 1993;13:1755–1762.
59. Nordoy A, Bonaa KH, Niilsen H, et al: Effects of simvastatin and omega-3 fatty acids on plasma lipoproteins and lipid peroxidation in patients with combined hyperlipidaemia. *J Intern Med* 1998;243:163–170.
60. Nordoy A, Hansen JB, Brox J, Svensson B: Effects of atorvastatin and omega-3 fatty acids on LDL subfractions and postprandial hyperlipemia in patients with combined hyperlipemia. *Nutrition Metab Cardiovasc Dis* 2001;11:7–16.
61. Davidson MH, Stein EA, Bays HE, et al: Efficacy and tolerability of adding prescription omega-3 fatty acids 4 g/day to simvastatin 40 mg/day in hypertriglyceridemic patients: An 8-week, randomized, double-blind, placebo-controlled study. *Clin Ther* 2007;29:1354–1367.
62. Autsin M, Hokanson J, Edwards K: Hypertriglyceridemia as a cardiovascular risk factor. *Am J Cardiol* 1998;81:7B–12B.
63. Castelli WP, Garrison RJ, Wilson PF, et al: Incidence of coronary heart disease and lipoprotein cholesterol levels: the Framingham Study. *JAMA* 1986;256:2835–2838.
64. Despres JP, Lemieux I, Dagenais GR, et al: HDL cholesterol as a marker of coronary heart disease risk: the Quebec cardiovascular study. *Atherosclerosis* 2000;153:263–272.
65. Austin M, Rodriguez B, McKnight B, et al: Low-density lipoprotein particle size, triglycerides, and high-density lipoprotein cholesterol as risk factors for coronary heart disease in older Japanese-American men. *Am J Cardiol* 2000;86:412–416.
66. Goldbourt U, Medalie J: High-density lipoprotein cholesterol and incidence of coronary heart disease: the Israeli Ischemic Heart Disease Study. *Am J Epidemiol* 1979;109:296–308.
67. Backer G, Bacquer D, Kornitzer M: Epidemiological aspects of high-density lipoprotein cholesterol. *Atherosclerosis* 1998;137: S1–S6.
68. Rywik S, Manolio T, Pajak A, et al: Association of lipids and lipoprotein level with total mortality and mortality caused by cardiovascular and cancer diseases (Poland and United States Collaborative Study on Cardiovascular Epidemiology). *Am J Cardiol* 1999;84:540–548.
69. Davidson MH, Clark JA, Glass LM, Kanumalla A: Statin safety: an appraisal from the adverse event reporting system. *Am J Cardiol* 2006;97(suppl):32C–43C.
70. Alsheikh-Ali AA, Karas RH: Increases in HDL cholesterol are the strongest predictors of risk reduction in lipid intervention trials [abstract 3754]. *Circulation* 2004;110(suppl):III-813.
71. Jones PH, Davidson MH: Reporting rate of rhabdomyolysis with fenofibrate + statin versus gemfibrozil + any statin. *Am J Cardiol* 2005;1:120–122.

72. Alsheikh-Ali AA, Kuvin JT, Karas RH: Risk of adverse events with fibrates. *Am J Cardiol* 2004;94:935–938.
73. Lipids in Diabetes Study (LDS): Combination statin and fibrate therapy in type 2 diabetes: results from the Lipids in Diabetes Study. *Diabetes* 2003;52:1:A74.
74. Davidson MH: Reducing residual risk for patients on statin therapy: the potential role of combination therapy. *Am J Cardiol* 2005;96(suppl):3K–13K.
75. Pearson TA, Laurora I, Chu H, Kafonek S: The Lipid Treatment Assessment Project (L-TAP): a multicenter survey to evaluate the percentages of dyslipidemic patients receiving lipid-lowering therapy and achieving low-density lipoprotein cholesterol goals. *Arch Intern Med* 2000;160:459–467.

CHAPTER 30

Low-Density Lipoprotein Apheresis

Patrick M. Moriarty

INTRODUCTION

Familial hypercholesterolemia (FH) is a clinical syndrome characterized by elevated plasma concentrations of low-density lipoprotein (LDL) cholesterol, xanthomas, and an increased risk of premature cardiovascular disease (CVD). FH is one of the most common monogenic disorders, with a frequency of 1:500 (10 million worldwide). Patients refractory to dietary and combined medical management require alternative measures for the elimination of plasma LDL. One method, defined as LDL-apheresis, is the extracorporeal removal of these pathogenic lipoproteins.

APHERESIS HISTORY

Bloodletting, a practice originally performed to remove the bad humors from the body, was initiated by the Egyptians around 1000 BC and lasted until the end of the 19th century.[1] Apheresis (Greek for "to take away") is an extracorporeal procedure in which blood passes through an apparatus and its basic components (red blood cells [RBCs], plasma, and plasma proteins) can be separated and removed from the body. The procedure was developed in 1914[2] but did not gain acceptance in the medical field until World War II, when there was an increased demand for plasma. Apheresis may be applied therapeutically for curing, preventing, or relieving the symptoms of diseases.

There are two major types of apheresis devices: centrifugation and membrane separation. Centrifugal apheresis (plasma exchange) spins blood in a chamber and with centrifugal forces divides the heavier weighted elements from the lighter ones, resulting in the separation of RBCs to the bottom, plasma to the top, and white blood cells to the middle (Fig. 30-1). The nonselectiveness of centrifugal devices results in the discarding of plasma and the replacement of it with donor plasma or saline with proteins such as albumin. Membrane apheresis, developed in 1978,[3] uses semiselective or specific plasma–cell separation by such methods as filtration, adsorption, or precipitation.

The application of apheresis for treating FH was first published in a case study by de Gennes et al in 1967.[4] In 1975, Thompson et al demonstrated that plasma exchange therapy for patients with FH resulted in a reduction of anginal symptoms and an influx of tissue cholesterol into the plasma.[5] In 1980, Thompson et al proved that the long-term use (2–3 years) of plasma exchange for patients with FH was associated with the resolution of xanthomas and stabilization of aortocoronary lesions in comparison with untreated FH siblings.[6] The 1980s marked the initiation of advanced apheresis technology for the specific removal of plasma cholesterol.

LOW-DENSITY LIPOPROTEIN—APHERESIS SYSTEMS

There are presently five different specific or semiselective LDL-apheresis systems commercially available: (1) membrane differential filtration (Fig. 30-2), (2) immunoadsorption (IA; Plasmaselect, Teterrow, Germany) (Fig. 30-3), (3) heparin-induced extracorporeal LDL precipitation (HELP; Melsungen, Germany) (Fig. 30-4), (4) dextran sulfate LDL adsorption (DSA; Liposorber LA-15 system; Kaneka, Osaka, Japan) (Fig. 30-5), and (5) hemoperfusion (direct adsorption of lipoproteins [DALI]; Fresenius, St. Wendel, Germany) (Fig. 30-6). The first four methods require the separation of plasma from the RBC, while hemoperfusion allows direct adsorption of the lipoproteins from whole blood.

To achieve anticoagulation, all five devices initiate therapy with a heparin bolus (2000–4000 IU) followed by a continuous infusion of 1500 IU/hour, except for the DALI system, which

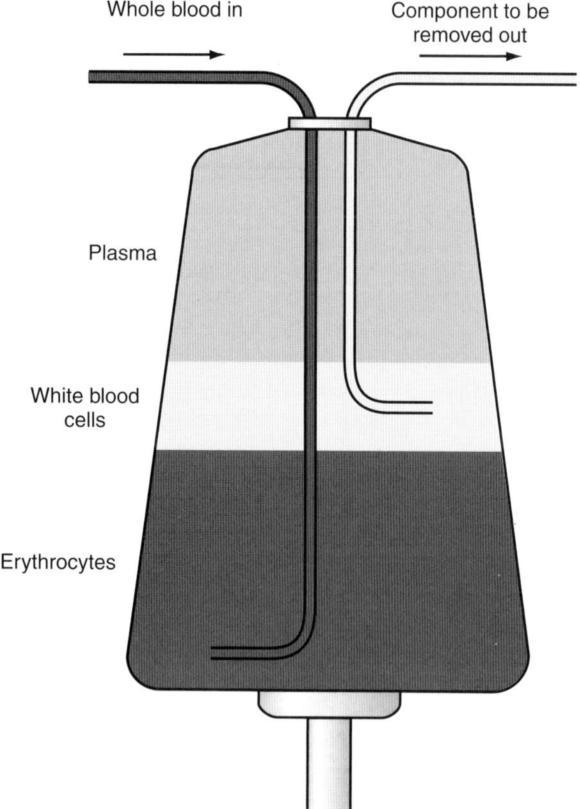

FIGURE 30-1 Centrifugal apheresis (plasma exchange).

uses a citrate solution for anticoagulation after the heparin bolus. All treatments are performed through a peripheral anticubital venous access (16- to 18-gauge needles), or occasionally patients may require placement of an arteriovenous fistula. At a flow rate of 40 to 100 mL/minute, 2000 to 10,000 mL of plasma may be treated in the course of a procedure (6000 mL of whole blood for hemoperfusion). During therapy, only 300 to 600 mL of plasma or blood is found extracorporeal at one time. Treatments lasting 2 to 4 hours (1.5–3 hours patient time and 1 hour nursing time for pre- and post-session) are scheduled weekly, biweekly, or longer, depending on baseline lipid levels and the response to therapy.

Membrane Filtration

In 1980, Agishi et al developed double membrane filtration (cascade filtration) apheresis.[7] The semiselective process involves elimination of atherogenic lipoproteins based on particle size and geometric properties. The system contains two hollow filters with different pore sizes. The first filter separates the plasma from whole blood. Plasma and proteins with a diameter smaller than 15 nm (albumin, high-density lipoprotein [HDL] cholesterol and immunoglobulins) are filtered through the pores of the second filter and returned to the patient together with the blood cells. Occasionally, an artificial membrane formed by cryogel can develop on the second filter and reduce its pore size, resulting in the retention of smaller proteins. Recent technology advances such as warming the plasma, adding a new lipid filtration membrane (Lipidfilter EC-50; Asahi Medical, Tokyo, Japan), and using a filtering machine (Octo Nova, Diamed; Cologne, Germany) have resulted in a decrease of unspecific protein loss.

Immunoadsorption

In 1981, Stoffel et al developed the first LDL-apheresis system for the specific removal of apolipoprotein (apo) B–containing lipoproteins.[8] The device contains two columns of Sepharose gel coupled with polyclonal sheep apoB-100 antibodies.[9] During an adsorption cycle (a total of six cycles), 1000 mL of plasma passes through one column while the other column is regenerated with a glycerin buffer (pH 2.8) and rinsed with a saline solution. The columns can be cleansed, stored, and reused up to 60 times. Another variation of IA is the Procard (Moscow, Russia) system, which uses sheep anti-lipoprotein(a) [Lp(a)] antibodies for the specific removal of Lp(a).[10] Recently, a fibrinogen adsorption

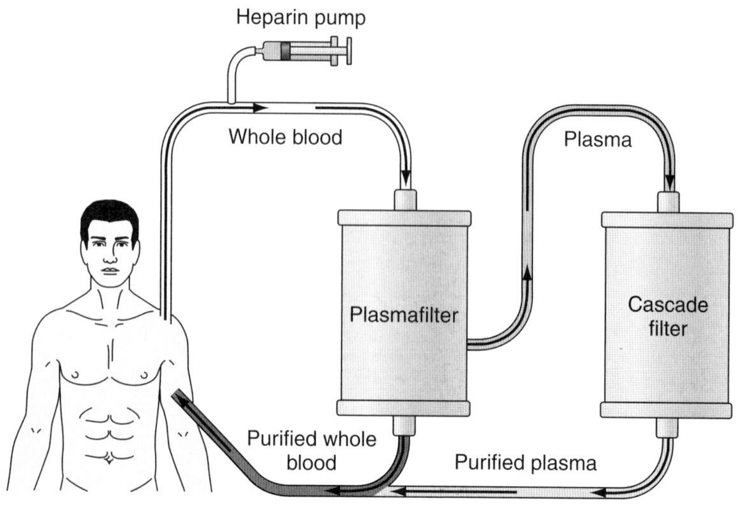

FIGURE 30-2 Membrane differentiation filtration.

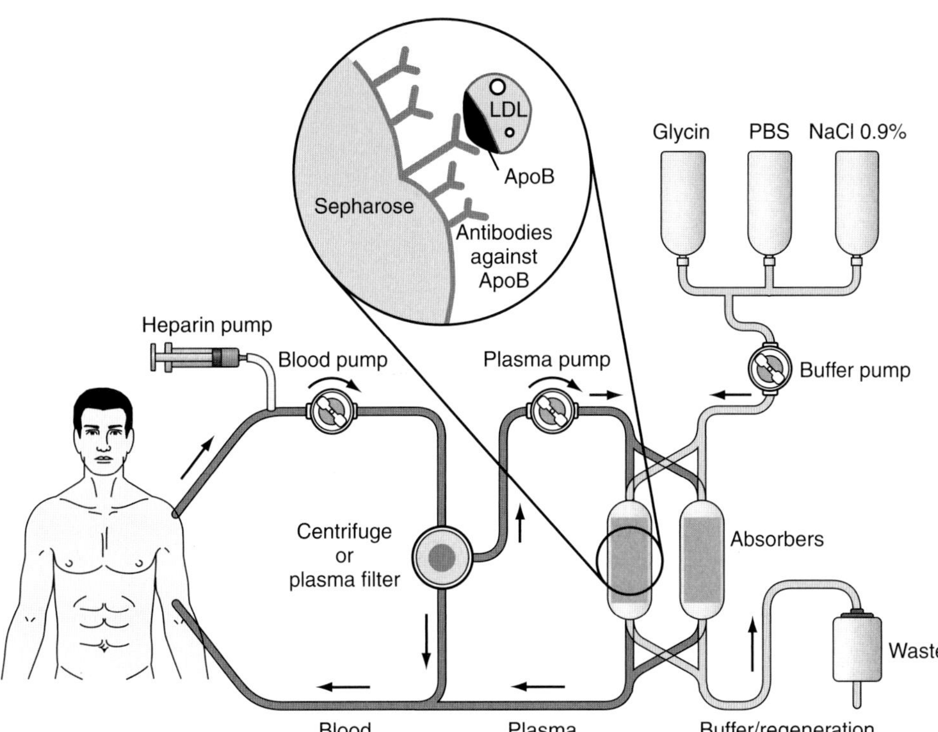

FIGURE 30-3 Immunoadsorption.

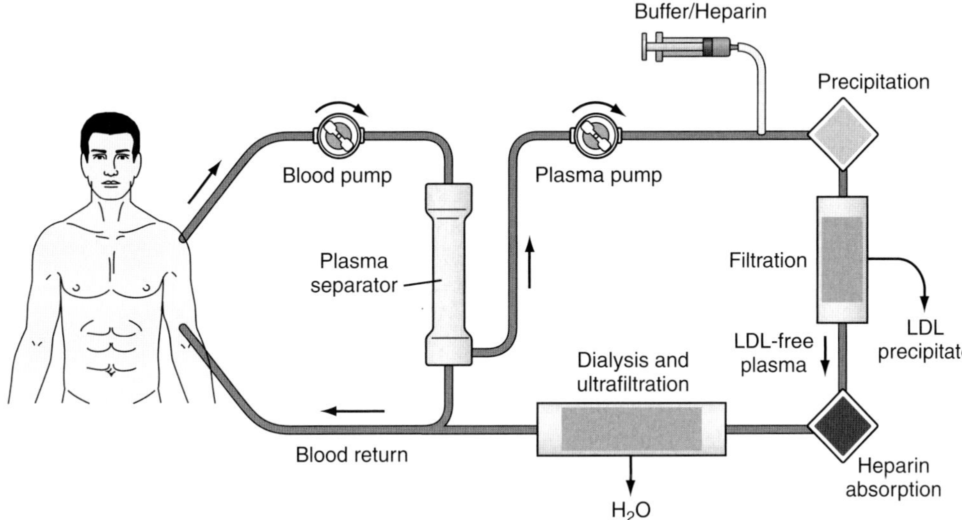

FIGURE 30-4 Heparin-induced extracorporeal LDL precipitation.

system (Rheosorb) was developed to reduce plasma and blood viscosity and improve microvascular flow. The antibodies on the column are replaced with a specific peptide that has a high affinity for fibrinogen.[11]

Heparin-Induced Extracorporeal Low-Density Lipoprotein Precipitation

In 1983, Wieland and Seidel introduced the HELP Secura system.[12] After separation, the plasma is mixed 1:1 with a 0.3 M acetate buffer (pH 4.8) solution containing heparin at a concentration of 100 U/mL. Precipitation of heparin and LDL occurs when the plasma buffer solution reaches an approximate pH of 5.2. The mechanism for the specific removal of lipoproteins is attributed to the negatively charged heparin precipitating with the positively charged apoB of LDL cholesterol, very-low-density lipoprotein (VLDL), and Lp(a). HDL cholesterol, having a negative charged membrane,[13] is normally spared from the precipitation process. The residual heparin in the LDL free plasma is adsorbed by a diethylaminoethyl cellulose filter. The physiologic pH of the plasma and the removal of excess fluid is achieved by dialysis and ultrafiltration. A newer version of HELP (Futura) delivers the dialysate without the need for the dialysis unit or precipitate recirculation. These changes have simplified its use and reduced the setup time of the machine.[14]

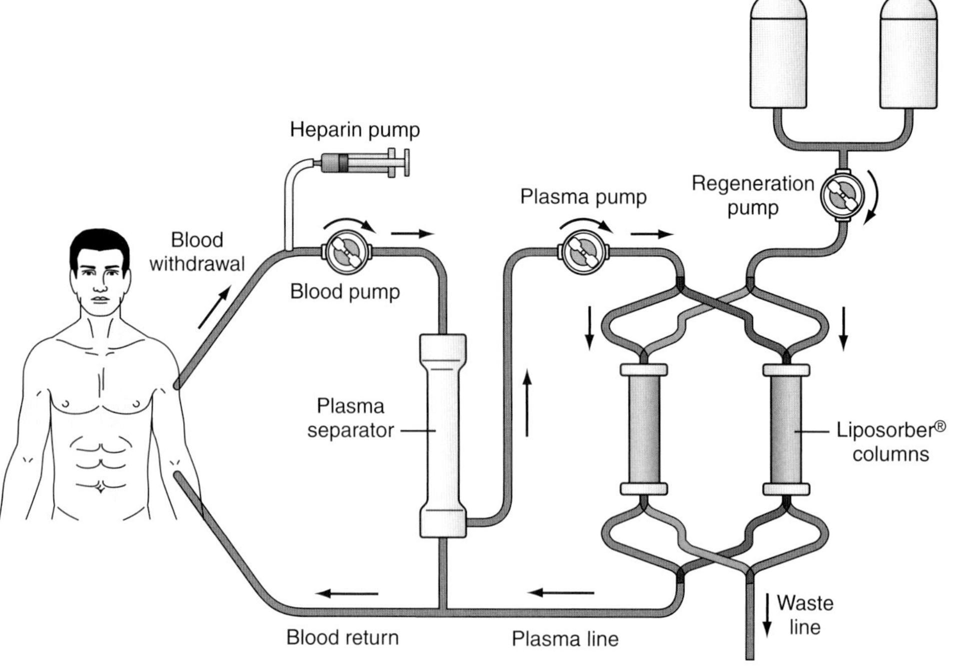

FIGURE 30-5 Dextran sulfate LDL adsorption.

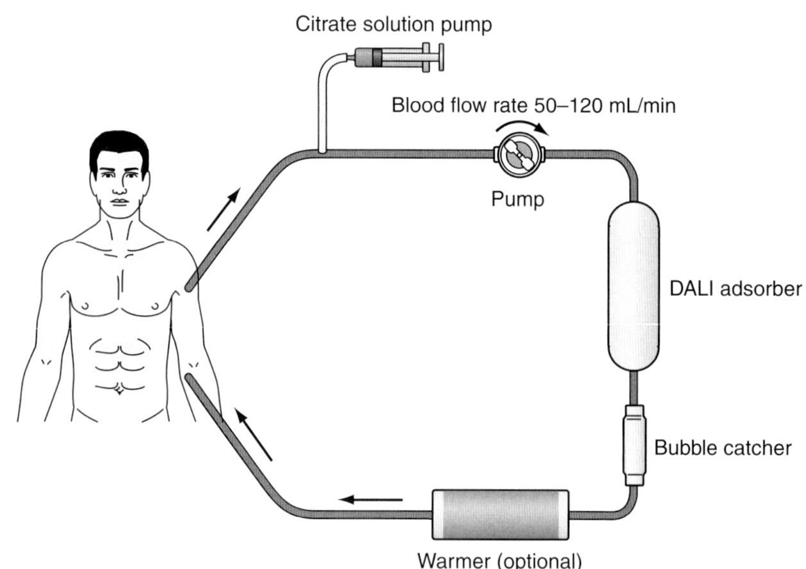

FIGURE 30-6 Hemoperfusion (direct adsorption of lipoproteins).

Dextran Sulfate Low-Density Lipoprotein Adsorption

In 1987, Mabuchi et al reported on the DSA system (LA-15).[15] Plasma is exposed to a column of cellulose beads coated with dextran sulfate cellulose. Similar to the HELP system, LDL, VLDL, and Lp(a) are removed through an electrostatic interaction of the polyanionic dextran sulfate ligands and the positively charged apoB–containing lipoproteins. The machine contains two dextran sulfate columns. After the first column is exposed to 500 mL of plasma, it is then cleansed and regenerated with a solution containing 4.1% sodium chloride. During the first column's rinsing process, plasma flow is redirected to the second column. Like the HELP system, most HDL is retained in the plasma.

Hemoperfusion

In 1993 the DALI blood perfusion system (Fresenius; St. Wendel, Germany), in which LDL is removed from whole blood without plasma separation, was first described by Bosch.[16] Blood is perfused through a column of polyacrylate-coated polyacrylamide beads. The beads contain negatively charged polyanions that interact with the cationic apoB moiety of LDL, VLDL, and Lp(a) in a similar fashion as the HELP and DSA systems.

In 2002, Kaneka developed a whole blood LDL-apheresis system (KLD01).[17] The mechanism for apoB–containing lipoprotein reduction is similar to that of the DSA, except the adsorber bead size has increased from 170 to 240 μm, resulting in minimal side effects in terms of blood cell activation and RBC loss.[18]

LIPID CHANGES

Table 30-1, based on multiple clinical studies, lists the range for acute mean changes in plasma lipids following LDL-apheresis. On average, more than 60% of apoB–containing lipoproteins are immediately reduced following a single procedure. Generally, the more elevated the baseline lipid level and quantity of treated plasma/blood then the greater the reduction of apoB–containing lipoproteins. Posttreatment recovery of LDL and Lp(a) ranges from 8 to 13 days.[19] Simultaneous lipid-lowering therapy, such as HMG-CoA reductase inhibitors (statins), enhances the efficacy of LDL-apheresis, even in homozygous patients with FH.[20] Long-term therapy may result in a 20% to 40% reduction of preapheresis LDL levels.[21,22] In addition to the quantitative changes of apoB–containing lipoproteins, LDL-apheresis can alter the composition of plasma LDL. Elevated circulating levels of oxidized LDL (ox-LDL)[23] and small dense LDL[24] have been associated with increased risk of CVD. LDL-apheresis significantly lowers ox-LDL[25] and decreases small dense LDL, while the total percentage of large buoyant LDL increases after treatment.[26] Despite the quantitative and qualitative changes to LDL, regular apheresis therapy does not alter kinetic parameters of apoB metabolism.[27]

The acute reduction of HDL after LDL-apheresis averages around 10% to 15% and has been attributed to membrane filtration (MF), hemodilution, activation of hepatic triglyceride lipase (HTGL), or decreased activity of lecithin:cholesterol acyltransferase (LCAT).[9] Several studies have revealed a greater acute reduction of total HDL than of apoA-I, the primary HDL apolipoprotein involved in reverse cholesterol transport, following a session of LDL-apheresis.[28,29] The difference in HDL and apoA-I levels following LDL-apheresis may represent a qualitative change in the composition of HDL. A recent study found that most HDL removed during LDL-apheresis was of the proinflammatory type[30] as measured by the inability of HDL to inhibit LDL-induced monocyte chemotactic activity.[31] Normally, HDL returns to pretreatment levels in 24 hours,[19] while long-term therapy will preserve or enhance the baseline level.[32] Despite the acute reductions of HDL, LDL-apheresis significantly lowers LDL/HDL ratios in converse to nonselective plasma exchanges, which raises LDL/HDL and reduces by equal amounts HDL and apoA-I.[28]

The acute reduction of triglycerides has been credited to the apoB moiety of VLDL or the activation of HTGL or lipoprotein lipase caused by the high-dose heparin used for anticoagulation.[33] Triglycerides, similarly to HDL, rebound within 24 hours.[19]

LDL-apheresis acutely lowers other apolipoproteins such as apoC-III and apoE by 40% to 50%.[34a]

Lp(a) is an inherited risk factor for atherosclerosis, myocardial infarction, stroke, and restenosis.[35] LDL-apheresis is the only treatment able to consistently reduce Lp(a) levels by more than 50%.[36]

CONTRAINDICATIONS, ADVERSE EVENTS, AND LIMITATIONS

Since 1996, only the DSA and HELP systems have received approval for clinical practice in North America. LDL-apheresis systems are contraindicated in patients for whom the use of heparin would cause excessive or uncontrolled anticoagulation or for whom adequate anticoagulation cannot be safely achieved, and in patients with a known hypersensitivity to heparin or ethylene oxide (DSA). In cases of sensitivity to heparin, the DSA system has used nafamostat mesilate, a broad-spectrum synthetic protease inhibitor, as an alternative anticoagulant.[37]

The occurrence of adverse events with LDL-apheresis is low and typical of procedures involving the circulation of blood outside the body.[38] Besides hypotension (<2%), the most common adverse event seen with apheresis is the inability to obtain venous access. The incidence of all other adverse events (flushing/blotching, chest pain, anemia, abdominal discomfort, hemolysis, and arrhythmia) are less than 1%.[22,39]

An uncommon but serious anaphylactoid reaction can occur in patients taking antihypertensive angiotensin-converting enzyme inhibitors (ACEI) who are receiving treatment with either the DSA or DALI machines.[40,41] Plasma bradykinin, a potent vasodilator, is produced by the DSA and DALI procedures through the activation of

TABLE 30-1 Acute Percent Lipid Changes Reductions Following LDL-Apheresis

	MF[16,34,41]	IA[15,41,94,97]	HELP[34,41,94,108]	DSA[15,16,24,41,96,97]	HP[15,24,41,96,97]
Total cholesterol	43%-57%	49%-68%	42%-54%	48%-68%	49%-61%
LDL cholesterol	42%-62%	54%-82%	55%-61%	49%-85%	53%-76%
HDL cholesterol	6%-42%	7%-27%	0%-19%	4%-32%	5%-31%
Lp(a)	53%-60%	51%-72%	55%-68%	19%-70%	28%-74%
Triglycerides	37%-57%	34%-49%	20%-61%	26%-64%	29%-40%

High variation of values may be partially the result of differences in treated plasma and blood volumes.

DSA, dextran sulfate LDL adsorption; HELP, heparin-induced extracorporeal LDL precipitation; HDL, high-density lipoprotein; HP, hemoperfusion; IA, immunoadsorption; LDL, low-density lipoprotein; LP(a), lipoprotein(a); MF, membrane differential filtration.

the intrinsic coagulation pathway (factors IV and XI, prekallikrein, high-molecular-weight kininogen),[42,43] and ACEI increases plasma bradykinin levels by inhibiting their metabolism. Because of the potential hypotensive reaction, ACEI usage is contraindicated in patients using either the DSA or DALI systems. Patients may abstain from ACEI at least 24 hours before therapy or switch to an angiotensin receptor blocker.

The amount of plasma/blood treated with the MF, IA, DSA, and DALI systems is unrestricted, whereas HELP, because of its limited-capacity precipitate filter, only processes approximately 3000 mL. The IM system may develop an autoimmune reaction consisting of fevers and hypotension, which is thought to be mediated during the procedure by heterophile antibodies developed against sheep antibodies (SAAL, SD 1986). The DALI system columns must be flushed before treatments with a rinsing fluid containing positively charged electrolytes to prevent derangement of the patient's electrolytes.[31] Elevated plasma levels of fibrinogen are a risk factor for atherosclerosis.[44] The mechanism of its effects on the vascular system has been linked to hemorheology, inflammation, and coagulation. While all apheresis devices reduce plasma fibrinogen, the HELP and MF systems remove significantly more fibrinogen (65%) than the other LDL-apheresis devices (10% to 20%).

CLINICAL TRIALS

Until the late 1990s, the benefit of LDL-apheresis for patients with FH and CVD was investigated through long-term analysis of angiographic changes in the coronary vessels.[45–49] The shortage of qualified candidates and the ethical dilemma of sham therapy has restricted the implementation of randomized, double-blinded, placebo-controlled trials.

In 1998, two clinical event outcome trials confirmed the effectiveness of long-term LDL-apheresis therapy for the prevention of CVD. The Hokuriko study, the largest and longest nonrandomized trial demonstrating the clinical benefits of LDL-apheresis, examined long-term (6 years) safety and efficacy of LDL-apheresis plus combination lipid-lowering therapy (low-dose statin plus probucol and resin or fibrate) for 43 heterozygous patients with FH compared with 87 heterozygous FH patients on similar combination lipid-lowering medications.[50] Kaplan–Meier analyses of the coronary events, including nonfatal myocardial infarction, percutaneous transluminal coronary angioplasty, coronary artery bypass grafting, and death from coronary heart disease, found that the event rate was 72% lower in the LDL-apheresis group (10%) compared with the drug-only group (36%) ($P = 0.0088$) resulting in a number needed to treat of four patients to prevent a coronary event (Fig. 30-7). The Liposorber Study Group examined long-term effects of LDL-apheresis (DSA) for 49 patients with FH (10 homozygotes and 39 heterozygotes) and LDL cholesterol levels greater than 160 mg/dL despite aggressive diet and combination drug therapy.[22] After 5 years of therapy, the rate of cardiovascular events (cardiac death, coronary revascularization, myocardial infarction, or cerebrovascular events) with LDL-apheresis was 3.5 per 1000 patient-months compared with 6.3 per

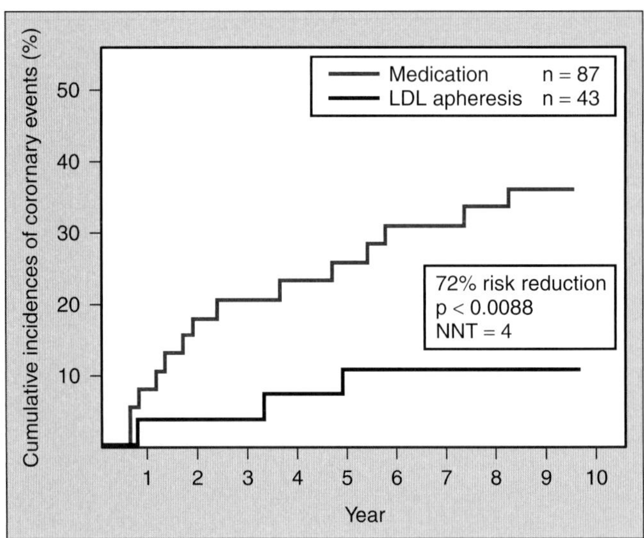

FIGURE 30-7 Kaplan–Meier curves for endpoints in reduction of coronary events.

1000 patient-months for the 5 years before initiating LDL-apheresis.

Observations of other cardiovascular effects related to LDL-apheresis therapy beyond event reduction have included immediate improvement of endothelial function,[51] coronary vasodilatation,[52] microvascular flow,[53] and myocardial perfusion.[54]

QUALIFICATION AND REIMBURSEMENT

LDL-apheresis is universally covered by private health insurers, Medicare, and other government payers. As indicated by the Food and Drug Administration, LDL-apheresis may be considered medically necessary when patients have failed previous treatment plans consisting of diet and maximum drug therapy (defined as a trial of drugs from at least two separate classes of hypolipidemic agents) for at least 6 months in addition to any one of the following criteria (Table 30-2): (1) homozygous FH (LDL cholesterol >500 mg/dL); (2) functional heterozygous FH with LDL greater than or equal to 200 mg/dL and documented coronary artery disease (i.e., history of myocardial infarction, coronary artery bypass surgery, percutaneous transluminal angioplasty or alternative revascularization procedure, or progressive angina documented by exercise or nonexercise test); or (3) FH with LDL cholesterol greater than or equal to 300 mg/dL. Reimbursement for

TABLE 30-2 Food and Drug Administration Criteria Required for LDL-Apheresis

Patient Characteristic	LDL Cholesterol (mg/dL)
Homozygous FH	≥500
Heterozygous FH and failure of medical therapy	≥300
Heterozygous FH with documented coronary disease and failure of medical therapy	≥200

FH, familial hypercholesterolemia; LDL, low-density lipoprotein.

LDL-apheresis in the hospital or outpatient setting can be highly variable ($2000 to $4000 per session), depending on the insurer and the location in the United States. A team effort is required by the patient, medical staff, and health care provider for the initiation and maintenance of an LDL-apheresis program. If only 1% of all patients with FH were intolerant to medical management, then the potential worldwide number of qualified LDL-apheresis candidates could be estimated at 100,000. Presently, there are less than 400 patients in North America receiving LDL-apheresis therapy. The DSA system is recommended for children with FH only if they weigh more than 15 kg and are older than 5 years of age, while the HELP system suggests that a patient's weight be greater than 37 kg before initiating therapy. Though not recommended, case studies have demonstrated LDL-apheresis safety and effectiveness for women with FH throughout their pregnancies.[55]

ALTERATION OF VASCULAR MARKERS

In addition to the considerable drop in lipids, LDL-apheresis can modify a number of markers associated with vascular disease (Table 30-3). Plasma markers of inflammation have been linked to atherosclerosis and CVD.[56] LDL-apheresis acutely reduces markers of vascular inflammation such as lipoprotein-associated phospholipase A_2 (Lp-PLA_2),[57] fibrinogen, E-selectin, vascular cellular adhesion molecule–1 (VCAM-1), intercellular adhesion molecule–1 (ICAM-1),[58] monocyte chemoattractant protein–1 (MCP-1), lipopolysaccharide-binding protein (LBP),[59,60] matrix metalloproteinase–9 (MMP-9), tissue inhibitor of metalloproteinase–1 (TMP-1),[61] and C-reactive protein (CRP).[62–65] Most plasma inflammatory markers return to baseline levels within 24 hours, which is probably dependent on the magnitude of their reduction and the plasma-life of the particular protein. A number of proteins (Lp-PLA_2, fibrinogen, and CRP), after multiple treatments of LDL-apheresis, remain lowered by 20% to 50%.[57,66,67]

LDL-apheresis therapy can acutely lower coagulation factors such as tissue factor, soluble CD40 ligand, homocysteine, fibrinogen,[59] and von Willebrand factor.[41] The percent reduction of clotting factors is dependent on the system. HELP primarily inhibits the extrinsic pathway (factors II, III, VII, X) through precipitation, while DALI and DSA interfere with the intrinsic pathway (prekallikrein, high-molecular-weight kinogen, factors XI and XII) by binding to the negatively charged adsorbers.[68,69] Markers that promote the fibrinolytic cascade, such as plasminogen, protein S, protein C, and antithrombin, are immediately reduced following LDL-apheresis.[43,70] Despite the removal of plasma thrombotic and fibrinolytic mediators, no serious clotting or bleeding complication has occurred from LDL-apheresis.

Hemorheology, particularly blood viscosity and its major determinants, is associated with CVD and early atherosclerosis.[71] Mediators of blood viscosity (in addition to hematocrit, shear forces, and temperature) include RBC deformability, RBC aggregation, and plasma viscosity. LDL-apheresis, after one treatment, lowers blood viscosity by more than 20%[72] and maintains this reduction for at least 7 days.[73]

TABLE 30-3 Acute Changes to Vascular Markers Following LDL-Apheresis

Marker	Acute changes (%)
Proinflammatory:	
MCP-1	−15 to −18
MMP-9	−20
TIMP-1	−30
LBP	−27
Lp-PLA_2	−22
VCAM-1	−10 to −20
ICAM-1	−10 to −16
E-selectin	−6 to −31
Fibrinogen	−10 to −65
Oxidized LDL	−65
CRP	−10 to −80
Vascular Function:	
Nitric oxide	25 to 45
VEGF	15
IGF-I	−37
Bradykinin	0 or >2000
ET-1	−15 to −75
PGI_2	300
Thrombotic	
Tissue factor	−26
Von Willebrand factor	−29 to −56
Thrombin	−55
Factor V	−57 to −74
Factor VII	−4 to −36
Factor XI	−27 to 82
Factor XII	−32 to 73
sCD40L	−16
Homocysteine	−15 to −25
Fibrinogen	−10 to −65
Fibrinolytic:	
Plasminogen	−23 to −50
Protein S	−11 to −35
Protein C	−32 to −48
Antithrombin	−11 to −25
Hemorheology:	
Plasma viscosity	−11 to −18
Blood viscosity	−5 to −15
RBC aggregation	−31 to −52
RBC deformability	45
Fibrinogen	−10 to −65

High variation of values may be partially the result of differences in treated plasma and blood volumes.

Data from references 28, 58, 59, 67, 78, 126–134.

CRP, C-reactive protein; ET-1, endothelin-1; ICAM-1, intercellular adhesion molecule–1; IGF-1, insulin-like growth factor–1; LBP, lipopolysaccharide-binding protein; Lp-PLA_2, lipoprotein-associated phospholipase A_2; MCP-1, monocyte chemoattractant protein–1; MMP-9, matrix metalloproteinase–9; PGI_2, prostaglandin I_2; RBC, red blood cell; sCD40L, soluble CD40 ligand; sCD430L, soluble CD430 ligand; TIMP-1, tissue inhibitor of metalloproteinase-1; VCAM-1, vascular cellular adhesion molecule-1 VEGF, vascular endotheliol growth factor.

The improvement of blood rheology by LDL-apheresis is related to changes in RBC aggregation/deformability and plasma viscosity.[74,75]

Immediate alterations of vasoreactive substances such as nitric oxide,[76] bradykinin,[77] prostaglandin I_2 (PGI_2),[78] insulin-like growth factor (IGF),[67] and endothelin[79] are observed after a session of LDL-apheresis. Vascular endothelial growth factor (VEGF), a mediator of vascular permeability, remains significantly elevated 3 months after the last treatment of LDL-apheresis.[67]

The influence on blood viscosity, endothelial function, and vasoreactive mediators by LDL-apheresis most likely assists in the rapid recovery of myocardial blood flow and the minimum coronary resistance seen in patients with CVD.[80]

ALTERNATIVE CLINICAL APPLICATIONS

Therapeutic apheresis can be used when standard therapy has failed or for complex diseases in which pathologic components of the blood or plasma need to be removed. LDL-apheresis, because of its effects on lipids, inflammation, coagulation, rheology, and vasoreactivity, has been used in certain vascular diseases not necessarily related to dyslipidemia (Table 30-4). This section reviews published clinical data on the alternative uses of LDL-apheresis.

Peripheral Vascular Disease

Peripheral vascular disease (PVD) is associated with reduced blood flow and is most often caused by stenosis or thrombosis of the major arteries of the lower limbs. The LDL Apheresis Atherosclerosis Regression Study (LAARS) used biweekly apheresis (DSA) plus simvastatin 40 mg/d or simvastatin 40 mg/d alone on 42 patients with FH, CVD, and PVD for 2 years.[81] Results revealed that, unlike simvastatin monotherapy, LDL-apheresis decreased stenosis of the aortotibial tract and decreased mean carotid intima–media thickness. In a study of 28 patients with PVD (15 with diabetes and 19 receiving hemodialysis), multiple treatments of LDL apheresis (10 in 5 weeks) led to an increase in ankle-brachial pressure index (ABI) (from 0.69 to 0.85) and significant improvements in walking distance (82%), claudication (54%), and foot ulcers (14%).[60] Earlier work by the same researchers suggested that the beneficial effects of LDL-apheresis for patients without FH (mean baseline LDL 94 mg/dL) and with ischemic limb was not associated with LDL reduction but perhaps alterations of other vascular markers (VEGF, IGF-1, CRP, and fibrinogen).[67] These studies and others[67,78,82,83] have convinced the Japanese health insurance system to approve LDL-apheresis for the treatment of drug resistant hyperlipidemia and PVD (Table 30-5).

TABLE 30-4	Alternative Applications of LDL-Apheresis
Peripheral vascular disease	
Cerebral vascular disease	
Acute coronary syndrome	
Cardiac transplantation	
Renal disease	
Sudden idiopathic hearing loss	
Ocular microcirculatory disturbances	
Pre-eclampsia	

Cerebral Vascular Disease

Stroke, the third most common cause of death, is usually ischemic in nature and linked to atherosclerosis.[84] Inflammation, particularly CRP, plays an important role in the early onset of the disease.[85] Initiation of aggressive statin therapy within 72 hours for patients with acute coronary syndrome may reduce the risk of cerebral vascular events by 50%.[86] The influence of LDL-apheresis on the cerebrovascular system was indirectly analyzed[87] by measuring the CO_2 reactivity (a marker of cerebral vasoreactivity) in patients with CHD and hyperlipidemia. Following a treatment of LDL-apheresis, the Co_2 reactivity was improved by almost 40% ($P < 0.05$). In another study, LDL-apheresis therapies (2 times over 8 days) for 48 patients with either acute embolic stroke or multi-infarct dementia and baseline LDL levels of 160 mg/dL resulted in significant improvement ($P < 0.05$) in the Mathew scale and Mini-Mental State Examination when compared with the control group.[88] Apheresis also produced immediate and significant reductions of rheologic markers (fibrinogen 34%, blood viscosity 17%, plasma viscosity 16%, and red cell transit time 17%).

Cardiac Transplantation

Cardiac transplant (CTX) patients have complications such as hyperlipidemia, rejection crisis, and hypertension, resulting in an acceleration of atherosclerosis and death.[42,89] Lowering cholesterol in CTX patients with statins can reduce mortality and morbidity.[90] Chronic LDL-apheresis treatments for CTX patients with cardiac allograft vasculopathy (CAV) and LDL

TABLE 30-5	Japanese Health Insurance Coverage of LDL-Apheresis Use for Patients with Peripheral Vascular Disease
1. Symptom classified as II or higher according to Fontaine's grading system	
2. Drug-resistant hyperlipemia; pharmacologic therapy has failed to lower total cholesterol to ≤200 mg/dL, LDL cholesterol to ≤140 mg/dL	
3. Surgical therapy unavailable because of occlusion of arteries below the popliteal artery, extended occlusions, etc.	
4. Insufficient efficacy of conventional pharmacologic therapy	

When peripheral vascular disease meets all of four conditions, then health insurance covers the cost of LDL-apheresis for courses of 10 runs each to be given within 3-month periods.

levels greater than 150 mg/dL, despite statin therapy, significantly increases coronary mean lumen diameter.[43,91] Patients with CTX and CAV who receive LDL-apheresis therapy increase their intramuscular (anterior tibial) partial pressure ($pO2$) by more than 150%, to values similar to those in healthy subjects.[92] A 3.6-year study comparing the development of CAV in patients with CTX ($N = 10$) on statin therapy (LDL = 130 mg/dL) or CTX patients ($N = 10$) receiving statins and weekly LDL-apheresis (LDL = 235 mg/dL) confirmed a significant ($P = 0.006$) prevention (10% versus 70%) of CAV in the LDL-apheresis group.[45,93] The authors attributed their results to the simultaneous reduction of LDL (48%), fibrinogen (35%), and Lp(a) (47%).

Renal Disease

Diabetic nephropathy is the leading cause of end-stage renal disease. The application of LDL-apheresis (DSA; 12 times in 8 weeks) for patients with long-standing type 2 diabetes and nephrotic syndrome, in comparison with controls, resulted in a significant reduction of blood urea nitrogen, urinary protein excretion, podocytes, and plasma creatinine levels, with an increase of creatinine clearance.[94] LDL-apheresis (DSA) treatments for patients with steroid-resistant nephrotic syndrome significantly lowered urinary protein and increased serum albumin when compared with a steroid-treated control group.[95] The National Health Insurance Program in Japan has approved LDL-apheresis (12 times over a 12-week period) for patients with a diagnosis of the nephrotic syndrome who are resistant to conventional drug therapy and have a total cholesterol level greater than 250 mg/dL.

Acute Coronary Syndrome

Defined as unstable angina or non-ST elevation myocardial infarction, acute coronary syndrome accounted for 1.6 million inpatient hospital discharges in 2004.[96] Factors associated with acute coronary syndrome include increased coagulation, inflammation, vasoconstriction, and viscosity.[97] Recent studies suggest that early intensive statin therapy for patients with acute coronary syndrome could reduce future CVD events, and the apparent benefit may be related to the pleiotropic effects of statins.[98] A prospective trial investigated whether LDL-apheresis (DSA) therapy immediately before and 5 days after coronary angioplasty in nine patients with CHD and total cholesterol below 200 mg/dL would be effective for preventing restenosis, in comparison with a similar control group of 27 patients after 4 months.[99] Follow-up angiogram demonstrated that the rate of restenosis was lower in the LDL-apheresis group (0%) than in the control group (30%). In addition, none of the treated patients had any adverse events related to the procedure. At the end of the trial, serum cholesterol had returned to pretreatment levels. Case studies examining the benefit of single or multiple treatments of LDL-apheresis for patients with acute coronary syndrome discovered clinical improvement with significant reduction of lipids, inflammatory markers, and cardio-specific isoenzymes without any adverse effects.[100]

The potential acute clinical benefit of LDL-apheresis for patients with acute coronary syndrome may be related to the procedures' effects on rheology. During increased cardiac demand, the capillaries, which have little vasodilatation capability because of their lack of elastic/muscle tissue, replace the arterioles for management of vascular resistance.[101] If vascular resistance $= [(8 \bullet l)/(\pi \bullet r^4)] \times \eta$, where l is length, r is the radius, and η is viscosity, then during cardiac stress the resistance to flow will be dictated in large part by the viscosity of the blood.

Ocular Microcirculatory Disturbances

Nonarteritic acute ischemic anterior optic neuropathy (NAION), characterized by a sudden loss of vision, is the most common acute optic neuropathy in patients older than 50 years of age.[102] The pathophysiologic mechanism is not fully understood, but risk factors include atherosclerosis, diabetes, and increased blood viscosity.[103,104] No present therapy has gained acceptance because of the lack of benefit.[105] Initial studies using LDL-apheresis (HELP) for patients with NAION have demonstrated stabilization and improvement of visual acuity following a series of treatments.[106,107] A prospective, controlled study examined the effects of LDL-apheresis (HELP) on 11 patients with NAION and LDL levels of 144 mg/dL.[108] After three treatments over a 17-day period, all of the patients had improved visual acuity ($P = 0.002$), in contrast to the control group ($P = 0.0001$), whose visual acuity declined.

Age-related macular degeneration (AMD) is the leading cause of blindness in persons older than 60 years of age.[109–111] The exact cause of AMD is unknown, but inflammatory markers such as CRP and fibrinogen are considered risk factors.[111] In a multicenter, prospective, randomized, double-masked, placebo-controlled trial, 43 patients with AMD were treated with LDL-apheresis (MF) or sham therapy (8 times over a 10-week period).[112] One-year follow-up demonstrated that the treated patients had significant ($P = 0.001$) improvement of their visual acuity compared with the control group.

Sudden Idiopathic Hearing Loss

Idiopathic sudden hearing loss (ISHL) with or without tinnitus is a condition that affects 20 out of 100,000 persons per year.[113] Assumed etiologies for ISHL include viral, vascular, or autoimmune diseases. Risk factors consist of elevated levels of fibrinogen or cholesterol, which may indicate a pathology related to increased rheology causing an alteration of microvascular blood flow, local hypoperfusion, and hearing loss.[114] Spontaneous recovery occurs in 50% to 70% of the patients afflicted with ISHL,[115] while the remaining develop permanent partial or complete deafness. Present therapeutic options include steroids and plasma expanders. Based on the hypothesis of decreased microvascular flow, LDL-apheresis therapy has been applied for patients with ISHL. Several uncontrolled studies using different LDL-apheresis devices (MF and IA) have demonstrated a 90% partial to complete recovery of hearing.[116,117] One controlled multicenter study involving 201 patients with sudden-onset of unilateral sensorineural hearing loss revealed that a treatment of LDL-apheresis (HELP) was as effective as conventional therapy (10 days of IV treatment with high-dose prednisolone and hydroxyethyl-starch) and could be used as an alternative therapy, particularly in patients with elevated fibrinogen (>295 mg/dL) and LDL (>134 mg/dL) levels.[118]

Pre-eclampsia

Pre-eclampsia, the leading cause of maternal death worldwide, is a poorly understood disease of pregnancy.[119] Generalized maternal endothelial cell dysfunction has been considered the pathophysiologic process.[120] Certain risk factors include ox-LDL,[121] CRP,[122] fibrinogen,[123] and Lp(a).[124] Early delivery, the treatment for pre-eclampsia, may result in fetal growth retardation, infant morbidity, and death. A recent study examined the feasibility of LDL-apheresis (HELP) treatments for patients with pre-eclampsia.[125] Nine pre-eclamptic patients, with mean LDL levels of 140 mg/dL, were treated on average three times with HELP apheresis. Clinical outcome revealed that the treated patients extended their pregnancies by 17.7 days (3–49 days) in comparison with the untreated pre-eclamptic patients. HELP apheresis also reduced maternal plasma markers of inflammation, coagulation, and viscosity without overt maternal or neonatal side effects.

SUMMARY

LDL-apheresis is a safe and effective procedure for the lowering of plasma cholesterol and the reduction of cardiovascular events in patients with uncontrolled hypercholesterolemia. The multiple and immediate changes to the vascular system by LDL-apheresis may warrant its alternative implementation for other acute and chronic vascular diseases. These potential applications for LDL-apheresis need to be validated by further scientific research.

REFERENCES

1. Ventura HO, Mehra MR: Bloodletting as a cure for dropsy: heart failure down the ages. [Erratum appears in J Card Fail. 2005;11(5):404.] *J Card Fail* 2005;11(4):247–252.
2. Abel JJ, Rowntree LG, Turner BB: Plasma removal with return of corpuscles (plasmaphaeresis). The Journal of Pharmacology and experimental therapeutics Vol. V. No. 6, July, 1914. *Trans Sci* 1990;11(2):166–177.
3. Solomon BA, Castino F, Lysaght MJ, et al: Continuous flow membrane filtration of plasma from whole blood. *Trans Am Soc Artif Intern Organs* 1978;24:21–26.
4. de Gennes JL, Touraine R, Maunand B, et al: Homozygous cutaneo-tendinous forms of hypercholesteremic xanthomatosis in an exemplary familial case. Trial of plasmapheresis ans heroic treatment. *Bull Mem Soc Med Hop Paris* 1967;118(15):1377–1402.
5. Thompson GR, Lowenthal R, Myant NB: Plasma exchange in the management of homozygous familial hypercholesterolaemia. *Lancet* 1975;1(7918):1208–1211.
6. Thompson GR, Myant NB, Kilpatrick D, et al: Assessment of long-term plasma exchange for familial hypercholesterolaemia. *Br Heart J* 1980;43(6):680–688.
7. Agishi T, Kaneko I, Hasuo Y, et al: Double filtration plasmapheresis. *Trans Am Soc Artif Intern Organs* 1980;26:406–411.
8. Stoffel W, Borberg, Grevev: Application of specific extracorporeal removal of low-density lipoprotein in familial hypercholesterolaemia. *Lancet* 1981;2(8254):1005–1007.
9. Richter WO, Jacob EG, Ritter MM, et al: Three-year treatment of familial heterozygous hypercholesterolemia by extracorporeal low-density lipoprotein immunoadsorption with polyclonal apolipoprotein B antibodies. *Metabolism* 1993;42(7):888–894.
10. Pokrovsky SN, Sussekov AV, Adamova IY, et al: Development of immunosorbents for apoB-containing lipoproteins apheresis. *Artif Organs* 1995;19(6):500–505.
11. Koll R, Klinkmann J, Richter W: RheoSorb: a specific adsorber for fibrinogen elimination in clinical situations with impaired rheology. *Artif Organs* 2002;26(2):145–151.
12. Wieland H, Seidel D: A simple specific method for precipitation of low-density lipoproteins. *J Lipid Res* 1983;24(7):904–909.
13. Davidson WS, Sparks DL, Lund-Katz S, Phillips MC: The molecular basis for the difference in charge between pre-beta- and alpha-migrating high-density lipoproteins. *J Biol Chem* 1994;269(12):8959–8965.
14. Susca M: Heparin-induced extracorporeal low-density lipoprotein precipitation futura, a new modification of HELP apheresis: technique and first clinical results. *Ther Apher* 2001;5(5):387–393.
15. Mabuchi H, Michishita I, Takeda M, et al: A new low-density lipoprotein apheresis system using two dextran sulfate cellulose columns in an automated column regenerating unit (LDL continuous apheresis). *Atherosclerosis* 1987;68(1-2):19–25.
16. Bosch T, Schmidt B, Blumenstein M, et al: Lipid apheresis by hemoperfusion: *in vitro* efficacy and *ex vivo* biocompatibility of a new low-density lipoprotein adsorber compatible with human whole blood. *Artif Organs* 1993;17(7):640–652.
17. Otto C, Geiss HC, Laubach E, Schwandt P: Effects of direct adsorption of lipoproteins apheresis on lipoproteins, low-density lipoprotein subtypes, and hemorheology in hypercholesterolemic patients with coronary artery disease. *Ther Apher* 2002;6(2):130–135.
18. Kobayashi A, Nakatani M, Furuyoshi S, Tani N: *In vitro* evaluation of dextran sulfate cellulose beads for whole blood infusion low-density lipoprotein-hemoperfusion. *Ther Apher* 2002;6(5):365–371.
19. Kroon AA, van't Hof MA, Fuss-Lejeune MM, et al: The rebound of lipoproteins after LDL-apheresis. Kinetics and estimation of mean lipoprotein levels. *Atherosclerosis* 2000;152(2):519–526.
20. Marais AD, Naoumova RP, Firth JC, et al: Decreased production of low-density lipoprotein by atorvastatin after apheresis in homozygous familial hypercholesterolemia. *J Lipid Res* 1997;38(10):2071–2078.
21. Pfohl M, Naoumova RP, Klass C, et al: Acute and chronic effects on cholesterol biosynthesis of LDL-apheresis with or without concomitant HMG-CoA reductase inhibitor therapy. *J Lipid Res* 1994;35(11):1946–1955.
22. Gordon BR, Kelsey SF, Dau PC, et al: Long-term effects of low-density lipoprotein apheresis using an automated dextran sulfate cellulose adsorption system. Liposorber Study Group. *Am J Cardiol* 1998;81(4):407–411.
23. Holvoet P, Mertens A, Verhamme P, et al: Circulating oxidized LDL is a useful marker for identifying patients with coronary artery disease. *Arterioscler Thromb Vasc Biol* 2001;21(5):844–848.
24. St-Pierre AC, Ruel IL, Cantin B, et al: Comparison of various electrophoretic characteristics of LDL particles and their relationship to the risk of ischemic heart disease. *Circulation* 2001;104(19):2295–2299.
25. Napoli C, Ambrosio G, Scarpato N, et al: Decreased low-density lipoprotein oxidation after repeated selective apheresis in homozygous familial hypercholesterolemia. *Am Heart J* 1997;133(5):585–595.
26. Schamberger B, Geiss HC, Ritter MM, et al: Influence of LDL apheresis on LDL subtypes in patients with coronary heart disease and severe hyperlipoproteinemia. *J Lipid Res* 2000;41:727–733.

27. Parhofer KG, Barrett PH, Demant T, et al: Effects of weekly LDL-apheresis on metabolic parameters of apolipoprotein B in heterozygous familial hypercholesterolemia. *J Lipid Res* 1996;37(11):2383–2393.
28. Hershcovici T, Schechner V, Orlin J, et al: Effect of different LDL-apheresis methods on parameters involved in atherosclerosis. *J Clin Apher* 2004;19(2):90–97.
29. Schechner V, Berliner S, Shapira I, et al: Comparative analysis between dextran sulfate adsorption and direct adsorption of lipoproteins in their capability to reduce erythrocyte adhesiveness/aggregation in the peripheral blood. *Ther Apher Dial* 2004;8(1):39–44.
30. Opole IO, Belmont JM, Kumar A, Moriarty PM, Effect of low-density lipoprotein apheresis on inflammatory and noninflammatory high-density lipoprotein cholesterol. *Am J Cardiol* 2007;100:1416–1418.
31. Navab M, Ananthramaiah GM, Reddy ST, et al: The double jeopardy of HDL. *Ann Med* 2005;37(3):173–178.
32. Schmaldienst S, Banyai S, Stuinig TM, et al: Prospective randomised cross-over comparison of three LDL-apheresis systems in statin pretreated patients with familial hypercholesterolaemia. *Atherosclerosis* 2000;151(2):493–499.
33. Richter WO, Donner MG, Schwandt P: Short- and long-term effects on serum lipoproteins by three different techniques of apheresis. *Artif Organs* 1996;20(4):311–317.
34. Geiss HC, Bremer S, Barrett PH et al: *In vivo* metabolism of LDL subfractions in patients with heterozygous FH on statin therapy: rebound analysis of LDL subfractions after LDL apheresis. *J Lipid Res* 2004;45(8):1459–1467.
34a. Le NA, Dutton J-A, Moriarty P, Brown WV: Acute changes in oxidative and inflammatory markers with LDL apheresis [abstract]. *Circulation* 2006;114:II-111.
35. Keller C: Apheresis in coronary heart disease with elevated Lp (a): a review of Lp (a) as a risk factor and its management. *Ther Apher Dial* 2007;11(1):2–8.
36. Bambauer R: Is lipoprotein(a)-apheresis useful? *Ther Apher Dial* 2005;9(2):142–147.
37. Kojima S, Shiba M, Kuramochi M et al: Effect of nafamostat mesilate on bradykinin generation and hemodynamics during LDL apheresis. *Artif Organs* 1995;19(2):135–139.
38. Schuff-Werner P: Clinical long-term results of H.E.L.P.-apheresis. *Z Kardiol* 2003;92(Suppl 3):III28–III29.
39. Bosch T, Gahr S, Belschner U, et al: Direct adsorption of low-density lipoprotein by DALI-LDL-apheresis: Results of a prospective long-term multicenter follow-up covering 12,291 sessions. *Ther Apher Dial* 2006;10(3):210–218.
40. Koga N, Nagano T, Sato T, Kagasawa K: Anaphylactoid reactions and bradykinin generation in patients treated with LDL-apheresis and an ACE inhibitor. *ASAIO J* 1993;39(3):M288–M291.
41. Bosch T, Keller C: Clinical effects of direct adsorption of lipoprotein apheresis: beyond cholesterol reduction. *Ther Apher Dial* 2003;7(3):341–344.
42. Johansen HT, BuØo L, Karlsrud TS, Aasen AO: Dextran sulphate activation of the contact system in plasma and ascites. *Thromb Res* 1994;76(4):363–371.
43. Julius U, Siegert G, Gromeier S: Intraindividual comparison of the impact of two selective apheresis methods (DALI and HELP) on the coagulation system. *Int J Artif Organs* 2000;23(3):199–206.
43a. Gordon BR, Sloan BJ, Parker TS, et al: Humoral immune response following extracorporeal immunoadsorption of patients with hypercholesterolemia. *Transfusion* 1990;30:327–332.
44. Tataru MC, Schulte H, von Eckardstein A, et al: Plasma fibrinogen in relation to the severity of arteriosclerosis in patients with stable angina pectoris after myocardial infarction. *Coron Artery Dis* 2001;12(3):157–165.
45. Tatami R, Inove N, Itoh H, et al: Regression of coronary atherosclerosis by combined LDL-apheresis and lipid-lowering drug therapy in patients with familial hypercholesterolemia: a multicenter study. The LARS Investigators. *Atherosclerosis* 1992;95(1):1–13.
46. Waidner T, Franzen D, Voelker W, et al: The effect of LDL apheresis on progression of coronary artery disease in patients with familial hypercholesterolemia. Results of a multicenter LDL apheresis study. *Clin Investig* 1994;72(11):858–863.
47. Schuff-Werner P, Gohlke H, Bartmann U, et al: The HELP-LDL-apheresis multicenter study, an angiographically assessed trial on the role of LDL-apheresis in the secondary prevention of coronary heart disease. II. Final evaluation of the effect of regular treatment on LDL cholesterol plasma concentration and the course of coronary heart disease. *Eur J Clin Invest* 1994;24: 724–732.
48. Thompson GR, Maherum, Matthews S, et al: Familial Hypercholesterolaemia Regression Study: a randomised trial of low-density-lipoprotein apheresis. [See comment.] *Lancet* 1995;345(8953):811–816.
49. Kroon AA, Aengevaeren WR, van der Werf T, et al: LDL-Apheresis Atherosclerosis Regression Study (LAARS). Effect of aggressive versus conventional lipid lowering treatment on coronary atherosclerosis. *Circulation* 1996;93(10):1826–1835.
50. Mabuchi H, Koizumi J, Shimizu M, et al: Long-term efficacy of low-density lipoprotein apheresis on coronary heart disease in familial hypercholesterolemia. Hokuriku-FH-LDL-Apheresis Study Group. *Am J Cardiol* 1998;82(12):1489–1495.
51. Tamai O, Matsuoka H, Itabe H, et al: Single LDL apheresis improves endothelium-dependent vasodilatation in hypercholesterolemic humans. *Circulation* 1997;95:76–82.
52. Igarashi K, Tsuji M, Nishimura M, Horimoto M: Improvement of endothelium-dependent coronary vasodilation after a single LDL apheresis in patients with hypercholesterolemia. *J Clin Apher* 2004;19(1):11–16.
53. Sato M, Amano I: Changes in oxidative stress and microcirculation by low-density lipoprotein apheresis. *Ther Apher Dial* 2003;7(4):419–424.
54. Kobayashi K, Yamashita K, Tasaki H, et al: Evaluation of improved coronary flow velocity reserve using transthoracic Doppler echocardiography after single LDL apheresis. *Ther Apher Dial* 2004;8(5):383–389.
55. Klingel R, Göhlen B, Schwarting A, et al: Differential indication of lipoprotein apheresis during pregnancy. *Ther Apher Dial* 2003;7(3):359–364.
56. de Ferranti SD, Rifai N: C-reactive protein: a nontraditional serum marker of cardiovascular risk. *Cardiovasc Pathol* 2007;16(1):14–21.
57. Moriarty PM, Gibson CA: Effect of low-density lipoprotein apheresis on lipoprotein-associated phospholipase A2. *Am J Cardiol* 2005;95(10):1246–1247.
58. Empen K, Otto C, Brödl VC, Parhofer KG: The effects of three different LDL-apheresis methods on the plasma concentrations of E-selectin, VCAM-1, and ICAM-1. *J Clin Apher* 2002;17(1):38–43.
59. Wang Y, Blessing F, Walli AK, et al: Effects of heparin-mediated extracorporeal low-density lipoprotein precipitation beyond lowering proatherogenic lipoproteins—reduction of circulating proinflammatory and procoagulatory markers. *Atherosclerosis* 2004;175(1):145–150.
60. Kobayashi S, Moriya H, Maesato K, et al: LDL-apheresis improves peripheral arterial occlusive disease with an implication for anti-inflammatory effects. *J Clin Apher* 2005;20(4):239–243.
61. Nakamura T, Matsuda T, Suzuki Y, Ueda Y, koicle H: Effects of low-density lipoprotein apheresis on plasma matrix metalloproteinase-9 and serum tissue inhibitor of metalloproteinase-1 levels in diabetic hemodialysis patients with arteriosclerosis obliterans. *ASAIO J* 2003;49(4):430–434.
62. Kobayashi J, Katsube S, Shimoda M, et al. Single LDL apheresis improves serum remnant-like particle-cholesterol, C-reactive protein, and malondialdehyde-modified-low-density lipoprotein concentrations in Japanese hypercholesterolemic subjects. *Clin Chim Acta* 2002;321(1-2):107–112.
63. Kojima S, Shida M, Yokoyama H: Changes in C-reactive protein plasma levels during low-density lipoprotein apheresis. *Ther Apher Dial* 2003;7(4):431–434.
64. Otto C, Geiss HC, Empen K, Parhofer KG: Long-term reduction of C-reactive protein concentration by regular LDL apheresis. *Atherosclerosis* 2004;174(1):151–156.
65. Wieland E, Schettler V, Armstrong VW: Highly effective reduction of C-reactive protein in patients with coronary heart disease by extracorporeal low-density lipoprotein apheresis. *Atherosclerosis* 2002;162(1):187–191.
66. Moriarty PM, Gibson CA, Shih J, Matias MS: C-reactive protein and other markers of inflammation among patients undergoing HELP LDL apheresis. *Atherosclerosis* 2001;158(2):495–498.
67. Kobayashi S, Moriya H, Negishi K, et al: LDL-apheresis up-regulates VEGF and IGF-I in patients with ischemic limb. [See comment.] *J Clin Apher* 2003;18(3):115–119.
68. Jovin IS, Taborski U, Muller-Berghaus G: Analysis of the long-term efficacy and selectivity of immunoadsorption columns for low-density lipoprotein apheresis. *ASAIO J* 2000;46(3): 298–300.

69. Knisel W, Di Nicuolo A, Pfohl M, et al: Different effects of two methods of low-density lipoprotein apheresis on the coagulation and fibrinolytic systems. [See comment.] *J Intern Med* 1993;234(5):479–487.
70. Jaeger BR: Evidence for maximal treatment of atherosclerosis: drastic reduction of cholesterol and fibrinogen restores vascular homeostatis. *Ther Apher* 2001;5(3):207–211.
71. Angelkort B, Amann B, Lawall H: Hemorheology and hemostatis in vascular disease. A pathophysiological review. *Clin Hemorheol Microcirc* 2002;26:145–154.
72. Moriarty PM, Gibson CA, Kensey KR, Hogenaver W: Effect of low-density lipoprotein cholesterol apheresis on blood viscosity. *Am J Cardiol* 2004;93(8):1044–1046.
73. Rubba P, Iannuzzi A, Postiglione A, et al: Hemodynamic changes in the peripheral circulation after repeat low-density lipoprotein apheresis in familial hypercholesterolemia. *Circulation* 1990;81:610–616.
74. Schuff-Werner P, Schütz E, Seyde WC, et al: Improved haemorheology associated with a reduction in plasma fibrinogen and LDL in patients being treated by heparin-induced extracorporeal LDL precipitation (HELP). *Eur J Clin Invest* 1989;19(1):30–37.
75. Iannuzzi A, Bianciardi G, Faccenda F, et al: Correction of erythrocyte shape abnormalities in familial hypercholesterolemia after LDL-apheresis: does it influence cerebral hemodynamics? *Heart Vessels* 1997;12:234–240.
76. Tasaki H: Low-density lipoprotein apheresis in the prevention of recurrent coronary heart disease: a review. *Ther Apher Dial* 2003;7(4):408–412.
77. Krieter DH, Steinke J, Kerkhoff M, et al: Contact activation in low-density lipoprotein apheresis systems. *Artif Organs* 2005;29(1):47–52.
78. Mii S, Mori A, Sakata H, et al: LDL apheresis for arteriosclerosis obliterans with occluded bypass graft: change in prostacyclin and effect on ischemic symptoms. *Angiology* 1998;49(3):175–180.
79. Nakamura T, Vshiyama C, Osada S, et al: Effect of low-density lipoprotein apheresis on plasma endothelin-1 levels in diabetic hemodialysis patients with arteriosclerosis obliterans. *J Diabetes Complications* 2003;17(6):349–354.
80. Mellwig KP, Baller D, Gleichmann U, et al: Improvement of coronary vasodilatation capacity through single LDL apheresis. *Atherosclerosis* 1998;139(1):173–178.
81. Kroon AA, van Asten WN, Stalenhoef AF: Effect of apheresis of low-density lipoprotein on peripheral vascular disease in hypercholesterolemic patients with coronary artery disease. *Ann Intern Med* 1996;125(12):945–954.
82. Takagi M, Yamada T, Yamaguchi H, et al: The role of low-density lipoprotein apheresis as postoperative care of bypass grafting for chronic arterial occlusion. *Cardiovasc Surg* 1996;4(4):459–465.
83. Walzl B, Walzl M, Lechner P, et al: Heparin-induced extracorporeal LDL precipitation (HELP): a new therapeutic intervention in cerebrovascular diseases and peripheral arterial occlusive disease. *Wien Med Wochenschr* 1993;143(22):563–570.
84. Goldstein LB, Adams R, Becker K, et al: Primary prevention of ischemic stroke: a statement for healthcare professionals from the Stroke Council of the American Heart Association. [See comment.] *Stroke* 2001;32(1):280–299.
85. Smith CJ, Emsley HC, Gavin CM, et al: Peak plasma interleukin-6 and other peripheral markers of inflammation in the first week of ischaemic stroke correlate with brain infarct volume, stroke severity and long-term outcome. *BMC Neurol* 2004;4(1):2.
86. Schwartz GG, Olsson AG, Ezekowitz MD, et al: Effects of atorvastatin on early recurrent ischemic events in acute coronary syndromes: The MIRACL study: a randomized controlled trial. [See comment][summary for patients in Curr Cardiol Rep 2002;4(6):485; PMID: 12379168]. *JAMA* 2001;285(13):1711–1718.
87. Pfefferkorn T, Knüppel HP, Jaeger BR, et al: Increased cerebral CO_2 reactivity after Heparin-mediated Extracorporeal LDL Precipitation (HELP) in patients with coronary heart disease and hyperlipidemia. *Stroke* 1999;30:1802–1806.
88. Walzl M, Lechner H, Walzl B, Schied G: Improved neurological recovery of cerebral infarctions after plasmapheretic reduction of lipids and fibrinogen. [See comment.] *Stroke* 1993;24(10): 1447–1451.
89. Wenke K: Management of hyperlipidaemia associated with heart transplantation. *Drugs* 2004;64(10):1053–1068.
90. Mehra MR, Raval NY: Metaanalysis of statins and survival in *de novo* cardiac transplantation. *Transplant Proc* 2004;36(5): 1539–1541.
91. Park JW, Merz M, Braun P: Regression of transplant coronary artery disease during chronic low-density lipoprotein-apheresis. *J Heart Lung Transplant* 1997;16(3):290–297.
92. Matschke K, Mrowietz C, Sternitzky R, et al: Effect of LDL apheresis on oxygen tension in skeletal muscle in patients with cardiac allograft vasculopathy and severe lipid disorder. *Clin Hemorheol Microcirc* 2004;30(3-4):263–271.
93. Jaeger BR, Meiser B, Nagel D, et al: Aggressive lowering of fibrinogen and cholesterol in the prevention of graft vessel disease after heart transplantation. *Circulation* 1997;96(Suppl 9): II-154–II-158.
94. Nakamura T, Kawagoe Y, Ogawa H, et al: Effect of low-density lipoprotein apheresis on urinary protein and podocyte excretion in patients with nephrotic syndrome due to diabetic nephropathy. *Am J Kidney Dis* 2005;45(1):48–53.
95. Muso E, Mune M, Fujii Y, et al: Significantly rapid relief from steroid-resistant nephrotic syndrome by LDL apheresis compared with steroid monotherapy. *Nephron* 2001;89(4): 408–415.
96. Heart Disease and Stroke Statistics—2007 Update: A Report From the American Heart Association Statistics Committee and Stroke Statistics Subcommittee. 2007:e69–e171.
97. Stone PH, Stone PH: Triggering myocardial infarction. [See comment.] *N Engl J Med* 2004;351(17):1716–1718.
98. Ray KK, Cannon CP, Ganz P: Beyond lipid lowering: What have we learned about the benefits of statins from the acute coronary syndromes trials? *Am J Cardiol* 2006;98(11A):18P–25P.
99. Adachi H, Niwa A, Shinoda T: Prevention of restenosis after coronary angioplasty with low-density lipoprotein apheresis. *Artif Organs* 1995;19(12):1243–1247.
100. Jaeger BR, Kreuzer E, Knez A, et al: Case reports on emergency treatment of cardiovascular syndromes through heparin-mediated low-density lipoprotein/fibrinogen precipitation: a new approach to augment cerebral and myocardial salvage. *Ther Apher* 2002;6(5):394–398.
101. Rim S-J, Leong-Poi H, Lindner JR, et al: Decrease in coronary blood flow reserve during hyperlipidemia is secondary to an increase in blood viscosity. *Circulation* 2001;104:2704–2709.
102. Buono LM, Foroozan R, Sergott RC, et al: Nonarteritic anterior ischemic optic neuropathy. *Curr Opin Ophthalmol* 2002;13(6): 357–361.
103. Beatty S, Au Eong KG : Acute occlusion of the retinal arteries: current concepts and recent advances in diagnosis and management. *J Accid Emerg Med* 2000;17(5):324–329.
104. Williamson TH, Rumley A, Lowe GD: Blood viscosity, coagulation, and activated protein C resistance in central retinal vein occlusion: a population controlled study. [See comment.] *Br J Ophthalmol* 1996;80(3):203–208.
105. Fraser S, Siriwardena D: Interventions for acute non-arteritic central retinal artery occlusion. *Cochrane Database of Syst Rev* 2002;(1):CD001989.
106. Walzl M, Lechner P, Walzl B, et al: First experiences with the heparin-induced extracorporeal low-density lipoprotein precipitation in the treatment of critical limb ischaemia: a new therapeutical approach? *Haemostasis* 1993;23(5): 237–243.
107. Moriarty PM, Whitaker TJ: Treatment of acute occlusion of the retinal artery by LDL-apheresis. *J Clin Apher* 2005;20(2):88–92.
108. Ramunni A, Giancipoli G, Guerriero S, et al: LDL-apheresis accelerates the recovery of nonarteritic acute anterior ischemic optic neuropathy. *Ther Apher Dial* 2005;9(1):53–58.
109. Friedman DS, O'Colmain BJ, Münoz B, et al: Prevalence of age-related macular degeneration in the United States. [See comment.] *Arch Ophthalmol* 2004;122(4):564–572.
110. Tan JS, Mitchell P, Rochtenina E, et al: Statins and the long-term risk of incident age-related macular degeneration: The Blue Mountains Eye Study. *Am J Ophthalmol* 2007;143(4): 685–687.
111. Schaumberg DA, Christen WG, Buring JE, et al: High-sensitivity C-reactive protein, other markers of inflammation, and the incidence of macular degeneration in women. *Arch Ophthalmol* 2007;125(3):300–305.
112. Pulido JS and Multicenter Investigation of Rheopheresis for AMD (MIRA-1) Study Group: Multicenter prospective, randomized, double-masked, placebo-controlled study of Rheopheresis to treat nonexudative age-related macular degeneration: interim analysis. *Trans Am Ophthalmol Soc* 2002;100:85–106; discussion 106–107.

113. Nakashima T, Itoh A, Misawa H, Ohno Y: Clinicoepidemiologic features of sudden deafness diagnosed and treated at university hospitals in Japan. *Otolaryngol Head Neck Surg* 2000;123(5):593–597.
114. Zheng S, Jiang R, Fan M: Hemorheological disorders in patients with sudden deafness. *Sheng Wu Yi Xue Gong Cheng Xue Za Zhi* 14(1):11–14.
115. Heiden C, Porzsolt F, Biesinger E, et al: Spontaneous remission of sudden deafness. *HNO* 2000;48(8):621–623.
116. Ullrich H, Kleinjung T, Steffens T, et al: Improved treatment of sudden hearing loss by specific fibrinogen aphaeresis. *J Clin Apher* 2004;19(2):71–78.
117. Balletshofer BM, Stock J, Rittig K, et al: Acute effect of rheopheresis on peripheral endothelial dysfunction in patients suffering from sudden hearing loss. *Ther Apher Dial* 2005;9(5):385–390.
118. Suckfull M, and G. Hearing Loss Study: Fibrinogen and LDL apheresis in treatment of sudden hearing loss: A randomised multicentre trial. [Erratum appears in Lancet 2003;361(9372): 1916.] *Lancet* 2002;360(9348):1811–1817.
119. Saftlas AF, Olson DR, Franks AL, et al: Epidemiology of preeclampsia and eclampsia in the United States, 1979–1986. [See comment.] *Am J Obstet Gynecol* 1990;163 (2):460–465.
120. Roberts JM, Taylor RN, Musci TJ, et al: Preeclampsia: an endothelial cell disorder. [See comment.] *Am J Obstet Gynecol* 1989;161(5):1200–1204.
121. Qiu C, Kivipelto M, Agüero-Torres H, et al: Oxidized low-density lipoprotein (Oxidized LDL) and the risk of preeclampsia. *Physiol Res* 2006;55(5):491–500.
122. Garcia RG, Celedón J, Sierra-Laguado J, et al: Raised C-reactive protein and impaired flow-mediated vasodilation precede the development of preeclampsia. *Am J Hypertens* 2007;20(1): 98–103.
123. Ustün Y, Engin-Ustün Y, Kamaci M: Association of fibrinogen and C-reactive protein with severity of preeclampsia. *Eur J Obstet Gynecol Reprod Biol* 2005;121(2):154–158.
124. Wang J, Mimuro S, Lahoud R, et al: Elevated levels of lipoprotein(a) in women with preeclampsia. [See comment.] *Am J Obstet Gynecol* 1998;178(1 Pt 1):146–149.
125. Wang Y, Walli AK, Schulze A, et al: Heparin-mediated extracorporeal low-density lipoprotein precipitation as a possible therapeutic approach in preeclampsia. *Transfus Apher Sci* 2006;35(2):103–110.
126. Grutzmacher P, Landgraf H, Esser R, et al: *In vivo* rheologic effects of lipid apheresis techniques: comparison of dextran sulfate LDL adsorption and heparin-induced LDL precipitation. *ASAIO Trans* 1990;36:M327–M330.
127. Thompson GR: LDL apheresis. *Atherosclerosis* 2003;167(1): 1–13.
128. Nakamura T, Ushi Yama C, Oscda S, et al: Effect of low-density lipoprotein apheresis on plasma endothelin-1 levels in diabetic hemodialysis patients with arteriosclerosis obliterans. *J Diabetes Complications* 2003;17(6):349–354.
129. Kojima S, Ogi M, Sugi T, et al: Changes in plasma levels of nitric oxide derivative during low-density lipoprotein apheresis. *Ther Apher* 1997;1(4):356–361.
130. Schaumann D, Welch-Wichary M, Voss A, et al: Prospective cross-over comparisons of three low-density lipoprotein (LDL)-apheresis methods in patients with familial hypercholesterolaemia. *Eur J Clin Invest* 1996;26(11):1033–1038.
131. Julius U, Metzler W, Pietsch J, et al: Intraindividual comparison of two extracorporeal LDL apheresis methods: lipidfiltration and HELP. *International Journal of Artif Organs* 2002;25(12):1180–1188.
132. Geiss HC, Parhofer KG, Donner MG, et al: Low-density lipoprotein apheresis by membrane differential filtration (cascade filtration). *Ther Apher* 1999;3(3):199–202.
133. Blaha M: Adhesive selectin molecules MCP-1 and endothelin-1 during long-lasting LDL-apheresis in familial hyperlipoproteinemia. *Ther Apher* 2005;9(3):A29.
134. Spieker LE, Ruschitzka F, Badimon JJ, et al: Shear stress-dependent platelet function after LDL cholesterol apheresis. *Thromb Res* 2004;113(6):395–398.

CHAPTER 31

Nutriceuticals and Functional Foods for Cholesterol Reduction

David J. A. Jenkins, Andrea R. Josse, Julia M. W. Wong, Tri H. Nguyen, and Cyril W. C. Kendall

INTRODUCTION

Over the years, a number of foods or food components, in addition to the fatty acids, have had cardioprotective properties ascribed to them, in large measure based on their effects on serum lipids. Foremost among these have been viscous fibers and plant sterols, which are recommended by the National Cholesterol Education Program Adult Treatment Panel III (NCEP ATP III) to improve the effectiveness of lipid-lowering diets.[1] To these, soy protein and nuts have also been added as foods for which the Food and Drug Administration (FDA) permits a health claim to be made for cardiovascular risk reduction through the lowering of low-density lipoprotein (LDL) cholesterol.[2,3] There has also been significant interest in Quorn derived from mycoprotein[4,5] and in garlic, especially the allicin component.[6,7] Policosanols from Cuban sugar cane[8–10] and conjugated linoleic acid[11,12] have also been explored for cardioprotective properties. Red rice yeast has clearly been demonstrated to lower serum cholesterol and contains a natural source of lovastatin (an HMG-CoA reductase inhibitor that decreases endogenous cholesterol production) produced by the yeast.[13] These are some of the most prominent functional foods and nutriceuticals with lipid-lowering and cardioprotective properties. However, their use as single therapeutic entities has been considered of marginal interest in light of the dramatically successful outcome of statins on both blood lipid reduction and coronary heart disease (CHD) endpoints.[14–17] While no single functional food can achieve the lipid reductions observed with statins, when used in combination these cholesterol-lowering foods and food components, through additive effects, can achieve large reductions in LDL cholesterol, in some instances not greatly different from first-generation statins.

The current review will first focus on the effects on blood lipids of the individual foods or food components with cholesterol-lowering properties. The cholesterol-lowering potential of these foods used in combination with statins will then be discussed.

PLANT STEROLS

Plant sterols are the plant's equivalent of cholesterol. They are found in significant quantities in vegetable oils, nuts, seeds, and leafy vegetables. In most instances, the chief components are β-sitosterol, campesterol, and stigmasterol.[18,19] More recently, pine wood has been used as an inexpensive source of plant sterols.[20] The material has been called Tall oil and it is extracted from wood resin.[21]

Early studies by Grundy and colleagues established plant sterols as hypocholesterolemic agents. Large doses (3 g/day) of relatively insoluble material were given.[22] The mechanism of action appeared to be the reduction of cholesterol absorption.[18,22] With the development of techniques for solubilizing plant sterols in fats, it became apparent that much lower doses of plant sterols were required to reduce serum cholesterol when the material was solubilized in margarine.[23,24] In a meta-analysis by Law, near maximum cholesterol reductions of 10% were obtained at doses of plant sterols of 2 g/day.[25] Sterols may also be hydrogenated to stanols, sitosterol to sitostanol, campesterol to campestanol, and so on. These hydrogenated sterols are thought to be more effective than the nonhydrogenated sterols in lowering cholesterol.[26] However, more recent data suggest their potency is comparable.[23,24] It was also recognized that stanols were less readily absorbed than sterols and resulted in almost negligible rises in blood levels after feeding significant doses.[27]

Although plant sterols have been recognized by the FDA as deserving health claim status for CHD risk reduction[28] and NCEP ATP III recommends them for cholesterol reduction,[1] concerns have been raised over their safety.[29] It has been suggested that they may limit fat-soluble vitamin absorption, and although serum reductions in fat-soluble vitamins are seen, these reductions are of small magnitude and are unlikely to be of significance in individuals whose diets are adequate.[29,30] More seriously, the issue has been raised that higher levels of plant sterols may relate to CHD.[31] It is true that those who are homozygous for the ATP-binding cassette half transporter G5/8 polymorphism are hyperabsorbers of sterols in general (cholesterol and plant sterols)[32–34] and may have advanced artery disease at an early age.[35,36] Although no direct measure of the prevalence of sitosterolemia has been undertaken, it is estimated that there are approximately 50 to 80 confirmed cases worldwide.[36] Nevertheless, the more common heterozygotes do not appear to hyperabsorb sterols, and their serum levels are not greatly influenced by environmental factors.[37] Furthermore, there does not appear to be a relation between serum levels of plant sterols and evidence of arteriosclerosis indicated by coronary artery calcification.[38] Finally, it appears that statin therapy is associated with increased serum levels of plant sterols, possibly secondary to increased overall sterol absorption. As yet, the degree to which plant sterols are elevated has not been implicated in reducing the efficacy of statins in CHD risk reduction.

As a result of the efficacy of plant sterols in reducing serum cholesterol and the ease with which they can be consumed, they have become a significant component of the functional food approach to blood lipid control.

VISCOUS FIBER

Early studies indicated that viscous fibers such as pectin reduced serum cholesterol and that insoluble particulate fibers such as wheat bran were largely without effect.[39–41] The cholesterol-lowering effect was associated with increased bile acid output, and an analogy was drawn with cholestyramine, the anion exchange resin that lowers cholesterol by diverting cholesterol to hepatic bile acid synthesis.[42] The mechanism by which fibers induce an increase in bile acid loss appears to be through physical entrapment rather than chemical binding; hence its dependency on viscosity. In the 20th century, a variety of viscous fiber sources have attracted interest in this respect, including guar gum, oat and barley β-glucan, psyllium, and konjac mannan.[43–47] Cohort studies have also suggested that soluble fiber sources (which include viscous fiber), as opposed to insoluble fiber sources, are most closely related to protection from heart disease.[48] Trials of viscous fiber have usually demonstrated modest falls in serum LDL cholesterol on the order of 7% to 9%,[49,50] although some meta-analyses appear to indicate smaller effects.[44] Studies have also suggested that the addition of viscous fiber to statin treatment is equivalent to doubling the dose of a statin,[51] a finding that could be predicted from the dose–response curve for statins, which tends to flatten shortly after the therapeutic dose is reached.

The problem with viscous fiber foods is the palatability of the food products and a possible increase in flatulence resulting from colonic fiber fermentation. Effective doses are in the 5- to 10-g/day range, doses at which symptoms are usually tolerable. Less well fermented fibers such as psyllium appear useful in those who are troubled by flatus. Common high fiber foods include oat bran and whole oats; barley; psyllium powder; flax seed coat; purified fibers such as guar gum, pectin, and konjac mannan; vegetables such as eggplant and okra; and fruit such as persimmon.

Some fibers are also susceptible to degradation with processing or during storage, and oat β-glucan is particularly sensitive in this respect, possibly related to β-gluconase in cereal foods with changes in state, including reduced solubility when baked goods are frozen.

SOY PROTEIN

Early studies by Sirtori et al established the therapeutic potential of soy protein in the management of hypercholesterolemia.[52] By 1995, Anderson was able to review 38 studies with a total of 564 patients who had been involved in studies of soy on blood lipids.[53] The meta-analysis indicated a 12.9% reduction in LDL cholesterol in subjects who consumed an average of 47 g/day of soy protein. Subsequent meta-analyses have shown more modest reductions,[54–57] and the American Heart Association (AHA) advisory on soy concluded that for more recent studies of soy protein, the LDL cholesterol reduction was as low as 3%.[58] In this analysis, most studies provided soy protein in the 20- to 50-g/day range (18 of 23 studies); five studies were higher with one study providing 133 g of soy protein per day.[58] However, this analysis also included highly processed and heat treated soy in cereal flakes.[59] The effect of high temperature on protein in the presence of carbohydrate has been little studied in terms of its effect on cholesterol lowering but may also be undesirable from the standpoint of the production of advanced glycation endproducts (AGEs).[60] There has also been debate over whether the isoflavones are part of the reason for the hypocholesterolemic effect of soy,[61,62] or whether it is the essential amino acids that raise cholesterol[63,64] or peptide components,[64] especially the 7S globulin fraction,[65] that is responsible for lowering LDL cholesterol. Certainly isolated isoflavones in capsules have not proved very effective in reducing cholesterol, but soy-enriched pasta consumption has been shown to reduce serum total and LDL cholesterol by 7.3% and 8.6%, respectively.[66] The precise mechanism by which soy lowers serum cholesterol is not entirely clear. Carroll concluded that the lack of excess essential amino acids in soy was an advantage, while the excess essential amino acids in many animal protein sources enhanced hepatic cholesterol biosynthesis.[64] On the other hand, demonstration of the inhibitory effect of 7S soy globulin on synthesis of apolipoprotein B by hepG2 cells *in vitro* has also been used to indicate a potential protein-associated reason for the beneficial effect of soy proteins in hyperlipidemia.[65]

Even if soy protein in the diet reduces LDL cholesterol by only 3% to 6%, the displacement of foods rich in saturated fat and cholesterol may well be worth another 3% to 6% in LDL cholesterol reduction. The effective LDL cholesterol reduction with soy in everyday life as opposed to artificially controlled experimental studies could be 6% to 12% when substitution for meat and full-fat dairy products is taken into account. Such LDL cholesterol reduction would certainly make a useful contribution to a cholesterol-lowering dietary portfolio.

NUTS

Nuts, including the legume peanuts, are the most recent addition to the foods for which the FDA permit a heart disease risk reduction health claim.[3] In general, nuts were previously proscribed for patients with heart disease because they were considered high fat and fattening. However, over the last decade, a significant number of major cohort studies have reported that increased nut consumption (≥2 to 5 servings per week) may reduce the risk of heart disease by 35% or more (Table 31-1).[67–72] Furthermore, clinical studies on individual nuts, including almonds, walnuts, pistachios, hazelnuts, pecans, and macadamias, have demonstrated reductions in serum LDL cholesterol, although most studies have been on almonds and walnuts (Table 31-2).[73–89] Not only have reductions in LDL cholesterol been reported, but also reductions have been seen in oxidized LDL and the total cholesterol/high-density lipoprotein (HDL) cholesterol ratio, along with increases in HDL cholesterol.[79] Furthermore, the concern that nuts cause a significant weight gain has not been borne out, and a number of studies have even indicated that nuts may be part of a successful weight loss program,[90–93] possibly because of incomplete absorption and excretion of a significant amount of fat.[94] Almonds have also been shown to modify lipids favorably in diabetes and to have beneficial effects on glucose and oxidation products postprandially.[95,96] The current data therefore provide a very different picture about the intake of nuts than was generally accepted 1 to 2 decades ago.

The mechanisms by which nuts reduce serum cholesterol may be several, depending on their content of monounsaturated fat, plant sterols, vegetable protein, and other phytochemicals. Walnuts, in addition, have omega-3 fatty acids (α-linolenic acids [ALA]) which may benefit CHD risk by nonlipid mechanisms.[97]

The lipid-lowering effect of nuts, their high palatability, and the ease with which a handful of nuts (1 oz or 28 g) can be taken in the diet makes these foods a useful part of the cholesterol-lowering diet.

TABLE 31-1 Nuts and Coronary Heart Disease Risk: Epidemiologic Studies

Study	Endpoints	Nut Consumption	Relative Risk
Iowa Women's Health[69]	Total CHD	≥4 times per week	0.60
Seventh Day Adventists[70]	CHD	≥5 times per week	0.45
Nurses' Health[71]	Total CHD	≥5 times per week	0.65
CARE[68]	Total CHD	≥2 times per week	0.75
Physicians' Health[67]	Total cardiac death	N/A	Inverse linear relationship

CARE, Cholesterol and Recurrent Events; CHD, coronary heart disease.

OTHER FOODS OR FOOD COMPONENTS WITH CHOLESTEROL-LOWERING PROPERTIES

A number of foods and food components have been identified in recent years that may favorably modify lipid risk factors, although the research on the scientific or regulatory acceptance has been less uniform. These foods or food components include red rice yeast, Quorn (mycoprotein), garlic, polycosanols, and conjugated linoleic acid.

Red Rice Yeast

The red rice yeast produces a statin (lovastatin) in the process of fermenting rice.[98] It has been part of traditional Chinese medicine and has undergone formal testing in the West. The data indicate that significant LDL cholesterol reductions of 22% can be obtained with 2.4 g of red rice yeast.[13] Interestingly, it caused no change in liver or muscle enzymes and therefore appears different from what is usually observed with common statin drugs.[99] For reasons which are not altogether clear, the FDA has not accepted red rice yeast for public sale in the United States, although it is available in health food outlets in Canada.

Quorn (Mycoprotein)

The mycoprotein Quorn, like the protein from soy, has also been shown to lower serum cholesterol. It is not known whether the mechanism is similar to that of soy, including the presence of 7S globulin or a reduction in surplus essential amino acids. However, reductions of 9% have been noted for 191 g/day intakes of Quorn in a metabolic study.[5] The respective figures for an *ad libitum* study were a 21% reduction with 108 g/day of Quorn.[4] The use of Quorn seems to have been largely restricted to European countries where concerns over genetically modified soy exist, and as yet, it has been little used in North America. This situation may change as additional vegetable proteins to substitute for soy are sourced.

Garlic

Allicin, the active ingredient in garlic, has long been known to lower serum cholesterol, and a significant number of studies of garlic in various forms have demonstrated modest reductions in LDL cholesterol.[6,7] Although it is claimed that odorless preparations of garlic are effective, most successful studies use garlic with the

TABLE 31-2 Nuts and Coronary Heart Disease Risk: Clinical Studies

Authors	Nut Consumed	Background Diet	Outcome
Sabate et al, 1993[85]	Walnuts	NCEP Step 1 (30% fat)	↓ LDL
Spiller et al, 1998[86]	Almonds	Olive oil (30% fat)	↓ LDL
Chisholm et al, 1998[74]	Walnuts	Low-fat (30% fat)	↓ LDL
Edwards et al, 1999[76]	Pistachios	High-fat (37% fat)	↓ LDL
Morgan et al, 2000[83]	Pecans	Self-selected without nuts	↓ LDL
Curb et al, 2000[75]	Macadamia	AHA (30% fat)	↓ LDL
Zambon et al, 2000[89]	Walnuts	Mediterranean (31% fat)	↓ LDL
Rajaram et al, 2001[84]	Pecans	NCEP Step 1 (30% fat)	↓ LDL
Almario et al, 2001[73]	Walnuts	Low-fat (20% fat)	↓ LDL
Iwamoto et al, 2002[78]	Walnuts	Japanese (25% fat)	↓ LDL
Lovejoy et al, 2002[81]	Almonds	Self-selected without nuts	↓ LDL
Jenkins et al, 2003[79]	Almonds	NCEP Step 2 (<10% saturated fat)	↓ LDL
Garg et al, 2003[77]	Macadamia	Self-selected without nuts (31% fat)	↓ LDL
Spiller et al, 2003[87]	Almonds	Heart-healthy (35% fat)	↓ LDL
Tapsell et al, 2004[88]	Walnuts	Low-fat (30% fat)	↓ LDL
Kocyigit et al, 2006[80]	Pistachios	Self-selected without nuts	↓ LDL
Mercanligil et al, 2007[82]	Hazelnuts	Self-selected without nuts (low-fat)	↓ LDL

AHA, American Heart Association, LDL, low-density lipoprotein; NCEP, National Cholesterol Education Program.

distinctive odor that is easily apparent on the skins of garlic eaters. In two studies, 900 mg of garlic and 9.6 mg of allicin were reported to lower LDL cholesterol by 14.2%[6] and 6.6%,[7] respectively. However, several studies have also shown garlic to have no effect on serum lipids and lipoproteins in humans.[100–105] Garlic has not been reported to have any side effects of note, apart from the odor that many people find offensive in garlic eaters. Therefore, garlic may fit into the cholesterol-lowering diet, especially in countries with a high proportion of garlic eaters.

Policosanols

Policosanols are long-chain aliphatic alcohols that are found in natural sources including beeswax and sugar cane. The original interest was in policosanols from sugar cane from Cuba. A significant number of reports from a small group of Cuban investigators suggested that the effects of policosanols were potent in reducing serum cholesterol.[8,9,106] Castano et al demonstrated that 10 mg/day of policosanols taken for 12 weeks lowered LDL cholesterol by 24.4% in older patients with type II hypercholesterolemia and high coronary risk.[8] However, a Canadian study with a similar dose showed that 10 mg/day of sugar cane policosanols resulted in no significant difference in lipid parameters after a 28-day crossover trial in 21 subjects with hypercholesterolemia.[10] Furthermore, all studies from outside Cuba have failed to confirm the cholesterol-lowering effect of policosanols.[107–110] Unless a significant reversal in the current trend is seen, it does not appear that policosanols will be recommended as part of the strategy to lower serum lipids.

Conjugated Linoleic Acid

The *cis*-9,*trans*-11 and the *trans*-10,*cis*-12 isomers of conjugated linoleic acid (CLA) are produced by bacteria in the rumen of herbivores using linoleic acid as the substrate. Consequently, CLA is found in dairy products and meat at relatively low concentrations. It can also be produced commercially in large quantities by the action of sodium hydroxide on linoleic acid. A number of health benefits have been ascribed to CLA, with the *cis*-9,*trans*-11 isomer related most closely to reductions of CHD[110] and the *trans*-10,*cis*-12 isomer to cancer risk reduction.[111] Most studies have involved rodents, and the few studies in humans have not allowed definitive conclusions to be drawn, although it has been said that healthy weight maintenance, but not weight loss, may be assisted.[11,12] More work will have to be undertaken in humans to establish clear indications before the use of CLA can be recommended in clinical situations.

THE NEED TO IMPROVE THE EFFECTIVENESS OF DIET

Although a number of dietary options are available to improve serum lipid risk factors, individually their effects are small. Furthermore, the simple restriction of saturated fat and dietary cholesterol, although it has the potential to achieve significant lipid reductions under metabolically controlled conditions,[112] has often proved difficult to achieve in the general population. With the increased success of statins in reducing LDL cholesterol and cardiac events, as shown in the early trials (Table 31-3),[14–17] the guidelines for high-risk individuals were revised downward so that the new target was

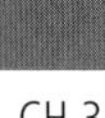

TABLE 31-3 Some Early Statin Intervention Trials

Trial	N	% Drop in LDL Cholesterol	Events	versus Placebo
WOSCOPS[117] (pravastatin)	6595	26%	MI, CHD death	30% fewer events
AFCAPS/TexCAPS[14] (lovastatin)	6605	25%	MI, CHD death	36% fewer events
PROSPER[16] (pravastatin)	5804	34%	MI, CHD death, CVA	13% fewer events
HPS (simvastatin)[15]	20,536	35%	Nonfatal MI, CHD death	26% fewer events

AFCAPS/TexCAPS, Air Force/Texas Coronary Atherosclerosis Prevention Study; CHD, coronary heart disease; CVA, cerebrovascular accident, HPS, Heart Protection Study; LDL, low-density lipoprotein; MI, myacordiol infarction; PROSPER, Prospective Study of Pravastatin in the Elderly of Risk; WOSCOPS, West of Scotland Coronary Prevention Study.

70 mg/dL (or 1.89 mmol/L) as opposed to 100 mg/dL (or 2.00 mmol/L).[113,114] The emphasis was therefore on drug therapy, although the combination or portfolio approach to diet was also mentioned.[115]

ORIGINS OF THE COMBINATION APPROACH TO DIET THERAPY

Even before the current update of the NCEP ATP III guidelines, it was apparent that a large population of middle aged men and postmenopausal women would require drug therapy to control their LDL cholesterol. In fact, it is estimated that half the men in the West of Scotland Coronary Prevention Study would benefit from statin therapy.[116,117] The question therefore arises as to whether there is a serious mismatch between ancient human genes and the contemporary Western diet and lifestyle. To test this hypothesis, a series of studies were undertaken to determine the effect of more primitive diets on the blood lipid response of contemporary humans.

Two weeks on an isocaloric diet of fruit, vegetables, and nuts reduced LDL cholesterol by 35% in a group of 10 normocholesterolemic and moderately hypercholesterolemic men and women.[45] This diet was constructed to reproduce the type of diet eaten by human ancestors at the end of the Miocene epoch about 5 million years ago, a time, it was reasoned, that would have captured many of the evolutionary pressures that have shaped the human genome. This diet was high volume, requiring the subjects to consume 5.5 kg of food per day per 70 kg of body weight. In the long term, the volume of such a diet would provide a natural barrier to consumption and would contrast markedly with contemporary energy-dense diets that, in combination with low physical activity, are associated with the current increased prevalence of obesity. The diet was high in vegetable protein (93 g/day), dietary fiber (143 g/day), plant sterols (1 g/day), and nuts (64 g/day of almonds and hazelnuts) based on a 2000-kcal diet. Ironically, the group of four food classes or food components covered the four categories for which the FDA now permits heart disease risk reduction health claims based on their cholesterol-lowering potential.[2, 3, 28,118,119] The recognition by the FDA of cholesterol-lowering foods is supported by NCEP ATP III recommendations to enhance the cholesterol-lowering potential of the diet with viscous fiber and plant sterols.[120] These two endorsements of functional foods, together with the demonstration of the magnitude of the lipid-lowering effect of the ancestral diet high in cholesterol-reducing elements, has encouraged the use of "combination" or "dietary portfolio" approaches to the dietary control of elevated serum cholesterol.

THE "COMBINATION" OR "DIETARY PORTFOLIO" APPROACH TO CHOLESTEROL REDUCTION

Although all diets by definition are combinations of foods, it is only comparatively recently that a number of foods with cholesterol-lowering properties have been used together in a simple diet by intent. The impetus to combine foods was the lack of effect of diet strategies when applied singly by comparison with the comparatively large and consistent effect in lowering serum cholesterol seen with statins. Furthermore, the repeated demonstration that the reduction in LDL cholesterol was also associated with similar percentage reductions in CHD has caused many of those responsible for lipid control in clinical situations to consider that diet could only be a possible adjunct to pharmacologic therapy but never the primary treatment.

However, recognition that soy, viscous fiber, plant sterols, and nuts (almonds) could each lower LDL cholesterol by 5% or more and that a good low–saturated fat, low-cholesterol diet by itself could result in a further 10% cholesterol reduction indicated that it was therapeutically possible to reduce serum LDL cholesterol by approximately 30% (Table 31-4), similar to a first generation statin.[121] A series of metabolically controlled studies demonstrated that this could be achieved[122,123] and that the reduction in LDL cholesterol was only 2% to 3% less than that achieved in the same group of subjects taking a first-generation statin, lovastatin (20 mg).[124] Furthermore, not only was there a benefit in terms of LDL cholesterol, but also C-reactive protein (CRP), a nonlipid risk factor for CHD,[125] was reduced.

A significant challenge was whether this dietary approach could be sustained in the long term when subjects were not provided with the foods to be consumed. Data from a 1-year study indicated a 13.6% reduction in LDL cholesterol and a 12.7% reduction in the ratio of total cholesterol to HDL cholesterol, with one third of the subjects showing LDL cholesterol reductions of greater than 20%, which was similar to what they achieved with a statin.[126] The variation in effect seen in the group may

TABLE 31-4 Combining the Cholesterol-Lowering Components of the Dietary Portfolio

		% LDL Reduction
NCEP Step 2 diet		10%
Portfolio Diet components	Viscous fiber	5%
	Vegetable protein	5%
	Plant sterols	5%
	Nuts (almonds)	5%
Total		30%

LDL, low-density lipoprotein; NCEP, National Cholesterol Education Program.

TABLE 31-5 Foods Recommended or Allowed on the Dietary Portfolio Based on a 2000-kcal Diet

Food Group and Quantity	Servings	Examples of Servings	Types of Foods
Viscous fiber (20 g/day)	7 per day (3 g/serving)	½ cup dry oat bran 1 slice oat bran specialty bread (50 g) ¼ cup dry barley 2 tsp (3.5 g) psyllium husk	Oat bran, oat meal, rolled oats, oat bran breads, barley, psyllium-containing cereals
	(1 g/serving)	½ cup okra 2 cups eggplant	Okra, eggplant
Soy protein (45 g/day)	7 per day (6.25 g/serving)	1 cup lite or fortified soy beverage ¼ cup extra-firm low-fat tofu 4 soy deli slices 1 soy burger 1 soy hot dog	Soy beverage, tofu, soy meat analogues, soy beans
Other vegetable proteins (12–16 g/day)	1 per day (8–16 g/serving)	½ cup cooked beans, lentils, or chick peas 1 cup instant lentil soup or instant vegetarian chili	Black/kidney/white beans; yellow/red/green lentils; split peas, black-eyed peas
Plant sterols (2 g/day)	5 per day (0.4 g/serving)	5 tsp plant sterol margarine	Flora Pro-activ, Take Control
Nuts—almonds (42 g/day)	1.5 per day (28 g/serving)	28 g almonds	Almonds
Fruits and vegetables	10	1 cup raw leafy vegetable ½ cup cooked vegetable ¾ cup vegetable or fruit juice 1 medium fruit ¼ cup dried fruit ½ cup fresh, frozen, or canned fruit	Tomatoes, carrots, green peas, squash, broccoli, collards, kale, spinach, artichokes, green beans, sweet potatoes, apricots, bananas, dates, grapes, oranges, orange juice, grapefruit, mangoes, melons, peaches, pineapples, prunes, raisins, strawberries, tangerines
High-MUFA oils and margarines (20 g/day)	4 per day (5 g/serving)	1 tsp margarine 1 tsp oil	Olive, canola; plant sterol 'lite' margarine
Sweets	2 (10 g/serving)	1½ tsp strawberry jam	Sugar, double-fruit jam
Not Encouraged: Fat-free or low-fat dairy foods	0 or ≤2 per week	1 cup milk, 1 cup yogurt, ½ cup cheese	Skim milk, low-fat yogurt, fat-free cheese, or fat-free cottage cheese
Egg whites and egg substitutes	0 or ≤3 whole egg equivalent per week	50 g egg white or egg substitutes	Egg white, egg substitutes, egg replacements
Poultry and fish	0 or ≤3 per week	85 g cooked poultry or fish	White poultry meat, no skin, any fish
Red meats	0 per week	85 g cooked meat	Lean or extra-lean red meats

MUFA, monounsaturated fatty acids.

have been influenced by genetic differences, but a far larger influence appeared to be compliance, because the same subjects who did well or badly in the long term did uniformly well when provided with the metabolically controlled diets.[126] In addition to an LDL cholesterol decrease, a lowering was also seen in blood pressure, from 122/74 mm Hg at baseline to 118/72 mm Hg at 1 year.[127] In subjects with higher blood pressure, reductions similar to those seen on the Dietary Approaches to Stop Hypertension (DASH) diet were also observed.[128] Furthermore, there were hematologic changes at 1 year that were indicative of a reduced CHD risk: notably, a reduction in white blood cell count and the neutrophil-to-lymphocyte ratio,[129] which would go along with lower CRP levels.

TABLE 31-6 Daily Checklist for the Required Portfolio Diet Components Based on a 2000-kcal Diet

Required Components (Quantity)	Required Servings per Day	Examples of Servings	Monday	Tuesday	Wednesday	Thursday	Friday	Saturday	Sunday	Your Total Servings per Week
Viscous fiber	7 (⅓ serving)	Oat bran (dry)—½ cup Oat bran bread—1 slice Barley (dry)—¼ cup Psyllium husk—2 tsp Okra (frozen)—½ cup Eggplant (raw)—2 cups								
Soy protein	7	Soy beverage (light)—1 cup Soy beverage (fortified)—1 cup Tofu (extra firm, low fat)—¼ cup Soy deli slices—4 slices Soy burgers—1 whole Soy hot dogs—1 whole								
Plant sterols	5	Pro-activ spread—1 tsp								
Nuts—almonds	1.5	Almonds—1 handful or 24 nuts								
Ideal daily servings			20.5	20.5	20.5	20.5	20.5	20.5	20.5	
Your daily servings										

PORTFOLIO: PRACTICAL APPLICATION

A number of lessons were learned from the 1-year diet. First, the closer the diet was to a vegan diet, the better the effect. However, at the end of the year, only a few subjects were on a fully vegan diet. Nevertheless, the meat and saturated fat intake for the group was greatly reduced, with red meat cut to one forth and saturated fat at 6% or less.[126] The detailed dietary advice that was given is shown in Table 31-5, with a checklist (Table 31-6) that individuals can complete on a weekly basis to ensure they reach targets for portfolio component intakes. Eating out is also a problem, and participants were given a number of useful tips that could be used both when eating out and eating at home (Table 31-7).

SIMILAR COMBINATION APPROACHES

A number of studies of combination diets have shown converging results. A more modest series of dietary changes in a study by Gardner et al resulted in significant reductions in LDL cholesterol (0.36 mmol/L; 9.3%) in comparison with a standard, adequate, low-fat diet.[130] This study also included soy protein, nuts, and some sources of viscous fiber with a reduction in overall meat intake.

A larger study by Bland focusing on plant sterols and soy also showed a range of cardiovascular protective changes, including a significant reduction in LDL cholesterol of 14.8% and triglycerides of 44.8%.[131] Combination therapy is common in pharmacologic treatment of disease, and diet appears to benefit from the same approach.

TABLE 31-7 Tips for Eating Out or Eating at Home
Vegetarian restaurants are your best bet when trying to follow the Dietary Portfolio; Chinese and Indian restaurants may be useful in this respect. But even in a regular restaurant, the following tips may help you make a better choice.
o Try choosing dishes made with tofu (bean curd).
o Try predominantly vegetable dishes (vegetable rolls/wraps, stir-fries, curries, sandwiches).
o Dishes with beans as a main or secondary ingredient are good choices.
o Try a dish containing eggplant and/or okra.
o Try items made with chick peas (hummus) or lentils (Indian dahl).
o Veggie burgers can be a good choice (choose soy burgers if possible).
o Salads with a variety of vegetables and *legumes (beans, lentils, chickpeas)* are good choices.
o Soups with barley, beans, and a variety of vegetables are good choices.
o Fruits, fruit ices (gelato), and soy-based smoothies/juices/yogurt are good dessert choices.
o Try soy milk or soy shakes.
o Try barley (boiled) as a replacement for potatoes or rice.
o For best results, we recommend a **vegan** diet with adequate amounts of oat bran, barley, okra, eggplant, soy and soy products, nuts, legumes, and plant sterol-enriched margarine.

CONCLUSION

Diet treatment still cannot replace the use of drugs, but at least it can increase the number of patients whose lipids are successfully controlled by diet. It might also allow drugs to be used at a dose below that at which the risk of side effects increases dramatically.

More general experience of combination diets on blood lipid reduction is required. It will then be necessary to use this dietary intervention to determine its effect on major secondary endpoints related to CHD.

REFERENCES

1. Expert Panel on Detection, Evaluation, and Treatment of High Blood Cholesterol in Adults: Executive Summary of The Third Report of The National Cholesterol Education Program (NCEP) Expert Panel on Detection, Evaluation, and Treatment of High Blood Cholesterol In Adults (Adult Treatment Panel III). *JAMA* 2001;285:2486–2497.
2. US-FDA: United States Food and Drug Administration. FDA Final Rule for Food Labeling: Health Claims: Soy Protein and Coronary Heart Disease (Federal Register 64 57699–57733). 1999.
3. US-FDA: United States Food and Drug Administration. Food Labeling: Health Claims: Nuts & Heart Disease (Federal Register Docket No. 02P-0505). 2003.
4. Turnbull WH, Leeds AR, Edwards DG: Mycoprotein reduces blood lipids in free-living subjects. *Am J Clin Nutr* 1992;55: 415–419.
5. Turnbull WH, Leeds AR, Edwards GD: Effect of mycoprotein on blood lipids. *Am J Clin Nutr* 1990;52:646–650.
6. Adler AJ, Holub BJ: Effect of garlic and fish-oil supplementation on serum lipid and lipoprotein concentrations in hypercholesterolemic men. *Am J Clin Nutr* 1997;65:445–450.
7. Kannar D, Wattanapenpaiboon N, Savige GS, et al: Hypocholesterolemic effect of an enteric-coated garlic supplement. *J Am Coll Nutr* 2001;20:225–231.
8. Castano G, Mas R, Fernandez JC, et al: Effects of policosanol in older patients with type II hypercholesterolemia and high coronary risk. *J Gerontol A Biol Sci Med Sci* 2001;56:M186–M192.
9. Castano G, Mas R, Fernandez L, et al: Effects of policosanol 20 versus 40 mg/day in the treatment of patients with type II hypercholesterolemia: a 6-month double-blind study. *Int J Clin Pharmacol Res* 2001;21:43–57.
10. Kassis AN, Jones PJ: Lack of cholesterol-lowering efficacy of Cuban sugar cane policosanols in hypercholesterolemic persons. *Am J Clin Nutr* 2006;84:1003–1008.
11. Salas-Salvado J, Marquez-Sandoval F, Bullo M: Conjugated linoleic acid intake in humans: a systematic review focusing on its effect on body composition, glucose, and lipid metabolism. *Crit Rev Food Sci Nutr* 2006;46:479–488.
12. Wang YW, Jones PJ: Conjugated linoleic acid and obesity control: efficacy and mechanisms. *Int J Obes Relat Metab Disord* 2004;28:941–955.
13. Heber D, Yip I, Ashley JM, et al: Cholesterol-lowering effects of a proprietary Chinese red-yeast-rice dietary supplement. *Am J Clin Nutr* 1999;69:231–236.
14. Downs JR, Clearfield M, Weis S, et al: Primary prevention of acute coronary events with lovastatin in men and women with average cholesterol levels: results of AFCAPS/TexCAPS. Air Force/Texas Coronary Atherosclerosis Prevention Study. 1998;*JAMA* 279:1615–1622.
15. Heart Protection Society Collaborative Group: MRC/BHF Heart Protection Study of cholesterol lowering with simvastatin in 20,536 high-risk individuals: a randomised placebo-controlled trial. *Lancet* 2002;360:7–22.
16. Shepherd J, Blauw GJ, Murphy MB, et al: Pravastatin in elderly individuals at risk of vascular disease (PROSPER): a randomised controlled trial. *Lancet* 2002;360:1623–1630.
17. Shepherd J, Cobbe SM, Ford I, et al: Prevention of coronary heart disease with pravastatin in men with hypercholesterolemia. West of Scotland Coronary Prevention Study Group. *N Engl J Med* 1995;333:1301–1307.

18. Jones PJ, MacDougall DE, Ntanios F, et al: Dietary phytosterols as cholesterol-lowering agents in humans. *Can J Physiol Pharmacol* 1997;75:217–227.
19. Patch CS, Tapsell LC, Williams PG, et al: Plant sterols as dietary adjuvants in the reduction of cardiovascular risk: theory and evidence. *Vasc Health Risk Manag* 2006;2:157–162.
20. Plat J, Mensink RP: Vegetable oil based versus wood based stanol ester mixtures: effects on serum lipids and hemostatic factors in non-hypercholesterolemic subjects. *Atherosclerosis* 2000;148:101–112.
21. Jones PJ, Howell T, MacDougall DE, et al: Short-term administration of tall oil phytosterols improves plasma lipid profiles in subjects with different cholesterol levels. *Metabolism* 1998;47: 751–756.
22. Lees AM, Mok HY, Lees RS, et al: Plant sterols as cholesterol-lowering agents: clinical trials in patients with hypercholesterolemia and studies of sterol balance. *Atherosclerosis* 1977;28: 325–338.
23. Fransen HP, de Jong N, Wolfs M, et al: Customary use of plant sterol and plant stanol enriched margarine is associated with changes in serum plant sterol and stanol concentrations in humans. *J Nutr* 2007;137:1301–1306.
24. Hallikainen MA, Sarkkinen ES, Gylling H, et al: Comparison of the effects of plant sterol ester and plant stanol ester-enriched margarines in lowering serum cholesterol concentrations in hypercholesterolaemic subjects on a low-fat diet. *Eur J Clin Nutr* 2000;54:715–725.
25. Law M: Plant sterol and stanol margarines and health. *BMJ* 2000;320:861–864.
26. Miettinen TA, Gylling H: Plant stanol and sterol esters in prevention of cardiovascular diseases. *Ann Med* 2004;36:126–134.
27. Jones PJ, Raeini-Sarjaz M, Ntanios FY, et al: Modulation of plasma lipid levels and cholesterol kinetics by phytosterol versus phytostanol esters. *J Lipid Res* 2000;41:697–705.
28. US-FDA: United States Food and Drug Administration. FDA Authorizes New coronary Heart Disease Health Claim for Plant Sterol and Plant Stanol Esters (Docket No. 001-1275, OOP-1276). 2000.
29. Berger A, Jones PJ, Abumweis SS: Plant sterols: factors affecting their efficacy and safety as functional food ingredients. *Lipids Health Dis* 2004;3:5.
30. Noakes M, Clifton P, Ntanios F, et al: An increase in dietary carotenoids when consuming plant sterols or stanols is effective in maintaining plasma carotenoid concentrations. *Am J Clin Nutr* 2002;75:79–86.
31. Assmann G, Cullen P, Erbey J, et al: Plasma sitosterol elevations are associated with an increased incidence of coronary events in men: results of a nested case–control analysis of the Prospective Cardiovascular Munster (PROCAM) study. *Nutr Metab Cardiovasc Dis* 2006;16:13–21.
32. Hubacek JA, Berge KE, Cohen JC, et al: Mutations in ATP-cassette binding proteins G5 (ABCG5) and G8 (ABCG8) causing sitosterolemia. *Hum Mutat* 2001;18:359–360.
33. Miwa K, Inazu A, Kobayashi J, et al: ATP-binding cassette transporter G8 M429V polymorphism as a novel genetic marker of higher cholesterol absorption in hypercholesterolaemic Japanese subjects. *Clin Sci (Lond)* 2005;109:183–188.
34. Weggemans RM, Zock PL, Tai ES, et al: ATP binding cassette G5 C1950G polymorphism may affect blood cholesterol concentrations in humans. *Clin Genet* 2002;62:226–229.
35. Salen G, Shefer S, Nguyen L, et al: Sitosterolemia. *J Lipid Res* 1992;33:945–955.
36. Sudhop T, von Bergmann K: Sitosterolemia—a rare disease. Are elevated plant sterols an additional risk factor? *Z Kardiol* 2004;93:921–928.
37. Kwiterovich PO Jr, Chen SC, Virgil DG, et al: Response of obligate heterozygotes for phytosterolemia to a low-fat diet and to a plant sterol ester dietary challenge. *J Lipid Res* 2003;44: 1143–1155.
38. Wilund KR, Yu L, Xu F, et al: No association between plasma levels of plant sterols and atherosclerosis in mice and men. *Arterioscler Thromb Vasc Biol* 2004;24:2326–2332.
39. Jenkins DJ, Newton C, Leeds AR, et al: Effect of pectin, guar gum, and wheat fibre on serum-cholesterol. *Lancet* 1975;1: 1116–1117.
40. Kay RM, Truswell AS: Effect of citrus pectin on blood lipids and fecal steroid excretion in man. *Am J Clin Nutr* 1977;30: 171–175.
41. Palmer GH, Dixon DG: Effect of pectin dose on serum cholesterol levels. *Am J Clin Nutr* 1966;18:437–442.
42. Daggy BP, O'Connell NC, Jerdack GR, et al: Additive hypocholesterolemic effect of psyllium and cholestyramine in the hamster: influence on fecal sterol and bile acid profiles. *J Lipid Res* 1997;38:491–502.
43. Arvill A, Bodin L: Effect of short-term ingestion of konjac glucomannan on serum cholesterol in healthy men. *Am J Clin Nutr* 1995;61:585–589.
44. Brown L, Rosner B, Willett WW, et al: Cholesterol-lowering effects of dietary fiber: a meta-analysis. *Am J Clin Nutr* 1999;69:30–42.
45. Jenkins DJ, Kendall CW, Popovich DG, et al: Effect of a very-high-fiber vegetable, fruit, and nut diet on serum lipids and colonic function. *Metabolism* 2001;50:494–503.
46. Ripsin CM, Keenan JM, Jacobs DR Jr, et al: Oat products and lipid lowering. A meta-analysis. *JAMA* 1992;267:3317–3325.
47. Truswell AS: Meta-analysis of the cholesterol-lowering effects of dietary fiber. *Am J Clin Nutr* 1999;70:942–943.
48. Pereira MA, O'Reilly E, Augustsson K, et al: Dietary fiber and risk of coronary heart disease: a pooled analysis of cohort studies. *Arch Intern Med* 2004;164:370–376.
49. Anderson JW, Allgood LD, Lawrence A, et al: Cholesterol-lowering effects of psyllium intake adjunctive to diet therapy in men and women with hypercholesterolemia: meta-analysis of 8 controlled trials. *Am J Clin Nutr* 2000;71:472–479.
50. Olson BH, Anderson SM, Becker MP, et al: Psyllium-enriched cereals lower blood total cholesterol and LDL cholesterol, but not HDL cholesterol, in hypercholesterolemic adults: results of a meta-analysis. *J Nutr* 1997;127:1973-1980.
51. Moreyra AE, Wilson AC, Koraym A: Effect of combining psyllium fiber with simvastatin in lowering cholesterol. *Arch Intern Med* 2005;165:1161–1166.
52. Sirtori CR, Agradi E, Conti F, et al: Soybean-protein diet in the treatment of type-II hyperlipoproteinaemia. *Lancet* 1977;1: 275–277.
53. Anderson JW, Johnstone BM, Cook-Newell ME: Meta-analysis of the effects of soy protein intake on serum lipids. *N Engl J Med* 1995;333:276–282.
54. Reynolds K, Chin A, Lees KA, et al: A meta-analysis of the effect of soy protein supplementation on serum lipids. *Am J Cardiol* 2006;98:633–640.
55. Taku K, Umegaki K, Sato Y, et al: Soy isoflavones lower serum total and LDL cholesterol in humans: a meta-analysis of 11 randomized controlled trials. *Am J Clin Nutr* 2007;85:1148–1156.
56. Zhan S, Ho SC: Meta-analysis of the effects of soy protein containing isoflavones on the lipid profile. *Am J Clin Nutr* 2005;81:397–408.
57. Zhuo XG, Melby MK, Watanabe S: Soy isoflavone intake lowers serum LDL cholesterol: a meta-analysis of 8 randomized controlled trials in humans. *J Nutr* 2004;134:2395–2400.
58. Sacks FM, Lichtenstein A, Van Horn L, et al: Soy protein, isoflavones, and cardiovascular health: an American Heart Association Science Advisory for professionals from the Nutrition Committee. *Circulation* 2006;113:1034–1044.
59. Jenkins DJ, Kendall CW, Vidgen E, et al: Effect of soy-based breakfast cereal on blood lipids and oxidized low-density lipoprotein. *Metabolism* 2000;49:1496–1500.
60. Negrean M, Stirban A, Stratmann B, et al: Effects of low- and high-advanced glycation endproduct meals on macro- and microvascular endothelial function and oxidative stress in patients with type 2 diabetes mellitus. *Am J Clin Nutr* 2007;85:1236–1243.
61. Crouse JR 3rd, Morgan T, Terry JG, et al: A randomized trial comparing the effect of casein with that of soy protein containing varying amounts of isoflavones on plasma concentrations of lipids and lipoproteins. *Arch Intern Med* 1999;159:2070–2076.
62. Gardner CD, Newell KA, Cherin R, et al: The effect of soy protein with or without isoflavones relative to milk protein on plasma lipids in hypercholesterolemic postmenopausal women. *Am J Clin Nutr* 2001;73:728–735.
63. Carroll KK: Dietary protein, cholesterolemia and atherosclerosis. *CMAJ* 1992;147:900.
64. Carroll KK: Review of clinical studies on cholesterol-lowering response to soy protein. *J Am Diet Assoc* 1991;91:820–827.
65. Lovati MR, Manzoni C, Gianazza E, et al: Soy protein peptides regulate cholesterol homeostasis in Hep G2 cells. *J Nutr* 2000;130:2543–2549.

66. Sadler MJ: Soy and Health 2006. Clinical evidence—dietetic application. British Nutrition Foundation: *Nutrition Bulletin* 2007;32:85–90.
67. Albert CM, Gaziano JM, Willett WW, Socks FM: Nut consumption and decreased risk of sudden cardiac death in the Physicians' Health Study. *Arch Intern Med* 2002;162:1382–1387.
68. Brown L, Rosner B, Willett WW, Socks FM: Nut consumption and risk of recurrent coronary heart disease. *FASEB* 1999;13:A538.
69. Ellsworth JL, Kushi LH, Folsom AR: Frequent nut intake and risk of death from coronary heart disease and all causes in postmenopausal women: the Iowa Women's Health Study. *Nutr Metab Cardiovasc Dis* 2001;11:372–377.
70. Fraser GE, Sabate J, Beeson WL, et al: A possible protective effect of nut consumption on risk of coronary heart disease. The Adventist Health Study. *Arch Intern Med* 1992;152:1416–1424.
71. Hu FB, Stampfer MJ, Manson JE, et al: Frequent nut consumption and risk of coronary heart disease in women: prospective cohort study. *BMJ* 1998;317:1341–1345.
72. Kris-Etherton PM, Zhao G, Binkoski AE, et al: The effects of nuts on coronary heart disease risk. *Nutr Rev* 2001;59:103–111.
73. Almario RU, Vonghavaravat V, Wong R, et al: Effects of walnut consumption on plasma fatty acids and lipoproteins in combined hyperlipidemia. *Am J Clin Nutr* 2001;74:72–79.
74. Chisholm A, Mann J, Skeaff M, et al: A diet rich in walnuts favourably influences plasma fatty acid profile in moderately hyperlipidaemic subjects. *Eur J Clin Nutr* 1998;52:12–16.
75. Curb JD, Wergowske G, Dobbs JC, et al: Serum lipid effects of a high-monounsaturated fat diet based on macadamia nuts. *Arch Intern Med* 2000;160:1154–1158.
76. Edwards K, Kwaw I, Matud J, et al: Effect of pistachio nuts on serum lipid levels in patients with moderate hypercholesterolemia. *J Am Coll Nutr* 1999;18:229–232.
77. Garg ML, Blake RJ, Wills RB: Macadamia nut consumption lowers plasma total and LDL cholesterol levels in hypercholesterolemic men. *J Nutr* 2003;133:1060–1063.
78. Iwamoto M, Imaizumi K, Sato M, et al: Serum lipid profiles in Japanese women and men during consumption of walnuts. *Eur J Clin Nutr* 2002;56:629–637.
79. Jenkins DJ, Kendall CW, Marchie A, et al: Dose response of almonds on coronary heart disease risk factors: blood lipids, oxidized low-density lipoproteins, lipoprotein(a), homocysteine, and pulmonary nitric oxide: a randomized, controlled, crossover trial. *Circulation* 2002;106:1327–1332.
80. Kocyigit A, Koylu AA, Keles H: Effects of pistachio nuts consumption on plasma lipid profile and oxidative status in healthy volunteers. *Nutr Metab Cardiovasc Dis* 2006;16:202–209.
81. Lovejoy JC, Most MM, Lefevre M, et al: Effect of diets enriched in almonds on insulin action and serum lipids in adults with normal glucose tolerance or type 2 diabetes. *Am J Clin Nutr* 2002;76:1000–1006.
82. Mercanligil SM, Arslan P, Alasalvar C, et al: Effects of hazelnut-enriched diet on plasma cholesterol and lipoprotein profiles in hypercholesterolemic adult men. *Eur J Clin Nutr* 2007;61: 212–220.
83. Morgan WA, Clayshulte BJ: Pecans lower low-density lipoprotein cholesterol in people with normal lipid levels. *J Am Diet Assoc* 2000;100:312–318.
84. Rajaram S, Burke K, Connell B, et al: A monounsaturated fatty acid-rich pecan-enriched diet favorably alters the serum lipid profile of healthy men and women. *J Nutr* 2001;131:2275–2279.
85. Sabate J, Fraser GE, Burke K, et al: Effects of walnuts on serum lipid levels and blood pressure in normal men. *N Engl J Med* 1993;328:603–607.
86. Spiller GA, Jenkins DA, Bosello O, et al: Nuts and plasma lipids: an almond-based diet lowers LDL cholesterol while preserving HDL cholesterol. *J Am Coll Nutr* 1998;17:285–290.
87. Spiller GA, Miller A, Olivera K, et al: Effects of plant-based diets high in raw or roasted almonds, or roasted almond butter on serum lipoproteins in humans. *J Am Coll Nutr* 2003;22:195–200.
88. Tapsell LC, Gillen LJ, Patch CS, et al: Including walnuts in a low-fat/modified-fat diet improves HDL cholesterol-to-total cholesterol ratios in patients with type 2 diabetes. *Diabetes Care* 2004;27:2777–2783.
89. Zambon D, Sabate J, Munoz S, et al: Substituting walnuts for monounsaturated fat improves the serum lipid profile of hypercholesterolemic men and women. A randomized crossover trial. *Ann Intern Med* 2000;132:538–546.
90. Foster GD, Wyatt HR, Hill JO, et al: A randomized trial of a low-carbohydrate diet for obesity. *N Engl J Med* 2003;348:2082–2090.
91. Rajaram S, Sabate J: Nuts, body weight and insulin resistance. *Br J Nutr* 2006;96(Suppl 2):S79–S86.
92. Sabate J, Cordero-Macintyre Z, Siapco G, et al: Does regular walnut consumption lead to weight gain? *Br J Nutr* 2005;94:859–864.
93. Wong JM, Kendall CW, Esfahani A, et al: Effectiveness of a vegan based high soy protein diet on weight loss and serum lipids. *FASEB J* 2007;21:111.8.
94. Ellis PR, Kendall CW, Ren Y, et al: Role of cell walls in the bioaccessibility of lipids in almond seeds. *Am J Clin Nutr* 2004;80:604–613.
95. Jenkins DJ, Kendall CW, Josse AR, et al: Almonds decrease postprandial glycemia, insulinemia, and oxidative damage in healthy individuals. *J Nutr* 2006;136:2987–2992.
96. Josse AR, Kendall CW, Augustin LS, et al: Almonds and postprandial glycemia—a dose-response study. *Metabolism* 2007;56:400–404.
97. Mozaffarian D: Does alpha-linolenic acid intake reduce the risk of coronary heart disease? A review of the evidence. *Altern Ther Health Med* 2005;11:24–30; quiz 31, 79.
98. Endo A: Monacolin K, a new hypocholesterolemic agent produced by a Monascus species. *J Antibiot (Tokyo)* 1979;32: 852–854.
99. Pasternak RC, Smith SC Jr, Bairey-Merz CN, et al: ACC/AHA/NHLBI clinical advisory on the use and safety of statins. *Stroke* 2002;33:2337–2341.
100. Berthold HK, Sudhop T, von Bergmann K: Effect of a garlic oil preparation on serum lipoproteins and cholesterol metabolism: a randomized controlled trial. *JAMA* 1998;279:1900–1902.
101. Gardner CD, Chatterjee LM, Carlson JJ: The effect of a garlic preparation on plasma lipid levels in moderately hypercholesterolemic adults. *Atherosclerosis* 2001;154:213–220.
102. Gardner CD, Lawson LD, Block E, et al: Effect of raw garlic vs commercial garlic supplements on plasma lipid concentrations in adults with moderate hypercholesterolemia: a randomized clinical trial. *Arch Intern Med* 2007;167:346–353.
103. Isaacsohn JL, Moser M, Stein EA, et al: Garlic powder and plasma lipids and lipoproteins: a multicenter, randomized, placebo-controlled trial. *Arch Intern Med* 1998;158:1189–1194.
104. Superko HR, Krauss RM: Garlic powder, effect on plasma lipids, postprandial lipemia, low-density lipoprotein particle size, high-density lipoprotein subclass distribution and lipoprotein(a). *J Am Coll Cardiol* 2000;35:321–326.
105. Turner B, Molgaard C, Marckmann P: Effect of garlic (Allium sativum) powder tablets on serum lipids, blood pressure and arterial stiffness in normo-lipidaemic volunteers: a randomised, double-blind, placebo-controlled trial. *Br J Nutr* 2004;92:701–706.
106. Castano G, Fernandez L, Mas R, et al: Effects of addition of policosanol to omega-3 fatty acid therapy on the lipid profile of patients with type II hypercholesterolaemia. *Drugs R D* 2005;6:207–219.
107. Berthold HK, Unverdorben S, Degenhardt R, et al: Effect of policosanol on lipid levels among patients with hypercholesterolemia or combined hyperlipidemia: a randomized controlled trial. *JAMA* 2006;295:2262–2269.
108. Cubeddu LX, Cubeddu RJ, Heimowitz T, et al: Comparative lipid-lowering effects of policosanol and atorvastatin: a randomized, parallel, double-blind, placebo-controlled trial. *Am Heart J* 2006;152:982.e1–5.
109. Dulin MF, Hatcher LF, Sasser HC, et al: Policosanol is ineffective in the treatment of hypercholesterolemia: a randomized controlled trial. *Am J Clin Nutr* 2006;84:1543–1548.
110. Tricon S, Burdge GC, Kew S, et al: Opposing effects of cis-9,trans-11 and trans-10,cis-12 conjugated linoleic acid on blood lipids in healthy humans. *Am J Clin Nutr* 2004;80:614–620.
111. Cho HJ, Kim EJ, Lim SS, et al: Trans-10,cis-12, not cis-9,trans-11, conjugated linoleic acid inhibits G1-S progression in HT-29 human colon cancer cells. *J Nutr* 2006;136:893–898.
112. Schaefer EJ, Lichtenstein AH, Lamon-Fava S, et al: Effects of National Cholesterol Education Program Step 2 diets relatively high or relatively low in fish-derived fatty acids on plasma lipoproteins in middle-aged and elderly subjects. *Am J Clin Nutr* 1996;63:234–241.

113. McPherson R, Frohlich J, Fodor G, et al: Canadian Cardiovascular Society position statement—recommendations for the diagnosis and treatment of dyslipidemia and prevention of cardiovascular disease. *Can J Cardiol* 2006;22:913–927.
114. Yan AT, Yan RT, Tan M, et al: Contemporary management of dyslipidemia in high-risk patients: targets still not met. *Am J Med* 2006;119:676–683.
115. Grundy SM, Cleeman JI, Merz CN, et al: Implications of recent clinical trials for the National Cholesterol Education Program Adult Treatment Panel III guidelines. *Circulation* 2004;110: 227–239.
116. Gotto AM Jr, Grundy SM: Lowering LDL cholesterol: questions from recent meta-analyses and subset analyses of clinical trial data issues from the Interdisciplinary Council on Reducing the Risk for Coronary Heart Disease, ninth Council meeting. *Circulation* 1999;99:E1–E7.
117. WOSCOPS: Influence of pravastatin and plasma lipids on clinical events in the West of Scotland Coronary Prevention Study (WOSCOPS). *Circulation* 1998;97:1440–1445.
118. US-FDA: United States Food and Drug Administration. Food Labeling: Health Claims: Soluble Fiber from Whole Oats and Risk of Coronary Heart Disease (Docket No. 95P-0197:15343–15344). 2001.
119. US-FDA: United States Food and Drug Administration. Food Labeling: Health Claims: Soluble Fiber from Certain Foods and Coronary Heart Disease (Docket No. 96P-0338). 1998.
120. National Cholesterol Education Program (NCEP) Expert Panel on Detection, Evaluation, and Treatment of High Blood Cholesterol in Adults (Adult Treatment Panel III): Third Report of the National Cholesterol Education Program (NCEP) Expert Panel on Detection, Evaluation, and Treatment of High Blood Cholesterol in Adults (Adult Treatment Panel III) final report. *Circulation* 2002;106:3143–3421.
121. Jenkins DJ, Kendall CW, Faulkner D, et al: A dietary portfolio approach to cholesterol reduction: combined effects of plant sterols, vegetable proteins, and viscous fibers in hypercholesterolemia. *Metabolism* 2002;51:1596–1604.
122. Jenkins DJ, Kendall CW, Marchie A, et al: The effect of combining plant sterols, soy protein, viscous fibers, and almonds in treating hypercholesterolemia. *Metabolism* 2003;52:1478–1483.
123. Jenkins DJ, Kendall CW, Marchie A, et al: Effects of a dietary portfolio of cholesterol-lowering foods vs lovastatin on serum lipids and C-reactive protein. *JAMA* 2003;290:502–510.
124. Jenkins DJ, Kendall CW, Marchie A, et al: Direct comparison of a dietary portfolio of cholesterol-lowering foods with a statin in hypercholesterolemic participants. *Am J Clin Nutr* 2005;81:380–387.
125. Ridker PM, Morrow DA: C-reactive protein, inflammation, and coronary risk. *Cardiol Clin* 2003;21:315–325.
126. Jenkins DJ, Kendall CW, Faulkner DA, et al: Assessment of the longer-term effects of a dietary portfolio of cholesterol-lowering foods in hypercholesterolemia. *Am J Clin Nutr* 2006;83: 582–591.
127. Jenkins DJ, Kendall CW, Faulkner DA, et al: Long-term effects of a plant-based dietary portfolio of cholesterol-lowering foods on blood pressure. *Eur J Clin Nutr* 2008;62(6):781–788.
128. Appel LJ, Moore TJ, Obarzanek E, et al: A clinical trial of the effects of dietary patterns on blood pressure. DASH Collaborative Research Group. *N Engl J Med* 1997;336:1117–1124.
129. Jenkins DJ, Kendall CW, Nguyen TH, et al: Effect on hematologic risk factors for coronary heart disease of a cholesterol reducing diet. *Eur J Clin Nutr* 2007;61:483–492.
130. Gardner CD, Coulston A, Chatterjee L, et al: The effect of a plant-based diet on plasma lipids in hypercholesterolemic adults: a randomized trial. *Ann Intern Med* 2005;142:725–733.
131. Lukaczer D, Liska DJ, Lerman RH, et al: Effect of a low glycemic index diet with soy protein and phytosterols on CVD risk factors in postmenopausal women. *Nutrition* 2006;22:104–113.

CHAPTER 32

Evolving Targets of Therapy

Philip Barter

INTRODUCTION

It has long been recognized that plasma lipids and lipoproteins play a fundamental role in the development of atherosclerosis. It is also widely accepted that strategies that treat lipid disorders, whether by lifestyle approaches or the use of lipid-modifying medications, translate into a reduction in the risk of the cardiovascular events caused by atherosclerosis. With the advent of agents such as statins that have the capacity to reduce the concentration of atherogenic lipoproteins to relatively low levels, it has become possible to achieve substantial reductions in risk for most people.

This chapter addresses several issues. Which plasma lipid fractions should be therapeutic targets, and what levels should be achieved for maximal benefit? Should the goals differ in different people? And what is the strength of the evidence supporting lipid surrogates as therapeutic targets?

LOW-DENSITY LIPOPROTEINS

The concentration of low-density lipoprotein (LDL) cholesterol has been shown consistently in large epidemiological studies to be a powerful predictor of future cardiovascular events.[1,2] Furthermore, therapies such as those with statins that reduce the level of LDL cholesterol reduce the risk of future cardiovascular events in what is one of the most proven cases in modern medicine.

Clinical endpoint trials with statins (Table 32-1) have been conducted in settings of primary prevention in people without manifest cardiovascular disease at entry into the trial[3–9] and in settings of secondary prevention in those with manifest cardiovascular disease.[3,9–15] Lowering the concentration of LDL cholesterol reduces fatal and nonfatal myocardial infarction, stroke, unstable angina, and the need to have revascularization procedures. The cardiovascular benefits associated with LDL cholesterol lowering have been demonstrated beyond all reasonable doubt in men and women, in people with and without manifest cardiovascular disease before commencing therapy, in young and old people, in those with acute coronary syndromes,[16] in those who previously had ischemic strokes,[15] in those with diabetes[3,7] or the metabolic syndrome,[17] and in those with hypertension.[5] The results of these trials have been amazingly consistent.

A recent meta-analysis of data from 90,056 participants in 14 randomized trials of statins concluded that for each 40-mg/dL (1.0-mmol/L) reduction in LDL cholesterol, there is a 12% reduction in all-cause mortality, a 23% reduction in the occurrence of myocardial infarction or coronary-related death, a 24% reduction in the need for coronary revascularization, and a 17% reduction in the rate of fatal or nonfatal stroke (Fig. 32-1).[18] All of these reductions were highly significant. This analysis also concluded that the reduction in major vascular events is proportional to the magnitude of the reduction in LDL cholesterol.

Thus, LDL cholesterol is now completely accepted as a target for therapy designed to reduce cardiovascular risk.

There is mounting evidence that the risk of having a cardiovascular event when treated with lipid-lowering agents is a direct function of the concentration of LDL cholesterol that is achieved.[19] This is independent of the pretreatment level, with significant benefits of lipid lowering apparent in high-risk people even when the baseline level of LDL cholesterol is low.[3] To date, the trials reported have not identified a lower threshold below which LDL cholesterol reduction is no longer of value.

Many current guidelines recommend an LDL cholesterol target of less than 100 mg/dL (2.6 mmol/L) in people at high cardiovascular risk,[20,21] although in the light of more recent

TABLE 32-1 Clinical Endpoint Trials with Statins

Trial	Drug	N and Gender	Age (years)	Follow-up (years)	Primary Endpoint
Primary Prevention					
WOSCOPS	Pravastatin	6595 male	45–64	4.9	CHD events
AFCAPS/TexCAPS	Lovastatin	5608 male, 997 female	45–73	5.2	CHD events
ASCOT-LLA	Atorvastatin	8363 male, 1942 female	40–79	3.3	CHD death and MI
ALLHAT-LLT	Pravastatin	5304 male, 5051 female	>55	4.8	All-cause mortality
Primary plus Secondary Prevention					
HPS	Simvastatin	15,454 male, 5082 female	40–80	5.0	Vascular events
PROSPER	Pravastatin	2804 male, 3000 female	70–82	3.2	CHD death, MI, stroke
Secondary Prevention					
4S	Simvastatin	3617 male, 827 female	35–70	5.4	Total mortality
CARE	Pravastatin	3583 male, 576 female	21–75	5.0	CHD events
LIPID	Pravastatin	7498 male, 1516 female	31–75	6.0	CHD mortality
PROVE IT	Atorvastatin, Pravastatin	3251 male, 911 female	Mean 58	2.0	Death, MI, UAP, revascularization, stroke
TNT	Atorvastatin 10 vs 80 mg	8099 male, 2002 female	Mean 61	4.9	Major cardiovascular events
IDEAL	Atorvastatin, Pravastatin	7187 male, 1701 female	Mean 62	4.8	Major cardiovascular events

CHD, coronary heart disease; MI, myocardial infarction; UAP, unstable angina pectoris.

evidence, the National Cholesterol Education Program Adult Treatment Panel III (NCEP ATP III) guidelines were updated with the recommendation that an LDL cholesterol target of less than 70 mg/dL (1.8 mmol/L) be considered as a serious option in high-risk individuals.[19] Importantly, support for this view is mounting. For example, the Reversal of Atherosclerosis with Aggressive Lipid Lowering (REVERSAL) trial in people with existing coronary artery disease compared the effects of aggressive therapy that achieved an LDL cholesterol concentration of 79 mg/dL (2.05 mmol/L) with the effects of more moderate therapy that achieved an LDL cholesterol level of 110 mg/dL (2.85 mmol/L).[22] There was significantly less progression of coronary atherosclerosis in the aggressively treated patients. The Pravastatin or Atorvastatin Evaluation and Infection Therapy (PROVE IT) trial in patients with acute coronary syndromes again compared aggressive and moderate LDL cholesterol lowering.[16] Aggressive therapy with 80 mg atorvastatin daily achieved an average LDL cholesterol level of 62 mg/dL (1.60 mmol/L), while moderate therapy with 40 mg pravastatin daily achieved an average LDL cholesterol level of 95 mg/dL (2.5 mmol/L). The aggressively treated group had a statistically significant 16% lower rate of cardiovascular events ($P < 0.005$).

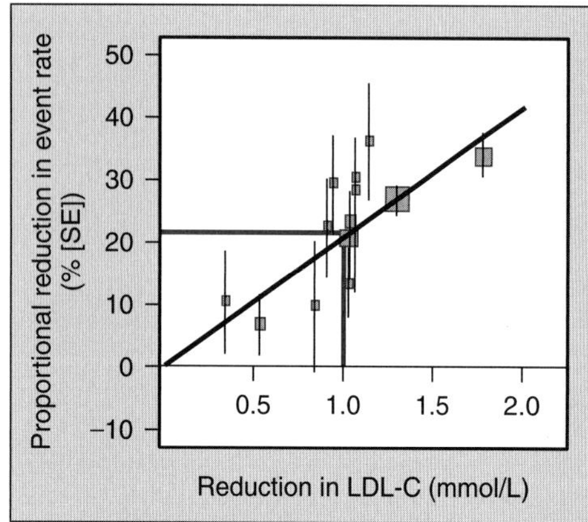

FIGURE 32-1 Meta-analysis of 14 trials (n = 90,056) demonstrating reduction in major vascular events with statin therapy. LDL-C, low-density lipoprotein cholesterol. *(From Ref. 18.)*

The "lower is better" hypothesis received further support from the Treatment to New Targets (TNT) trial, which involved more than 10,000 patients with stable coronary heart disease (CHD).[12] Atorvastatin at a dose of 10 mg or 80 mg per day achieved mean LDL cholesterol levels of 101 mg/dL (2.6 mmol/L) and 77 mg/dL (2.0 mmol/L), respectively, in the two treatment groups. The major cardiovascular event rate was 22% lower in the aggressively treated than in the less-aggressively treated group ($P < 0.001$). A similar result was observed in the more recently reported Incremental Decrease in End Points through Aggressive Lipid Lowering (IDEAL) trial, in which the effects of low-dose simvastatin were compared with the effects of high-dose atorvastatin.[13] The low-dose simvastatin group achieved an LDL cholesterol level of 104 mg/dL (2.7 mmol/L) compared with 84 mg/dL (2.2 mmol/L) in the high-dose atorvastatin group. Reduction in the primary endpoint (major coronary events) was not statistically significant (11%, P = 0.07). However, the occurrence of major cardiovascular events (the primary endpoint in TNT) was 13% lower in the aggressively treated group than in the less-aggressively treated group, and this was statistically significant (P = 0.02).

The results of these trials support an LDL cholesterol target of somewhere between 70 and 80 mg/dL

(1.8–2.1 mmol/L) in people at high risk of having a cardiovascular event (Fig. 32-2). It is highly likely that the results of future trials will support even lower LDL cholesterol targets in high-risk people. Whether these very low LDL cholesterol levels should be the target in all people is less certain. The benefits of aggressive LDL cholesterol–lowering therapy in lower-risk people must be balanced against the potential risks and costs of embarking on long-term, high-dose statin therapy. In lower-risk people, it may be argued (as is the case in many national guidelines) that the LDL cholesterol target should be less than 100 mg/dL (2.6 mmol/L).

NON–HIGH-DENSITY LIPOPROTEIN CHOLESTEROL

LDLs are not the only atherogenic lipoproteins in plasma.[23] Triglyceride-rich lipoproteins such as very-low-density lipoproteins (VLDLs) and chylomicrons (especially the partially catabolized remnants of these lipoproteins) are potentially atherogenic but are not captured by assessment of LDL cholesterol. This has led to the suggestion that it is preferable to use some measure of the level of all atherogenic lipoproteins as an indicator of risk and as a target for therapy. One practical way to do this is to measure the non–high-density lipoprotein (non-HDL) cholesterol concentration. This captures the cholesterol contained in all potentially atherogenic lipoproteins. The concentration of non-HDL cholesterol is very simple to compute, being the difference between the plasma total cholesterol concentration and the HDL cholesterol concentration.

Non-HDL cholesterol was included as a secondary target in people with elevated triglyceride in the report of the NCEP ATP III,[20] but the main focus of these guidelines has continued to be LDL cholesterol. One reason is that the evidence supporting non-HDL cholesterol as a primary target for therapy is less than that for LDL cholesterol. However, evidence in support of non-HDL cholesterol is mounting, with several population studies showing that this measure may be superior to LDL cholesterol as a predictor of future cardiovascular events.[24–30] The most compelling case for considering non-HDL cholesterol as a target has emerged from a recent analysis of the combined data set from the TNT[12] and IDEAL[13] studies in which a total of 18,889 patients with established CHD were assigned to usual-dose or high-dose statin treatment and followed up for a median of just under 5 years. In univariate analysis, both LDL cholesterol and non-HDL cholesterol were strongly and significantly associated with major cardiovascular event occurrence. However, after adjustment for non-HDL cholesterol, the significant relationship between LDL cholesterol and cardiovascular events was lost, whereas the on-treatment level of non-HDL cholesterol remained predictive of events after adjustment for LDL cholesterol levels. In patients with LDL cholesterol below 100 mg/dL (2.6 mmol/L), non-HDL cholesterol (but not LDL cholesterol) remained a significant predictor of major cardiovascular events.[30a]

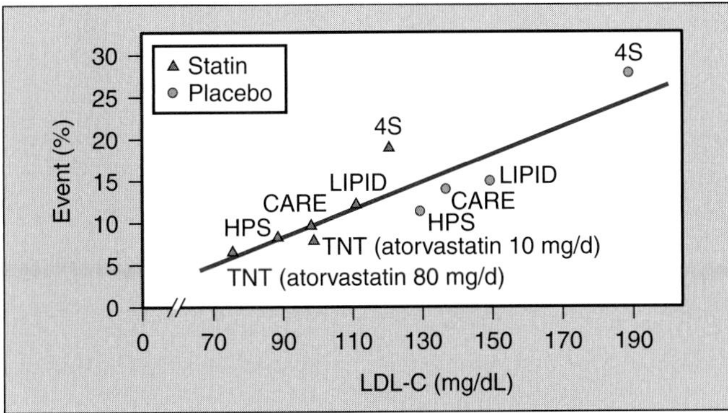

FIGURE 32-2 Relation between low-density lipoprotein cholesterol (LDL-C) on treatment and clinical event rates in major statin trials. *(From Ref. 12.)*

It is most likely that non-HDL cholesterol will eventually replace LDL cholesterol as the primary target for cholesterol-lowering therapy. On the basis of available evidence, it is reasonable to recommend a non-HDL cholesterol target of less than 100 mg/dL (2.6 mmol/L) in very high-risk people and less than 130 mg/dL (3.4 mmol/L) in those at lower risk.

APOLIPOPROTEIN B

Another measure of the concentration of all atherogenic lipoproteins is apolipoprotein (apo) B. Because chylomicrons and their remnants, VLDLs and their remnants, and LDLs all contain one molecule of apoB per particle,[31,32] it follows that the concentration of apoB provides a direct measure of the concentration of all atherogenic lipoprotein particles.

ApoB may also be superior to LDL cholesterol as a measure of the atherogenic potential of the LDL fraction even in people who have very low levels of chylomicrons and VLDLs. LDLs vary in size from large, cholesterol-rich particles to smaller particles that contain less cholesterol. Consider two people: one whose LDL particles are large and the other whose LDL particles are small. They may have the same concentration of LDL cholesterol but very different concentrations of LDL particles. For any given concentration of LDL cholesterol, the person with smaller LDLs will have a higher LDL particle concentration than someone whose LDL particles are larger (Fig. 32-3). Add to this the possibility that smaller LDL particles may be more susceptible to oxidative modification and thus be more atherogenic,[33,34] and it follows that the estimation of cardiovascular risk based solely on the level of LDL cholesterol will be an underestimate in people whose LDL particles are small. The importance of this is highlighted by the fact that people with type 2 diabetes tend to have LDL particles that are smaller than their counterparts without diabetes or the metabolic syndrome.[35]

Thus, the concentration of apoB as a measure of atherogenic lipoprotein particle concentration should theoretically be superior to LDL cholesterol concentration as an indicator of cardiovascular risk and a better surrogate as a target for therapy.

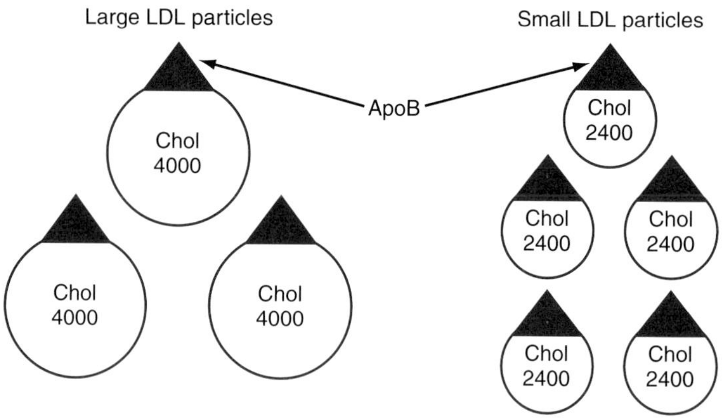

FIGURE 32-3 Schematic diagram showing that for a given amount of cholesterol (Chol) in the low-density lipoprotein (LDL) fraction, there are more LDL particles in someone whose LDL particles are small than in someone whose particles are large. Apo, apolipoprotein.

The concentration of apoB has been shown in several studies to be highly predictive of future cardiovascular events, with some studies identifying apoB levels as more predictive than LDL cholesterol.[29,30,36–41] In the analysis of the combined TNT and IDEAL studies, the on-treatment level of apoB was clearly superior to that of LDL cholesterol as a predictor of cardiovascular events, but it was not superior to non-HDL cholesterol.[30a]

Whether non-HDL cholesterol will, in time, be replaced by apoB as a predictor of cardiovascular risk and as a target for therapy will depend on future research that compares the predictive power of the two measures. It is possible that apoB will eventually win out on the grounds that the non-HDL cholesterol may still underestimate the concentration of atherogenic lipoproteins in people with type 2 diabetes and the metabolic syndrome, in whom there is a preponderance of small dense LDL particles.

On the basis of available evidence, it is reasonable to recommend an apoB target of less than 80 mg/dL in very high-risk people and less than 90 mg/dL in those at lower risk.[41a,41b]

HIGH-DENSITY LIPOPROTEINS

In marked contrast to the proatherogenicity of LDLs and the remnants of chylomicrons and VLDLs, HDLs are antiatherogenic. An inverse relationship between the level of HDL cholesterol and the risk of developing premature CHD has been a consistent finding in large-scale prospective population studies.[42–48] In some of these studies, the level of HDL cholesterol has been the single most powerful lipid predictor of future cardiovascular events.[49] A low level of HDL cholesterol increases cardiovascular risk regardless of whether the LDL cholesterol is high, average, or low, while a high level of HDL cholesterol reduces risk even when the LDL cholesterol is high.[49]

The importance of HDL cholesterol as a potential therapeutic target has been strengthened by the observation that a low level of HDL cholesterol remains highly predictive of cardiovascular events in people who are well treated with statins,[50–52] even when the LDL cholesterol has been reduced to levels below 70 mg/dL (1.7 mmol/L) (Fig. 32-4).[53]

Studies in several animal models have demonstrated that HDL-raising interventions inhibit the development of atherosclerosis.[54–58] In humans, however, the evidence that HDL-raising interventions are protective is mostly circumstantial.

In the Lipid Research Clinics Coronary Primary Prevention Trial using cholestyramine as the active agent, a reduction in CHD events correlated positively with changes in LDL cholesterol levels and negatively with changes in HDL cholesterol. For every 1% increase in the concentration of HDL cholesterol in this study, there was a 0.6% reduction in CHD events that was independent of the changes in LDL cholesterol levels.[59]

The relationship between changes in HDL cholesterol and CHD events in the statin trials is unclear, possibly because it is obscured by the major reductions

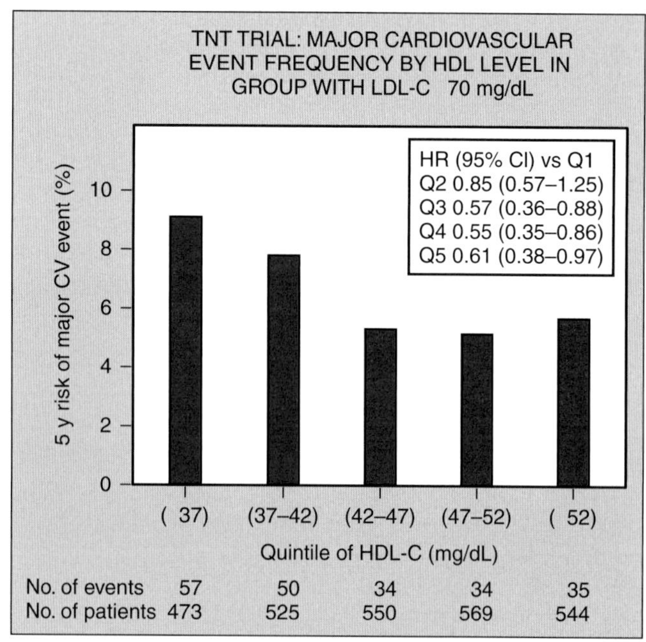

FIGURE 32-4 Multivariate analysis of the relationship between major cardiovascular events and quintiles of HDL cholesterol (HDL-C) levels. Covariates in the multivariate analysis were treatment, sex, age, smoking status, body mass index, systolic blood pressure, fasting glucose, triglyceride (at month 3), baseline LDL cholesterol (LDL-C), and presence or absence of diabetes, myocardial infarction, cardiovascular disease, and hypertension. *(From Ref. 53.)*

in LDL cholesterol. Despite this, the HDL cholesterol increase with simvastatin in the Scandinavian Simvastatin Survival Study (4S) was a significant (although weak) predictor of benefit,[50] and in the Air Force/Texas Coronary Atherosclerosis Prevention Study (AFCAPS/TexCAPS) with lovastatin, the level of apoA-I at 1 year was also predictive of benefit.[60] In contrast, the increase in HDL cholesterol induced by pravastatin in the West of Scotland Coronary Prevention Study (WOSCOPS), Cholesterol and Recurrent Events (CARE), and Long-Term Intervention with Pravastatin in Ischaemic Disease (LIPID) did not correlate significantly with the reduction in CHD events.[52,61]

The results of fibrate trials have been mixed (Table 32-2).[62–66] In the Helsinki Heart Study, which used gemfibrozil as the active agent, it was concluded that a 1% increase in HDL cholesterol was associated with a 2% to 3% decrease in CHD events that was independent of changes in levels of LDL cholesterol.[67] In the Veterans Affairs HDL Intervention Trial (VA-HIT) study the on-treatment HDL cholesterol level was predictive of CHD events in both the active and placebo groups. Multivariate regression analysis showed that, of all of the variables measured, the increase in HDL cholesterol was the only one that predicted benefit.[68] The Bezafibrate Infarction Prevention (BIP) study, another secondary prevention study, used bezafibrate as the active agent. In this study, there was no significant effect of bezafibrate on the primary outcome (the combined incidence of nonfatal myocardial infarction or death from CHD) despite an 18% increase in concentration of HDL cholesterol in the treated group.[65] The Fenofibrate Intervention and Event Lowering in Diabetes (FIELD) study, conducted in people with type 2 diabetes, used fenofibrate as the active agent. This study added little to the argument, because fenofibrate treatment resulted in an HDL cholesterol increase of less than 2%, which may have been one of the reasons why the primary endpoint of this study was reduced by only 11% and was not statistically significant.[66]

Studies with niacin add strong circumstantial support to the view that raising the level of HDL cholesterol is protective. Niacin has long been used as a lipid-modifying agent. It lowers plasma triglyceride by 40% to 50%, lowers LDL cholesterol by 10% to 15%, and increases HDL cholesterol by up to 30%.[69] When coadministered with statins, niacin promotes significant angiographic regression of atheromatous plaque and reduces clinical cardiovascular events.[70–72]

The most compelling evidence of a direct benefit of HDL raising in humans has been provided by a small study in which humans with documented coronary atherosclerosis received intravenous injections of a synthetic HDL preparation. As little as five injections given at weekly intervals resulted in a statistically significant reduction in the atheroma burden in the coronary arteries as assessed by intravascular ultrasound.[73] While the study included only a small number of subjects, the result was consistent with a profound protective action of HDL and has provided a powerful incentive to conduct further research.

There is a need for additional research to determine whether the putative benefits of raising HDL cholesterol in humans are dependent on the mechanism of the HDL-raising therapy and on the specific HDL subpopulations that are raised. There is also a need to determine whether the concentration of HDL cholesterol is the best measure of the protective function of these lipoproteins. It is possible that an increase in a minor subpopulation of highly functional HDL particles (with little change in the total HDL cholesterol level) may be more effective than a larger increase of less functional particles.[74] However, there is currently insufficient knowledge to make recommendations related either to which HDL subpopulation(s) should be targeted or to what HDL function should be used as a measure of cardioprotective potential.

However, despite the fact that the evidence is still mainly circumstantial, it is reasonable at this time to regard HDL cholesterol as a therapeutic target in high-risk people and to recommend interventions designed to achieve a level of greater than 40 mg/dL in men and greater than 50 mg/dL in women.

APOLIPOPROTEIN A-I

Whereas the atherogenic lipoproteins (LDLs, VLDLs, and chylomicrons) contain one molecule of apoB per particle, HDL particles contain anywhere from two to four molecules of apoA-I.[75] They may also contain substantial amounts of other apolipoproteins, such as apoA-II, apoA-IV, and apoE. It is apparent, therefore, that the concentration of apoA-I does not equate with the HDL particle concentration. Despite this, there have been reports suggesting that the concentration of apoA-I has a power to predict cardiovascular events that is as great as or even superior to that of HDL cholesterol.[76]

TABLE 32-2 Clinical Endpoint Trials with Fibrates

Trial	Primary or Secondary	Drug	N and Gender	Age (years)	Follow-up (years)	Primary Endpoint
WHO	Primary	Clofibrate	10,627 male	30–59	5.3	CHD events
HHS	Primary	Gemfibrozil	4081 male	40–55	5.0	CHD events
VA-HIT	Secondary	Gemfibrozil	2531 male	<74	5.1	CHD events
BIP	Secondary	Bezafibrate	2825 male, 165 female	45–74	6.2	CHD events
FIELD	Primary and secondary	Fenofibrate	6138 male, 3657 female	Mean 62	5.0	CHD plus nonfatal MI

CHD, coronary heart disease; MI, myocardial infarction.

However, there is insufficient evidence at this time to recommend apoA-I as a target for therapy.

RATIOS

A number of population studies have identified various lipid and lipoprotein ratios as robust predictors of cardiovascular events. These ratios include total plasma cholesterol/HDL cholesterol and apoB/apoA-I. Both of these ratios provide estimates of the relative concentrations of atherogenic and antiatherogenic lipoproteins. The total cholesterol/HDL cholesterol ratio has been shown in population studies to be predictive of future cardiovascular events, with a power greater than either component of the ratio alone.[77] The other measure that reflects the relative amounts of proatherogenic and antiatherogenic particles is the ratio of apoB to apoA-I. This ratio has received much attention since publication of the Apolipoprotein-related Mortality Risk (AMORIS)[38,78] and INTERHEART[79] studies, in which it was an extremely powerful predictor of events. A potential advantage of using such a ratio is that a practicing clinician needs to act on the basis of only a single number rather than two numbers. However, a ratio that is predictive in a large-scale epidemiological study may be less informative as a risk predictor in individual patients. Furthermore, defining risk on the basis of a ratio does not inform about which component of the ratio (or whether both) should be the main target of therapy designed to reduce cardiovascular risk.

On the basis of the current evidence, it is likely that the apoB/apoA-I ratio will (in time) be incorporated into risk engines that predict cardiovascular risk, but it is uncertain whether this ratio will ever be used to guide therapy or be considered as a specific therapeutic target.

TRIGLYCERIDE

The concentration of plasma triglyceride has been shown in a number of studies to be predictive of future cardiovascular events, independent of the levels of other lipid subfractions.[80,81] Three of the larger prospective studies that have had the ability to investigate the relationships between triglyceride and cardiovascular event rates are the Framingham Heart Study,[82] the Prospective Cardiovascular Münster (PROCAM) study,[83] and the Helsinki Heart Study (placebo group).[67] In these studies, the level of plasma triglyceride was predictive of cardiovascular events only in those who also had an elevated level of LDL cholesterol, a low level of HDL cholesterol, or both. To date, however, there is no definitive evidence that reducing the level of plasma triglyceride translates into a reduction in cardiovascular events.

Triglyceride per se appears not to be atherogenic, as evidenced by the absence of an increased CHD risk in patients with a deficiency of lipoprotein lipase, in whom plasma triglyceride levels may be very high (often >2000 mg/dL). It is possible that the observed positive relationship between plasma triglyceride and cardiovascular risk is because an elevated level of plasma triglyceride in some people reflects an accumulation of the atherogenic remnants of chylomicrons and VLDLs. These particles are rich in both triglyceride and cholesterol and appear to be at least as atherogenic as LDLs.

Fibrates, niacin, and statins all reduce plasma triglyceride levels to some extent. In the case of statins, the positive benefits of the LDL cholesterol lowering make it difficult to determine whether the reduction in triglyceride levels plays any part in the reduction of cardiovascular risk. Similarly, the ability of niacin to raise HDL cholesterol and lower LDL cholesterol limits any conclusions that can be drawn about the benefits of the accompanying reduction in triglyceride levels. Fibrates are highly effective in reducing plasma triglyceride, while having only a modest ability to increase the level of HDL cholesterol and little ability to reduce LDL cholesterol levels. The relationship between triglyceride lowering and cardiovascular risk has been assessed in several trials using fibrates as the active agent. While the presence of an elevated level of triglyceride identifies people who derive a disproportionately large reduction in cardiovascular events when treated with a fibrate,[67,68] these benefits are unrelated to the degree of the fibrate-induced triglyceride reduction.[67,68]

Thus, at this time, the presence of elevated plasma triglyceride supports the use of fibrates to reduce cardiovascular risk, but there is no current evidence to support plasma triglyceride as a therapeutic target.

LOW-DENSITY LIPOPROTEIN PARTICLE SIZE

LDL particles exist in a spectrum of sizes, with evidence that populations of smaller LDLs are more susceptible to oxidation and other modifications and may thus be more atherogenic than larger LDL particles.[33,34] Small dense LDLs are especially prominent in people with elevated levels of plasma triglyceride[35] and may be secondary to cholesteryl ester transfer protein (CETP)–mediated exchanges of cholesteryl esters and triglyceride between LDLs and VLDLs. It is possible that the concentration of small dense LDLs correlates with cardiovascular risk only by virtue of the fact that in someone with small dense LDLs, the LDL particle concentration is higher than predicted from the concentration of LDL cholesterol.[35] Small dense LDL levels may well lose their predictive power if adjusted for LDL particle concentration as assessed by the level of apoB. It should also be noted that people with small dense LDLs frequently have diabetes or the metabolic syndrome and that the small dense LDLs may be secondary to elevated levels of plasma triglyceride, which are frequently observed in such people.

At present, there is no strong evidence to support the measurement of LDL particle size either for risk assessment or as a potential therapeutic target.

HIGH-DENSITY LIPOPROTEIN SUBPOPULATIONS

The HDL fraction in human plasma is heterogeneous in terms of shape, size, density, composition, and surface charge.[75] When isolated on the basis of density by ultracentrifugation, human HDLs separate into two major subfractions, HDL_2 and HDL_3. Nondenaturing polyacrylamide gradient gel electrophoresis separates HDLs on the basis of particle size into at least five distinct subpopulations. HDLs can also be divided into two main subpopulations on the basis of their apolipoprotein composition. One subpopulation comprises HDLs that contain apoA-I but not apoA-II (A-I HDL, or LpA-I), while another comprises particles that contain both apoA-I and apoA-II (A-I/A-II HDL, or LpA-I/A-II). ApoA-I is divided approximately equally between A-I HDL and A-I/A-II HDL in most subjects, while almost all of the apoA-II is in A-I/A-II HDL. When subjected to agarose gel electrophoresis, HDLs have either α, pre-α, pre-β, or γ migration. The α-migrating particles are spherical lipoproteins and account for the major proportion of HDL in plasma. They include the HDL_2 and HDL_3 subfractions as well as A-I HDL and A-I/A-II HDL subpopulations. Pre-β-HDLs are either lipid-poor apoA-I or discoidal particles consisting of two or three molecules of apoA-I complexed with phospholipids and possibly a small amount of unesterified cholesterol. γ HDLs contain apoE and no apoA-I.

Results of some human population studies and some transgenic animal studies have raised the possibility that A-I HDL may be superior to A-I/A-II HDL in its ability to protect against atherosclerosis,[84,85] although other studies have suggested that the protection conferred by A-I HDL and A-I/A-II HDL is comparable.[86] It has been reported that populations of larger HDL are more protective than smaller HDL,[87] while it has been suggested by others that minor subpopulations of discoidal, pre-β–migrating HDL are superior to spherical, α-migrating HDL in their ability to inhibit atherosclerosis because such particles are the preferred acceptors of cholesterol released from cells by the ATP-binding cassette (ABC) A1 transporter.[88] However, the discovery that another transporter, ABCG1, promotes cholesterol efflux from cells to large HDL particles[89,90] supports the epidemiological finding that larger HDL particles are also protective.

Overall, it may be concluded that the evidence linking protection against CHD to specific HDL subpopulations in humans is conflicting and confusing. It remains unknown whether the cardioprotective effects of HDLs are influenced by their apolipoprotein composition, size, density, or electrophoretic mobility.

It is thus premature to consider any particular HDL subpopulation as a therapeutic target.

CONCLUSIONS

The concentration of LDL cholesterol is a well-proven predictor of cardiovascular risk, and the evidence supporting it as a target of therapy is robust. However, evidence is mounting that non-HDL cholesterol and/or apoB may be superior to LDL cholesterol as a predictor of risk and should perhaps replace LDL cholesterol as the main target for lipid-lowering therapy. The concentration of HDL cholesterol is also a powerful (inverse) predictor of cardiovascular risk, which is independent of the level of LDL cholesterol. It is highly likely that HDL cholesterol will, in time, be considered as a therapeutic target that is as important as LDL cholesterol, non-HDL cholesterol, and apoB. The situation with plasma triglyceride is less clear. While the triglyceride level predicts cardiovascular risk, there is no evidence that reducing its level reduces the risk. Thus, at this time, triglyceride should be considered as a predictor of risk but not necessarily a target for therapy. The case for considering lipoprotein particle size and lipid ratios as targets for therapy must await further research.

REFERENCES

1. Gordon T, Kannel WB, Castelli WP, Dawber TR: Lipoproteins, cardiovascular disease, and death. The Framingham study. *Arch Intern Med* 1981;141:1128–1131.
2. Kannel WB, Neaton JD, Wentworth D, et al.: Overall and coronary heart disease mortality rates in relation to major risk factors in 325,348 men screened for the MRFIT. Multiple Risk Factor Intervention Trial. *Am Heart J* 1986;112:825–836.
3. Heart Protection Study Collaborative Group: MRC/BHF Heart Protection Study of cholesterol lowering with simvastatin in 20,536 high-risk individuals: a randomised placebo-controlled trial. *Lancet* 2002;360:7–22.
4. Downs JR, Clearfield M, Weis S, et al.: Primary prevention of acute coronary events with lovastatin in men and women with average cholesterol levels: Results of AFCAPS/TexCAPS. Air Force/Texas Coronary Atherosclerosis Prevention Study. *JAMA* 1998;279:1615–1622.
5. Sever PS, Dahlof B, Poulter NR, et al.: Prevention of coronary and stroke events with atorvastatin in hypertensive patients who have average or lower-than-average cholesterol concentrations, in the Anglo-Scandinavian Cardiac Outcomes Trial—Lipid Lowering Arm (ASCOT-LLA): a multicentre randomised controlled trial. *Lancet* 2003;361:1149–1158.
6. Shepherd J, Cobbe SM, Ford I, et al.: Prevention of coronary heart disease with pravastatin in men with hypercholesterolemia. West of Scotland Coronary Prevention Study Group. *N Engl J Med* 1995;333:1301–1307.
7. Colhoun HM, Betteridge DJ, Durrington PN, et al.: Primary prevention of cardiovascular disease with atorvastatin in type 2 diabetes in the Collaborative Atorvastatin Diabetes Study (CARDS): multicentre randomised placebo-controlled trial. *Lancet* 2004;364:685–696.
8. ALLHAT Officers and Coordinators for the ALLHAT Collaborative Research Group: Major outcomes in moderately hypercholesterolemic, hypertensive patients randomized to pravastatin vs usual care: the Antihypertensive and Lipid-Lowering Treatment to Prevent Heart Attack Trial (ALLHAT-LLT). *JAMA* 2002;288:2998–3007.
9. Shepherd J, Blauw GJ, Murphy MB, et al.: Pravastatin in elderly individuals at risk of vascular disease (PROSPER): a randomised controlled trial. *Lancet* 2002;360:1623–1630.
10. Scandinavian Simvastatin Survival Study Group: Randomised trial of cholesterol lowering in 4444 patients with coronary heart disease: the Scandinavian Simvastatin Survival Study (4S). *Lancet* 1994;344:1383–1389.
11. The Long-Term Intervention with Pravastatin in Ischaemic Disease (LIPID) Study Group: Prevention of cardiovascular events and death with pravastatin in patients with coronary heart disease and a broad range of initial cholesterol levels. *N Engl J Med* 1998;339:1349–1357.
12. LaRosa JC, Grundy SM, Waters DD, et al.: Intensive lipid lowering with atorvastatin in patients with stable coronary disease. *N Engl J Med* 2005;352:1425–1435.
13. Pedersen TR, Faergeman O, Kastelein JJ, et al.: High-dose atorvastatin vs usual-dose simvastatin for secondary prevention after myocardial infarction: the IDEAL study: a randomized controlled trial. *JAMA* 2005;294:2437–2445.
14. Sacks FM, Pfeffer MA, Moye LA, et al.: The effect of pravastatin on coronary events after myocardial infarction in patients with average cholesterol levels. *N Engl J Med* 1996;335:1001–1009.
15. Amarenco P, Bogousslavsky J, Callahan A III, et al.: High-dose atorvastatin after stroke or transient ischemic attack. *N Engl J Med* 2006;355:549–559.
16. Cannon CP, Braunwald E, McCabe CH, et al.: Intensive versus moderate lipid lowering with statins after acute coronary syndromes. *N Engl J Med* 2004;350:1495–1504.

17. Deedwania P, Barter P, Carmena R, et al.: Reduction of low-density lipoprotein cholesterol in patients with coronary heart disease and metabolic syndrome: analysis of the Treating to New Targets study. *Lancet* 2006;368:919–928.
18. Baigent C, Keech A, Kearney PM, et al.: Efficacy and safety of cholesterol-lowering treatment: prospective meta-analysis of data from 90,056 participants in 14 randomised trials of statins. *Lancet* 2005;366:1267–1278.
19. Grundy SM, Cleeman JI, Merz CN, et al.: Implications of recent clinical trials for the National Cholesterol Education Program Adult Treatment Panel III guidelines. *Circulation* 2004;110: 227–239.
20. Expert Panel on Detection, Evaluation, and Treatment of High Blood Cholesterol in Adults: Executive Summary of The Third Report of The National Cholesterol Education Program (NCEP) Expert Panel on Detection, Evaluation, and Treatment of High Blood Cholesterol in Adults (Adult Treatment Panel III). *JAMA* 2001;285:2486–2497.
21. De Backer G, Ambrosioni E, Borch-Johnsen K, et al.: European guidelines on cardiovascular disease prevention in clinical practice. Third Joint Task Force of European and other Societies on Cardiovascular Disease Prevention in Clinical Practice (constituted by representatives of eight societies and by invited experts). *Atherosclerosis* 2004;173:381–391.
22. Nissen SE, Tuzcu EM, Schoenhagen P, et al.: Effect of intensive compared with moderate lipid-lowering therapy on progression of coronary atherosclerosis: a randomized controlled trial. *JAMA* 2004;291:1071–1080.
23. Havel RJ: Role of triglyceride-rich lipoproteins in progression of atherosclerosis. *Circulation* 1990;81:694–696.
24. Liu J, Sempos CT, Donahue RP, et al.: Non-high-density lipoprotein and very-low-density lipoprotein cholesterol and their risk predictive values in coronary heart disease. *Am J Cardiol* 2006;98:1363–1368.
25. Rallidis LS, Pitsavos C, Panagiotakos DB, et al.: Non-high-density lipoprotein cholesterol is the best discriminator of myocardial infarction in young individuals. *Atherosclerosis* 2005;179: 305–309.
26. Bittner V, Hardison R, Kelsey SF, et al.: Non-high-density lipoprotein cholesterol levels predict five-year outcome in the Bypass Angioplasty Revascularization Investigation (BARI). *Circulation* 2002;106:2537–2542.
27. von Muhlen D, Langer RD, Barrett-Connor E: Sex and time differences in the associations of non-high-density lipoprotein cholesterol versus other lipid and lipoprotein factors in the prediction of cardiovascular death (The Rancho Bernardo Study). *Am J Cardiol* 2003;91:1311–1315.
28. Farwell WR, Sesso HD, Buring JE, Gaziano JM: Non-high-density lipoprotein cholesterol versus low-density lipoprotein cholesterol as a risk factor for a first nonfatal myocardial infarction. *Am J Cardiol* 2005;96:1129–1134.
29. Ridker PM, Rifai N, Cook NR, et al.: Non-HDL cholesterol, apolipoproteins A-I and B100, standard lipid measures, lipid ratios, and CRP as risk factors for cardiovascular disease in women. *JAMA* 2005;294:326–333.
30. Pischon T, Girman CJ, Sacks FM, et al.: Non-high-density lipoprotein cholesterol and apolipoprotein B in the prediction of coronary heart disease in men. *Circulation* 2005;112:3375–3383.
30a. Kastelein JJ, van der Steeg WA, Holme I, et al.: Lipids, apolipoproteins, and their ratios in relation to cardiovascular events with statin treatment. *Circulation* 2008;117:3002–3009.
31. Chapman MJ, Laplaud PM, Luc G, et al.: Further resolution of the low-density lipoprotein spectrum in normal human plasma: physicochemical characteristics of discrete subspecies separated by density gradient ultracentrifugation. *J Lipid Res* 1988;29:442–458.
32. Elovson J, Chatterton JE, Bell GT, et al.: Plasma very low-density lipoproteins contain a single molecule of apolipoprotein B. *J Lipid Res* 1988;29:1461–1473.
33. de Graaf J, Hak-Lemmers HL, Hectors MP, et al.: Enhanced susceptibility to in vitro oxidation of the dense low-density lipoprotein subfraction in healthy subjects. *Arterioscler Thromb* 1991;11:298–306.
34. Tribble DL, Holl LG, Wood PD, Krauss RM: Variations in oxidative susceptibility among six low-density lipoprotein subfractions of differing density and particle size. *Atherosclerosis* 1992;93:189–199.
35. Sniderman AD, Scantlebury T, Cianflone K: Hypertriglyceridemic hyperapob: the unappreciated atherogenic dyslipoproteinemia in type 2 diabetes mellitus. *Ann Intern Med* 2001;135:447–459.
36. Everett BM, Kurth T, Buring JE, Ridker PM: The relative strength of C-reactive protein and lipid levels as determinants of ischemic stroke compared with coronary heart disease in women. *J Am Coll Cardiol* 2006;48:2235–2242.
37. Benn M, Nordestgaard BG, Jensen GB, Tybjaerg-Hansen A: Improving prediction of ischemic cardiovascular disease in the general population using apolipoprotein B: the Copenhagen City Heart Study. *Arterioscler Thromb Vasc Biol* 2007;27:661–670.
38. Walldius G, Jungner I, Holme I, et al.: High apolipoprotein B, low apolipoprotein A-I, and improvement in the prediction of fatal myocardial infarction (AMORIS study): a prospective study. *Lancet* 2001;358:2026–2033.
39. St-Pierre AC, Cantin B, Dagenais GR, et al.: Apolipoprotein-B, low-density lipoprotein cholesterol, and the long-term risk of coronary heart disease in men. *Am J Cardiol* 2006;97:997–1001.
40. Hsia SH, Pan D, Berookim P, Lee ML: A population-based, cross-sectional comparison of lipid-related indexes for symptoms of atherosclerotic disease. *Am J Cardiol* 2006;98:1047–1052.
41. Shai I, Rimm EB, Hankinson SE, et al.: Multivariate assessment of lipid parameters as predictors of coronary heart disease among postmenopausal women: potential implications for clinical guidelines. *Circulation* 2004;110:2824–2830.
41a. Brunzell JD, Davidson M, Furberg CD, et al.: Lipoprotein managemnet in patients with cardiometabolic risk: consensus conference report from the American Diabetes Association and the American College of Cardiology Foundation. *J AM Coll Cardiol* 2008;51:1512–1524.
41b. Ballantyne CM, Raichlen JS, Cain VA: Statin therapy alters the relationship between apolipoprotein B and low-density lipoprotein cholesterol and non-high-density lipoprotein cholesterol targets in high-risk patients: the MERCURY II (Measuring Effective Reductions in Cholesterol Using Rosuvastatin) trial. *J AM Coll Cardiol* 2008;52:626–632.
42. Gordon DJ, Knoke J, Probstfield JL, et al.: High-density lipoprotein cholesterol and coronary heart disease in hypercholesterolemic men: the Lipid Research Clinics Coronary Primary Prevention Trial. *Circulation* 1986;74:1217–1225.
43. Enger SC, Hjermann I, Foss OP, et al.: High-density lipoprotein cholesterol and myocardial infarction or sudden coronary death: a prospective case–control study in middle-aged men of the Oslo study. *Artery* 1979;5:170–181.
44. Miller NE, Thelle DS, Forde OH, Mjos OD: The Tromso heart-study. High-density lipoprotein and coronary heart-disease: a prospective case–control study. *Lancet* 1977;1:965–968.
45. Miller M, Seidler A, Kwiterovich PO, Pearson TA: Long-term predictors of subsequent cardiovascular events with coronary artery disease and 'desirable' levels of plasma total cholesterol. *Circulation* 1992;86:1165–1170.
46. Gordon DJ, Probstfield JL, Garrison RJ, et al.: High-density lipoprotein cholesterol and cardiovascular disease. Four prospective American studies. *Circulation* 1989;79:8–15.
47. Jacobs DR Jr, Mebane IL, Bangdiwala SI, et al.: High-density lipoprotein cholesterol as a predictor of cardiovascular disease mortality in men and women: the follow-up study of the Lipid Research Clinics Prevalence Study. *Am J Epidemiol* 1990;131: 32–47.
48. Pekkanen J, Linn S, Heiss G, et al.: Ten-year mortality from cardiovascular disease in relation to cholesterol level among men with and without preexisting cardiovascular disease. *N Engl J Med* 1990;322:1700–1707.
49. Gordon T, Castelli WP, Hjortland MC, et al.: High-density lipoprotein as a protective factor against coronary heart disease. The Framingham Study. *Am J Med* 1977;62:707–714.
50. Pedersen TR, Olsson AG, Faergeman O, et al.: Lipoprotein changes and reduction in the incidence of major coronary heart disease events in the Scandinavian Simvastatin Survival Study (4S). *Circulation* 1998;97:1453–1460.
51. Simes RJ, Marschner IC, Hunt D, et al.: Relationship between lipid levels and clinical outcomes in the Long-term Intervention with Pravastatin in Ischemic Disease (LIPID) Trial: to what extent is the reduction in coronary events with pravastatin explained by on-study lipid levels? *Circulation* 2002;105: 1162–1169.

52. Sacks FM, Tonkin AM, Shepherd J, et al.: Effect of pravastatin on coronary disease events in subgroups defined by coronary risk factors: the Prospective Pravastatin Pooling Project. *Circulation* 2000;102:1893–1900.
53. Barter P, Gotto AM, LaRosa JC, et al.: HDL cholesterol, very low levels of LDL cholesterol, and cardiovascular events. *N Engl J Med* 2007;357:1301–1310.
54. Badimon JJ, Badimon L, Fuster V: Regression of atherosclerotic lesions by high-density lipoprotein plasma fraction in the cholesterol-fed rabbit. *J Clin Invest* 1990;85:1234–1241.
55. Paszty C, Maeda N, Verstuyft J, Rubin EM: Apolipoprotein AI transgene corrects apolipoprotein E deficiency-induced atherosclerosis in mice. *J Clin Invest* 1994;94:899–903.
56. Rubin EM, Krauss RM, Spangler EA, et al.: Inhibition of early atherogenesis in transgenic mice by human apolipoprotein AI. *Nature* 1991;353:265–267.
57. Plump AS, Scott CJ, Breslow JL: Human apolipoprotein A-I gene expression increases high-density lipoprotein and suppresses atherosclerosis in the apolipoprotein E-deficient mouse. *Proc Natl Acad Sci USA* 1994;91:9607–9611.
58. Hoeg JM, Santamarina-Fojo S, Berard AM, et al.: Overexpression of lecithin:cholesterol acyltransferase in transgenic rabbits prevents diet-induced atherosclerosis. *Proc Natl Acad Sci USA* 1996;93:11448–11453.
59. The Lipid Research Clinics Coronary Primary Prevention Trial results. I. Reduction in incidence of coronary heart disease. *JAMA* 1984;251:351–364.
60. Gotto AM Jr, Whitney E, Stein EA, et al.: Relation between baseline and on-treatment lipid parameters and first acute major coronary events in the Air Force/Texas Coronary Atherosclerosis Prevention Study (AFCAPS/TexCAPS). *Circulation* 2000;101: 477–484.
61. West of Scotland Coronary Prevention Study Group: Influence of pravastatin and plasma lipids on clinical events in the West of Scotland Coronary Prevention Study (WOSCOPS). *Circulation* 1998;97:1440–1445.
62. A co-operative trial in the primary prevention of ischaemic heart disease using clofibrate. Report from the Committee of Principal Investigators. *Br Heart J* 1978;40:1069–1118.
63. Frick MH, Elo O, Haapa K, et al.: Helsinki Heart Study: primary-prevention trial with gemfibrozil in middle-aged men with dyslipidemia. Safety of treatment, changes in risk factors, and incidence of coronary heart disease. *N Engl J Med* 1987;317: 1237–1245.
64. Rubins HB, Robins SJ, Collins D, et al.: Gemfibrozil for the secondary prevention of coronary heart disease in men with low levels of high-density lipoprotein cholesterol. Veterans Affairs High-Density Lipoprotein Cholesterol Intervention Trial Study Group. *N Engl J Med* 1999;341:410–418.
65. Secondary prevention by raising HDL cholesterol and reducing triglycerides in patients with coronary artery disease: the Bezafibrate Infarction Prevention (BIP) study. *Circulation* 2000;102:21–27.
66. Keech A, Simes RJ, Barter P, et al.: Effects of long-term fenofibrate therapy on cardiovascular events in 9795 people with type 2 diabetes mellitus (the FIELD study): randomised controlled trial. *Lancet* 2005;366:1849–1861.
67. Manninen V, Tenkanen L, Koskinen P, et al.: Joint effects of serum triglyceride and LDL cholesterol and HDL cholesterol concentrations on coronary heart disease risk in the Helsinki Heart Study. Implications for treatment. *Circulation* 1992;85:37–45.
68. Robins SJ, Collins D, Wittes JT, et al.: Relation of gemfibrozil treatment and lipid levels with major coronary events: VA-HIT: a randomized controlled trial. *JAMA* 2001;285:1585–1591.
69. Carlson LA: Niaspan, the prolonged release preparation of nicotinic acid (niacin), the broad-spectrum lipid drug. *Int J Clin Pract* 2004;58:706–713.
70. Brown G, Albers JJ, Fisher LD, et al.: Regression of coronary artery disease as a result of intensive lipid-lowering therapy in men with high levels of apolipoprotein B. *N Engl J Med* 1990;323:1289–1298.
71. Brown BG, Zhao XQ, Chait A, et al.: Simvastatin and niacin, antioxidant vitamins, or the combination for the prevention of coronary disease. *N Engl J Med* 2001;345:1583–1592.
72. Taylor AJ, Sullenberger LE, Lee HJ, et al.: Arterial Biology for the Investigation of the Treatment Effects of Reducing Cholesterol (ARBITER) 2: a double-blind, placebo-controlled study of extended-release niacin on atherosclerosis progression in secondary prevention patients treated with statins. *Circulation* 2004;110:3512–3517.
73. Nissen SE, Tsunoda T, Tuzcu EM, et al.: Effect of recombinant ApoA-I_{milano} on coronary atherosclerosis in patients with acute coronary syndromes: a randomized controlled trial. *JAMA* 2003;290:2292–2300.
74. Barter PJ, Rye KA: Relationship between the concentration and antiatherogenic activity of high-density lipoproteins. *Curr Opin Lipidol* 2006;17:399–403.
75. Rye KA, Clay MA, Barter PJ: Remodelling of high-density lipoproteins by plasma factors. *Atherosclerosis* 1999;145:227–238.
76. Florvall G, Basu S, Larsson A: Apolipoprotein A1 is a stronger prognostic marker than are HDL and LDL cholesterol for cardiovascular disease and mortality in elderly men. *J Gerontol A Biol Sci Med Sci* 2006;61:1262–1266.
77. Lu W, Resnick HE, Jablonski KA, et al.: Non-HDL cholesterol as a predictor of cardiovascular disease in type 2 diabetes: the strong heart study. *Diabetes Care* 2003;26:16–23.
78. Walldius G, Jungner I: The apoB/apoA-I ratio: a strong, new risk factor for cardiovascular disease and a target for lipid-lowering therapy—A review of the evidence. *J Intern Med* 2006;259:493–519.
79. Yusuf S, Hawken S, Ounpuu S, et al.: Effect of potentially modifiable risk factors associated with myocardial infarction in 52 countries (the INTERHEART study): case–control study. *Lancet* 2004;364:937–952.
80. Austin MA: Plasma triglyceride and coronary heart disease. *Arterioscler Thromb* 1991;11:2–14.
81. Sprecher DL, Pearce GL, Cosgrove DM, et al.: Relation of serum triglyceride levels to survival after coronary artery bypass grafting. *Am J Cardiol* 2000;86:285–288.
82. Castelli WP, Garrison RJ, Wilson PW, et al.: Incidence of coronary heart disease and lipoprotein cholesterol levels. The Framingham Study. *JAMA* 1986;256:2835–2838.
83. Assmann G, Cullen P, Schulte H: The Munster Heart Study (PROCAM). Results of follow-up at 8 years. *Eur Heart J* 1998;19(Suppl A):A2–A11.
84. Warden CH, Hedrick CC, Qiao JH, et al.: Atherosclerosis in transgenic mice overexpressing apolipoprotein A-II. *Science* 1993;261:469–472.
85. Amouyel P, Isorez D, Bard JM, et al.: Parental history of early myocardial infarction is associated with decreased levels of lipoparticle AI in adolescents. *Arterioscler Thromb* 1993;13: 1640–1644.
86. Tailleux A, Bouly M, Luc G, et al.: Decreased susceptibility to diet-induced atherosclerosis in human apolipoprotein A-II transgenic mice. *Arterioscler Thromb Vasc Biol* 2000;20: 2453–2458.
87. Miller NE: Associations of high-density lipoprotein subclasses and apolipoproteins with ischemic heart disease and coronary atherosclerosis. *Am Heart J* 1987;113:589–597.
88. Castro GR, Fielding CJ: Early incorporation of cell-derived cholesterol into pre-beta-migrating high-density lipoprotein. *Biochemistry* 1988;27:25–29.
89. Wang N, Lan D, Chen W, et al.: ATP-binding cassette transporters G1 and G4 mediate cellular cholesterol efflux to high-density lipoproteins. *Proc Natl Acad Sci USA* 2004;101: 9774–9779.
90. Nakamura K, Kennedy MA, Baldan A, et al.: Expression and regulation of multiple murine ATP-binding cassette transporter G1 mRNAs/isoforms that stimulate cellular cholesterol efflux to high-density lipoprotein. *J Biol Chem* 2004;279:45980.

CHAPTER 33

Modulation of Biomarkers of Inflammation

Ishwarlal Jialal and Sridevi Devaraj

INTRODUCTION

Cardiovascular disease (CVD) is the leading cause of morbidity and mortality in the United States. Inflammation plays a pivotal role in all phases of atherosclerosis, from the nascent fatty streak lesion to the culmination in acute coronary syndromes (ACS). There are numerous inflammatory markers that have been shown in various studies to predict cardiovascular events.[1,2] These include cell adhesion molecules, cytokines, chemokines, lipoprotein-associated phospholipase A_2 (Lp-PLA$_2$), myeloperoxidase (MPO), acute-phase reactants such as fibrinogen, serum amyloid A, and C-reactive protein (CRP), and so on. In this brief review, we focus on the most studied inflammatory markers (CRP, MPO, and Lp-PLA$_2$) and examine the modulation of inflammation with diet and pharmacotherapy.

C-REACTIVE PROTEIN

Biochemistry and Biology

CRP is the prototypic marker of inflammation in humans. CRP is a member of the pentraxin family. It comprises five noncovalently associated protomers of 206 amino acids, each arranged symmetrically around a central pore, and has a molecular weight of 118,000 Da.[3,4] It is a nonglycosylated protein in humans, and the gene has been mapped to chromosome 1. Twin studies have shown a highly heritable component to baseline levels of CRP. The general consensus is that the production of CRP is predominantly under the control of interleukin-6 (IL-6). However, IL-1 and tumor necrosis factor (TNF) may also contribute to the hepatic synthesis and secretion of CRP. CRP has a half-life of approximately 19 hours, and this appears to be constant in health and disease. Thus, the sole determinant of CRP levels is the synthetic rate. Its ligand-binding site contains two ligated calcium ions, and it binds phosphocholine and small ribonucleoproteins. To date, in leukocytes and endothelial cells, it has been shown to bind Fc-γ receptors I and II, and its function appears to be to clear apoptotic and necrotic cells via opsonophagocytosis.[3,4]

Much recent data challenge the dogma that CRP is exclusively produced by the liver. Indeed, cogent data suggest that it is produced in the atherosclerotic lesion (especially by endothelial cells, smooth muscle cells [SMCs], and macrophages), the kidney, neurons, alveolar macrophages, and adipose tissue.[5]

High-Sensitivity C-Reactive Protein and Cardiovascular Risk

Numerous studies from various parts of the world have clearly established that CRP predicts future risk for CVD in apparently healthy persons, independent of established risk factors in most studies.[6,7] In the studies to date, CRP has been shown to predict myocardial infarction (MI), coronary artery disease (CAD) death, stroke, peripheral artery disease, sudden death, and so on. In the Women's Health Study, Ridker and colleagues have shown that CRP is additive to low-density lipoprotein (LDL) cholesterol and the Framingham 10-year risk score in predicting future CVD in healthy American women.[8] Thus, based on these data, the American Heart Association and Centers for Disease Control and Prevention have issued a statement recommending that CRP be used as a risk marker for CVD in individuals with a Framingham risk score between 10% and 20%.[9] In these recommendations, CRP levels less than 1 mg/L were considered low risk, levels of 1 to 3 mg/L were considered average risk, and levels greater than 3 mg/L were considered high risk for CVD. With regard to risk assessment, if the value on two occasions 1 month apart is in the same category (i.e., <1, 1 to 3, or 3 to 10 mg/L), this can be taken as reliable evidence with regard to low, average, or high risk for subsequent CVD. However, if the CRP level is greater than 10 mg/L, then CRP cannot be used to assess cardiovascular risk, and other active inflammatory processes (e.g., trauma, infection, etc.) should be excluded. Thus, when using CRP to assess cardiovascular risk in primary prevention, one needs to adopt the high-sensitivity CRP (hsCRP) assay, and the patient should be free from any kind of acute inflammation such as infection, trauma, and so on for at least 2 weeks.

C-Reactive Protein and Atherothrombosis

In addition to CRP's being a cardiovascular risk marker, several lines of evidence point to a proatherogenic, prothrombotic role for CRP via effects on endothelial cells, vascular SMCs (VSMCs), and monocyte/macrophages, as reviewed previously (Table 33-1).[4,5]

C-Reactive Protein and Endothelium

Endothelial cell dysfunction is a key early event in atherogenesis. CRP levels correlate inversely with endothelial vasoreactivity.[4,5] Furthermore, the incubation of human endothelial cells with CRP induced the expression of adhesion molecules, which translated into a biological effect (i.e., increased monocyte–endothelial cell adhesion).[10]

TABLE 33-1 Proatherogenic Effects of C-Reactive Protein

Endothelium
Increased adhesion molecules: ICAM, VCAM, E-selectin
Promotes monocyte-endothelial cell adhesion under static and shear stress
Inhibits eNOS activity via uncoupling and prostacyclin release via nitration of prostaglandin synthase
Induces IL-8 expression via NF-κB
Up-regulates CD40/CD40L expression
Promotes PAI-1 activity via Rho kinase and NF-κB
Decreases tPA via up-regulation of IL-1 and TNF
Reduces endothelial progenitor cell number
Increases expression of MMP-1 and MMP-10 via up-regulation of MAPK
Smooth Muscle Cells
Up-regulates angiotensin-I receptor expression
Promotes VSMC migration and proliferation
Increases ROS production and neointimal proliferation
Monocyte/Macrophages
Induces tissue factor antigen and activity
Increases expression of proinflammatory cytokines
Promotes oxidized LDL uptake
Up-regulates MCP-1–mediated chemotaxis via up-regulation of CCR2
Decreases LPS-induced IL-10 via inhibition of adenyl cyclase
Up-regulates MMP-1 via Fc-γ receptor II and ERK

CCR2, chemokine (C-C motif) receptor 2; eNOS, endothelial nitric oxide synthase; ERK, extracellular receptor kinase; ICAM, intercellular adhesion molecule; IL, interleukin; LDL, low-density lipoprotein; LPS, lipopolysaccharide; MAPK, mitogen-activated protein kinase; MCP-1, monocyte chemoattractant protein-1; MMP, Matrix metalloproteinase; NF-κB, nuclear factor-κB; ROS, reactive oxygen species; TNF, tumor necrosis factor; tPA. tissue plasminogen activator; VCAM, vascular cell adhesion molecule; VSMC, vascular smooth muscle cell.

CRP has been demonstrated to promote monocyte–endothelial cell adhesion. It has also been recently demonstrated that CRP not only promotes nuclear factor–κB–dependent (NF-κB–dependent) adhesion of monocytes to endothelial cells under static conditions, but that this effect also occurs under more clinically relevant shear flow conditions and is inhibited by antibodies to the Fc-γ receptors CD32 and CD64.[10,11]

Two groups have shown that CRP inhibits endothelial nitric oxide synthese (eNOS) activity and bioactivity.[10,12] CRP has been shown to reduce both mRNA and protein for eNOS. Qamirani and colleagues showed that CRP inhibits endothelium-dependent nitric oxide (NO)–mediated dilation in coronary arterioles by producing superoxide from NADPH oxidase via p38 kinase activation.[13] More recently, it was shown that the inhibition of eNOS by CRP was mediated via the Fc-γ receptors, and data from Shaul's group suggest that FcRIIB mediates CRP inhibition of eNOS synthase via PP2A.[14,15] It has been recently shown that human CRP promotes eNOS uncoupling via the activation of NADPH oxidase (p47phox) and the reduction of the availability of tetrahydrobiopterin; this was reversed by antibodies to the Fc-γ receptors CD32 and CD64.[15a] Furthermore, in support of the *in vitro* findings, three groups have independently shown that human CRP transgenic mice exhibit decreased eNOS activity.[15–17] Another important product of endothelial cells is prostacyclin, a potent vasodilator, inhibitor of platelet aggregation, and inhibitor of SMC proliferation. CRP decreases prostacyclin levels in endothelial cells through increased nitration of prostacyclin synthase (PGIS) activity.[4,5] CRP also promotes the release of endothelin-1, another potent vasoconstrictor.[4,5]

Several reports suggest that CRP activates the NF-κB signal transduction pathway in endothelial cells. Degradation of inhibitory NF-κB–α (IκB-α), but not IκB-β, seems to be the major pathway leading to NF-κB nuclear translocation and activation induced by CRP. It has been shown previously that CRP induces the chemokine IL-8, and this is mediated via up-regulation of NF-κB activity in human aortic endothelial cells (HAEC).[18]

A major advance in the field was the demonstration that binding and internalization of CRP by Fc-γ receptors mediate biological effects in endothelial cells.[14] Saturable binding of CRP was obtained at 60 minutes with a CRP concentration between 100 and 150 μg/mL and Kd of 88 nM. Also, binding and internalization of biotinylated CRP was confirmed by fluorescence microscopy and CRP colocalized with CD32 and CD64. Most importantly, a stimulatory effect of CRP was shown. There was an increase in IL-8 as well as an inhibitory effect of CRP (i.e., the decrease in prostacyclin was abrogated with antibodies to CD32 and CD64). Taken together, these data provide the critical insight that CRP mediates its biological effects in endothelial cells via binding and internalization through Fc-γ receptors CD32 and CD64. In addition, CRP enhances lectin-like oxidized LDL receptor–1 (LOX-1) mRNA and protein in HAEC.[4,5] The CD40/CD40 ligand (CD40L) signaling dyad has emerged as a critical cellular hub for oxidative stress, matrix degradation, and plaque rupture. Lin and colleagues have demonstrated a direct effect of CRP to up-regulate CD40/CD40L expression in endothelial cells.[19]

CRP also significantly reduces endothelial progenitor cell (EPC) number, inhibits the expression of the endothelial cell–specific markers Tie-2, endothelial cell–lectin, and vascular endothelial–cadherin, significantly increases EPC apoptosis, and impairs EPC-induced angiogenesis.[20] EPC-induced angiogenesis was dependent on the presence of NO, and CRP treatment caused a decrease in eNOS mRNA expression by EPCs.

In addition to the effects of CRP on endothelial NO and prostaglandin I_2 (PGI_2) release, which are known to be inhibitors of coagulation and thrombosis, CRP can inhibit fibrinolysis via effects on plasminogen activator inhibitor–1 (PAI-1) and tissue plasminogen activator (tPA).[4,5] It was demonstrated that CRP increases PAI-1 expression in HAEC. This was confirmed in bovine aortic endothelial cells, in which the authors reported that CRP activates Rho/Rho-kinase signaling, which in turn activates NF-κB activity, resulting in increased PAI-1 expression.[4,5] More recently, it was demonstrated that CRP decreases tPA in aortic endothelial cells.[4,5] Endothelial cells exposed to CRP exhibited a profound reduction in tPA antigen and activity. CRP increased IL-1β and TNF-α. Neutralization of both IL-1β and TNF-α reversed the inhibition of tPA by CRP. Furthermore, in volunteers who had high CRP levels, euglobulin clot lysis time was significantly increased compared with those who had low CRP levels, providing further evidence that high CRP levels are associated with a procoagulant state. Human CRP transgenic mice have also exhibited increased thrombotic occlusion in the femoral artery after injury.[21]

C-Reactive Protein and Smooth Muscle Cells

CRP markedly up-regulates angiotensin-I receptor (AT1-R) mRNA and protein expression and increases AT1-R number on VSMCs. CRP has been shown to promote VSMC migration and proliferation *in vitro,* increased reactive oxygen species production, and increased neointimal proliferation.[22]

C-Reactive Protein and Monocyte/Macrophages

In monocyte/macrophages, at least two groups have shown that CRP induces tissue factor antigen and activity.[4,5] Ballou and colleagues showed that the incubation of human monocytes with CRP significantly increased levels of IL-1β, TNF-α, and IL-6.[4,5] A single report has shown increased CD11b expression on monocytes incubated with CRP, and this resulted in increased adhesion of these monocytes to lipopolysaccharide (LPS)–activated human umbilical vein endothelial cells.[23] CRP induced the phosphorylation of Syk and an increase in [Ca(2+)](i), both of which were inhibitable by the Syk-specific antagonist piceatannol. While there has been a report that CRP promotes uptake of native LDL, the Witztum group recently demonstrated in an elegant study that CRP promotes the uptake of oxidized but not native LDL because of certain unexposed phosphocholine epitopes on oxidized LDL.[24]

Lim and colleagues have demonstrated that p38 inhibition attenuates the proinflammatory response to CRP by human peripheral blood mononuclear cells.[25] CRP-induced p38 kinase activity in human mononuclear cells was blocked by treatment with an inhibitor of p38 kinase. These results indicate that an important relationship exists between p38 mitogen-activated protein kinase (MAPK) signaling and CRP-induced proinflammatory and prothrombotic activities in human mononuclear cells.

In human monocytes, Han and colleagues demonstrated that CRP up-regulated monocyte chemoattractant protein–1 (MCP-1)–mediated chemotaxis through up-regulating CC chemokine receptor–2 expression in human monocytes.[26] In addition, CRP has been shown to alter the balance of inflammatory cytokines released from monocytes/macrophages. An important effect of CRP on the anti-inflammatory cytokine IL-10 has been recently demonstrated. Because monocytes/macrophages are the major source of IL-10, the effect of CRP on LPS-induced IL-10 secretion in human monocyte-derived macrophages (HMDMs) was tested. Incubation of HMDMs with azide-free CRP (25 μg/mL) significantly decreased LPS-induced IL-10 mRNA (500 ng/mL) and intracellular and secreted IL-10 *in vitro* via inhibition of adenyl cyclase. Furthermore, human CRP delivered to Sprague-Dawley rats decreased plasma IL-10 levels.[27]

Effects of C-Reactive Protein on Matrix Metalloproteinases

Matrix metalloproteinases (MMPs) have been widely implicated in the development of plaque instability and rupture. Recently, Montero and colleagues demonstrated that CRP increased levels of MMP-1 and MMP-10 in human endothelial cells without any significant change in the tissue inhibitor of MMP (TIMP).[28] They also showed that CRP treatment resulted in an increase in MMP activity. Furthermore, specific inhibition of p38 MAPK or MEK abolished the CRP induction of MMP-1, whereas blockade of MMP-10 induction required the simultaneous blockade of p38 MAPK and c-Jun N-terminal kinase (JNK) pathways. In patients with CRP levels greater than 3 mg/L, compared with patients with lower levels of CRP, both MMP-1 and MMP-10 levels were elevated after adjusting for confounding variables. Finally, CRP and MMP colocalized in the endothelial layer and macrophage-rich areas of advanced atherosclerotic plaques. Similar findings have been reported in macrophages, wherein CRP increased production of MMP-1 through the Fc-γ receptor II, CD32, via extracellular receptor kinase (ERK) activation. Doronzo and colleagues evaluated the effects of CRP on the synthesis and release of MMP-2, which is known to play a critical role in plaque instabilization and vascular remodeling.[29] CRP up-regulated MMP-2 mRNA expression. MMP-2 synthesis and activity were increased by 1 to 10 mg/L of CRP starting from an 8-hour incubation. The effect was prevented by exposure to PD98059. CRP did not modify TIMP-2 mRNA expression, protein synthesis, or secretion. Taken together, CRP may directly influence the integrity of the extracellular matrix and tip the balance in favor of matrix degradation with eventual predisposition to rupture.

C-Reactive Protein's Effects Are Not Related to Contamination with Azide and Lipopolysaccharide

Recent reports suggest that CRP-induced effects are artifacts attributable to the presence of contaminants (LPS and azide) in commercial CRP. Different strategies have been used to show that CRP's effects are not the result of contamination: Trypsinized or boiled CRP failed to have the effects of native CRP; the addition of polymixin B did not abrogate CRP's effects; antibodies to CD32 and 64 are able to block CRP's effects; and most convincingly, it has been shown that knocking out TLR4 (ligand for LPS) fails to abrogate CRP's effects.[30]

Autocrine and Paracrine Role of C-Reactive Protein in Atherosclerosis

There is an emerging body of evidence to suggest that CRP may alter vascular homeostasis through an autocrine and/or paracrine mechanism. Although CRP was initially thought to be produced solely from the liver, recent evidence suggests that CRP may be released from endothelial cells, VSMCs, and even adipocytes.[4,5] Yasojima and colleagues provided cogent evidence that CRP mRNA in atheroma was 10 times greater than in the normal vessel.[4,5] Kobayashi and colleagues have shown, in 39 directed coronary atherectomy samples, using antisense riboprobe, that CRP is present in the coronary atheroma.[4,5] This has been confirmed by other groups. Sattler and colleagues have documented CRP protein and mRNA using techniques of western blotting, immunohistochemistry, and real-time reverse transcriptase–polymerase chain reaction (RT-PCR) in plaques obtained from patients undergoing carotid endarterectomy ($n = 41$). Furthermore, the CRP staining was in plaque shoulders, microvessels, or borders, mainly in foam cells and endothelial cells. CRP staining in plaque strongly colocalized with NF-κB activation. Inoue and colleagues demonstrated the local release of CRP from vulnerable plaques and coronary arterial walls injured by stenting.[32]

The role of CRP as a local factor involved in atherothrombosis was strengthened by observations indicating that human arterial endothelial cells produce CRP. The presence of CRP mRNA was detected by RT-PCR and *in situ* hybridization, intracellular protein was detected by Western blot, and secreted protein was detected by ELISA.[32] Coincubation with the cytokines IL-1, IL-6, and TNF alone and in combination showed that the most potent agonist for CRP production from HAEC is the combination of IL-1 and IL-6 ($P < 0.05$). To mimic the *in vivo* situation, we examined whether VSMC-conditioned media and/or macrophage-conditioned media (MCM) could augment CRP production by HAEC. While VSMC-conditioned media had no effect, incubation with MCM resulted in a significant twofold increase in the synthesis of both intracellular and secreted CRP. The effect of MCM could be reversed by inhibiting both IL-1 and IL-6. The recent observations that CRP is produced in aortic endothelid cells and that secreted CRP could be augmented 100-fold with human MCM incubated with endothelial cells argues for paracrine and autocrine loops in the atheroma that could result in exceedingly high CRP concentrations in microdomains. Indeed, plasma CRP levels ranging from 20 to 64 mg/L have been reported in patients with ACS, and levels appear to be higher and predict poorer outcomes in aortic sinus samples.[4,5]

C-Reactive Protein and Atherothrombosis: Effects *in Vivo* in Animal Models and Humans

The transgenic expression of human CRP in animals may accelerate atherosclerosis and increase thrombosis. In apolipoprotein E–deficient (apoE−/−) mice, transgenic CRP expression produced 34% larger aortic atherosclerotic lesions. These lesions were associated with AT1-R, vascular cell adhesion molecule–1 (VCAM-1), and collagen expression.[33] In another study, human transgenic CRP mice were more likely than wild-type animals to develop full thrombotic occlusion of the femoral artery within 28 days after transluminal wire injury (75% vs. 17%, $P < 0.05$). Moreover, the time to clot formation after arterial photochemical injury was shorter in transgenic CRP mice as compared with wild-type mice (33 versus 59 minutes, $P < 0.05$).[21] Bisoendial and Stroes demonstrated a marked activation of inflammation and coagulation after infusion of CRP in humans (1.25 mg/kg recombinant human CRP [rhCRP] or diluent, respectively). CRP concentrations rose after rhCRP infusion from 1.9 (0.3–8.5) to 23.9 (20.5–28.1) mg/L, and subsequently both inflammation and coagulation were activated. CRP infusion resulted in an increase in vWFAg, E-selectin, IL-6, and IL-8, with a trend toward monocytic CD11b and CD18 up-regulation. After 8 hours, both serum amyloid A protein and $sPLA_2$ concentrations rose significantly. There was also a threefold increase in prothrombin F1 +2 ng/mL concentrations 4 hours after rhCRP infusion and a marked increase in D-dimer concentrations and PAI-1 release. Even a short-term increase from a single bolus, obtaining concentrations that are pathophysiologically relevant, induces endothelial cell activation, elicits an acute systemic inflammatory response, and activates the coagulation cascade. This striking sequence of events indicates that CRP, beyond its predictive value, probably also has a causal relation to the occurrence of cardiovascular events.

If CRP contributes to plaque instability and the genesis of ACS, then modulating CRP in the setting of ACS may prove beneficial. In this regard, exciting new data are emerging. In both the Pravastatin or Atorvastatin Evaluation and Infection (PROVE IT) and A to Z studies, concomitant reduction of LDL and CRP with statin therapy resulted in a greater benefit in cardiovascular endpoints.[34] Also, in patients with chronic CAD (Reversal of Atherosclerosis with Aggressive Lipid Lowering (REVERSAL) study, intensive treatment with statins resulted in the greatest benefit, and reductions of hsCRP and LDL cholesterol below the median were associated with slower disease progression.[34] In the appropriate animal model, human CRP has been shown to induce MI and increase stroke volume. Recently, Pepys and colleagues demonstrated that administration of 1,6-bis(phosphocholine)-hexane to rats undergoing acute MI abrogated the increase in infarct size and the cardiac dysfunction produced by injection of human CRP after coronary ligation.[35] These studies further support the notion that CRP might be an active participant in atherothrombosis and the genesis of ACS. However, these exciting preliminary findings need to be confirmed in future studies.

Modulation of C-Reactive Protein

CRP levels can be modulated nutritionally and by using pharmacotherapy (Table 33-2).

Nutritional Modulation

Several studies investigated the effects of weight loss on CRP levels and other inflammatory proteins such as the cytokines IL-6 and TNF-α in obesity, obesity with hyperinsulinemia, diabetes, and rheumatoid arthritis.

Weight loss achieved through different diets (low-fat, high-protein, or hypocaloric) in combination with exercise or nutritional counseling, ranging from 3 to 15 kg, has been shown to result in concomitant reduction of CRP levels by 7% to 48%. The duration of the diet programs ranged from 1 week to 2 years. We have recently reviewed the literature and documented that there is a significant positive correlation between weight loss and the percentage reduction of CRP levels from pooled data from several dietary intervention trials.[36,37] In addition, all of the studies investigating the effect of gastric surgery on CRP observed significantly decreased CRP levels after weight loss.

The meal modulation of inflammatory status as a therapeutic approach toward attenuating atherogenic inflammatory activities in obese women has been relatively well studied. In an effort to determine the effects of lifestyle changes on markers of systemic vascular inflammation and insulin resistance, a randomized single-blind trial was conducted in 120 premenopausal obese women (body mass index [BMI] ≥30 kg/m^2) aged 20 to 46 years without diabetes, hypertension, or hyperlipidemia. The intervention group (n = 60) adhered to a low-energy Mediterranean-style diet (foods rich in complex carbohydrates, monounsaturated fat, and fiber; a lower ratio of omega-6 to omega-3 fatty acids) and increased physical activity. The control group (n = 60) was given general information about healthy food choices and exercise. BMI decreased more in the intervention group than in controls, as did serum concentrations of IL-6, IL-18, and CRP, while adiponectin levels increased significantly. In multivariate analyses, changes in free fatty acid (FFA) and adiponectin levels were independently associated with changes in insulin sensitivity.[52,53] The same group of authors further investigated the effects of a Mediterranean-style diet on endothelial function and vascular inflammatory markers in 180 patients (99 men and 81 women) with the metabolic syndrome (as defined by the National Cholesterol Education Program Adult Treatment Panel III [NCEP ATP III]) who were randomized equally to the intervention and placebo groups for a period of 2 years. The patients in the intervention group were instructed to follow a Mediterranean-style diet and received detailed advice about how to increase daily consumption of whole grains, fruits, vegetables, nuts, and olive oil; patients in the control group (n = 90) followed a prudent diet (carbohydrates, 50%–60%; proteins, 15%–20%; total fat, <30%). Compared with the patients consuming the control diet, the patients adhering to the intervention diet had significantly reduced serum concentrations of hsCRP and IL-6, as well as decreased insulin resistance, whereas adiponectin levels increased significantly. However, IL-18 was not significantly decreased. Endothelial function scores improved in the intervention group but remained stable in the control group. In addition, a 2-year follow-up revealed that only 40 patients in the intervention group still had features of the metabolic syndrome, compared with 78 patients in the control group. Hence, it was concluded that a Mediterranean-style diet might be effective in reducing the prevalence of the metabolic syndrome and its associated inflammation and cardiovascular risk.

Jenkins and colleagues[37a] further documented the anti-inflammatory effects of a dietary portfolio treatment in hyperlipidemic adults in whom a combination of soy proteins, viscous fiber, plant sterols, and almonds lowered CRP by 28.2%. The anti-inflammatory effect was equivalent to low-dose statin therapy. Also, the changes in circulating CRP after weight reduction were examined in relation to the parameters relevant to the metabolic syndrome in obese females (n = 40, ages 25–35 years). These subjects participated in an intervention program of dietary education and supervised physical activity for a period of 9 weeks. Anthropologic parameters and biochemical measurements included CRP, plasma lipoproteins, IL-6, and adiponectin analysis before and after the intervention. BMI, plasma FFAs, and fasting insulin decreased by more than 7%, 30%, and 15%, respectively. High-density lipoprotein (HDL) increased by 8% without any significant change in either LDL or triglycericles. Subcutaneous and visceral adipose tissue mass decreased by 12% and 18%. CRP decreased by 30%; however, IL-6 and adiponectin remained unchanged. In linear regression analysis, the changes in plasma hsCRP concentrations were associated with the baseline hsCRP

TABLE 33-2 Modulation of C-Reactive Protein
Nutritional Modulation Weight loss (hypocaloric diets/Mediterranen-style diet/intensive lifestyle intervention/gastric surgery)
α-linolenic acid
Plant sterols
α-tocopherol (>400 IU RRR-AT/day)
Pharmacotherapy HMG-CoA reductase inhibitors—statins
PPAR-γ agonists—thiazolidinediones
Metformin
PPAR-α agonists—fibrates
Ezetimibe-statin combination
Endocannabinoid (CB_1) receptor blocker—rimonabant

concentration, with the changes in triacylglycerols and FFA concentrations, and with waist circumference. In this study, it appeared that the decrease in hsCRP concentration after weight reduction was not mediated by decreases in circulating IL-6 or adiponectin concentrations; however, the changes in hsCRP were related to the changes in waist circumference and plasma triacylglycerol and FFA levels.

Dansinger and colleagues[37b] compared the effectiveness of four popular diets (Atkins, Zone, Weight Watchers, and Ornish) for weight loss and cardiac risk reduction by carrying out a single-center randomized trial in 160 obese adults (mean BMI, 35 kg/m^2; ages 22–72 years) with hypertension, dyslipidemia, or fasting hyperglycemia. The participants were randomly assigned to either Atkins (carbohydrate restriction, $n = 40$), Zone (macronutrient balance, $n = 40$), Weight Watchers (calorie restriction, $n = 40$), or Ornish (fat restriction, $n = 40$) diet groups for 2 months on specified diets followed by subsequent selection of their own levels of dietary adherence. Mean (SD) weight loss at 1 year was 2.1 (4.8) kg for Atkins (21 [53%] of 40 participants completed, $P = 0.009$), 3.2 (6.0) kg for Zone (26 [65%] of 40 completed, $P = 0.002$), 3.0 (4.9) kg for Weight Watchers (26 [65%] of 40 completed, $P < 0.001$), and 3.3 (7.3) kg for Ornish (20 [50%] of 40 completed, $P = 0.007$). For each diet, decreasing levels of total/HDL cholesterol, CRP, and insulin were significantly associated with weight loss (mean $r = 0.36$, 0.37, and 0.39, respectively), with no significant difference between diets. Thus, it is apparent that each popular diet modestly reduced body weight and several cardiac risk factors at 1 year with concomitant reduction in CRP.

The Diabetes Prevention Program was a randomized clinical trial testing strategies to prevent or delay the development of type 2 diabetes in high-risk individuals with elevated fasting plasma glucose concentrations and impaired glucose tolerance. A total of 3234 participants were randomized to one of three intervention groups—an intensive lifestyle intervention focusing on a healthy diet and exercise and two masked medication treatment groups, metformin or placebo, combined with standard diet and exercise recommendations—and followed for 3 to 5 years. Metformin reduced CRP in women compared with the placebo group. In men, the median changes in CRP from baseline to 1 year were −33% in the lifestyle group, −7% in the metformin group, and +5% in the placebo group. In women, the changes in CRP from baseline to follow-up were −29% in the lifestyle group, −14% in the metformin group, and 0% in the placebo group. In the lifestyle group, weight loss rather than increased physical activity accounted for most of the changes in CRP. This reduction in CRP occurred despite only a 7% decline in weight achieved at 6 months. This was the first long-term large trial to show that lifestyle intervention (reducing caloric intake by 500 calories/day and exercising for 150 minutes/week) results in a significant (58%) decrease in the incidence of diabetes and a significant reduction in CRP levels.[38]

Gastric surgery, a known strategy for weight loss in morbidly obese individuals, has also been shown to decrease CRP levels. The three studies we have reviewed on gastric surgery effects on CRP by Kopp and colleagues, Laimer and colleagues, and Hanusch-Enserer and colleagues, which were done mostly in women, observed large mean body weight changes of approximately 31, 44, and 44 kg, respectively. Laimer and colleagues' subjects had a BMI of 42 kg/m^2 at baseline. Kopp and colleagues' subjects had baseline BMI of 49 ± 7 kg/m^2, and Hanusch-Enserer and colleagues' subjects' baseline BMI was 50 ± 10 kg/m^2. These baseline BMIs are much higher than those of the subjects in the diet studies, and accordingly, CRP levels decreased more dramatically. CRP levels in subjects decreased by 71% in Kopp and colleagues' study (from 8.6 to 2.5 mg/L), by 70% in subjects in Laimer and colleagues' study (from 13.3 to 4.0 mg/L), and by 29% in Hanusch-Enserer and colleagues' study (from 12 ± 8 to 8.5 ± 6.9 mg/L).

A recent meta-analysis of 33 different weight loss studies (lifestyle and surgical interventions) demonstrated that for each 1 kg of weight loss, the mean change in CRP level was −0.13 mg/L (weighted Pearson correlation, $r = 0.85$). The weighted correlation for weight and change in CRP level with lifestyle interventions alone was 0.30 (slope, 0.06).[39]

In summary, weight loss achieved through gastric surgery or diet programs results in a reduction of CRP levels. The magnitude of change in CRP seems to depend on the baseline characteristics of the subjects. Those who have a higher baseline BMI, and thus higher baseline CRP levels, have greater decreases in CRP. The individual nutrients/factors that account for this reduction in CRP have, however, not been identified.

Dietary Fatty Acids and C-Reactive Protein

Intervention trials with *trans* fatty acids have been somewhat conflicting. CRP levels increased with *trans* fatty acid substitution in a high-fat diet (39% fat) in healthy subjects, whereas a 6% substitution of *trans* fatty acids in a standard-fat diet (30% fat) showed no effects on CRP in moderately hypercholesterolemic subjects, while TNF-α and IL-6 levels increased. Because a high-fat diet (59% fat) has also been shown to promote inflammation in healthy patients and patients with type 2 diabetes, the level of dietary fat may influence the proinflammatory actions of saturated or *trans* fatty acids, which, in turn, may exert differential effects on acute-phase proteins and inflammatory cytokines.[36,37]

Monounsaturated Fatty Acids

The Lyon Diet Heart Study[39a] demonstrated the cardioprotective effects of a Mediterranean diet on composite measures of coronary recurrence rates after a first MI, but it did not measure biomarkers of inflammation in these subjects. While the authors ascribe part of the benefit to α-linolenic acid (ALA), the role of the individual dietary factors (oleic acid, ALA, or antioxidants) in the Mediterranean diet in modulating inflammation is not yet defined.[36,37] Esposito and colleagues[39b] reported the anti-inflammatory effects of a Mediterranean-style diet in patients with the metabolic syndrome and without CVD who randomly received instructions to follow either a control diet or the Mediterranean-style diet. Though the macronutrient compositions of the two diets were similar (carbohydrates 50%–60%, proteins 15%–20%, total fat <30%), the patients consuming the Mediterranean-style diet had higher intakes of fruits, vegetables, nuts, whole grains, and olive oil in comparison with the control group. These patients showed a concomitant decrease in serum concentrations of hsCRP and cytokines (IL-6, IL-7, and IL-18; $P < 0.05$) and decreased insulin resistance compared with the control group. However, Michalsen and colleagues[39c] reported null effects with a Mediterranean diet in patients with medically treated CAD on biomarkers of inflammation. Thus, a Mediterranean-style diet, high in oleic acid or monounsaturated fatty acid content, fiber, and antioxidants, may reduce inflammation and corresponding coronary events in middle-aged adults; however, its effects in patients with heart disease need further investigation.

Polyunsaturated Fatty Acids

The relationship between dietary n-3 polyunsaturated fatty acids (PUFAs) (ALA, eicosapentaenoic acid [EPA], and docosahexaenoic acid [DHA]) and inflammation has been relatively well studied. Epidemiologic studies indicate that there is an inverse association between dietary ALA and risk of MI.[36,37] Randomized trials have reported anti-inflammatory effects of ALA. With regard to n-3 PUFA and CRP, although some epidemiologic studies have shown an inverse correlation between dietary fish or fish oil (EPA and DHA) consumption and biomarkers of inflammation, most intervention trials have failed to demonstrate an anti-inflammatory effect.

Pharmacotherapy and C-Reactive Protein

Drugs that have been shown to result in decreased CRP levels include metformin, fibrates, thiazolidinediones (TZDs), statins, and rimonabant.

Metformin

Twenty nonobese women with polycystic ovarian syndrome were randomized to receive either metformin (500 mg twice daily for 3 months, then 1000 mg twice daily for 3 months) or ethinyl estradiol (35 μg)–cyproterone acetate (2 mg) oral contraceptive pills. During metformin treatment, serum CRP levels decreased significantly from 3.08 ± 0.7 mg/L to 1.52 ± 0.26 mg/L at 6 months in the whole study population ($P = 0.006$) and especially in obese subjects ($P < 0.001$).[40]

The Diabetes Prevention Program clinical trial studied the effect of an intensive lifestyle intervention or metformin on progression to diabetes relative to placebo in 3234 adults with impaired glucose tolerance followed for 3 to 5 years. The effects of these interventions on CRP and fibrinogen at 12 months were examined in this report. Metformin reduced CRP in men (−7%) and women (−14%) compared with placebo.[38]

Thiazolidinediones, Fibrates, and C-Reactive Protein

Previous clinical studies in patients with type 2 diabetes have shown that the peroxisome proliferator–activated receptor–γ (PPAR-γ) agonists or TZDs pioglitazone and rosiglitazone significantly reduced plasma CRP levels.[41–43] Within a week, TZDs have been shown to reduce plasma CRP levels by 30%, while the corresponding effect of statins was only 14%.[41–43] In addition, Satoh and colleagues demonstrated that pioglitazone treatment of patients with type 2 diabetes resulted in a significant reduction of CRP levels in both responders and nonresponders, classified according to the reduction in hemoglobin A1c levels.[43a] These findings provided initial evidence that the potential antiatherogenic effects of TZDs are independent of their antidiabetic actions. Furthermore, rosiglitazone treatment has been shown to reduce CRP levels in nondiabetic patients with CAD, in nondiabetic hypertensive patients, and in nondiabetic and diabetic obese patients.[41–43] Because adipocytes have been proposed to be the missing link between insulin resistance and CVD, the TZD-mediated decrease in CRP levels in obese subjects may have important implications for treatment strategies in this high-risk population.

PPAR-α agonists, such as fibrates, attenuate the expression of inflammatory proteins of the acute phase *in vivo,* including fibrinogen, CRP, and IL-6. Furthermore, Després and colleagues confirmed the efficacy of gemfibrozil (600 mg twice daily for 6 months) in the reduction of CRP levels (~32%), with no effect on IL-6 and TNF levels in abdominally obese patients with MetS.[45] In patients with hypercholesterolemia, fibrates decreased IL-6 and CD40L as well as MCP-1.[44–47] Furthermore, in a study of dyslipidemic obese patients (with features of metabolic syndrome), fibrates resulted in significant reductions of CRP.[44–47] Thus, in addition to their favorable effects on lipid profiles, evidence is mounting that benefits may also stem from the anti-inflammatory and antiatherosclerotic properties of the PPAR-α agonists. In patients with angiographically established atherosclerosis, fenofibrate treatment decreased the circulating levels of IL-6 and lowered the plasma levels of CRP and fibrinogen.[44–47] In addition, fenofibrate treatment significantly reduced plasma interferon and TNF levels in patients with type IIb hyperlipoproteinemia.[47] Similar effects were observed in hypertriglyceridemic patients after bezafibrate administration.[44–47] Fenofibrate treatment also led to a reduction in intercellular adhesion molecule–1 (ICAM-1), MCP-1, and α2-macroglobulin and plasminogen plasma levels in patients with hyperlipoproteinemia.[47]

In summary, PPAR-α agonists are as effective as other classes of lipid-lowering drugs (e.g., statins) in lowering CRP plasma levels *in vivo.* In patients with different forms of dyslipidemia and CAD, fibrates, especially fenofibrate, have been shown to decrease CRP levels. These changes are not correlated with changes in lipid or fibrinogen levels. None of these studies reported an association between the fibrate effects on triglyceride, HDL cholesterol (or LDL cholesterol) and the decrease in CRP levels.

Statins and C-Reactive Protein

Several studies have shown that statin therapy lowers CRP levels independent of its lipid-lowering effects.

In the Cholesterol and Recurrent Events (CARE) study, which tested the effect of pravastatin on patients with total cholesterol levels less than 6.2 mmol/L, it was shown that the greatest benefit was achieved in the group with the highest hsCRP (54% reduction in cardiovascular events compared with 25% in the lowest quartile for hsCRP).[47a] In the Air Force/Texas Coronary Atherosclerosis Prevention Study (AFCAPS/TexCAPS), a primary prevention trial, lovastatin therapy (20–40 mg daily) decreased CRP levels by 14% ($P < 0.001$),[47b] and this effect was independent of its lipid-lowering effects and resulted in a 37% reduction in incident major coronary events. If either the baseline LDL cholesterol or CRP was over the median, lovastatin decreased relative risk significantly; however, if both were below the median, then the effect failed to reach statistical significance. Thus, this study showed that in persons with LDL cholesterol below the median (149 mg/dL) and hsCRP levels above the median (1.6 mg/L), lovastatin conferred a benefit, but if both were below the median, there was no benefit from statin therapy. This further underscores the usefulness of measurement of CRP in deciding on drug therapy. We showed in the first prospective randomized, double-blind crossover study in patients with combined hyperlipidemia (LDL >130 mg/dL, triglycerides 200–600 mg/dL) that 6-week therapy with three commonly prescribed statins, simvastatin (20 mg/day), atorvastatin (10 mg/day), and pravastatin (40 mg/day), resulted in a significant reduction in hsCRP levels (Fig. 33-1).[47c] There were no significant differences in the magnitude of the reduction in hsCRP with the three statins, suggesting a class effect. In this study, we failed to show a significant correlation with regard to LDL cholesterol reduction and hsCRP reduction, in agreement with the CARE study, suggesting that the effects of statins might be pleiotropic.

In the Diabetes Atorvastatin Lipid Intervention (DALI) study the dose–response effect of atorvastatin (10 and 80 mg) for 30 weeks compared with placebo in patients with type 2 diabetes and dyslipidemia but without CAD was reported.[47d] While atorvastatin 80 mg/day resulted in a significant decrease in CRP levels (47% reduction), atorvastatin 10 mg/day had significant effects only in patients with baseline CRP levels greater than 3 mg/L. This reduction in CRP was independent of effects on lipid lowering or changes in IL-6 levels. Furthermore, the effect of atorvastatin 80 mg/day on CRP levels was more potent than that of atorvastatin 10 mg/day or placebo. These findings suggest a dose–response effect, which needs to be confirmed in future studies.

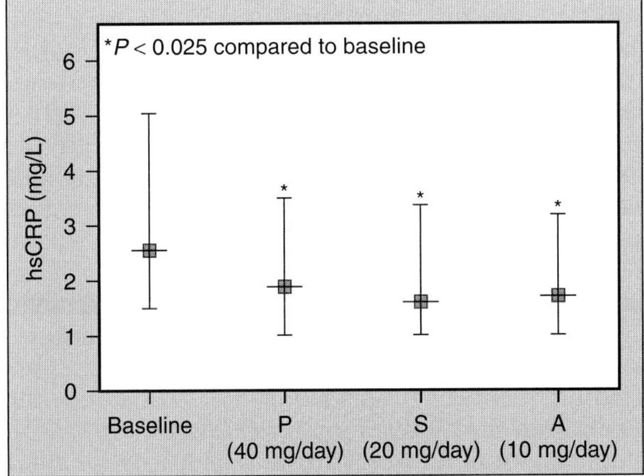

FIGURE 33-1 Effect of statin therapy on high sensitivity C-reactive protein (hs-CRP) levels. *(From Ref. 47c.)*
A, atorvastatin; P, pravastatin; S, simvastatin.

The Atorvastatin vs Simvastatin on Atherosclerosis Progression (ASAP) study was a 2-year randomized double-blind trial with 325 hypercholesterolemic patients treated with atorvastatin 80 mg/day or simvastatin 40 mg/day, respectively. Both statins reduced hsCRP levels, with atorvastatin being significantly better than simvastatin at the doses used. No correlations were observed between hsCRP levels and change in lipids; however, significant associations were seen in the change in intima–media thickness (IMT) progression and the extent of CRP reduction.[47e]

Another trial, Arterial Biology for the Investigation of the Treatment Effects of Reducing Cholesterol (ARBITER), was a randomized clinical trial of 161 patients at intermediate risk for CAD who were administered either pravastatin (40 mg/day) or atorvastatin (80 mg/day). It also reported that long-term treatment with atorvastatin resulted in significant lowering of hsCRP compared with pravastatin (12 months, $P < 0.005$) and greater benefit on IMT progression.[47f]

The A to Z trial compared initiation of an intensive statin regimen (40 mg/day of simvastatin for 1 month followed by 80 mg/day thereafter) with delayed initiation (placebo for 4 months followed by 20 mg/day simvastatin) in patients with high-risk ACS.[47g] During follow-up for at least 6 months and up to 24 months, the study showed a favorable trend but failed to demonstrate a significant reduction in the prespecified primary composite endpoint of cardiovascular death, nonfatal MI, readmission for ACS, and stroke ($P = 0.14$). A recent reanalysis of the trial showed that patients with hsCRP levels greater than 3 mg/L at 30 days and at 4 months after ACS had significantly higher 2-year mortality rates than those with hsCRP levels of 1 to 3 mg/L or hsCRP levels less than 1 mg/L ($P < 0.0001$).[34] Furthermore, patients allocated to early intensive statin therapy were more likely to achieve hsCRP levels of less than 1 mg/L at 30 days ($P = 0.028$) and 4 months ($P < 0.0001$). Thus, this study showed that achieved levels of hsCRP at 30 days and 4 months after ACS are independently associated with long-term survival and that patients on aggressive statin therapy are more likely to achieve lower levels of hsCRP. Recently, several studies conducted in patients with ACS indicated the utility of early intensive therapy with statins in providing benefits in the setting of ACS.[48]

The Myocardial Ischemia Reduction with Aggressive Cholesterol Lowering (MIRACL) trial showed that in patients with unstable angina or Q-wave MI, compared with placebo, atorvastatin (80 mg/day for 16 weeks) initiated 24 to 96 hours after hospital admission significantly reduced the risk of the primary combined endpoint. Also, there was a significantly greater reduction in CRP levels with atorvastatin, −83% versus −74%, ($P < 0.0001$) but not IL-6.[48a] Reductions in CRP and serum amyloid A were observed in patients with unstable angina and non–Q-wave MI, with initial LDL cholesterol less than 125 mg/dL or greater than or equal to 125 mg/dL, indicating an anti-inflammatory effect independent of LDL cholesterol or troponin -I levels.

The PROVE IT trial compared initiation of a standard statin regimen (40 mg/day of pravastatin) with an intensive regimen (80 mg/day of atorvastatin) in patients hospitalized with ACS.[48b] In patients with

ACS, compared with pravastatin (40 mg/day), atorvastatin (80 mg/day) resulted in a 16% reduction in the primary endpoint ($P < 0.0005$). Also, in these patients, there was a greater reduction in CRP levels with atorvastatin compared with pravastatin (levels on treatment: 1.3 and 2.1 mg/L, respectively). When patients were divided into categories based on final hsCRP and LDL cholesterol levels achieved, those with hsCRP levels reduced to less than 2 mg/L had fewer recurrent events, regardless of the LDL cholesterol level achieved by statin therapy. Also, the patients at the highest risk were those in whom both LDL cholesterol and hsCRP remained elevated despite statin therapy. In fact, the greatest benefit was achieved in those patients that achieved concomitant reductions in both CRP (<2 mg/L) and LDL cholesterol (<70 mg/dL) levels.[48c]

In the REVERSAL trial, in patients with CAD, atorvastatin (80 mg/day) resulted in a significant reduction in the progression of coronary atherosclerosis by intravascular ultrasound compared with pravastatin (40 mg/day). The investigators ascribed the benefit to the reductions in both atherogenic lipoproteins and CRP levels.[48d] Irrespective of statin use, the greatest benefit with regard to atheroma volume was in patients who achieved a CRP and LDL cholesterol level below the median. These observations underscore the importance of both lipid lowering and inflammation reduction by statins in the treatment of atherosclerosis.

Thus, recent trials have demonstrated that early intensive therapy with statins resulted in improved clinical outcomes as compared with delayed statin therapy. The benefit of intensive therapy is likely related to the dual effect of LDL and CRP reduction. Findings from the recent studies suggest that to maximize the benefit of statin therapy, physicians may need to monitor hsCRP levels in addition to LDL cholesterol levels for secondary prevention of CAD.

In addition, the cholesterol absorption inhibitor ezetimibe in conjunction with simvastatin has been shown to significantly reduce median hsCRP levels compared with simvastatin alone (−34.8% vs. −18.2%, $P < 0.01$). While ezetimibe alone failed to significantly reduce hsCRP levels, incremental reductions were observed at each simvastatin dose level with combination therapy. Thus, while ezetimibe monotherapy does not lower CRP, when ezetimibe is added to statins there is a greater reduction in CRP levels. Thus, coadministration of ezetimibe with simvastatin offers an attractive strategy for combined benefits on the lipid profile and inflammation.

Rimonabant and C-Reactive Protein

The newly discovered endocannabinoid system contributes to the physiologic regulation of energy balance, food intake, and lipid and glucose metabolism through both central and peripheral effects. This system consists of endogenous ligands and two types of G-protein–coupled receptors: cannabinoid receptor type 1 (CB_1), which is located in the brain and in a variety of peripheral tissues (e.g., adipose tissue, the gastro intestinol tract, heart, lung, liver) and CB_2, which is in the immune system. CB_1 receptor inhibition holds promise as a possible treatment target for high-risk overweight or obese subjects. The pharmacologic blockade of CB_1 receptors with the selective antagonist rimonabant [N-piperidineo-5-(4-chlorophenyl)-1-(2,4-dichlorophenyl)-4-methyl-3-pyrazole-carboxamide, also known as SR 141716] reduces food intake and induces weight loss in mice and rats.[49–51] These findings suggest a physiologic role for the hypothalamic CB_1 receptor in the control of appetite. Recent randomized double-blind placebo-controlled trials investigated the effect of rimonabant (a CB_1 receptor blocker) on different parameters in overweight/obese patients. The Rimonabant in Obesity (RIO)–Lipids study was a multicenter, double-blind placebo-controlled trial of 1036 overweight or obese patients with dyslipidemia (high triglycerides and/or high total cholesterol/HDL ratio) and a BMI of 27 to 40kg/m^2 who were randomized to receive, for 1 year, 20 mg/day or 5 mg/day rimonabant or placebo, along with a reduced-calorie diet. Patients in the high-dose rimonabant group lost an average of 20 lb, compared with only 5 lb in the placebo group ($P < 0.001$). The percentage of patients who lost more than 10% of their body weight was 44.3% ($P < 0.001$ vs. placebo), 16.3%, and 10.3% in the rimonabant 20 mg and 5 mg and placebo groups, respectively. The number of patients in the rimonabant 20 mg group classified as having metabolic syndrome was reduced from 52.9% at baseline to 25.8% at 1 year ($P < 0.0001$ vs. placebo). Rimonabant 20 mg was associated with significant reductions in waist circumference, triglycerides (9.1% decrease), and CRP (12% decrease) and an increase in HDL cholesterol (15% increase) (all $P < 0.01$ versus placebo).[51a] However, to date, this drug has not been approved by the Food and Drug Administration in the United States.

MYELOPEROXIDASE

Biochemistry and Biology

MPO is a member of the heme peroxidase family that is released from azurophilic granules in neutrophils and monocytes in response to inflammatory stimuli.[52–54] MPO catalyzes the reaction of hydrogen peroxide with chloride ions to produce the cytotoxic oxidant hypochlorous acid (HOCl). MPO is a potent NO scavenger, a catalytic sink for NO. In turn, these diffusible oxidants mediate lipid peroxidation and promote oxidant stress at sites of inflammation. Because MPO is a highly cationic protein, it can adhere to endothelial cells and leukocytes after its release with retention of its peroxidase activity.[52–54] Moreover, MPO binds to LDL and HDL under physiologically relevant conditions and may promote their oxidation while limiting the ability of antioxidants to scavenge the reactive oxygen and nitrogen species (Table 33-3).[52–54]

HOCl and the reactive nitrogen species modify apolB, the primary protein constituent of LDL, which results in a form that binds to scavenger receptors on macrophages and can be readily internalized, thereby promoting foam cell formation. MPO also catalyzes the nitration and chlorination of apoA-I, the primary protein constituent of HDL, thereby impairing its ability to mediate cholesterol efflux from macrophages and making HDL more susceptible to degradation.[52–54] Thus,

TABLE 33-3 Myeloperoxidase and Atherosclerosis
Potent NO scavenger
Promotes nitration and chlorination of proteins
Increases cholesterol uptake and promotes formation of dysfunctional HDL
Increases MPO-modified proteins in atherosclerotic lesions
Promotes leukocyte chemotaxis
Induces SMC apoptosis
Up-regulates MMP and tissue factor

HDL, high-density lipoprotein; MMP, Matrix metalloproteinase; MPO, myeloperoxidase; NO, nitric oxide; SMC, smooth muscle cell.

MPO has a major impact on the cholesterol content of the arterial wall: it increases cholesterol uptake by modifying LDL and promotes the formation of dysfunctional HDL. Evidence of MPO-modified lipoproteins has been found in human atherosclerotic lesions. The production of 3-chlorotyrosine in LDL is a specific marker of MPO-mediated oxidation of LDL via HOCl.[52–54] The level of 3-chlorotyrosine–modified LDL was six times higher in atherosclerotic tissue than in normal aortic intima and 30 times higher than in circulating LDL. Immunohistochemical staining for HOCl-modified LDL in atherosclerotic lesions was predominantly associated with monocytes/macrophages, SMCs, and endothelial cells, particularly in the arterial intima. Pronounced staining for HOCl-modified LDL was detected in human atheroma and advanced lesions, which colocalized with staining for MPO, but it was not detected in a lesion-prone area of normal aorta. The level of 3-chlorotyrosine–modified HDL in atherosclerotic lesions was eight times higher than in circulating HDL.[52–54] Also, immunohistochemical analysis showed that apoA-I colocalized with HOCl epitopes in atherosclerotic tissue. Together, these results show that MPO catalyzes LDL and HDL oxidation in human atherosclerotic lesions.

Thus, MPO is a potent catalytic sink for NO, it promotes leukocyte chemotaxis, the formation of atherogenic LDL and dysfunctional HDL, and SMC apoptosis, and it up-regulates proteases such as MMP and tissue factor.

Myeloperoxidase and Cardiovascular Risk

MPO levels were associated with CAD risk in a case–control study involving 158 patients with established CAD and 175 control subjects without angiographically significant CAD. MPO levels in leukocytes and blood were significantly higher in the CAD patients than in control subjects (both $P < 0.001$). The risk of CAD increased with increasing quartile of leukocyte MPO ($P < 0.05$) and blood MPO ($P < 0.001$). Patients in the highest quartile of blood MPO were at approximately 20 times higher risk of CAD than those in the lowest quartile, even after adjustment for traditional cardiovascular risk factors, Framingham Risk Score, and leukocyte count ($P < 0.001$).[52–54]

Further evidence that MPO is a cardiovascular risk factor was obtained by measuring MPO-modified lipoproteins in serum. Nitrotyrosine and chlorotyrosine levels in apoB and apoA-I were measured in 44 healthy volunteers and 45 consecutive patients with CVD who received preventive cardiology care. The patients had 2.2 times higher nitrotyrosine levels in apoB ($P = 0.001$) and 1.44 times higher nitrotyrosine levels in apoA-I ($P = 0.005$) than did the healthy controls. Moreover, the patients with CVD had 2.7 times higher chlorotyrosine levels in apoA-I ($P < 0.001$) and also showed a trend for having higher chlorotyrosine levels in apoB ($P = 0.24$).[52–54] Similarly, in a case–control study of 100 CAD patients and 108 controls, protein-bound nitrotyrosine levels were nearly 2 times higher in the CAD patients than in the healthy controls (9.1 vs. 5.2 μmol/mol; $P < 0.001$). Moreover, subjects in the highest nitrotyrosine quartile were at 4.4 times higher risk of CAD as compared with those in the lowest quartile after adjusting for Framingham Risk Score and CRP level (95% confidence interval [CI], 1.8 to 10.6; $P < 0.001$).[52–54] Thus, these studies suggest that plasma levels of MPO and MPO-catalyzed products are independent predictors of CAD risk.

Plasma MPO was also able to predict short-term cardiovascular risk in a study of 604 consecutive patients presenting to an emergency department with chest pain.[52–54] MPO levels correlated weakly with peak troponin T levels ($r = 0.21$, $P < 0.001$) and CRP levels ($r = 0.10$, $P = 0.01$). Patients in the highest quartile of MPO had 3.9 times higher risk (95% CI, 2.2 to 6.8; $P < 0.01$) than did those in the lowest quartile. The risk of major cardiovascular events at 30 days and 6 months also increased linearly with increasing quartile of MPO, even among those who were persistently negative for troponin T ($P < 0.001$ for trend). At both time points, the risk of cardiovascular events in the highest quartile was 4.7 times higher than in the lowest quartile (95% CI, 2.8 to 7.7; $P < 0.01$). In comparison, CRP was less sensitive at predicting outcome, but did not discriminate risk in troponin T–negative patients. On multivariate analysis that included adjustment for CRP and clinical history, MPO remained an independent risk factor of adverse outcomes. Similarly, in a study of 1090 patients with ACS, MPO independently predicted 6-month cardiovascular risk and was particularly effective in identifying at-risk patients with low troponin T levels.[52–55] These data show that MPO is predictive of short-term cardiovascular risk in patients presenting with chest pain or ACS, even among those without evidence by troponin T of myocardial necrosis. In a hospital-based population of 298 subjects, a strong inverse relation between brachial artery flow–mediated dilation and increasing quartile of serum MPO level was observed (11.0% ± 6.0%, 9.4% ± 5.3%, 8.6% ± 5.8%, and 6.4% ± 4.5% for quartiles 1 through 4, respectively; $P < 0.001$ for trend). Using the median as a cutpoint to define endothelial dysfunction, increasing quartile of MPO predicted endothelial dysfunction after adjustment for classic CVD risk factors, CRP levels, prevalence of cardiovascular disease, and ongoing treatment with cardiovascular medications (adds ratio, 6.4; 95% CI, 2.6 to 16; $P = 0.001$ for highest versus lowest quartile).

However, the caveat for MPO measurement in cardiovascular risk is that it is an enzyme and thus it is preferable to measure enzymatic activity rather than MPO mass, and gas chromatrography/mass spectrometry

(GC/MS) is the method of choice for the measurement of signatures of MPO activity such as dityrosine, chlorotyrosine, and nitrotyrosine.

Modulation of Myeloperoxidase

Regular endurance exercise, which is known to be cardioprotective, could beneficially affect MPO. Thirty-two subjects (age 31–68 years, 56% males) with elevated cardiovascular risk, including 10 patients with CAD, volunteered for supervised 12-week endurance training (196 ± 15 min/week). Their fitness, evaluated by 2-km test runs, improved significantly after training (17.3 ± 0.8 vs. 15.7 ± 0.9 minutes, $P < 0.001$). ADMA (pre: 0.94 ± 0.03 vs. post: 0.75 ± 0.04 μM/L) and MPO (pre: 296.8 ± 22.2 vs. post: 185.7 ± 19.5 ng/mL) serum levels decreased significantly by 17.6 ± 4.6% and 28.5 ± 7.5%, respectively, after training (both $p < 0.001$). Their down-regulation was inversely correlated (ADMA: $r = -0.609$, $P < 0.001$; MPO: $r = -0.437$, $P = 0.014$) with the up-regulation of plasma cGMP levels (pre: 1.6 ± 0.12 vs. post: 2.21 ± 0.2 μM/mL, $P = 0.001$) reflecting NO production. These changes may result in numerous antiatherosclerotic effects such as the improvement of NO bioavailability, the reduction of oxidative stress, and lipid peroxidation.

Statin therapy results in decreased MPO gene expression in macrophages. Shishebor and colleagues examined the effect of a 12-week administration of atorvastatin therapy on MPO in patients with hypercholesterolemia and no known CAD.[52–54] Statin therapy elicited significant reductions in plasma protein content of the MPO specific product chlorotyrosine, the product of NO-derived oxidants nitrotyrosine and the oxidative cross-link dityrosine (reductions in mean levels of 30%, 25% and 32%, respectively; $P < 0.001$ each). Statin-induced reductions in these species were again similar in magnitude to, but independent of, reductions in total cholesterol and apoB-100 (25% and 29%, respectively; $P < 0.001$ each). However, this was not a placebo-controlled study. Recently, atorvastatin (10 mg/day) also significantly decreased MPO levels in patients with ACS. These findings suggest that MPO and NO–dependent oxidation reactions may have effects on oxidant stress in atherosclerosis, and that measurement of oxidant markers may have utility in monitoring therapeutic regimens.

LIPOPROTEIN-ASSOCIATED PHOSPHOLIPASE A_2

Biochemistry and Biology

Lp-PLA_2, also known as platelet-activating factor acetylhydrolase (PAF-AH), was initially identified as the enzyme responsible for hydrolyzing and inactivating the proinflammatory phospholipid PAF.[56–58] Lp-PLA_2 in plasma is predominantly bound to LDL, with the remaining amount bound to HDL and very-low-density lipoprotein (VLDL). It preferentially cleaves oxidized phospholipids by hydrolyzing the *sn*-2 fatty acid on oxidized LDL, resulting in the generation of lysophosphatidylcholine and oxidized FFAs, both of which are proatherogenic and contribute to the cytotoxic effects of oxidized LDL on macrophages. Lp-PLA_2 is expressed in macrophage-rich regions of early to advanced atherosclerotic lesions. Macrophages and T cells appear to be the primary sources of Lp-PLA_2 in these lesions. Stafforini and colleagues have also demonstrated that increased Lp-PLA_2 activity contributes to increased F_2-isoprostanes.[58a]

However, the high specificity of Lp-PLA_2 to polar phospholipids raises the question of whether hydrolysis of PAF-like phospholipids in oxidized LDL by Lp-PLA_2 actually attenuates their proinflammatory properties.

Lipoprotein-Associated Phospholipase A_2 and Cardiovascular Risk

Several studies have shown that Lp-PLA_2 is generally associated with LDL cholesterol and apoB but not with hsCRP or other markers. After adjusting for other risk factors, these studies provide some evidence that Lp-PLA_2 may be an independent CAD risk factor.

Lp-PLA_2 activity in blood was determined by an enzymatic assay in 3148 patients who were hospitalized for coronary angiography.[56–58] Of these, 2524 patients had angiographically confirmed CAD and the remaining 694 subjects served as controls. Lp-PLA_2 activity showed the strongest correlations with LDL cholesterol ($r = 0.517$, $P < 0.001$) and apoB ($r = 0.644$, $P < 0.001$) and weaker but significant correlations with other lipid parameters, white blood cells, and serum amyloid A (all $P < 0.001$). Lp-PLA_2 activity did not correlate with hsCRP ($r = 0.001$, $P = 0.95$), nor did it predict CAD risk in the entire study cohort. However, separate analyses were conducted for the 1630 patients who were not taking lipid-lowering therapy. In this subgroup, the highest quartile of Lp-PLA_2 activity was associated with a 2.21-fold greater risk of CAD (95% CI, 1.65 to 2.96; $P < 0.001$) than the lowest quartile. Lp-PLA_2 remained an independent risk factor after adjusting for other factors (1.85 times higher CAD risk; 95% CI, 1.23 to 2.78; $P = 0.003$). Thus, Lp-PLA_2 was independently associated with CAD risk in patients not taking lipid-lowering drugs in this study.

In the West of Scotland Coronary Prevention Study (WOSCOPS), 580 men with a coronary event during follow-up were each matched for age and smoking status with two control subjects who had not had a coronary event.[58b] Lp-PLA_2 levels were weakly correlated with LDL cholesterol ($r = 0.21$, $P < 0.001$) and fibrinogen ($r = 0.086$, $P < 0.01$) in this cohort. Lp-PLA_2 levels were significantly associated with increased risk of the composite endpoint of nonfatal MI, cardiac death, or first revascularization, with each 0.52-mg/L increase in Lp-PLA_2 increasing risk by 20% ($P < 0.001$). This risk estimate was unaffected by adjustment for CRP, white cell count, or fibrinogen ($P = 0.002$) or for age, systolic blood pressure, LDL cholesterol, or HDL cholesterol ($P = 0.005$). When grouped according to quintiles of Lp-PLA_2, patients in the highest quintile had a 1.8-fold higher cardiovascular risk than did those in the lowest quintile after adjustment for the other factors.

In the Atherosclerosis Risk in Communities (ARIC) study, in 608 patients with a CAD event (nonfatal MI, CAD death, or revascularization) and 740 controls, Lp-PLA_2 correlated with LDL cholesterol ($r = 0.36$,

$P < 0.0001$) and inversely with HDL cholesterol ($r = -0.33$, $P < 0.0001$) but not with hsCRP, BMI, or blood pressure.[58c] After adjusting for age, sex, and race, patients in the highest tertile of Lp-PLA$_2$ had a 1.8-fold greater risk of CAD (95% CI, 1.33 to 2.38) than did those in the lowest tertile. However, when additional adjustments were made for smoking status, systolic blood pressure, LDL cholesterol, HDL cholesterol, diabetes, and hsCRP, Lp-PLA$_2$ no longer significantly predicted CAD risk. When the analysis focused solely on individuals with LDL cholesterol levels less than 130 mg/dL, both Lp-PLA$_2$ and hsCRP independently predicted CAD risk. The highest tertile of Lp-PLA$_2$ was associated with a 2.08-fold higher risk (95% CI, 1.20 to 3.62), whereas hsCRP levels greater than 3 mg/L were associated with a 1.76-fold higher risk (95% CI, 1.02 to 3.03). Notably, the increased risk associated with these markers was seen only in patients who had both high Lp-PLA$_2$ and high hsCRP. This study suggests that measurement of Lp-PLA$_2$ and hsCRP may be additive for identifying patients with low LDL cholesterol who are at high CAD risk.

In addition to its association with CAD, Lp-PLA$_2$ activity has been shown to be an independent predictor of ischemic stroke in the general population in prospective population-based studies.[58d,58e] Subjects in the highest quartile had an approximately doubled risk of a future ischemic stroke compared with those in the lowest quartile. Because total cholesterol is not associated with risk of stroke, the association between Lp-PLA$_2$ activity and stroke suggests that Lp-PLA$_2$, although carried by LDL, may convey a different risk. Another study showed that Lp-PLA$_2$ concentrations were associated with the presence of stable CAD, independently of other biochemical markers. This suggests that Lp-PLA$_2$ may be a novel independent risk marker for CAD.

It should be noted that different Lp-PLA$_2$ assays were used in these studies, and enzyme mass or activity were measured. The availability of a commercial ELISA may help to improve comparisons in future studies. There is also a relatively low correlation ($r = 0.36$) between Lp-PLA$_2$ mass and activity in recent studies, which has raised the question as to what is being measured in the different assays. Also, 20% to 30% of LpPLA$_2$ resides in HDL and is thus anti-inflammatory in nature. Furthermore, as detailed by Zalewski and colleagues, Lp-PLA$_2$ is not a useful biomarker in ACS.[58] Controversy also exists with regard to the proinflammatory effects of Lp-PLA$_2$ because it hydrolyzes PL in oxidized LDL and PAF.

Modulation of Lipoprotein-Associated Phospholipase A$_2$

The Pravastatin Inflammation/CRP Evaluation (PRINCE) evaluated the effect of pravastatin 40 mg daily versus placebo on Lp-PLA$_2$ levels among 481 subjects free of CVD who were randomized to pravastatin ($n = 246$) or placebo ($n = 235$). After 12 weeks, Lp-PLA$_2$ levels decreased by 22.1% among participants treated with pravastatin and by 7.8% among those randomized to placebo ($P < 0.001$). In this study, Lp-PLA$_2$ levels were significantly reduced at 12 weeks by pravastatin, an effect that was significantly related to LDL cholesterol reduction accounting for about 6% of the variability in this response. Moreover, the pravastatin-induced reduction in Lp-PLA$_2$ was no longer significant after taking LDL cholesterol into account.[58f]

In the PROVE IT trial, plasma levels of Lp-PLA$_2$ activity were measured at baseline ($n = 3648$) and 30 days ($n = 3265$) in patients randomized to atorvastatin 80 mg/day or pravastatin 40 mg/day after ACS. The primary endpoint was death, MI, unstable angina, revascularization, or stroke (mean follow-up 24 months). Overall, mean levels of Lp-PLA$_2$ were lower at 30 days of follow-up than at baseline (35.7 vs. 40.9 nmol/min/mL $P < 0.001$). In particular, treatment with atorvastatin 80 mg/day was associated with a 20% reduction in Lp-PLA$_2$ activity ($P < 0.001$), whereas Lp-PLA$_2$ rose 3.6% with pravastatin 40 mg/day ($P < 0.001$). Patients with 30-day Lp-PLA$_2$ activity in the highest quintile were at significantly increased risk of recurrent cardiovascular events compared with those in the lowest quintile (26.4% vs. 17.6%; P trend $= 0.002$). After adjustment for cardiac risk factors, treatments, achieved LDL, and CRP, Lp-PLA$_2$ activity in the highest quintile remained independently associated with a higher risk of recurrent cardiovascular events (adjusted hazard ratio, 1.33; 95% CI 1.01 to 1.74). At 30 days after ACS, Lp-PLA$_2$ activity was significantly lowered with high-dose statin therapy and was associated with an increased risk of cardiovascular events independent of CRP and LDL cholesterol levels.[58g]

CONCLUSIONS

Epidemiologic studies provide convincing evidence that biomarkers of inflammation are predictive of increased cardiovascular risk in otherwise apparently healthy individuals. Future and ongoing prospective studies will decide whether therapeutic strategies that specifically reduce an inflammation biomarker produce the desired risk reduction for cardiovascular events and death. Until then, LDL cholesterol remains the primary focus of treatment as in the current NCEP ATP III guidelines. The additional measurement of biomarkers of inflammation may be most prudent in patients at intermediate cardiovascular risk who would benefit from a more intensive intervention. Recently, Grundy and colleagues suggested that a reasonable therapeutic goal in moderately high risk primary prevention is LDL cholesterol levels less than 100 mg/dL. CRP level greater than 3 mg/L may be useful in determining intensity of therapy in intermediate-risk patients.

Because CRP portends a worse morbidity and mortality after ACS and targeting CRP in a coronary ligation model prevented an increase in infarct size, this could provide a fertile area of investigation for strategies directed at reducing CRP. Finally, while we focused on the three best studied biomarkers (hsCRP, MPO, and Lp-PLA$_2$), one cannot rule out the importance in the future of modulating IL-6, IL-18, MMPs, sCD40L, and so on.[59]

REFERENCES

1. Libby P: Inflammation in atherosclerosis. *Nature* 2002;420(6917):868–874.
2. Myers GL, Rifai N, Tracy RP, et al: CDC/AHA Workshop on Markers of Inflammation and Cardiovascular Disease: Application to Clinical and Public Health Practice: report from the laboratory science discussion group. *Circulation* 2004;110(25):e545–e549.

3. Thompson D, Pepys MB, Wood SP: The physiological structure of human C-reactive protein and its complex with phosphocholine. *Structure* 1999;7(2):169–177.
4. Venugopal SK, Devaraj S, Jialal I: Effect of C-reactive protein on vascular cells: evidence for a proinflammatory, proatherogenic role. *Curr Opin Nephrol Hypertens* 2005;14(1):33–37.
5. Verma S, Devaraj S, Jialal I: Is C-reactive protein an innocent bystander or proatherogenic culprit? C-reactive protein promotes atherothrombosis. *Circulation* 2006;113(17):2135–2150.
6. Bassuk SS, Rifai N, Ridker PM: High-sensitivity C-reactive protein: clinical importance. *Curr Probl Cardiol* 2004;29(8):439–493.
7. Verma S, Szmitko PE, Ridker PM: C-reactive protein comes of age. *Nat Clin Pract Cardiovasc Med* 2005;2(1):29–36.
8. Ridker PM, Buring JE, Shih J, et al: Prospective study of C-reactive protein and the risk of future cardiovascular events among apparently healthy women. *Circulation* 1998;98(8):731–733.
9. Pearson TA, Mensah GA, Alexander RW, et al: Markers of inflammation and cardiovascular disease: application to clinical and public health practice: a statement for healthcare professionals from the Centers for Disease Control and Prevention and the American Heart Association. *Circulation* 2003;107(3):499–511.
10. Venugopal SK, Devaraj S, Yuhanna I, et al: Demonstration that C-reactive protein decreases eNOS expression and bioactivity in human aortic endothelial cells. *Circulation* 2002;106(12):1439–1441.
11. Devaraj S, Davis B, Simon SI, Jialal I: CRP promotes monocyte-endothelial cell adhesion via Fcgamma receptors in human aortic endothelial cells under static and shear flow conditions. *Am J Physiol Heart Circ Physiol* 2006;291(3):H1170–H1176.
12. Verma S, Wang CH, Li SH, et al: A self-fulfilling prophecy: C-reactive protein attenuates nitric oxide production and inhibits angiogenesis. *Circulation* 2002;106(8):913–919.
13. Qamirani E, Ren Y, Kuo L, Hein TW: C-reactive protein inhibits endothelium-dependent NO-mediated dilation in coronary arterioles by activating p38 kinase and NAD(P)H oxidase. *Arterioscler Thromb Vasc Biol* 2005;25(5):995–1001.
14. Devaraj S, Du Clos TW, Jialal I: Binding and internalization of C-reactive protein by Fcgamma receptors on human aortic endothelial cells mediates biological effects. *Arterioscler Thromb Vasc Biol* 2005;25(7):1359–1363.
15. Mineo C, Gormley AK, Yuhanna IS, et al: FcgammaRIIB mediates C-reactive protein inhibition of endothelial NO synthase. *Circ Res* 2005;97(11):1124–1131.
15a. Singh V, Devaraj S, Vasquez-Vivar J, Jialal I: C-reactive protein decreases endothelial nitric oxide synthase activity via uncoupling. *J Mol Cell Cardiol* 2007; 43: 780–791.
16. Grad E, Golomb M, Mor Yosef I, et al: Transgenic expression of human C-reactive protein suppresses endothelial nitric oxide synthase expression and bioactivity following vascular injury. *Am J Physiol Heart Circ Physiol* 2007;293:H489–H495 (Epub ahead of print).
17. Schwartz R, Osborne-Lawrence S, Hahner L, et al: C-reactive protein downregulates endothelial NO synthase and attenuates reendothelialization *in vivo* in mice. *Circ Res* 2007;100(10):1452–1459.
18. Devaraj S, Kumaresan PR, Jialal I: Effect of C-reactive protein on chemokine expression in human aortic endothelial cells. *J Mol Cell Cardiol* 2004;36(3):405–410.
19. Lin R, Liu J, Gan W, Yang G: C-reactive protein-induced expression of CD40-CD40L and the effect of lovastatin and fenofibrate on it in human vascular endothelial cells. *Biol Pharm Bull* 2004;27(10):1537–1543.
20. Verma S, Kuliszewski MA, Li SH, et al: C-reactive protein attenuates endothelial progenitor cell survival, differentiation, and function: further evidence of a mechanistic link between C-reactive protein and cardiovascular disease. *Circulation* 2004;109(17):2058–2067.
21. Danenberg HD, Szalai AJ, Swaminathan RV, et al: Increased thrombosis after arterial injury in human C-reactive protein-transgenic mice. *Circulation* 2003;108(5):512–515.
22. Wang CH, Li SH, Weisel RD, et al: C-reactive protein upregulates angiotensin type 1 receptors in vascular smooth muscle. *Circulation* 2003;107(13):1783–1790.
23. Woollard KJ, Fisch C, Newby R, Griffiths HR: C-reactive protein mediates CD11b expression in monocytes through the non-receptor tyrosine kinase, Syk, and calcium mobilization but not through cytosolic peroxides. *Inflamm Res* 2005;54(12):485–492.
24. Chang MK, Binder CJ, Torzewski M, Witztum JL: C-reactive protein binds to both oxidized LDL and apoptotic cells through recognition of a common ligand: phosphorylcholine of oxidized phospholipids. *Proc Natl Acad Sci USA* 2002;99(20):13043–13048.
25. Lim MY, Wang H, Kapoun AM, et al: p38 Inhibition attenuates the pro-inflammatory response to C-reactive protein by human peripheral blood mononuclear cells. *J Mol Cell Cardiol* 2004;37(6):1111–1114.
26. Han KH, Hong KH, Park JH, et al: C-reactive protein promotes monocyte chemoattractant protein-1–mediated chemotaxis through upregulating CC chemokine receptor 2 expression in human monocytes. *Circulation* 2004;109(21):2566–2571.
27. Singh U, Devaraj S, Dasu MR, et al: C-reactive protein decreases interleukin-10 secretion in activated human monocyte-derived macrophages via inhibition of cyclic AMP production. *Arterioscler Thromb Vasc Biol* 2006;26(11):2469–2475.
28. Montero I, Orbe J, Varo N, et al: C-reactive protein induces matrix metalloproteinase-1 and -10 in human endothelial cells: implications for clinical and subclinical atherosclerosis. *J Am Coll Cardiol* 2006;47(7):1369–1378.
29. Doronzo G, Russo I, Mattiello L, et al: C-reactive protein increases matrix metalloproteinase-2 expression and activity in cultured human vascular smooth muscle cells. *J Lab Clin Med* 2005;146(5):287–298.
30. Dasu MR, Devaraj S, Du Clos TW, Jialal I: The biological effects of CRP are not attributable to endotoxin contamination: evidence from TLR4 knockdown human aortic endothelial cells. *J Lipid Res* 2007;48(3):509–512.
31. Sattler KJ, Woodrum JE, Galili O, et al: Concurrent treatment with renin-angiotensin system blockers and acetylsalicylic acid reduces nuclear factor kappaB activation and C-reactive protein expression in human carotid artery plaques. *Stroke* 2005;36(1):14–20.
32. Venugopal SK, Devaraj S, Jialal I: Macrophage conditioned medium induces the expression of C-reactive protein in human aortic endothelial cells: potential for paracrine/autocrine effects. *Am J Pathol* 2005;166(4):1265–1271.
33. Paul A, Ko KW, Li L, et al: C-reactive protein accelerates the progression of atherosclerosis in apolipoprotein E-deficient mice. *Circulation* 2004;109(5):647–655.
33a. Bisoendial RJ, Kastelein JJ, Levels JH, et al. Activation of inflammation and coagulation after infusion of C-reactive protein in humans. *Circ Res* 2005;96:714–716.
34. Devaraj S, Rogers J, Jialal I: Statins and biomarkers of inflammation. *Curr Atheroscler Rep* 2007;9(1):33–41.
35. Pepys MB, Hirschfield GM, Tennent GA, et al: Targeting C-reactive protein for the treatment of cardiovascular disease. *Nature* 2006;440(7088):1217–1221.
36. Devaraj S, Kasim-Karakas S, Jialal I: The effect of weight loss and dietary fatty acids on inflammation. *Curr Atheroscler Rep* 2006;8(6):477–486.
37. Basu A, Devaraj S, Jialal I: Dietary factors that promote or retard inflammation. *Arterioscler Thromb Vasc Biol* 2006;26(5):995–1001.
37a. Jenkins DJ, Kendall CW, Marchie A, et al: Effects of a dietary portfolio of cholesterol-lowering foods vs lovastatin on serum lipids and C-reactive protein. *JAMA* 2003;290:502–510.
37b. Dansinger ML, Gleason JA, Griffith JL, et al: Comparison of the Atkins, Ornish, Weight Watchers, and Zone diets for weight loss and heart disease risk reduction: A randomized trial. *JAMA* 2005;293:43–53.
38. Haffner S, Temprosa M, Crandall J, et al: Diabetes Prevention Program Research Group. Intensive lifestyle intervention or metformin on inflammation and coagulation in participants with impaired glucose tolerance. *Diabetes* 2005;54(5):1566–1572.
38a. Kopp HP, Kopp CW, Festa A, et al: Impact of weight loss on inflammatory proteins and their association with the insulin resistance syndrome in morbidly obese patients. *Arterioscler Thromb Vasc Biol* 2003;23:1042–1047.
38b. Laimer M, Ebenbichler CF, Kaser S, et al: Markers of chronic inflammation and obesity: A prospective study on the reversibility of this association in middle-aged women undergoing weight loss by surgical intervention. *Int J Obes Relat Metab Disord* 2002;26:659–662.
38c. Hanusch-Enserer U, Cauza E, Spak M, et al: Acute-phase response and immunological markers in morbid obese patients and patients following adjustable gastric banding. *Int J Obes Relat Metab Disord* 2003;27:355–361.

39. Selvin E, Paynter NP, Erlinger TP: The effect of weight loss on C-reactive protein: a systematic review. *Arch Intern Med* 2007;167(1):31–39.

39a. de Lorgeril M, Salen P, Martin JL, et al: Mediterranean diet, traditional risk factors, and the rate of cardiovascular complications after myocardial infarction: Final report of the Lyon Diet Heart Study. *Circulation* 1999;99:779–785.

39b. Esposito K, Marfella R, Ciotola M, et al: Effect of a mediterranean-style diet on endothelial dysfunction and markers of vascular inflammation in the metabolic syndrome: A randomized trial. *JAMA* 2004;292:1440–1446.

39c. Michalsen A, Lehmann N, Pithan C, et al: Mediterranean diet has no effect on markers of inflammation and metabolic risk factors in patients with coronary artery disease. *Eur J Clin Nutr* 2006;60:478–485.

40. Morin-Papunen L, Rautio K, Ruokonen A, et al: Metformin reduces serum C-reactive protein levels in women with polycystic ovary syndrome. *J Clin Endocrinol Metab* 2003;88(10):4649–4654.

41. Consoli A, Devangelio E: Thiazolidinediones and inflammation. *Lupus* 2005;14(9):794–797.

42. Blaschke F, Spanheimer R, Khan M, Law RE: Vascular effects of TZDs: new implications. *Vascul Pharmacol* 2006;45:3–18.

43. Haffner SM: Pre-diabetes, insulin resistance, inflammation and CVD risk. *Diabetes Res Clin Pract* 2003;61(Suppl 1):S9–S18.

43a. Satoh N, Ogawa Y, Usui T, et al: Antiatherogenic effect of pioglitazone in type 2 diabetic patients irrespective of the responsiveness to its antidiabetic effect. *Diabetes Care* 2003;26:2493–2499.

44. Rizos E, Kostoula A, Elisaf M, Mikhailidis DP: Effect of ciprofibrate on C-reactive protein and fibrinogen levels. *Angiology* 2002;53(3):273–277.

45. Després JP, Lemieux I, Robins SJ: Role of fibric acid derivatives in the management of risk factors for coronary heart disease. *Drugs* 2004;64(19):2177–2198.

46. Wang TD, Chen WJ, Lin JW, et al: Efficacy of fenofibrate and simvastatin on endothelial function and inflammatory markers in patients with combined hyperlipidemia: relations with baseline lipid profiles. *Atherosclerosis* 2003;170(2):315–323.

47. Gelman L, Fruchart JC, Auwerx J: An update on the mechanisms of action of the peroxisome proliferator-activated receptors (PPARs) and their roles in inflammation and cancer. *Cell Mol Life Sci* 1999;55(6–7):932–943.

47a. Ridker PM, Rifai N, Pfeffer MA, et al: Inflammation, pravastatin, and the risk of coronary events after myocardial infarction in patients with average cholesterol levels. Cholesterol and Recurrent Events (CARE) Investigators. *Circulation* 1998;98:839–844.

47b. Ridker PM, Rifai N, Clearfield M, et al: Measurement of C-reactive protein for the targeting of statin therapy in the primary prevention of acute coronary events. *N Engl J Med* 2001;344:1959–1965.

47c. Jialal I, Stein D, Balis D, et al: Effect of hydroxymethyl glutaryl coenzyme a reductase inhibitor therapy on high sensitive C-reactive protein levels. *Circulation* 2001;103:1933–1935.

47d. Dallinga-Thie GM, Berk-Planken II, Bootsma AH, Jansen H: Atorvastatin decreases apolipoprotein C-III in apolipoprotein B-containing lipoprotein and HDL in type 2 diabetes: A potential mechanism to lower plasma triglycerides. *Diabetes Care* 2004;27:1358–1364.

47e. van Wissen S, Trip MD, Smilde TJ, et al: Differential hs-CRP reduction in patients with familial hypercholesterolemia treated with aggressive or conventional statin therapy. *Atherosclerosis* 2002;165:361–366.

47f. Taylor AJ, Kent SM, Flaherty PJ, et al: ARBITER: Arterial Biology for the Investigation of the Treatment Effects of Reducing Cholesterol: A randomized trial comparing the effects of atorvastatin and pravastatin on carotid intima medial thickness. *Circulation* 2002;106:2055–2060.

47g. de Lemos JA, Blazing MA, Wiviott SD, et al: Early intensive vs a delayed conservative simvastatin strategy in patients with acute coronary syndromes: Phase Z of the A to Z trial. *JAMA* 2004;292:1307–1316.

48. Jialal I, Devaraj S: Statins and acute cardiovascular syndromes. *Curr Opin Lipidol* 2007;18(5):610–612.

48a. Kinlay S, Schwartz GG, Olsson AG, et al: High-dose atorvastatin enhances the decline in inflammatory markers in patients with acute coronary syndromes in the MIRACL study. *Circulation* 2003;108:1560–1566.

48b. Cannon CP, Braunwald E, McCabe CH, et al: Intensive versus moderate lipid lowering with statins after acute coronary syndromes. *N Engl J Med* 2004;350:1495–1504.

48c. Ridker PM, Cannon CP, Morrow D, et al: C-reactive protein levels and outcomes after statin therapy. *N Engl J Med* 2005;352:20–28.

48d. Nissen SE, Tuzcu EM, Schoenhagen P, et al: Statin therapy, LDL cholesterol, C-reactive protein, and coronary artery disease. *N Engl J Med* 2005;352:29–38.

49. Kakafika AI, Mikhailidis DP, Karagiannis A, Athyros VG: The role of endocannabinoid system blockade in the treatment of the metabolic syndrome. *J Clin Pharmacol* 2007;47(5):642–652.

50. Despres JP, Lemieux I, Almeras N: Contribution of CB1 blockade to the management of high-risk abdominal obesity. *Int J Obes* (Lond) 2006;30(Suppl 1):S44–S52.

51. Pi-Sunyer FX, Aronne LJ, Heshmati HM, et al: RIO-North America Study Group. Effect of rimonabant, a cannabinoid-1 receptor blocker, on weight and cardiometabolic risk factors in overweight or obese patients: RIO-North America: a randomized controlled trial. *JAMA* 2006;295(7):761–775.

51a. Després JP, Golay A, Sjöström L: Effects of rimonabant on metabolic risk factors in overweight patients with dyslipidemia. *N Engl J Med* 2005;353:2121–2134.

52. Carr AC, Myzak MC, Stocker R, et al: Myeloperoxidase binds to low-density lipoprotein: potential implications for atherosclerosis. *FEBS Lett* 2005;487(2):176–180.

53. Nambi V: The use of myeloperoxidase as a risk marker for atherosclerosis. *Curr Atheroscler Rep* 2005;7(2):127–131.

54. Nicholls SJ, Hazen SL: Myeloperoxidase and cardiovascular disease. *Arterioscler Thromb Vasc Biol* 2005;25(6):1102–1011.

55. Baldus S, Heeschen C, Meinertz T, et al: Myeloperoxidase serum levels predict risk in patients with acute coronary syndromes. *Circulation* 2003;108(12):1440–1445.

56. Sudhir K: Lipoprotein-associated phospholipase A2, vascular inflammation and cardiovascular risk prediction. *Vasc Health Risk Manag* 2006;2(2):153–156.

57. Jenny NS: Lipoprotein-associated phospholipase A2: novel biomarker and causal mediator of atherosclerosis? *Arterioscler Thromb Vasc Biol* 2006;26(11):2417–2418.

58. Zalewski A, Nelson JJ, Hegg L, Macphee C: Lp-PLA2: a new kid on the block. *Clin Chem* 2006;52(9):1645–1650.

58a. Stafforini DM, Sheller JR, Blackwell TS, et al: Release of free F_2-isoprostanes from esterified phospholipids is catalyzed by intracellular and plasma platelet-activating factor acetylhydrolases. *J Biol Chem* 2006;281:4616–4623.

58b. Packard CJ, O'Reilly DS, Caslake MJ, et al: Lipoprotein-associated phospholipase A2 as an independent predictor of coronary heart disease. *N Engl J Med* 2000;343:1148–1155.

58c. Ballantyne CM, Hoogeveen RC, Bang H, et al: Lipoprotein-associated phospholipase A_2, high-sensitivity C-reactive protein, and risk for incident coronary heart disease in middle-aged men and women in the Atherosclerosis Risk in Communities (ARIC) study. *Circulation* 2004;109:837–842.

58d. Oei HH, van der Meer IM, Hofman A, et al: Lipoprotein-associated phospholipase A2 activity is associated with risk of coronary heart disease and ischemic stroke: The Rotterdam Study. *Circulation* 2005;111:570–575.

58e. Ballantyne CM, Hoogeveen RC, Bang H, et al: Lipoprotein-associated phospholipase A2, high-sensitivity C-reactive protein, and risk for incident ischemic stroke in middle-aged men and women in the Atherosclerosis Risk in Communities (ARIC) study. *Arch Intern Med* 2005;165:2479–2484.

58f. Albert MA, Danielson E, Rifai N, Ridker PM: Effect of statin therapy on C-reactive protein levels: The Pravastatin Inflammation/CRP Evaluation (PRINCE): A randomized trial and cohort study. *JAMA* 2001;286:64–70.

58g. O'Donoghue M, Morrow DA, Sabatine MS, et al: Lipoprotein-associated phospholipase A_2 and its association with cardiovascular outcomes in patients with acute coronary syndromes in the PROVE IT-TIMI 22 (PRavastatin Or atorVastatin Evaluation and Infection Therapy–Thrombolysis In Myocardial Infarction) trial. *Circulation* 2006;113:1745–1752.

59. Jialal I: Role of biomarkers of inflammation and cardiovascular disease/atherosclerosis. *Crit Pathw Cardiol* 2006; 5:191–210.

CHAPTER 34

Invasive Imaging Modalities and Atherosclerosis: The Role of Intravascular Ultrasound

Stephen J. Nicholls and Steven E. Nissen

INTRODUCTION

For nearly fifty years, coronary angiography has been widely used to detect and quantify atherosclerotic coronary artery disease (CAD). Angiography has guided the use of a range of medical and revascularization therapies. Serial quantitative coronary angiography has evaluated the impact of medical therapies on the rate of progression of obstructive disease. While this approach has demonstrated that modification of established risk factors attenuates disease progression, the magnitude of this effect is less than the impact that these therapies exert on clinical events. Angiography portrays a two-dimensional silhouette of the arterial lumen and does not visualize the vessel wall, the site in which plaque accumulates. The use of imaging modalities that directly evaluate the artery wall provides the opportunity to assess the impact of medical therapies on changes in atherosclerotic burden.

INTRAVASCULAR ULTRASOUND

Technological advances in intravascular ultrasound (IVUS) permit the placement of high frequency (30–40 MHz) ultrasound transducers within the coronary arteries. High-frequency ultrasound transducers in close proximity to the endothelial surface result in the generation of high-resolution cross-sectional tomographic images of the entire vessel wall (Fig. 34-1). Ultrasonic imaging within the coronary arteries demonstrates the full extent of atherosclerotic plaque within the artery wall. As a result, IVUS often demonstrates the presence of extensive atherosclerosis in segments that appear normal or only minimally diseased on angiography.[1] The discord between atherosclerotic burden and the degree of obstructive disease reflects the ability of the artery wall to change its size and shape, which is termed remodeling. As initially described on the basis of necropsy specimens, the artery wall typically undergoes expansion of the external elastic membrane (EEM) in response to early accumulation of atherosclerotic plaque.[2] Lumen contraction does not usually occur until later in the process, at which time extensive atherosclerosis is present within the coronary arteries. As a result, abnormalities on angiography, which visualizes the lumen, do not reflect the true burden of atherosclerotic disease in the artery wall.

IVUS has been used to investigate factors that influence the natural history of plaque formation and its clinical complications. In addition to demonstrating that coronary atherosclerosis is more extensive than suggested by angiographic techniques, ultrasonic imaging has also revealed that atherosclerosis is typically present at a younger age than traditionally thought. In a series of 262 heart transplant recipients, IVUS performed shortly after transplantation revealed the presence of macroscopic atheroma in the apparently healthy coronary arteries of nearly one in six teenage donors. The prevalence of coronary atheroma rises exponentially with subsequent increases in donor age.[3]

A large number of ultrasonic studies have further characterized the patterns of arterial wall remodeling originally observed in pathology reports.[4] Variable patterns of remodeling are reported to predominate in the setting of different clinical presentations. Culprit lesions in the setting of acute myocardial infarction are typically accompanied by expansive remodeling. In contrast, patients with stable clinical syndromes are more likely to undergo constrictive

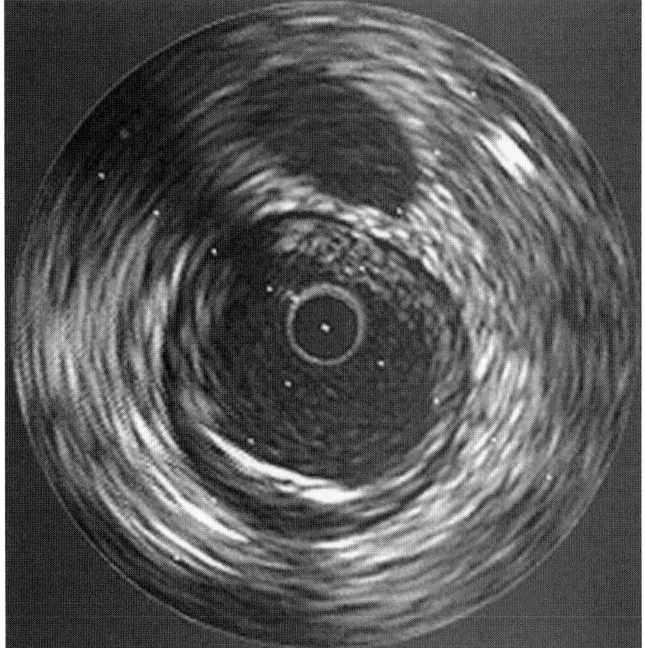

FIGURE 34-1 Tomographic cross-sectional Imaging of the arterial wall generated by intravascular ultrasound. Typical artifact resulting from the presence of the guidewire obscures the artery wall at 11 o'clock.

remodeling at the site of their culprit lesion.[5] This is consistent with the finding that patients with expansive remodeling at the site of the culprit lesion have elevated levels of matrix metalloproteinases, factors involved in the promotion of plaque rupture.[6] In further investigations of patients with acute ischemic syndromes, IVUS demonstrated the presence of multiple sites of plaque rupture throughout the coronary arterial tree, which is consistent with the systemic nature of the disease process.[7] IVUS has also characterized the factors that promote restenosis after percutaneous interventions[8] and the development of neointimal hyperplasia in the coronary arteries after heart transplantation.[9]

USE OF INTRAVASCULAR ULTRASOUND TO MONITOR ATHEROSCLEROTIC BURDEN

Planimetry of the leading edges of the lumen and EEM, in accordance with consensus guidelines for IVUS by the American College of Cardiology and European Society of Cardiology,[10] permits calculation of the area occupied by atheroma (Fig. 34-2). Given that the thickness of the arterial media is negligible (< 500 microns) the area between these leading edges is regarded as atherosclerotic plaque.

$$Plaque_{area}\,(mm^2) = EEM_{area} - Lumen_{area}$$

Automatic pullback devices permit continuous acquisition of images during withdrawal of the ultrasound transducer through an arterial segment at a constant rate (typically 0.5 mm/second) (Fig. 34-3). Summation of plaque areas from each measured image within the segment determines the volume of plaque.

$$Total\ Atheroma\ Volume\,(TAV, mm^3) = \Sigma(EEM_{area} - Lumen_{area})$$

The definition of arterial segments based on the fixed anatomic location of side branches results in significant heterogeneity of the vessel length evaluated. To control for this difference between subjects in clinical trials, TAV is normalized by multiplying the mean plaque area within a given arterial segment by the median number of evaluable images in the entire study population.

$$Normalized\ TAV\,(mm^3) = \frac{\Sigma(EEM_{area} - Lumen_{area})}{Number\ of\ Images\ in\ Pullback} \times Median\ Number\ of\ Images$$

Alternatively, the extent of atherosclerosis is expressed as the percent atheroma volume (PAV), which represents the proportion of the vessel wall occupied by atherosclerotic plaque.

$$PAV = \frac{\Sigma(EEM_{area} - Lumen_{area})}{\Sigma(EEM_{area})} \times 100$$

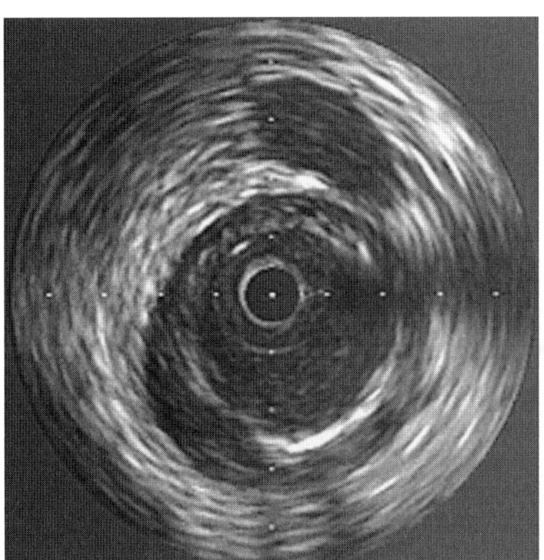

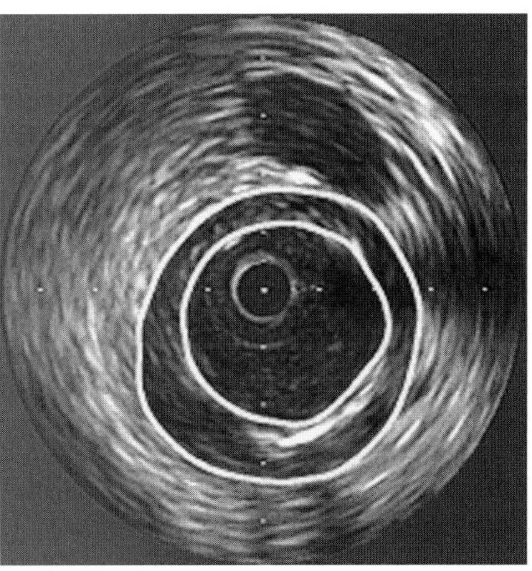

FIGURE 34-2 Typical measurements derived from a cross-sectional image of the artery wall. The leading edges of the lumen *(inner circle)* and external elastic membrane *(outer circle)* are defined by either manual planimetry or automatic edge detection software packages. The area between the leading edges represents atherosclerotic plaque.

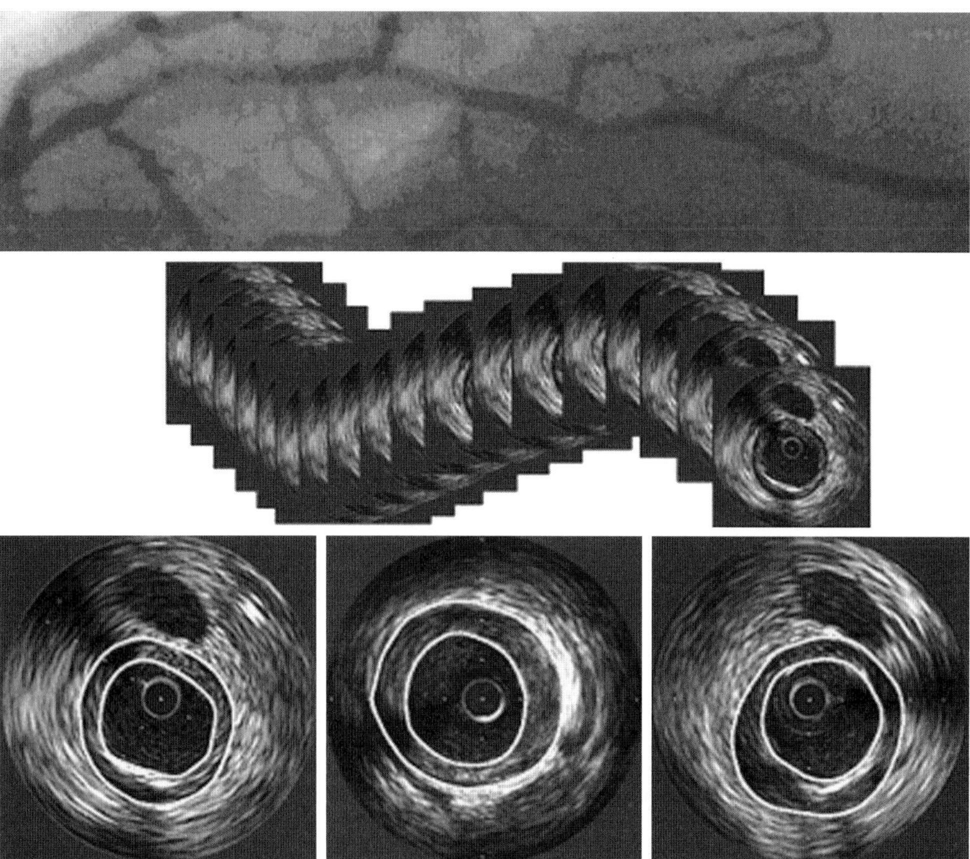

FIGURE 34-3 The ultrasound transducer continuously images during the withdrawal of the catheter from a distal site in the artery *(upper panel)*. This generates a series of cross-sectional images of the artery wall *(middle panel)*. Images spaced precisely 1 mm apart are selected for measurement *(lower panels)*.

Additional measurements obtained from ultrasonic images include changes in plaque volume in the 10-mm segment containing the greatest amount of disease, maximum and minimum plaque thickness, and the degree of calcification. Serial IVUS has been used to evaluate the impact of a number of medical therapies that target either established risk factors or pathologic events implicated in the formation of atherosclerotic plaque (Figs. 34-4 and 34-5).

LOWERING LEVELS OF LOW-DENSITY LIPOPROTEIN CHOLESTEROL

The pivotal role of cholesterol in promoting the formation and propagation of atherosclerosis is well established. Lowering levels of low-density lipoprotein (LDL) cholesterol in large placebo-controlled trials consistently reduces the rate of clinical events.[11–16] As a result, lowering LDL cholesterol is the primary goal of guidelines for lipid modification. While inhibitors of 3-hydroxy-3-methylglutaryl coenzyme A reductase (statins) have become increasingly prescribed, their optimal use in management remains to be defined. It is uncertain whether there exists a low enough level of LDL cholesterol below which incremental benefit is not observed. The impact of lowering LDL cholesterol on established atherosclerotic plaque remains to be established. The ability to evaluate an arterial segment at different time points with IVUS has provided important insights about the relationship between lowering LDL cholesterol and the natural history of atheroma progression.

Several groups have found no significant relationship between levels of LDL cholesterol and plaque burden, either at a single site or throughout an arterial segment.[17,18] In contrast, LDL cholesterol levels predict the rate of disease progression. In a cohort of 60 patients who underwent ultrasonic assessment of the most diseased site in the left main coronary artery at two different time points spaced 18 months apart, levels of LDL cholesterol correlated positively with changes in plaque area ($r = 0.41$, $P < 0.0001$) and inversely with lumen area ($r = -0.32$, $P < 0.01$).[18] Recent analysis revealed that the relationship between LDL cholesterol and the rate of plaque progression was observed at all ages.[19] These findings suggested that lowering LDL cholesterol might have a beneficial impact on the rate of disease progression.

Several investigators have studied the impact of lowering LDL cholesterol with apheresis on the rate of disease progression using quantitative coronary angiography. After anecdotal reports of disease regression,[20,21] clinical trials were conducted to evaluate the impact of combining apheresis with medical therapy, yielding equivocal results.[22,23] In particular, there was no definitive evidence that LDL apheresis had an incremental influence on angiographic progression. In the Low-density Lipoprotein-Apheresis Coronary Morphology and Reserve Trial (LACMART),[24] 18 patients with familial hypercholesterolemia were treated with lipid-lowering medications alone or in combination with LDL apheresis for 12 months. Treatment with

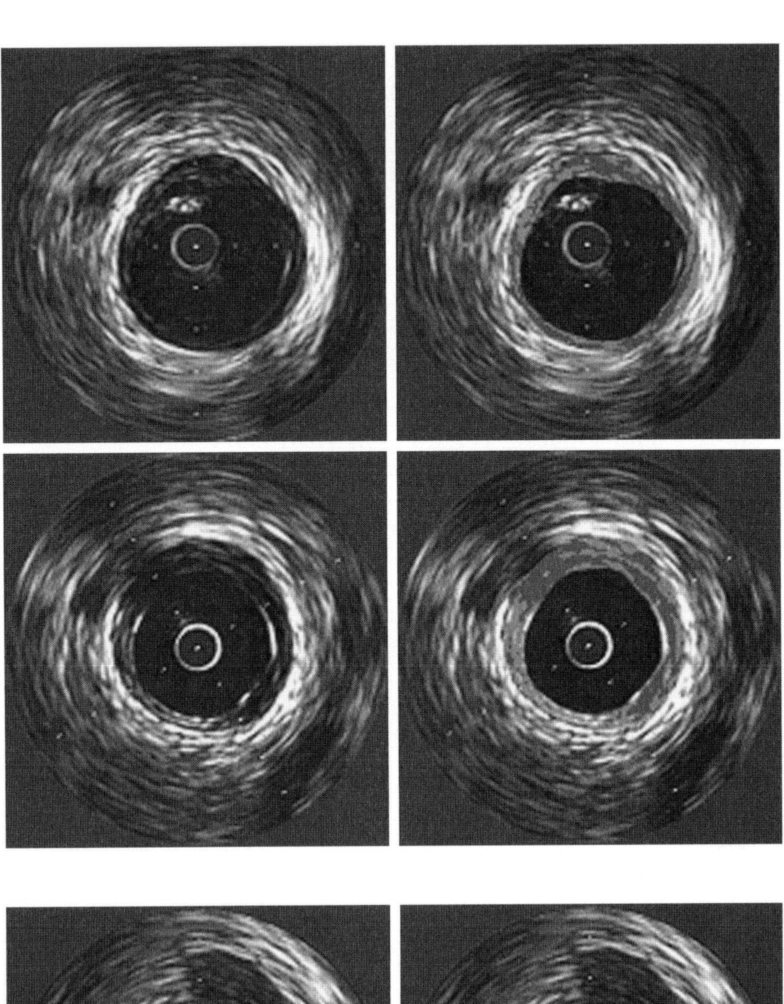

FIGURE 34-4 Illustrative example of the progression of coronary atherosclerosis. Increasing atheroma area *(shaded area)* at matched sites at baseline *(upper panels)* and follow-up *(lower panels)*.

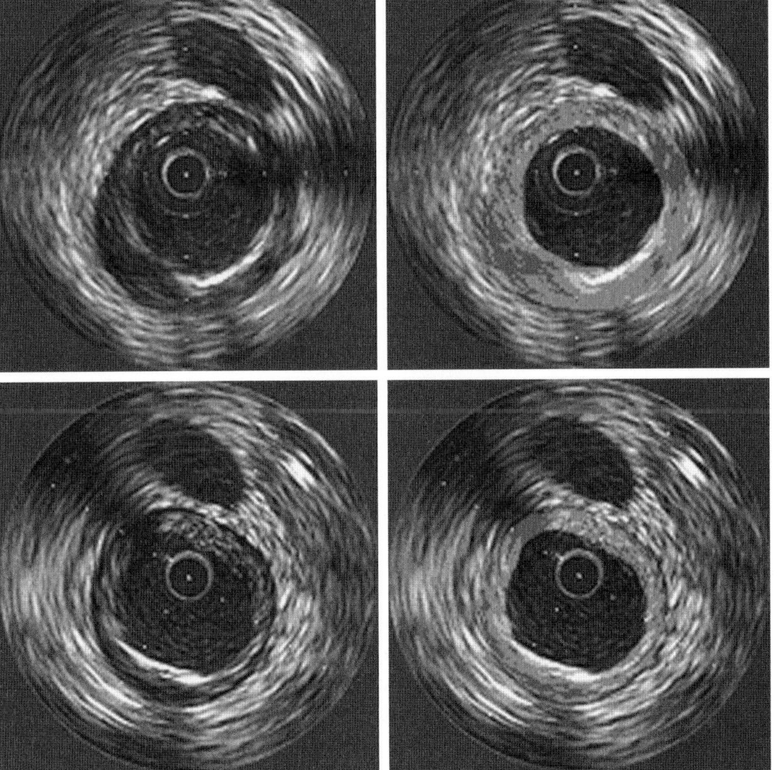

FIGURE 34-5 Illustrative example of the regression of coronary atherosclerosis. Decreasing atheroma area *(shaded area)* at matched sites at baseline *(upper panels)* and follow-up *(lower panels)*.

apheresis resulted in a 34.3% reduction in LDL cholesterol, a finding associated with a significant reduction in plaque area and an increase in minimum lumen diameter. These findings suggested that intensive lowering of LDL cholesterol could promote atheroma regression.

A number of investigators subsequently endeavored to determine whether intensive lowering of LDL cholesterol with medical therapy had a beneficial impact on plaque progression, by assessing serial changes in atheroma volume on IVUS. In the German Atorvastatin Investigation (GAIN), 131 patients with angiographic CAD participated in an open-label comparison of treatment with atorvastatin or usual care for 12 months.[25] The greater lowering of LDL cholesterol observed in patients treated with atorvastatin (86 versus 140 mg/dL) was not associated with attenuation of plaque progression. Intensive lowering of LDL cholesterol was associated with an increase in a calculated hyperechogenicity index, suggesting a favorable impact on plaque composition.

The Reversal of Atherosclerosis with Aggressive Lipid Lowering (REVERSAL) trial randomized 502 patients with angiographic CAD and an LDL cholesterol level between 125 and 210 mg/dL to treatment with an intensive (atorvastatin 80 mg/day) or moderate (pravastatin 40 mg/day) lipid-lowering strategy for 18 months.[26] More ntensive lowering of LDL cholesterol (79 versus 110 mg/dL) was associated with a significant impact on the serial change in plaque volume. While atheroma volume increased by 2.7% in patients treated with pravastatin, consistent with plaque progression, there was no significant difference between baseline and follow-up (−0.4%) in patients treated with atorvastatin. This suggested that intensive lowering of LDL cholesterol could halt the natural history of plaque progression.

While a direct relationship was observed between changes in LDL cholesterol and atheroma volume, a difference was noted between treatment groups. Patients treated with pravastatin required an additional 30 mg/dL lowering of LDL cholesterol to achieve the same impact on plaque progression. This suggested that factors in addition to lowering LDL cholesterol contributed to the beneficial impact of high-dose atorvastatin. Findings of greater lowering of the inflammatory marker C-reactive protein (CRP) in patients treated with atorvastatin (36% versus 5%) and a direct relationship between changes in CRP and atheroma volume suggest that anti-inflammatory properties may have contributed to the beneficial impact of high-dose atorvastatin on plaque progression.[27]

The influence of an intensive lipid-lowering strategy on plaque progression complemented observations from the Pravastatin or Atorvastatin Evaluation and Infection Therapy (PROVE IT) study, which demonstrated that treatment with atorvastatin 80 mg/day was associated with a significant reduction in clinical events compared with pravastatin 40 mg/day in patients with an acute coronary syndrome.[28] In subsequent analyses, it was reported that the rates of plaque progression[27] and clinical events[29] were lowest in patients who demonstrated the greatest lowering of both LDL cholesterol and CRP. These findings provide support for the concept that potential pleiotropic properties of statins contribute to their benefit *in vivo.*

The analysis of the major clinical trials that used serial IVUS measurements revealed a direct relationship between achieved levels of LDL cholesterol and changes in PAV. It remained to be determined whether further lowering of LDL cholesterol could promote plaque regression. In A Study to Evaluate the Effect of Rosuvastatin on Intravascular Ultrasound–Derived Coronary Atheroma Burden (ASTEROID), 349 patients underwent serial IVUS evaluation before and after 24 months of treatment with rosuvastatin 40 mg/day.[30] Rosuvastatin lowered LDL cholesterol by 53% to 60.8 mg/dL and raised high-density lipoprotein (HDL) cholesterol by 14.7% to 49 mg/dL, resulting in a 58.5% reduction of the LDL cholesterol/HDL cholesterol ratio to 1.3. These profound effects on plasma lipids were associated with significant reductions in all indices of atheroma burden, which is consistent with plaque regression. Depending on the parameter used, 63% to 78% of patients demonstrated some evidence of regression. Subgroup analysis revealed that only patients who achieved an LDL cholesterol level of less than 70 mg/dL demonstrated significant reductions in atheroma burden. These findings provide important insights to suggest that high-dose statin therapy resulting in very low levels of LDL cholesterol and modest elevations in HDL cholesterol could promote regression of coronary atherosclerosis.

The finding that lowering LDL cholesterol with a statin could promote plaque regression supported early reports from small cohorts of subjects studied with serial IVUS. In the Early Statin Treatment in Patients with Acute Coronary Syndrome (ESTABLISH) study, 70 Japanese patients hospitalized for an acute coronary syndrome were randomized to treatment with an intensive lipid-lowering strategy (atorvastatin 20 mg/day) or placebo following percutaneous coronary intervention for 6 months.[31] A 41.7% reduction in LDL cholesterol levels with atorvastatin was associated with a significant 13.1% reduction in atheroma volume. In contrast, the 0.7% increase in LDL cholesterol in the placebo group was accompanied by an 8.7% increase in plaque volume, which is consistent with disease progression.

In a similar finding, Danish investigators demonstrated regression of coronary atherosclerosis in a small cohort ($n = 40$) of male patients with hypercholesterolemia and established CAD.[32] Patients were treated with a lipid-lowering diet for 3 months, followed by simvastatin 40 mg/day for 12 months. Simvastatin therapy lowered LDL cholesterol by 42.6%, which was associated with a 6.3% reduction in atheroma volume. The findings of regression in these two small patient cohorts were observed in much shorter arterial segments than typically evaluated in clinical trials that use serial monitoring by IVUS. Regardless, the totality of evidence suggests that the effective lowering of levels of LDL cholesterol has a beneficial impact on the natural history of atherosclerotic plaque progression.

PROMOTING BIOLOGICAL ACTIVITY OF HIGH-DENSITY LIPOPROTEINS

Epidemiological[33] and animal[34] studies have established that HDL protects against the development of atherosclerosis. Promoting the biological activity of HDL induces regression of established lesions in animal models of atherosclerosis.[35] This activity is likely to result from a number of functional properties of HDL. In addition to its pivotal role in promoting cholesterol efflux and facilitating reverse cholesterol transport, HDL has also been reported to inhibit inflammatory, oxidative, apoptotic, and thrombotic events implicated in atherosclerosis.[36] Current therapeutic approaches raise levels of HDL cholesterol to a modest degree. Serial IVUS has been used in a number of important clinical trials that assessed the efficacy of emerging therapeutic strategies to promote the protective properties of HDL.

The mutant protein apolipoprotein A-I_{Milano} (AIM) has been proposed to possess enhanced protective properties.[37] Despite having low levels of HDL cholesterol, AIM carriers appear to be protected from atherosclerotic cardiovascular disease.[37] Based on the profound antiatherosclerotic effects in animal models,[38,39] serial IVUS was used to evaluate the impact of infusing AIM in humans. A cohort of 47 patients, within 2 weeks of an acute coronary syndrome, were randomized to receive weekly intravenous infusions of saline or either low-dose (15 mg/kg) or high-dose (45 mg/kg) AIM complexed with phospholipids (ETC-216).[40] IVUS performed within 2 weeks of the final infusion revealed that administration of either dose of AIM resulted in a significant 4.2% reduction in atheroma volume compared with baseline. Subsequent analysis revealed a more substantial regression (11.2%) in the regions containing the greatest amount of plaque, suggesting that the major impact was likely to be observed at the site of large, lipid-rich lesions.[41] The observation that regression was accompanied by contraction of the EEM, with no change in lumen dimensions,[41] provides further support for the concept that monitoring the effect of medical therapies on atherosclerotic plaque requires imaging modalities that visualize the entire artery wall. While these results hold exciting promise for the concept that acute infusional HDL therapy could promote rapid removal of cholesterol from the artery wall, they await further validation in large-scale clinical trials. Furthermore, the impact of this therapeutic approach on clinical event outcomes remains to be determined.

Considerable debate has focused on whether AIM possesses more protective properties than wild-type apoA-I. The Effect of rHDL on Atherosclerosis-Safety and Efficacy (ERASE) investigators performed a similar study, in which reconstituted HDL (rHDL) particles (CSL-111) containing wild-type apoA-I isolated from human plasma were infused.[42] A total of 183 patients were randomized to receive weekly infusions of saline or rHDL containing 40 or 80 mg/kg of protein for 4 weeks. Because of liver enzyme abnormalities, the high-dose group was discontinued. Infusing CSL-111 resulted in a 3.4% reduction in plaque volume, which is consistent with regression. This was associated with a favorable impact on a plaque characterization index, suggesting stabilization, and on obstructive disease on angiography. While the development of both forms of rHDL infusions requires more robust clinical trial validation, they provide excitement for the potential utility of infusional therapy in patients with acute ischemic syndromes.

The marked benefit of infusing rHDL in humans was observed without altering systemic levels of HDL cholesterol. This has important implications for the development of new therapies to promote HDL function. Considerable attention has focused on the development of therapeutic measures to elevate HDL cholesterol levels. While existing therapies raise HDL cholesterol by only modest amounts, this appears to have a beneficial impact. A recent pooled analysis of patients treated with statins in clinical trials that used serial IVUS assessments of atheroma burden revealed that an increasing level of HDL cholesterol is an independent predictor of the impact of statin therapy on the rate of disease progression.[43] The combination of effective lowering of LDL cholesterol and modest raising of HDL cholesterol (greater than 7.5%) resulted in the greatest plaque regression.

The most advanced experimental approach to effectively raise levels of HDL cholesterol has involved the development of chemical inhibitors of cholesteryl ester transfer protein (CETP). The findings that CETP inhibitors prevent lesion formation in animal models[44] and raise HDL cholesterol levels by more than 50% in humans[45] stimulated the search to characterize their impact on the rate of plaque progression. In the Investigation of Lipid Level management using coronary UltraSound To assess Reduction of Atherosclerosis by CETP Inhibition and HDL Elevation (ILLUSTRATE), 991 patients underwent treatment with atorvastatin (mean dose: 23 mg/day) to achieve LDL cholesterol levels of less than 100 mg/dL before randomization to additional treatment with torcetrapib 60 mg/day or placebo.[46] Torcetrapib administration raised HDL cholesterol by 61%, to 72.1 mg/dL, and lowered LDL cholesterol by 20%, to 70.1 mg/dL, resulting in an LDL cholesterol/HDL cholesterol ratio of 0.93. Torcetrapib also raised systolic blood pressure by 4.6 mm Hg. The lack of difference between treatment groups with regard to the primary endpoint (the change in PAV) suggested that torcetrapib therapy did not have a beneficial impact on the rate of plaque progression. While the small difference between treatment groups in favor of torcetrapib with regard to the reduction in atheroma volume throughout the whole arterial segment was significant, there was no difference observed in the most diseased 10-mm segment. A number of additional observations further highlight the lack of efficacy of torcetrapib. The rate of plaque progression, in terms of the change in PAV, was much greater than that typically observed at LDL cholesterol levels of 71 mg/dL (Fig. 34-6). In addition, the reduction in TAV with

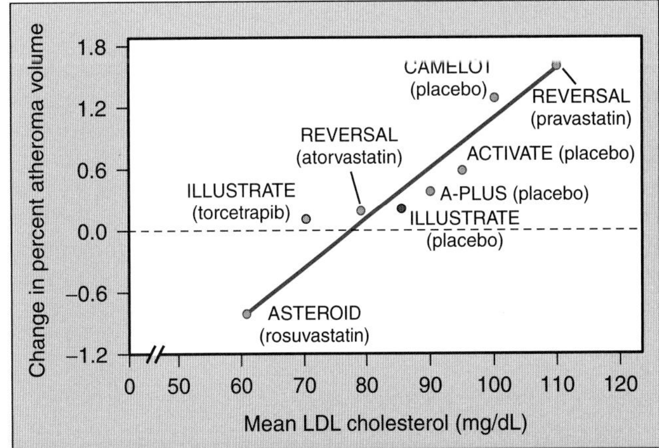

FIGURE 34-6 Relationship between the change in percent atheroma volume and LDL cholesterol in regression–progression trials using intravascular ultrasonography. ACTIVATE, ACAT Intravascular Atherosclerosis Treatment Evaluation; A-PLUS, Avasimibe and Progression of Lesions on Ultrasound; ASTEROID, A Study to Evaluate the Effect of Rosuvastatin on Intravascular Ultrasound-Derived Coronary Atheroma Burden; CAMELOT, Comparison of Amlodipine vs. Enalapril to Limit Occurrences of Thrombosis; ILLUSTRATE, Investigation of Lipid Level Management Using Coronary Ultrasound to Assess Reduction of Atherosclerosis by CETP Inhibition and HDL Elevation; LDL, Low-density lipoprotein; REVERSAL, Reversal of Atherosclerosis with Aggressive Lipid Lowering. *(From Ref. 46.)*

substantial HDL cholesterol raising after 24 months of treatment with torcetrapib was less than that observed after five weekly infusions of rHDL containing AIM.[40] The findings complemented the lack of a beneficial impact on the progression of carotid intimal–media thickness and the lack of efficacy in a large clinical events trial.[47] It remains to be determined whether the lack of efficacy with torcetrapib reflects a problem with the molecule or the generation of dysfunctional HDL particles as a result of CETP inhibition.

INHIBITION OF CHOLESTEROL ESTERIFICATION

The uptake of esterified cholesterol by macrophages to become foam cells is the pivotal step in the formation and propagation of atherosclerotic plaque. In addition to lowering systemic levels of LDL cholesterol, inhibiting cholesterol esterification has been proposed as a potential therapeutic strategy.[48] Inhibitors of acyl–coenzymA: cholesterol acyltransferase (ACAT) have a beneficial impact on lesion formation in atherogenic animal models.[48] Serial IVUS has demonstrated that two pharmacologic inhibitors of ACAT do not have a favorable impact on progression of coronary atherosclerosis in humans.

In the Avasimibe and Progression of Lesions on UltraSound (A-PLUS) study, 509 patients were treated with avasimibe or placebo for 18 months.[49] There was no difference between the groups with regard to the change in TAV. Levels of LDL cholesterol were higher in patients treated with avasimibe, which is consistent with the ability of avasimibe to induce cytochrome P450 3A4 and statin metabolism. The ACAT Intravascular Atherosclerosis Treatment Evaluation (ACTIVATE) subsequently investigated the impact of pactimibe, an ACAT inhibitor with no influence on the metabolism of concomitant statin therapy.[50] A total of 408 patients were treated with pactimibe or placebo for 24 months. There was no difference between the groups with regard to plasma lipids and the primary endpoint, which was the change in PAV. A significant difference was observed between treatment groups, in favor of placebo, with regard to the change in atheroma volume throughout the entire length of artery evaluated and the 10-mm segment containing the greatest amount of plaque at baseline. This suggested that ACAT inhibition with pactimibe may have a detrimental impact on the progression of atherosclerotic plaque. Because of these findings, it appears that nonselective ACAT inhibition is unlikely to be an effective therapeutic strategy to prevent atherosclerotic cardiovascular disease.

LIMITATIONS AND FUTURE DIRECTIONS

While ultrasonic imaging within the coronary arteries has characterized the natural history of atherosclerosis, a number of important caveats should be noted. Because IVUS requires invasive catheterization, its use is currently limited to the patient who requires coronary angiography for clinical indications. As a result, the findings of regression–progression studies can only be directly applied to the setting of the patient with established CAD. The precision needed to study atherosclerotic plaque depends critically on the quality of the images that are generated. High-quality imaging is limited by a number of artifacts, including the presence of calcium, arterial side branches, and nonuniform rotational deformities that result from the frictional drag on the catheter. Technological advances in catheter imaging and the greater experience of operators participating in clinical trials have made a substantial impact on the ability to provide high-resolution imaging on a serial basis. Clinical trials typically involve the evaluation of a single coronary artery. It is not known whether the impact of medical therapies is homogeneous throughout the coronary arterial tree.

Conventional IVUS permits a substantial characterization of plaque composition. However, the broad distinctions among fibrotic, echolucent, and calcific regions lack the precision required to make accurate assessments in serial changes in plaque components. A number of observations from gray scale ultrasound suggest that medical therapies have a favorable impact on plaque composition. In studies involving the use of statin therapy[26] or infusions of rHDL,[40] the greatest degree of regression is observed in the 10-mm segment containing the most plaque at baseline, a region that is likely to contain more lipid. As a result, the regression is likely to involve the removal of lipid from the artery wall. The benefit of high-dose atorvastatin is also likely to be derived from a reduction in the inflammatory milieu of atherosclerotic plaque. In a post hoc analysis of the REVERSAL study, the benefit of high-dose atorvastatin was primarily observed in obese patients. Given that the degree of LDL cholesterol lowering was less and CRP lowering was greater in obese patients treated with atorvastatin compared with nonobese patients, the greater impact on plaque progression is likely to involve a reduction in the inflammatory components of plaque.[51] Furthermore, the recent observation that more-calcified lesions are less likely to undergo either regression or progression[52] has important implications for understanding which plaque components are likely to contribute to changes in atheroma volume on serial evaluation.

Analysis of radiofrequency backscatter has been reported to characterize plaque composition, with good correlation to findings on histology in *ex vivo* coronary artery samples (Fig. 34-7).[53] Preliminary studies of a small cohort of Japanese patients with established CAD demonstrated that 6 months of statin therapy resulted in an increase in fibrotic and a decrease in lipidic content of atherosclerotic plaque.[54] Future large-scale studies using serial IVUS evaluations of coronary arteries are likely to incorporate an analysis of plaque composition to gain further insight into the impact of medical therapies on the artery wall.

The requirement for invasive catheterization limits the use of IVUS to patients with CAD established on angiography performed for a clinical indication. Accordingly, the results of regression–progression trials can be directly applied only to the setting of secondary prevention of the patient with established disease. Technological advances in a number of imaging modalities permit the artery wall to be visualized in a

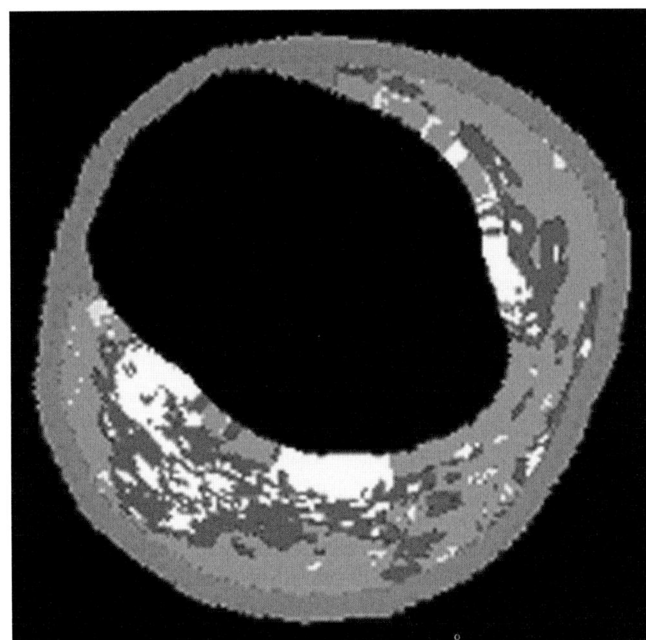

FIGURE 34-7 Illustrative example of tissue map of atherosclerotic plaque generated by radiofrequency backscatter of intravascular ultrasound.

noninvasive fashion. Preliminary studies with magnetic resonance imaging demonstrate a favorable impact of lipid-modifying therapies on atheroma within the walls of the aorta and carotid arteries.[55] Further improvements in resolution are necessary to enable the precise imaging of the coronary arteries required to evaluate the impact of medical therapies on atherosclerotic CAD.

A major challenge for the use of all atherosclerosis imaging modalities is the ability to translate the impact of therapies on plaque progression to clinical outcome. An early study demonstrated that the degree of progression of atherosclerosis at the most diseased site in the left main coronary artery predicted the prospective risk of clinical events.[56] A number of lines of evidence suggest that observations from IVUS studies complement the findings of clinical event trials. Direct relationships are observed between achieved levels of LDL cholesterol and both the rate of atheroma progression[26] and clinical event rates.[57] Using the same therapeutic regimens, the REVERSAL[26] and PROVE IT[28] studies demonstrated that high-dose atorvastatin has a beneficial impact on both plaque progression and clinical events. Similarly, atorvastatin had a beneficial impact in placebo-controlled trials of patients with acute coronary syndromes with regard to both the impact on atherosclerotic plaque (ESTABLISH)[31] and clinical events (Myocardial Ischemia Reduction with Aggressive Cholesterol Lowering [MIRACL]) study.[58] The finding that modest elevations in levels of HDL cholesterol independently predict the impact of statins on plaque progression[43] complements the report that small increases in levels of HDL cholesterol with atorvastatin predict decreases in clinical event rates.[59]

The complementary findings have also been demonstrated with non-ipid-modifying therapies in the setting of clinical trials that have embedded serial IVUS evaluations. In the Comparison of Amlodipine versus Enalapril to Limit Occurrences of Thrombosis (CAMELOT) study, administration of amlodipine had the greatest impact on plaque progression and a composite of clinical events.[60] Administration of the immunomodulatory agent everolimus reduced the progression of vasculopathy and the rates of clinical events in heart transplant recipients.[61] Further evidence supporting the correlation of serial changes in atheroma volume with clinical outcome will provide further impetus for the monitoring of plaque progression in the development of new therapies.

SUMMARY

Advances in IVUS permit the characterization of coronary atherosclerosis in the *in vivo* setting. The ability to image arterial segments at different points in time has defined the clinical factors that influence the natural history of atherosclerosis. More recently, serial IVUS has been used in clinical trials to assess the impact of medical therapies. These studies have primarily found that intensively lowering levels of LDL cholesterol or promoting the biological activity of HDL has a profound impact on the rate of atheroma progression. Furthermore, intensive medical modification of established lipid risk factors can promote the regression of a pathologic process that developed within the artery wall over a number of decades. The direct link between the impact of these therapies on atherosclerotic plaque and clinical outcome remains to be defined.

REFERENCES

1. Mintz GS, Painter JA, Pichard AD, et al: Atherosclerosis in angiographically “normal” coronary artery reference segments: an intravascular ultrasound study with clinical correlations. *J Am Coll Cardiol* 1995;25:1479–1485.
2. Glagov S, Weisenberg E, Zarins CK, et al: Compensatory enlargement of human atherosclerotic coronary arteries. *N Engl J Med* 1987;316:1371–1375.
3. Tuzcu EM, Kapadia SR, Tutar E, et al: High prevalence of coronary atherosclerosis in asymptomatic teenagers and young adults: evidence from intravascular ultrasound. *Circulation* 2001;103:2705–2710.
4. Schoenhagen P, Ziada KM, Vince DG, et al: Arterial remodeling and coronary artery disease: the concept of “dilated” versus “obstructive” coronary atherosclerosis. *J Am Coll Cardiol* 2001;38:297–306.
5. Schoenhagen P, Ziada KM, Kapadia SR, et al: Extent and direction of arterial remodeling in stable versus unstable coronary syndromes: an intravascular ultrasound study. *Circulation* 2000;101:598–603.
6. Schoenhagen P, Vince DG, Ziada KM, et al: Relation of matrix-metalloproteinase 3 found in coronary lesion samples retrieved by directional coronary atherectomy to intravascular ultrasound observations on coronary remodeling. *Am J Cardiol* 2002;89:1354–1359.
7. Schoenhagen P, Stone GW, Nissen SE, et al: Coronary plaque morphology and frequency of ulceration distant from culprit lesions in patients with unstable and stable presentation. *Arterioscler Thromb Vasc Biol* 2003;23:1895–1900.
8. Mintz GS, Kent KM, Pichard AD, et al: Intravascular ultrasound insights into mechanisms of stenosis formation and restenosis. *Cardiol Clin* 1997;15:17–29.
9. Kapadia SR, Nissen SE, Tuzcu EM: Impact of intravascular ultrasound in understanding transplant coronary artery disease. *Curr Opin Cardiol* 1999;14:140–150.

10. Mintz GS, Nissen SE, Anderson WD, et al: American College of Cardiology Clinical Expert Consensus Document on Standards for Acquisition, Measurement and Reporting of Intravascular Ultrasound Studies (IVUS). A report of the American College of Cardiology Task Force on Clinical Expert Consensus Documents. *J Am Coll Cardiol* 2001;37:1478–1492.
11. Randomised trial of cholesterol lowering in 4444 patients with coronary heart disease: The Scandinavian Simvastatin Survival Study (4S). *Lancet* 1994;344:1383–1389.
12. Prevention of cardiovascular events and death with pravastatin in patients with coronary heart disease and a broad range of initial cholesterol levels. The Long-Term Intervention with Pravastatin in Ischaemic Disease (LIPID) Study Group. *N Engl J Med* 1998;339:1349–1357.
13. Heart Protection Study Collaborative Group: MRC/BHF Heart Protection Study of cholesterol lowering with simvastatin in 20,536 high-risk individuals: a randomised placebo-controlled trial. *Lancet* 2002;360:7–22.
14. Downs JR, Clearfield M, Weis S, et al: Primary prevention of acute coronary events with lovastatin in men and women with average cholesterol levels: results of AFcaps/Texcaps. AirForce/Texas Coronary Atherosclerosis Prevention Study. *JAMA* 1998;279:1615–1622.
15. Sacks FM, Pfeffer MA, Moye LA, et al: The effect of pravastatin on coronary events after myocardial infarction in patients with average cholesterol levels. Cholesterol and Recurrent Events Trial investigators. *N Engl J Med* 1996;335:1001–1009.
16. Shepherd J, Cobbe SM, Ford I, et al: Prevention of coronary heart disease with pravastatin in men with hypercholesterolemia. West of Scotland Coronary Prevention Study Group. *N Engl J Med* 1995;333:1301–1307.
17. Nicholls SJ, Tuzcu EM, Crowe T, et al: Relationship between cardiovascular risk factors and atherosclerotic disease burden measured by intravascular ultrasound. *J Am Coll Cardiol* 2006;47:1967–1975.
18. von Birgelen C, Hartmann M, Mintz GS, et al: Relation between progression and regression of atherosclerotic left main coronary artery disease and serum cholesterol levels as assessed with serial long-term (> or =12 months) follow-up intravascular ultrasound. *Circulation* 2003;108:2757–2762.
19. Hartmann M, von Birgelen C, Mintz GS, et al: Relation between plaque progression and low-density lipoprotein cholesterol during aging as assessed with serial long-term (> or =12 months) follow-up intravascular ultrasound of the left main coronary artery. *Am J Cardiol* 2006;98:1419–1423.
20. Koga N, Iwata Y: Pathological and angiographic regression of coronary atherosclerosis by LDL-apheresis in a patient with familial hypercholesterolemia. *Atherosclerosis* 1991;90:9–21.
21. Kitabatake A, Sato H, Hori M, et al: Coronary atherosclerosis reduced in patients with familial hypercholesterolemia after intensive cholesterol lowering with low-density lipoprotein-apheresis: 1-year follow-up study. The Osaka LDL-Apheresis Multicenter Trial Group. *Clin Ther* 1994;16:416–428.
22. Thompson GR, Maher VM, Matthews S, et al: Familial Hypercholesterolaemia Regression Study: a randomised trial of low-density-lipoprotein apheresis. *Lancet* 1995;345:811–816.
23. Kroon AA, Aengevaeren WR, van der Werf T, et al: LDL-Apheresis Atherosclerosis Regression Study (LAARS). Effect of aggressive versus conventional lipid lowering treatment on coronary atherosclerosis. *Circulation* 1996;93:1826–1835.
24. Matsuzaki M, Hiramori K, Imaizumi T, et al: Intravascular ultrasound evaluation of coronary plaque regression by low-density lipoprotein-apheresis in familial hypercholesterolemia: The Low-density Lipoprotein-Apheresis Coronary Morphology and Reserve Trial (LACMART). *J Am Coll Cardiol* 2002;40:220–227.
25. Schartl M, Bocksch W, Koschyk DH, et al: Use of intravascular ultrasound to compare effects of different strategies of lipid-lowering therapy on plaque volume and composition in patients with coronary artery disease. *Circulation* 2001;104:387–392.
26. Nissen SE, Tuzcu EM, Schoenhagen P, et al: Effect of intensive compared with moderate lipid-lowering therapy on progression of coronary atherosclerosis: a randomized controlled trial. *JAMA* 2004;291:1071–1080.
27. Nissen SE, Tuzcu EM, Schoenhagen P, et al: Statin therapy, LDL cholesterol, C-reactive protein, and coronary artery disease. *N Engl J Med* 2005;352:29–38.
28. Cannon CP, Braunwald E, McCabe CH, et al: Intensive versus moderate lipid lowering with statins after acute coronary syndromes. *N Engl J Med* 2004;350:1495–1504.
29. Ridker PM, Cannon CP, Morrow D, et al: C-reactive protein levels and outcomes after statin therapy. *N Engl J Med* 2005;352:20–28.
30. Nissen SE, Nicholls SJ, Sipahi I, et al: Effect of very high-intensity statin therapy on regression of coronary atherosclerosis: the ASTEROID trial. *JAMA* 2006;295:1556–1565.
31. Okazaki S, Yokoyama T, Miyauchi K, et al: Early statin treatment in patients with acute coronary syndrome: demonstration of the beneficial effect on atherosclerotic lesions by serial volumetric intravascular ultrasound analysis during half a year after coronary event: the ESTABLISH Study. *Circulation* 2004;110:1061–1068.
32. Jensen LO, Thayssen P, Pedersen KE, et al: Regression of coronary atherosclerosis by simvastatin: a serial intravascular ultrasound study. *Circulation* 2004;110:265–270.
33. Gordon T, Castelli WP, Hjortland MC, et al: High-density lipoprotein as a protective factor against coronary heart disease. The Framingham Study. *Am J Med* 1977;62:707–714.
34. Badimon JJ, Badimon L, Fuster V: Regression of atherosclerotic lesions by high-density lipoprotein plasma fraction in the cholesterol-fed rabbit. *J Clin Invest* 1990;85:1234–1241.
35. Nicholls SJ, Cutri B, Worthley SG, et al: Impact of short-term administration of high-density lipoproteins and atorvastatin on atherosclerosis in rabbits. *Arterioscler Thromb Vasc Biol* 2005;25:2416–2421.
36. Barter PJ, Nicholls S, Rye KA, et al: Antiinflammatory properties of HDL. *Circ Res* 2004;95:764–772.
37. Sirtori CR, Calabresi L, Franceschini G, et al: Cardiovascular status of carriers of the apolipoprotein A-I(Milano) mutant: the Limone sul Garda study. *Circulation* 2001;103:1949–1954.
38. Shah PK, Nilsson J, Kaul S, et al: Effects of recombinant apolipoprotein A-I(Milano) on aortic atherosclerosis in apolipoprotein E-deficient mice. *Circulation* 1998;97:780–785.
39. Shah PK, Yano J, Reyes O, et al: High-dose recombinant apolipoprotein A-IMilano mobilizes tissue cholesterol and rapidly reduces plaque lipid and macrophage content in apolipoprotein E-deficient mice. *Circulation* 2001;103:3047–3050.
40. Nissen SE, Tsunoda T, Tuzcu EM, et al: Effect of recombinant ApoA-I Milano on coronary atherosclerosis in patients with acute coronary syndromes: a randomized controlled trial. *JAMA* 2003;290:2292–2300.
41. Nicholls SJ, Tuzcu EM, Sipahi I, et al: Relationship between atheroma regression and change in lumen size after infusion of apolipoprotein A-I Milano. *J Am Coll Cardiol* 2006;47:992–997.
42. Tardif JC, Gregoire J, L'Allier PL, et al: Effects of reconstituted high-density lipoprotein infusions on coronary atherosclerosis: a randomized controlled trial. *JAMA* 2007;297:1675–1682.
43. Nicholls SJ, Tuzcu EM, Sipahi I, et al: Statins, high-density lipoprotein cholesterol, and regression of coronary atherosclerosis. *JAMA* 2007;297:499–508.
44. Okamoto H, Yonemori F, Wakitani K, et al: A cholesteryl ester transfer protein inhibitor attenuates atherosclerosis in rabbits. *Nature* 2000;406:203–207.
45. Brousseau ME, Schaefer EJ, Wolfe ML, et al: Effects of an inhibitor of cholesteryl ester transfer protein on HDL cholesterol. *N Engl J Med* 2004;350:1505–1515.
46. Nissen SE, Tardif JC, Nicholls SJ, et al: Effect of torcetrapib on the progression of coronary atherosclerosis. *N Engl J Med* 2007;356:1304–1316.
47. Kastelein JJ, van Leuven SI, Burgess L, et al: Effect of torcetrapib on carotid atherosclerosis in familial hypercholesterolemia. *N Engl J Med* 2007;356:1620–1630.
48. Rudel LL, Lee RG, Parini P: ACAT2 is a target for treatment of coronary heart disease associated with hypercholesterolemia. *Arterioscler Thromb Vasc Biol* 2005;25:1112–1118.
49. Tardif JC, Gregoire J, L'Allier PL, et al: Effects of the acyl coenzyme A:cholesterol acyltransferase inhibitor avasimibe on human atherosclerotic lesions. *Circulation* 2004;110:3372–3377.
50. Nissen SE, Tuzcu EM, Brewer HB, et al: Effect of ACAT inhibition on the progression of coronary atherosclerosis. *N Engl J Med* 2006;354:1253–1263.
51. Nicholls SJ, Tuzcu EM, Sipahi I, et al: Effects of obesity on lipid-lowering, anti-inflammatory, and antiatherosclerotic benefits of atorvastatin or pravastatin in patients with coronary artery disease (from the REVERSAL Study). *Am J Cardiol* 2006;97:1553–1557.

52. Nicholls SJ, Tuzcu EM, Wolski K, et al: Coronary artery calcification and changes in atheroma burden in response to established medical therapies. *J Am Coll Cardiol* 2007;49:263–270.
53. Nair A, Kuban BD, Tuzcu EM, et al: Coronary plaque classification with intravascular ultrasound radiofrequency data analysis. *Circulation* 2002;106:2200–2206.
54. Kawasaki M, Sano K, Okubo M, et al: Volumetric quantitative analysis of tissue characteristics of coronary plaques after statin therapy using three-dimensional integrated backscatter intravascular ultrasound. *J Am Coll Cardiol* 2005;45:1946–1953.
55. Corti R, Fuster V, Fayad ZA, et al: Lipid lowering by simvastatin induces regression of human atherosclerotic lesions: two years' follow-up by high-resolution noninvasive magnetic resonance imaging. *Circulation* 2002;106:2884–2887.
56. von Birgelen C, Hartmann M, Mintz GS, et al: Relationship between cardiovascular risk as predicted by established risk scores versus plaque progression as measured by serial intravascular ultrasound in left main coronary arteries. *Circulation* 2004;110:1579–1585.
57. Baigent C, Keech A, Kearney PM, et al: Efficacy and safety of cholesterol-lowering treatment: prospective meta-analysis of data from 90,056 participants in 14 randomised trials of statins. *Lancet* 2005;366:1267–1278.
58. Schwartz GG, Olsson AG, Ezekowitz MD, et al: Effects of atorvastatin on early recurrent ischemic events in acute coronary syndromes: the MIRACL study: a randomized controlled trial. *JAMA* 2001;285:1711–1718.
59. Athyros VG, Mikhailidis DP, Papageorgiou AA, et al: Effect of atorvastatin on high-density lipoprotein cholesterol and its relationship with coronary events: a subgroup analysis of the GREek Atorvastatin and Coronary-heart-disease Evaluation (GREACE) Study. *Curr Med Res Opin* 2004;20:627–637.
60. Nissen SE, Tuzcu EM, Libby P, et al: Effect of antihypertensive agents on cardiovascular events in patients with coronary disease and normal blood pressure: the CAMELOT study: a randomized controlled trial. *JAMA* 2004;292:2217–2225.
61. Eisen HJ, Tuzcu EM, Dorent R, et al: Everolimus for the prevention of allograft rejection and vasculopathy in cardiac-transplant recipients. *N Engl J Med* 2003;349:847–858.

CHAPTER 35

Noninvasive Imaging Modalities and Atherosclerosis: The Role of Ultrasound

Vijay Nambi and Christie M. Ballantyne

The use of surrogate measures to monitor atherosclerosis, although frequent in clinical trials, has not yet found routine use in clinical practice. The rapid advances in imaging technology combined with the advances in proteomics and genomics will, however, likely lead to a more routine use of imaging in risk assessment, disease monitoring, and "personalizing" medicine in the future. Among the various imaging technologies available, ultrasound represents the safest and the most comfortable modality for any given individual. Here we review the use of external ultrasound in monitoring atherosclerosis.

MONITORING ATHEROSCLEROSIS: CONSIDERATIONS FOR ULTRASOUND IMAGING

Given that atherosclerosis is a disease of the vessel wall, imaging the vessel wall remains the ideal way to track the progression or regression of atherosclerosis. The carotid arteries are well suited for imaging to track the progression of atherosclerosis for several reasons. Because they are superficial and have limited movement,[1] the carotid arteries (especially the common carotid artery) are easy to image noninvasively and provide the possibility of high-quality images with excellent resolution. Also, of the peripheral arteries (i.e., outside of the aorta), the carotid arteries are among the larger in caliber and, therefore, are easier to visualize and analyze. In addition, the carotid bifurcation provides a naturally occurring landmark that can be easily identified for reproducibility. Finally, atherosclerotic deposits in the carotid artery are common.

Measurement of carotid intima–media thickness (CIMT) has been the method of choice for ultrasound monitoring of atherosclerosis. As discussed elsewhere in this book (see Chapter 16), measurement of CIMT has been associated in numerous studies with both coronary and cerebrovascular disease, and with the respective clinical outcomes of myocardial infarction and stroke.[2–7] In addition, CIMT has been used successfully in many studies (reviewed later) as a surrogate to monitor the effect of various therapies on atherosclerosis.

Espeland and colleagues[8] evaluated whether CIMT satisfies criteria to be considered a good surrogate for cardiovascular events, specifically with respect to clinical trials using 3-hydroxy-3-methylglutaryl–coenzyme A reductase inhibitors (statins). Based on their meta-analysis, they concluded that CIMT progression may account for at least some of the treatment effects attributable to statin therapy. Further, they noted that the majority of the criteria for surrogacy that Boissel and coauthors[9] and Prentice[10] established were clearly met for the use of CIMT progression as a surrogate for cardiovascular endpoints in statin trials, although not necessarily in trials of other agents.[8] The U.S. Food and Drug Administration (FDA) has accepted CIMT as a measure to monitor the progression of atherosclerosis in clinical trials.[11]

LIMITATIONS TO THE USE OF CAROTID INTIMA–MEDIA THICKNESS IN ATHEROSCLEROTIC IMAGING

Although CIMT has been used successfully in a number of clinical trials to demonstrate the antiatherosclerotic efficacy of several therapies, several important issues must be considered (Fig. 35-1). Given that the annual change in CIMT is on the order of ~0.01 mm, small errors in measurement can be significant. Also, as with any ultrasound test, measurement of CIMT is highly operator dependent. Several measures, including use of the Meijer's arc (to ensure that repeat measurements are performed at the same angle) and image overlay, are used to limit technician error and improve reproducibility. In addition, several programs for automatic measurement of CIMT have also been developed to limit errors in measurement.

Atherosclerotic deposits occur in the subintimal region, whereas CIMT, as the name suggests, is a measure of both the intima and media of the arterial wall. The intimal layer is thought to contribute only ~2.5% of the IMT in normal arteries, whereas in more diseased arteries, it may contribute only ~20% of the IMT.[12] Hence, diseases that cause medial hypertrophy, such as hypertension, may have a greater influence on IMT progression and not accurately reflect the true atherosclerotic burden. In addition, atherosclerosis may be focal, and the mean CIMT of multiple segments may not reflect the presence of the focal atherosclerotic deposits.

The protocols to measure CIMT have not been well standardized. Clinical trials have used changes in mean CIMT of various segments of the carotid arteries (common, bulb, and internal) alone and in combination as endpoints. Therefore, in interpreting trials that use CIMT, one must always look at the endpoint used and the measurements considered. In addition, although CIMT can be measured from the near and far walls of the carotid arteries, because of technical considerations, the far wall measurements are likely to be more accurate (Fig. 35-2).[13,14] Furthermore, CIMT should be measured consistently in the same phase of the cardiac cycle (diastole) using electrocardiographic gating and/or systolic and diastolic dimensions, because systolic lumen expansion and thinning of the CIMT will occur.[15,16] Other issues to consider include the ultrasound settings such as the gain and the dynamic range.[17] Bots and coworkers[18] concluded that the use of the mean of the maximum CIMT from multiple segments would be the optimal primary endpoint for clinical trials. However, Wikstrand[13] reports that the error in measurement of ten measurements over a 10-mm segment would be less than with one measurement, and that the overall precision would increase when more than one image from an arterial segment is recorded and a mean value is calculated. Wikstrand also suggests that a composite mean of 10-mm sections from the far wall of the common carotid artery and the carotid artery bulb be used as the primary variable of interest.

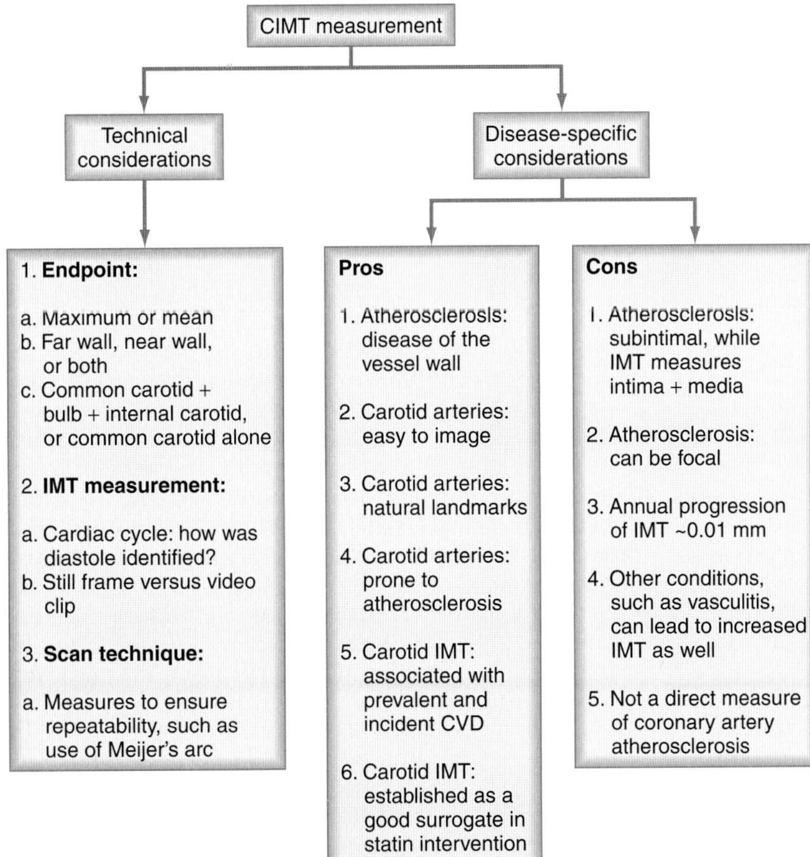

FIGURE 35-1 Considerations in using carotid intima–media thickness (IMT) in clinical trials. CVD, cardiovascular disease.

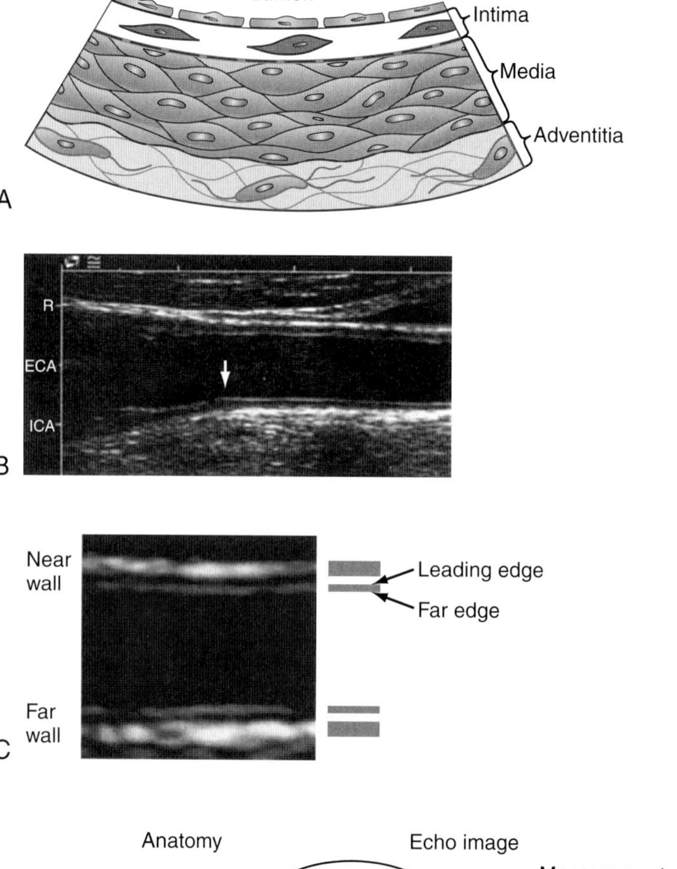

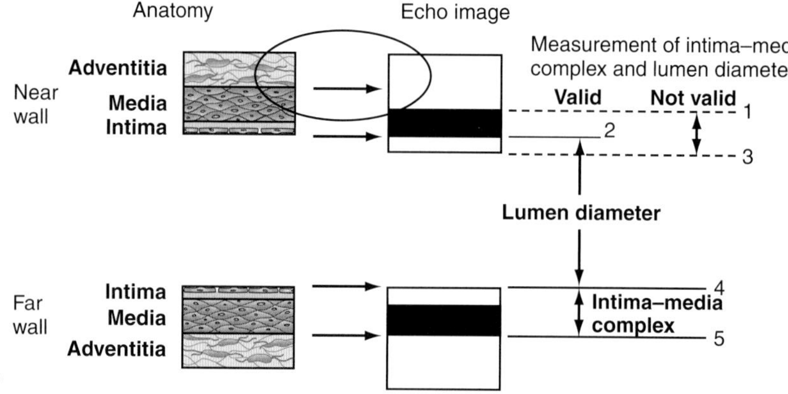

FIGURE 35-2 Ultrasound assessment of the carotid arteries. ***A,*** Arterial wall. ***B,*** Carotid ultrasonogram; *arrow* designates transition from common carotid artery to carotid artery bulb. ***C,*** Leading edge and far edge of near wall intima–lumen interface, common carotid artery segment. ***D,*** Anatomic correlates to echoes from a carotid artery: 1 = far edge of near wall adventitia echo; 2 = leading edge of echo from near wall intima–lumen interface; 3 = far edge of echo from near wall intima–lumen interface; 4 = leading edge of echo from far wall lumen–intima interface; 5 = leading edge of echo from far wall media–adventitia interface. *(Reprinted from Wikstrand,[13] by permission.) ECA, external carotid artery; ICA, internal carotid artery.*

Despite the limitations, CIMT remains a good surrogate to image and track atherosclerosis.

USE OF CAROTID INTIMA–MEDIA THICKNESS IN CLINICAL TRIALS

Since the late 1980s, several trials have used CIMT as the primary endpoint to examine the effect of various therapies that treat risk factors associated with atherosclerosis. Among trials of lipid-lowering therapies, the Cholesterol Lowering Atherosclerosis Study (CLAS) was the first to use CIMT to monitor atherosclerosis.[19] CLAS was a randomized, placebo-controlled trial of colestipol plus niacin in addition to diet in nonsmoking men with previous coronary bypass surgery. In addition to coronary and femoral angiography components, a pilot study of standardized B-mode carotid ultrasound studied 78 individuals who had ultrasound examinations at baseline and at 2 and 4 years. Treatment with colestipol and niacin resulted in the reduction of the CIMT of the far wall of the right common carotid artery (measured using an automated boundary detection program over 120 points); the mean CIMT decreased from 0.65 mm at baseline to 0.60 mm at 4 years in the combination therapy group and increased from 0.61 mm at baseline to 0.66 mm at 4 years in the placebo group. The differences between the active treatment and placebo groups were statistically significant at both 2 and 4 years ($P < 0.0001$). Since then, a number of studies have examined the effects of other lipid-lowering therapies, including statin therapy, on CIMT progression measured in various segments of the carotid arteries.

Trials of Statin Monotherapy

Studies of statins compared with placebo include the Asymptomatic Carotid Artery Progression Study (ACAPS),[20] Pravastatin, Lipids and Atherosclerosis in the

Carotid Arteries (PLAC II),[21] Kuopio Atherosclerosis Prevention Study (KAPS),[22] Monitored Atherosclerosis Regression Study (MARS),[23] Carotid Atherosclerosis Italian Ultrasound Study (CAIUS),[24] Regression Growth Evaluation Statin Study (REGRESS),[25] Long-Term Intervention with Pravastatin in Ischaemic Disease (LIPID) Atherosclerosis Substudy,[26] and the Beta-Blocker Cholesterol-Lowering Asymptomatic Plaque Study (BCAPS).[27]

Whereas most trials of statin monotherapy have found greater benefit on CIMT with statin than placebo (Table 35-1), no benefit was reported in the Cerivastatin in Diabetes (CERDIA) trial,[28] in which 250 patients with type 2 diabetes were randomized to statin (initially cerivastatin 0.4 mg; subsequently changed to simvastatin 20 mg after the withdrawal of cerivastatin from the market) or placebo. At 2 years, no significant difference was found in the primary endpoint of mean common CIMT between treatment groups, although low-density lipoprotein (LDL) cholesterol decreased by 25% in the statin group and increased by 8% in the placebo group. However, a significant reduction was found in cardiovascular events in the statin therapy group, although there were only 14 cardiovascular events in all (2 in the statin group as opposed to 12 in the placebo group; $P = 0.006$).

More recently, the Measuring Effects on Intima–Media Thickness: An Evaluation of Rosuvastatin (METEOR) study[29] enrolled "low-risk" patients who were not candidates for lipid-altering therapy based on the U.S. National Cholesterol Education Program Adult Treatment Panel III (NCEP ATP III) guidelines[30] and had age as the only coronary heart disease (CHD) risk factor or 10-year Framingham risk score less than 10%, increased LDL cholesterol level, and baseline maximum CIMT of 1.2 to 3.5 mm. Patients were randomized in a 5:2 ratio to receive rosuvastatin 40 mg daily or placebo. Over a 2-year period, the primary endpoint of annualized rate of change in maximum CIMT based on all scans performed during the study period from each of the 12 carotid artery sites (near and far walls of the right and left common carotid artery, carotid bulb, and internal carotid artery) was −0.0014 mm/year (95% confidence interval [CI], −0.0041 to 0.0014 mm/year) for the rosuvastatin group versus 0.0131 mm/year (95% CI, 0.0087 to 0.0174 mm/year) for the placebo group ($P < 0.001$). These results suggest that, although statin therapy did not lead to a significant regression of atherosclerosis in these patients with low Framingham risk score, it did lead to a significant reduction in the rate of progression of atherosclerosis (−0.0145 mm [95% CI, −0.0196 to −0.0093]; $P < 0.001$). Among the various prespecified secondary endpoints, the maximum CIMT of the common carotid arteries was significantly reduced (−0.0038 mm/year [95% CI, −0.0064 to −0.0013; $P < 0.001$). The mean LDL cholesterol level attained with rosuvastatin in this study was 78 mg/dL, compared with 152 mg/dL with placebo. Whether significant reductions in LDL cholesterol that retarded the progression of atherosclerosis even in a low risk group translate to clinical benefit will need to be studied carefully in the future.

Overall, these studies consistently showed that statin therapy was superior to placebo in reducing atherosclerotic progression assessed by CIMT. REGRESS, LIPID, and MARS showed significant regression with statin treatment compared with no change or progression in the placebo group, and PLAC II and METEOR showed significantly reduced progression in the mean of the maximum CIMT in the statin group compared with placebo. Meta-analyses of statin trials have suggested that statin therapy is associated with relative reduction in CIMT compared with placebo; Espeland and colleagues[8] reported that CIMT progression was reduced by 0.012 mm/year (95% CI, −0.016 to −0.007 mm/year) with statin therapy (Fig. 35-3).

The effects of two different statins on CIMT were compared in the Atorvastatin versus Simvastatin on

TABLE 35-1 Placebo-Controlled Trials of Statin Monotherapy with Carotid Intima–Media Thickness End Points

Study	Patients	n	Follow-up, Yr	Statin, mg/day	CIMT Measure	Mean CIMT Change, mm/yr		
						Statin	Placebo	*P*
ACAPS[20]	Asymptomatic, moderately increased LDL cholesterol	919	3	Lovastatin 20–40	Mean maximum	−0.009	0.006	0.001
BCAPS[27]	Asymptomatic, moderately increased LDL cholesterol	793	3	Fluvastatin 40	Far wall CCA	0.011	0.036	0.002
CAIUS[24]	Asymptomatic, moderately increased LDL cholesterol	305	3	Pravastatin 40	Mean maximum	−0.0043	0.0089	<0.0007
KAPS[22]	Asymptomatic, increased LDL cholesterol	447	3	Pravastatin 40	CCA, bulb combined	0.017	0.031	0.005
LIPID[26]	CAD, moderately increased LDL cholesterol	522	4	Pravastatin 40	Far wall CCA	−0.014	0.048	<0.0001
MARS[23]	CAD, moderately increased LDL cholesterol	188	2	Lovastatin 20–40	Far wall CCA	−0.038	0.019	<0.001
PLAC II[21]	CAD, increased LDL cholesterol	151	3	Pravastatin 10–40	Mean CCA	0.0295	0.0456	0.03
REGRESS[25]	CAD, moderately increased LDL cholesterol	255	2	Pravastatin 40	CCA, bulb, ICA and femoral combined	−0.05	0	0.0085

From Ref. 1, with permission.

ACAPS, Asymptomatic Carotid Artery Progression Study; BCAPS, Beta-Blocker Cholesterol-Lowering Asymptomatic Plaque Study; CAD, coronary artery disease; CAIUS, Carotid Atherosclerosis Italian Ultrasound Study; CCA, common carotid artery; CIMT, carotid intima-media thickness; FAST, Fukuoka Atherosclerosis Trial; ICA, internal carotid artery; KAPS, Kuopio Atherosclerosis Prevention Study; LDL, low-density lipoprotein; LIPID, Long-Term Intervention with Pravastatin in Ischaemic Disease Atherosclerosis Substudy; MARS, Monitored Atherosclerosis Regression Study; PLAC II, Pravastatin, Lipids and Atherosclerosis in the Carotid Arteries; REGRESS, Regression Growth Evaluation Statin Study.

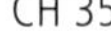

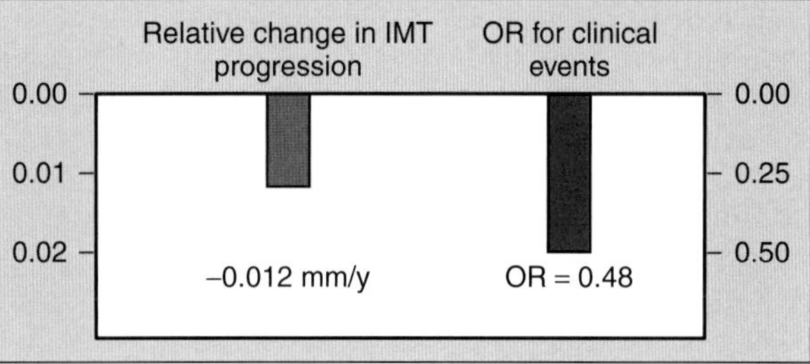

FIGURE 35-3 Relative change in carotid intima–media thickness (CIMT) progression as a surrogate for cardiovascular events: pooled estimate from Asymptomatic Carotid Artery Progression Study (ACAPS),[20] Kuopio Atherosclerosis Prevention Study (KAPS),[22] Pravastatin, Lipids and Atherosclerosis in the Carotid Arteries (PLAC II),[21] Carotid Atherosclerosis Italian Ultrasound Study (CAIUS),[24] Regression Growth Evaluation Statin Study (REGRESS),[25] Beta-Blocker Cholesterol-Lowering Asymptomatic Plaque Study (BCAPS),[27] and Fukuoka Atherosclerosis Trial (FAST).[74] *(Data from Ref. 8.)* OR, odds ratio.

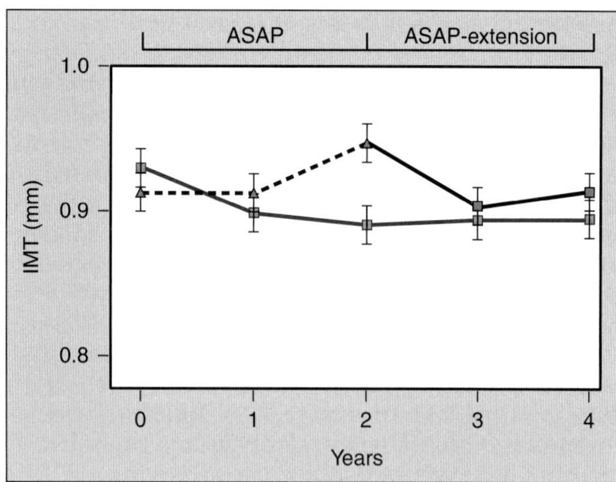

FIGURE 35-4 Changes in intima–media thickness (IMT) (mean ± standard error) in the Atorvastatin versus Simvastatin on Atherosclerosis Progression (ASAP) study extension phase. *Squares* represent atorvastatin; *triangles* represent simvastatin. *(Reprinted from Ref. 32, with permission.)*

Atherosclerosis Progression (ASAP) trial,[31] in which 325 individuals (aged 30–70 years) with heterozygous familial hypercholesterolemia were randomized to receive aggressive lipid-lowering therapy with atorvastatin 80 mg/day or conventional lipid-lowering therapy with simvastatin 40 mg/day. Over a follow-up period of 2 years, the primary endpoint of change in mean CIMT (combined measurements of the common and internal carotid arteries and the carotid bifurcation on both sides) significantly decreased by 0.031 mm in the atorvastatin group (95% CI, −0.007 to −0.055; $P = 0.0017$) but significantly increased by 0.036 mm (95% CI, 0.014 to 0.058; $P = 0.0005$) in the simvastatin group; the difference between the two groups was also significant ($P = 0.0001$). The LDL cholesterol reduction in the atorvastatin group (51%, from 309 mg/dL at baseline to 150 mg/dL at 2 years) was also significantly greater than the LDL cholesterol reduction in the simvastatin group (41%, from 322 to 186 mg/dL; $P = 0.0001$ for the difference between treatment groups).[31] In an extension study of ASAP,[32] 255 of the 280 individuals who completed the ASAP protocol were treated with open-label atorvastatin 80 mg/day and followed for an additional 2 years. At the end of this period, those individuals who were taking atorvastatin in the original ASAP study and continued taking atorvastatin in the extension phase had no change in CIMT (0.89 mm at the start of the extension vs. 0.90 mm at the completion of the extension; $P = 0.57$), whereas those who were taking simvastatin in the original ASAP study and started atorvastatin therapy in the extension phase had significant regression of CIMT (0.95 mm at the start vs. 0.92 mm at the completion of the extension; $P = 0.01$) (Fig. 35-4), suggesting that after maximal therapy with statins, further regression may be difficult to achieve.[32]

The effects of different intensities of statin therapy on CIMT were also examined in the Arterial Biology for the Investigation of the Treatment Effects of Reducing Cholesterol (ARBITER) study,[33] in which 161 individuals with CHD were randomized to receive atorvastatin 80 mg or pravastatin 40 mg. At 12-month follow-up, the primary end point of change in the mean CIMT of the far wall of the common carotid artery indicated regression in the atorvastatin group (−0.034 ± 0.021 mm), whereas CIMT remained stable in the pravastatin group (change of 0.025 ± 0.017 mm). Mean LDL cholesterol was reduced to 76 mg/dL (49% reduction) in the atorvastatin group and to 110 mg/dL (27% reduction) in the pravastatin group. On further analysis,[34] the investigators reported that changes in CIMT were directly related to final LDL cholesterol level on therapy. Individuals with final LDL cholesterol in the lowest quartile (<70 mg/dL) had mean regression (mean CIMT decrease of 0.06 ± 0.17 mm), whereas individuals with final LDL cholesterol in the highest quartile (≥114 mg/dL) had mean progression (mean CIMT increase of 0.06 ± 0.09 mm). Regression was observed in 61% of patients with final LDL cholesterol in the lowest quartile but in only 29% of patients with final LDL cholesterol in the highest quartile. The finding of ARBITER that lower LDL cholesterol level in patients with CHD was associated with improved outcome is consistent with evidence from clinical trials that examined clinical events as the primary end point,[35–39] which led to the updated NCEP ATP III guidelines recommending an optional LDL cholesterol goal of less than 70 mg/dL in individuals at very high risk with CHD or CHD risk equivalent.[40] Overall, based on these trials, it appears that statin therapy arrests or retards the progression of atherosclerosis. In studies that compared different intensities of statin therapy, higher efficacy statins seemed to have the greatest effect.

Trials of Statin Combination Therapy

Other studies have used CIMT to compare the effects of statin monotherapy with those of statin combined with other agents. The effect of adding niacin to statins was compared with that of statin monotherapy in the Arterial Biology for the Investigation of the Treatment Effects of Reducing Cholesterol (ARBITER) 2 study,[41] in which 167 individuals with CHD and high-density lipoprotein (HDL) cholesterol levels less than 45 mg/dL who were already receiving statin therapy were randomized to receive extended-release niacin (1000 mg) or placebo in addition to statin. After 12 months, the group randomized to niacin had a 21% increase in HDL cholesterol and no change in mean common CIMT (0.014 ± 0.104 mm; $P = 0.23$), whereas the mean common CIMT significantly increased in the placebo group (0.044 ± 0.100 mm; $P < 0.001$). However, the change in mean common CIMT was not significantly different ($P = 0.08$) between the two groups. Of the individuals who completed the ARBITER 2 study, 130 consented to participate in the open-label ARBITER 3 study,[42] in which niacin therapy was continued in patients randomized to niacin in ARBITER 2 and initiated in patients randomized to placebo in ARBITER 2. At the completion of this additional 1 year of follow-up, individuals who converted from placebo in ARBITER 2 to niacin therapy in ARBITER 3 ($n = 47$) had significant regression in CIMT (−0.095 ± 0.019; $P < 0.001$ versus during the placebo phase), whereas those who converted from blinded to open-label therapy with niacin ($n = 57$) had further regression in the mean common CIMT (−0.041 ± 0.021; $P < 0.001$). Currently, niacin in combination with statin is being compared with ezetimibe in combination with statin in the ARBITER 6 study.[43]

Another HDL cholesterol–increasing strategy that has been assessed by CIMT in clinical trials in combination with statin therapy is cholesteryl ester transfer protein (CETP) inhibition. The Rating Atherosclerotic Disease Change by Imaging with a New CETP Inhibitor (RADIANCE) studies evaluated the effect of torcetrapib added to atorvastatin on CIMT progression. In RADIANCE 1,[44] 850 patients with heterozygous familial hypercholesterolemia were randomized to either atorvastatin monotherapy (20–80 mg, titrated to reduce LDL cholesterol to goal; mean dose, 56.5 mg) or atorvastatin combined with 60 mg torcetrapib for 2 years. Although combination therapy resulted in significantly greater increases in HDL cholesterol (54% increase vs. 2.5% increase with atorvastatin monotherapy) and significantly greater decreases in LDL cholesterol (14% decrease vs. an increase of 6% with monotherapy), there was no difference in the primary endpoint of yearly change in maximum CIMT for 12 segments (0.0047 ± 0.0028 mm/year vs. 0.0053 ± 0.0028 mm/year with monotherapy; $P = 0.87$ for the difference). The secondary endpoint of annualized change in mean common carotid IMT, however, showed a decrease of 0.0014 mm/year in the atorvastatin-only group, compared with an increase of 0.0038 mm/year in the torcetrapib/atorvastatin group ($P = 0.005$). Furthermore, patients receiving combination therapy had significantly increased incidence of hypertensive adverse events. RADIANCE 2[45] enrolled 752 individuals with mixed dyslipidemia and randomized them to receive 60 mg torcetrapib or placebo added onto baseline therapy with atorvastatin 20 to 80 mg, titrated to reduce LDL cholesterol to NCEP ATP III–established goals based on estimated cardiovascular risk (mean dose, 13.3 mg). Individuals randomized to torcetrapib plus atorvastatin had a 63% increase in HDL cholesterol and an 18% decrease in LDL cholesterol compared with those randomized to placebo plus atorvastatin. However, no change occurred in the primary endpoint of the yearly rate of change in the maximum CIMT for 12 segments: maximum CIMT increased by 0.025 ± 0.005 mm/year in patients receiving torcetrapib with atorvastatin and 0.030 ± 0.005 mm/year in those receiving atorvastatin alone (difference, −0.005 [95% CI, −0.018 to 0.008] mm/year; $P = 0.46$). Patients receiving combination therapy also had significantly greater and significantly more frequent increases in systolic blood pressure. The lack of improvement in CIMT with torcetrapib reported in RADIANCE 1 and RADIANCE 2 was also consistent with the results of the Investigation of Lipid Level Management Using Coronary Ultrasound to Assess Reduction of Atherosclerosis by CETP Inhibition and HDL Elevation (ILLUSTRATE),[46] which did not show a significant difference in CHD progression assessed by coronary intravascular ultrasound between atorvastatin monotherapy or atorvastatin in combination with torcetrapib, and the Investigation of Lipid Level Management to Understand Its Impact in Atherosclerotic Events (ILLUMINATE),[47] in which the addition of torcetrapib to atorvastatin resulted in a significantly increased risk for cardiovascular events (hazard ratio, 1.25 [95% CI, 1.09 to 1.44]; $P = 0.001$) and death (hazard ratio, 1.58 [95% CI, 1.14 to 2.19]; $P = 0.006$), leading to early termination of the study and discontinuation of development of torcetrapib.

Ezetimibe was combined with statin therapy in the Ezetimibe and Simvastatin in Hypercholesterolemia Enhances Atherosclerosis Regression study (ENHANCE),[48] in which 2-year change in the mean CIMT of the far walls of the left and right common carotid arteries, carotid bulbs, and internal carotid arteries was compared in 720 patients with familial hypercholesterolemia randomized to receive simvastatin 80 mg alone or the combination of simvastatin 80 mg plus ezetimibe 10 mg. Although LDL cholesterol reduction (56% in combination therapy vs. 39% with simvastatin monotherapy) and C-reactive protein reduction were significantly greater with combination therapy, the primary endpoint of mean change in CIMT was not different between treatment groups. The mean CIMT at baseline was 0.70 ± 0.13 in the simvastatin monotherapy arm and 0.69 ± 0.13 in the simvastatin + ezetimibe arm. At the end of the study period, the mean CIMT increased by 0.0058 ± 0.0037 mm in the simvastatin group and 0.0111 ± 0.0038 mm in the combined therapy group; the difference between the two groups was not statistically different ($P = 0.29$). This study generated controversy because despite greater reductions in LDL cholesterol and C-reactive protein, there was no difference in CIMT between the two groups, calling into question the effectiveness of ezetimibe and also raising questions about the use of surrogate markers. Although the actual answer as to why there was not a greater response to the combination therapy may not be known until the results of the clinical outcomes trial Improved Reduction of Outcomes: Vytorin Efficacy International Trial (IMPROVE IT)[49] are published, several important factors should be considered. First, the *patient population enrolled* should be considered. The baseline CIMT was less than in prior studies in individuals with familial hypercholesterolemia such as ASAP (Table 35-2), ~80% of ENHANCE patients were already receiving statin therapy at baseline, and there was little progression in the control group with simvastatin 80 mg. Interestingly, a previous study in patients with heterozygous familial hypercholesterolemia that also used simvastatin 80 mg but included patients with a much thicker CIMT showed significant regression; mean combined far wall IMT of

TABLE 35-2 Differences between Atorvastatin versus Simvastatin on Atherosclerosis Progression and Ezetimibe and Simvastatin in Hypercholesterolemia Enhances Atherosclerosis Regression Trials

	ASAP[31]		ENHANCE[48]	
	Atorvastatin	Simvastatin	Simvastatin	Simvastatin + Ezetimibe
Baseline TC, mg/dL (mean ± SD)	386 ± 72	397 ± 81	400 ± 68	400 ± 68
Baseline LDL cholesterol, mg/dL (mean ± SD)	309 ± 71	322 ± 78	318 ± 66	319 ± 65
Baseline HDL cholesterol, mg/dL (mean ± SD)	46 ± 12	45 ± 11	47 ± 13	47 ± 11
Change in LDL cholesterol, %	−50.5	−41.2	−39.1	−55.6
Change HDL cholesterol, %	13.2	13.4	7.8	10.2
Prior statin use, %	71	71	82	81
Baseline CIMT, mm (Mean ± SD)				
Composite*	0.93 ± 0.20	0.92 ± 0.18	0.70 ± 0.13	0.69 ± 0.13
CCA	0.86 ± 0.16	0.87 ± 0.18	0.68 ± 0.16	0.67 ± 0.16
ICA	0.84 ± 0.37	0.82 ± 0.29	0.61 ± 0.17	0.62 ± 0.17
Bulb	1.09 ± 0.32	1.07 ± 0.26	0.80 ± 0.20	0.79 ± 0.22
Difference in CIMT between Baseline and 24 Months, mm				
	Mean Change (95% CI)		*Least-Square Mean ± SE*	
Composite*	−0.031 (−0.055 to −0.007)	0.036 (0.014 to 0.058)	0.0058 ± 0.0037	0.0111 ± 0.0038
CCA	−0.041 (−0.062 to −0.020)	−0.018 (−0.034 to 0.002)	0.0024 ± 0.0043	0.0019 ± 0.0044
ICA	−0.032 (−0.082 to −0.018)	0.088 (0.002 to 0.174)	−0.0007 ± 0.0064	0.0099 ± 0.0065
Bulb	−0.022 (−0.062 to 0.018)	0.062 (0.026 to 0.098)	0.0062 ± 0.0069	0.0144 ± 0.0070

*ASAP: distal portion of anterior and posterior wall of CCA, anterior and posterior wall of carotid bifurcation, proximal portion of posterior wall of ICA; ENHANCE: right and left CCA, carotid bulbs, and ICA.

ASAP, Atorvastatin versus Simvastatin on Atherosclerosis Progression; CCA, common carotid artery; CI, confidence interval; CIMT, carotid intima-media thickness; ENHANCE, Ezetimibe and Simvastatin in Hypercholesterolemia Enhances Atherosclerosis Regression; HDL, high-density lipoprotein; ICA, internal carotid artery; LDL cholesterol, low-density lipoprotein cholesterol; SD, standard deviation; SE, standard error; TC, total cholesterol.

the carotid and femoral arteries decreased from 1.07 mm (95% CI, 1.05 to 1.09 mm) at baseline to 0.99 mm (95% CI, 0.97 to 1.01 mm) at 2 years, representing a 0.081-mm regression (95% CI for the difference −0.109 to −0.053 mm).[50] Thus, it may be more difficult to show benefit of therapy and in particular regression of atherosclerosis if CIMT is close to normal and not thick at baseline. The second factor to be considered is *technical issues.* CIMT measurements in ENHANCE used single-frame images rather than video clips, which can potentially increase errors in the CIMT measurement because the image analyzer is dependent on the technologist and the image provided to him/her; no electrocardiographic gating was used, which is important in helping to identify diastole ("R" wave of the electrocardiographic tracing), although M-mode use allowed for identification of diastole. The third factor to consider is *failure of therapy.* It is possible that incremental LDL cholesterol lowering with ezetimibe does not provide the additional clinical benefit expected with further LDL cholesterol lowering. In summary, the patient population tested, technical considerations relevant to measurement of IMT, the amount of disease and progression in the comparator groups, and the incremental efficacy of therapy compared with usual care must all be considered in designing and interpreting clinical trials with CIMT as the primary endpoint.

Trials of Other Agents

In addition to statin therapy, other lipid-regulating agents have been studied for their effects on CIMT. Bezafibrate was compared with placebo in 164 patients with diabetes and no known cardiovascular disease in the St. Mary's, Ealing, Northwick Park Diabetes Cardiovascular Disease Prevention (SENDCAP) study.[51] The primary endpoint of change in the mean of the maximum CIMT at 3-year follow-up was not significantly different between treatment groups, although the bezafibrate group had significantly greater improvements in total cholesterol (−7% vs. −0.3%), HDL cholesterol (6% vs. −2%), and triglycerides (−32% vs. 4%) than placebo and fewer cardiovascular events, although, like in CERDIA, the number of events were small. The change in LDL cholesterol was not significantly different between treatment groups (−9.6% with bezafibrate vs. 0.6% with placebo; $P = 0.06$).

The effect on CIMT of therapies that treat other risk factors associated with atherosclerosis have also been examined, including therapies for diabetes,[52–62] hypertension,[27,63–71] and antiplatelet therapies.[72]

Recently, Howard and coauthors[73] reported the results of an open-label, blinded-to-endpoint 3-year trial in which 499 American Indian men and women older than 40 years with diabetes and no prior cardiovascular events were randomized to receive aggressive therapy, with an

LDL cholesterol target level of ≤70 mg/dL (statin therapy followed by ezetimibe if needed) and a systolic blood pressure target of ≤115 mm Hg, or to receive conventional therapy, with an LDL cholesterol target level of ≤100 mg/dL and target systolic blood pressure of ≤130 mm Hg. The primary endpoint of progression of atherosclerosis measured by mean common CIMT indicated regression in the aggressive therapy group and progression in the conventional therapy group (−0.012 vs. 0.038 mm, respectively; $P < 0.001$), suggesting that more aggressive LDL cholesterol and blood pressure targets may arrest atherosclerosis in American Indians with diabetes. However, although the combined reduction of LDL cholesterol and systolic blood pressure likely contributed to the regression of CIMT, the relative contribution of each these parameters is not known. Although several therapies have been shown to regress/stabilize CIMT, the critical aspect to consider is whether this stabilization of carotid atherosclerosis translates into a reduction in cardiovascular morbidity and mortality.

Association of Carotid Intima–Media Thickness and Clinical Events in Clinical Trials

Although, as noted earlier, CIMT has been associated with cardiovascular events in observational epidemiologic studies,[2–7] only limited information is available on the relation of CIMT changes and incident cardiovascular events in interventional trials. Trials with CIMT as the primary endpoint are not designed specifically to detect statistically significant differences in clinical events, which generally requires larger study populations and longer follow-up. However, a number of trials have reported improvements in both CIMT and cardiovascular events with statin therapy (ACAPS,[20] PLAC II,[21] REGRESS,[25] BCAPS,[27] CERDIA,[28] KAPS,[22] CAIUS,[24] Fukuoka Atherosclerosis Trial [FAST][74]).

The relation between CIMT and coronary events was examined in long-term follow-up (8.8 years) from CLAS,[75] in which each 0.03-mm/year increase in CIMT for the entire study population was associated with relative risks of 2.2 (95% CI, 1.4 to 3.6) for nonfatal myocardial infarction or coronary death and 3.1 (95% CI, 2.1 to 4.5) for any coronary event (nonfatal myocardial infarction, coronary death, or coronary revascularization). In addition to change in CIMT, the absolute CIMT at 2 years was also associated with clinical coronary events. Incidence of nonfatal myocardial infarction, coronary death, and coronary artery revascularization was reduced in the group assigned to colestipol and niacin therapy ($P = 0.01$; relative risk, 0.41); however, this relationship was lost ($P > 0.2$; relative risk, 1.1) when the on-study (end of trial) CIMT progression was included in the model.

Espeland and colleagues[8] concluded, based on a meta-analysis of seven statin trials with both CIMT and clinical event outcomes, that statin therapy was associated with an average reduction in CIMT of 0.012 mm/year (95% CI, −0.016 to −0.007) compared with placebo, and that in these trials there was a significant reduction in the odds for a cardiovascular event (odds ratio, 0.46 [95% CI, 0.30 to 0.78)] for patients receiving statin therapy (see Fig. 35-3). They further observed that when IMT progression was added as a covariate to the regression models, the relative odds ratio for cardiovascular events increased to 0.64 and was not statistically significant ($P = 0.13$), suggesting that changes in IMT explained, in part, the effect of statins on cardiovascular events.

Similarly, Amarenco and coworkers[76] performed a meta-analysis and examined the effect of statins on stroke and CIMT. They reported that the stroke reduction effect of statins was closely related to the LDL cholesterol lowering. Each 10% reduction of LDL cholesterol was shown to be associated with ~15% reduction in stroke (95% CI, 6.7 to 23.6) and a 0.73% per year reduction in CIMT (95% CI, 0.27 to 1.19). They also noted a strong correlation between LDL cholesterol lowering and CIMT reduction ($r = 0.65$; $P = 0.004$) (Fig. 35-5).

BEYOND CAROTID INTIMA–MEDIA THICKNESS

Presence of plaque on a carotid ultrasound examination has been associated with traditional cardiovascular risk factors including age, systolic blood pressure, use of tobacco, ratio of total cholesterol to HDL cholesterol, and body mass index or weight.[77–82] Studies have also shown that the presence of plaque in the carotid artery is associated with the presence of CHD[83,84] and with incident myocardial infarction or cardiovascular death.[85–92]

Although the presence of plaque is strongly associated with CIMT,[77,93] some individuals who have "thinner" CIMT have plaque, and some individuals have "thick" CIMT without plaque. It is thought that "thick" CIMT may be a precursor for plaque development, and although this is most likely the case, conditions such as vasculitis may lead to increased CIMT without being related to the process of atherosclerosis. In contrast, atherosclerotic plaque, as the name implies, is related solely to atherosclerosis. However, the definition of plaque is not standardized. Some studies have classified plaque as a focal widening relative to adjacent segments with protrusion into the lumen,[85–87] whereas

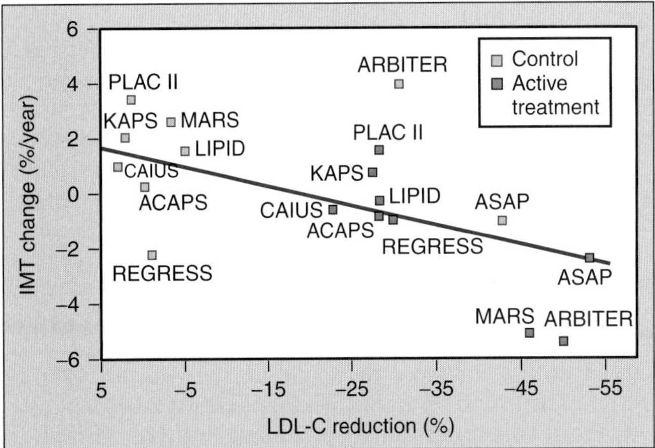

FIGURE 35-5 Relationship between low-density lipoprotein cholesterol (LDL-C) reduction and intima–media thickness (IMT) change. *(Reprinted from Ref. 76, with permission.)*

others have used CIMT values (e.g., >1.5 mm) to define plaque.[92] Furthermore, other issues such as calcification in the plaque, which renders plaque difficult to image with ultrasound, and plaque eccentricity, which requires evaluation at multiple angles to image plaque adequately, must be considered.[94] However, the relatively greater annual change in plaque area[12,95] may allow for recruitment of individuals with more rapid progression, and the possibility of plaque characterization may provide additional parameters for evaluation in clinical trials.

Quantification of plaque volume using three-dimensional (3-D) reconstruction of ultrasound images has been performed by some investigators[92,96,97] and may permit investigators to study the effect of therapies on plaque volume rather than on the thickness of the carotid artery, although this can be challenging. The recent introduction of real-time 3-D imaging may allow for more accurate estimation of plaque volume. The real-time 3-D transducer has a motor incorporated within it that allows the computer to calculate the exact distance and time of sweep, allowing for accurate rendering of the 3-D images. Furthermore, it will allow superior visualization of the data by permitting visualization in orthogonal planes.

Attempts at plaque characterization using ultrasound dates back to the mid 1980s, when plaque was identified as homogeneous or heterogeneous.[98,99] Subsequently, suggestions were made that echogenicity of a plaque should be standardized against three reference structures: flowing blood for anechogenicity, sternocleidomastoid muscle for isoechogenicity, and the adjacent transverse apophysis of the cervical vertebrae or the bright far wall media–adventitia interface for hyperechogenicity.[100,101] Anechogenic plaques are thought to represent either necrotic or hemorrhagic lesions, whereas echogenic appearance of the plaque represents a predominantly fibrotic tissue. However, such characterization had a high rate of interoperator and intraoperator variability.[102] Integrated backscatter signals have been used to characterize plaque components.[103–106]

Other methods to characterize plaque have included the use of computer-aided analysis,[107] a more operator-independent assessment of plaque that resulted in the estimation of the grayscale median, which is the frequency distribution of gray values of the pixels within the plaque that are used as the measure of echogenicity. Comparisons between the different instruments were initially difficult because of the different settings but have since been improved by normalizing images by using digital image processing and by using blood and adventitia as references.[107] Although such characterization correlated closely with clinical symptoms in some studies, the correlation with histology has not been consistent.[108–112] This is likely because conventional 2-D techniques are not very accurate because they are limited to a subjective selection of a particular ultrasound image that needs to be representative of the plaque structure.[113] A stratified grayscale median measurement combined with color mapping was shown to correlate well with histopathologic components; however, the study was performed in only 28 patients with stroke.[114] The use of the more accurate ultrasound imaging that is now available may enable further improvements in characterization of plaque.

Another advancement in ultrasound-based analysis of atherosclerosis is the use of contrast agents. Ultrasonic contrast agents are microbubbles of gas that are enveloped by a shell of various substances such as albumin and lipid polymer, and are strong reflectors of acoustic energy. These contrast agents have been shown to improve the resolution of both the near wall and far wall in CIMT measurement,[115,116] and have been described to identify plaque vasa vasorum, a marker of plaque instability.[117] Another potential use of ultrasound contrast that is being actively evaluated is the noninvasive imaging of molecular or cellular processes. Because the ultrasound contrast bubbles are pure intravascular tracers, novel contrast agents that target events that are important in the pathophysiology of atherosclerosis, such as inflammation, thrombus formation, and angiogenesis, have been developed and are being studied.[118] The same approach may also provide a method for effective drug delivery. Although recent FDA "black box warnings" about potential side effects of contrast agents may limit their immediate use in clinical trials, further advances and additional data may enable the use of contrast-enhanced ultrasound to monitor atherosclerosis in the future.

SUMMARY

CIMT has been used effectively as a surrogate marker to monitor the progression of atherosclerosis and to monitor the effect of various antiatherosclerosis therapies. However, several key issues should be considered in using CIMT as a surrogate, including the method used in the measurement of CIMT, the primary endpoint, and the population studied. Overall, currently, it seems that the far wall of the common carotid artery may be the most reliable segment to track. Future advances will likely focus on improving our ability to estimate plaque volume and characterize plaque morphology.

CONCLUSION

Ultrasound imaging is the safest and most comfortable imaging modality available. It has been used effectively and reliably in clinical trials to monitor progression of atherosclerosis. Currently, ultrasound may be useful in improving risk assessment in "intermediate-risk" patients[119] (see Chapter 16). Despite limitations, advancements in technology and standardization of protocols will improve the utility of ultrasound in clinical trials and perhaps in clinical practice in the future.

REFERENCES

1. Bots ML: Carotid intima–media thickness as a surrogate marker for cardiovascular disease in intervention studies. *Curr Med Res Opin* 2006;22:2181–2190.
2. Chambless LE, Heiss G, Folsom AR, et al: Association of coronary heart disease incidence with carotid arterial wall thickness and major risk factors: The Atherosclerosis Risk in Communities (ARIC) Study, 1987-1993. *Am J Epidemiol* 1997;146:483–494.

3. Bots ML, Hoes AW, Koudstaal PJ, et al: Common carotid intima–media thickness and risk of stroke and myocardial infarction: The Rotterdam Study. *Circulation* 1997;96:1432–1437.
4. O'Leary DH, Polak JF, Kronmal RA, et al; Cardiovascular Health Study Collaborative Research Group: carotid-artery intima and media thickness as a risk factor for myocardial infarction and stroke in older adults. *N Engl J Med* 1999;340:14–22.
5. Chambless LE, Folsom AR, Clegg LX, et al: Carotid wall thickness is predictive of incident clinical stroke: The Atherosclerosis Risk in Communities (ARIC) study. *Am J Epidemiol* 2000;151: 478–487.
6. del Sol AI, Moons KG, Hollander M, et al: Is carotid intima–media thickness useful in cardiovascular disease risk assessment? *The Rotterdam Study. Stroke* 2001;32:1532–1538.
7. Lorenz MW, Markus HS, Bots ML, et al: Prediction of clinical cardiovascular events with carotid intima–media thickness: a systematic review and meta-analysis. *Circulation* 2007;115: 459–467.
8. Espeland MA, O'Leary DH, Terry JG, et al: Carotid intimal–media thickness as a surrogate for cardiovascular disease events in trials of HMG-CoA reductase inhibitors. *Curr Control Trials Cardiovasc Med* 2005;6:3.
9. Boissel JP, Collet JP, Moleur P, Haugh M: Surrogate endpoints: a basis for a rational approach. *Eur J Clin Pharmacol* 1992;43: 235–244.
10. Prentice RL: Surrogate endpoints in clinical trials: definition and operational criteria. *Stat Med* 1989;8:431–440.
11. Black DM: Documenting regression of atherosclerosis: practical approaches in drug development. *Am J Cardiol* 2002;89:1B–3B.
12. Spence JD: Ultrasound measurement of carotid plaque as a surrogate outcome for coronary artery disease. *Am J Cardiol* 2002;89:10B–16B.
13. Wikstrand J: Methodological considerations of ultrasound measurement of carotid artery intima–media thickness and lumen diameter. *Clin Physiol Funct Imaging* 2007;27:341–345.
14. Roman MJ, Naqvi TZ, Gardin JM, et al: Clinical application of noninvasive vascular ultrasound in cardiovascular risk stratification: a report from the American Society of Echocardiography and the Society of Vascular Medicine and Biology. *J Am Soc Echocardiogr* 2006;19:943–954.
15. Devereux RB, Waeber B, Roman MJ: Conclusions on the measurement of arterial wall thickness: anatomic, physiologic and methodologic considerations. *J Hypertens Suppl* 1992;10:S119–S121.
16. Tardy Y, Hayoz D, Mignot JP, et al: Dynamic non-invasive measurements of arterial diameter and wall thickness. *J Hypertens Suppl* 1992;10:S105–S109.
17. Potter K, Reed CJ, Green DJ, et al: Ultrasound settings significantly alter arterial lumen and wall thickness measurements. *Cardiovasc Ultrasound* 2008;6:6.
18. Bots ML, Evans GW, Riley WA, Grobbee DE: Carotid intima–media thickness measurements in intervention studies: design options, progression rates, and sample size considerations: a point of view. *Stroke* 2003;34:2985–2994.
19. Blankenhorn DH, Selzer RH, Crawford DW, et al: Beneficial effects of colestipol–niacin therapy on the common carotid artery: Two- and four-year reduction of intima–media thickness measured by ultrasound. *Circulation* 1993;88:20–28.
20. Furberg CD, Adams HP Jr, Applegate WB, et al; for the Asymptomatic Carotid Artery Progression Study (ACAPS) Research Group: Effect of lovastatin on early carotid atherosclerosis and cardiovascular events. *Circulation* 1994;90:1679–1687.
21. Crouse JR III, Byington RP, Bond MG, et al: Pravastatin, lipids, and atherosclerosis in the carotid arteries (PLAC-II). *Am J Cardiol* 1995;75:455–459.
22. Salonen R, Nyyssonen K, Porkkala E, et al: Kuopio Atherosclerosis Prevention Study (KAPS): a population-based primary preventive trial of the effect of LDL lowering on atherosclerotic progression in carotid and femoral arteries. *Circulation* 1995;92:1758–1764.
23. Hodis HN, Mack WJ, LaBree L, et al: Reduction in carotid arterial wall thickness using lovastatin and dietary therapy: a randomized controlled clinical trial. *Ann Intern Med* 1996;124:548–556.
24. Mercuri M, Bond MG, Sirtori CR, et al: Pravastatin reduces carotid intima–media thickness progression in an asymptomatic hypercholesterolemic Mediterranean population: The Carotid Atherosclerosis Italian Ultrasound Study. *Am J Med* 1996;101: 627–634.
25. de Groot E, Jukema JW, Montauban van Swijndregt AD, et al: B-mode ultrasound assessment of pravastatin treatment effect on carotid and femoral artery walls and its correlations with coronary arteriographic findings: a report of the Regression Growth Evaluation Statin Study (REGRESS). *J Am Coll Cardiol* 1998;31:1561–1567.
26. MacMahon S, Sharpe N, Gamble G, et al; on behalf of the LIPID Trial Research Group: Effects of lowering average of below-average cholesterol levels on the progression of carotid atherosclerosis: results of the LIPID Atherosclerosis Substudy. *Circulation* 1998;97:1784–1790.
27. Hedblad B, Wikstrand J, Janzon L, et al: Low-dose metoprolol CR/XL and fluvastatin slow progression of carotid intima–media thickness: main results from the Beta-Blocker Cholesterol-Lowering Asymptomatic Plaque Study (BCAPS). *Circulation* 2001;103:1721–1726.
28. Beishuizen ED, van de Ree MA, Jukema JW, et al: Two-year statin therapy does not alter the progression of intima–media thickness in patients with type 2 diabetes without manifest cardiovascular disease. *Diabetes Care* 2004;27:2887–2892.
29. Crouse JR 3rd, Raichlen JS, Riley WA, et al: Effect of rosuvastatin on progression of carotid intima–media thickness in low-risk individuals with subclinical atherosclerosis: The METEOR Trial. *JAMA* 2007;297:1344–1353.
30. Expert Panel on Detection, Evaluation, and Treatment of High Blood Cholesterol in Adults. Executive summary of the third report of the National Cholesterol Education Program (NCEP) Expert Panel on Detection, Evaluation, and Treatment of High Blood Cholesterol in Adults (Adult Treatment Panel III). *JAMA* 2001;285:2486–2497.
31. Smilde TJ, van Wissen S, Wollersheim H, et al: Effect of aggressive versus conventional lipid lowering on atherosclerosis progression in familial hypercholesterolaemia (ASAP): a prospective, randomised, double-blind trial. *Lancet* 2001;357:577–581.
32. van Wissen S, Smilde TJ, Trip MD, et al: Long-term safety and efficacy of high-dose atorvastatin treatment in patients with familial hypercholesterolemia. *Am J Cardiol* 2005;95:264–266.
33. Taylor AJ, Kent SM, Flaherty PJ, et al: ARBITER: Arterial Biology for the Investigation of the Treatment Effects of Reducing Cholesterol: a randomized trial comparing the effects of atorvastatin and pravastatin on carotid intima medial thickness. *Circulation* 2002;106:2055–2060.
34. Kent SM, Coyle LC, Flaherty PJ, et al: Marked low-density lipoprotein cholesterol reduction below current National Cholesterol Education Program targets provides the greatest reduction in carotid atherosclerosis. *Clin Cardiol* 2004;27:17–21.
35. Heart Protection Study Collaborative Group: MRC/BHF Heart Protection Study of cholesterol lowering with simvastatin in 20 536 high-risk individuals: a randomised placebo-controlled trial. *Lancet* 2002;360:7–22.
36. Shepherd J, Blauw GJ, Murphy MB, et al: Pravastatin in elderly individuals at risk of vascular disease (PROSPER): a randomised controlled trial. *Lancet* 2002;360:1623–1630.
37. Sever PS, Dahlof B, Poulter NR, et al; for the ASCOT Investigators: Prevention of coronary and stroke events with atorvastatin in hypertensive patients who have average or lower-than-average cholesterol concentrations, in the Anglo-Scandinavian Cardiac Outcomes Trial—Lipid Lowering Arm (ASCOT-LLA): a multicentre randomised controlled trial. *Lancet* 2003;361:1149–1158.
38. Cannon CP, Braunwald E, McCabe CH, et al; for the Pravastatin or Atorvastatin Evaluation and Infection Therapy–Thrombolysis in Myocardial Infarction 22 Investigators: Comparison of intensive and moderate lipid lowering with statins after acute coronary syndromes. *N Engl J Med* 2004;350:1495–1504.
39. LaRosa JC, Grundy SM, Waters DD; for the Treating to New Targets (TNT) Investigators: Intensive lipid lowering with atorvastatin in patients with stable coronary disease. *N Engl J Med* 2005;352:1425–1435.
40. Grundy SM, Cleeman JI, Bairey Merz CN, et al; for the Coordinating Committee of the National Cholesterol Education Program: Implications of recent clinical trials for the National Cholesterol Education Program Adult Treatment Panel III guidelines. *Circulation* 2004;110:227–239.
41. Taylor AJ, Sullenberger LE, Lee HJ, et al: Arterial Biology for the Investigation of the Treatment Effects of Reducing Cholesterol (ARBITER) 2: a double-blind, placebo-controlled study of extended-release niacin on atherosclerosis progression in

secondary prevention patients treated with statins. *Circulation* 2004;110:3512–3517.
42. Taylor AJ, Lee HJ, Sullenberger LE: The effect of 24 months of combination statin and extended-release niacin on carotid intima–media thickness: ARBITER 3. *Curr Med Res Opin* 2006;22:2243–2250.
43. Devine PJ, Turco MA, Taylor AJ: Design and rationale of the ARBITER 6 trial (Arterial Biology for the Investigation of the Treatment Effects of Reducing Cholesterol)-6-HDL and LDL Treatment Strategies in Atherosclerosis (HALTS). *Cardiovasc Drugs Ther* 2007;21:221–225.
44. Kastelein JJ, van Leuven SI, Burgess L, et al; for the RADIANCE 1 Investigators: Effect of torcetrapib on carotid atherosclerosis in familial hypercholesterolemia. *N Engl J Med* 2007;356:1620–1630.
45. Bots ML, Visseren FL, Evans GW, et al; for the RADIANCE 2 Investigators: Torcetrapib and carotid intima–media thickness in mixed dyslipidaemia (RADIANCE 2 study): a randomised, double-blind trial. *Lancet* 2007;370:153–160.
46. Nissen SE, Tardif JC, Nicholls SJ, et al; for the ILLUSTRATE Investigators: Effect of torcetrapib on the progression of coronary atherosclerosis. *N Engl J Med* 2007;356:1304–1316.
47. Barter PJ, Caulfield M, Eriksson M, et al; for the ILLUMINATE Investigators: Effects of torcetrapib in patients at high risk for coronary events. *N Engl J Med* 2007;357:2109–2122.
48. Kastelein JJ, Akdim F, Stroes ES, et al: Simvastatin with or without ezetimibe in familial hypercholesterolemia. *N Engl J Med* 2008;358:1431–1443.
49. IMPROVE-IT: Examining outcomes in subjects with acute coronary syndrome: vytorin (ezetimibe/simvastatin) vs simvastatin (study P04103). Available at: http://clinicaltrials.gov/ct/show/NCT00202878. Accessed November 8, 2006.
50. Nolting PR, de Groot E, Zwinderman AH, et al: Regression of carotid and femoral artery intima–media thickness in familial hypercholesterolemia: treatment with simvastatin. *Arch Intern Med* 2003;163:1837–1841.
51. Elkeles RS, Diamond JR, Poulter C, et al: Cardiovascular outcomes in type 2 diabetes: a double-blind placebo-controlled study of bezafibrate: The St. Mary's, Ealing, Northwick Park Diabetes Cardiovascular Disease Prevention (SENDCAP) Study. *Diabetes Care* 1998;21:641–648.
52. Yokoyama H, Katakami N, Yamasaki Y: Recent advances of intervention to inhibit progression of carotid intima–media thickness in patients with type 2 diabetes mellitus. *Stroke* 2006;37:2420–2427.
53. Langenfeld MR, Forst T, Hohberg C, et al: Pioglitazone decreases carotid intima–media thickness independently of glycemic control in patients with type 2 diabetes mellitus: results from a controlled randomized study. *Circulation* 2005;111:2525–2531.
54. Yamasaki Y, Katakami N, Hayaishi-Okano R, et al: α-Glucosidase inhibitor reduces the progression of carotid intima–media thickness. *Diabetes Res Clin Pract* 2005;67:204–210.
55. Katakami N, Yamasaki Y, Hayaishi-Okano R, et al: Metformin or gliclazide, rather than glibenclamide, attenuate progression of carotid intima–media thickness in subjects with type 2 diabetes. *Diabetologia* 2004;47:1906–1913.
56. Esposito K, Giugliano D, Nappo F, Marfella R: Regression of carotid atherosclerosis by control of postprandial hyperglycemia in type 2 diabetes mellitus. *Circulation* 2004;110:214–219.
57. Hanefeld M, Chiasson JL, Koehler C, et al: Acarbose slows progression of intima–media thickness of the carotid arteries in subjects with impaired glucose tolerance. *Stroke* 2004;35:1073–1078.
58. Mazzone T, Meyer PM, Feinstein SB, et al: Effect of pioglitazone compared with glimepiride on carotid intima–media thickness in type 2 diabetes: a randomized trial. *JAMA* 2006;296:2572–2581.
59. Satoh N, Ogawa Y, Usui T, et al: Antiatherogenic effect of pioglitazone in type 2 diabetic patients irrespective of the responsiveness to its antidiabetic effect. *Diabetes Care* 2003;26:2493–2499.
60. Koshiyama H, Shimono D, Kuwamura N, et al: Rapid communication: inhibitory effect of pioglitazone on carotid arterial wall thickness in type 2 diabetes. *J Clin Endocrinol Metab* 2001;86:3452–3456.
61. Minamikawa J, Tanaka S, Yamauchi M, et al: Potent inhibitory effect of troglitazone on carotid arterial wall thickness in type 2 diabetes. *J Clin Endocrinol Metab* 1998;83:1818–1820.
62. Hodis HN, Mack WJ, Zheng L, et al: Effect of peroxisome proliferator-activated receptor γ agonist treatment on subclinical atherosclerosis in patients with insulin-requiring type 2 diabetes. *Diabetes Care* 2006;29:1545–1553.
63. Pontremoli R, Viazzi F, Ravera M, et al: Long term effect of nifedipine GITS and lisinopril on subclinical organ damage in patients with essential hypertension. *J Nephrol* 2001;14:19–26.
64. Simon A, Gariepy J, Moyse D, Levenson J: Differential effects of nifedipine and co-amilozide on the progression of early carotid wall changes. *Circulation* 2001;103:2949–2954.
65. Terpstra WF, May JF, Smit AJ, et al: Effects of nifedipine on carotid and femoral arterial wall thickness in previously untreated hypertensive patients. *Blood Press Suppl* 2003;1:22–29.
66. Borhani NO, Mercuri M, Borhani PA, et al: Final outcome results of the Multicenter Isradipine Diuretic Atherosclerosis Study (MIDAS): a randomized controlled trial. *JAMA* 1996;276:785–791.
67. Hosomi N, Mizushige K, Ohyama H, et al: Angiotensin-converting enzyme inhibition with enalapril slows progressive intima–media thickening of the common carotid artery in patients with non-insulin-dependent diabetes mellitus. *Stroke* 2001;32:1539–1545.
68. Zanchetti A, Crepaldi G, Bond MG, et al: Different effects of antihypertensive regimens based on fosinopril or hydrochlorothiazide with or without lipid lowering by pravastatin on progression of asymptomatic carotid atherosclerosis: Principal results of PHYLLIS—a randomized double-blind trial. *Stroke* 2004;35:2807–2812.
69. Uchiyama-Tanaka Y, Mori Y, Kishimoto N, et al: Comparison of the effects of quinapril and losartan on carotid artery intima–media thickness in patients with mild-to-moderate arterial hypertension. *Kidney Blood Press Res* 2005;28:111–116.
70. MacMahon S, Sharpe N, Gamble G, et al; for the PART-2 Collaborative Research Group: Randomized, placebo-controlled trial of the angiotensin-converting enzyme inhibitor, ramipril, in patients with coronary or other occlusive arterial disease. *J Am Coll Cardiol* 2000;36:438–443.
71. Daskalopoulou SS, Daskalopoulos ME, Perrea D, et al: Carotid artery atherosclerosis: what is the evidence for drug action? *Curr Pharm Des* 2007;13:1141–1159.
72. Kodama M, Yamasaki Y, Sakamoto K, et al: Antiplatelet drugs attenuate progression of carotid intima–media thickness in subjects with type 2 diabetes. *Thromb Res* 2000;97:239–245.
73. Howard BV, Roman MJ, Devereux RB, et al: Effect of lower targets for blood pressure and LDL cholesterol on atherosclerosis in diabetes: the SANDS randomized trial. *JAMA* 2008;299:1678–1689.
74. Sawayama Y, Shimizu C, Maeda N, et al: Effects of probucol and pravastatin on common carotid atherosclerosis in patients with asymptomatic hypercholesterolemia: Fukuoka Atherosclerosis Trial (FAST). *J Am Coll Cardiol* 2002;39:610–616.
75. Hodis HN, Mack WJ, LaBree L, et al: The role of carotid arterial intima–media thickness in predicting clinical coronary events. *Ann Intern Med* 1998;128:262–269.
76. Amarenco P, Labreuche J, Lavallee P, Touboul PJ: Statins in stroke prevention and carotid atherosclerosis: systematic review and up-to-date meta-analysis. *Stroke* 2004;35:2902–2909.
77. Bonithon-Kopp C, Touboul PJ, Berr C, et al: Relation of intima–media thickness to atherosclerotic plaques in carotid arteries: The Vascular Aging (EVA) Study. *Arterioscler Thromb Vasc Biol* 1996;16:310–316.
78. Mannami T, Konishi M, Baba S, et al: Prevalence of asymptomatic carotid atherosclerotic lesions detected by high-resolution ultrasonography and its relation to cardiovascular risk factors in the general population of a Japanese city: the Suita study. *Stroke* 1997;28:518–525.
79. Aminbakhsh A, Frohlich J, Mancini GB: Detection of early atherosclerosis with B mode carotid ultrasonography: assessment of a new quantitative approach. *Clin Invest Med* 1999;22:265–274.
80. Sun Y, Lin CH, Lu CJ, et al: Carotid atherosclerosis, intima–media thickness and risk factors—an analysis of 1781 asymptomatic subjects in Taiwan. *Atherosclerosis* 2002;164:89–94.
81. Ebrahim S, Papacosta O, Whincup P, et al: Carotid plaque, intima–media thickness, cardiovascular risk factors, and prevalent cardiovascular disease in men and women: the British Regional Heart Study. *Stroke* 1999;30:841–850.
82. Homma S, Hirose N, Ishida H, et al: Carotid plaque and intima–media thickness assessed by B-mode ultrasonography in subjects ranging from young adults to centenarians. *Stroke* 2001;32:830–835.

83. Young W, Gofman JW, Tandy R, et al: The quantitation of atherosclerosis. II. Quantitative aspects of the relationship of blood pressure and atherosclerosis. *Am J Cardiol* 1960;6:294–299.
84. Mitchell JR, Schwartz CJ: Relationship between arterial disease in different sites: a study of the aorta and coronary, carotid, and iliac arteries. *Br Med J* 1962;1:1293–1301.
85. Salonen JT, Salonen R: Ultrasonographically assessed carotid morphology and the risk of coronary heart disease. *Arterioscler Thromb* 1991;11:1245–1249.
86. van der Meer IM, Bots ML, Hofman A, et al: Predictive value of noninvasive measures of atherosclerosis for incident myocardial infarction: The Rotterdam Study. *Circulation* 2004;109:1089–1094.
87. Störk S, van den Beld AW, von Schacky C, et al: Carotid artery plaque burden, stiffness, and mortality risk in elderly men: a prospective, population-based cohort study. *Circulation* 2004;110:344–348.
88. Rosvall M, Janzon L, Berglund G, et al: Incident coronary events and case fatality in relation to common carotid intima–media thickness. *J Intern Med* 2005;257:430–437.
89. Belcaro G, Nicolaides AN, Ramaswami G, et al: Carotid and femoral ultrasound morphology screening and cardiovascular events in low risk subjects: a 10-year follow-up study (the CAFES-CAVE study). *Atherosclerosis* 2001;156:379–387.
90. Hunt KJ, Sharrett AR, Chambless LE, et al: Acoustic shadowing on B-mode ultrasound of the carotid artery predicts CHD. *Ultrasound Med Biol* 2001;27:357–365.
91. Wattanakit K, Folsom AR, Chambless LE, Nieto FJ: Risk factors for cardiovascular event recurrence in the Atherosclerosis Risk in Communities (ARIC) study. *Am Heart J* 2005;149:606–612.
92. Spence JD, Eliasziw M, DiCicco M, et al: Carotid plaque area: a tool for targeting evaluating vascular preventive therapy. *Stroke* 2002;33:2916–2922.
93. Wyman RA, Mays ME, McBride PE, Stein JH: Ultrasound-detected carotid plaque as a predictor of cardiovascular events. *Vasc Med* 2006;11:123–130.
94. Stein JH, Korcarz CE, Hurst RT, et al: Use of carotid ultrasound to identify subclinical vascular disease and evaluate cardiovascular disease risk: a consensus statement from the American Society of Echocardiography Carotid Intima–Media Thickness Task Force. Endorsed by the Society for Vascular Medicine. *J Am Soc Echocardiogr* 2008;21:93–111; quiz 89–90.
95. Barnett PA, Spence JD, Manuck SB, Jennings JR: Psychological stress and the progression of carotid artery disease. *J Hypertens* 1997;15:49–55.
96. Ainsworth CD, Blake CC, Tamayo A, et al: 3D ultrasound measurement of change in carotid plaque volume: a tool for rapid evaluation of new therapies. *Stroke* 2005;36:1904–1909.
97. Landry A, Spence JD, Fenster A: Measurement of carotid plaque volume by 3-dimensional ultrasound. *Stroke* 2004;35:864–869.
98. Reilly LM, Lusby RJ, Hughes L, et al: Carotid plaque histology using real-time ultrasonography: clinical and therapeutic implications. *Am J Surg* 1983;146:188–193.
99. Sztajzel R: Ultrasonographic assessment of the morphological characteristics of the carotid plaque. *Swiss Med Wkly* 2005;135:635–643.
100. Baud JM, Delanoy P, Coordinateurs de l'Etude AFFCA: Reproducibilit ultrasonore dans la characterization des plaques carotides. In: de Bray JM, Baud JM, Dauzat M, et al. (eds): Plaques Carotides: Diagnostic, Evaluation, Prognostic. Montpellier, France: Sauramps Medical, 1997, pp 289–292.
101. Joakimsen O, Bonaa KH, Stensland-Bugge E: Reproducibility of ultrasound assessment of carotid plaque occurrence, thickness, and morphology: The Tromsø Study. *Stroke* 1997;28:2201–2207.
102. Polak JF, Shemanski L, O'Leary DH, et al; for the Cardiovascular Health Study: Hypoechoic plaque at US of the carotid artery: an independent risk factor for incident stroke in adults aged 65 years or older. *Radiology* 1998;208:649–654.
103. Kawasaki M, Ito Y, Yokoyama H, et al: Assessment of arterial medial characteristics in human carotid arteries using integrated backscatter ultrasound and its histological implications. *Atherosclerosis* 2005;180:145–154.
104. Yokoyama H, Kawasaki M, Ito Y, et al: Effects of fluvastatin on the carotid arterial media as assessed by integrated backscatter ultrasound compared with pulse-wave velocity. *J Am Coll Cardiol* 2005;46:2031–2037.
105. Kawasaki M, Takatsu H, Noda T, et al: Noninvasive quantitative tissue characterization and two-dimensional color-coded map of human atherosclerotic lesions using ultrasound integrated backscatter: comparison between histology and integrated backscatter images. *J Am Coll Cardiol* 2001;38:486–492.
106. Kawasaki M, Takatsu H, Noda T, et al: *In vivo* quantitative tissue characterization of human coronary arterial plaques by use of integrated backscatter intravascular ultrasound and comparison with angioscopic findings. *Circulation* 2002;105:2487–2492.
107. el-Barghouty N, Geroulakos G, Nicolaides A, et al: Computer-assisted carotid plaque characterisation. *Eur J Vasc Endovasc Surg* 1995;9:389–393.
108. El-Barghouty NM, Levine T, Ladva S, et al: Histological verification of computerised carotid plaque characterisation. *Eur J Vasc Endovasc Surg* 1996;11:414–416.
109. Matsagas MI, Vasdekis SN, Gugulakis AG, et al: Computer-assisted ultrasonographic analysis of carotid plaques in relation to cerebrovascular symptoms, cerebral infarction, and histology. *Ann Vasc Surg* 2000;14:130–137.
110. Grønholdt ML, Nordestgaard BG, Bentzon J, et al: Macrophages are associated with lipid-rich carotid artery plaques, echolucency on B-mode imaging, and elevated plasma lipid levels. *J Vasc Surg* 2002;35:137–145.
111. Denzel C, Balzer K, Muller KM, et al: Relative value of normalized sonographic *in vitro* analysis of arteriosclerotic plaques of internal carotid artery. *Stroke* 2003;34:1901–1906.
112. Lovett JK, Redgrave JN, Rothwell PM: A critical appraisal of the performance, reporting, and interpretation of studies comparing carotid plaque imaging with histology. *Stroke* 2005;36:1091–1097.
113. Seabra JC, Sanches JM, Pedro LM, Fernandes JF: Carotid plaque 3D compound imaging and echo-morphology analysis: a Bayesian approach. *Conf Proc IEEE Eng Med Biol Soc* 2007;1:763–766.
114. Sztajzel R, Momjian S, Momjian-Mayor I, et al: Stratified gray-scale median analysis and color mapping of the carotid plaque: correlation with endarterectomy specimen histology of 28 patients. *Stroke* 2005;36:741–745.
115. Macioch JE, Katsamakis CD, Robin J, et al: Effect of contrast enhancement on measurement of carotid artery intimal medial thickness. *Vasc Med* 2004;9:7–12.
116. Shah F, Balan P, Weinberg M, et al: Contrast-enhanced ultrasound imaging of atherosclerotic carotid plaque neovascularization: a new surrogate marker of atherosclerosis? *Vasc Med* 2007;12:291–297.
117. Feinstein SB: Contrast ultrasound imaging of the carotid artery vasa vasorum and atherosclerotic plaque neovascularization. *J Am Coll Cardiol* 2006;48:236–243.
118. Lindner JR: Microbubbles in medical imaging: current applications and future directions. *Nat Rev Drug Discov* 2004;3:527–532.
119. Nambi V, Chambless L, Folsom AR, et al: Carotid intima–media thickness improves coronary heart disease risk prediction in the Atherosclerosis Risk In Communities (ARIC) Study. *Circulation* 2007;116:II-809.

CHAPTER 36

Noninvasive Imaging Modalities and Atherosclerosis: The Role of Magnetic Resonance Imaging and Positron Emission Tomography Imaging

Kelly S. Myers, James H. F. Rudd, and Zahi A. Fayad

INTRODUCTION

Atherosclerosis and its clinical consequences now reach far beyond the Western world. It is predicted to replace infection and malnutrition as the leading cause of death by 2010.[1] Our knowledge of the pathology of atherosclerosis and its risk factors and genetic predispositions has advanced tremendously over the last two decades. The initiation, progression, and complications of the disease are closely linked with inflammation.[2] Crucially, the risk of clinical events such as myocardial infarction, stroke, and transient ischemic attack (TIA) may be predicted by the level of inflammation in the plaque, mainly in the form of activated macrophages.

Encouragingly, treatment options for atherosclerosis have also evolved to keep pace with our deeper understanding of its biology. Interventional coronary techniques such as stenting and bypass surgery relieve symptoms and improve mortality in certain population groups. However, recent debates about the long-term safety of drug-eluting stents[3] and the realization that intensive medical therapy (as opposed to percutaneous coronary intervention) may be the most appropriate treatment for low- to moderate-risk individuals[4] means that identifying such patients has taken on increased importance. Established methods of stratifying patients include the use of scoring systems, such as Framingham, which sum risk factors to give an estimated chance of cardiovascular events over the following 10 years. Risk scoring in this way can be refined and marginally improved by the addition of measurements of circulating biomarkers (such as C-reactive protein) into the risk prediction algorithm.[5] Imaging may help in this role by identifying patients who may already have manifestations of subclinical atherosclerosis,[6,7] including coronary artery calcification,[8] expansion of the carotid artery intima–media thickness,' or occult peripheral vascular disease.[10] This chapter focuses on two novel imaging modalities—magnetic resonance imaging (MRI) and[11] fluorodeoxyglucose positron emission tomography (FDG PET), which are complementary techniques.

MAGNETIC RESONANCE IMAGING

MRI has emerged as one of the most promising noninvasive imaging modalities for the assessment of atherosclerotic plaque. In contrast to x-ray angiography, MRI is able to characterize the vessel wall, providing information about fibrosis, calcification, hemorrhage deposits, and lipid cores within individual plaques. This is an important distinction because while the stenotic lesions detected by x-ray angiography are most often the cause of stable angina, most acute coronary events are caused by smaller plaques that must be characterized on a molecular level. With the use of specific contrast agents that target molecular components of atherosclerosis, MRI may further characterize the arterial wall on a biologic level with the detection of activated macrophages, fibrin, and integrins.

The lack of ionizing radiation with MRI allows the technique to be safely repeated in patients over time and permits the tracking of disease progression. Additionally, MRI has a high spatial resolution (<1 mm), which is necessary to image the coronary vessels, though a poor temporal resolution makes coronary imaging more challenging. MRI may delineate plaque components more easily in larger vessels such as the aorta and carotid arteries, and thus more clinical studies have focused on these regions. Although the use of MRI of plaque has become more widespread, image acquisition remains a lengthy process, and there is not yet an accepted, user-independent image analysis software.[11] These limitations have continued to improve in recent years, allowing MRI to further its potential in the future of plaque imaging.

PLAQUE IMAGING WITH MAGNETIC RESONANCE IMAGING

Magnetic Resonance Imaging Techniques

MRI acquires images by using strong magnets to apply radiofrequency pulses that affect the alignment of protons in tissues. When the protons return to their equilibrium state, they release energy and their spins dephase at specific rates that can be measured. These rates are known as T1 and T2, respectively, and are dependent on the composition of the tissue. The contribution of T1 and T2 in an image can be controlled during image acquisition to create a T1 or T2 image. The contribution of both parameters may be lowered such that the image reflects the water or lipid proton densities; this is called a proton density–weighted (PDW) image. Time-of-flight (TOF), or bright-blood imaging, is an additional technique used to intensify the signal from flowing blood. Alternatively, a black-blood sequence, which is a double inversion recovery sequence, may be used to null the signal from the blood, allowing the arterial wall to be easily visualized. Magnetization prepared rapid gradient echo (MPRAGE) is another sequence that allows for rapid acquisition with T1-weighted dominance. These different contrasts allow MRI to separate tissues based on their chemical and physical composition.[12–14] The signal intensity of different plaque components varies with the sequence used, and MRI of atherosclerotic plaques uses a combination of these inherent contrasts to best characterize the plaque and vessel wall (Figs. 36-1 and 36-2).

Specifically, T2 has been shown to detect early intimal thickening, distinguish media from adventitia in the arterial wall, and delineate the fibrous cap and lipid core of a plaque.[15,16] Using sequences that combine T1, T2, PDW, and TOF contrasts, including rapid image acquisition sequences such as MPRAGE, an MR scan can further characterize plaque to identify structure, calcifications, necrotic cores, and recent hemorrhages.[13,14] Several common parameters are consistently obtained from an MRI of an artery or plaque (Table 36-1).

The choice of coils during image acquisition can affect the signal-to-noise ratio (SNR) of the obtained images. Ideally, multiple phased-array receiver coils are placed circumferentially on the body surface close to the artery to allow for an improved SNR. The carotid arteries are ideal for MRI, as they are close to the surface without significant motion, allowing for a resolution as high as 400 μm to be achieved in this region. Various groups have developed special coils to increase the SNR.[14,17,18] Blaimer et al. used multiple coils to maintain the SNR while decreasing scan time.[19] Some groups have investigated the use of intravascular coils to further increase the SNR of the images.[20,21] Although studies using intravascular coils have shown promising correlations with histology, the development of the technique will likely be hindered by its invasive nature and the dissipation of heat from the coils.[22]

MRI of the coronary arteries poses several technical challenges because of the small vessel size, cardiac and respiratory motion artifacts, the tortuous path of the vessels, and noise from the surrounding epicardial fat. Although a few groups have shown the feasibility of coronary MRI,[23,24] further technical developments are necessary to fully detect and characterize coronary artery lesions.

Validation

Two anatomic measurements derived from MRI of plaque are vessel wall area and vessel wall thickness. These measurements are highly reproducible between scans and readers in the aorta and carotid arteries.[25–28] In attempts to eliminate interobserver variability in MR image analysis, several groups are developing software for automated detection of the vessel wall. One group has compared vessel wall thickness and inner and outer wall dimensions as detected by automated software versus expert manual tracing and has found a high correlation ($r = 0.85$–0.99) between the values in the carotid and aortic arteries.[29,30]

MRI plaque parameters have been correlated with parameters from other imaging modalities as well. Human aortic plaque thickness, composition, and extent correlated well between MRI and transesophageal echocardiography *in vivo*.[24,31] Another study found a strong correlation between carotid wall thickness as measured by ultrasound and MRI.[32,33]

Individual plaque components detected by MRI have been validated with histology in animal models and in humans. In mice, the size, shape, and appearance of aortic plaques on MRI correlated with their measurements and American Heart Association (AHA) classification by histology.[34] MR detection of fibrous and lipid components[35] as well as lesion fissures, necrotic cores, and fibrous caps[36] have been validated in rabbit aortas.

Several groups have correlated human carotid artery plaque components on MRI with histology. Specifically, *in vivo* measurements of a carotid plaque's fibrous cap,[14,37–39] lipid core,[14,39] necrotic core,[40] intimal tissue calcification,[14] thrombotic components,[14] intraplaque hemorrhage,[14,40,41] and vessel wall area[42] as assessed by MRI have all correlated with histologic findings. Cai et al. found that carotid plaque characteristics on MRI *in vivo* could accurately identify a plaque's AHA classification.[43] MRI of carotid endarterectomy specimens had 100% sensitivity for calcified, fibrocellular, fibrocellular plus lipid, fibrous cap, and lipid core components of plaque and 84% sensitivity for thrombus. The specificity for fibrous cap, lipid core, and thrombus components was 100%, and the specificity for fibrocellular plus lipid components was 95%.[44] Another group found that when looking at human carotids *in vivo*, MRI had a 85% sensitivity and 92% specificity for lipid and acute intraplaque hemorrhage.[40]

Computer programs using cluster analysis and logistic stepwise regression models have recently been

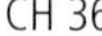

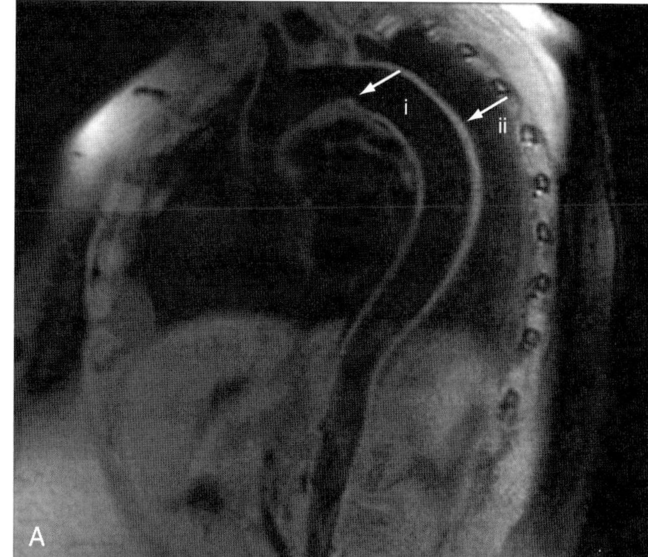

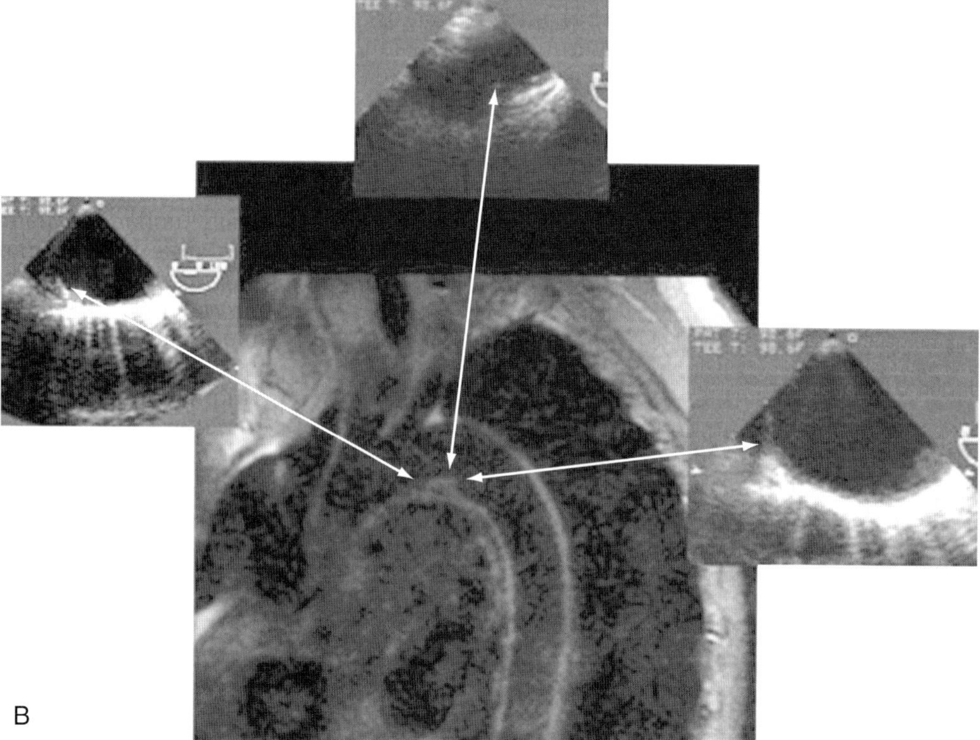

FIGURE 36-1 ***(A)*** Sagittal view of (i) atherosclerotic plaque in the aortic arch and (ii) wall thickening of the thoracic aorta, visualized by a black-blood magnetic resonance imaging (MRI) sequence using a combination of endogenous contrasts. ***(B)*** The aortic arch plaque is confirmed by transesophageal ultrasound.

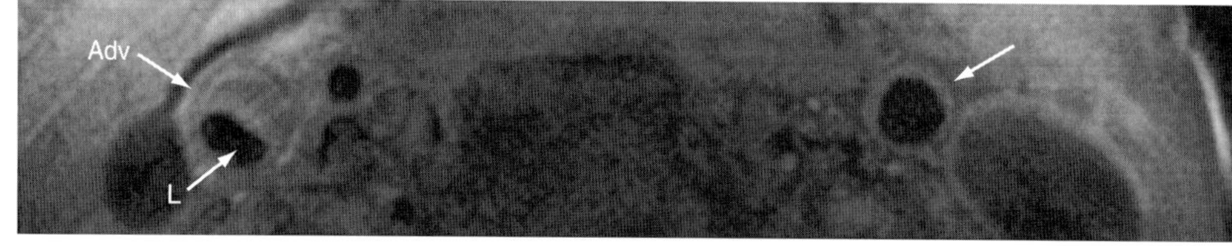

FIGURE 36-2 Plaque in the right common carotid artery *(top left arrow)* as detected by magnetic resonance imaging with no visible plaque in the left common carotid *(right arrow)*. Acquisition using a black-blood proton density–weighted (PDW) sequence *(top)* allows for visualization of the lumen (L) and the adventitia (Adv). A T2-weighted image *(bottom)* shows delineation of the lipid core (LC) and fibrous cap (FC).

TABLE 36-1 Common Magnetic Resonance Imaging–Derived Parameters of Atherosclerotic Disease

Vessel wall area (VWA)
Vessel wall thickness (VWT)
Vessel wall volume (VWV)
Total vessel area (TVA)
Plaque characterization
Lipid-rich necrotic core Fibrous cap Hemorrhage Calcification

investigated for their use in the automated detection of various plaque components.[45,46] In one study, results obtained from cluster analysis correlated well with the AHA's plaque classification types I to IV.[46]

CLINICAL CORRELATIONS WITH MAGNETIC RESONANCE IMAGING

Plaque Parameters and Risk Factors

Many studies have correlated arterial wall and plaque characteristics with known risk factors for cardiovascular disease. One study looked at an offspring cohort from the Framingham Heart Study who had no clinical signs or symptoms of coronary artery disease.[47] Thirty-eight percent of women and 41% of men were found to have evidence of aortic atherosclerosis, the prevalence of which significantly correlated with Framingham Coronary Risk Score.[47] Another study recruited 196 subjects without clinical cardiovascular disease and found that the mean and maximum aortic wall thickness correlated with age and male sex. The group also found that the maximum aorta wall thickness was significantly greater in African Americans compared to Caucasians.[48] In a separate study, young smokers were found to have decreased aortic distensibility and decreased flow-mediated vasodilation as detected by MRI when compared with nonsmokers.[49]

In higher-risk populations, aortic wall thickness measured by MRI has been correlated with several known risk factors for cardiovascular disease. Taniguchi et al. looked at MRI characteristics of aortic plaque in 102 subjects awaiting coronary catheterization. Plaques were detected more often in subjects with elevated low-density lipoprotein (LDL) or a history of smoking. Plaque thickness correlated with age, the presence of coronary artery disease, systolic hypertension, and elevated high-sensitivity C-reactive protein or fibrinogen.[50] Subjects with homozygous familial hypercholesterolemia have also been found to have increased aortic wall thickness.[51]

MRI characteristics of the carotid arteries have not always been found to be correlated with the same risk factors as aortic parameters have. No significant difference in vessel wall thickness was found in the symptomatic versus asymptomatic carotid arteries of 23 subjects with unilateral carotid disease.[52] However, the symptomatic carotid artery did have a higher incidence of fibrous cap rupture, juxtaluminal hemorrhage or thrombus, type I hemorrhage, and complicated AHA type VI lesions as well as larger amounts of hemorrhage and loose matrix.[52] The affected side also had smaller lumen areas and a lower incidence of uncomplicated AHA type IV and V lesions.[52] In a study of 28 elderly subjects, carotid artery wall thickness did not correlate with high-density lipoprotein (HDL) or LDL, although a correlation between lipid core volume and HDL levels was found.[53]

Two studies have looked at the MRI characteristics of carotid artery plaques in subjects with symptomatic carotid disease. Yuan et al.[54] compared the characteristics of fibrous caps in carotid artery plaques between 28 subjects with a recent TIA or stroke and 25 subjects with asymptomatic carotid stenosis. Seventy percent of all ruptured fibrous caps versus 9% of all thick fibrous caps were found in subjects with a recent TIA or stroke, making subjects with a ruptured cap 23 times more likely than those with a thick cap to have had a recent TIA or stroke.[54] In a study of 41 subjects with symptomatic carotid disease, subjects with lipid cores in their carotid plaque by MRI had ipsilateral cerebral infarctions more often than those without lipid cores (68% vs. 31%).[55]

Plaque Parameters Associated with Future Events

Prospective studies have also been done to investigate characteristics of carotid artery plaque on MRI that are associated with disease progression and future cardiovascular events. One group enrolled 154 subjects with asymptomatic carotid stenosis of 50% to 79% and performed an MRI at baseline. Subjects were followed clinically every 3 months for an average of 38.2 months, during which 12 ipsilateral cerebrovascular events occurred. Carotid plaque MRI parameters on the baseline scan that were significantly associated with the occurrence of a future event were the presence of a thin or ruptured fibrous cap (hazard ratio, 17.0), intraplaque hemorrhage (hazard ratio, 5.2), larger mean intraplaque hemorrhage area (hazard ratio for a 10-mm^2 increase, 2.6), larger maximum percent of lipid-rich/necrotic core (hazard ratio for 10% increase, 1.6), and larger maximum wall thickness (hazard ratio for a 1-mm increase, 1.6).[56] Another study performed carotid MRI on 53 subjects within 7 days of a second cerebrovascular accident. Subjects with vulnerable carotid lesions, as defined by eccentric shape and heterogeneous signal on MRI corresponding to AHA plaque types IV, V, and VI, had an eight times greater risk of a third cerebrovascular accident compared to those without vulnerable lesions (24% vs. 3%).[57] The knowledge of such risk factors for future events may allow for early detection and intervention of high-risk carotid plaques.

CONTRAST AGENTS IN MAGNETIC RESONANCE IMAGING

Dynamic Contrast-Enhanced Magnetic Resonance Imaging

Dynamic contrast-enhanced (DCE) MRI of atherosclerotic plaques looks at the rate at which plaque components are enhanced following an injection of the contrast agent gadolinium. Ten or more images are acquired at the same location over time, and a differential equation that describes the rate of contrast enhancement on the MR images is used to analyze the region. This type of imaging is applicable to plaques because different plaque components have various tissue permeabilities and blood supplies, and therefore receive contrast at different rates. Applying the differential equation to plaque images obtained by DCE MRI allows for the solving of two variables in the equation, and some studies have correlated these variables with histologic findings of plaque inflammation and neovasculature.[58,59]

Targeted Molecular Contrast Agents

Recently, there has been an increasing interest in the investigation of specific molecular targeted contrast agents. The development of these targeted agents would allow MRI to provide not only structural information about a plaque, but biologic information as well. Several groups have investigated the use of small particles of iron oxide (SPIO) (diameter 50–500 nm) and ultrasmall particles of iron oxide (USPIO) (diameter <50 nm), both of which accumulate in macrophages.[60] This is a sensible target since there is an association between the presence of macrophages in the arterial wall and the site of plaque rupture.[61] Other investigated targets include the fibrin of a thrombus,[62–64] the $\alpha_v\beta_3$-integrin expressed on neovessels,[65,66] lipid cores through the use of recombinant HDL nanoparticles,[67] fibronectin in the vasovasorum of plaques,[68] glycoprotein IV found in injured arterial lesions,[69] and the macrophage scavenger receptor.[70]

PLAQUE MAGNETIC RESONANCE IMAGING AND DRUG TRIALS

Validity of Magnetic Resonance Imaging for Drug Trials

The hypothesis that MRI could be used to follow plaque progression was first investigated in rabbits by McConnell. Thirty-one rabbits with balloon injury and 4 months of a high-cholesterol diet underwent an MRI and were subsequently assigned to continued high-cholesterol diet or low-cholesterol diet for an additional 16 months. MRI at 20 months compared to 4 months showed increased wall thickness and luminal stenosis in the high-cholesterol group and a decrease of the same parameters in the low-cholesterol group, demonstrating the ability of MRI to detect progression and regression of disease.[71] In a different study, aortic atherosclerotic lesions were induced in 18 New Zealand white rabbits by balloon injury and cholesterol feeding. The rabbits were then imaged with MRI, underwent 12 weeks of continued high-cholesterol diet and then 12 weeks of normal diet. MR imaging was repeated every 3 months and showed increasing wall volume during the continued high-cholesterol diet and decreasing wall volume during the normal diet phase, again confirming that MR could detect disease progression and regression.[72] Knowing that MRI is able to detect changes in plaque parameters over time, along with its proven validation with histology and reproducibility, make it a promising modality for tracking of disease in drug trials. Given low interscan variability, power calculations show that a study with 14 participants in each group could detect a 5% change in the wall/outer wall ratio of the artery, a 10% change in wall volume, and a 20% change in percent of lipid-rich/necrotic core components with 80% power.[28]

Several studies have looked at the response to carotid and aortic lesions *in vivo* to treatment with statins (Table 36-2). One study performed MRI of the carotid arteries in 68 asymptomatic subjects with at least 50% stenosis at 0 and 18 months. The rate of increase per year in carotid wall area was significantly lower in those taking statins compared with the nonstatin group (1.2% vs. 4.4%).[73] In one case–control study, eight subjects with coronary artery disease who had taken intensive lipid-lowering treatment (niacin 2.5 g/day, lovastatin 40 mg/day, and colestipol 20 mg/day) for 10 years were matched for age, LDL, and triglycerides with eight subjects with coronary artery disease who had never been treated with lipid-lowering drugs. MRI of the most diseased portion of the carotid artery in the treated group compared with the nontreated group showed significantly less lipid core area (0.7 mm^2 vs. 10.2 mm^2) and lipid composition (1% vs. 17%). There were trends toward increased luminal area and decreased plaque area in the treated group, but these differences were not statistically significant.[74]

One study was able to detect changes in thoracic aortic plaque volume and lumen in response to statin treatment as early as 6 months.[75] This study, however, used both surface and transesophageal coils during image acquisition, and other studies using surface coils alone have detected changes only as early as 12 months.[76] Plaques in the aorta and carotid arteries of hypercholesterolemic subjects showed continued decreases in vessel wall thickness and vessel wall area after 18 and 24 months of statin treatment, justifying long-term treatment.[77] In fact, decreases in aortic and carotid artery vessel wall area and maximum vessel wall thickness ranged from 8% to 11% after 12 months of statin treatment, but were 16% to 19% after 24 months of treatment.[77]

In addition to length of treatment, the impact of increased doses of statin on plaque progression has been investigated. One study randomized 40 hypercholesterolemic patients to receive 5 or 20 mg/day of atorvastatin for 12 months, and MRI of the aorta was performed at baseline and 12 months. In the thoracic aorta, the 20-mg group had significantly greater reductions in vessel wall thickness and area compared with the 5-mg/day group, although in the abdominal aorta no reduction in vessel parameters was seen for the 20-mg group and a significant increase in vessel wall thickness and area was observed in the 5-mg group.[78] However, 5 mg/day of atorvastatin is lower than the minimum prescribed dose of 10 mg and may not have represented a therapeutic dose. This concept was further investigated in another study in which 51 hypercholesterolemic subjects were randomized to 20 or 80 mg daily of simvastatin. MRI of aortic and carotid lesions at 12 months compared to baseline showed no difference in vessel parameters between the two groups, although both groups showed significant decreases in vessel wall area in the aorta and carotid arteries at 12 months.[79]

TABLE 36-2 Studies Using Magnetic Resonance Imaging to Detect Plaque Regression in Response to Medical Therapy

Study	Patient Population	n	Design	Intervention	Outcome	Result
Carotid:						
Zhao, 2001[74]	CAD + 10 years aggressive lipid-lowering treatment *or* CAD + newly diagnosed hyperlipidemia, age-, LDL- and TG-matched	8 8	Case-control	None	Carotid VWA: treated group vs. untreated group; percent lipid area in plaque; treated group vs. untreated group	VWA: NS percent lipid: +1% vs. +17%**
Saam, 2006[73]	>50% carotid stenosis, asymptomatic, including subjects on and off statins	68	Longitudinal	None	Percent change in VWA baseline vs. 18 months: overall vs. baseline; those on statins vs. not on statins	VWA: +2.2%*** +1.4% vs. +4.4%**
Carotid and aorta:						
Corti, 2001[76]	Hyperlipidemic, documented aortic or carotid plaque by ultrasound	18	Longitudinal	20–80 mg simvastatin × 12 months	Percent change in carotid LA, VWA and maximum VWT: baseline vs. 6 and 12 months	6 months: no changes; 12 months: changes in VWA (–15%)*** and VWT (–11%)**
					Percent change in aortic LA, VWA, and maximum VWT: baseline vs. 6 and 12 months	6 months: no changes; 12 months: changes in VWA (–8%)*** and VWT (–9%)***
Corti, 2002[77]	Untreated hyperlipidemia, documented aortic or carotid plaque by ultrasound	21	Longitudinal	20–80 mg simvastatin × 2 years	Change in carotid LA, VWA, maximum VWT: baseline vs. 6, 12, and 24 months	6 months: no changes; 12 months: changes in VWA (–11%)** and VWT (–18%)**; 24 months: increase in LA (+5%)*** and further decreases in VWA (–18%)*** and VWT (–19%)*** from baseline
					Change in aortic LA, VWA, maximum VWT: baseline vs. 6, 12, and 24 months	6 months: no changes; 12 months: changes in VWA (–11%)***; 24 months: increase in LA (+6%)*** and further decreases in VWA (–16%)*** and VWT (–16%)*** from baseline
Corti, 2006[79]	Newly diagnosed hyperlipidemia, documented aortic or carotid plaque by ultrasound	51	Randomized controlled trial	20 mg simvastatin *or* 80 mg simvastatin	Change in carotid LA, VWA, and maximum VWT: baseline vs. 6, 12, and 24 months for both groups	No difference between groups; 6 months: no changes; 12 months: –14% in VWA and –10% in VWT in both groups; 24 months: +5% in LA in both groups, further decreases in VWA (–18%) and VWT (–17%)
					Change in aortic LA, VWA, and maximum VWT: baseline vs. 6, 12, and 24 months for both groups	No difference between groups 6 months: no changes; 12 months: –10% in VWA and –9% in VWT in both groups; 24 months: +6% in LA in both groups, further decreases in VWA (–15%) and VWT (–15%)

Continued

TABLE 36-2 Studies Using Magnetic Resonance Imaging to Detect Plaque Regression in Response to Medical Therapy—cont'd

Study	Patient Population	n	Design	Intervention	Outcome	Result
Aorta:						
Yonemura, 2005[78]	Hyperlipidemic	40	Randomized controlled trial	5 mg atorvastatin *or* 20 mg atorvastatin	Thoracic aorta: percent change in LA, VWA, and maximum VWT: baseline vs. 12 months for both groups	Significant difference in all parameters between 5-mg and 20-mg groups: LA, 0% (NS) vs. +5%***; VWA, +4% (NS) vs. -18%***; VWT, +1% (NS) vs. -12%***
					Abdominal aorta: percent change in LA, VWA, and maximum VWT: baseline vs. 12 months for both groups	Significant difference in all parameters between 5-mg and 20-mg groups: LA, -3% vs. 0% (NS)***; VWA, +12% vs. +3% (NS)***; VWT, +5% vs. -1% (NS)***
Lima, 2004[75]	Hyperlipidemic	27	Randomized controlled trial	20–80 mg simvastatin × 6 months	Using combined transesophageal/ surface coil: percent change in aortic plaque volume and luminal volume; baseline vs. 6 months	Plaque volume: −12%*; luminal volume, NS
Ayaori, 2006[80]	Hyperlipidemic	22	Nonrandomized controlled trial	400 mg bezafibrate (n = 14) *or* placebo (n = 8)	Thoracic aorta: percent change in LA, VWA, and VWT, baseline vs. 1 year for both groups	Bezafibrate vs. placebo: LA, no changes for either group; VWA, -6% vs. +5%***; VWT, -3% vs. 0%***
					Abdominal aorta: percent change in LA, VWA, and VWT; baseline vs. 1 year for both groups	Bezafibrate vs. placebo: LA, +3% vs. 0%*; VWA, -8% vs. +6%**; VWT, -5% vs. +2%**

*$p < 0.05$; **$p < 0.01$; ***$p < 0.001$.
LA, luminal area; NS, not significant.

The effect of fibrates on aortic plaques has also been investigated. In a nonrandomized prospective study, dyslipidemia subjects who took 400 mg daily of bezafibrate had significantly reduced vessel wall areas in the thoracic and abdominal aorta compared to baseline, while dyslipidemic subjects who chose not to take bezafibrate showed a nonsignificant increase in vessel wall area.[80]

FLUORODEOXYGLUCOSE POSITRON EMISSION TOMOGRAPHY IMAGING

FDG PET is a nuclear imaging technique that provides unique insight into the metabolic activity of tissue. It relies on the fact that FDG, which is an analog of glucose, is taken up into cells in proportion to their metabolic activity. Once inside the cell, FDG cannot be metabolized further and becomes trapped. After FDG is tagged with a positron-emitting ^{18}F moiety, a PET scanner can localize and quantify the distribution of the FDG within the body with high sensitivity but limited spatial resolution. To improve localization, an anatomic image is required, usually in the form of computed tomography (CT) scanning. Increasingly, the two separate scanners are combined into a hybrid PET/CT system, an arrangement that ensures more accurate co-registration of images than is obtained with separate scanners.

FDG PET is already established in clinical oncology practice for the detection of malignant disease and monitoring its response to treatment.[81] Atherosclerosis imaging with FDG PET was first conceived in 2002, with the publication of a prospective study using FDG PET to image metabolic activity within carotid atherosclerosis as a marker of plaque inflammation.[82] Eight patients with TIA were imaged shortly after symptoms. Significantly more FDG accumulated within symptomatic plaques than asymptomatic lesions, and autoradiography of excised plaques after surgery confirmed that FDG had entered plaque macrophages (Figs. 36-3 and 36-4). Tawakol and colleagues recently confirmed a strong positive correlation between carotid plaque FDG uptake and macrophage content in a similar patient cohort with severe carotid stenosis.[83]

Other arteries, including the vertebral arteries[84] and aorta,[85] have now been successfully imaged with this

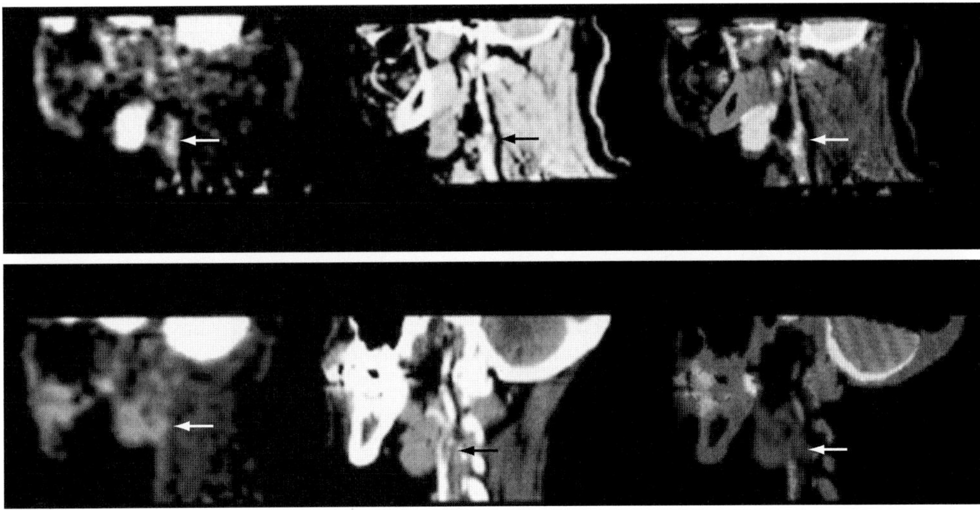

FIGURE 36-3 Sagittal positron emission tomography (PET) (left), computed tomography (CT) *(middle)*, and fused PET/CT *(right)* images of a subject with unilateral symptomatic carotid artery stenosis. There was high fluorodeoxygloucose (FDG) uptake in the symptomatic carotid artery *(upper row with arrows denoting carotid plaque)* compared with low FDG uptake on the asymptomatic side *(lower row with arrows denoting carotid plaque)*. (From Ref. 82, with permission.)

technique. One exciting recent development has been the visualization of coronary artery plaque inflammation by Dunphy et al.[85] This had previously been considered very unlikely to work because the signal from the myocardium would overpower the signal from arterial FDG uptake. But, either fortuitously or with dietary manipulation, myocardial FDG uptake can be suppressed to such a degree that the arterial signal becomes apparent. Other arteries, such as the iliac and femoral arteries, are now being imaged as part of multicenter trials of drug therapy and plaque characterization.

As plaque FDG imaging becomes more established, researchers have begun to study the association between plaque inflammation, cardiovascular risk factors,[86] and serum biomarkers[87] that are associated with elevated risk of atherosclerosis. In one study, there appeared to be a stepwise increase in carotid inflammation as patients accumulated more elements of the metabolic syndrome, such as hypertension, insulin resistance, and increasing waist circumference,[86] while

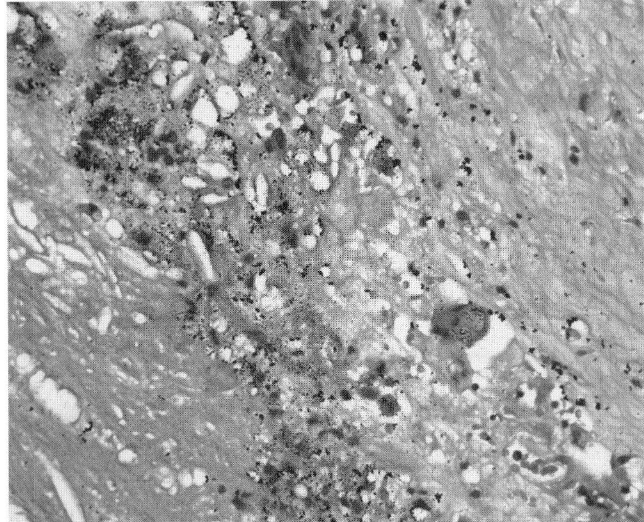

FIGURE 36-4 20× magnification of tritiated deoxyglucose autoradiography of symptomatic carotid artery plaque, showing the accumulation of silver grains predominantly in macrophages at the lipid core/fibrous cap border.

other recent work has highlighted an association between carotid plaque FDG uptake and the serum marker of inflammation matrix metalloproteinase–1.[87] This is not entirely unexpected, as the histologic evidence data from animal studies confirming this association are increasing.[88–90]

In terms of using FDG PET imaging to track regression of atherosclerotic inflammation, two studies are described. The first was an animal study that showed that inflammation can be reduced by 3 months of treatment with the agent probucol, and that such reduction can be imaged successfully using FDG PET in atherosclerotic rabbits.[91] In the first human study of its kind,[92] FDG PET was used in patients with cancer to track a reduction in carotid plaque inflammation resulting from 3 months of treatment with simvastatin 40 mg daily. There was significantly more inflammation reduction seen in the statin group than in the patients on diet alone (Fig. 36-5). This study was important because it showed that the effect of a drug could be detected noninvasively after only 12 weeks of therapy; this can be compared to MRI studies, in which typically 1 year of treatment would be required before MRI could document a change in plaque structure (area of plaque, thickness of fibrous cap, etc.). This study highlights the fact that FDG PET can detect functional change in plaque biology (inflammation reduction) at a time when structural change has not yet become apparent.

Further work needs to be done before FDG PET imaging of atherosclerosis can fulfill more of the roles described above. For example, if the technique is to be used to evaluate new drugs, the reproducibility of the plaque FDG signal must be assessed. Additionally, for multicenter trials of drugs, values for inter- and intra-observer agreement must be defined. Such work is already under way, and early results suggest that this functional technique might be a valuable addition to currently available "anatomic" imaging techniques. Other issues to be addressed include radiation dose reduction; this might be achieved through the use of combined PET/MRI scanners. Finally, the use of more-macrophage-specific tracers might allow visualization

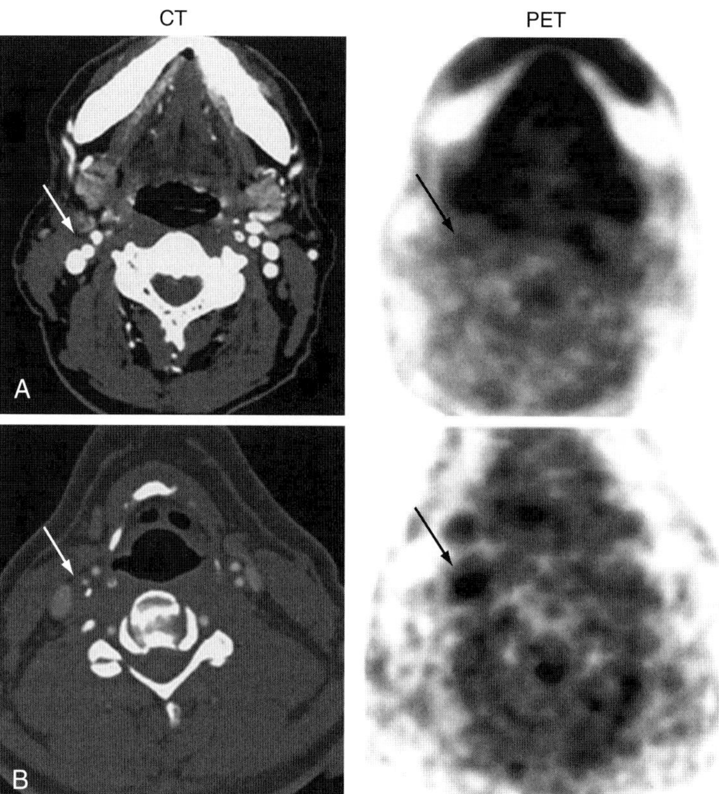

FIGURE 36-5 Axial computed tomography (CT) *(left)* and positron emission tomography (PET) *(right)* images at the level of subsequent carotid endarterectomy in two subjects, with arrows showing carotid plaque in all images. Subject **A** *(upper row)* had high fluorodeoxyglucose (FDG) uptake in the carotid artery with the excised plaque showing high macrophage content, whereas subject **B** *(lower row)* had low FDG uptake in the carotid artery with the excised plaque showing limited macrophage content. (From Ref. 83, with permission.)

of the coronary arteries. At present, the coronary circulation presents a special challenge because of the invariably high uptake of FDG by the surrounding myocardial muscle. Novel tracers or dietary and metabolic manipulation of the patient prior to imaging might allow coronary plaque inflammation quantification to become a reality.

CONCLUSIONS

The detection of high-risk plaques is important not only for the early diagnosis and treatment of those at risk, but also to further our understanding of the disease and provide an endpoint for the development of anti-atherosclerosis drugs. Both MRI and FDG PET have demonstrated the ability to characterize atherosclerotic plaques. MRI is especially practical since it has a high spatial resolution, and its lack of ionizing radiation allows for serial imaging. MRI has been shown to provide morphological information about atherosclerotic plaques and the arterial wall with a high degree of sensitivity and reproducibility. In addition, the ongoing development of specific molecular targeted contrast agents may provide functional information about the disease as well. MRI has been shown to track progression and regression of atherosclerotic disease, with some studies demonstrating the ability of MRI to detect arterial changes in response to antiatherosclerotic drugs. FDG PET has shown the unique ability to detect inflammation within atherosclerotic plaques. Current research in determining the optimal techniques and reproducibility of FDG PET in the imaging of atherosclerotic plaques will allow for further investigation of its application. Such complementary characteristics of MRI and FDG PET facilitate their potential as future modalities to diagnosis and monitor atherosclerotic disease.

REFERENCES

1. Rosamond W, Flegal K, Friday G, et al: Heart Disease and Stroke Statistics—2007 update: a report from the American Heart Association Statistics Committee and Stroke Statistics Subcommittee. *Circulation* 2007;115:e69–e171.
2. Ross R: Atherosclerosis—an inflammatory disease. *N Engl J Med* 1999;340:115–126.
3. Lagerqvist B, James S, Stenestrand U, et al: Long-term outcomes with drug-eluting stents versus bare-metal stents in Sweden. *N Engl J Med* 2007;356:1009–1019.
4. Boden WE, O'Rourke RA, Teo KK, et al: Optimal medical therapy with or without PCI for stable coronary disease. *N Engl J Med* 2007;356:1503–1516.
5. Cooper J, Miller G, Humpries S: A comparison of the PROCAM and Framingham point-scoring systems for estimation of individual risk of coronary heart disease in the Second Northwick Park Heart Study. *Atherosclerosis* 2005;181:93–100.
6. Greenland P, LaBree L, Azen S, et al: Coronary artery calcium score combined with Framingham score for risk prediction in asymptomatic individuals. *JAMA* 2004;291:210–215.
7. Greenland P, Smith SJ, Grundy S: Improving coronary heart disease risk assessment in asymptomatic people: role of traditional risk factors and noninvasive cardiovascular tests. *Circulation* 2001;104:1863–1867.

8. Bellasi A, Raggi P: Diagnostic and prognostic value of coronary artery calcium screening. *Curr Opin Cardiol* 2005;20:375–380.
9. Tzou W, Douglas P, Srinivasan SR, et al: Increased subclinical atherosclerosis in young adults with metabolic syndrome: the Bogalusa Heart Study. *J Am Coll Cardiol* 2005;46:457–463.
10. Feringa H, Bax J, van Waning V, et al: The long-term prognostic value of the resting and postexercise ankle-brachial index. *Arch Intern Med* 2006;166:529–535.
11. Corti R: Noninvasive imaging of atherosclerotic vessels by MRI for clinical assessment of effectiveness of therapy. *Pharmacol Ther* 2006;110:57–70.
12. Choudhury R, Fuster V, Fayad Z, et al: Molecular, cellular and functional imaging of atherosclerosis. *Nat Rev Drug Discov* 2004;3(11):913–925.
13. Fayad Z, Fuster V: Characterization of atherosclerotic plaques by magnetic resonance imaging. *Ann N Y Acad Sci* 2000;902: 173–186.
14. Toussaint J, LaMuraglia G, Southern J, et al: Magnetic resonance images lipid, fibrous, calcified, hemorrhagic and thrombotic components of human atherosclerosis *in vivo*. *Circulation* 1996;94(5):932–938.
15. Martin A, Gotlieb A, Henkelman R: High resolution MR imaging of human arteries. *J Magn Reson Imaging* 1995;5:93–100.
16. Toussaint J, Southern J, Fuster V, Kantor H: T2-weighted contrast for NMR characterization of human atherosclerosis. *Arterioscler Thromb Vasc Biol* 1995;15:1533–1542.
17. Buehrer M, Huber M, Wiesinger F, et al: Coil setup optimization for 2D-SENSE whole-heart coronary imaging. *Magn Reson Med* 2006;55:460–464.
18. Hadley J, Roberts J, Goodrich K, et al: Relative RF coil performance in carotid imaging. *Magn Reson Imaging* 2005;23:629–639.
19. Blaimer M, Breuer F, Mueller M, et al: SMASH, SENSE, PILS, GRAPPA: how to choose the optimal method. *Top Magn Reson Imaging* 2004;15:223–236.
20. Correia L, Atalar E, Kelemen M, et al: Intravascular magnetic resonance imaging of aortic atherosclerotic plaque composition. *Arterioscler Thromb Vasc Biol* 1997;17:3626–3632.
21. Rogers W, Prichard J, Hu Y, et al: Characterization of signal properties in atherosclerotic plaque components by intravascular MRI. *Arterioscler Thromb Vasc Biol* 2000;20:1824–1830.
22. Wilensky R, Song H, Ferrari V: Role of magnetic resonance and intravascular magnetic resonance in the detection of vulnerable plaques. *J Am Coll Cardiol* 2006;47(8 Suppl):C48–C56.
23. Botnar R, Stuber M, Kissinger K, et al: Noninvasive coronary vessel wall and plaque imaging with magnetic resonance imaging. *Circulation* 2000;102:2582–2587.
24. Fayad Z, Fuster V, Fallon J, et al: Noninvasive *in vivo* human coronary artery lumen and wall imaging using black-blood magnetic resonance imaging. *Circulation* 2000;102(5):506–510.
25. Corti R, Fuster V, Badimon J, et al: New understanding of atherosclerosis (clinically and experimentally) with evolving MRI technology *in vivo*. *Ann N Y Acd Sci* 2001;947:181–195.
26. Corti R, Fuster V, Fayad Z, et al: Effects of aggressive versus conventional lipid-lowering therapy by simvastatin on human atherosclerotic lesions: a prospective, randomized, double-blind trial with high-resolution magnetic resonance imaging. *J Am Coll Cardiol* 2001;46(1):106–112.
27. Dehnavi R, Doornbos J, Tamsma J, et al: Assessment of the carotid artery by MRI at 3T: a study on reproducibility. *J Magn Reson Imaging* 2007;25(5):1035–1043.
28. Saam T, Kerwin W, Chu B, et al: Sample size calculation for clinical trials using magnetic resonance imaging for the quantitative assessment of carotid atherosclerosis. *J Cardiovasc Magn Reson* 2005;7(5):799–808.
29. Adame I, de Koning P, Lelieveldt B, et al: An integrated automated analysis method for quantifying vessel stenosis and plaque burden from carotid MRI images: combined postprocessing of MRA and vessel wall MR. *Stroke* 2006;37(8):2162–2164.
30. Adame I, van der Geest R, Bluemke D, et al: Automatic vessel wall contour detection and quantification of wall thickness in *in-vivo* MR images of the human aorta. *J Magn Reson Imaging* 2006;24(3):595–602.
31. Fayad Z, Nahar T, Fallon J, et al: *In vivo* magnetic resonance evaluation of atherosclerotic plaques in the human thoracic aorta: a comparison with transesophageal echocardiography. *Circulation* 2000;101(21):2503–2509.
32. Crowe L, Ariff B, Keegan J, et al: Comparison between three-dimensional volume-selective turbo spin-echo imaging and two-dimensional ultrasound for assessing carotid artery structure and function. *J Magn Reson Imaging* 2005;21(3):282–289.
33. Underhill H, Kerwin W, Hatsukami T, Yuan C, et al: Automated measurement of mean wall thickness in the common carotid artery by MRI: a comparison to intima-media thickness by B-mode ultrasound. *J Magn Reson Imaging* 2006;24(2):379–387.
34. Fayad Z, Fallon J, Shinnar M, et al: Noninvasive *in vivo* high-resolution magnetic resonance imaging of atherosclerotic lesions in genetically engineered mice. *Circulation* 1998;98(15): 1541–1547.
35. Helft G, Worthley S, Fuster V, et al: Atherosclerotic aortic component quantification by noninvasive magnetic resonance imaging: an *in vivo* study in rabbits. *J Am Coll Cardiol* 2001;37(4):1149–1154.
36. Skinner M, Yuan C, Mitsumori L, et al: Serial magnetic resonance imaging of experimental atherosclerosis detects lesion fine structure, progression and complications *in vivo*. *Nat Med* 1995;1(1):69–73.
37. Hatsukami T, Ross R, Polissar N, Yuan C: Visualization of fibrous cap thickness and rupture in human atherosclerotic carotid plaque *in vivo* with high-resolution magnetic resonance imaging. *Circulation* 2000;102(9):959–964.
38. Mitsumori L, Hatsukami T, Ferguson M, et al: *In vivo* accuracy of multisequence MR imaging for identifying unstable fibrous caps in advanced human carotid plaques. *J Magn Reson Imaging* 2003;17:410–420.
39. Trivedi R, U-King-Im J, Graves M, et al: MRI-derived measurements of fibrous-cap and lipid-core thickness: the potential for identifying vulnerable carotid plaques *in vivo*. *Neuroradiology* 2004;46:738–743.
40. Yuan C, Mitsumori L, Ferguson M, et al: *In vivo* accuracy of multispectral magnetic resonance imaging for identifying lipid-rich necrotic cores and intraplaque hemorrhage in advanced human carotid plaques. *Circulation* 2001;104(17):2051–2056.
41. Chu B, Kampschulte A, Ferguson M, et al: Hemorrhage in the atherosclerotic carotid plaque: a high-resolution MRI study. *Stroke* 2004;35(5):1079–1084.
42. Yuan C, Beach K, Smith L Jr, Hatsukami T: Measurement of atherosclerotic carotid plaque size *in vivo* using high resolution magnetic resonance imaging. *Circulation* 1998;98(24): 2666–2671.
43. Cai J, Hatsukami T, Ferguson M, et al: Classification of human carotid atherosclerotic lesions with *in vivo* mutlicontrast magnetic resonance imaging. *Circulation* 2002;106(11):1368–1373.
44. Shinnar M, Fallon J, Wehrli S, et al: The diagnostic accuracy of *ex vivo* MRI for human atherosclerotic plaque characterization. *Arterioscler Thromb Vasc Biol* 1999;19(11):2756–2761.
45. Cappendijk V, Cleutjens K, Kessels A, et al: Assessment of human atherosclerotic carotid plaque components with multisequence MR imaging: Initial experience. *Radiology* 2005;234(2): 487–492.
46. Itskovich V, Samber D, Mani V, et al: Quantification of human atherosclerotic plaques using spatially enhanced cluster analysis of multicontrast-weighted magnetic resonance images. *Magn Reson Med* 2004;52(3):515–523.
47. Jaffer F, O'Donnell C, Larson M, et al: Age and sex distribution of subclinical aortic atherosclerosis: a magnetic resonance imaging examination of the Framingham Heart Study. *Arterioscler Thromb Vasc Biol* 2002;22(5):849–854.
48. Li A, Kamel I, Rando F, et al: Using MRI to assess aortic wall thickness in the multiethnic study of atherosclerosis: distribution by race, sex, and age. *AJR Am J Roentgenol* 2004;182(3): 593–597.
49. Wiesmann F, Petersen S, Leeson P, et al: Global impairment of brachial, carotid, and aortic vascular function in young smokers: direct quantification by high-resolution magnetic resonance imaging. *J Am Coll Cardiol* 2004;44(10):2056–2064.
50. Taniguchi H, Momiyama Y, Fayad Z, et al: *In vivo* magnetic resonance evaluation of associations between aortic atherosclerosis and both risk factors and coronary artery disease in patients referred for coronary angiography. *Am Heart J* 2004;148(1):137–143.
51. Summers R, Andrasko-Bourgeois J, Feuerstein I, et al: Evaluation of the aortic root by MRI: insights from patients with homozygous familial hypercholesterolemia. *Circulation* 1998;98(6):509–518.
52. Saam T, Cai J, Ma L, et al: Comparison of symptomatic and asymptomatic atherosclerotic carotid plaque features with *in vivo* MR imaging. *Radiology* 2006;240(2):464–472.

53. Desai M, Rodriguez A, Wasserman B, et al: Association of cholesterol subfractions and carotid lipid core measured by MRI. *Arterioscler Thromb Vasc Biol* 2005;25(6):e110–e111.
54. Yuan C, Zhang S, Polissar N, et al: Identification of fibrous cap rupture with magnetic resonance imaging is highly associated with recent transient ischemic attack or stroke. *Circulation* 2002;105(2):181–185.
55. Ouhlous M, Flach H, de Weert T, et al: Carotid plaque composition and cerebral infarction: MR imaging study. *AJNR Am J Neuroradiol* 2005;26(5):1044–1049.
56. Takaya N, Yuan C, Chu B, et al: Presence of intraplaque hemorrhage stimulates progression of carotid atherosclerotic plaques: a high-resolution magnetic resonance imaging study. *Circulation* 2005;111(21):2768–2775.
57. Lin K, Zhang Z, Detrano R, et al: Carotid vulnerable lesions are related to accelerated recurrence for cerebral infarction magnetic resonance imaging study. *Acad Radiol* 2006;13(10):1180–1186.
58. Kerwin W, Hooker A, Spilker M, et al: Quantitative magnetic resonance imaging analysis of neovasculature volume in carotid atherosclerotic plaque. *Circulation* 2003;107(6):851–856.
59. Kerwin W, O'Brien K, Ferguson M, et al: Inflammation in carotid atherosclerotic plaque: a dynamic contrast-enhanced MR imaging study. *Radiology* 2006;241(2):459–468.
60. Schmitz S, Taupitz M, Wagner S, et al: Iron-oxide-enhanced magnetic resonance imaging of atherosclerotic plaques: postmortem analysis of accuracy, inter-observer agreement, and pitfalls. *Radiology* 2002;37:405–411.
61. Kolodgie F, Burke A, Farb A, et al: The thin-cap fibroatheroma: a type of vulnerable plaque. The major precursor lesion to acute coronary syndromes. *Curr Opin Cardiol* 2001;16:285–292.
62. Botnar R, Buecker A, Wiethoff A, et al: *In vivo* magnetic resonance imaging of coronary thrombosis using a fibrin-binding molecular magnetic resonance contrast agent. *Circulation* 2004;110(11):1463–1466.
63. Winter P, Caruthers S, Yu X, et al: Improved molecular imaging contrast agent for detection of human thrombus. *Magn Reson Med* 2003;50(2):411–416.
64. Yu X, Song S, Chen J, et al: High-resolution MRI characterization of human thrombus using a novel fibrin-targeted paramagnetic nanoparticle contrast agent. *Magn Reson Med* 2000;44(6):867–872.
65. Lanza G, Winter P, Caruthers S, et al: Magnetic resonance molecular imaging with nanoparticles. *J Nucl Cardiol* 2004;11(6):733–743.
66. Winter P, Morawski A, Caruthers S, et al: Molecular imaging of angiogenesis in early-stage atherosclerosis with alpha(v) beta3-integrin-targeted nanoparticles. *Circulation* 2003;108(18):2270–2274.
67. Frias J, Williams K, Fisher E, et al: Recombinant HDL-like nanoparticles: a specific contrast agent for MRI of atherosclerotic plaques. *J Am Chem Soc* 2004;126(50):16315–16317.
68. Matter C, Schuler P, Alessi P, et al: Molecular imaging of atherosclerotic plaques using a human antibody against the extra-domain B of fibronectin. *Circ Res* 2004;95(12):1225–1233.
69. Gawaz M, Konrad I, Hauser A, et al: Non-invasive imaging of glycoprotein VI binding to injured arterial lesions. *Thromb Haemost* 2005;93(5):910–913.
70. Amirbekian V, Lipinski M, Briley-Saebo K, et al: Detecting and assessing macrophages *in vivo* to evaluate atherosclerosis noninvasively using molecular MRI. *Proc Natl Acad Sci U S A* 2007;104(3):961–966.
71. McConnell M, Aikawa M, Maier S, et al: MRI of rabbit atherosclerosis in response to dietary cholesterol lowering. *Arterioscler Thromb Vasc Biol* 1999;19(8):1956–1959.
72. Hegyi L, Hockings P, Benson M, et al: Short-term arterial remodelling in the aortae of cholesterol fed New Zealand white rabbits shown *in vivo* by high-resolution magnetic resonance imaging—implications for human pathology. *Pathol Oncol Res* 2004;10(3):159–165.
73. Saam T, Yuan C, Chu B, et al: Predictors of carotid atherosclerotic plaque progression as measured by noninvasive magnetic resonance imaging. *Atherosclerosis* 2006.
74. Zhao X, Yuan C, Hatsukami T, et al: Effects of prolonged intensive lipid-lowering therapy on the characteristics of carotid atherosclerotic plaques *in vivo* by MRI: a case–control study. *Arterioscler Thromb Vasc Biol* 2001;21(10):1623–1629.
75. Lima J, Desai M, Steen H, et al: Statin-induced cholesterol lowering and plaque regression after 6 months of magnetic resonance imaging-monitored therapy. *Circulation* 2004;110(16):2336–2341.
76. Corti R, Fayad Z, Fuster V, et al: Effects of lipid-lowering by simvastatin on human atherosclerotic lesions: a longitudinal study by high-resolution, noninvasive magnetic resonance imaging. *Circulation* 2001;104(3):249–252.
77. Corti R, Fuster V, Fayad Z, et al: Lipid lowering by simvastatin induces regression of human atherosclerotic lesions: two years' follow-up by high-resolution noninvasive magnetic resonance imaging. *Circulation* 2002;106(23):2884–2887.
78. Yonemura A, Momiyama Y, Fayad Z, et al: Effect of lipid-lowering therapy with atorvastatin on atherosclerotic aortic plaques detected by noninvasive magnetic resonance imaging. *J Am Coll Cardiol* 2005;45(5):733–742.
79. Corti R, Fuster V, Fayad Z, et al: Effects of aggressive versus conventional lipid-lowering therapy by simvastatin on human atherosclerotic lesions: a prospective, randomized, double-blind trial with high-resolution magnetic resonance imaging. *J Am Coll Cardiol* 2006;46(1):106–112.
80. Ayaori M, Momiyama Y, Fayad Z, et al: Effect of bezafibrate therapy on atherosclerotic aortic plaques detected by MRI in dyslipidemic patients with hypertriglyceridemia. *Atherosclerosis* 2006.
81. Avril N, Weber W: Monitoring response to treatment in patients utilizing PET. *Radiol Clin North Am* 2005;43:189–204.
82. Rudd J, Warburton E, Fryer Tal, et al: Imaging atherosclerotic plaque inflammation with [18F]-fluorodeoxyglucose positron emission tomography. *Circulation* 2002;105:2708–2711.
83. Tawakol A, Migrino R, Bashian Gal, et al: *In vivo* 18F-fluorodeoxyglucose positron emission tomography imaging provides a noninvasive measure of carotid plaque inflammation in patients. *J Am Coll Cardiol* 2006;48:1818–1824.
84. Davies J, Rudd J, Fryer Tal, et al: Identification of culprit lesions after transient ischemic attack by combined 18F fluorodeoxyglucose positron-emission tomography and high-resolution magnetic resonance imaging. Stroke 2005;36:2642–2647.
85. Dunphy M, Freiman A, Larson S, et al: Association of vascular 18F-FDG uptake with vascular calcification. *J Nucl Med* 2005;46:1278–1284.
86. Tahara N, Kai H, Yamagishi Sal, et al: Vascular inflammation evaluated by [18F]-fluorodeoxyglucose positron emission tomography is associated with the metabolic syndrome. *J Am Coll Cardiol* 2007;49:1533–1539.
87. Wu Y, Kao H, Chen Mal, et al: Characterization of plaques using 18F-FDG PET/CT in patients with carotid atherosclerosis and correlation with matrix metalloproteinase-1. *J Nucl Med* 2007;48:227–233.
88. Ogawa M, Ishino S, Mukai Tal, et al: (18)F-FDG accumulation in atherosclerotic plaques: immunohistochemical and PET imaging study. *J Nucl Med* 2004;45:1245–1250.
89. Tawakol A, Migrino R, Hoffman Ual, et al: Noninvasive *in vivo* measurement of vascular inflammation with F-18 fluorodeoxyglucose positron emission tomography. *J Nucl Cardiol* 2005;12:294–301.
90. Zhang Z, Machac J, Helft Gal, et al: Non-invasive imaging of atherosclerotic plaque macrophage in a rabbit model with F-18 FDG PET: a histopathological correlation. *BMC Nucl Med* 2006;6:3.
91. Ogawa M, Magata Y, Kato Tal, et al: Application of 18F-FDG PET for monitoring the therapeutic effect of antiinflammatory drugs on stabilization of vulnerable atherosclerotic plaques. *J Nucl Med* 2006;47:1845–1850.
92. Tahara N, Kai H, Ishibashi Mal, et al: Simvastatin attenuates plaque inflammation: evaluation by fluorodeoxyglucose positron emission tomography. *J Am Coll Cardiol* 2006;48:1825–1831.

CHAPTER 37

Special Patient Populations: Diabetes and Metabolic Syndrome

Salila Kurra, Tina J. Chahil, and Henry N. Ginsberg

HISTORY OF METABOLIC SYNDROME AND ITS RELATIONSHIP TO INSULIN RESISTANCE AND DIABETES MELLITUS

Metabolic syndrome (MetS), a term that describes a group of cardiovascular and metabolic risk factors, has received a great deal of attention both in the lay and scientific press. It has previously been known by several other names, including Syndrome X, Reaven's syndrome, the Deadly Quartet, and the more revealing term, insulin resistance (IR) syndrome. It is interesting to note that more than 80 years ago, Kylin described the clustering of diabetes mellitus (DM), gout, and hypertension in individuals.[1] Later in the 20th century, French physician Jean Vague made the observation that upper-body obesity appeared to predispose to DM and heart disease, while lower-body obesity did not have those associations.[2] He noted that a "male" pattern of body fat distribution, which he referred to as android obesity, was more likely to be associated with DM and cardiovascular disease (CVD). Gerald Reaven's seminal paper went into further detail regarding the classification and clinical importance of a clustering of metabolic abnormalities that he termed *Syndrome X*.[3] His definition included resistance to insulin-stimulated glucose uptake, glucose intolerance, hyperinsulinemia, increased plasma levels of very-low-density lipoprotein (VLDL) triglyceride (TG), decreased plasma high-density lipoprotein (HDL) cholesterol concentration, and hypertension. Reaven postulated that these risk factors, occurring in the same individual, "may be of enormous importance in the genesis of CAD [coronary artery disease]." Moreover, he attributed the etiology of this cluster of risk factors to underlying IR.

Since the original description of this syndrome, several organizations and groups have made modifications to the definition of this cluster of risk factors (Table 37-1). In 1998, the World Health Organization (WHO) proposed criteria[4] that required the presence of DM, impaired glucose tolerance (IGT), impaired fasting glucose (IFG), or IR, and any two of the following criteria:

- Blood pressure (BP) ≥140/90 mm Hg
- Dyslipidemia: TG ≥1.7 mmol/L (150 mg/dL), and/or HDL cholesterol <0.9 mmol/L (35 mg/dL) in men, <1.0 mmol/L (39 mg/dL) in women
- Central obesity: waist-to-hip ratio >0.9 in men, >0.85 in women, and/or body mass index (BMI) >30 kg/m^2
- Microalbuminuria: urinary albumin excretion rate ≥20 μg/min or albumin-to-creatinine ratio ≥30 mg/g.

The European Group for the Study of Insulin Resistance (EGIR) (1999)[5] offered a modification of the WHO classification that both eliminated individuals with DM and required IR or fasting hyperinsulinemia, the latter defined as the top 25% of the fasting plasma insulin values among individuals without DM, and two or more of the following:

- Fasting plasma glucose ≥6.1 mmol/L (110 mg/dL)
- Hypertension: BP ≥140/90 mm Hg or treated for hypertension
- Dyslipidemia: TG >2.0 mmol/L (177 mg/dL) and/or HDL cholesterol <1.0 mmol/L (39 mg/dL) or treated for dyslipidemia
- Central obesity: waist circumference ≥94 cm (37 in) in men, ≥80 cm (31.5 in) in women

In 2001, the National Cholesterol Education Program Adult Treatment Panel III (NCEP ATP III) published further and important modifications,[6]

TABLE 37-1 Metabolic Syndrome Definitions

	WHO, 1998[4]	EGIR, 1999[5]	NCEP ATP III, 2001[6]	IDF, 2005[8]
Diagnostic criteria	Insulin resistance + ≥2:	Insulin resistance + ≥2:	≥3:	Obesity + ≥2:
Blood pressure	≥140/90 mm Hg	≥140/90 mm Hg or treatment for HTN	≥130/85 mm Hg	SBP ≥130 mm Hg or DBP ≥85 mm Hg or treatment for HTN
TG*	≥150 mg/dL	>177 mg/dL or treatment for dyslipidemia	≥150 mg/dL	>150 mg/dL or treatment for HTG
HDL cholesterol*	<35 mg/dL in men, <39 mg/dL in women	<39 mg/dL or treatment for dyslipidemia	<40 mg/dL in men, <50 mg/dL in women	<40 mg/dL in men, <50 mg/dL in women, or treatment for low HDL cholesterol
Central obesity	WHR >0.9 in men, >0.85 in women; and/or BMI >30 kg/m^2	Waist ≥94 cm in men, ≥80 cm in women	Waist >102 cm in men, >88 cm in women	Waist ≥94 cm in men,† ≥80 cm in women†
Microalbuminuria	Urinary albumin excretion rate ≥20 μg/min or albumin/creatinine ratio ≥30 mg/g			
Fasting plasma glucose		≥110 mg/dL	≥110 mg/dL‡	≥100 mg/dL or type 2 DM
Insulin resistance	Required: DM, IGT, IFG, or insulin resistance	Required: insulin resistance or hyperinsulinemia (top 25% for non-DM)		

*TG and/or HDL cholesterol included in single criterion "dyslipidemia" in WHO and EGIR; counted as separate criteria in NCEP ATP III and IDF.
†In Europids, Sub-Saharan Africans, or Eastern Mediterranean and Middle Eastern (Arab) men and women; ≥90 cm and ≥80 cm, respectively, in South Asian, Chinese, or South and Central American men and women; ≥85 cm and ≥90 cm, respectively, in Japanese men and women.
‡Subsequently changed to ≥100 mg/dL.[25]
BMI, body mass index; DBP, diastolic blood pressure; DM, diabetes mellitus; HDL, high-density lipoprotein; HTG, hypertriglyceridemia; HTN, hypertension; IFG, impaired fasting glucose; IGT, impaired glucose tolerance; SBP, systolic blood pressure; TG, triglycerides; WHR, waist/hip ratio.

requiring at least three of the following criteria for the clinical identification of the MetS:

- Abdominal obesity: waist circumference >102 cm (40 in) in men, >88 cm (35 in) in women
- TG ≥150 mg/dL (1.7 mmol/L)
- HDL cholesterol <40 mg/dL in men, <50 mg/dL in women
- BP ≥130/85 mm Hg
- Fasting plasma glucose ≥110 mg/dL

Of note, the NCEP ATP III criteria do not include any direct assessment of, or requirement for, the presence of IR. The NCEP ATP III guidelines focused on the cluster of cardiovascular (CV) risk factors rather than the underlying metabolic abnormalities causing the cluster. In doing so, the NCEP ATP III criteria might be viewed as diminishing the risk of diabetes in people with the MetS. As with any proposed guidelines; there was controversy. In September 2005, a joint statement from the American Diabetes Association (ADA) and the European Association for the Study of Diabetes (EASD) evaluated the utility of the term "MetS."[7] Their conclusion was that too much critically important information was missing to warrant its designation as a syndrome. They went on to say that clinicians should evaluate and treat all CVD risk factors without regard to whether a patient meets criteria for diagnosis of the MetS. However, other authors have reached the opposite conclusion.

Most recently, in 2005, the International Diabetes Federation (IDF)[8] published a worldwide consensus definition of the MetS that requires central obesity (defined as waist circumference ≥94 cm [37 in] for Europid men and ≥80 cm [31.5 in] for Europid women, with ethnicity-specific values for other groups; see Table 37-1) in addition to any two of the following four criteria:

- Raised TG level: >150 mg/dL, or specific treatment for this lipid abnormality
- Reduced HDL cholesterol: <40 mg/dL in men, <50 mg/dL in women, or specific treatment for this lipid abnormality
- Raised BP: systolic BP ≥130 mm Hg or diastolic BP ≥85 mm Hg, or treatment of previously diagnosed hypertension
- Raised fasting plasma glucose: ≥100 mg/dL, or previously diagnosed type 2 DM (T2DM). (If fasting glucose is >100 mg/dL, an oral glucose tolerance test [OGTT] is strongly recommended but is not necessary to define presence of the syndrome.)

EPIDEMIOLOGY OF THE METABOLIC SYNDROME AND ITS RELATIONSHIP TO CARDIOVASCULAR DISEASE

For the purposes of this chapter, we will be referring to the NCEP ATP III criteria when the MetS is mentioned, unless we specifically note otherwise. Recent data suggest that in the United States, 64 million individuals aged >20 years and older have MetS, and its prevalence is increasing. The unadjusted prevalence of the MetS was 23.1% in the National Health and Nutrition Examination Survey (NHANES) III (1988–1994) and 26.7% in NHANES 1999–2000.[9] In spite of the increasing prevalence of the MetS, there is still debate about whether it is a real syndrome or just a compilation of risk factors, and, specifically, the debate centers on whether this cluster of conditions conveys a greater CV risk than each of the components themselves.

A recent paper by Stern et al. followed 1709 San Antonio Heart Study (SAHS) participants with no DM at baseline for a 7.5-year period, and 1353 Mexico City Diabetes Study (MCDS) participants, also without baseline DM, for 6.5 years.[10] The authors evaluated the effectiveness of the MetS as defined by the NCEP ATP III criteria for predicting CV events or the development of T2DM. The MetS was less effective at predicting CVD than the Framingham Risk Score and less effective at predicting T2DM than the Diabetes Risk Score. Thus, the authors concluded that the MetS is a less effective predictor of CV events and T2DM than models that already exist.

On the other hand, a recent systematic review and meta-analysis of longitudinal studies evaluating the MetS and risk of incident CV events and death by Gami et al.[11] suggests that people with the MetS are at increased risk of CV events. This analysis drew from a large number of longitudinal studies that included 172,573 subjects. The investigators concluded that the MetS confers CV risk beyond that which is associated with its component risk factors. However, as with most meta-analyses, not all studies were represented. One such study by Alexander et al.[12] analyzed NHANES data for people older than 50 years of age and demonstrated that while the MetS was a strong univariate predictor of prevalent coronary heart disease (CHD), it was not predictive in a multivariate analysis using the components of the MetS. A study by Sundström et al.[13] of a Swedish cohort followed between the ages of 50 and 70 years for CV mortality also showed no predictive power of the MetS beyond its components.

Although the pathophysiology underlying type 1 DM (T1DM) is different from that of T2DM, both diseases lead to microvascular and macrovascular complications.[14] Of interest in this regard is whether an association between T1DM and the MetS exists. Purnell et al.[15] observed that in the Diabetes Control and Complications Trial (DCCT),[16] a landmark study of individuals with T1DM, increased weight gain in the intensive treatment group was associated with more dyslipidemia and hypertension. In a recent paper, Kilpatrick et al.[17] found that baseline evidence of IR (but not the MetS) predicted greater incidence of both micro- and macro-vascular disease in the DCCT population. In addition, they observed increasing prevalence of the MetS as the DCCT study progressed, particularly in the intensively treated group. In support of the importance of IR in the development of macrovascular complications in T1DM, Orchard et al.[18] reported that measures of IR, but not glycemia, predicted CVD events in their cohort followed for 10 years. On the other hand, intensive glucose lowering in the DCCT reduced the risk of any CVD event by 42% and the risk of nonfatal myocardial infarction (MI), stroke, or death from CVD by 57%.[19]

DYSLIPIDEMIA IN INSULIN RESISTANCE AND TYPE 2 DIABETES MELLITUS

As noted above, and despite controversy, many physicians and scientists consider IR to be the hallmark of T2DM, and the central unifying principle of the MetS[7,20–22]; this is evident in the requirement of IR as the core abnormality in the definitions of the MetS as separately established by the WHO, the EGIR, and the American Association of Clinical Endocrinologists (AACE).[5,23–25] In contrast, IR is a listed, but nonessential, feature of the MetS, according to the NCEP ATP III and IDF definitions of the MetS.[6,8] Nevertheless, insulin sensitivity and the MetS are closely correlated, and the majority of individuals with the MetS are insulin resistant to some degree. An analysis of the NHANES III data revealed that more than 85% of the population older than 50 years of age with the MetS by NCEP ATP III criteria had IR, as defined by IFG, IGT, or DM. Conversely, 69% of the population with IFG and 86% of the population with DM were found to have the MetS.[26,27]

It is also clear that IR is closely tied to abnormal lipid and lipoprotein metabolism.[28–30] Abundant evidence has demonstrated the existence of a characteristic set of lipid and lipoprotein abnormalities accompanying the presence of IR, even in the absence of frank hyperglycemia or abnormal glucose tolerance. This atherogenic dyslipidemia is characterized by low plasma levels of HDL cholesterol and elevations in plasma TG levels compared with levels seen in individuals who are not insulin resistant. Additionally, an increase in the proportion of low-density lipoprotein (LDL) particles that are small, dense, and cholesteryl ester (CE) poor is a prominent feature of this disordered lipid phenotype. This latter finding, described as the pattern B subclass of LDL,[31] is nonetheless largely accompanied by similar plasma LDL cholesterol levels as those seen in individuals with normal glucose tolerance (NGT). Furthermore, total cholesterol levels in insulin-resistant individuals are generally comparable to levels in people who are insulin sensitive, reinforcing the need for quantitative and qualitative lipoprotein measures in the assessment of CVD risk.[29,32–43] Of note, the lipid derangements seen with IR progressively worsen across a continuum of declining glucose tolerance, from NGT through IGT and T2DM.[40,44] An analysis of individuals in the Framingham Offspring Study further demonstrated that even among individuals with NGT, stratification by glucose tolerance status reveals a worsening lipid phenotype with increasing IR (Fig. 37-1). Hence, individuals with NGT who are relatively insulin resistant display the atherogenic lipid phenotype prior to the onset of clinically evident glucose intolerance.[45] Importantly, evidence from the Insulin Resistance Atherosclerosis Study (IRAS) and others suggests that the relationship between IR and dyslipidemia extends across major ethnic groups, including African and Hispanic Americans.[35,46] Additionally, substantial data support differential effects of IR and T2DM on dyslipidemia in women compared to men. Among women, IR and T2DM seem to exert a greater negative impact on several CVD risk factors, including TG and HDL cholesterol levels and LDL particle size. This may, at least in part, account for the increased CHD risk observed in women with T2DM compared with their male counterparts.[33,36,37,46–48]

IR is also associated with increases in VLDL particle number and VLDL TG concentration, and a predominance of larger, more buoyant $VLDL_1$ particles. In contrast, HDL particle number and size decrease in the face of increasing IR.[29,35,40,49–51] Plasma levels of

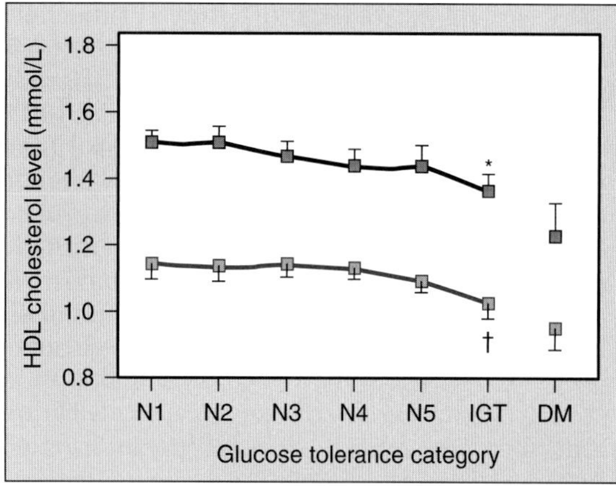

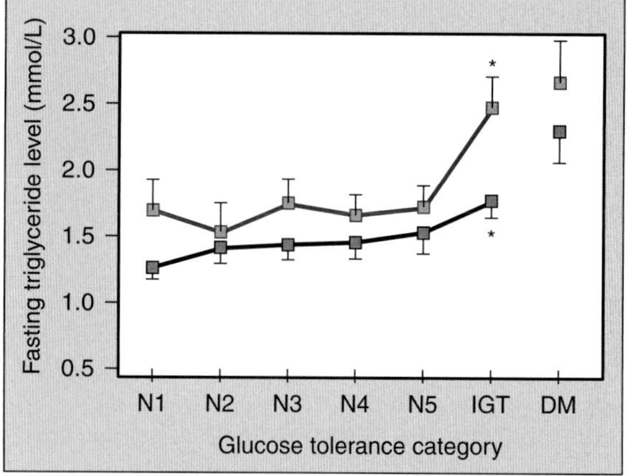

FIGURE 37-1 Distribution of lipid levels by glucose tolerance category in the Framingham Offspring Study. Mean plasma levels of high-density lipoprotein (HDL) cholesterol (left) and triglyceride (right) and 95% confidence intervals (error bars) among women (black squares and lines) and men (red squares and lines) are given for each glucose tolerance category: from the lowest quintile (N1) to the highest quintile (N5) of fasting plasma glucose level among participants with normal glucose tolerance (NGT); imparied glucose tolerance (IGT); and previously undiagnosed diabetes mellitus (DM). Means are multivariable adjusted. $^{*}P < 0.001$; $^{\dagger}P = 0.003$ for trend from the lowest quintile of normal fasting glucose level to IGT. Reprinted from Ref. 45, with permission.

apolipoprotein (apo) B-100, the defining protein of the atherogenic lipoprotein series, which includes VLDL, intermediate-density lipoproteins (IDL), and LDL, are increased in the setting of IR.[30] This is particularly true when hypertriglyceridemia is also present, as is usually the case in individuals with IR or T2DM. Total apoB levels are highly correlated with non-HDL cholesterol levels, the latter equaling the sum of cholesterol in VLDL, IDL, and LDL particles. In contrast, plasma levels of apoA-I, the surface protein associated with HDL particles, are reduced with IR.[30]

The derangements in lipid and lipoprotein physiology discussed thus far occur in the context of the fasting state. Importantly however, IR and T2DM are also associated with disordered postprandial lipid metabolism.[52] Although the severity of postprandial hyperlipidemia is typically closely related to the fasting plasma TG level,[52–57] postprandial dyslipidemia has been demonstrated in people with T2DM even in the setting of normal fasting TG levels and optimal blood glucose control.[55,56,58] Although postprandial dyslipidemia has been associated with increased CVD prevalence in individuals without diabetes,[52,59,60] this relationship has not been well characterized in people with IR or T2DM.[52,53,61]

NORMAL LIPOPROTEIN METABOLISM AND ABNORMALITIES ASSOCIATED WITH INSULIN RESISTANCE AND TYPE 2 DIABETES MELLITUS

The presence of IR exerts profound changes on lipid and lipoprotein physiology. These complex interactions are better appreciated in the context of an understanding of normal lipid and lipoprotein metabolism. Although normal lipoprotein metabolism is addressed in detail Chapter 1, the presentation in this chapter will combine normal lipoprotein physiology with the alterations present in individuals with IR and/or T2DM (Fig. 37-2).

Lipoproteins are macromolecular complexes consisting of core lipids, mainly TG and CEs, and surface phospholipids, free cholesterol, and one or more apolipoproteins. Five distinct major classes of lipoproteins have been characterized based on physical characteristics, including separation by ultracentrifugation, molecular weight, diameter, and chemical composition. Lipoprotein subclasses have been further defined based on subtle differences in physical and chemical properties. Notably, in addition to providing structural stability, the surface apolipoproteins impart critical functions to their respective lipoprotein particles.[62,63]

In the postprandial state, dietary TGs and CEs are assembled into chylomicrons in enterocytes of the small intestine. Assembly and secretion of chylomicrons, which are the largest and most TG-enriched lipoprotein particles, require the presence of apoB-48, a surface protein unique to these particles. The assembly and secretion of chylomicrons by the enterocyte is in several ways analogous to VLDL assembly and secretion by the hepatocyte: whereas apoB-100 is the prototypic surface protein associated with VLDL, IDL, and LDL, apoB-48, a truncated form of apoB-100, characterizes chylomicrons. Microsomal triglyceride transfer protein (MTP) packages apoB-48 with core lipids and is essential to the formation of chylomicrons. These newly assembled particles, also carrying apoA-I and apoA-IV, are secreted into the lymphatic system and eventually enter the venous circulation.[53,62–65] Studies in animal models of IR and/or diabetes have demonstrated increased intestinal secretion of apoB-48–containing lipoproteins, accompanied by increased expression, mass, and activity of intestinal MTP.[66–70] In one such model, a fructose-fed hamster with IR and dyslipidemia, intestinal lipoprotein overproduction was also associated with an increase in intestinal *de novo* lipogenesis, likely mediated through activation of a major transcription factor, the sterol response element–binding protein–1c (SREBP-1c).[68–70] Treatment with an insulin-sensitizing agent, rosiglitazone, reduced intestinal lipoprotein production in two separate models of IR and dyslipidemia.[71,72] A recent study of men with varying degrees of IR, but without DM, demonstrated increased intestinal production of apoB-48–containing TG-rich lipoprotein (TRL) particles.[54] Moreover, this has also been recently shown in subjects with T2DM.[73] A

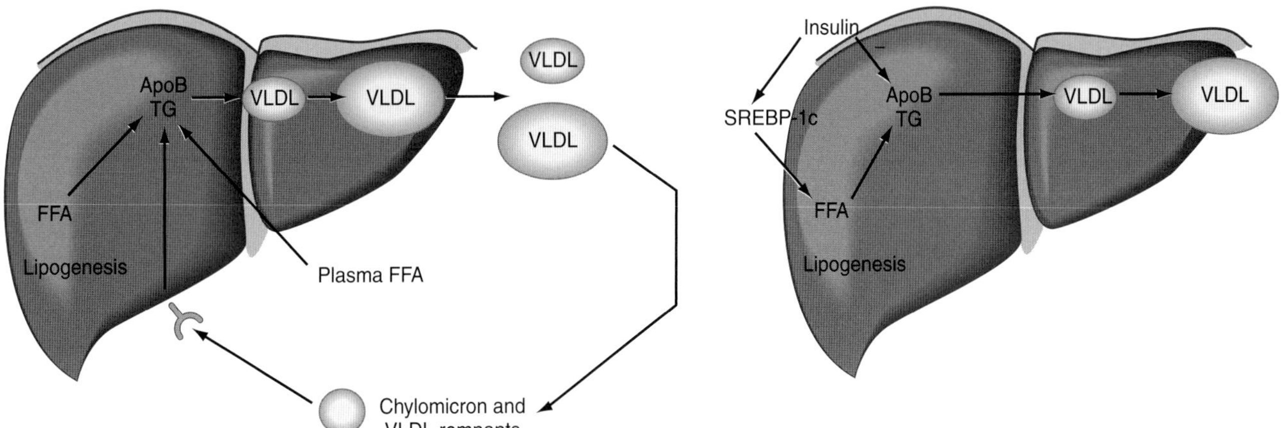

FIGURE 37-2 (A). Regulation of very-low-density lipoprotein (VLDL) assembly and secretion by three sources of triglyceride (TG). There are three major sources of hepatic TG, the main substrate regulating VLDL apolipoprotein (apo) B secretion. They are plasma free fatty acids (FFA), which are albumin bound and derived mainly from lipolysis of TG in adipose tissue; TG fatty acids that are delivered to the hepatocytes by endocytosis of chylomicron and VLDL remnants; and fatty acids that are synthesized by *de novo* hepatic lipogenesis. In the setting of insulin resistance and hyperinsulinemia, fatty acid flux through the plasma to the liver is increased; peripheral removal of chylomicron and VLDL TG by lipolysis is reduced, leaving TG-enriched remnant particles for hepatic uptake; and *de novo* hepatic lipogenesis is increased. All three sources of TG may contribute to the increased VLDL secretion present in individuals with insulin resistance. (B) Effects of insulin and hepatic insulin resístance on VLDL assembly and secretion. Insulin regulates the balance between VLDL secretion and hepatic steatosis by stimulating both *de novo* hepatic lipogenesis, through activation of transcription factor sterol response element–binding protein–1c (SREBP-1c), and the degradation of apoB. Hepatic insulin resistance does not seem to affect lipogenesis but does impair insulin-mediated apoB degradation. Therefore, if plasma hyperinsulinemia is accompanied by modest hepatic insulin resistance, then both lipogenesis and apoB degradation will be increased, leading to the development of hepatic steatosis. However, in the presence of plasma hyperinsulinemia and severe hepatic insulin resistance, lipogenesis will still be increased, but apoB degradation will be impaired, leading to more VLDL secretion. The latter situcation could reduce the risk of developing hepatic steatosis but exacerbate the dyslipidemia. This relationship between lipogenesis and apoB degradation is further modulated by FFAs taken up from the plasma by the liver, and by the TG content of chylomicron and VLDL remnant particles returning to the liver. Reprinted from Ref. 87, with permission.

separate study, comparing individuals with or without T2DM, demonstrated increased intestinal expression of MTP in people with T2DM.[74] Furthermore, treatment with inhibitors of 3-hydroxy-3-methylglutaryl–coenzyme A (HMG-CoA) reductase, the rate-limiting enzyme in cholesterol biosynthesis, was associated with lower MTP mRNA levels both in individuals with and those without T2DM in that study. This effect was possibly mediated through decreased activation of a positive sterol response element in the promoter region of the MTP gene.[74,75]

After entering the plasma, chylomicrons acquire apoC-I, apoC-II, and apoC-III from the surface of HDL particles. Chylomicron clearance is largely mediated through hydrolysis of core TGs by adipose tissue–derived lipoprotein lipase (LPL) in a process that requires apoC-II as an activator of LPL. In contrast, apoC-III can inhibit LPL-mediated lipolysis. The breakdown of chylomicron TG releases fatty acids (FAs), which are taken up by the local tissue, and produces chylomicron remnant particles. These remnants acquire apoE from HDL particles and are also enriched in CEs derived from exchange of core lipids with LDL and HDL, the latter process being mediated by cholesteryl ester transfer protein (CETP). Ultimately, chylomicron remnant particles are cleared mainly by hepatic uptake through the interactions of apoE with the hepatic LDL receptor, the LDL receptor–related protein (LRP), and/or cell-surface heparan sulfate proteoglycans. Additionally, hepatic lipase (HL) further hydrolyzes chylomicron remnant particle TG and may augment uptake by the liver. ApoC-I and apoC-III modulate chylomicron clearance by the liver by interfering in the binding of apoE to its receptors.[53,63–65,76,77]

IR adversely affects chylomicron and remnant particle metabolism at several steps. IR and T2DM are associated with modestly decreased LPL activity and an increase in apoC-III relative to apoC-II levels. Increased apoC-III secretion into plasma has been demonstrated in individuals with IR and hypertriglyceridemia.[78,79] The resulting effect is impaired LPL-mediated lipolysis of chylomicron TG as well as decreased hepatic uptake of remnant particles. This decrease in chylomicron clearance is further exacerbated by hepatic overproduction of TG-rich VLDL particles as a consequence of IR.[30] Increased numbers of VLDL particles subsequently compete with chylomicrons for LPL-mediated lipolysis. The net effect is an increase in circulating TRLs, which are known to be particularly atherogenic.[51,65,80,81]

While the postprandial state is largely characterized by intestinal chylomicron production, hepatic VLDL assembly and secretion predominate during the fasting state. This process is initiated in the hepatocyte rough endoplasmic reticulum (ER), where apoB-100 is constitutively synthesized. Utilization of nascent apoB-100 for the assembly and secretion of VLDL is, to a large extent, limited by substrate availability, namely TG.[82] Decreased availability of core lipids and/or insufficient MTP activity can lead to both co- and post-translational degradation of apoB-100. However, in the presence of adequate TG, apoB-100 is progressively lipidated through the actions of hepatic MTP, and the newly assembled VLDL particle is transported to the Golgi apparatus, where it may undergo further lipidation before secretion into plasma. The size of the nascent VLDL particle is also determined by TG availability, with a predominance of larger, more buoyant, TG-rich $VLDL_1$, and fewer smaller, denser $VLDL_2$ particles produced in the presence of excess hepatocyte TG. Insulin also exerts a major regulatory effect on this process through its ability to target apoB-100 for post-translational degradation; in the presence of IR, this effect may be significantly diminished. The combination of IR and excess hepatic TG availability results in increased hepatic secretion of both apoB-100 and TG.[51,80,83–85] This process is complicated, however, by the systemic hyperinsulinemia present in most individuals with IR; the balance of plasma insulin levels and the degree of hepatic IR, together with hepatic TG availability, will determine whether apoB-100 is degraded or secreted as VLDL. Further complicating this scheme is the ER stress that develops in the presence of IR and fatty liver[86]; we have unpublished data demonstrating that apoB-100 degradation may be increased by ER stress, leading to less hepatic VLDL secretion and greater steatosis.

As VLDL assembly and secretion are highly dependent on TG availability, FA contribution to the hepatic TG pool is an important driver of this process. Three major sources of FAs have been described: circulating free FAs (FFAs) from the peripheral tissues, notably from adipose tissue, FAs derived from chylomicron and VLDL remnant uptake by the liver, and FAs obtained through *de novo* hepatic lipogenesis. In the presence of IR and hyperinsulinemia, increased hepatic FA availability results from alterations in all three sources.[87,88] First, increased FA flux to the liver occurs as a result of IR in adipocytes. We have observed increased hepatic secretion of apoB-containing lipoproteins resulting from infusion of albumin-bound FAs in mice,[89] and similar results have been demonstrated in humans.[90] Second, the enhanced postprandial lipemia and overproduction of TG-rich VLDL particles in the fasting state combine to produce elevated levels of apoB-48– and apoB-100–containing remnant particles carrying TG that is available for hepatic uptake.[65,80] *De novo* lipogenesis, the third source of hepatic TG, is likely up-regulated via insulin-mediated stimulation of SREBP-1c, a major lipogenic transcription factor. Importantly, this effect of insulin appears to occur normally despite hepatic resistance to the effects of insulin on carbohydrate metabolism.[91] If there is concomitant hyperglycemia, there will also be induction of another transcription factor, carbohydrate responsive element–binding protein (ChREBP), which also activates genes required for lipogenesis.[85,87] Interestingly, the hepatic expression of another nuclear transcription factor, peroxisome proliferator–activated receptor–γ (PPAR-γ), is increased in a number of mouse models of IR and dyslipidemia,[92] as well as in humans with hepatic steatosis. In humans, nonalcoholic fatty liver disease (NAFLD), which is closely associated with IR, is characterized by increased hepatic TG derived from *de novo* lipogenesis.[93]

Once secreted, the fate of VLDL particles initially parallels that of chylomicrons in the postprandial state; namely, hydrolysis of VLDL TG by LPL in a process modulated by the relative proportions of apoC-II and apoC-III. Lipolysis of core TG yields smaller, denser VLDL remnants usually referred to as IDL; the efficiency of this process is impaired in the setting of IR. The eventual hepatic uptake of VLDL remnants is mediated by the same pathways involved in chylomicron particle uptake. However, unlike chylomicron remnants, VLDL remnants may also undergo further catabolism to yield LDL particles. HL is thought to play an important role in this process. However, despite the increased levels of HL observed with IR and T2DM, conversion of VLDL to LDL is typically reduced. LDL particles are primarily composed of core CEs associated with surface apoB-100. As with VLDL remnants and IDL, clearance of LDL occurs mainly through hepatic LDL receptor–mediated uptake. IR is associated with a reduction in LDL receptors, thereby limiting removal of these particles from the circulation.[63,77,80,94,95]

Importantly, circulating LDL can participate in CETP-mediated exchange of its core CE for VLDL or chylomicron TG, resulting in a TG-enriched, CE-depleted LDL particle. This transfer may be increased if LDL particles are not efficiently cleared by hepatic LDL receptors. Subsequent lipolysis of the TG-enriched LDL particle by LPL or HL produces small dense LDL. As expected, the hypertriglyceridemia typically seen with IR or T2DM is strongly related to the presence of small dense LDL. Furthermore, it has been proposed that the large $VLDL_1$ particles that predominate in the setting of hypertriglyceridemia are avid acceptors of CEs from HDL, also through a process mediated by CETP, and that these CE-enriched particles then preferentially undergo catabolism to give rise to small dense LDL.[63,96–100] In addition, the increased HL activity observed in T2DM could play an important role in the production of small dense LDL particles.[63,101]

The HDL class differs considerably in structure and function from the lipoproteins discussed thus far. The formation of HDL begins with the secretion by the liver and intestine of cholesterol-poor phospholipid discs containing surface apoA-I. Cellular transfer of intracellular or plasma membrane cholesterol to these nascent particles occurs via the transport protein, ATP-binding cassette transporter A1 (ABCA1). This transfer is coupled with cholesterol esterification by the enzyme lecithin:cholesterol acyltransferase (LCAT), accompanied by movement of the product CEs to the core of the maturing HDL_3 particle. ApoA-I mediates this process through its ability to activate LCAT. Repeated cycles of this process, together with transfer of cell cholesterol to the maturing HDL particle via ATP-binding cassette transporter G1 (ABCG1) and scavenger receptor class B type I (SR-BI), give rise to mature, CE-rich HDL_2. Mature HDL particles can deliver both free and esterified cholesterol to the liver via interaction with SR-BI.[30,102] This process of reverse cholesterol transport (RCT) from the peripheral tissues and, notably, from cholesterol-laden tissue macrophages, with eventual hepatic uptake and metabolism, is a critical function of HDL.[102,103] The fate of apoA-I is less certain, but it is known that significant quantities are taken up and degraded by the kidneys and liver. If CETP-mediated exchange of core lipids is increased, as is the case in IR with dyslipidemia, apoA-I affinity for the small HDL particles that result from HL-mediated lipolysis of TG-rich HDL is decreased. This leads to dissociation of apoA-I from the small HDL and clearance of free apoA-I by the kidney.[63,101–103]

In the presence of IR or T2DM, multiple factors acting in concert result in lower levels of HDL cholesterol and apoA-I. As already discussed, these include enhanced postprandial lipemia, hepatic overproduction of TG-rich VLDL, and decreased LPL-mediated lipolysis; all of these abnormalities result in increased numbers of TRLs available for CETP-mediated interactions with HDL. Added to this is increased HL activity in IR, which, together with increased CETP-mediated exchange of core lipids, leads to smaller and fewer HDL particles. The decrease in HDL particles available for participation in RCT may be critical to the atherogenicity of the dyslipidemia associated with IR or T2DM.[87,100–103]

THERAPEUTIC APPROACHES TO THE DYSLIPIDEMIA OF INSULIN RESISTANCE AND TYPE 2 DIABETES MELLITUS

Rationale for Treating LDL

Over the past 50 years, results from epidemiologic studies, animal models, and clinical trials have clearly demonstrated that elevated LDL cholesterol is a major risk factor for CV morbidity and mortality.[6,104] In addition, it has been demonstrated that aggressively lowering LDL cholesterol levels can decrease CV risk.[105–108] As a result, many investigators are interested in determining the appropriate amount of LDL cholesterol reduction needed to substantially decrease CV risk. It is important to remember that all individuals do not have the same absolute CV risk, and as a result, LDL cholesterol goals must be adjusted to accommodate each individual's absolute risk.[6] Major risk factors known to increase CV risk that should be assessed when determining LDL cholesterol goals include cigarette smoking, hypertension (BP ≥140/90 mm Hg or treatment with an antihypertensive medication), low HDL cholesterol (<40 mg/dL for both men and women), family history of premature CHD (<55 years in male first-degree relatives; <65 years in female first-degree relatives), and age (men ≥45 years; women ≥55 years). Using these risk factors, patients can be stratified into three risk categories. The highest risk category is CHD or CHD risk equivalent; this category includes patients with known CHD, other clinical forms of atherosclerotic disease (such as peripheral artery disease, abdominal aortic aneurysm, and symptomatic carotid artery disease), DM, and/or a 10-year Framingham risk for major coronary events greater than 20%. As a result, their lipid treatment goals are aggressive and they should be targeted to achieve an LDL cholesterol of less than 100 mg/dL (Table 37-2). The second category of patients includes those patients who have two or more major risk factors and a 10-year Framingham risk for CHD that is 10% to 20%. As a result, their treatment goal is less aggressive and their LDL cholesterol goal is less than 130 mg/dL. The third category consists of persons having zero to one risk factors and a 10-year risk less than 10%; their LDL cholesterol goal is less than 160 mg/dL.

TABLE 37-2 National Cholesterol Education Program Adult Treatment Panel III Lipid Goals and Therapeutic Considerations for Patients with Diabetic Dyslipidemia

Goals LDL cholesterol <100 mg/dL; <70 mg/dL optional goal for very-high-risk patients
Non-HDL cholesterol <130 mg/dL if TG ≥200 mg/dL
Therapeutic considerations Initiate TLC
Intensively treat nonlipid risk factors (hypertension, cigarette smoking, hyperglycemia)
If TG ≥200 mg/dL, consider fibrate or niacin (alone or with statin*) to achieve non-HDL cholesterol goal
If niacin is used, use relatively low doses (<3 g/day)
In patients with baseline LDL cholesterol ≥130 mg/dL
Many diabetic patients (type 1 or 2) will require LDL cholesterol–lowering drug therapy (statins usually first choice) in addition to TLC
Clinical judgment is required in type 1 diabetes to determine intensity of LDL cholesterol–lowering therapy
In patients with type 2 diabetes, treatment of atherogenic dyslipidemia (high TG, low HDL, small LDL) should generally be delayed until LDL cholesterol goal has been achieved
In patients with baseline LDL cholesterol 100–129 mg/dL
Consider intensifying TLC
Consider using LDL cholesterol–lowering drug
Consider using drug therapy to lower TG or raise HDL cholesterol
Control nonlipid risk factors
In patients with on-treatment LDL cholesterol 100–129 mg/dL
Intensify TLC
If TG <200 mg/dL, consider intensifying LDL cholesterol–lowering therapy (such as increasing statin dose or combining statin with bile acid sequestrant)

*The combination of statin plus fibrate may increase risk for myopathy. Patients should be instructed to be aware of the signs and symptoms of myopathy and report these immediately to their physician.

HDL, high-density lipoprotein; LDL, low-density lipoprotein; NCEP ATP III, National Cholesterol Education Program Adult Treatment Panel III; TG, triglycerides; TLC, therapeutic lifestyle changes.

From Refs. 109 and 121, with permission.

Recently, there has been a push to drive LDL cholesterol goals lower and lower with the hopes that this will lead to an improvement in CV outcomes. In fact, the NCEP issued a "white paper" suggesting an even lower LDL cholesterol goal of less than 70 mg/dL for patients at very high CV risk.[109] The Treating to New Targets (TNT) study demonstrated that intensive therapy with atorvastatin 80 mg compared with atorvastatin 10 mg significantly reduced the rate of major CV events by 22%. In TNT, the end-of-treatment mean LDL cholesterol levels were 98.6 mg/dL and 77 mg/dL with atorvastatin 10 mg and 80 mg, respectively.[108] The Incremental Decrease in End Points through Aggressive Lipid Lowering (IDEAL) study was similar in design to TNT and compared simvastatin 20 mg with atorvastatin 80 mg.[110] Although IDEAL did not show a significant benefit of treatment with a higher dose of statin for the overall endpoint (P=0.07), numerous secondary endpoints were statistically different in favor of high-dose treatment, and the overall view is that IDEAL generally supported the results from TNT. The results of the Pravastatin or Atorvastatin Evaluation and Infection Therapy–Thrombolysis in Myocardial Infarction 22 (PROVE IT–TIMI 22) study,[111] in which patients with acute coronary syndrome who had their mean LDL cholesterol level reduced to 62 mg/dL fared better than those patients whose mean LDL cholesterol was 95 mg/dL, support the TNT results.

In TNT, individuals with the MetS had a similar benefit from more aggressive LDL cholesterol lowering as did those without the MetS; nevertheless, participants with the MetS in either treatment group had more events than did their counterparts without the MetS.[112] Additionally, post hoc analyses of other statin studies have shown a benefit in MetS or "MetS-like" subgroups.[105,113–115] Statin trials have also been conducted specifically in patients with T2DM. In the Collaborative Atorvastatin Diabetes Study (CARDS), treatment with atorvastatin resulted in a significant reduction in major CV events irrespective of pretreatment cholesterol levels.[116] On the other hand, the Atorvastatin Study for Prevention of Coronary Heart Disease Endpoints in Non-Insulin-Dependent Diabetes Mellitus (ASPEN), which randomized patients with T2DM to receive 10 mg of atorvastatin or placebo in a 4-year study, did not demonstrate a significant reduction in the primary composite endpoint of CV death with atorvastatin treatment.[117]

It is important to note that the NCEP ATP III guidelines did not place patients with the MetS into any specific risk category; their risk is determined by the number of risk factors that they carry as well as whether they have clinical CVD. Some individuals with the MetS will fall into the CHD risk equivalent class, but others will not. However, the "white paper" categorized individuals with the combination of the MetS and CVD as being very high risk and requiring, therefore, an LDL cholesterol goal of less than 70 mg/dL.[109] Additionally, although the NCEP ATP III defined DM as a CHD risk equivalent condition,[6] there are several studies showing that patients with T2DM without established CHD do not have a 10-year CHD risk greater than 20%.[118–120] The best approach, therefore, is to take all of an individual's risk factors into account rather than simply classifying him/her based on a single diagnosis such as DM or MetS.

Rationale for Treating HDL and TG

While LDL cholesterol remains the primary target of Lipid-modifying therapy for the primary and secondary prevention of CVD in the general population and among people with DM, HDL cholesterol and TG are given high importance, especially in higher-risk individuals.[6] Epidemiologic and clinical trial evidence has clearly demonstrated the presence of elevated TG levels and decreased HDL cholesterol with IR, in the presence or absence of T2DM.[29,32–45] As defined by the NCEP ATP III, the MetS dyslipidemia is characterized by TG levels of 150 mg/dL or higher and HDL cholesterol less than 40 mg/dL in men and less than 50 mg/dL in women.[121] Additionally, the NCEP ATP III guidelines state that when TG levels are modestly or greatly elevated (200–499 mg/dL), non-HDL cholesterol should be a secondary goal of therapy. Non-HDL cholesterol (total cholesterol – HDL cholesterol) is considered a surrogate marker for the apoB-100–containing lipoproteins, and thus is believed by many to be a good predictor of atherogenic potential.[122–126] Non-HDL cholesterol goals are set at 30 mg/dL higher than the LDL cholesterol goal for each level of risk; in the case of most individuals with T2DM, the non-HDL cholesterol target is less than 130 mg/dL.[121] Alternatively, in the case of either normotriglyceridemia (TG $<$150 mg/dL), or mildly elevated TG levels (TG 150–199 mg/dL), raising low HDL cholesterol should be considered; however, the NCEP ATP III does not set specific HDL cholesterol goals, nor does it set target TG levels. The ADA also emphasizes the prime importance of attaining target LDL cholesterol levels, but employs a different approach to the management of TGs and HDL cholesterol (Table 37-3). The ADA guidelines recommend lowering TG levels to less than 150 mg/dL and include gender-specific HDL cholesterol goals; namely, more than 40 mg/dL in men and more than 50 mg/dL in women.[127,128]

The rationale for treatment to improve HDL cholesterol levels in people with IR or T2DM is grounded in evidence from numerous epidemiologic studies in which low HDL cholesterol is an independent predictor of CHD morbidity and mortality. Notably, this effect has been observed in studies involving large numbers of people with IR or T2DM.[34,37,129–134] Evidence from prospective intervention trials and secondary analyses has suggested a benefit of raising HDL cholesterol levels on the risk of CHD events, independent of changes in other lipid and nonlipid risk factors.[135,136] Of note, a post hoc analysis of the Bezafibrate Infarction Prevention (BIP) Study focusing on the subgroup of participants with the MetS revealed a reduced incidence in MI associated with significant improvements in HDL cholesterol and TG levels.[137] Furthermore, in that analysis, a cardiac mortality benefit was demonstrated among subjects having "augmented" (i.e., four or five) features of the MetS, as defined by the NCEP ATP III. More-definitive conclusions will require evidence from prospective clinical trials. In the Veterans Affairs HDL Intervention Trial (VA-HIT), in which increases in HDL cholesterol were predictive of reductions

TABLE 37-3 American Diabetes Association Dyslipidemia Treatment Goals and Recommendations for Adults with Diabetes

Treatment goals
LDL cholesterol
In patients without overt CVD
Primary goal is LDL cholesterol <100 mg/dL
Statin therapy to decrease LDL cholesterol by 30%–40% in patients >40 years of age regardless of baseline LDL cholesterol
In patients with overt CVD
Treat with statin to decrease LDL cholesterol by 30%–40%.
Option: Treat with high-dose statin to reduce LDL cholesterol to <70 mg/dL
Decrease TG to <150 mg/dL
Increase HDL cholesterol to >40 mg/dL; consider increasing HDL cholesterol to >50 mg/dL in women
Treatment recommendations
Medical nutrition therapy
Weight loss in overweight and obese individuals
Diet with reduced intake of total fat (~30% of total calories), saturated fat (<7% of total calories), and *trans* fatty acids (minimal); cholesterol <200 mg/day
Increased exercise
Smoking cessation
Pharmacologic therapy
Statin therapy to decrease LDL cholesterol
Fibrate therapy to decrease TG and increase HDL cholesterol
Combination therapy with statin and another agent if necessary to achieve lipid targets

From Ref. 127, with permission.

in CV endpoints in the group treated with gemfibrozil,[136] the greatest overall benefit of treatment was observed in subgroups with IR, with or without T2DM.[138,139]

In contrast to the evidence supporting an inverse relationship between HDL cholesterol levels and CHD morbidity and mortality, the data regarding the independent effects of plasma TG levels on CHD risk are more controversial. Part of the difficulty stems from the close interrelationships between levels of TGs and the atherogenic apoB-containing lipoproteins.[140,141] TG levels have nevertheless been shown to predict CHD risk in observational studies.[142–144] In several clinical trials, stratification of individuals by TG and HDL cholesterol levels has revealed higher-risk subgroups with dyslipidemia that have benefited most from LDL cholesterol lowering interventions with respect to CHD risk reduction.[112,115,145] However, no clinical trials thus far have demonstrated an independent relationship between TG lowering and CHD risk reduction, including VA-HIT, in which TG levels fell by 31%.[135,136]

As mentioned earlier, it is worth noting that postprandial lipemia has been associated with CHD in individuals without DM, whereas the evidence is less convincing or absent in individuals with IR or DM.[52,53] Data from one cross-sectional study do not support an association between postprandial lipemia and the presence of CHD among people with T2DM.[61] Another small study suggests that postprandial numbers of small remnant particles may contribute to the severity of angiographic CHD in T2DM.[146] Larger prospective studies are needed before recommendations can be made regarding the potential utility of postprandial hyperlipidemia as a predictor of CV risk in IR or DM. This, along with the lack of simple, clinically useful uniform measures of postprandial lipemia, explains the lack of guidelines for therapy of postprandial hyperlipidemia.

Treatment Options

Diet and Lifestyle Modification

It has long been known by clinicians, investigators, and lay people alike that appropriate lifestyle interventions involving diet and exercise can lead to weight loss; since obesity is a major contributor to the MetS and T2DM, weight loss should provide significant benefits to individuals with these problems. Indeed, in the Diabetes Prevention Program,[147] about 6% weight loss and the addition of 2 hours of exercise per week was associated with a 58% reduction in the incidence of new T2DM in a group with IGT. Similar results were obtained with weight loss and exercise in a study conducted in Finland.[148] Recently, the 1-year results of Look AHEAD (Action for Health in Diabetes), a study of weight loss and diet in overweight and obese individuals, reported that intensive lifestyle intervention resulted in clinically significant weight loss in people with T2DM.[149] Participants in the intensive lifestyle intervention group achieved an average loss of 8.6% of initial body weight and a 21% improvement in CV fitness. These participants had a significantly greater decrease in the number of medicines used to treat their DM and BP as well as a greater improvement in glycemic control when compared with participants receiving only diabetes support and education.

In addition to simply reducing caloric intake, interventions that alter the nutrient composition of the diet may have benefits on risk factors for CVD and T2DM. There has been much debate, however, both in the popular press and in the medical community, regarding which diet strategy is most effective for both weight loss and reductions in CV risk. A study by Foster et al.[150] suggested that although a low-carbohydrate, high-protein, high-fat diet produced a greater weight loss at 6 months than did a low-calorie, high-carbohydrate, low-fat diet, the difference was no longer significant at 1 year. When compared with a low-fat diet, the low-carbohydrate diet actually reduced some components of the MetS and risk factors for CHD (serum TG and serum HDL cholesterol), but not others (BP, insulin sensitivity, and serum LDL cholesterol). In a very similar study, Samaha et al. presented data that demonstrated that severely obese subjects with a high prevalence of the MetS or DM lost more weight during 6 months on a carbohydrate-restricted diet than on a calorie- and fat-restricted diet. Even after adjustments were made for weight loss, participants on the carbohydrate-restricted diet had a relative improvement in insulin sensitivity and TG levels.[151] A randomized trial by Dansinger et al. further explored the effectiveness of different popular diets: Atkins, Zone, Weight Watchers, and Ornish.

At the end of 1 year, there were no significant differences in achieved weight loss between the diets; all diets led to about 2 kg of weight loss. Importantly, those subjects with better adherence to any of the diets had greater weight loss and improvements in their CV risk profiles.[152] The conclusions, which are consistent with previous data, suggest that low-carbohydrate diets increase HDL cholesterol, and diets low in saturated fat decrease LDL cholesterol. In contrast, a recent trial at Stanford University Medical School compared four weight-loss diets (Atkins, Zone, LEARN, and Ornish) and observed statistically significant differences among diet groups for both weight loss and CV risk factors at 12 months. Participants assigned to follow the lowest-carbohydrate diet, the Atkins diet, lost more weight and had more favorable overall metabolic effects at 12 months than those assigned to follow the other diets. However, the question of whether altering macronutrient composition without achieving weight loss can lead to changes in CV risk profile needs further elucidation.[153]

Lichtenstein[154] considered the individual effects of different dietary macronutrients on CV risk factors in an iso-weight setting. In the setting of stable body weight, replacement of dietary carbohydrate with fat resulted in lower TG and VLDL cholesterol concentrations, higher HDL cholesterol concentration, and a lower total cholesterol/HDL cholesterol ratio. Earlier studies had demonstrated similar effects of high-carbohydrate diets in subjects with or without diabetes.[155,156] On the other hand, Chandalia et al.[157] showed that increasing fiber in a high-carbohydrate diet abrogated the effects of that diet on plasma TG and HDL cholesterol levels. Most recently, the Diet Effects on Lipids and Thrombogenic Activity (DELTA) study demonstrated that a diet with higher carbohydrate and increased fiber was associated with a modest but significant increase in plasma TG levels and a small but significant reduction in HDL cholesterol levels compared with a diet in which 8% of the carbohydrate was replaced with monounsaturated fatty acids in subjects with the dyslipidemia of the MetS.[158]

Conclusions that may be drawn from these diet interventions must be considered with the following caveat: We do not know if the changes that we see in plasma TG levels and, in particular, in HDL cholesterol concentrations, are indicative of changes in risk for CVD. We are, in fact, extrapolating from large epidemiologic databases that show that increased TG and reduced HDL cholesterol levels are associated with increased CV risk; this extrapolation remains to be proven in a clinical trial with dietary intervention.

Pharmacologic Therapy

Before discussing in detail specific pharmacologic therapies, it is important to note that improving glycemic control in T2DM can result in mild to modest improvement in the dyslipidemia of diabetes. This is particularly true for hypertriglyceridemia in the setting of poor glycemic control; furthermore, the degree of TG lowering may be related to the magnitude of improvement in glycemia. Concomitant with optimization of glucose control, therapeutic lifestyle changes (TLC), including dietary modification, weight reduction, and regular physical activity, should be initiated prior to, or simultaneously with, pharmacologic therapy. Pharmacologic therapy for dyslipidemia should be considered in the context of these changes.[121,127]

3-Hydroxy-3-Methylglutaryl–Coenzyme A (HMG-CoA) Reductase Inhibitors. The HMG-CoA reductase inhibitors, or "statins," are the most extensively studied group of lipid-modifying agents.[159] They are the most effective pharmacologic agents for reducing LDL cholesterol concentrations and should be considered first-line therapy for this purpose, both in individuals with and in individuals without T2DM.[121,127,160] Several agents are available for clinical use, including lovastatin, fluvastatin, pravastatin, simvastatin, atorvastatin, and rosuvastatin. As a class, they produce LDL cholesterol reductions of 18% to 55%, with more modest changes in HDL cholesterol and TG levels (5%–15% elevations and 7%–30% reductions, respectively).[121,161]

Statins achieve their LDL cholesterol–lowering effect through inhibition of HMG-CoA reductase, the rate-limiting enzyme in cholesterol biosynthesis. Decreased hepatic cholesterol in turn causes up-regulation of hepatic LDL receptors and increased LDL particle clearance. There is also evidence for reduction in VLDL levels with statin therapy. In individuals with the dyslipidemia of IR or T2DM, statins have been shown to reduce the hepatic assembly and secretion of apoB-containing lipoproteins; this may or may not be accompanied by increased clearance of VLDL and LDL particles from the circulation. Moreover, some data suggest that statins reduce VLDL TG secretion; however, the mechanism for this is unclear.[121,127,161] These agents may also lower apoC-III levels, thereby enhancing lipolysis of TRL particles, as suggested in an analysis of the Diabetes Atorvastatin Lipid Intervention (DALI) study.[162]

Many clinical trial data support the effectiveness of statin therapy in primary and secondary CV risk reduction in the general population with hypercholesterolemia and in people with DM (Table 37-4), although the body of evidence for primary prevention of CVD in individuals with DM is smaller.[128,159] Furthermore, the relative beneficial effects of statins are similar in individuals with or without DM.[160] CARDS, a primary prevention study of 2838 participants with T2DM, demonstrated a statistically significant 37% reduction in major CV events among participants on low-dose atorvastatin treatment.[116] Moreover, this effect did not differ by pretreatment cholesterol levels; participants having baseline LDL cholesterol levels lower than 120 mg/dL had similar treatment benefits as those with higher pretreatment LDL cholesterol. The Medical Research Council/British Heart Foundation Heart Protection Study (MRC/BHF HPS) included a large cohort of participants with T2DM, approximately half of whom had no evidence of existing coronary or other occlusive arterial disease.[163] Simvastatin therapy produced substantial reductions in the risk of coronary events, stroke, and revascularizations in participants with DM, irrespective of pre-existing occlusive arterial disease or lipid concentrations. Similar to the CARDS findings, the treatment benefit in the MRC/BHF HPS extended even to participants with relatively normal baseline LDL

TABLE 37-4 Major Placebo-Controlled Clinical Trials of Statin Therapy in Patients with Type 2 Diabetes Millitus

Trial	*n* (DM)	Statin, mg/day	Years	Change from Baseline, %			CHD Event* Rate		RRR, %	*P* for RRR	ARR, %	NNT
				LDL Cholesterol	TG	HDL Cholesterol	Statin	Placebo				
Secondary prevention												
4S[113]	202	Simvastatin 20–40	5.4†	-36	-11	+7	22.9	45.4	55	0.002	22.5	4
4S reanalysis[114]	483	Simvastatin 20–40	5.4†	~-36	~-11	~+6	23.5	37.5	42	0.001	14.0	7
CARE[105]	586	Pravastatin 40	5.0‡	-27	-13	+4	17.7	20.4	13	NS	2.7	37
LIPID[167]	1077	Pravastatin 40	6.0‡	~-28	~-19	~+4	19.6	23.4	19	0.11	3.8	26
IFG	940	Pravastatin 40	6.0‡				11.8	17.8	36	0.009	6.0	17
HPS[163]	5963	Simvastatin 40	4.8‡	-28	-13	+1	9.4	12.6	27	<0.0001	4.9	20
Primary prevention												
ASCOT[164]	2532	Atorvastatin 10	3.3†	-36	-16	+2	9.6	11.4	16	NS	1.8	56
CARDS[116]	2838	Atorvastatin 10	3.9†	-31	-17	-9	5.8	9.0	37	0.001	3.2	31
4D[166]	1255	Atorvastatin 20	4.0‡	-42	NA	NA	38	37	8	0.37	—	—

*CHD death or nonfatal myocardial infarction except in Collaborative Atorvastatin Diabetes Study (CARDS) (also unstable angina and nonfatal cardiac arrest) and German Diabetes and Dialysis Study (4D) (also stroke).

†Median follow-up.

‡Mean follow-up.

Adapted with permission from Ginsberg.[161] Copyright 2006, The Endocrine Society.

ARR, absolute risk reduction; CHD, coronary heart disease; DM, diabetes mellitus; IFG, impaired fasting glucose; NA, not available; NNT, number needed to treat to prevent one event; NS, not significant; RRR, relative risk reduction.

cholesterol levels, defined by the investigators as lower than 116 mg/dL. Nevertheless, other major trials that included large numbers of individuals with T2DM did not confirm these findings. As noted earlier in this chapter, ASPEN, which included primary and secondary prevention participants, did not demonstrate a significant reduction in the primary composite endpoint with atorvastatin.[117] The negative finding was attributed to certain features of the study design, as well as to changes in lipid treatment guidelines during the course of the study that necessitated protocol changes. Similarly, statin therapy did not impart a benefit with regard to coronary events in the subgroup of participants with T2DM in the Anglo-Scandinavian Cardiac Outcomes Trial–Lipid-Lowering Arm (ASCOT-LLA).[164] The lack of benefit was ascribed to a low coronary event rate, a result stemming in part from the early cessation of the trial because of a marked benefit of statin therapy in the general study population. In the nonblinded Antihypertensive and Lipid-Lowering Treatment to Prevent Heart Attack Trial–Lipid-Lowering Trial (ALLHAT-LLT), the lack of effect with pravastatin therapy in participants with T2DM is believed to be due to the high use of lipid-lowering therapy in the "usual care" control group, resulting in a smaller differential in LDL cholesterol levels between the statin and control groups compared with that seen in other large statin trials.[165] Finally, the German Diabetes and Dialysis Study evaluated participants with T2DM and end-stage renal disease; treatment with atorvastatin did not confer a statistically significant benefit over placebo therapy.[166] What role, then, do statins play in the prevention of CVD in individuals with DM but without overt CVD? Recently, a joint statement from the American Heart Association and the ADA addressed this issue. Of note, the recommendations addressed one particularly interesting subgroup of people; namely, individuals with baseline LDL cholesterol levels less than 100 mg/dL. In these patients, the decision to begin statin therapy should take into account age and CVD risk. Specifically, the initiation of statins in individuals with DM who are over the age of 40 years and have at least one major CVD risk factor may be appropriate in this setting and should be based on clinical judgment.[128]

In contrast to studies of statins for the primary prevention of CVD in individuals with DM, the data with regard to secondary prevention of CV events are very robust. The MRC/BHF HPS provided strong evidence supporting the benefit of simvastatin in reducing the risk of CVD in individuals with DM and pre-existing occlusive arterial disease.[163] Further support was added by a subgroup analysis of the Long-Term Intervention with Pravastatin in Ischaemic Disease (LIPID) trial, which demonstrated a reduction in CV events, including stroke, in participants with IFG or T2DM and established CHD.[167] Moreover, the absolute risk reductions seen in those with IFG or T2DM were greater than those seen in the overall study population. These findings supported the results of post hoc analyses of participants with IFG or DM in the Scandinavian Simvastatin Survival Study (4S).[114,168] Another post hoc analysis demonstrated an increased risk of CHD events and greater benefit with simvastatin therapy among 4S participants with low HDL cholesterol and elevated TG accompanying elevated LDL cholesterol levels at baseline, compared with participants with isolated elevations in pretreatment LDL cholesterol.[115] A separate analysis demonstrated similar relative risk reduction and greater absolute risk reduction in participants meeting the NCEP ATP III criteria for the MetS, after excluding participants with DM.[113] The Cholesterol and Recurrent Events (CARE) trial demonstrated a beneficial effect of pravastatin treatment on coronary outcomes in the overall study population[169] as well as in the subgroups with DM or IFG, the latter being defined in that study by fasting glucose levels between 110 and 125 mg/dL.[105] Finally, a post hoc analysis of the TNT study that examined those participants who met the NCEP ATP III criteria for the MetS, but excluded individuals with T2DM, suggested an incremental benefit of high-dose atorvastatin therapy in this group.[112]

The greatest value of statin therapy in the treatment of the dyslipidemia of T2DM may be in its potential for combination therapy with other lipid-modifying agents. In patients with T2DM who have CVD or multiple poorly controlled risk factors (and defined, therefore, as very high risk), LDL cholesterol lowering to levels below 70 mg/dL may be an appropriate goal.[109] This very low level of LDL cholesterol may be attained through up-titration of statin doses or through combination with other agents, such as plant stanol and sterol esters, bile acid–binding resins, and inhibitors of enteral cholesterol absorption. The addition of statins to niacin or PPAR-α agonists can produce significant reductions in TG and increases in HDL cholesterol levels, thereby improving all of the major lipid parameters commonly affected by IR and T2DM.[121,127,161] However, it is very important to recognize that there have been no randomized, double-blind, prospective trials of the effects of combination therapies on CVD outcomes.

Nicotinic Acid. For slightly over five decades, nicotinic acid (niacin) has been the most potent HDL cholesterol–raising pharmacologic agent available. Furthermore, it is unique in its favorable effects on all major aspects of the atherogenic lipid profile, namely, HDL cholesterol, TGs, and LDL cholesterol.[170,171] These effects of niacin are thought to be mediated through several major mechanisms. First, niacin exhibits high-affinity binding to a G-protein–coupled receptor found on adipocytes.[172] Activation of the nicotinic acid receptor results in down-regulation of the activity of the enzyme hormone-sensitive lipase (HSL), thereby decreasing lipolysis and resulting in increased sequestering of FA in adipose tissue. It is believed that the consequent reduction in plasma levels of nonesterified fatty acids (NEFAs) leads to a decrease in hepatic production of TG-rich VLDL particles, and hence, lower levels of circulating TRLs. The dual effects of decreases in plasma NEFAs and TG-enriched lipoproteins lead to less CETP-mediated exchange of LDL CE for TG in TRLs, leading to a shift in LDL particle composition from small dense LDL to less atherogenic larger, more buoyant LDL particles. HDL particles also undergo favorable quantitative and qualitative changes as a consequence of treatment with niacin. Niacin treatment results in increased numbers of larger HDL particles and a decrease in the fractional catabolic rate of apoA-I.[173,174]

Niacin is available in short-acting and extended-release forms and is typically associated with increases in HDL cholesterol of 15% to 35%, with 20% to 35%

reductions in TG levels.[121,170] In contrast, it has a more modest effect on LDL cholesterol levels, with reductions in the range of 10% to 20%. For this reason, it is not recommended as first-line therapy for LDL cholesterol lowering. It is, however, suggested for use as monotherapy in individuals with the atherogenic lipid phenotype but without concomitant elevations of LDL cholesterol. For people who exhibit elevated LDL cholesterol in addition to abnormal HDL cholesterol and TG levels, niacin can be used in combination with other agents that are more effective at lowering LDL cholesterol, especially the HMG-CoA reductase inhibitors. Niacin can also reduce levels of lipoprotein(a) between 15% to 25%; moreover, it is the only agent that significantly lowers levels of this atherogenic lipoprotein.[121]

Only one study, the Coronary Drug Project (CDP), has examined the effects of niacin monotherapy on CV outcomes; treatment in this study resulted in reductions in nonfatal recurrent MI and long-term total mortality.[175] Despite favorable lipoprotein effects and trial data, the clinical use of niacin has been limited, especially in individuals with IR or T2DM. This is due largely to concerns over its association with glucose intolerance and hyperglycemia, particularly at higher doses.[171,176] The basis for these adverse effects on carbohydrate metabolism appears to result from niacin-induced IR.[177] Induction of IR by niacin is surprising, given its ability to suppress FA release from adipose tissue. However, studies in nonhuman primates indicate that niacin-induced IR is not associated with changes in plasma FA levels.[178] The relevance of niacin-induced IR vis-à-vis CV risk was addressed in a post hoc analysis of the CDP, in which participants were stratified by baseline glycemic status and by change in glycemia during the first year of treatment.[179] Treatment with niacin reduced the risk of recurrent MI and CHD death in study participants at all levels of baseline fasting plasma glucose, including those meeting criteria for DM. Benefits from niacin therapy were also maintained in participants who exhibited the greatest increases in fasting plasma glucose or 1-hour post challenge glucose levels relative to participants who exhibited lesser increases in these parameters. Another post hoc analysis of the CDP compared the effects of niacin on clinical outcomes in study participants with or without the MetS. The reductions in recurrent nonfatal MI and long-term total mortality achieved with niacin treatment were similar in both groups of participants.[180]

There have been two large prospective studies of the safety and efficacy of niacin therapy in T2DM.[181,182] These studies indicated that adjustment of glycemic medications in previously well-controlled patients with T2DM results in maintenance of glycemic control during treatment with niacin. On the other hand, it is common experience that patients with IFG, a frequent concomitant of the MetS, can develop frank diabetes after initiation of niacin therapy. Two large trials of the efficacy of niacin in combination with a statin versus statin therapy alone, the Atherothrombosis Intervention in Metabolic Syndrome with Low HDL/High Triglycerides and Impact on Global Health Outcomes (AIM-HIGH) and the Heart Protection Study 2–Treatment of HDL to Reduce the Incidence of Vascular Events (HPS2-THRIVE), will provide critical data regarding the issue of niacin and IR.[177]

In summary, niacin is an excellent lipid-altering agent that has been shown to reduce CV events and death in a large secondary prevention trial. Its use in patients with the MetS and/or T2DM also appears to reduce CV risk; however, careful monitoring of glycemic control in these individuals is required.[171] In patients with T2DM, adjustment of diabetes medications may be needed to maintain optimal glycemic control[127]; in people with the MetS, conversion to DM is a possible outcome of niacin therapy.

Bile Acid Sequestrants. The bile acid sequestrants represent another class of agents that have long been used in the management of lipid disorders.[183,184] In the United States, currently available drugs in this category include cholestyramine, colestipol, and colesevelam. These agents function mainly to lower LDL cholesterol through their actions in the intestine, where they bind bile acids, thereby reducing the return of cholesterol to the liver. This results in increased diversion of hepatic cholesterol to the bile acid synthesis pathway and consequent lowering of hepatic cholesterol content. The decrease in hepatic cholesterol leads to up-regulation of hepatic LDL receptors, which in turn lowers LDL cholesterol levels. Typical improvements seen with bile acid sequestrant therapy include 15% to 30% reductions in LDL cholesterol and smaller increases in HDL cholesterol, on the order of 3% to 5%. In some cases, therapy with agents in this class increases hepatic VLDL production, thereby increasing plasma TG levels and worsening hypertriglyceridemia. These drugs should, therefore, be avoided in individuals with severe hypertriglyceridemia (TG >400 mg/dL), and caution should be exercised when considering bile acid sequestrants for LDL cholesterol lowering in patients with moderately elevated TG levels (TG >200 mg/dL), a group that encompasses a considerable number of people with the MetS and/or T2DM. In addition, bile acid sequestrants should be avoided in patients with DM complicated by autonomic neuropathy and constipation, because of the gastrointestinal side effects associated with these drugs, particularly cholestyramine and colestipol.[121,183,184]

The Lipid Research Clinics Coronary Primary Prevention Trial (LRC-CPPT) demonstrated the beneficial effects of monotherapy with a bile acid sequestrant on CV endpoints in severely hypercholesterolemic individuals.[185–187] The National Heart, Lung, and Blood Institute (NHLBI) Type II Coronary Intervention Study, a secondary prevention trial, added to these data by suggesting a positive relationship between cholestyramine therapy and decreased angiographic progression of CHD in people with hyperlipoproteinemia.[188,189] There is, however, a relative lack of studies of bile acid sequestrant therapy specifically in individuals with the MetS or T2DM. The likely coexistence of elevated TG levels in these particular groups of people makes bile acid–binding resins a seemingly less desirable choice for therapy. However, a small randomized, double-blind, crossover study of the effects of cholestyramine therapy in individuals with T2DM has shed some light on this issue.[190] Participants in this study had elevated fasting LDL cholesterol levels (>130 mg/dL) and either normal or moderately elevated plasma TGs (<150 mg/dL or 150–300 mg/dL, respectively). Treatment with cholestyramine resulted in similar responses among study participants, irrespective of baseline TG levels. Compared with placebo, cholestyramine treatment resulted in a statistically significant 28% reduction in LDL cholesterol. However, it also caused a 13.5% increase in plasma TG, although none of the participants developed marked elevations in TG levels, defined by the investigators as greater than 500 mg/dL. The increase in TGs was not associated with any change in VLDL cholesterol concentration, hence suggesting an increase in VLDL particle size. Importantly, HDL cholesterol levels were not affected by the elevation in TGs.

Recently, preclinical studies of the role of farnesoid X receptor (FXR) in the regulation of carbohydrate metabolism have raised interest in the glucose-lowering effects of bile acid sequestrants.[191] Of note, glucose levels improved in participants with T2DM treated with cholestyramine in the study described above,[190] and similar results, with reductions in hemoglobin A1c (HbA1c) levels, were demonstrated in a recent study with colesevelam.[192] Further investigation is required to elucidate the potential role for bile acid sequestrants in the management of dyslipidemia among individuals with DM or the MetS.

Cholesterol Absorption Inhibitors. Ezetimibe is the first available agent in a new class of molecules that interferes with cholesterol absorption by selectively inhibiting the uptake of cholesterol from the intestinal lumen at the level of the brush border of the enterocyte. In October 2002, ezetimibe was approved by the U.S. Food and Drug Administration for the treatment of hypercholesterolemia after being evaluated in several studies, including a multicenter, randomized, double-blind, placebo-controlled trial that demonstrated that 10 mg of ezetimibe compared with placebo caused statistically significant decreases in LDL cholesterol levels.[193] Ezetimibe decreases LDL cholesterol levels in the range of 17% to 20%.[194] It has small effects on TG and HDL cholesterol levels; these are significant in some, but not all, studies. Studies in individuals without DM have demonstrated that combined therapy with ezetimibe and a statin produces greater reductions in LDL cholesterol and TG levels, and greater increases in HDL cholesterol, than either therapy alone.[195,196] Several studies have specifically examined the effects of ezetimibe when added to statin therapy in individuals with the MetS and/or T2DM[197–199]; the results were similar to those observed in groups without DM. To date, there have been no reports of trials showing reduced CV events with ezetimibe, either as monotherapy or in combination with statin therapy.

PPARα Agonists. PPAR-α is a protein that, as a heterodimer with another protein, retinoid X receptor (RXR), binds to specific DNA sequences in the promoters of genes and activates them. PPAR-α is mainly expressed in the liver and activates genes important for hepatic lipid and lipoprotein metabolism.[200] The natural ligands for PPAR-α are likely to be FAs or their derivatives. Fibrates are pharmacologic PPARα agonists, two of which, gemfibrozil and fenofibrate, are available in the United States. Typically, TG levels are reduced by 35% to 50% and HDL cholesterol levels are increased by 10% to 20% with fibrate treatment; greater changes are seen with more extreme baseline abnormalities.[201,202] Three major fibrate monotherapy studies with CV events as the major outcome have included some participants with the MetS and/or T2DM. In the Helsinki Heart Study (HHS), a primary prevention study of hypercholesterolemic subjects, gemfibrozil treatment was associated with increases in HDL cholesterol, reductions in total, LDL, and non-HDL cholesterol and TGs, and a 35% fall in CV events in the overall study.[203] In HHS, there was a very small group of patients with T2DM who had similar relative benefits from gemfibrozil treatment.[204] In addition, participants with high LDL cholesterol/HDL cholesterol ratios (>5) and higher TG levels (>200 mg/dL) had the highest event rates and the greatest benefit from fibrate therapy.[145] In VA-HIT, a secondary prevention study of men with "normal" LDL cholesterol levels (112 mg/dL), moderately elevated TG levels (160 mg/dL) and very low levels of HDL cholesterol (32 mg/dL), gemfibrozil treatment was associated with a 7% increase in HDL cholesterol, a 31% reduction in TG levels, and a 22% reduction in MI or CHD death.[205] Of note, approximately 25% of the participants had T2DM, and they had significantly higher CV event rates but benefited equally in relative terms.[138] Importantly, about 25% of the VA-HIT participants met criteria for IR, defined in that study as the top tertile of IR by homeostasis model assessment (HOMA), with or without concomitant DM; this group had most of the CV events and benefited most from fibrate treatment.[139] Although these studies support the use of gemfibrozil therapy, particularly in subjects with the MetS or T2DM, its use is limited because most of those individuals will already be treated with statins, and gemfibrozil increases the risk of statin-associated myositis when the two are used in combination.

The latter problem raised expectations for the results of the Fenofibrate Intervention and Event Lowering in Diabetes (FIELD) study, because pharmacokinetic studies indicated that fenofibrate might be used in combination with statins without an increase in the risk of myositis.[206] FIELD was a monotherapy study in individuals with T2DM that enrolled both primary and secondary prevention participants; 80% of the participants were categorized as primary prevention.[120] Unfortunately, fenofibrate did not significantly reduce the risk of the primary outcome of coronary events (CHD death and nonfatal MI) compared to placebo; nonfatal MI was reduced, but CHD death was unchanged. A secondary analysis with a wider range of endpoints was significantly reduced in the fenofibrate-treated group, but the degree of reduction was modest and not close to the level of benefit seen with gemfibrozil. A potential confounder of the FIELD study was an imbalanced statin "drop-in"; by the end of the study, nearly 40% of subjects in the placebo group had been exposed to statins, while only 20% of the fenofibrate group were treated with statins at some point in the study. Overall, however, we are left with this conundrum: gemfibrozil raises serum statin levels significantly more than fenofibrate, and as a result, the risk of myopathy is lower with fenofibrate and statin combinations.[207,208] However, gemfibrozil monotherapy has demonstrated efficacy in patients with the MetS and/or T2DM, while fenofibrate has not yet been shown to have similar benefit.

Combination Therapy with Lipid-Altering Agents. There have been numerous publications from trials of combination lipid therapy in participants with the MetS and/or T2DM. These include studies with statins and niacin,[209,210] statins and ezetimibe,[197–199] statins and bile acid sequestrants,[211] and statins and fibrates.[212,213] However, there are no large, randomized, double-blind trials focused on the efficacy of such combinations in reducing CV events. The HDL Atherosclerosis Treatment Study (HATS)[214] and the Arterial Biology for the Investigation of the Treatment Effects of Reducing Cholesterol (ARBITER) 2 trial[215] suggest a benefit of statin plus niacin therapy on atherosclerosis progression, but HATS did not compare combination treatment with statin alone, and ARBITER 2 was a small study that did not have statistical power to compare combination therapy directly with statin alone. Several CV outcomes trials are under way, including AIM-HIGH and HPS2-THRIVE, which compare niacin plus statin versus statin alone, Improved Reduction of Outcomes: Vytorin Efficacy International Trial (IMPROVE IT), which compares ezetimibe plus statin versus statin alone, and the Action to Control Cardiovascular Risk in Diabetes (ACCORD) study, which compares fenofibrate plus statin versus statin alone. Until the results of these studies are reported, combination therapy of statin plus any other agent must be used with the knowledge that changing blood lipid levels does not necessarily translate into improved CV outcomes.

REFERENCES

1. Kylin E: Studien ueber das Hypertonie-Hyperglyka "mie-Hyperuika" miesyndrom. *Zentralbl Innere Med* 1923;44:105–127.
2. Vague J: The degree of masculine differentiation of obesities: a factor determining predisposition to diabetes, atherosclerosis, gout, and uric calculous disease. Am J Clin Nutr 1956;4:20–34.
3. Reaven GM: Role of insulin resistance in human disease. *Diabetes* 1988;37:1595–1607.
4. Alberti KGMM, Zimmet PZ: Definition, diagnosis and classification of diabetes mellitus and its complications Part 1: diagnosis and classification of diabetes mellitus Provisional Report of a WHO Consultation. *Diab Med* 1998;15:539–553.
5. Balkau B, Charles MA, for the European Group for the Study of Insulin Resistance (EGIR): Comment on the provisional report from the WHO consultation. *Diabet Med* 1999;16:442–443.
6. Expert Panel on Detection, Evaluation, and Treatment of High Blood Cholesterol in Adults: Executive summary of the third report of the NCEP expert panel on detection, evaluation, and treatment of high cholesterol in adults (adult treatment panel III). *JAMA* 2001;285:2486–2497.
7. Kahn R, Buse J, Ferrannini E, Stern M, American Diabetes Association, European Association for the Study of Diabetes: The metabolic syndrome: time for a critical appraisal: joint statement from the American Diabetes Association and the European Association for the Study of Diabetes. *Diabetes Care* 2005;28:2289–2304.
8. Alberti KG, Zimmet P, Shaw J, IDF Epidemiology Task Force Consensus Group: The metabolic syndrome—a new worldwide definition. *Lancet* 2005;366:1059–1062.
9. Ford ES, Giles WH, Mokdad AH: Increasing prevalence of the metabolic syndrome among U.S. adults. *Diabetes Care* 2004;10:2444–2449,
10. Stern MP, Williams K, Gonzalez-Villalpando C: Does the metabolic syndrome improve identification of individuals at risk of type 2 diabetes and/or cardiovascular disease? *Diabetes Care* 2004;27:2676–2681.
11. Gami AS, Witt BJ, Howard DE, et al.: Metabolic syndrome and risk of incident cardiovascular events and death: a systematic review and meta-analysis of longitudinal studies. *J Am Coll Cardiol* 2007;49:403–414.
12. Alexander CM, Landsman PB, Teutsch SM, Haffner SM: NCEP-defined metabolic syndrome, diabetes, and prevalence of coronary heart disease among NHANES III participants age 50 years and older. *Diabetes* 2003;52:1210–1214.
13. Sundström J, Vallhagen E, Riserus U, et al.: Risk associated with the metabolic syndrome versus the sum of its individual components. *Diabetes Care* 2006;29:1673.
14. Nathan DM: Long-term complications of diabetes mellitus. *N Engl J Med* 1993;328:1676–1685.
15. Purnell JQ, Hokanson JE, Marcovina SM, Steffes MW, Cleary PA, Brunzell JD: Effect of excessive weight gain with intensive therapy of type 1 diabetes on lipid levels and blood pressure: results from the DCCT. *JAMA* 1998;280:140–146.
16. Diabetes Control and Complications Trial Research Group: The effect of intensive treatment of diabetes on the development and progression of long-term complications in insulin-dependent diabetes mellitus. *N Engl J Med* 1993;329:977–986.
17. Kilpatrick ES, Rigby AS, Atkin SL: Insulin resistance, the metabolic syndrome, and complication risk in type 1 diabetes. *Diabetes Care* 2007;30:707–712.
18. Orchard TJ, Olson JC, Erbey JR, et al.: Insulin resistance-related factors, but not glycemia, predict coronary artery disease in type 1 diabetes. *Diabetes Care* 2003;26:1374–1379.
19. Nathan DM, Cleary PA, Backlund JY, et al.: Intensive diabetes treatment and cardiovascular disease in patients with type 1 diabetes. *N Engl J Med* 2005;353:2643–2653.
20. Reaven GM: Role of insulin resistance in human disease (Syndrome X): an expanded definition. *Annu Rev Med* 1993; 44:121–131.
21. Eckel RH, Grundy SM, Zimmet PZ: The metabolic syndrome. *Lancet* 2005;365:1415–1428.
22. Reaven GM: The metabolic syndrome: is this diagnosis necessary? *Am J Clinical Nutr* 2006;83:1237–1247.
23. World Health Organization: Definition, diagnosis and classification of diabetes mellitus and its complications. Report of a WHO consultation. Geneva: World Health Organization, 1999.
24. The European Group for the Study of Insulin Resistance (EGIR): Frequency of the WHO metabolic syndrome in European cohorts, and an alternative definition of an insulin resistance syndrome. *Diabetes Metab* 2002;28:364–376.
25. Grundy SM, Brewer HB, Jr, Cleeman JI, et al.: Definition of metabolic syndrome. Report of the National Heart, Lung, and Blood Institute/American Heart Association Conference on Scientific Issues Related to Definition. *Circulation* 2004;109: 433–438.
26. Hanley AJ, Wagenknecht LE, D'Agostino RB Jr, et al.: Identification of subjects with insulin resistance and B-cell dysfunction using alternative definitions of the metabolic syndrome. *Diabetes* 2003;52:2740–2747.
27. Alexander CM, Landsman PB, Grundy SM: Metabolic syndrome and hyperglycemia: congruence and divergence. *Am J Cardiol* 2006;98:982–985.
28. Binnert C, Genoud M, and Seematter G: Glucose-induced insulin secretion in dyslipidemic and normolipidemic patients with normal glucose tolerance. *Diabetes Care* 2005;28:1225–1227.
29. Laakso M, Sarlund H, Mykkanen L: Insulin resistance is associated with lipid and lipoprotein abnormalities in subjects with varying degrees of glucose tolerance. *Arteriosclerosis* 1990;10: 223–231.
30. Chahil TJ, Ginsberg GN: Diabetic dyslipidemia. *Endocrinol Metab Clin N Am* 2006;35:491–510.
31. Austin MA, Breslow JL, Hennekens CH, Buring JE, Krauss RM: Low-density lipoprotein subclass patterns and risk of myocardial infarction. *JAMA* 1988;260:1917–1921.
32. Haffner SM, Stern MP, Hazuda HP, Mitchell BD, Patterson JK: Cardiovascular risk factors in confirmed prediabetic individuals. Does the clock for coronary heart disease start ticking before the onset of clinical diabetes? *JAMA* 1990;263:2893–2898.
33. Siegel RD, Cupples A, Schaefer EJ, Wilson PWF: Lipoproteins, apolipoproteins, and low-density lipoprotein size among diabetics in the Framingham Offspring Study. *Metabolism* 1996;45:1267–1272.
34. Niskanen L, Turpeinen A, Penttila I, Uusitupa M: Hyperglycemia and compositional lipoprotein abnormalities as predictors of cardiovascular mortality in type 2 diabetes. A 15-year follow-up from the time of diagnosis. *Diabetes Care* 1998;21:1861–1869.
35. Howard BV, Mayer-Davis EJ, Goff D, et al.: Relationships between insulin resistance and lipoproteins in nondiabetic African Americans, Hispanics, and non-Hispanic whites: The Insulin Resistance Atherosclerosis Study. *Metabolism* 1998;47: 1174–1179.
36. Howard BV, Cowan LD, Go O, Welty TK, Robbins DC, Lee ET: Adverse effects of diabetes on multiple cardiovascular disease risk factors in women. *Diabetes Care* 1998;21:1258–1265.
37. Juutilainen A, Kortelainen S, Lehto S, et al.: Gender difference in the impact of type 2 diabetes on coronary heart disease risk. *Diabetes Care* 2004;27:2898–2904.

38. Wei M, Gaskill SP, Haffner SM, Stern MP: Effects of diabetes and level of glycemia on all-cause and cardiovascular mortality. The San Antonio Heart Study. *Diabetes Care* 1998;21:1167–1172.
39. Resnick HE, Harris MI, Brock DB, Harris TB: American Diabetes Association diabetes dagnostic criteria, advancing age, and cardiovascular disease risk profiles. Results from the Third National Health and Nutrition Examination Survey. *Diabetes Care* 2000;23:176–180.
40. Goff DC Jr, D'Agostino RB Jr, Haffner SM, Otvos JD: Insulin resistance and adiposity influence lipoprotein size and subclass concentrations. Results from the Insulin Resistance Atherosclerosis Study. *Metabolism* 2005;54:264–270.
41. Haffner SM, D'Agostino R Jr, Mykkanen L, et al.: Insulin sensitivity in subjects with type 2 diabetes. Relationship to cardiovascular risk factors: The Insulin Resistance Atherosclerosis Study. *Diabetes Care* 1999;22:562–568.
42. Haffner SM: Lipoprotein disorders associated with type 2 diabetes mellitus and insulin resistance. Am J Cardiol 2002;90:55i–61i.
43. Haffner SM, Mykkanen L, and Festa A: Insulin-resistant subjects have more atherogenic risk factors than insulin-sensitive prediabetic subjects. Implications for preventing coronary heart disease during the prediabetic state. *Circulation* 2000;101:975–980.
44. Goff DC Jr, D'Agostino RB Jr, Haffner SM, Saad MF, Wagenknecht LE: Lipoprotein concentrations and carotid atherosclerosis by diabetes status: results from the Insulin Resistance Atherosclerosis Study. *Diabetes Care* 2000;23:1006–1011.
45. Meigs JB, Nathan DM, Wilson PW.F, et al.: Metabolic risk factors worsen continuously across the spectrum of nondiabetic glucose tolerance: The Framingham Offspring Study. *Ann Intern Med* 1998;128:524–533.
46. Haffner SM, Miettinen H, and Stern MP: Relatively more atherogenic coronary heart disease risk factors in prediabetic women than in prediabetic men. *Diabetologia* 1997;40:711–717.
47. Haffner SM, Mykkanen L, and Stern MP: Greater effect of diabetes on LDL size in women than in men. *Diabetes Care* 1994;17: 1164–1171.
48. Haffner SM: The prediabetic problem: development of non-insulin-dependent diabetes mellitus and related abnormalities. *J Diabetes Complications* 1997;11:69–76.
49. Festa A, Williams K, Hanley AJ, et al.: Nuclear magnetic resonance lipoprotein abnormalities in prediabetic subjects in the Insulin Resistance Atherosclerosis Study. *Circulation* 2005;111: 3465–3472.
50. Garvey WT, Kwon S, Zheng D, et al.: Effects of insulin resistance and type 2 diabetes on lipoprotein subclass particle size and concentration determined by nuclear magnetic resonance. *Diabetes* 2003;52:453–462.
51. Taskinen MR: Diabetic dyslipidaemia: from basic research to clinical practice. *Diabetologia* 2003;46:733–749.
52. Ginsberg HN, Illingworth DR: Postprandial dyslipidemia: an atherogenic disorder common in patients with diabetes. *Am J Cardiol* 2001;88:9H–15H.
53. Tomkin GH, Owens D: Abnormalities in Apo B-containing lipoproteins in diabetes and atherosclerosis. *Diabetes Metab Res Rev* 2001;17:27–43.
54. Duez H, Lamarche B, Uffelman KD, Valero R, Cohn JS, Lewis GF: Hyperinsulinemia is associated with increased production rate of intestinal apolipoprotein B48 containing lipoproteins in humans. *Arterioscler Thromb Vasc Biol* 2006;26: 1357–1363.
55. Annuzzi G, De Natale C, Iovine C, et al.: Insulin resistance is independently associated with postprandial alterations of triglyceride-rich lipoproteins in type 2 diabetes mellitus. *Arterioscler Thromb Vasc Biol* 2004;24:2397.
56. Chen Y-D, Swami S, Skowronski R, et al.: Differences in postprandial lipemia between patients with normal glucose tolerance and noninsulin-dependent diabetes mellitus. *J Clin Endocrinol Metab* 1993;76:172–177.
57. Jeppesen J, Hollenbeck CB, Zhou MY, et al.: Relation between insulin resistance, hyperinsulinemia, postheparin plasma lipoprotein lipase activity, and postprandial lipemia. *Arterioscler Thromb Vasc Biol* 1995;15:320–324.
58. Rivellese AA, De Natale C, Di Marino L, et al.: Exogenous and endogenous postprandial lipid abnormalities in type 2 diabetic patients with optimal blood glucose control and optimal fasting triglyceride levels. *J Clin Endocrinol Metab* 2004;89:2153–2159.
59. Ginsberg HN, Jones J, Blaner WS, et al.: Association of postprandial triglyceride and retinyl palmitate responses with newly diagnosed exercise-induced myocardial ischemia in middle-aged men and women. *Arteriosc Thromb Vasc Biol* 1995;15:1829–1838.
60. Sharret AR, Chambless LE, Heiss G, Paton CC, Patsch W: Association of postprandial triglyceride and retinyl palmitate responses with asymptomatic carotid artery atherosclerosis in middle-aged men and women. *Arterioscler Thromb Vasc Biol* 1995;15:2122–2129.
61. Syvanne M, Hilden H, Taskinen M-R: Abnormal metabolism of postprandial lipoproteins in patients with non–insulin-dependent diabetes mellitus is not related to coronary artery disease. *J Lipid Res* 1994;35:15–26.
62. Gotto Jr AM, Pownall HJ, Havel RJ: Introduction to the plasma lipoproteins. *Methods Enzymol* 1986;128:3–41.
63. Ginsberg HN: Lipoprotein physiology. *Endocrinol Metab Clin North Am* 1998;27:503–519.
64. Havel RJ: Lipid transport function of lipoproteins in blood plasma. *Am J Physiol* 1987;253:E1–E5.
65. de Man FH, Cabezas MC, Van Barlingen HHJJ, ErkelensDW, De Bruin TWA: Triglyceride-rich lipoproteins in non–insulin dependent diabetes mellitus: post-prandial metabolism and relation to premature atherosclerosis. *Eur J Clin Invest* 1996;26:89–108.
66. Phillips C, Bennett A, Anderton K: Intestinal rather than hepatic microsomal triglyceride transfer protein as a cause of postprandial dyslipidemia in diabetes. *Metabolism* 2002;51:847–852.
67. Phillips C, Owens D, Collins P, Tomkin GH: Microsomal triglyceride transfer protein: does insulin resistance play a role in the regulation of chylomicron assembly? *Atherosclerosis* 2002;160:355–360.
68. Haidari M, Leung N, Mahbub F: Fasting and postprandial overproduction of intestinally derived lipoproteins in an animal model of insulin resistance. *J Biol Chem* 2002;277:31646–31655.
69. Federico LM, Naples M, Taylor D, Adeli K: Intestinal insulin resistance and aberrant production of apolipoprotein B48 lipoproteins in an animal model of insulin resistance and metabolic dyslipidemia. Evidence foir activation of protein tyrosine phosphatase-1B, extracellular signal–related kinase and sterol regulatory element-binding protein-1c in the fructose-fed hamster. *Diabetes* 2006;55:1316–1326.
70. Guo Q, Avramoglu RK, Adeli K: Intestinal assembly and secretion of highly dense/lipid-poor apolipoprotein B48-containing lipoprotein particles in the fasting state: evidence for induction by insulin resistance and exogenous fatty acids. *Metabolism* 2005;54:689–697.
71. Lewis GF, Uffelman K, Naples M: Intestinal lipoprotein overproduction, a newly recognized component of insulin resistance, is ameliorated by the insulin sensitizer rosiglitazone: studies in the fructose-fed syrian golden hamster. *Endocrinology* 2005;146: 247–255.
72. Leung N, Naples M, Uffelman K: Rosiglitazone improves intestinal lipoprotein overproduction in the fat-fed syrian golden hamster, and animal model of nutritionally-induced insulin resistance. *Atherosclerosis* 2004;174:235–241.
73. Hogue J-C, Lamarche B, Trembley AJ, et al.: Evidence of increased secretion of apolipoprotein B-48 containing lipoproteins in subjects with type 2 diabetes. *J Lipid Res* 2007;48:1336–1342.
74. Phillips C, Mullan K, Owens D, Tomkin GH: Intestinal microsomal triglyceride transfer protein in type 2 diabetic and non-diabetic subjects: the relationship to triglyceride-rich postprandial lipoprotein composition. *Atherosclerosis* 2006;187:57–64.
75. Lally S, Tan CY, Owens D, Tomkin GH: Messenger RNA levels of genes involved in dysregulation of postprandial lipoproteins in type 2 diabetes: the role of Niemann-Pick C1-Like 1, ATP-binding cassette, transporters G5 and G8 and of microsomal triglyceride transfer protein. *Diabetologia* 2006;49:1008–1016.
76. Golderg IJ: Clinical review 124, diabetic dyslipidemia: causes and consequences. *J Clin Endocrinol Metab* 2001;86:965–971.
77. Mahley RW, Ji ZS: Remnant lipoprotein metabolism: key pathways involving cell-surface heparan sulfate proteoglycans and apolipoprotein. *J Lipid Res* 1999;40:1–16.
78. Cohn JS, Patterson BW, Uffelman KD, Davignon J, Steiner G: Rate of production of plasma and very-low-density lipoprotein (VLDL) apolipoprotein C-III is strongly related to the concentration and level of production of VLDL triglyceride in male subjects with different body weights and levels of insulin sensitivity. *J Clin Endocrinol Metab* 2004;89:3949–3955.

79. Nagashima K, Lopez C, Donovan D, et al.: Effects of the PPAR agonist pioglitazone on lipoprotein metabolism in patients with type 2 diabetes mellitus. *J Clin Invest* 2005;115:1323–1332.
80. Ginsberg HN, Zhang Y-L, Hernandez-Ono A: Regulation of plasma triglycerides in insulin resistance and diabetes. *Arch Med Res* 2005;36:232–240.
81. Krauss RM: Atherogenicity of triglyceride-rich lipoproteins. *Am J Cardiol* 1998;81:13B–17B.
82. Fisher EA, Ginsberg HN: Complexity in the secretory pathway: the assembly and secretion of apolipoprotein B-containing lipoproteins. *J Biol Chem* 2002;277:17377–17380.
83. Avramoglu RK, Basciano H, Adeli K: Lipid and lipoprotein dysregulation in insulin resistant states. *Clin Chim Acta* 2006;368:1–19.
84. Adiels M, Boren J, Caslake MJ, et al.: Overproduction of VDLD1 driven by hyperglycemia is a dominant feature of diabetic dyslipidemia. *Arterioscler Thromb Vasc Biol* 2005;25: 1697–1703.
85. Adiels M, Olofsson S-O, Taskinen M-R, Boren J: Diabetic dyslipidemia. *Curr Opin Lipidol* 2006;17:238–246.
86. Ozcan U, Cao Q, Yilmaz E, et al.: Endoplasmic reticulum stress links obesity, insulin action, and type 2 diabetes. *Science* 2004;306:457–461.
87. Ginsberg HN, Zhang Y-L, Hernandez-Ono A: A metabolic syndrome: focus on dyslipidemia. *Obesity* 2006;14:41S–49S.
88. Ginsberg HN, Yu Y-H: Adipocyte signaling and lipid homeostasis. Sequelae of insulin-resistant adipose tissue. *Circ Res* 2005;96:1042–1052.
89. Zhang Y-L, Hernandez-Ono A, Ko C, Yasunaga K, Huang L-S, Ginsberg HN: Regulation of hepatic apolipoprotein B-lipoprotein assembly and secretion by the availability of fatty acids: 1: differential effects of delivering fatty acids via albumin or remnant-like emulsion particles. *J Biol Chem* 2004;279: 19362–19374.
90. Lewis GF, Uffelman KD, Szeto LW, Weller B, Steiner G: Interaction between free fatty acids and insulin in the acute control of very-low-density lipoprotein production in humans. *J Clin Invest* 1995;95:158–166.
91. Shimomura I, Matsuda M, Hammer RE, Bashmakov Y, Brown MS, Goldstein JL: Decreased IRS-2 and increased SREBP-1c lead to mixed insulin resistance and sensitivity in livers of lipodystrophic and ob/ob mice. *Mol Cell* 2000;6:77–86.
92. Zhang YL, Hernandez-Ono A, Siri P, et al.: Aberrant hepatic expression of PPARgamma2 stimulates hepatic lipogenesis in a mouse model of obesity, insulin resistance, dyslipidemia, and hepatic steatosis. *J Biol Chem* 2006;281:37603–37615.
93. Donnelly KL, Smith CI, Schwarzenberg SJ, Jessurun J, Boldt MD, Parks EJ: Sources of fatty acids stored in liver and secreted via lipoprotein in patients with nonalcoholic fatty liver disease. *J Clin Invest* 2005;115:1139–1142.
94. Jong MC, Hofker MH, Havekes LM: Role of ApoCs in lipoprotein metabolism. Functional differences betwen ApoC1, ApoC2, and ApoC3. *Artheroscler Thromb Vasc Biol* 1999;19:472–484.
95. Shachter NS: Apolipoproteins C I and C III as important modulators of lipoprotein metabolism. *Curr Opin Lipidol* 2001;12:297–304.
96. Krauss RM, Siri PW: Metabolic abnormalities: triglyceride and low-density lipoprotein. *Endocrinol Metab Clinic North Am* 2004;33:405–415.
97. Guerin M, Le Goff W, Lassel TS, et al.: Proatherogenic role of elevated CE transfer from HDL to $VLDL_1$ and dense LDL in type 2 diabetes. Impact of the degree of triglyceridemia. *Arterioscler Thromb Vasc Biol* 2001;21:282–288.
98. Tan KC, Cooper MB, Ling KL, et al.: Fasting and posptrandial determinants for the occurrence of small dense LDL species in non-insulin-dependent diabetic patients with and without hypertriglyceridaemia: the involvement of insulin, insulin precursor species and insulin resistance. *Atherosclerosis* 1995;113:273–287.
99. Jones RJ, Owens D, Brennan C, Collins PB, Johnson A, Tomkin GH: Increased esterification of cholesterol and transfer of cholesteryl ester to apo B-containing lipoproteins in Type 2 diabetes: relationship to serum lipoproteins A-I and A-II. *Atherosclerosis* 1996;119:151–157.
100. Riemens S, van Tol A, Sluiter W, Dullaart R: Elevated plasma cholesteryl ester transfer in NIDDM: relationships with apolipoprotein B-containing lipoproteins and phospholipid transfer protein. *Atherosclerosis* 1998;140:71–79.
101. Deeb SS, Zambon A, Carr MC, et al.: Hepatic lipase and dyslipidemia: interactions among genetic variants, obesity, gender, and diet. *J Lipid Res* 2003;44:1279–1286.
102. Lewis GF, Radar DJ: New insights into the regulation of HDL. Metabolism and reverse cholesterol transport. *Circ Res* 2005;96:1221–1232.
103. Borggreve SE, De Vries R, Dullaart RP: Alterations in high-density lipoprotein metabolism and reverse cholesterol transport in insulin resistance and type 2 diabetes mellitus: role of lipolytic enzymes, lecithin:cholesterol acyltransferase and lipid transfer proteins. *Eur J Clin Invest* 2003;33:1051–1069.
104. The Expert Panel: Report of the National Cholesterol Education Program Expert Panel on detection, evaluation, and treatment of high blood cholesterol in adults. *Arch Intern Med* 1998;148:36–69.
105. Goldberg RB, Mellies MJ, Sacks FM, et al.: Cardiovascular events and their reduction with pravastatin in diabetic and glucose-intolerant myocardial infarction survivors with average cholesterol levels: subgroup analyses in the cholesterol and recurrent events (CARE) trial. The Care Investigators. *Circulation* 1998;98:2513–2519.
106. Pedersen TR, Simvastatin Survival Study Group: Randomised trial of cholesterol lowering in 4444 patients with coronary heart disease: The Scandinavian Simvastatin Survival Study (4S). *Lancet* 1994;344:1383–1389.
107. Heart Protection Study Collaborative Group: MRC/BHF heart protection study of cholesterol lowering with simvastatin in 20,536 high-risk individuals: a randomised placebo-controlled trial. *Lancet* 2002;360:7–22.
108. LaRosa JC, Grundy SM, Waters DD, et al.: Intensive lipid lowering with atorvastatin in patients with stable coronary disease. *N Engl J Med* 2005;352:1425–1435.
109. Grundy SM, Cleeman JI, Merz CN, et al.: Implications of recent clinical trials for the National Cholesterol Education Program Adult Treatment Panel III Guidelines. *Circulation* 2004;110:227–239.
110. Pedersen TR, Faergeman O, Kastelein JJ, et al.: High-dose atorvastatin vs usual-dose simvastatin for secondary prevention after myocardial infarction. The IDEAL study: a randomized controlled trial. *JAMA* 2005;294:2437–2445.
111. Cannon CP, Braunwald E, McCabe CH, et al.: Intensive versus moderate lipid lowering with statins after acute coronary syndromes. *N Engl J Med* 2004;350:1495–1504.
112. Deedwania P, Barter P, Carmena R, for theTreating to New Targets Investigators: Reduction of low-density lipoprotein cholesterol in patients with coronary heart disease and metabolic syndrome: analysis of the treating to New Targets Study. *Lancet* 2006;368:919–928.
113. Pyorala K, Ballantyne CM, Gumbiner B, for the Scandinavian Simvastatin Survival Study Group: Reduction of cardiovascular events by simvastatin in nondiabetic coronary heart disease patients with and without the metabolic syndrome. Subgroup Analyses of the Scandinavian Simvastatin Survival Study (4S). *Diabetes Care* 2004;27:1735–1740.
114. Haffner SM, Alexander CM, Cook TJ, for the Scandinavian Simvastatin Survival Study Group: Reduced coronary events in simvastatin-treated patients with coronary heart disease and diabetes or impaired fasting glucose levels. Subgroup analyses in the Scandinavian Simvastatin Survival Study. *Arch Intern Med* 1999;159:2661–2667.
115. Ballantyne CM, Olsson AG, Cook TJ, Mercuri MF, Pedersen TR, Kjekshus J: Influence of low high-density lipoprotein cholesterol and elevated triglyceride on coronary heart disease events and response to simvastatin therapy in 4S. *Circulation* 2001;104:3046–3051.
116. Colhoun HM, Betteridge DJ, Durrington PN, et al.: Primary prevention of cardiovascular disease with atorvastatin in type 2 diabetes in the Collaborative Atorvastatin Diabetes Study (CARDS): multicentre randomised placebo-controlled trial. *Lancet* 2004;364:685–696.
117. Knopp RH, D'Emden M, Smilde JG, Pocock SJ: Efficacy and safety of atorvastatin in the prevention of cardiobascular end points in subjects with type 2 diabetes. *Diabetes Care* 2006;29:1478–1485.
118. Lee CD, Folsom AR, Pankow JS, Brancati FL: Cardiovascular events in diabetic and nondiabetic adults with or without history of myocardial infarction. *Circulation* 2004;109: 855–860.

119. Evans JMM, Wang J, Morris AD: Comparison of cardiovascular risk between patients with type 2 diabetes and those who had had a myocardial infarction: cross sectional and cohort studies. *BMJ* 2002;324:939–942.
120. Keech A, Simes RJ, Barter P: Effects of long-term fenofibrate therapy on cardiovascular events in 9795 people with type 2 diabetes mellitus (the FIELD study): randomised controlled trial. *Lancet* 2005;366:1849–1861.
121. National Cholesterol Education Program Third report of the National Cholesterol Education Program (NCEP) Expert Panel on Detection, Evaluation, and Treatment of High Blood Cholesterol in Adults (Adult Treatment Panel III) final report. *Circulation* 2002;106:3143–3421.
122. Xydakis AM, Ballantyne CM: Role of non-high-density lipoprotein cholesterol in prevention of cardiovascular disease: updated evidence from clinical trials. *Curr Opin Cardiol* 2003;18:503–509.
123. Grundy SM: Low-density lipoprotein, non-high-density lipoprotein, and apolipoprotein B as targets of lipid-lowering therapy. *Circulation* 2002;106:2526–2529.
124. Pischon T, Girman CJ, Sacks FM: Non-high-density lipoprotein cholesterol and apolipoprotein B in the prediction of coronary heart disease in men. *Circulation* 2005;112:3375–3383.
125. Jiang R, Schulze MB, Li T: Non-HDL cholesterol and apolipoprotein B predict cardiovascular disease events among men with type 2 diabetes. *Diabetes Care* 2004;27:1991–1997.
126. Schulze MB, Shai I, Manson JE: Joint role of non-HDL cholesterol and glycated haemoglobin in predicting future coronary heart disease events among women with type 2 diabetes. *Diabetologia* 2004;47:2129–2136.
127. American Diabetes Association: Standards of medical care in diabetes. *Diabetes Care* 2007;30:S4–S41.
128. Buse JB, Ginsberg HN, Bakris GL, et al.: Primary prevention of cardiovascular diseases in people with diabetes mellitus. A scientific statement from the American Heart Association and the American Diabetes Association. *Diabetes Care* 2007;30:162–172.
129. Turner RC, Millns H, Neil HA.W, Stratton IM, Manley SE, Matthews DR, Holman RR: Risk factors for coronary artery disease in non-insulin dependent diabetes mellitus: United Kingdom prospective diabetes study (UKPDS: 23). *BMJ* 1998; 316:823–828.
130. Drexel H, Aczel S, Marte T, et al.: Is atherosclerosis in diabetes and impaired fasting glucose driven by elevated LDL cholesterol or by decreased HDL cholesterol? *Diabetes Care* 2005;28:101–107.
131. Boden WE: High-density lipoprotein cholesterol as an independent risk factor in cardiovascular disease: Assessing the Data from Framingham to the Veterans Affairs High-Density Lipoprotein Intervention Trial. *Am J Cardiol* 2000;86: 19L-22L.
132. Gordon DJ, Probstfield JL, Garrison RJ, et al.: High-density lipoprotein cholesterol and cardiovascular disease: four prospective American studies. *Circulation* 1989;79:8–15.
133. Gotto AM Jr: High-density lipoprotein cholesterol and triglycerides as therapeutic targets for preventing and treating coronary artery disease. *Am Heart J* 2002;144:S33–S42.
134. Tenenbaum A, Fisman EZ, Motro M, Adler Y: Atherogenic dyslipidemia in metabolic syndrome and type 2 diabetes: therapeutic options beyond statins. *Cardiovasc Diabetol* 2006;5:20.
135. Manninen V, Elo MO, Frick MH, et al.: Alterations and decline in the incidence of coronary heart disease in the Helsinki Heart Study. *JAMA* 1988;260:641–651.
136. Robins SJ, Collins D, Wittes JT, et al.: Relation of gemfibrozil treatment and lipid levels with major coronary events. VA-HIT: a randomized controlled trial. *JAMA* 2001;285: 1585–1591.
137. Tenenbaum A, Motro M, Fisman EZ, Tanne D, Boyko V, Behar S: Bezafibrate for the secondary prevention of myocardial infarction in patients with metabolic syndrome. *Arch Intern Med* 2005;165:1154–1160.
138. Rubins Bloomfield H, Robins SJ, Collins D, et al.: Diabetes, plasma insulin, and cardiovascular disease. *Arch Intern Med* 2002;162:2597–2604.
139. Robins SJ, Rubins HB, Faas FH, et al.: Insulin resistance and cardiovascular events with low HDL cholesterol. *Diabetes Care* 2003;26:1513–1517.
140. Tkac I, Kimball BP, Lewis G, et al.: The severity of coronary atherosclerosis in type 2 diabetes mellitus is related to the number of circulating triglyceride-rich lipoprotein particles. *Arterioscler Thromb Vasc Biol* 1997;17:3633–3638.
141. Carmena R, Duriez P, Fruchart J-C: Atherogenic lipoprotein particles in atherosclerosis. *Circulation* 2004;109:III-2–III-7.
142. Hokanson JE, Austin MA: Plasma triglyceride level is a risk factor for cardiovascular disease independent of high-density lipoprotein cholesterol level: a meta-analysis of population-based prospective studies. *J Cardiovasc Risk* 1996;3:213–219.
143. Fuller JH, Stevens LK, Wang S-L, and the WHO Multinational Study Group: Risk factors for cardiovascular mortality and morbidity. The WHO Multinational Study of Vascular Disease in Diabetes. *Diabetologia* 2001;44:S54–S64.
144. Sarwar N, Danesh J, Eiriksdottir G, et al.: Triglycerides and the risk of coronary heart disease: 10,158 incident cases among 265,525 participants in 29 Western prospective studies. *Circulation* 2007;115:450–458.
145. Manninen V, Tenkanen L, Koskinen P, et al.: Joint effects of serum triglyceride and LDL cholesterol and HDL cholesterol concentrations on coronary heart disease risk in the Helsinki Heart Study. *Circulation* 1992;85:37–45.
146. Mero N, Malmstrom R, Steiner G, Taskinen M-R, Syvanne M: Postprandial metabolism of apolipoprotein B-48- and B-100–containing particles in type 2 diabetes mellitus: relations to angiographically verified severity of coronary artery disease. *Atherosclerosis* 2000;150:167–177.
147. Diabetes Prevention Program Research Group: Reduction in the incidence of type 2 diabetes with lifestyle intervention or metformin. *N Engl J Med* 2002;346:393–403.
148. Tuomilehto J, Lindstrom J, Eriksson JG, et al.: Prevention of type 2 diabetes mellitus by changes in lifestyle among subjects with impaired glucose tolerance. *N Engl J Med* 2001;344:1343–1350.
149. The Look AHEAD Research Group: Reduction in weight and cardiovascular disease risk factors in individuals with type 2 diabetes. *Diabetes Care* 2007;30:1374–1383.
150. Foster GD, Wyatt HR, Hill JO: A randomized trial of a low-carbohydrate diet for obesity. N Engl J Med 2003;348:2082–2090.
151. Samaha FF, Iqbal N, Seshadari P, et al.: A low-carbohydrate as compared with a low-fat diet in severe obesity. *N Engl J Med* 2003;348:2074–2081.
152. Dansinger ML, Gleason JA, Griffith JL: Comparison of the Atkins, Ornish, Weight Watchers, and Zone diets for weight loss and heart disease risk reduction: a randomized trial. *JAMA* 2005;293:43–53.
153. Gardner CD, Kiazand A, Alhassan S, et al.: Comparison of the Atkins, Zone, Ornish and LEARN diets for change in weight and related risk factors among overweight premenopausal women. The A to Z Weight Loss Study: a randomized trial. *JAMA* 2007;297:969–977.
154. Lichtenstein AH: Thematic review series: patient-oriented research. Dietary fat, carbohydrate, and protein: effects on plasma lipoprotein patterns. *J Lipid Res* 2006;47:1661–1667.
155. Garg A, Grundy SM, Koffler M: Effect of high carbohydrate intake on hyperglycemia, islet function, and plasma lipoproteins in NIDDM. *Diabetes Care* 1992;15:1572–1580.
156. Grundy SM, Nix D, Whelan MF, Franklin L: Comparison of three cholesterol-lowering diets in normolipidemic men. *JAMA* 1986;256:2351–2355.
157. Chandalia M, Garg A, Lutjohann D, von Bergmann K, Grundy SM, Brinkley LJ: Beneficial effects of high dietary fiber intake in patients with type 2 diabetes mellitus. *N Engl J Med* 2000;342:1392–1398.
158. Berglund L, Lefevre M, Ginsberg HN, et al.: Comparison of monounsaturated fat versus carbohydrate as replacement for saturated fat in subjects with a high metabolic risk profile: studies in the fasting and postprandial state. *Am J Clin Nutr* 2007;86:1611–1620.
159. Baigent C, Keech A, Kearney PM, for the Cholesterol Treatment Trialists' (CTT) Collaborators: Efficacy and Safety of cholesterol-lowering treatment: prospective meta-analysis of data from 90,056 participants in 14 randomised trials of statins. *Lancet* 2005;366:1267–1278.
160. Ryden L, Standl E, Bartnik M, et al.: Guidelines on diabetes, pre-diabetes, and cardiovascular diseases: Executive Summary. Task Force on Diabetes and Cardiovascular Diseases of the European Society of Cardiology (ESC) and the European Association for the Study of Diabetes (EASD). *Eur Heart J* 2007;28:88–136.

161. Ginsberg HN: Efficacy and mechanism of action of statins in the treatment of diabetic dyslipidemia. *J Clin Endocrinol Metab* 2006;91:383–392.
162. Dallinga-Thie GM, Berk-Planken II, Bootsma AH, Jansen H, Diabetes Atorvastatin Lipid Intervention (DALI) Study Group: Atorvastatin decreases apolipoprotein C-III in apolipoprotein B-containing lipoprotein and HDL in type 2 diabetes: a potential mechanism to lower plasma triglycerides. *Diabetes Care* 2004;27:1358–1364.
163. Heart Protection Study Collaborative Group: MRC/BHF heart protection study of cholesterol-lowering with simvastatin in 5,963 people with diabetes. *Lancet* 2005;361:2005–2016.
164. Sever PS, Poulter NR, Dahlof B, for the ASCOT Investigators: Reduction in cardiovascular events with atorvastatin in 2,532 patients with type 2 diabetes. Anglo-Scandinavian Cardiac Outcomes Trial-Lipid-Lowering Arm (ASCOT-LLA). *Diabetes Care* 2005;28:1151–1157.
165. ALLHAT Officers and Coordinators for the ALLHAT Collaborative Research Group: Major outcomes in moderately hypercholesterolemic, hypertensive patients randomized to pravastatin vs usual care. *JAMA* 2002;288:2998–3007.
166. Wanner C, Krane V, Marz W, for the German Diabetes and Dialysis Study Investigators: Atorvastatin in patients with type 2 diabetes mellitus undergoing hemodialysis. *N Engl J Med* 2005;353:238–248.
167. Keech A, Colquhoun D, Best J, et al.: Secondary prevention of cardiovascular events with long-term pravastatin in patients with diabetes or impaired fasting glucose: results from the LIPID trial. *Diabetes Care* 2003;26:2713–2721.
168. Pyorala K, Pedersen TR, Kjekshus J, Faergeman O, Olsson AG, Thorgeirsson G: Cholesterol lowering with simvastatin improves prognosis of diabetic patients with coronary heart disease. A subgroup analysis of the Scandinavian Simvastatin Survival Study (4S). *Diabetes Care* 1997;20:614–620.
169. Sacks FM, Pfeffer MA, Moye LA, et al.: The effect of pravastatin on coronary events after myocardial infarction in patients with average cholesterol levels. Cholesterol and recurrent events trial investigators. *N Engl J Med* 1996;335:1001–1009.
170. Carlson LA: Nicotinic acid: the broad-spectrum lipid drug. A 50th anniversary review. *J Intern Med* 2005;258:94–114.
171. Shepherd J, Betteridge J, Van Gaal L: Nicotinic acid in the management of dyslipidaemia associated with diabetes and metabolic syndrome: a position paper developed by a European Consensus Panel. *Curr Med Res Opin* 2005;21:665–682.
172. Karpe F, Frayn KN: The nicotinic acid receptor—a new mechanism for an old drug. *Lancet* 2004;363:1892–1894.
173. Blum CB, Levy RI, Eisenberg S, Hall M, Goebel RH, Berman M: High-density lipoprotein metabolism in man. *J Clin Invest* 1977;60:795–807.
174. Sheperd J, Packard CJ, Patsch JR, Gotto AM Jr, Taunton DO: Effects of nicotinic acid therapy on plasma high-density lipoprotein subfraction distribution and composition and on apolipoprotein A metabolism. *J Clin Invest* 1979;63:858–867.
175. Canner PL, Berge KG, Wenger NK, et al.: Fifteen year mortality in Coronary Drug Project patients: long-term benefit with niacin. *J Am Coll Cardiol* 1986;8:1245–1255.
176. Haffner SM, Goldberg RB: New strategies for the treatment of diabetic dyslipidemia. *Diabetes Care* 2002;25:1237–1239.
177. Ginsberg HN: Niacin in the metabolic syndrome: more risk than benefit? *Nat Clin Pract Endocrinol Metab* 2006;2:300–301.
178. Kahn SE, McCulloch DK, Schwartz MW, et al.: Effect of insulin resistance and hyperglycemia on proinsulin release in a primate model of diabetes mellitus. *J Clin Endocrinol Metab* 1992;74:192–197.
179. Canner PL, Furberg CD, Terrin ML, McGovern ME: Benefits of niacin by glycemic status in patients with healed myocardial infarction (from the Coronary Drug Project). *Am J Cardiol* 2005;95:254–257.
180. Canner PL, Furberg CD, McGovern ME: Benefits of niacin in patients with versus without the metabolic syndrome and healed myocardial infarction (from the Coronary Drug Project). *Am J Cardiol* 2006;97:477–479.
181. Elam MB, Hunninghake DB, Davis KB, et al.: Effect of niacin on lipid and lipoprotein levels and glycemic control in patients with diabetes and peripheral arterial disease. *JAMA* 2000;284:1263–1270.
182. Grundy SM, Vega GL, McGovern ME, et al.: Efficacy, safety and tolerability of once-daily niacin for the treatment of dyslipidemia associated with type 2 diabetes. *Arch Intern Med* 2002;162:1568–1576.
183. Ast M, Frishman WH: Bile acid sequestrants. *J Clin Pharmacol* 1990;30:99–106.
184. Davidson MH, Dillon MA, Gordon B, et al.: Colesevelam hydrochloride (Cholestagel). A new, potent bile acid sequestrant associated with a low incidence of gastrointestinal side effects. *Arch Intern Med* 1999;159:1893–1900.
185. Lipid Research Clinics Program: The Lipid Research Clinics Coronary Primary Prevention Trial results. I. Reduction in incidence of coronary heart disease. *JAMA* 1984;251:351–364.
186. Lipid Research Clinics Program: The Lipid Research Clinics Coronary Primary Prevention Trial results. II. The relationship of reduction in incidence of coronary heart disease to cholesterol lowering. *JAMA* 1984;251:365–374.
187. Gordon DJ, Knoke J, Probstfield JL, Superko R, Tyroler HA: High-density lipoprotein cholesterol and coronary heart disease in hypercholesterolemic men: The Lipid Research Clinics Coronary Primary Prevention Trial. *Circulation* 1986;74:1217–1225.
188. Brensike JF, Levy RI, Kelsey SF, et al.: Effects of therapy with cholestyramine on progression of coronary arteriosclerosis. Results of the NHLBI Type II Coronary Intervention Study. *Circulation* 1984;69:313–324.
189. Levy RI, Brensike JF, Epstein SE, et al.: The influence of changes in lipid values induced by cholestyramine and diet on progression of coronary artery disease: results of the NHLBI Type II Coronary Intervention Study. *Circulation* 1984;69:325–337.
190. Garg A, Grundy SM: Cholestyramine therapy for dyslipidemia in non-insulin dependent diabetes mellitus. A short-term, double-blind, crossover trial. *Ann Intern Med* 1994;121:416–422.
191. Staels B, Kuipers F: Bile acid sequestrants and the treatment of type 2 diabetes mellitus. *Drugs* 2007;67:1383–1392.
192. Zieve FJ, Kalin MF, Schwartz SI, et al.: Results of the glucose-lowering effect of WelChol Study (GLOWS): a randomized, double-blind, placebo-controlled pilot study evaluating the effect of colesevelam hydrochloride on glycemic control in subjects with type 2 diabetes. *Clin Ther* 2007;29:74–83.
193. Dujovne CA, Ettinger MP, McNeer JF: Efficacy and safety of a potent new selective cholesterol absorption inhibitor, ezetimibe, in patients with primary hypercholesterolemia. *Am J Cardiol* 2002;90:1092–1097.
194. Bays HE, Moore PB, Drehobl MA: Effectiveness and tolerability of ezetimibe in patients with primary hypercholesterolemia: pooled analysis of two phase II studies. *Clin Ther* 2001;23:1209–1230.
195. Davidson MH, McGarry T, Bettis R, et al.: Ezetimibe coadministered with simvastatin in patients with primary hypercholesterolemia. *J Am Coll Cardiol* 2002;40:2125–2134.
196. Ballantyne CM, Houri J, Notarbartolo a, et al.: Effect of ezetimibe coadministered with atorvastatin in 628 patients with primary hypercholesterolemia: a prospective, randomized, double-blind trial. *Circulation* 2003;107:2409–2415.
197. Denke M, Pearson T, McBride P, et al.: Ezetimibe added to ongoing statin therapy improves LDL cholesterol goal attainment and lipid profile in patients with diabetes or metabolic syndrome. *Diabetes Vasc Dis Res* 2006;3:93–102.
198. Goldberg RB, Guyton JR, Mazzone T, et al.: Ezetimibe/Simvastatin vs atorvastatin in patients with type 2 diabetes mellitus and hypercholesterolemia: The VYTAL Study. *Mayo Clin Proc* 2006;81:1579–1588.
199. Simons L, Tonkon M, Masana L, et al.: Effects of ezetimibe added to on-going statin therapy on the lipid profile of hypercholesterolemic patients with diabetes mellitus or metabolic syndrome. *Curr Med Res Opin* 2004;20:1437–1445.
200. Staels B, Dallongeville J, Auwerx J, Schoonjans K, Leitersdorf E, Fruchart J-C: Mechanism of action of fibrates on lipid and lipoprotein metabolism. *Circulation* 1998;98:2088–2093.
201. Fruchart J-C, Brewer HB Jr, Leitersdorf E: Consensus for the use of fibrates in the treatment of dyslipoproteinemia and coronary heart disease. Fibrate Consensus Group. *Am J Cardiol* 1998;81:912–917.
202. Rader DJ, Haffner SM: Role of fibrates in the management of hypertriglyceridemia. *Am J Cardiol* 1999;83:30F–35F.
203. Frick MH, Elo MO, Haapa K,et al.: Helsinki Heart Study: primary-prevention trial with gemfibrozil in middle-aged men with dyslipidemia. Safety of treatment, changes in risk factors, and incidence of coronary heart disease. *N Engl J Med* 1987;317:1237–1245.

204. Koskinen P, Manttari M, Manninen V, et al.: Coronary heart disease incidence in NIDDM patients in the Helsinki Heart Study. *Diabetes Care* 1992;15:820–825.
205. Rubins HB, Robins SJ, Collins D, et al.: Gemifibrozil for the secondary prevention of coronary heart disease in men with low levels of high-density lipoprotein cholesterol. Veterans Affairs High-Density Lipoprotein Cholesteroal Intervention Trial Study Group. *N Engl J Med* 1999;341:410–418.
206. McKenney JM, Davidson MH, Jacobson TA, Guyton JR, National Lipid Association Statin Safety Assessment Task Force: Final conclusions and recommendations of the National Lipid Association statin safety assesent task force. *Am J Cardiol* 2006;97: 89C–94C.
207. Rosenson RS: Current overview of statin-induced myopathy. *Am J Med* 2004;116:408–416.
208. Davidson MH, Armani A, McKenney JM, Jacobson TA: Safety considerations with fibrate therapy. *Am J Cardiol* 2007;99: 3C–18C.
209. Zhao XQ, Morse JS, Dowdy AA, et al.: Safety and tolerability of simvastatin plus niacin in patients with coronary artery disease and low high-density lipoprotein cholesterol (The HDL Atherosclerosis Treatment Study). *Am J Cardiol* 2004;93:307–312.
210. Guyton JR, Goldberg AC, Kreisberg RA, et al.: Effectiveness of once-nightly dosing of extended-release niacin alone and in combination for hypercholesterolemia. *Am J Cardiol* 1998;82:737–743.
211. Bays HE, Davidson M, Jones MR, Abby SL: Effects of colesevelam hydrochloride on low-density lipoprotein cholesterol and high-sensitivity C-reactive protein when added to statins in patients with hypercholesterolemia. *Am J Cardiol* 2006;97:1198–1205.
212. Grundy SM, Vega GL, Yuan Z, et al.: Effectiveness and tolerability of simvastatin plus fenofibrate for combined hyperlipidemia (the SAFARI Trial). *Am J Cardiol* 2005;95:462–468.
213. Athyros VG, Papageorgious AA, Athyrou V, et al.: Atorvastatin and micronized fenofibrate alone and in combination in type 2 diabetes with combined hyperlipidemia. *Diabetes Care* 2002;25:1198–1202.
214. Brown BG, Zhao X-Q, Chait A, et al.: Simvastatin and niacin, antioxidant vitamins, or the combination for the prevention of coronary disease. *N Engl J Med* 2001;345:1583–1592.
215. Taylor AJ, Sullenberger LE, Lee HJ, et al.: Arterial Biology for the Investigation of the Treatment Effects of Reducing Cholesterol (ARBITER) 2: a double-blind, placebo-controlled study of extended-release niacin on atherosclerosis progression in secondary prevention patients treated with statins. *Circulation* 2004;110:3512–3517.

CHAPTER 38

Special Patient Populations: Women and Elderly

Carl J. Lavie and Nanette K. Wenger

INTRODUCTION

Although cardiovascular disease (CVD) ranks as the leading cause of morbidity and mortality in the United States for both women and the elderly, preventive strategies, including lipid assessment and treatment, seem to be significantly underutilized in these populations.[1–3] We review evidence from epidemiologic and lipid intervention trials demonstrating the importance of lipid assessment and vigorous intervention, especially with statin therapy, in both female and elderly individuals.

WOMEN

Background Data

Worldwide and in the United States, CVD is the leading cause of death among women, accounting for almost one-third of all mortality.[2,4] Although in many countries, including the United States, more women than men died of CVD in almost every year during the past two decades, that fact remains largely unknown by the lay public and by clinicians. Typically, women cite cancers, specifically breast cancer, as their major threat to health. Nevertheless, the annual mortality of women from CVD is twice that for all cancers combined, and almost one in two women will die from CVD compared with 1 in 30 from breast cancer.[2,4]

There is considerable evidence that dyslipidemia, including elevated levels of total cholesterol (TC) and low-density lipoprotein (LDL) cholesterol,[2] increases CVD risk in women,[2,3] although these relationships are less prominent in elderly women.[2,5] In contrast, low levels of high-density lipoprotein (HDL) cholesterol and elevated levels of triglycerides (TGs) impart comparable risk in young and elderly women; these lipid fractions appear to be independent risk factors for coronary heart disease (CHD) events and mortality in women, although not in elderly men.[2,5] Despite this evidence, information from several studies that compared gender data demonstrated that men have their lipid values measured more often than women, and abnormal values also seem to be treated more aggressively in men, resulting in lower levels of LDL cholesterol in men.[2,6] In women enrolled in the Heart and Estrogen/Progestin Replacement Study (HERS; 1993), all of whom had established CHD, 63% failed to meet the National Cholesterol Education Program Adult Treatment Panel I (NCEP ATP I) 1988 LDL cholesterol goal of less than 130 mg/dL, and 91% failed to meet the NCEP ATP II (1993) LDL cholesterol goal of less than 100 mg/dL.[7] In a trial in patients with stable CHD (1994–1997), 31% of men and only 12% of women reached LDL cholesterol of less than 100 mg/dL.[8] In the recent Women's Ischemia Syndrome Evaluation (WISE) study, which enrolled women with chest pain and myocardial ischemia documented on noninvasive testing between 1996 and 2003, only 24% met their LDL cholesterol goals.[9] These studies and others document the overall less aggressive treatment of dyslipidemia in high-risk women, including those with documented CHD.[2–4]

Guidelines

Recent revised guidelines from both the NCEP ATP III[10] and the American Heart Association (AHA) evidence-based guidelines for CVD prevention in women[4] have new recommendations that may affect the management of dyslipidemia in women and increase the number of women eligible for intensive lipid therapy. Whereas the NCEP ATP II guidelines assumed a benefit of menopausal hormone therapy (HT) for lipid lowering in CHD prevention in women,[11] the NCEP

ATP III did not advise HT and recommended a similar treatment approach for women and men for both primary and secondary prevention.[10,12] However, considering that the onset of clinical evidence of CHD is typically 10 to 15 years later in women than men, NCEP ATP III has different age cut-offs for the genders; 55 years is the age considered a risk factor for women compared to 45 years for men, and family history of premature CHD is before age 65 years for women and before age 55 years for men.[12] In addition, compared to the AHA 2004 prevention guidelines for women,[13] the 2007 AHA update recommends a scheme for a general risk stratification approach to the female patient that classifies her as high risk, at risk, or optimal risk (Table 38-1).[4] In addition, the 2007 AHA update guideline focuses on the very high average lifetime risk for CVD in women (essentially 1 in 2) as opposed to a relatively narrow focus on short-term (10-year) risk of major CHD events emphasized by the Framingham global risk score and the new Reynolds Risk Score[14] (which reclassified 40%–50% of women at intermediate risk into higher- or lower-risk categories).[4,14,15] These changes in the guidelines will make more women candidates for more aggressive preventive therapies, including more vigorous lipid interventions.

Nonpharmacologic Therapies for Lipid Management

Therapeutic lifestyle changes (TLCs) are required for the optimal management of dyslipidemia in women, including dietary changes, increases in physical activity and exercise, and smoking cessation, all of which have been shown to reduce overall CVD risk factors and contribute to a decline in CHD.[1,2,4] Among 84,129 women in the Nurses' Health Study, 82% of CHD events were attributed to lack of adherence to lifestyle guidelines.[16] Tobacco use is a major preventable cause both of dyslipidemia and of CHD in women.[1] Cigarette consumption is inversely related to levels of HDL cholesterol and directly related to TC, LDL cholesterol, and TG levels. Although clinical studies support the benefits of diet and exercise in reducing dyslipidemia, in a study of 180 postmenopausal women and 197 men with low levels of HDL cholesterol and moderately elevated LDL cholesterol levels, the AHA Step 2 diet failed to significantly lower levels of LDL cholesterol in both women and men in the absence of aerobic exercise training.[17] We recently focused on the potential benefits of moderate alcohol consumption in preventive cardiology, recognizing that this represents a "razor-sharp, double-edged sword."[18] Moderate (e.g., one to two drinks per day) of alcohol consumption increases HDL cholesterol in women and may be cardioprotective, but because of other concerns (e.g., increased risk of breast cancer, liver disease, alcoholism), it is difficult to routinely recommend regular alcohol consumption to nondrinkers. The 2007 AHA women's prevention guidelines suggest limiting alcohol intake to one drink per day for women.[4] Finally, in addition to dietary restrictions in saturated fat, *trans* fatty acids, and cholesterol, aerobic exercise training, smoking cessation, and possibly small doses of alcohol, the NCEP ATP III recommends inclusion of plant sterols/stanols (2 g/day) and soluble fiber (10–25 g/day) in the diet.[1,4,12] Some studies have reported that increased intakes of soy or soy protein, especially as a replacement for animal protein, resulted in small, but at times, statistically significant, lipid improvements in women.[1,19]

We have published numerous studies on the benefits of cardiac rehabilitation and exercise training (CRET) programs, including the effects of this therapy in women[20–22] and the elderly.[23] Although our studies indicate that women with CHD, especially older women, have statistically higher levels of TC and LDL cholesterol, as well as HDL cholesterol, compared with men, both genders in general have statistically similar improvements in most CHD risk factors following CRET as TLC in secondary prevention.[20,21] On average, these patients have improvements in TC (–5%), TGs (–15%), HDL cholesterol (+6%), LDL cholesterol (–3%), and LDL cholesterol/HDL cholesterol ratio (–8%) following CRET, as well as significant improvements in many other CHD risk factors, such as estimated exercise capacity (+35%), metabolic syndrome prevalence (–37%), body mass index (BMI), and percent of body fat (–1.5% and –5%, respectively), inflammation (C-reactive protein [CRP]; –40%), and numerous other factors (autonomic function, blood viscosity and rheology, adverse psychological factors, and overall quality of life).[20–22,24] These data reinforce the CRET recommendations in the 2007 AHA's women's guidelines.[4]

TABLE 38-1 Classification of Cardiovascular Disease Risk in Women

Risk Status	Criteria
High risk	Established coronary heart disease Cerebrovascular disease Peripheral artery disease Abdominal aortic aneurysm End-stage or chronic renal disease Diabetes mellitus 10-year Framingham global risk >20%*
At risk	≥1 major risk factors for CVD, including: Cigarette smoking Poor diet Physical inactivity Obesity, especially central adiposity Family history of premature CVD (CVD at <55 years of age in male relative and <65 years of age in female relative) Hypertension Dyslipidemia Evidence of subclinical vascular disease (e.g., coronary calcification) Metabolic syndrome Poor exercise capacity on treadmill test and/or abnormal heart rate recovery after stopping exercise
Optimal risk	Framingham global risk <10% and a healthy lifestyle, with no risk factors

*Or at high risk on the basis of another population-adapted tool used to assess global risk.

Reproduced Ref. 4, with permission.

CVD, cardiovascular disease.

Menopausal Hormone Therapy

Considerable controversy persists on the exact roles of several components of HT and their role in treatment of dyslipidemia and prevention of CHD in women.[1]

Epidemiologic studies, mostly using estrogen therapy (ET), have demonstrated a consistent reduction of CHD in women receiving HT.[1] However, two randomized controlled trials in secondary prevention and one study in primary prevention have not supported benefits of HT.[1,25–27] HERS[25] was a large-scale randomized controlled trial with conjugated equine estrogen (CEE) and medroxyprogesterone acetate (MPA), which did not show benefit for nonfatal myocardial infarction (MI) or CHD death in 2763 women with established CHD. The Estrogen Replacement and Atherosclerosis (ERA) trial[26] also reported no benefit of either estrogen alone or with MPA on angiographic progression of atherosclerosis during a 3-year follow-up. The Women's Health Initiative (WHI) primary prevention trial[27] suggested that estrogen plus progestin HT may be associated with an increase in early CHD events, although the absolute number of events in this study was fairly low. Both unopposed estrogen and estrogen plus progestin increased the risk of stroke and venous thromboembolism.[1] Age at onset of HT may be important regarding its relative risk/benefit ratio. In a recent analysis from the WHI, women who initiated HT closer to menopause tended to have lower CHD and mortality, although the risk of stroke was elevated regardless of years since menopause.[28]

Further, the hormone composition and pattern and route of administration of HT may have a substantial effect on overall CVD risk. For example, in the Post-Menopausal Estrogen/Progestin Interventions (PEPI) trial,[29] the effect of CEE alone or in combination with either cyclic or continuous MPA or cyclic micronized progesterone (MP) versus placebo was evaluated in 875 healthy postmenopausal women. All HT regimens were superior to placebo in increasing HDL cholesterol. Although CEE alone exerted the most benefit in raising HDL cholesterol, the combination of CEE and MP had better HDL cholesterol effects than did CEE with MPA. All regimens exerted equal lowering of LDL cholesterol and fibrinogen levels. This study demonstrated the potential differences among various hormone regimens on CVD risk factors and suggested that natural progesterone had more favorable lipid effects than MPA. These regimens, as well as lower doses of estrogen (which may have similar lipid effects but less adverse effects on coagulation and inflammation), require further study in clinical trials. In addition, increases in the inflammatory marker CRP have occurred with oral estrogen, especially using moderate doses, but may not occur with topical therapy.[30]

Other nontraditional modes of HT have also been studied, including selective estrogen receptor modulators (SERMs) such as tamoxifen and raloxifene. These drug therapies have beneficial effects on LDL cholesterol, fibrinogen, and lipoprotein(a), as well as on bone minerals and lack of adverse effects on endometrium and breast tissue, but do not increase HDL cholesterol (or TGs). Like traditional HT, they have adverse effects on the potential for venous thromboembolism. In a recent major randomized controlled clinical trial, the SERM raloxifene did not reduce CHD events.[31]

What Is the Role of Lipid-Lowering Pharmacologic Therapy for CHD Prevention in Women?

Statins

The protective role of lipid-lowering therapy in women, especially with the 3-hydroxy-3-methylglutaryl–coenzyme A reductase inhibitors, or statins, is well established by major clinical trials using several statins; reductions in CVD risk ranged from 11% to 54% (Table 38-2).[2,32–41] Although the representation of women in most of these trials was small (averaging <20%), as was the number of major CHD events in women, the positive trend for benefit was consistent and large across all trials, which involved nearly 20,000 women. More importantly, the protective effect of various statins in these trials appeared to be equal to or greater than that observed for men. The reduction in risk of major CHD events in women ranged from 11% in the Long-term Intervention with Pravastatin Ischemic Disease (LIPID) study[35] to 54% in the Greek Atorvastatin and Coronary-Heart-Disease Evaluation (GREACE) trial.[40] There was no significant effect in women in the Prospective Study of Pravastatin in the Elderly at Risk (PROSPER)[37] or in the lipid lowering arm

TABLE 38-2 Major Lipid-Lowering Trials Using Statin Therapy for CHD Prevention

Study	Patients, *n*	Women, *n* (%)	Prevention Category	Drug	Year	Risk Reduction—Major CHD Events in Women, %
4S[33]	4444	827 (19)	Secondary	Simvastatin	1994	35
CARE[34]	4159	576 (14)	Secondary	Pravastatin	1996	46
LIPID[35]	9014	1516 (17)	Secondary	Pravastatin	1998	11
AFCAPS/TexCAPS[36]	6605	997 (15)	Primary	Lovastatin	1998	46
PROSPER[37]	5804	3000 (52)	Both	Pravastatin	2002	NS benefit for women
HPS[38]	20,536	5082 (25)	Primary	Simvastatin	2002	19
ALLHAT-LLT[39]	10,355	5051 (49)	Primary (HTN) (14% CHD)	Pravastatin	2002	Sex-specific data not reported; NS in total cohort
GREACE[40]	1600	344 (21)	Secondary	Atorvastatin	2002	54
ASCOT-LLA[41]	10,305	1942 (19)	Primary (HTN)	Atorvastatin	2003	NS benefit for women

CHD, coronary heart disease; HTN, hypertension; NS, not significant.
Adapted from Ref. 32.

of the Anglo-Scandinavian Cardiac Outcomes Trial (ASCOT).[41] There was no significant effect in the total cohort (men or women) in the lipid-lowering arm of the Antihypertensive and Lipid-Lowering Treatment to Prevent Heart Attack Trial (ALLHAT).[39] More recently, a major trial of a high dose (80 mg) versus a low dose (10 mg) of atorvastatin (Treating to New Targets [TNT]) showed equal protection against major CVD events with more-intensive therapy in women, statistically similar to men, without any rhabdomyolysis with 80 mg of atorvastatin.[42] However, there was slightly greater discontinuation of therapy in women than men (10% vs. 6.5%) and liver function test abnormalities (2.5% vs. 1%). Likewise, in patients with acute coronary syndromes (ACS) (4162 patients, 22% women), more-intensive lipid treatment with atorvastatin 80 mg versus pravastatin 40 mg also yielded similar benefits in women and men.[43]

In aggregate, these statin trials demonstrate the efficacy and safety of statin therapy, including more-intensive treatments, for protection against CHD and major CVD events in women. There are six major statins currently on the U.S. market (lovastatin, simvastatin, pravastatin, atorvastatin, fluvastatin, and rosuvastatin), with the first four having major clinical events trials that included women. In addition to significant reduction in LDL cholesterol and moderate improvements in HDL cholesterol and TGs, other potential beneficial effects of statins include improvements in endothelial function, plaque stabilization, anti-inflammatory effects, and antiplatelet effects, among others. These therapies are probably most effective in high-risk patients, such as for secondary prevention in women. It has been argued that treating young women with dyslipidemia with relatively few risk factors may not be cost-effective[1]; however, as mentioned previously, recent prevention guidelines focus on long-term as opposed to merely 10-year risk.[4,14,15] In addition, women carry a high short-term mortality rate associated with first CHD events (more than twice that for men), providing further ammunition for consideration to initiate statin therapy for both primary and secondary prevention of CVD in women.[1,4,44]

Nonstatin Pharmacologic Agents

Although several other forms of lipid therapy are available, including bile acid sequestrant resins, nicotinic acid or niacin, fibrates (gemfibrozil and fenofibrate), and ezetimibe, none of these therapies have reported clinical trial data for women.[1,2,4] Nevertheless, based on an accumulation of considerable prevention data in women as well as the clinical trial data for men, the current AHA cardiovascular prevention guidelines for women incorporate the use of these therapies to meet LDL cholesterol goals, and also to provide additional pharmacotherapy for women with high levels of non-HDL cholesterol (usually women with elevated levels of TGs and/or low levels of HDL cholesterol) as well as for women with persistent low levels of HDL cholesterol (Table 38-3).[4] Both the 2007 AHA prevention guidelines for women and the update to NCEP ATP III place greater emphasis on combining statins with other agents (e.g., ezetimibe) to further reduce LDL cholesterol and/or levels of CRP or with niacin or fibrates to improve levels of HDL cholesterol, non-HDL cholesterol, or TGs.[4,10] Finally, these other classes of agents may be required for the relatively large number of women (more than 10% by some estimates) who are either intolerant to statin therapy or, for some reason, refuse to comply with statin medications.[45]

Pregnancy: Special Considerations

Existing pharmacological therapies are not currently approved in pregnancy. Women with high TGs should be monitored during pregnancy since TGs can increase dramatically and cause pancreatitis, with high risk of mortality of both the fetus and mother.

TABLE 38-3 Guidelines for Prevention of Cardiovascular Disease in Women—Clinical Lipid Recommendations
Lipid and lipoprotein levels—optimal levels and lifestyle The following levels of lipids and lipoproteins in women should be encouraged through lifestyle approaches: LDL cholesterol <100 mg/dL, HDL cholesterol >50 mg/dL, triglycerides <150 mg/dL, and non-HDL cholesterol (total cholesterol minus HDL cholesterol) <130 mg/dL (*Class I, Level B*). If a women is at high risk or has hypercholesterolemia, intake of saturated fat should be <7% and cholesterol intake <200 mg/d (*Class I, Level B*).
Lipids—pharmacotherapy for LDL lowering, high-risk women Use LDL cholesterol-lowering drug therapy simultaneously with lifestyle therapy in women with CHD to achieve an LDL cholesterol <100 mg/dL (*Class I, Level A*) and similarly in women with other atherosclerotic CVD or diabetes mellitus or 10-year absolute risk >20% (*Class I, Level B*).
A reduction to <70 mg/dL is reasonable in very-high-risk women with CHD and may require an LDL-lowering drug combination (*Class IIa, Level B*).
Lipids—pharmacotherapy for LDL lowering, other at-risk women Use LDL cholesterol-lowering therapy if LDL cholesterol level is ≥130 mg/dL with lifestyle therapy and there are multiple risk factors and 10-year absolute risk 10% to 20% (*Class I, Level B*).
Use LDL cholesterol-lowering therapy if LDL cholesterol level is ≥160 mg/dL with lifestyle therapy and multiple risk factors even if 10-year absolute risk is <10% (*Class I, Level B*).
Use LDL cholesterol-lowering therapy if LDL level is ≥190 mg/dL regardless of the presence or absence of other risk factors or CVD on lifestyle therapy (*Class I, Level B*).
Lipids—pharmacotherapy for low HDL or elevated non-HDL, high-risk women Use niacin or fibrate therapy when HDL cholesterol is low or non-HDL cholesterol is elevated in high-risk women after LDL cholesterol goal is reached (*Class IIa, Level B*).
Lipids—pharmacotherapy for low HDL or elevated non-HDL, other at-risk women Consider niacin or fibrate therapy when HDL cholesterol is low or non-HDL cholesterol is elevated after LDL cholesterol goal is reached in women with multiple risk factors and a 10-year absolute risk of 10% to 20% (*Class IIb, Level B*).

Reprinted from Ref. 4, with permission.

ELDERLY

Background Data

Cardiovascular disease continues to be a major threat to the health of older patients, who account for more than 75% of total CHD mortality and well over 50% of all acute MIs in the United States.[3] Although CHD morbidity and mortality have declined in recent decades, the percent reduction of CHD events during this period is nearly 50% less among older patient groups. Despite the high prevalence of CVD, including both CHD and cerebrovascular disease, in the elderly population, there appears to be a strong age bias in the prevention and treatment of CVD, highly pertinent to the assessment and treatment of lipid disorders for primary and secondary prevention in the elderly.[3]

Dyslipidemia is prevalent at advanced age, even more so in elderly women than in elderly men.[2,5,21] Because the TC/HDL cholesterol ratio, which is a potent predictor of CHD events in the older population, declines progressively with advancing age in men but rises in women, this ratio is comparable in both genders by age 80, potentially partly explaining the narrowing gap in CHD incidence between genders with advanced age.[2,5]

The role of lipids and lipid subfractions in CHD prevention at elderly age have been somewhat controversial over the years, since some studies, including the Framingham Heart Study,[46] the Established Population for the Epidemiologic Study of the Elderly (EPESE),[47] and the Honolulu Heart Program,[48] did not show a statistical relationship between TC and all-cause CHD mortality in patients older than 70 years. This led some experts to discourage lipid treatment and primary prevention in the elderly. Although TC did not predict CHD in men older than 70 years in the Framingham Heart Study,[5,46] it continued to predict CHD in women well into the 9th decade. By contrast, several other studies found that lipid levels predicted CHD at elderly age,[5,49–52] and because of the increased attributable risk in the elderly population, lipid intervention may have greater impact for overall CVD reduction in older populations compared with younger groups, who have a lower prevalence of disease. Although various studies demonstrate markedly different effects of individual lipid fractions (e.g., TC, HDL cholesterol, TC/HDL cholesterol ratio, LDL cholesterol) in the elderly population, in aggregate these studies demonstrate the importance of dyslipidemia as a CHD and CVD risk factor at elderly age.[5]

Although the relative risk of high TC or low HDL cholesterol decreases somewhat with older age, the attributable risk is greater because of high CHD prevalence in older people.[3,5] Therefore, the diminished relative risk associated with dyslipidemia at advanced age is more than offset by the considerably greater absolute and attributable risk in the elderly population. Both TC and HDL cholesterol generally predict CHD death in the elderly, and a high TC/HDL cholesterol ratio appears to be the single lipid component that consistently predicts CHD in this population. The role of TGs as an independent risk factor remains controversial in many populations, including the elderly, but clearly low levels of HDL cholesterol, which are often associated with elevated TGs, predict CHD in older women.[5]

Nonpharmacologic Approaches

Although interventions in dyslipidemia for the elderly population have generally been directed toward statin therapy, which is discussed in more detail below, several other forms of therapy, including TLCs with vigorous nonpharmacologic approaches, such as CRET programs, can provide additional preventive treatment for the elderly.[23]

Numerous studies indicate the protective effects of increased fitness for CVD, which may be particularly applicable to elderly patients, who typically have lower levels of fitness than younger cohorts.[21,23] In addition to low levels of fitness, older CHD patients in our studies typically have lower BMI, higher percent of body fat, more hypertension, and overall lower function and quality-of-life scores. Elderly men typically have similar levels of LDL cholesterol as younger men, but have lower TGs and higher levels of HDL cholesterol compared with their younger CHD cohorts.[23] Elderly women with CHD usually have higher levels of LDL cholesterol than do other CHD patients.[21] Nevertheless, despite having higher levels of HDL cholesterol than younger patients, a substantial number of elderly CHD patients also have low levels of HDL cholesterol.[23,53]

We and others have demonstrated the marked benefits of formal CRET programs in the elderly, including studies of very elderly (≥70 years of age) and elderly women,[21,54] generally similar to benefits noted in younger patients. A recent study, however, suggested less impressive lipid improvements in a very deconditioned, sedentary elderly population.[55,56]

As was discussed regarding women, recent guidelines have recommended greater dietary consumption of plant stanols/sterols as well as soluble fiber.[1,4,12] Although generally increasing daily consumption of dietary fiber, especially soluble fiber, seems to be sound advice for all Americans, this may be particularly applicable to the elderly population, who have substantial colonic disease and constipation. Therefore, supplements of psyllium, oat bran, or guar gum given two to three times daily is probably the easiest and most practical way to obtain adequate dietary fiber consumption and can provide colonic protection as well as reductions in LDL cholesterol by up to 20% (generally 5%–10%) without significantly affecting (or only slightly reducing) levels of HDL cholesterol. This healthy nonpharmacologic therapy may provide sufficient treatment for many elderly patients with only slightly increased levels of TC and LDL cholesterol or for patients who need only mild additional lowering of LDL cholesterol after standard doses of statins. It may also limit the need for higher doses of statins and their potential toxicity in the elderly population.

Statins

Numerous large-scale studies, including both cohort studies and randomized controlled clinical trials involving thousands of patients, have established the efficacy and safety of statins in both primary and secondary CVD prevention.[57] Although there remains considerable underutilization of these medications in the elderly population, substantial evidence supports use of statins in the increasingly large group of elderly patients.[3,57]

Both observational data, including the LDS Hospital/University of Utah cohort study,[58] the Cardiovascular Health Study (CHS),[59] and a New York Medical College Study,[60] and several randomized controlled trials in large patient cohorts, including primary and secondary prevention, support the value of statin therapy in the elderly.[51] In 1250 women and 664 men in the CHS aged 65 years and older and free of CVD, during a 7.3-year follow-up those taking a statin had a 56% reduction in CVD events and a 44% reduction in the risk of all-cause mortality.[59] These benefits were noted in the entire elderly cohort as well as in those aged 75 and older. In the LDS Hospital/University of Utah cohort study of 7200 patients followed for 3.3 years, those under aged 65 years received statin therapy 28% of the time, those aged 65 to 79 years received statin 21% of the time, and those aged 80 and older received statins 20% of the time ($P < 0.001$ for trend).[58] Statin therapy was associated with reductions in mortality of 50% in those aged 80 and older, 41% in those aged 65 to 79 years, and 30% in those under age 65. In a study of 1410 patients with a mean age of 81 years with prior MI and an LDL cholesterol greater than 125 mg/dL, statin therapy was associated with an event reduction of more than 30%, even in the 9th and 10th decades of life.[60]

The randomized controlled trials that presented data in elderly subgroups compared to younger patients all showed either equal or greater benefits of statin therapy for CVD reduction in those aged 65 and older (Table 38-4). The majority of these studies, including the Scandinavian Simvastatin Survival Study (4S),[33] the Cholesterol and Recurrent Events (CARE)[34] trial, LIPID,[35] and the Pravastatin or Atorvastatin Evaluation and Infection Therapy (PROVE IT)[43,61] study, were secondary prevention trials; the Heart Protection Study (HPS)[38] and PROSPER[39] included patients in both primary and secondary prevention subgroups. All these studies demonstrated major CVD and CHD event reduction with the use of statins in patients aged 65 and older.[62] In a meta-analysis of 90,056 randomized patients in 14 clinical trials, CHD mortality, stroke, and revascularization rates were reduced by 26% among patients less than 65 years of age and 18% among those 65 years of age and older.[63] The absolute risk reduction for the combined endpoint of CHD death and nonfatal MI was identical in elderly and younger patients. Finally, in a large population-based study, lipid medications, usually statins, were associated with significant reductions in major clinical events and mortality in elderly individuals following coronary revascularization.[64] These very-large-scale clinical trials clearly demonstrate the marked benefits of statins in both primary and, particularly, secondary prevention in elderly patients. However, a large retrospective study of Medicare patients with acute MI demonstrated that the "young" elderly (aged 65 to 80 years) had significant mortality benefits when discharged on statins, but this was not the case in the very old (aged >80 years).[65]

High-Intensity Lipid Therapy Trials in Acute Coronary Syndrom and Stable Coronary Heart Disease

Although age-related data were not available in the Myocardial Ischemia Reduction with Aggressive Cholesterol Lowering (MIRACL),[66] TNT,[67] PROVE IT,[43,61] and the Z phase of the Aggrastat to Zocor (A to Z) Trial,[68] which studied high-intensity versus moderate-intensity lipid therapy in more than 4000 ACS patients each, demonstrated no significant differences between the relative event reduction noted in elderly compared with younger patients. In aggregate, all these trials support more intensive lipid treatment and lower levels of LDL cholesterol, with LDL cholesterol targets of less than 70 mg/dL, which currently seems reasonable in elderly patients with ACS and probably in elderly patients with stable CHD.

Effect of Statins on Stroke and Dementia

Neurological diseases, including stroke and dementia, are among the leading causes of morbidity and mortality in the elderly.[69,70] Stroke is the third leading cause of death and is the leading cause of long-term disability in the United States. Although stroke can affect people

TABLE 38-4 Results by Age from Major Statin Trials of Cardiovascular Disease Prevention

Study	Treatment; duration; % elderly	Risk reduction ≥65 years	Risk reduction <65 years
Secondary Prevention:			
4S (n = 4444)[33]	20–40 mg simvastatin; 5.4 years; 23% elderly	-34% death -43% CHD death -34% events	- 28% death -42% CHD death -35% events
CARE (n = 4159)[34]	40 mg pravastatin; 5 years; 31% elderly	-45% CHD death -23% events	-(NS) CHD death -19% events
LIPID (n = 9014)[35]	40 mg pravastatin; 5 years; 31% elderly	-21% death -21% CHD death -22% events	-24% death -24% CHD death -25% events
PROVE IT (n = 4162)[43]	80 mg atorvastatin vs. 40 mg pravastatin; 2 years; 30% elderly	-20% events	-21% events
Primary and Secondary Prevention:			
HPS (n = 20,536)[38]	40 mg simvastatin; 5 years; 52% elderly	-20% events	-24% events
PROSPER (n = 5804)[37]	40 mg pravastatin; 3.2 years; 100% elderly	-24% CHD death -19% events	

at any age, the overwhelming majority of strokes occur in older persons, making stroke prevention a major healthcare issue in the elderly population.

Although many major CHD risk factors overlap with stroke risk factors, including age, male gender, hypertension, diabetes, smoking, and physical inactivity, as well as advanced age, serum lipids have been demonstrated to be major risk factors for CHD but generally not for stroke (Fig. 38-1).[69,70] The Framingham Heart Study and other large epidemiologic studies, including 45 prospective observational cohorts totaling 450,000 individuals and representing a mean 16-year follow-up and a total of more than 13,000 strokes, failed to show an association between TC and the incidence of stroke.[69,71]

Despite the lack of epidemiologic association between TC and stroke, numerous statin trials, including several in the elderly, have demonstrated a strong effect of statin medications in reducing the risk of stroke.[69] For example, in CARE, stroke and transient ischemic attacks (TIAs) were reduced significantly by 26% with pravastatin, and stroke was reduced by 31% ($P = 0.03$) in the total cohort and by 40% ($P < 0.05$) in those older than 65 years.[57,72] In 4S, patients treated with simvastatin had a 28% reduction in combined stroke and TIA and a 24% reduction in stroke.[57,73] In LIPID, pravastatin reduced stroke risk by 19% ($P < 0.05$), with equivalent effects regardless of age.[35] In MIRACL, high-dose (80 mg) atorvastatin reduced stroke by more than 50% after only 4 months.[74] TIA and stroke were reduced significantly by 17% ($P = 0.02$) and 25% ($P < 0.0001$), respectively, with simvastatin in HPS.[38] In the ASCOT, low-dose atorvastatin (10 mg) reduced fatal and nonfatal stroke by 27% ($P = 0.02$) after 3.3 years.[41] In PROSPER, which included only elderly participants (70–82 years), TIA was reduced by 25% with pravastatin after 3 years.[37] Finally, in the Stroke Prevention by Aggressive Reduction of Cholesterol Levels (SPARCL), which studied 4731 patients (mean age 60 years) with prior stroke and LDL cholesterol 100 to 190 mg/dL, 80 mg of atorvastatin reduced subsequent stroke or TIA by 23% ($P < 0.001$) and produced a 35% reduction in CHD events ($P < 0.01$).[75] There was overall marked benefit despite a small increase in incidence of the more rare hemorrhagic stroke in atorvastatin-treated patients. In aggregate, these trials show the fairly marked beneficial effects of statins in the primary and secondary prevention of stroke and highlight the non–LDL cholesterol–lowering benefit of statins that may be particularly applicable to the elderly population.[69,70]

A major issue applicable to the elderly population, in addition to CHD and stroke, is dementia, which is now the fifth leading cause of death in the United States.[69,70] Although some early studies suggested that statins may reduce dementia, in recent years there has been considerable media attention, mainly generated by isolated case studies suggesting that statins may actually worsen memory loss and cognitive function.[70,76] However, data from more than 30,000 patients (mostly elderly) in two large-scale prospective randomized clinical trials, in HPS[38] with simvastatin 40 mg, and pravastatin 40 mg in PROSPER,[37] demonstrated that statins did not adversely affect cognitive function.[69,70,76] In addition, in one small proof-of-concept randomized, placebo-controlled trial in patients with mild to moderate Alzheimer's disease, atorvastatin 80 mg improved state-of-the art measures of cognition compared with placebo.[77] In addition, several case–control and cohort studies suggest that statins may lower the risk of Alzheimer's disease and dementia.[69,70,76] Given the profound effects of statins on reducing ischemic stroke, the weight of evidence suggests that solely by this mechanism, long-term results of statin therapy will likely provide long-term cognitive function benefits in the elderly population.

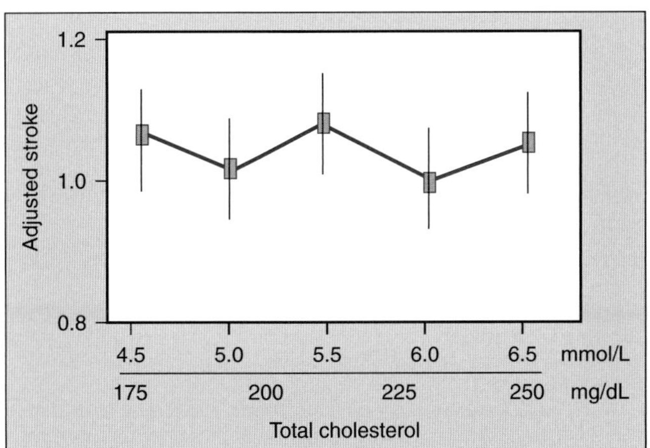

FIGURE 38-1 Serum cholesterol and stroke rate based on data from 45 prospective studies, 450,000 individuals, mean 16-year follow-up, and more than 13,000 strokes. Adapted from Ref. 71.

Safety of and Adherence to Statins in Elderly

Although statins are generally considered extremely safe and well tolerated in elderly patients, several factors might predispose elderly patients to statin-related adverse events (Tables 38-5 and 38-6).[78] It could be argued that many of these factors define the elderly population, making them the most likely group of patients susceptible to the major adverse effects of statin therapy. Given the high likelihood of multiple medication use in the elderly and the increased evidence supporting the benefits of statins in this population, a thorough knowledge of statin pharmacology, drug interactions, and safety considerations is necessary for selecting statins and concomitant medications in older persons.

TABLE 38-5 Factors That May Predispose Elderly Patients to Statin-Related Adverse Effects
Advanced age (especially in older elderly)
Female gender
Small body frame; frailty
Multisystem disease (especially chronic kidney disease and diabetes)
Perioperative periods
Excess alcohol consumption
Fatty liver disease
Hypothyroidism
Multiple medications (see Table 38-6)

Reprinted from Ref. 78, with permission.

TABLE 38-6 Commonly Used Medications by Elderly That Alter Cytochrome P450 Metabolism

3A4 Inhibitors	2C9 Inhibitors	2C19 Inhibitors
Amiodarone	Amiodarone	Gemfibrozil
Macrolide antibiotics	Fluconazole	Fluconazole
Azole antifungals	Metronidazole	Omeprazole
Cyclosporine	Fluoxetine	
Diltiazem/verapamil		
Protease inhibitors		
Large quantities of grapefruit juice		

Reprinted from Ref. 78, with permission.

Recent studies have demonstrated poor adherence rates for statin therapy in the elderly. In fact, in three large cohorts of elderly patients with ACS, with chronic CHD, or without CHD, statin adherence at 2 years was 40%, 35%, and 25% of patients, respectively, in these three groups.[62,79] In a study of 34,501 elderly patients prescribed statins, 60% compliance was noted with statins at 6 months compared with only 32% at 10 years.[80] In fact, fewer than 50% of patients of all ages prescribed statins are adherent 12 months after initiating treatment. These studies demonstrate that greater efforts are needed to promote better adherence to lipid medications, especially statins, to enhance statin therapy in preventive cardiology in the elderly.

Nonstatin Pharmacologic Therapies

Although interventions for dyslipidemia for the elderly population, as was discussed for women, generally have been directed toward statin therapy, several other forms of therapy can provide additional preventive treatment.[23] Other potent therapies (e.g., ezetimibe, niacin, and fibrates) are also available to treat dyslipidemia in elderly patients, either as monotherapy, or more commonly, combined with statins in high-risk elderly patients who either do not reach their LDL cholesterol goals on statin therapy alone or who have additional lipid disorders, including elevated TGs and/or low levels of HDL cholesterol. Only limited data are available on the use of these therapies in elderly patients, who may be at greater risk of drug interactions (especially combining statins with gemfibrozil)[23,78]; the risks versus benefits of these drug combinations must be considered, especially in high-risk elderly patients.

CONCLUSIONS

Despite the lack of age-specific data in many studies and the low number of women enrolled in the major clinical trials of lipid-lowering therapies as well as the relatively low overall major event rates for women, the available evidence on the risk-to-benefit ratio of statins supports their widespread use in both women and the elderly. Analysis of large, randomized controlled trials supports the use of vigorous lipid therapy in both women and the elderly, similar to these therapies given to men and younger patients. Further data are required about the long-term effects of statins and other lipid therapies, including the long-term risk of malignant diseases. In addition, effective methods for improving short- and long-term adherence rates to statins and other lipid therapies are needed for both women and elderly groups to maximize the long-term effectiveness of these therapies, as well as additional data on the efficacy and safety of drug combinations in these groups of patients.

REFERENCES

1. Mosca LJ: Contemporary management of hyperlipidemia in women. J Womens Health (Larchmt) 2002;11:423–432.
2. Wenger NK: Lipid abnormalities in women: data for risk, data for management. *Cardiol Rev* 2006;14:276–280.
3. Lavie CJ: Assessment and treatment of lipids in elderly persons. *Am J Geriatr Cardiol* 2004;13(3 supp 1):2–3.
4. Mosca L, Banka C, Benjamin E, et al: Evidence-based guidelines for cardiovascular disease prevention in women:2007 update. *Circulation* 2007;115:1481–1501.
5. Wenger N: Dyslipidemia as a risk factor at elderly age. *Am J Geriatr Cardiol* 2004;13(3 supp1):4–9.
6. Kim C, Hofer TP, Kerr EA: Review of evidence and explanations for suboptimal screening and treatment of dyslipidemia in women. A conceptual model. *J Gen Intern Med* 2003;18:854–863.
7. Schrott HG, Bittner V, Vittinghoff E, et al: Adherence to National Cholesterol Education Program treatment goals in postmenopausal women with heart disease. The Heart and Estrogen/progestin Replacement Study (HERS). *JAMA* 1997;277:1281–1286.
8. Miller M, Byington R, Hunninghake D, et al: Sex bias and underutilization of lipid-lowering therapy in patients with coronary artery disease at academic medical centers in the United States and Canada. Prospective Randomized Evaluation of the Vascular Effects of Norvasc Trial (PREVENT) Investigators. *Arch Intern Med* 2000;160:343–347.
9. Bittner V., Olson M, Kelsey SF et al: Effect of coronary angiography on use of lipid-lowering agents in women: a report from the Women's Ischemia Syndrome Evaluation (WISE) study. *Am J Cardiol* 2000;85:1083–1088.
10. Grundy SM, Cleeman JI, Merz CN, et al: Implications of recent clinical trials for the National Cholesterol Education Program Adult Treatment Panel III guidelines. National Heart, Lung and Blood Institute, American College of Cardiology Foundation, American Heart Association. *Circulation* 2004;110:227–239 (correction published in Circulation 2004;110:763).
11. Expert Panel on Detection, Evaluation and Treatment of High Blood Cholesterol in Adults: Summary of the Second Report of the National Cholesterol Education Program (NCEP) Expert Panel on Detection, Evaluation, and Treatment of High Blood Cholesterol in Adults (Adult Treatment Panel II). *JAMA* 1993;269:3015–3023.
12. Expert Panel on Detection, Evaluation and Treatment of High Blood Cholesterol in Adults: Executive summary of the Third Report of the National Cholesterol Education Program Expert Panel on Detection, Evaluation and Treatment of High Blood Cholesterol in Adults (Adult Treatment Panel III). *JAMA* 2001;285:2486–2497.
13. Mosca L, Appel LJ, Benjamin EJ, et al: Evidence-based guidelines for cardiovascular disease prevention in women. *Circulation* 2004;109:672–692.
14. Ridker PJ, Buring JE, Rifai N, Cook NR: Development and validation of improved algorithms for the assessment of global cardiovascular risk in women. *JAMA* 2007;297:611–619.
15. Blumenthal RS, Michos ED, Nasir K: Further improvements in CHD risk prediction for women. *JAMA* 2007;297:641–643.
16. Stampfer MJ, Hu FB, Manson JE, et al: Primary prevention of coronary heart disease in women through diet and lifestyle. *N Engl J Med* 2000;343:16–22.
17. Stefanick ML, Mackey S, Sheehan M, et al: Effects of diet and exercise in men and postmenopausal women with low levels of

HDL cholesterol and high levels of LDL cholesterol. *N Engl J Med* 1998;339:12–20.

18. O'Keefe JH, Bybee KA, Lavie CJ: Alcohol and cardiovascular health: the razor sharp double-edged sword. *J Am Coll Cardiol* 2007;50:1009–1014.
19. Crouse JR III, Morgan T, Terry JG, et al: A randomized trial comparing the effect of casein with that of soy protein containing varying amounts of isoflavones on plasma concentrations of lipids and lipoproteins. *Arch Intern Med* 1999;159: 2070–2076.
20. Lavie CJ, Milani RV: Effects of cardiac rehabilitation and exercise training on exercise capacity, coronary risk factors, behavioral characteristics, and quality of life in women. *Am J Cardiol* 1995;75:340–343.
21. Lavie CJ, Milani RV: Benefits of cardiac rehabilitation and exercise training in elderly women. *Am J Cardiol* 1997;79: 664–666.
22. Lavie CJ, Milani RV, Cassidy MM, Gilliland YE: Effects of cardiac rehabilitation and exercise training in women with depression. *Am J Cardiol* 1999;83:1480–1483.
23. Lavie CJ: Treatment of hyperlipidemia in elderly persons with exercise training, nonpharmacologic therapy, and drug combinations. *Am J Geriatr Cardiol* 2004;13(suppl 1):29–33.
24. Lavie CJ, Milani RV: Cardiac rehabilitation and exercise training programs in metabolic syndrome and diabetes. *J Cardiopulm Rehabil* 2005;25:59–66.
25. Hulley S, Grady D, Bush T, et al: Randomized trial of estrogen plus progestin for secondary prevention of coronary heart disease in postmenopausal women. Heart and Estrogen/Progestin Replacement Study (HERS) Research Group. *JAMA* 1998;280:605–613.
26. Herrington DM, Reeboussin DM, Brosnihan KB, et al: Effect of estrogen replacement on the progression of coronary artery atherosclerosis. *N Engl J Med* 2000;343:522–529.
27. The Women's Health Initiative Study Group: Design of the Women's Health Initiative clinical trial and observational study. *Controlled Clin Trials* 1998;19:61–109.
28. Rossouw JE, Prentice RL, Manson JE, et al: Postmenopausal hormone therapy and risk of cardiovascular disease by age and years since menopause. *JAMA* 2007;297(13):1465–1477.
29. The Writing Group for the PEPI Trial: Effects of estrogen or estrogen/progestein regimens on heart disease risk factors in postmenopausal women: The Post-Menopausal Estrogen/Progestin Interventions (PEPI) Trial. *JAMA* 1995;273:199–208.
30. Karine L, Emmanuel O, Gregoire LG, SARAH Investigators: Differential effects of oral and transdermal postmenopausal estrogen replacement therapies on C-reactive protein. *Thromb Haemost* 2003;90:124–131.
31. Barrett-Connor E, Mosca L, Collins P, et al: Effects of raloxifene on cardiovascular events and breast cancer in postmenopausal women. *N Engl J Med* 2006;355:125–137.
32. Wenger NK: Lipid abnormalities recognition and management. *Women and Heart Disease*. 2nd ed. London and New York: Taylor and Francis Group, 2005 pp 53–63.
33. Miettinen TA, Pyorala K, Olsson EG, et al: Cholesterol-lowering therapy in women and elderly patients with myocardial infarction or angina pectoris. Findings from the Scandinavian Simvastatin Survival Study (4S). Scandinavian Simvastatin Study Group. *Circulation* 1997;96:4211–4218.
34. Lewis SJ, Sacks FM, Mitchell JS, et al:Effect of pravastatin on cardiovascular events in women after myocardial infarction: The Cholesterol and Recurrent Events (CARE) Trial. *J Am Coll Cardiol* 1998;32:140–146.
35. The Long-Term Intervention with Pravastatin in Ischemic Disease (LIPID) Study Group: Prevention of cardiovascular events and death with pravastatin in patients with coronary heart disease and broad range of initial cholesterol levels. *N Engl J Med* 1998;339:1349–1357.
36. Downs JR, Clearfield M, Weis S, et al: Primary prevention of acute coronary events with lovastatin in men and women with average cholesterol levels. Results of AFCAPS/TexCAPS. *JAMA* 1998;279:1615–1622.
37. Shepherd J, Blauw GJ, Murphy MB, et al: Pravastatin in elderly individuals at risk of vascular disease (PROSPER): a randomized controlled trial. *Lancet* 2002;360:1623–1630.
38. Heart Protection Study Collaborative Group: MRCBHP Heart Protection Study of cholesterol lowering with simvastatin in 20,536 high-risk individuals: a randomized placebo controlled trial. *Lancet* 2002;360:7–22.
39. The ALLHAT Officers and Coordinators for the ALLHAT Collaborative Research Group: Major outcomes in moderately hypercholesterolemic, hypertensive patients randomized to pravastatin vs usual care. The Antihypertensive and Lipid-Lowering Treatment to Prevent Heart Attack Trial (ALLHAT-LLT). *JAMA* 2002;288:2998–3007.
40. Athyros VG, Papageorgious AA, Mercouris BR, et al: Treatment with atorvastatin to the National Cholesterol Educational Program Gol versus "usual" care in secondary coronary heart disease prevention. The GREek Atorvastatin and Coronary-heart disease Evaluation (GREACE) Study. *Curr Med Res Opin* 2002; 18:220–228.
41. Sever PS, Daholf B, Poulter NR, et al: Prevention of coronary and stroke events with atorvastatin in hypertensive patients who have average or lower than average cholesterol concentrations, in the Anglo-Scandinavian Cardiac Outcomes Trial-Lipid Lowering Arm (ASCOT-LLA): a multicentre randomized controlled trial. *Lancet* 2003;361:1149–1158.
42. Wenger NK, Lewis SJ, Welty FK, et al: Effect of 80 mg versus 10 mg of atorvastatin in women and men with stable coronary heart disease. TNT Steering Committee and Investigators. *Circulation* 2005;112(suppl II):II-819.
43. Cannon CP, Braunwald E, McCabe C, et al: Intensive versus moderate lipid lowering with statins after acute coronary syndromes. Pravastatin or Atorvastatin Evaluation and Infection Therapy-Thrombolysis in Myocardial infarction 22 Investigators. *N Engl J Med* 2004;350:1495–1504.
44. Vaccarino V, Parsons L, Every NR, et al: Sex-based differences in early mortality after myocardial infarction. National Registry of Myocardial Infarction 2 Participants. *N Engl J Med* 1999; 341:217–225.
45. Yilmaz MB, Pinar M, Naharci I, et al: Being well-informed about statin is associated with continuous adherence and reaching targets. *Cardiovasc Drugs Ther* 2005;19:437–440.
46. Kronmal RA, Cain KC, Ye Z, et al: Total serum cholesterol levels and mortality risk as a function of age: a report based on the Framingham Data. *Arch Intern Med* 1993;153:1065–1073.
47. Krumholz HM, Seeman TE, Merrill SS, et al: Lack of association between cholesterol and coronary heart disease mortality and morbidity and all-cause mortality in persons older than 70 years. *JAMA* 1994;272:1335–1340.
48. Schatz IJ, Masaki K, Yano K, et al: Cholesterol and all-cause mortality in elderly people from the Honolulu Heart Program: a cohort study. *Lancet* 2001;358:351–355.
49. Benefante R, Reed D: Is elevated serum cholesterol level a risk factor for coronary heart disease in the elderly? *JAMA* 1990; 263:393–396.
50. Barrett-Connor E, Suarez L, Khaw K, et al: Ischemic heart disease risk factors after age 50. *J Chronic Dis* 1984;37:903–908.
51. Castelli WP, Wilson WF, Levy D: Cardiovascular risk factors in the elderly. *Am J Cardiol* 1989;63:12H–19H.
52. Rubin SM, Sidney S, Black DM, et al: High blood cholesterol in elderly men and the excess risk of coronary heart disease. *Ann Intern Med* 1990;113:916–920.
53. Lavie CJ, Milani RV: High-density lipoprotein cholesterol and coronary risk in the elderly. *Cardiol Elder* 1994;2:251–252.
54. Lavie CJ, Milani RV: Effects of cardiac rehabilitation programs in very elderly patients >75 years of age. *Am J Cardiol* 1996; 78:675–677.
55. Boardley D, Fahlman M, Topp R, et al: The impact of exercise training on blood lipids in older adults. *Am J Geriatr Cardiol* 2007;16:30–35.
56. Lavie CJ, Milani RV: Aerobic and resistance exercise training in the elderly. *Am J Geriatr Cardiol* 2007;16:36–37.
57. Lewis S: Statin therapy in the elderly: observational and randomized controlled trials support event reduction. *Am J Geriatr Cardiol* 2004;13:10–16.
58. Maycock CA, Muhlestein JB, Horne BD, et al: Statin therapy is associated with reduced mortality across all age groups of individuals with significant coronary disease, including very elderly patients. *J Am Coll Cardiol* 2002;40:1777–1785.
59. Lemaitre RN, Psaty BM, Heckbert SR, et al: Therapy with hydroxymethylglutaryl coenzyme a reductase inhibitors (statins) and associated risk of incident cardiovascular events in older adults. Evidence from the Cardiovascular Health Study. *Arch Intern Med* 2002;162:1395–1400.
60. Aronow WS, Ahn C: Incidence of new coronary events in older persons with prior myocardial infarction and serum low-density

lipoprotein cholesterol 125 mg/dl treated with statins versus no lipid-lowering drug. *Am J Cardiol* 2002;89:67–69.

61. Ray KK, Bach RG, Cannon CP, et al: Benefits of achieving the NCEP optional LDL cholesterol goal among elderly patients with ACS. PROVE-IT-TIMI 22 Investigators. *Eur Heart J* 2006;27: 2310–2316.
62. Raffel OC, White HD: Drug insight: statin use in the elderly. *Nat Clin Pract* 2006;3:318–328.
63. Baigent C, Keech A, Kearney PM, et al: Efficacy and safety of cholesterol-lowering treatment: prospective meta-analysis of data from 90,056 participants in 14 randomised trials of statins. *Lancet* 2005;366:1267–1278.
64. Brophy J, Brassard P, Bourgault C: The benefit of cholesterol-lowering medications after coronary revascularization: a population study. *Am Heart J* 2005;150:282–286.
65. Foody JM, Rathore SS, Galusha D, et al: Hydroxymethylglutaryl-CoA reductase inhibitors in older persons with acute myocardial infarction: evidence for an age-statin interaction. *J Am Geriatr Soc* 2006;5:421–430.
66. Schwartz GG, Olsson G, Ezekowitz MD, et al: Effect of atorvastatin on early recurrent ischemic events in acute coronary syndromes: The MIRACL Study: a randomized controlled trial. Myocardial Ischemia Reduction with Aggressive Cholesterol Lowering (MIRACL) Study Investigators. *JAMA* 2002;285: 1711–1718.
67. Wenger NK, Lewis SJ, Herrington DM, et al: Effect of 80 mg versus 10 mg of atorvastatin in patients 65 years of age or older with stable coronary heart disease. *Ann Intern Med* 2007;147:1–9.
68. de Lemos JA, Blazing MA, Wiviott SD, et al: Early intensive versus a delayed conservative simvastatin strategy in patients with acute coronary syndromes: phase Z of the A to Z Trial. *JAMA* 2004;292:1307–1316.
69. Milani RV: Lipid and statin effects on stroke and dementia. *Am J Geriat Cardiol* 2004;13(suppl 1):25–28.
70. Courville KA, Lavie CJ, Milani RV: Lipid-lowering therapy for elderly patients at risk for coronary events and stroke. *Am Heart Hosp J* 2005:3:256–262.
71. Prospective Studies Collaboration. Cholesterol, diastolic blood pressure, and stroke: 13,000 strokes in 450,000 people in 45 prospective cohorts: *Lancet* 1995;346:1647–1653.
72. Lewis SJ, Moye LA, Sacks FM, et al: Effect of pravastatin on cardiovascular events in older patients with myocardial infarction and cholesterol levels in the average range. Results of the Cholesterol and Recurrent Events (CARE) Trial. *Ann Intern Med* 1998;129:681–689.
73. Miettinen TA, Pyorala K, Olsson AG, et al: Cholesterol lowering therapy in women and elderly patients with myocardial infarction or angina pectoris: findings from the Scandinavian Simvastatin Survival Study (4S). *Circulation* 1997;96:4211–4218.
74. Waters DD, Schwartz GG, Olsson AG, et al: Effects of atorvastatin on stroke in patients with unstable angina or non-Q-wave myocardial infarction. A Myocardial Ischemia Reduction with Aggressive Cholesterol Lowering (MIRACL) substudy. *Circulation* 2002;106:1690–1695.
75. The Stroke Prevention by Aggressive Reduction in Cholesterol Levels (SPARCL) Investigators: High-dose atorvastatin after stroke or transient ischemic attack. *N Engl J Med* 2006;355: 549–559.
76. Lavie CJ, Milani RV: Optimal lipids, statins, dementia. *J Am Coll Cardiol* 2005;45:964–965.
77. Sparks DL, Sabbagh M, Connor D, et al: Statin therapy in Alzheimer's disease. *Acta Neurol Scand Suppl* 2006;185:78–86.
78. Bottorff MB: Statin safety: what to know. *Am J Geriatr Cardiol* 2004;13(suppl 1):34–38.
79. Jackevicius CA, Mamdani M, Tu JV: Adherence with statin therapy in elderly patients with and without acute coronary syndromes. *JAMA* 2002;288:462–467.
80. Benner JS, Glynn RJ, Mogun H, et al: Long-term persistence in use of statin therapy in elderly patients. *JAMA* 2002;288: 455–461.

CHAPTER 39

Special Patient Populations: Acute Coronary Syndromes

Gregory G. Schwartz

DEFINITION, SCOPE OF PROBLEM, AND RISK OF RECURRENT EVENTS

Acute coronary syndrome (ACS), which encompasses unstable angina and acute myocardial infarction (AMI), is diagnosed on the basis of rapidly accelerating symptoms of myocardial ischemia coupled with objective evidence of acute ischemia from the electrocardiogram and/or elevated serum markers of myocardial injury. ACS continues to present a major challenge to clinicians because of its frequency and because of the subsequent high risk of recurrent ischemic cardiovascular events. In the United States alone, there are approximately 1.5 million annual hospital admissions for ACS[1]; the incidence of ACS is similar in other Western countries and is increasing in developing countries.[2] Despite recent advances in medical and interventional therapies, patients continue to face a strikingly high risk of early recurrent ischemic events after ACS. For example, after presentation with a non–ST-segment elevation ACS, the 6-month risk of death or recurrent nonfatal AMI is approximately 10% and the risk of death, AMI, or recurrent unstable ischemia is approximately 20%.[3–6] A common misconception among patients and physicians is that risk returns to a low level after successful percutaneous coronary intervention or bypass of the "culprit" lesion(s) presumed responsible for an ACS event. In fact, recent large trials have shown that revascularization of the presumed culprit lesion in ACS prevented at best only about 20% of recurrent ischemic events and in some cases afforded no benefit[6,7]; in either case, it is clear that risk remains high in the period following ACS, particularly in the first few months.[5,6] This is not a surprising observation if one considers that although revascularization procedures relieve angina that is due to coronary obstruction, the coronary lesion responsible for a future AMI most often will not be the most severe stenosis found on antecedent angiography[8]; in fact, plaque rupture is more likely among a larger number of less obstructive lesions than among a smaller number of more obstructive lesions. Thus, preventive strategies, including lipid management, assume critical importance after ACS. This chapter reviews the evidence supporting early and intensive lipid-modifying therapy after ACS.

EFFECT OF RECENT ACUTE CORONARY SYNDROME ON LIPID AND LIPOPROTEIN MEASUREMENTS

To determine the relationship between plasma lipids and lipoproteins and prognosis after ACS and to guide a rational approach to therapy, lipids and lipoproteins would be measured ideally under steady-state metabolic conditions. However, ACS is often accompanied by an acute systemic inflammatory response, manifest by fever, leukocytosis, elevation of the erythrocyte sedimentation rate, and an alteration in the profile of plasma proteins known as the acute-phase response. Some acute-phase reactants, such as C-reactive protein (CRP), increase in concentration, while (HDL) lipoprotein high-density and low-density lipoprotein (LDL) decrease, resulting in a decrease in HDL cholesterol and LDL cholesterol levels. The time course of lipoprotein changes after ACS has been characterized and reviewed by Rosenson.[9] Levels may begin to decrease within 24 hours after an ACS event, particularly among patients with more extensive myocardial necrosis.[10,11] The levels reach a nadir at approximately 1 week, and then gradually recover. A metabolic steady-state is usually reattained by 1 month following ACS.[12,13] The most pronounced changes seen after ACS are decreased levels of LDL cholesterol, with smaller decrements in HDL cholesterol; conversely, triglyceride and lipoprotein(a) [Lp(a)] rise.[9,11] The magnitude of changes in lipoprotein concentration is variable and is related to the extent of myocardial necrosis, with the largest changes generally observed after extensive transmural myocardial infarction and smaller to insignificant changes after limited infarction or unstable angina.[9,11] After extensive myocardial infarction, it is not uncommon to observe a nadir in LDL cholesterol that is 30% or more below baseline (Fig. 39-1).[9] Concurrent drug therapy may also influence lipid measurements after ACS; for example, initiation of β-blocker therapy may contribute to a rise in triglycerides. The practical implication of acute-phase effects on lipids and lipoproteins is that accurate measurements are best made as soon as possible after presentation and/or several weeks later. Nonetheless, it is fair to say that if LDL cholesterol levels are higher than desirable during the acute-phase response following ACS, they will almost certainly be undesirably high during metabolic steady state.

DO LEVELS OF LIPOPROTEINS AND LIPIDS INFLUENCE LONG- AND SHORT-TERM PROGNOSIS AFTER ACUTE CORONARY SYNDROME?

Previous chapters contain reviews of the strong epidemiologic data linking elevated levels of atherogenic lipoproteins, particularly LDL, and reduced levels of protective lipoproteins, particularly HDL, to the initial development of coronary heart disease. Similarly, in patients with established, stable coronary heart disease (e.g., patients with stable angina pectoris, remote myocardial infarction, or prior coronary revascularization), substantial evidence from observational studies and placebo-controlled trials of statins indicates that long-term prognosis is adversely affected by an atherogenic pattern of plasma lipoproteins.[14–18] Relationships between high LDL cholesterol, low HDL cholesterol, and cardiovascular risk persist among patients treated with statins in randomized trials.[15,16]

Do analogous relationships exist between atherogenic lipoproteins and cardiovascular events in the early period following ACS, when risk is especially high? Relatively few analyses have addressed this question directly. Prior to the statin era, the question was not investigated, largely because of difficulty in interpreting lipoprotein measurements made early after ACS, when metabolism is not at steady state. In the statin era, natural history studies became more difficult because of the prevailing use of these drugs in patients with coronary heart disease. Some important insights were obtained in an analysis by Olsson et al.[19] of relationships between lipoproteins measured 1 to 4 days after ACS and 4-month cardiovascular outcomes in 3086 patients participating in a placebo-controlled trial of atorvastatin. Treatment with atorvastatin reduced both LDL cholesterol levels and short-term risk of major adverse cardiovascular events. Surprisingly, however, in multivariate analyses incorporating both treatment assignment and lipoproteins, there was no relationship between LDL cholesterol or apolipoprotein (apo) B levels and event rates: For example, for each 1-mg/dL increase in LDL cholesterol measured 1 to 4 days after ACS (prior to assignment to statin or placebo), the hazard ratio for an ischemic cardiovascular event was 1.000, i.e., a null relationship (Fig. 39-2). Further supporting the lack of relationship between LDL cholesterol and short-term prognosis after ACS, an analysis restricted to the placebo group, reflecting natural history, demonstrated a hazard ratio of 1.001 per 1-mg/dL increase in LDL cholesterol, that is, again almost a null relationship. One might speculate that the absence of a relationship between LDL cholesterol and short-term risk is the result of two counterbalancing

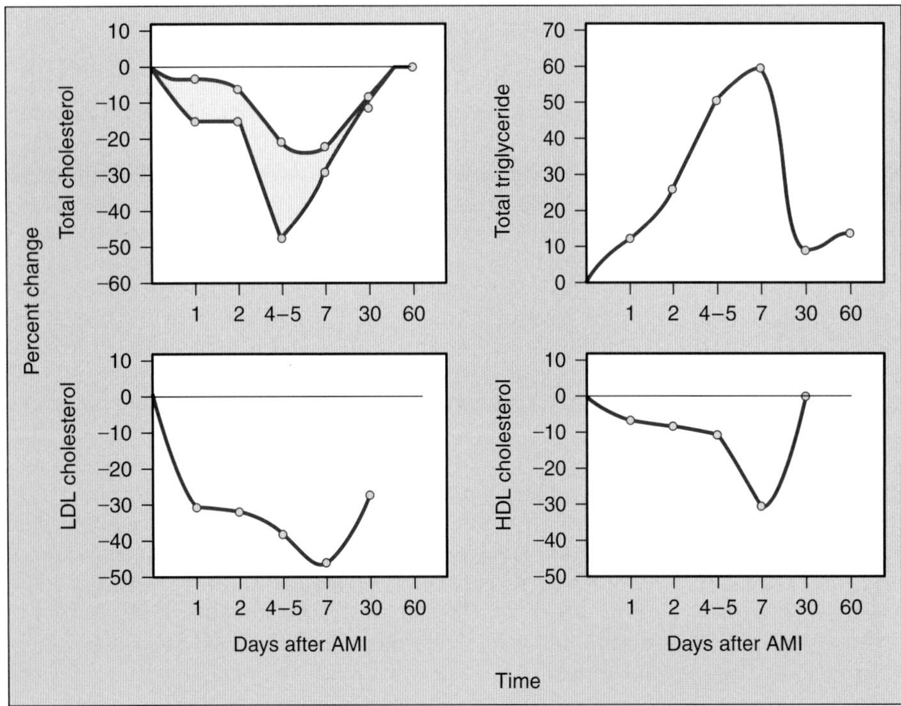

FIGURE 39-1 Effect of acute myocardial infarction on measurement of plasma lipids and lipoproteins. Time course of changes in cholesterol and triglycerides after completed acute myocardial infarction (AMI). For total cholesterol, the shaded region indicates the range of expected changes; for the other analytes, the graphs indicate the maximal expected changes after completed AMI. Total cholesterol and its subfractions begin to decline and triglycerides rise within the first day after AMI, with maximal changes occurring at approximately 1 week. Smaller changes in each analyte may occur after limited or aborted AMI LDL, low-density lipoprotein; HDL, high-density lipoprotein. (From Ref. 9, with permission.)

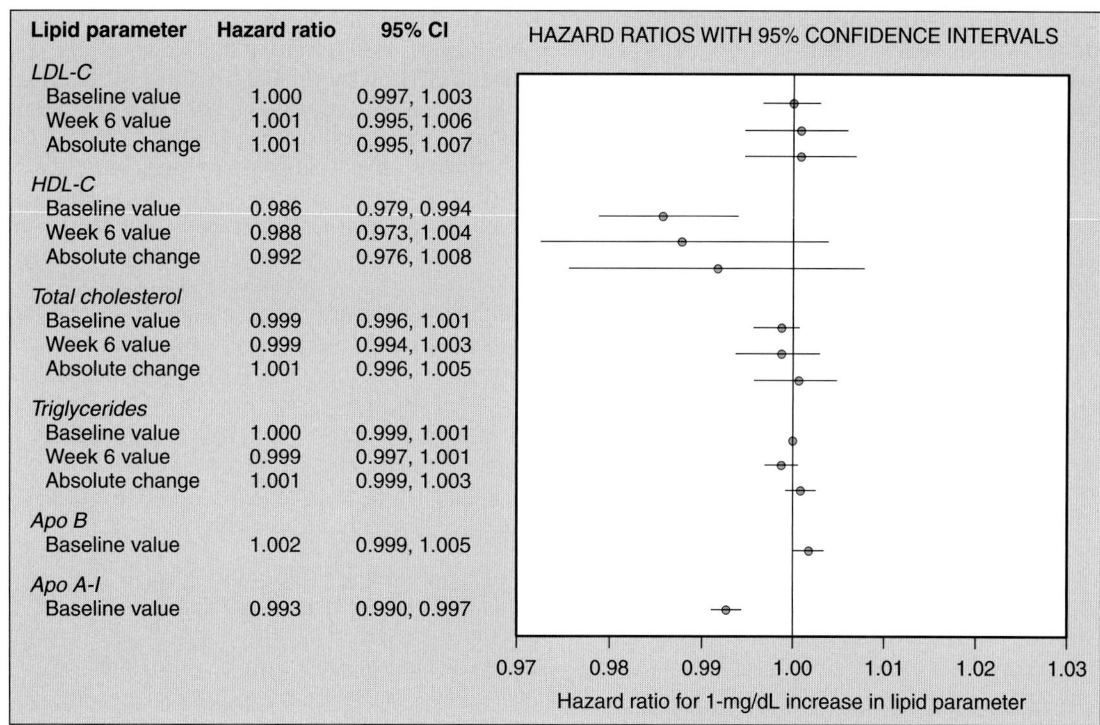

FIGURE 39-2 Relationship between risk of a recurrent cardiovascular event (death, myocardial infarction, cardiac arrest, or unstable angina) following acute coronary syndrome (ACS) and levels of lipids and lipoproteins. Data from the Myocardial Ischemia Reduction with Aggressive Cholesterol Lowering (MIRACL) trial that compared treatment with atorvastatin 80 mg/day or placebo for 16 weeks in 3086 patients with ACS. Each data point shows results of multivariate models that incorporated treatment assignment. Hazard ratios are expressed as the fractional change in risk per 1-mg/dL increase in the measured variable. Baseline refers to measurements before assignment to randomized treatment; week 6 refers to values obtained after 6 weeks of treatment with placebo or atorvastatin, and absolute change refers to the difference between week 6 and baseline values. There was no relationship between levels of total or low-density lipoprotein cholesterol (LDL-C), triglycerides, or apolipoprotein B, measured either at baseline or on assigned treatment, and short-term cardiovascular risk after ACS. In contrast, baseline levels of high-density lipoprotein cholesterol (HDL-C) and apolipoprotein A-I bore a significant inverse relationship to risk. (From Ref. 19, with permission.)

factors. On one hand, higher levels of LDL may be associated with increased risk through promotion of atherosclerosis, while on the other, lower levels of LDL may be associated with increased risk because patients with poorer prognosis because of larger infarcts have greater acute-phase depression of LDL. However, when Olsson et al. incorporated baseline troponin-I (as a surrogate for infarct size) in multivariate models relating lipoprotein levels to risk, there was still no evidence of a relationship between LDL measured shortly after ACS and short-term risk. In contrast to the neutral relationship of LDL cholesterol to short-term risk, higher concentrations of HDL cholesterol and/or apoA-I were favorably related to short-term prognosis after ACS. For every 1-mg/dL increment in HDL cholesterol, the 4-month risk of composite cardiovascular events declined by 1.4% (see Fig. 39-2). The strength of this relationship is comparable to that between HDL cholesterol and risk in long-term observational studies.[20] Similar findings were obtained in an observational analysis of 1032 patients with ACS who were treated with coronary stents.[21] In this cohort, the risk of major adverse cardiovascular events declined by 2.6% for every 1-mg/dL increase in HDL cholesterol measured during the index hospitalization, even after accounting for clinical covariates such as presence/absence of diabetes. These findings raise the question whether pharmacologic interventions to raise HDL cholesterol might reduce early risk after ACS.

EVIDENCE SUPPORTING EARLY AND INTENSIVE STATIN TREATMENT AFTER ACUTE CORONARY SYNDROME

Until recently, lipid-lowering drug therapy was viewed as a long-term strategy to reduce cardiovascular risk, rather than an intervention to be employed in the near-term management of patients after ACS. The conventional viewpoint was based on experimental and angiographic evidence that lipid lowering promotes gradual removal of lipid from atherosclerotic plaques, leading to gradual, modest regression of arterial stenoses. The conventional view was also based on landmark clinical trials that established the efficacy of statin treatment in reducing cardiovascular morbidity and mortality in patients with stable coronary heart disease. These landmark trials include the Scandinavian Simvastatin Survival Study (4S),[22] Cholesterol and Recurrent Events (CARE) study,[23] Long-Term Intervention with Pravastatin in Ischaemic Disease (LIPID) study,[24] and Heart Protection Study.[25] In each of these trials, patients with acute coronary syndrome within the preceding 3 to 6 months (i.e., within the highest-risk period) were excluded, and 1 to 2 years of statin treatment were required before a reduction in events could be discerned. The delayed benefit observed in initially stable patients led to an assumption that statin therapy would not produce early benefit in patients with recent ACS.

However, there are reasons to predict that statins could be beneficial in the early weeks and months after ACS. Delayed benefit of statin treatment in the landmark trials might reflect the fact that in a population of stable patients, a prolonged period of time is required to accrue a sufficient number of events that are modifiable by statin therapy. In contrast, in an ACS population, potentially modifiable events occur at a more rapid rate. Second, the landmark trials employed moderate-intensity statin treatment, such as pravastatin 40 mg daily or simvastatin 20 to 40 mg daily. It is possible that to achieve a benefit of statin therapy in the early period after ACS, high-intensity treatment is required (i.e., the highest doses and/or use of the most potent statins). Third, both experimental and clinical evidence indicate that statins have the potential to act rapidly to normalize the interface between bloodstream and vessel wall. Such effects may include anti-inflammatory actions, improvement in endothelial integrity and function, antithrombotic effects, and favorable plaque remodeling, and may not depend on concurrent reduction of LDL cholesterol.

Experimental Data Supporting Early Beneficial Effects of Statins

Anti-inflammatory effects of statins may be particularly important after ACS. While pathologic studies have shown that inflammatory infiltrates are prominent in the ruptured plaques responsible for ACS,[26] clinical studies have shown that heightened inflammation of coronary atheromas is not limited to an individual "culprit" lesion, but rather is widespread in the coronary arteries of patients with ACS. Such evidence includes studies that have detected elevated temperature of nonculprit coronary lesions by thermography[27] and abnormal activation of leukocytes in the coronary artery contralateral to the site of the culprit lesion in ACS[28] (Fig. 39-3). In addition, circulating levels of inflammatory markers, including but not limited to CRP, lipoprotein-associated phospholipase A_2 (Lp-PLA$_2$), soluble CD40 ligand (sCD40L) and intercellular adhesion molecule–1, are elevated after ACS and associated with adverse prognosis.[29–32] Statins exert rapid anti-inflammatory effects *in vitro*, and may act with similar rapidity *in vivo* after ACS. For example, in a study of 90 patients with ACS selected for high initial values of CRP,[33] treatment with atorvastatin 40 mg daily was associated with a mean decline in CRP of 43 mg/L by the time of hospital discharge (an average of 4 days after initiation of treatment), compared with a mean decline of 5 mg/L over the same period of time among patients treated with placebo.

Statins May Act Rapidly to Improve Vascular Endothelial Function

Atherosclerosis is associated with impaired coronary endothelial function, and this is particularly evident in patients with ACS.[34] Hyperlipidemia contributes to endothelial dysfunction by reducing expression and activity of nitric oxide synthase and by increasing catabolism of nitric oxide. Conversely, correction of hyperlipidemia with statins can partially restore endothelial function by up-regulating expression of endothelial nitric oxide synthase.[35] Moreover, statins promote mobilization of circulating endothelial progenitor cells that help to repair damaged endothelium.[36] Improvement in brachial artery endothelial function has been demonstrated in patients with ACS within 6 weeks of initiation of statin treatment[37] (Fig. 39-4). It has not been determined whether statin treatment affects coronary endothelial function with similar rapidity after ACS. The potential benefit of statins on endothelial function and mobilization of endothelial progenitor cells after ACS may be independent of a reduction of LDL cholesterol. Illustrating this point, Landmesser et al.[38] produced nearly identical reductions in LDL

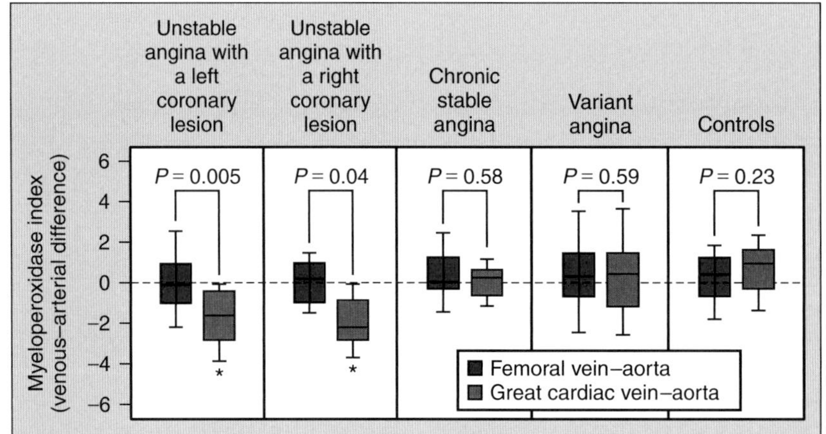

FIGURE 39-3 Evidence of widespread inflammation in the coronary circulation of patients with unstable coronary disease. Myeloperoxidase content of neutrophils was measured in blood from the aorta, femoral vein, and great cardiac vein (which drains the territory of the left coronary artery) in patients with unstable angina (n = 33), stable angina (n = 13), variant angina (n = 13), and normal controls (n = 6). Depletion of myeloperoxidase content across a vascular bed (indicated by negative values in the figure) is an indicator of neutrophil activation. Patients with unstable angina had greater transcoronary neutrophil activation than patients with stable angina, variant angina, or controls. As an internal control, there was no neutrophil myeloperoxidase gradient across the femoral circulation in any of the groups. When patients with unstable angina were subdivided into those with a left coronary and those with a right coronary culprit lesion, both subgroups demonstrated a similar myeloperoxidase gradient across the left coronary circulation. This finding suggests that vascular inflammation is widespread in the coronary circulation of patients with unstable angina, and not simply limited to the site of the culprit lesion for the acute event. (From Ref. 28, with permission.)

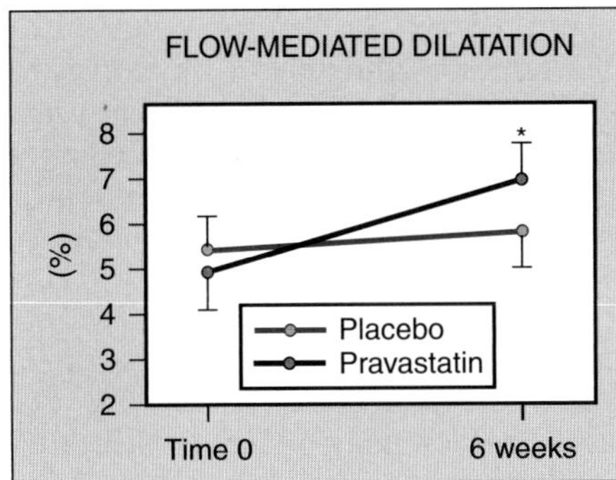

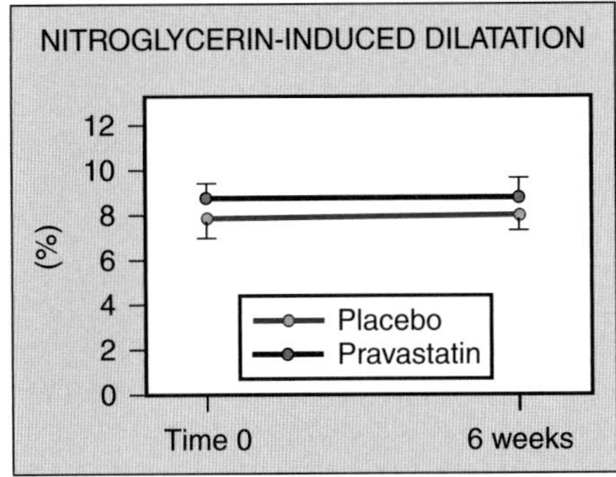

FIGURE 39-4 Six weeks of statin treatment improves endothelium-dependent, flow-mediated vasodilation in patients with acute coronary syndrome (ACS). Fifty-five patients with ACS were randomized prior to hospital discharge to receive treatment with pravastatin 40 mg daily or placebo for 6 weeks. Assessments of endothelium-dependent (flow-mediated) and endothelium-independent (nitroglycerin-induced) vasodilatation were made at baseline and at 6 weeks. Flow-mediated dilatation improved significantly (*) with statin treatment, indicating the potential for rapid improvement in peripheral arterial endothelial function after ACS. (From Ref. 37, with permission.)

cholesterol in two groups of patients with non-ischemic heart failure: One was treated with low-dose simvastatin and the other with ezetimibe. Radial artery endothelial function and the population of circulating endothelial progenitor cells increased in the statin group, but not in the ezetimibe group.

Statins may exert antithrombotic effects that are important after ACS. Thrombosis is involved in the pathogenesis of ACS. Hyperlipidemia promotes a prothrombotic state, and conversely, lipid-lowering may help to reverse a prothrombotic tendency. Hyperlipidemia may increase platelet activation by altering intracellular pH regulation,[39] may promote thrombosis through decreased production of nitric oxide by vascular endothelium, and may increase secretion of tissue factor by activated macrophages.[40] Conversely, treatment with a statin for 4 weeks has been shown to correct abnormal deposition of platelet thrombus on biological media,[41] the elaboration of tissue factor by activated macrophages,[42] and the production of thromboxane by platelets.[43] These *in vitro* observations occur in the absence of any changes in the lipid milieu. In sum, experimental data indicate rapid anti-inflammatory, endothelial-protectant, and anti-thrombotic effects of statins that might be clinically beneficial in the early period following ACS.

Recent data also indicate that lipid-regulating agents may promote rapid and favorable physical remodeling of atherosclerotic plaques after ACS, occurring within a much shorter time frame than previously thought possible from regression studies in animals and humans. Using intracoronary ultrasound, a reduction in plaque volume within 6 months of an ACS event was detected in 24 patients randomized to treatment with atorvastatin 20 mg daily, while plaque volume increased in 24 patients randomized to usual care[44] (Fig. 39-5). In the Reversal of Atherosclerosis with Aggressive Lipid Lowering (REVERSAL) trial in 500 patients with ACS, 18 months of high-intensity statin treatment with atorvastatin 80 mg daily resulted in slower progression of coronary atherosclerosis than moderate-intensity treatment with pravastatin 40 mg daily.[45] Similarly, two studies with intracoronary ultrasound have demonstrated favorable effects of HDL interventions on plaque morphology after ACS. A reduction in coronary plaque volume was detected within 5 weeks in ACS patients treated with infusions of recombinant apoA-I_{Milano}, compared with placebo infusions,[46] and favorable trends toward plaque regression after ACS were evident after four weekly infusions of reconstituted human HDL, compared with placebo.[47]

Observational Data Supporting Early Statin Treatment after Acute Coronary Syndrome

The clinical evidence supporting early statin therapy after ACS consists of observational analyses and randomized controlled trials. The former category generally supports a benefit of early statin therapy, but individual analyses vary widely in magnitude of estimated effect. A Swedish cohort of 20,000 patients who suffered first AMI was followed prospectively for 1 year. After adjusting for 42 covariates and a propensity score for statin use, prescription of a statin drug at hospital discharge was associated with a large reduction in 1-year mortality

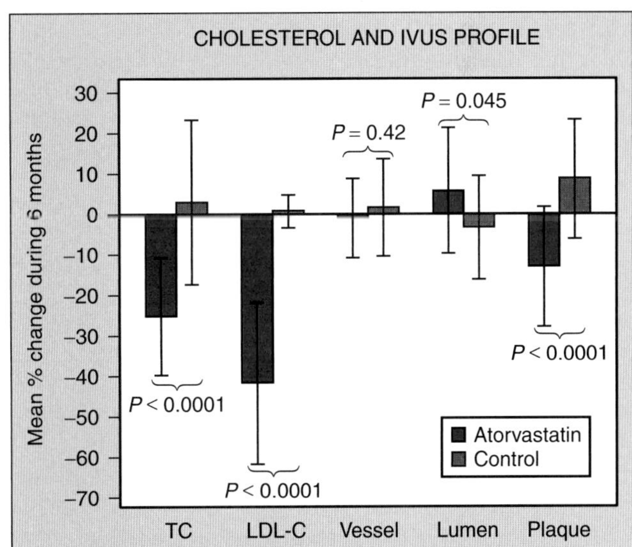

FIGURE 39-5 Improvement in plaque morphology with early statin treatment after acute coronary syndrome (ACS), as determined by intravascular ultrasound (IVUS). Forty-eight patients with ACS who underwent percutaneous coronary intervention were randomized to treatment with atorvastatin 20 mg daily or usual care for 6 months. Intravascular ultrasound examination was performed at baseline and at 6 months to determine the morphology of plaque at nonintervention sites in the culprit coronary artery. Compared with the control group at 6 months, lumen volume was greater and plaque volume was less in the atorvastatin group, indicating that statin treatment can produce rapid and favorable physical remodeling of coronary plaque after ACS. LDL-C, low-density lipoprotein cholesterol; TC, total cholesterol. (From Ref. 44, with permission.)

compared with discharge without statin treatment (relative risk, 0.75; $P = 0.001$).[48] Similar findings were obtained in a multivariate analysis of more than 20,000 patients with ACS enrolled in the Global Use of Streptokinase or t-PA for Occluded Coronary Arteries (GUSTO) IIb and Platelet Glycoprotein IIb/IIIa in Unstable Angina: Receptor Suppression Using Integrilin Therapy (PURSUIT) studies. Use of a lipid-lowering medication at hospital discharge was associated with an odds ratio of 0.67 ($P = 0.02$) for death at 6 months, compared with no lipid-lowering therapy.[49] In contrast, in an analysis of more than 12,000 patients with ACS in the Sirofiban versus Aspirin to Yield Maximum Protection from Ischemic Heart Events Post-Acute Coronary Syndromes (SYMPHONY) and second SYMPHONY trials, there was no apparent effect of early statin use on 1-year mortality (adjusted hazard ratio 0.99).[50]

Large databases have also been used to determine whether in-hospital initiation of statin treatment affects in-hospital outcomes. In an analysis of the National Registry of Myocardial Infarction,[51] data on in-hospital treatment and outcomes were collected in 17,000 patients who continued statin therapy they had received before index AMI hospitalization, 22,000 patients who initiated statin therapy within 24 hours of AMI hospitalization, and 126,000 patients who did not receive statin treatment. After adjustment for covariates and propensity scoring, the odds ratio for in-hospital mortality was 0.46 with continued statin therapy and 0.42 for newly started therapy, compared with no therapy. The Euro Heart Survey[52] compared outcomes in 1426 patients who received statins and survived the first 24 hours after ST elevation AMI with 6771 patients who did not receive statins and survived at least 24 hours. In multivariate analysis, 7-day mortality was significantly lower (hazard ratio, 0.34; 95% confidence interval 0.15–0.79) among treated patients. The Global Registry of Acute Coronary Events (GRACE)[53] examined outcomes in approximately 15,000 patients in 14 countries who were not treated with a statin prior to an index ACS event. Compared with patients who never received statin, in-hospital initiation of statin was associated with a relative risk of 0.87 for in-hospital death, reinfarction, or stroke. Thus, observational studies generally indicate benefit of early statin therapy after ACS, but provide varying estimates of the effect size. Because observational analyses are inherently limited by unaccounted differences between nonrandomized treatment groups, these analyses must be considered "hypothesis generating" and do not substitute for randomized, placebo-controlled trials to provide more conclusive testing of hypotheses.

Randomized Clinical Trials of Statins in Acute Coronary Syndrome

Six large randomized trials of statins in ACS have been conducted and are listed in Table 39-1. The Pravastatin Acute Coronary Treatment (PACT)[54] and the Prevention of Ischemic Events by Early Treatment with Cerivastatin (PRINCESS; unpublished, presented at European Society of Cardiology meeting in 2004) studies were terminated prematurely for administrative or regulatory reasons, and the Fluvastatin on Risk Diminishment after Acute Myocardial Infarction (FLORIDA) trial[55] was powered for a surrogate endpoint (ambulatory ischemia assessed by Holter monitor), rather than clinical events. As a result, these trials had inadequate power to detect differences in cardiovascular events between statin-treated and untreated patients.

Three other large trials provide the foundation for our current understanding of the role of statins after ACS. These are the Myocardial Ischemia Reduction with Aggressive Cholesterol Lowering (MIRACL),[56] A-to-Z,[13] and Pravastatin or Atorvastatin and Infection Therapy (PROVE IT) trials.[57] The MIRACL trial compared high-intensity statin treatment (atorvastatin 80 mg daily) with placebo for 4 months. PROVE IT compared two active treatments, high-intensity treatment with atorvastatin 80 mg daily and moderate-intensity treatment with pravastatin 40 mg, for 2 years. The A-to-Z trial had a two-phase design in which moderate-intensity statin treatment (simvastatin 40 mg daily) was first compared with placebo for 4 months, followed by transition of the two groups to high-intensity therapy (simvastatin 80 mg daily) or low-intensity therapy (simvastatin 20 mg daily), respectively, for a total treatment period of 2 years. The primary efficacy measure in each of these three trials was similar, but not identical, as indicated in Table 39-1. The trials also differed in the frequency of adjunctive coronary revascularization for the index ACS event. Such procedures were an exclusion criterion in MIRACL, and were performed in 44% and 69% of the patients in A-to-Z and PROVE IT, respectively. Another important difference between these trials is that MIRACL and A-to-Z excluded patients already treated with a statin at the time of the index ACS event, while 25% of the patients in PROVE IT fell into this category. None of the three trials imposed a lower limit on total or LDL cholesterol at baseline, and each had an upper limit of total cholesterol at randomization of 240 to 270 mg/dL.

In MIRACL, the 4-month composite efficacy measure of death, reinfarction, cardiac arrest, or recurrent unstable angina was reduced from 17.2% in the placebo group to 14.6% in the atorvastatin group ($P = 0.048$) (Figure 39-6A). Consistent benefit of atorvastatin 80 mg was observed in patients with metabolic syndrome[58] and in the elderly.[59] The most pronounced effects of atorvastatin 80 mg were on recurrent unstable angina (reduced by 26%) and stroke (reduced by 50% from 1.6% in the placebo group to 0.8% in the atorvastatin group, $P = 0.045$).[60] Although the confidence boundaries around this 50% reduction in stroke were wide, the 0.8% absolute reduction in stroke observed over 4 months with atorvastatin 80 mg in MIRACL compares favorably with a 1.9% absolute reduction in stroke observed over 5 years with atorvastatin 80 mg in the placebo-controlled Stroke Prevention by Aggressive Reduction in Cholesterol Levels (SPARCL) trial,[61] which included patients with prior stroke or transient ischemic attack. Overall, the MIRACL trial indicates that early and intensive statin therapy after ACS is an efficient as well as an effective intervention: The trial results lead to the estimate that 38 patients need to be treated for 4 months (a total of 13 patient-years of treatment) to prevent one death, reinfarction, or recurrence of unstable angina, and 125 patients need to be treated for 4 months (31 patient-years) to prevent one stroke.

TABLE 39-1 Major Randomized Controlled Trials of Statins after Acute Coronary Syndrome

Trial	Treatment A, Mean LDL Cholesterol	Treatment B, Mean LDL Cholesterol	Duration of Treatment	Patients Randomized, *n*	Primary Endpoint Definition	Results
MIRACL, 2001[56]	Placebo 135 mg/dL	Atorvastatin 80 mg 72 mg/dL	4 months	3086	Death, AMI, hospitalization for recurrent unstable myocardial ischemia, or cardiac arrest with resuscitation. Stroke was a secondary endpoint.	Atorvastatin reduced primary endpoint from 17.2% in placebo to 14.6% in atorvastatin group ($P = 0.048$). Strokes were reduced from 1.6 to 0.8% ($P = 0.045$).
FLORIDA, 2002[55]	Placebo 149 mg/dL	Fluvastatin 80 mg 103 mg/dL	1 year	540	Death, AMI, hospitalization for recurrent unstable myocardial ischemia, coronary revascularization, or ischemia on ambulatory ECG	No significant difference in primary endpoints. Major clinical events in 27.9% of placebo and 26.6% of fluvastatin groups
PROVE IT, 2004[57]	Pravastatin 40 mg 95 mg/dL	Atorvastatin 80 mg 62 mg/dL	2 years	4162	Death, AMI, hospitalization for recurrent unstable myocardial ischemia, coronary revascularization, or stroke	Fewer endpoints with atorvastatin (22.4%) than with pravastatin (26.3%, $P = 0.005$). Atorvastatin reduced death or AMI by 18% ($P = 0.06$)
A-to-Z, 2004[13]	Placebo 124 mg/dL* *followed by* simvastatin 20 mg 81 mg/dL*	Simvastatin 40 mg 62 mg/dL[a] *followed by* simvastatin 80 mg 66 mg/dL*	4 months 2 years	4496	Cardiovascular death, AMI, hospitalization for recurrent unstable myocardial ischemia, or stroke	No significant difference between groups. In the placebo-controlled phase (up to 4 months), primary endpoints occurred in 8.1% of placebo and 8.2% of simvastatin-treated patients. At 2 years, events occurred in 16.7% of the placebo → simvastatin 20 mg group and 14.4% of the simvastatin 40 mg → simvastatin 80 mg group ($P = 0.14$).
PACT, 2004[54]	Placebo On-treatment LDL cholesterol not measured	Pravastatin 20–40 mg On-treatment LDL cholesterol not measured	1 month	3408	Death, AMI, or hospitalization for recurrent unstable myocardial ischemia	No significant difference in primary endpoints, which occurred in 12.4% of placebo and 11.6% of pravastatin-treated patients.
PRINCESS, presented at European Society of Cardiology, 2004	Placebo 139 mg/dL	Cerivastatin 0.4 mg 97 mg/dL	3 months†	3605	Cardiovascular death, AMI, hospitalization for recurrent unstable myocardial ischemia or CHF, or stroke	No significant difference between groups. At 3 months, primary endpoints occurred in ~13.2% of placebo and ~11.8% of cerivastatin groups.

*Median values.

†Study was designed with a subsequent 18-month period in which both groups were to be treated with cerivastatin 0.4–0.8 mg/day. However, this was not accomplished due to early termination of study.

AMI, acute myocardial infarction; CHF, congestive heart failure; ECG, electrocardiogram.

Reprinted from Ref. 83, with permission

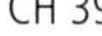

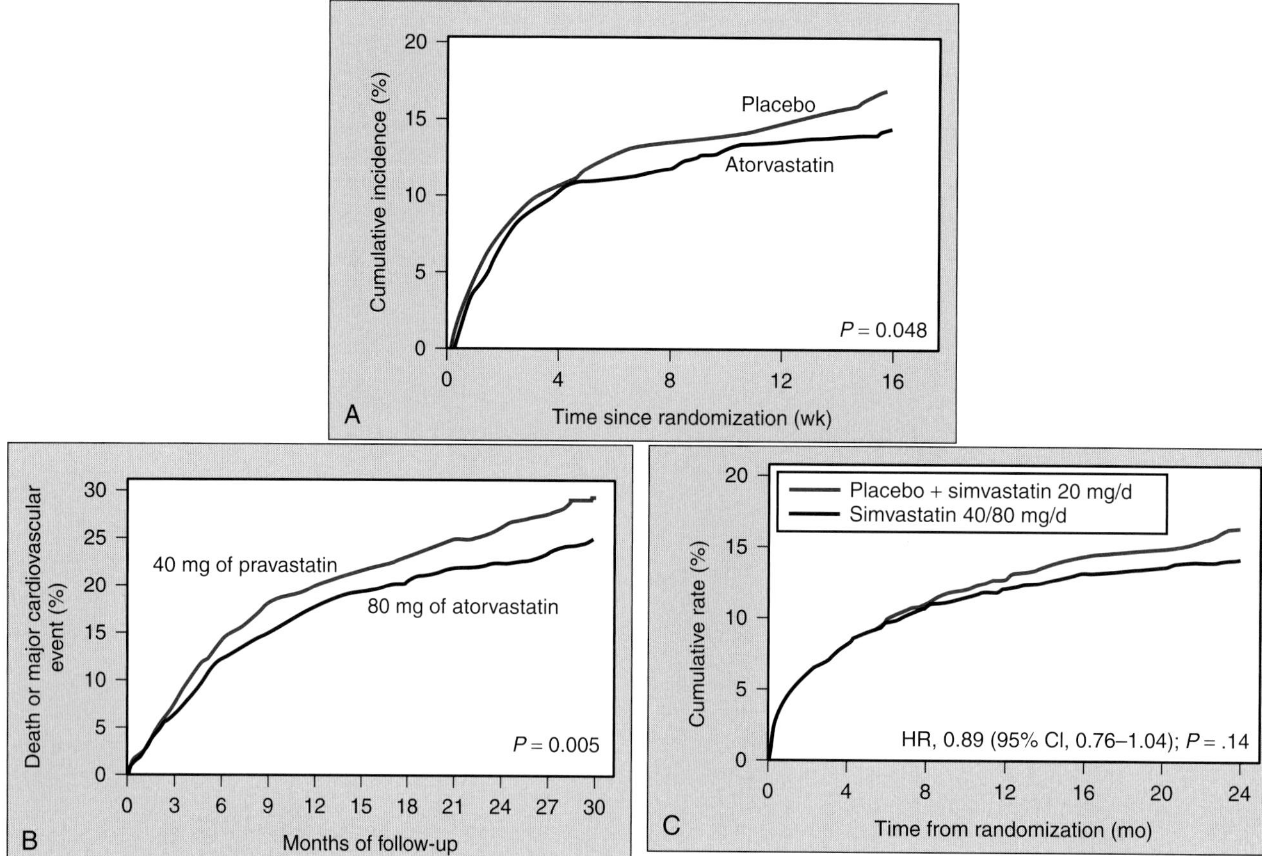

FIGURE 39-6 Key randomized trials that investigated the efficacy of early statin treatment after acute coronary syndrome (ACS). ***(A)*** The Myocardial Ischemia Reduction with Aggressive Cholesterol Lowering trial compared treatment with atorvastatin 80 mg daily versus placebo for 16 weeks in 3086 patients with ACS. The primary outcome measure, a composite of death, reinfarction, cardiac arrest, or recurrent unstable angina, was reduced from 17.4% in the placebo group to 14.6% in the atorvastatin group. Thus, this trial demonstrated that early, intensive statin treatment improves short-term clinical outcomes after ACS. ***(B)*** The Pravastatin or Atorvastatin Evaluation and Infection Therapy (PROVE IT) trial compared high-intensity treatment with atorvastatin 80 mg with moderate-intensity treatment with pravastatin 40 mg for 2 years in 4162 patients with ACS. The primary efficacy measure, a composite of death, reinfarction, stroke, recurrent unstable angina, and unanticipated myocardial revascularization, was reduced from 26.3% in the pravastatin group to 22.4% in the atorvastatin group. Thus, this trial demonstrated the superiority of high-intensity statin treatment over moderate-intensity statin treatment in the period following ACS. ***(C)*** The A-to-Z trial compared immediate moderate- to high-intensity treatment with simvastatin (40 mg daily for 4 months, 80 mg daily thereafter) with delayed, low-intensity treatment (placebo for 4 months, simvastatin 20 mg daily thereafter) for a total treatment period of up to 2 years in 4497 patients with ACS. The primary efficacy measure, a composite of death, reinfarction, stroke, or recurrent ACS, was nonsignificantly improved in the moderate- to high-intensity treatment group. However, a post hoc comparison of events occurring from 4 months to the end of the study (i.e., comparing simvastatin 80 mg to simvastatin 20 mg daily) showed improved outcomes in the high-intensity arm. Thus, the results of the A-to-Z trial also support early intensive statin treatment after ACS. (From Refs. 13, 56, and 57, with permission.)

In PROVE IT, the composite endpoint of death, reinfarction, stroke, recurrent unstable angina, or unanticipated coronary revascularization was reduced from 26.3% in the pravastatin 40 mg group to 22.4% in the atorvastatin 80 mg group at 2 years (p=0.005) (Fig. 39-6, Panel B). The difference in event rates between groups became statistically significant at 6 months. Thus, MIRACL demonstrated superiority of high-intensity statin treatment over placebo in a 4-month period following ACS, whereas PROVE IT demonstrated superiority of high-intensity statin treatment over moderate-intensity statin treatment over a 2-year period following ACS.

In contrast, the results of A-to-Z suggest that moderate-intensity treatment provides little or no benefit compared with placebo during the early period after ACS. During the 4-month placebo-controlled phase of A-to-Z, event rates were 8.2% in the simvastatin 40 mg group and 8.1% in the placebo group (Figure 39-6C). However, in the active comparator phase of A-to-Z, high-intensity statin treatment provided greater benefit than moderate-intensity treatment. Treatment with simvastatin 80 mg from 4 months to 2 years resulted in significantly fewer events compared with treatment with simvastatin 20 mg over this period of time.[13] Thus, A-to-Z also supports the efficacy of high-intensity statin treatment after ACS.

Is greater reduction in LDL cholesterol the mechanism by which intensive statin treatment reduces early recurrent events after ACS? Unfortunately, data from the three key randomized trials do not support such a simple explanation. In fact, at 4 months of randomized treatment in the A-to-Z trial, average LDL cholesterol concentration was 62 mg/dL in the simvastatin 40 mg group and 124 mg/dL in the placebo group, while at the same time point in the MIRACL trial, LDL cholesterol averaged 72 mg/dL in the atorvastatin 80 mg group and 135 mg/dL in the placebo group. Thus, the difference in LDL cholesterol between active treatment and placebo groups was nearly identical in both trials (62–63 mg/dL), but atorvastatin at 80 mg reduced clinical events in MIRACL while simvastatin 40 mg did not in A-to-Z. Moreover, analysis of MIRACL did not demonstrate a relationship between LDL cholesterol concentration during randomized treatment and risk of an ischemic event.[19] Thus, it appears that factors other than LDL cholesterol reduction determine whether statin therapy is beneficial in the early period after ACS.

There is evidence to suggest that anti-inflammatory effects of intensive statin treatment may be related to early clinical benefit after ACS. For example, treatment with atorvastatin, compared with placebo, was also associated with 35% lower CRP levels 4 months after ACS.[62] Similarly, CRP was reduced to a greater extent with atorvastatin 80 mg than with pravastatin 40 mg in the PROVE IT trial.[57] Other biomarkers also suggest that early anti-inflammatory effects of statins are important. Patients in the MIRACL trial with an initial plasma concentration of sCD40L above the 90th percentile of the study population who were assigned to placebo had significantly higher risk of a subsequent ischemic event, compared with patients with sCD40L concentrations at or below the 90th percentile assigned to placebo. However, the increased risk associated with high initial sCD40L was completely abrogated by atorvastatin treatment[63] (Fig. 39-7). In the PROVE IT trial, elevated levels of Lp-PLA$_2$ after 30 days of statin treatment following ACS were associated with poor prognosis, independent of LDL cholesterol and CRP levels. High-intensity treatment with atorvastatin 80 mg reduced Lp-PLA$_2$ to a greater extent than moderate-intensity treatment with pravastatin 40 mg daily.[30] Another potentially beneficial anti-inflammatory effect of early statin treatment after ACS involves mobilization and clearance of oxidized LDL,[64] as discussed in detail in Chapter 8.

In longer-term follow-up after ACS (i.e., 2 years), both reduction of LDL cholesterol and suppression of inflammation contribute to the benefit of statin therapy. An important conclusion from the PROVE IT trial was that achievement of LDL cholesterol less than 70 mg/dL and CRP less than 2 mg/L were independently related to a favorable prognosis.[65] Moreover, there did not appear to be a lower threshold for benefit with either analyte. Among patients in the atorvastatin 80 mg arm of the trial, there was a graded relationship between ranges of achieved LDL cholesterol (<40, 40–60, 60–80, and 80–100 mg/dL) and prognosis, with best prognosis among those with LDL cholesterol below 40 mg/dL[66] (Fig. 39-8). Similarly, patients who achieved CRP levels lower than 1 mg/L appeared to have a better prognosis than those who achieved levels lower than 2 mg/L.[65]

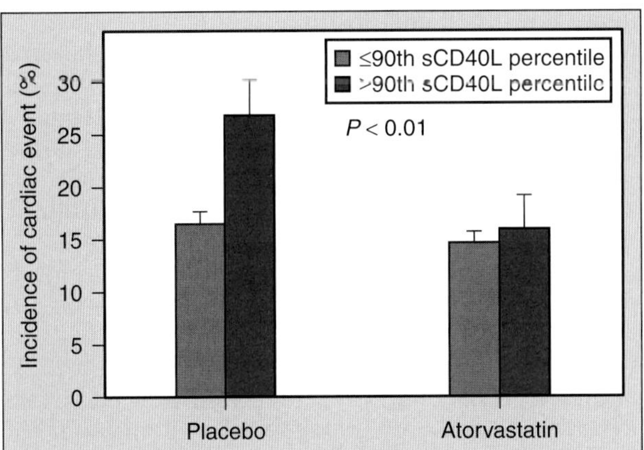

FIGURE 39-7 High concentrations of soluble CD40 ligand (sCD40L) predict short-term risk after acute coronary syndrome (ACS) and risk reduction with high-dose atorvastatin. The 16-week risk of an ischemic endpoint event in the Myocardial Ischemia Reduction with Aggressive Cholesterol Lowering (MIRACL) trial is plotted for initial levels of sCD40L dichotomized at the 90th percentile of the study population. Levels of sCD40L higher than the 90th percentile were associated with increased risk in the placebo group, but this risk was abrogated in the atorvastatin group. These data indicate that a highly proinflammatory state, as marked by sCD40L, identifies a group of high-risk patients who are likely to benefit from early intensive statin treatment after ACS. (From Ref. 63, with permission.)

SHOULD C-REACTIVE PROTEIN OR OTHER INFLAMMATORY MARKERS BE TARGETS OF THERAPY AFTER ACUTE CORONARY SYNDROME, IN ADDITION TO LOW-DENSITY LIPOPROTEIN CHOLESTEROL?

The role of inflammation in the pathogenesis of atherosclerosis, the relationship between risk after ACS and elevated levels of inflammatory markers such as CRP, and the effect of statins to lower CRP lead to the question of whether CRP (or other inflammatory biomarkers) should be primary targets of therapy in patients with ACS. Current data do not support such an approach, at least in regard to CRP. The conventional paradigm is that inflammation in the arterial wall leads to release of nanogram per liter quantities of inflammatory cytokines such as interleukins, which act on the liver to stimulate synthesis and release of milligram per liter quantities of CRP. Thus, the liver amplifies inflammatory stimuli from sites such as the vasculature, which are then reflected by circulating CRP concentrations. While this paradigm may explain the relation between atherosclerosis and elevated levels of CRP, the reduction of CRP with statin therapy may not necessarily reflect suppression of vascular inflammation. This is because statins exert direct effects on the liver to suppress CRP expression[67,68] (Fig. 39-9). Therefore, it is possible that reduction in CRP with statin

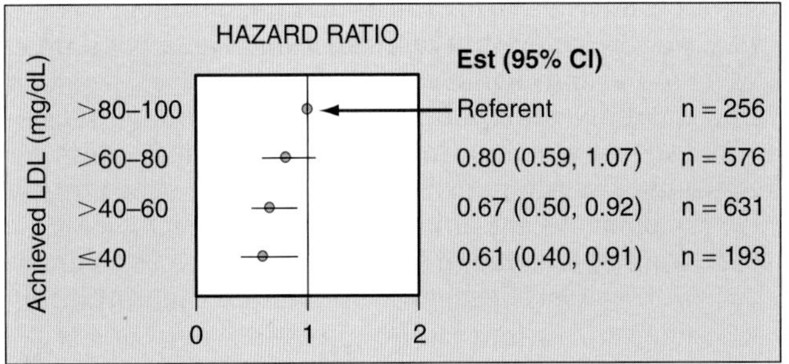

FIGURE 39-8 Relation between achieved low-density lipoprotein (LDL) cholesterol levels and clinical outcomes among patients treated with atorvastatin 80 mg daily in the PROVE IT trial. Hazard ratio of the primary endpoint (composite of death, myocardial infarction, stroke, unstable angina, or unanticipated revascularization) stratified by achieved LDL cholesterol. Data are adjusted for age, gender, baseline calculated LDL cholesterol, diabetes mellitus, and prior myocardial infarction. The r eferent group is patients with on-treatment LDL cholesterol 80 to 100 mg/dL. These data suggest that prognosis after ACS is inversely related to LDL cholesterol levels achieved on statin treatment, without a discernible lower limit of this relation. (From Ref. 66, with permission.)

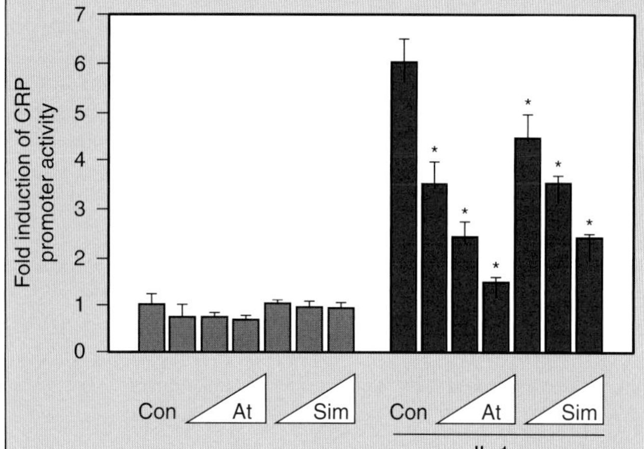

FIGURE 39-9 Statins act directly on liver to reduce C-reactive protein gene expression. Data show the activity of the promoter of C-reactive protein (CRP) in human hepatoma cells in culture, using a luciferase reporter gene. The reference value is the activity of the promoter without stimulation of the cells with interleukin-1α and without statin treatment. Under unstimulated conditions (left side of graph), neither atorvastatin nor simvastatin affect CRP promoter activity. With interleukin-1α stimulation (right side of graph), CRP promoter activity increases dramatically, but this response is suppressed in a dose-dependent fashion by exposure to atorvastatin or simvastatin at clinically relevant concentrations (1, 3, and 10 μM). These findings demonstrate that statins have the potential to act directly on liver to suppress CRP production. A potential implication is that a reduction in CRP observed in patients with ACS treated with statin may not necessarily reflect anti-inflammatory effects in the vasculature or other extrahepatic sites, but rather an effect in the liver. (From Ref. 67, with permission.)

therapy primarily reflects suppression of hepatic CRP production, rather than attenuation of vascular inflammation. On the other hand, CRP may play a direct role in atherothrombosis, in which case its suppression by statins may be beneficial irrespective of whether the primary effect is exerted in vessel wall or in liver. For example, immunohistologic and *in vitro* experimental studies demonstrate localization of CRP in atherosclerotic plaque and show that CRP exerts a variety of toxic effects on endothelial and vascular smooth muscle cells that would be expected to promote the atherosclerotic process.[69] In sum, CRP has been validated as a risk marker after ACS, but not yet as a primary target of therapy.

SAFETY OF INTENSIVE STATIN THERAPY

To this point, this chapter has focused on the efficacy of intensive statin treatment after ACS. However, any therapeutic decision must be based on a favorable balance between efficacy and safety. Serious adverse effects, particularly rhabdomyolysis, can occur with any statin drug at any dosage. However, atorvastatin 80 mg has proven to be remarkably safe in large clinical trials. In the combined atorvastatin 80 mg arms of the MIRACL, PROVE IT, Treating to New Targets (TNT),[70] Incremental Decrease in End Points through Aggressive Lipid Lowering (IDEAL),[71] and SPARCL trials, there were a total of six cases of rhabdomyolysis in 59,000 patient-years of assigned treatment, an incidence no higher than observed with placebo. In the A-to-Z trial, there were nine patients treated with simvastatin 80 mg daily who developed creatine kinase more than 10 times the upper limit of normal in association with muscle symptoms.[13] However, there are no head-to-head data to support the conclusion that atorvastatin 80 mg daily is safer than simvastatin 80 mg daily. While the vast majority of patients with ACS can be treated safely with high-dose statins, it is important to recognize factors that increase the risk of statin-induced rhabdomyolysis, including advanced age, renal or hepatic dysfunction, hypothyroidism, and small body mass, and to individualize treatment accordingly.

TRANSLATING CLINICAL TRIALS TO CLINICAL PRACTICE

Based in part on the data from MIRACL and PROVE IT, the National Cholesterol Education Program recommended an optional target for LDL cholesterol of less than 70 mg/dL in patients considered at very high risk for cardiovascular events, including those with recent ACS.[72] On the surface, this recommendation appears to be consistent with the findings of the clinical trials in which LDL cholesterol averaged 62 to 72 mg/dL in the atorvastatin 80 mg arms. However, it is important to recognize that the trials demonstrating efficacy of early, intensive statin therapy did not titrate dosage to achieve a specific LDL cholesterol target, but rather treated all assigned patients with the same dosage. Second, the PROVE IT trial found progressively lower risk with progressively lower achieved LDL cholesterol levels in the atorvastatin 80 mg arm, extending even to those patients with LDL cholesterol level less than 40 mg/dL. Therefore, it would appear to be illogical to attenuate the intensity of therapy to achieve an LDL cholesterol level of 70 mg/dL when a higher statin dosage might drive LDL even lower. Third, it is important to recognize that many patients with ACS present with relatively low levels of LDL cholesterol prior to treatment. For example, at steady state in the placebo group of A-to-Z, a quarter of patients had LDL cholesterol lower than 105 mg/dL.[13] Many of these patients could achieve an LDL cholesterol level of less than 70 mg/dL with lower doses of statins than those that have been proven to be effective in clinical trials, resulting in treatment that is not fully evidence based. Thus, given the data supporting both efficacy and safety of high-intensity statin treatment after ACS, at least with atorvastatin, it would be reasonable to apply this strategy of initiation of high-dose statin therapy to the majority of patients presenting with ACS, rather than titrating the intensity of statin treatment to achieve an LDL level of ~70 mg/dL.

WITHDRAWAL OF STATIN THERAPY

This and preceding chapters of this book have catalogued the strong evidence supporting the efficacy of statins in reducing cardiovascular risk. However, it is important to consider the potential consequences of withdrawal of statin therapy, which occurs commonly when patients are hospitalized for acute illness or when there is nonadherence to prescribed treatment. Is there a rebound increase in cardiovascular risk associated with statin withdrawal?

Experimental data suggest that this could be the case. Within a few days after stopping chronic statin therapy, flow-mediated arterial dilatation, platelet aggregability, and plasma levels of risk markers such as sCD40L interleukin-6 (IL-6), and CRP return to pre-treatment levels.[73–77] In some studies, cessation of statin therapy has led to rebound overshoot activation of G-proteins Rho and Rac, causing oxidative stress and suppression of nitric oxide bioavailability.[78,79]

Although in patients with stable coronary heart disease there was no observed increase in the incidence of ACS when chronic statin therapy was withdrawn for a period of 6 weeks,[80] in patients with ACS there is some evidence that interruption of chronic statin therapy could pose a clinically relevant risk. In an analysis of the National Registry of Myocardial Infarction,[51] 35% of patients on chronic statin therapy had treatment withdrawn during the first 24 hours of hospitalization for AMI. In multivariate analysis, these patients were at substantially higher risk for in-hospital complications, including death, compared with patients who continued to be treated with statins. In an analysis of the Platelet Receptor Inhibition in Ischemic Syndrome Management (PRISM) trial,[81,82] discontinuation of prior statin treatment at the time of hospitalization for ACS was associated with increased risk of death or reinfarction at 7 and 30 days ($P = 0.03$ and $P = 0.06$, respectively), compared with patients who continued statin treatment. Analysis of the GRACE registry[53] revealed discontinuation of prior statin treatment during hospitalization for ACS resulted in a risk of death, reinfarction, or stroke similar to that in patients who were never treated with statin, and greater than those who continued statin treatment in hospital. The practical message from these analyses is that whenever possible, statin therapy should not be interrupted in patients hospitalized for ACS. It remains to be determined whether initiation or interruption of statin therapy affects outcomes of patients hospitalized with other acute medical or surgical illnesses.

FUTURE DIRECTIONS

Despite the efficacy of early, intensive statin therapy, most of the residual risk after ACS persists despite this intervention. For example, in the PROVE IT trial, even though the majority of patients received percutaneous coronary revascularization for the index ACS event, thienopyridine antiplatelet agents, and other contemporary evidence-based treatments, patients in the atorvastatin 80 mg arm had a 2-year incidence of death, reinfarction, stroke, recurrent unstable angina, or unanticipated coronary revascularization of 22.4%. Thus, there is a pressing need to develop and validate additional strategies to reduce risk after ACS, including those that favorably modify lipoproteins. Potential approaches include raising HDL cholesterol with cholesteryl ester transport inhibitors or compounds that mimic the structure and function of apoA-I, adding a cholesterol absorption inhibitor to optimal use of statins, activating peroxisome proliferator–activated receptors, or antagonizing endocannabinoid receptors. Clinicians, investigators, and patients will eagerly await the outcomes of trials to test these approaches.

Acknowledgment

Supported by the Medical Research Service of the U.S. Department of Veterans Affairs.

REFERENCES

1. American Heart Association: 2002 Heart and Stroke Statistical Update. Dallas, TX: American Heart Association, 2002.
2. Abdallah MH, Arnaout S, Karrowni W, Dakik HA: The management of acute myocardial infarction in developing countries. *Int J Cardiol* 2006;111:189–94.
3. The Platelet Receptor Inhibition in Ischemic Syndrome Management in Patients Limited by Unstable Signs and Symptoms (PRISM-PLUS) Study Investigators: Inhibition of the platelet glycoprotein IIb/IIIa receptor with tirofiban in unstable angina and non-Q wave myocardial infarction. *N Engl J Med* 1998;338:1488–1497.
4. The Clopidogrel in Unstable Angina to Prevent Recurrent Events Trial Investigators: Effects of clopidogrel in addition to aspirin in patients with acute coronary syndromes without ST-segment elevation. *N Engl J Med* 2001;345:494–502.
5. Fragmin and Fast Revascularisation during Instability in Coronary Artery Disease (FRISC II) Investigators: Invasive compared with noninvasive treatment in unstable coronary-artery disease: FRISC II prospective randomised multicentre study. *Lancet* 1999;354:708–715.
6. Cannon CP, Weintraub WS, Demopoulos LA, et al: Comparison of early invasive and conservative strategies in patients with unstable coronary syndromes treated with the glycoprotein IIb/IIIa inhibitor tirofiban. *N Engl J Med* 2001;344:1879–1887.
7. de Winter RJ, Windhausen F, Cornel JH, et al: Early invasive versus selectively invasive management for acute coronary syndromes. *N Engl J Med* 2005;353:1095–1104.
8. Giroud D, Li JM, Urban P, et al: Relation of the site of acute myocardial infarction to the most severe coronary arterial stenosis at prior angiography. *Am J Cardiol* 1992;69:729–732.
9. Rosenson RS: Myocardial injury: the acute phase response and lipoprotein metabolism. *J Am Coll Cardiol* 1993;22:933–940.
10. Fresco C, Maggione AP, Signorini S, et al: Variations in lipoprotein levels after myocardial infarction and unstable angina: The LATIN trial. *Ital Heart J* 2002;3:587–592.
11. Henkin Y, Crystal E, Goldberg Y, et al: Usefulness of lipoprotein changes during acute coronary syndromes for predicting post-discharge lipoprotein levels. *Am J Cardiol* 2002;89:7–11.
12. Shephard MDS, Hester J, Walmsley RN, White GH: Variation in plasma apolipoprotein A-I and B concentrations following myocardial infarction. *Ann Clin Biochem* 1990;27:9–14.
13. de Lemos JA, Blazing MA, Wiviott SD, et al: Early intensive vs a delayed conservative simvastatin strategy in patients with acute coronary syndromes: phase Z of the A to Z trial. *JAMA* 2004;292:1307–1316.
14. Wong ND, Wilson PW, Kannel WB: Serum cholesterol as a prognostic factor after myocardial infarction: The Framingham study. *Ann Intern Med* 1991;115:687–693.
15. Simes RJ, Marschner IC, Hunt D, et al: Relationship between lipid levels and clinical outcomes in the Long-term Intervention with Pravastatin in Ischemic Disease (LIPID) trial: to what extent is the reduction in coronary events with pravastatin explained by on-study lipid levels? *Circulation* 2002;105:1162–1169.
16. Baigent C, Keech A, Kearney PM, et al: Efficacy and safety of cholesterol-lowering treatment: prospective meta-analysis of data from 90,056 participants in 14 randomised trials of statins. *Lancet* 2005;366:1267–1278.
17. Berge KG, Canner PL, Hainline A Jr: High-density lipoprotein cholesterol and prognosis after myocardial infarction. *Circulation* 1982;66:1176–1178.
18. Goldbourt U, Cohen L, Neufeld HN: High-density lipoprotein cholesterol: prognosis after myocardial infarction. The Israeli Ischemic Heart Disease Study. *Int J Epidemiol* 1986;15:51–55.
19. Olsson AG, Schwartz GG, Szarek M, et al: High-density lipoprotein, but not low-density lipoprotein cholesterol levels influence short-term prognosis after acute coronary syndrome: results from the MIRACL trial. *Eur Heart J* 2005;26:890–896.
20. Gordon T, Castelli WP, Hjortland MC, et al: High-density lipoprotein as a protective factor against coronary heart disease. The Framingham Study. *Am J Med* 1977;62:707–714.

21. Wolfram RM, Brewer HB, Xue Z, et al: Impact of low high-density lipoproteins on in-hospital events and one-year clinical outcomes in patients with non–ST-elevation myocardial infarction acute coronary syndrome treated with drug-eluting stent implantation. *Am J Cardiol* 2006;98:711–717.
22. Scandinavian Simvastatin Survival Study Group: Randomised trial of cholesterol lowering in 4444 patients with coronary heart disease: The Scandinavian Simvastatin Survival Study. *Lancet* 1994;344:1383–1389.
23. Sacks FM, Pfeffer MA, Moye LA, et al: The effect of pravastatin on coronary events after myocardial infarction in patients with average cholesterol levels. *N Engl J Med* 1996;335:1001–1009.
24. Long-Term Intervention with Pravastatin in Ischemic Disease (LIPID) Study Group: Prevention of cardiovascular events and death with pravastatin in patients with coronary heart disease and a broad range of initial cholesterol levels. *N Engl J Med* 1998;339:1349–1357.
25. Heart Protection Study Collaborative Group: MRC/BHF Heart Protection Study of cholesterol lowering with simvastatin in 20,536 high-risk individuals: a randomized placebo-controlled trial. *Lancet* 2002;360:7–22.
26. Moreno PR, Falk E, Palacios IF, et al: Macrophage infiltration in acute coronary syndromes. Implications for plaque rupture. *Circulation* 1994;90:775–778.
27. Toutouzas K, Drakopoulou M, Mitropoulos J, et al: Elevated plaque temperature in non-culprit *de novo* atheromatous lesions of patients with acute coronary syndromes. *J Am Coll Cardiol* 2006;47:301–306.
28. Buffon A, Biasucci LM, Liuzzo G, et al: Widespread coronary inflammation in unstable angina. *N Engl J Med* 2002;347:5–12.
29. Liuzzo G, Biasucci LM, Gallimore JR, et al: The prognostic value of C-reactive protein and serum amyloid A protein in severe unstable angina. *N Engl J Med* 1994;331:417–424.
30. O'Donoghue M, Morrow DA, Sabatine MS, et al: Lipoprotein-associated phospholipase A2 and its association with cardiovascular outcomes in patients with acute coronary syndromes in the PROVE IT-TIMI 22 trial. *Circulation* 2006;113:1745–1752.
31. Varo N, deLemos JA, Libby P, et al: Soluble CD40L. Risk prediction after acute coronary syndromes. *Circulation* 2003;108:1049–1052.
32. Ray KK, Morrow DA, Shui A, et al: Relation between soluble intercellular adhesion molecule-1, statin therapy, and long-term risk of clinical cardiovascular events in patients with previous acute coronary syndrome (from PROVE IT-TIMI 22). *Am J Cardiol* 2006;98:861–865.
33. Macin SM, Perna ER, Farias EF, et al: Atorvastatin has an important acute anti-inflammatory effect in patients with acute coronary syndrome: results of a randomized, double-blind, placebo-controlled study. *Am Heart J* 2005;149:451–457.
34. Bogaty P, Hackett D, Davies G, Maseri A: Vasoreactivity of the culprit lesion in unstable angina. *Circulation* 1994;90:5–11.
35. Laufs U, La Fata V, Plutzky J, Liao JK: Upregulation of endothelial nitric oxide synthase by HMG CoA reductase inhibitors. *Circulation* 1998;97:1129–1135.
36. Vasa M, Fichtlscherer S, Adler K, et al: Increase in circulating endothelial progenitor cells by statin therapy in patients with stable coronary artery disease. *Circulation* 2001;103:r21–r26.
37. Dupuis J, Tardif J-C, Cernacek P, Théroux P: Cholesterol reduction rapidly improves endothelial function after acute coronary syndromes. *Circulation* 1999;99:3227–3233.
38. Landmesser U, Bahlmann F, Mueller M, et al: Simvastatin versus ezetimibe: pleiotropic and lipid-lowering effects on endothelial function in humans. *Circulation* 2005;111:2356–2363.
39. Nofer J-R, Tepel M, Kehrel B, et al: Low-density lipoproteins inhibit the Na+/H+ antiport in human platelets: a novel mechanism enhancing platelet activity in hypercholesterolemia. *Circulation* 1997;95:1370–1377.
40. Rosenson RS, Lowe GDO: Effects of lipids and lipoproteins on thrombosis and rheology. *Atherosclerosis* 1998;140:271–280.
41. Lacoste L, Lam JYT, Hung J, et al: Hyperlipidemia and coronary disease: correction of the increased thrombogenic potential with cholesterol reduction. *Circulation* 1995;92:3172–3177.
42. Ferro D, Basili S, Alessandri C, et al: Inhibition of tissue-factor-mediated thrombin generation by simvastatin. *Atherosclerosis* 2000;149:111–116.
43. Notarbartolo A, Davi G, Averna M, et al: Inhibition of thromboxane biosynthesis and platelet function by simvastatin in type IIa hypercholesterolemia. *Arterioscler Thromb Vasc Biol* 1995;15:247–251.
44. Okazaki S, Yokoyama T, Miyauchi K, et al: Early statin treatment in patients with acute coronary syndrome: demonstration of the beneficial effect on atherosclerotic lesions by serial volumetric intravascular ultrasound analysis during half a year after coronary event: The ESTABLISH Study. *Circulation* 2004;110:1061–1068.
45. Nissen SE, Tuzcu EM, Schoenhagen P, et al: Effect of intensive compared with moderate lipid-lowering therapy on progression of coronary atherosclerosis: a randomized controlled trial. *JAMA* 2004;291:1071–1080.
46. Nissen SE, Tsunoda T, Tuzcu EM, et al: Effect of recombinant apo A-I Milano on coronary atherosclerosis in patients with acute coronary syndromes: a randomized controlled trial. *JAMA* 2003;290:2292–2300.
47. Tardif JC, Gregoire J, L'Allier PL, et al: Effects of reconstituted high-density lipoprotein infusions on coronary atherosclerosis: a randomized controlled trial. *JAMA* 2007;297:1675–1682.
48. Stenestrand U, Wallentin L, for the Swedish Register of Cardiac Intensive Care (RIKS-HIA): Early statin treatment following acute myocardial infarction and 1-year survival. *JAMA* 2001;285:430–436.
49. Aronow HD, Topol EJ, Roe MT, et al: Effect of lipid-lowering therapy on early mortality after acute coronary syndromes: an observational study. *Lancet* 2001;357:1063–1068.
50. Newby LK, Kristinsson A, Bhapkar MV, et al: Early statin initiation and outcomes in patients with acute coronary syndromes. *JAMA* 2002;287:3087–3095.
51. Fonorow GC, Wright RS, Spencer FA, et al: Effect of statin use within the first 24 hours of admission for acute myocardial infarction on early morbidity and mortality. *Am J Cardiol* 2005;96:611–616.
52. Lenderink T, Boersma E, Gitt AK, et al: Patients using statin treatment within 24 h after admission for ST-elevation acute coronary syndromes had lower mortality than non-users: a report from the first Euro Heart Survey on acute coronary syndromes. *Eur Heart J* 2006;27:1799–1804.
53. Spencer FA, Allegrone J, Goldberg RJ: Association of statin therapy with outcomes of acute coronary syndromes: The GRACE study. *Ann Intern Med* 2004;140:857–866.
54. Thompson PL, Meredith I, Amerena J, et al: Effect of pravastatin compared with placebo initiated within 24 hours of onset of acute myocardial infarction or unstable angina: The Pravastatin in Acute Coronary Treatment (PACT) trial. *Am Heart J* 2004;148:e2.
55. Liem AH, van Boven AJ, Veeger NJ, et al: Effect of fluvastatin on ischaemia following acute myocardial infarction: a randomized trial. *Eur Heart J* 2002;23:1931–1917.
56. Schwartz GG, Olsson AG, Ezekowitz MD, et al: Effects of atorvastatin on early recurrent ischemic events in acute coronary syndromes. The MIRACL study: a randomized controlled trial. *JAMA* 2001;85:1711–1718.
57. Cannon CP, Braunwald E, McCabe CH, et al: Intensive versus moderate lipid lowering with statins after acute coronary syndromes. *N Engl J Med* 2004;350:1495–1504.
58. Schwartz GG, Olsson AG, Szarek M, Sasiela WJ: Characteristics of metabolic syndrome: relation to short-term prognosis and effects of intensive statin therapy after acute coronary syndrome. An analysis of the MIRACL trial. *Diabetes Care* 2005;28:2508–2513.
59. Olsson AG, Schwartz GG, Szarek M, et al: Effects of high-dose atorvastatin in patients ≥65 years of age with acute coronary syndrome. *Am J Cardiol* 2007;99:632–635.
60. Waters DD, Schwartz GG, Olsson AG, et al: Effects of atorvastatin on stroke in patients with unstable angina or non-Q wave myocardial infarction: A Myocardial Ischemia Reduction with Aggressive Cholesterol Lowering (MIRACL) Substudy. *Circulation* 2002;106;1690–1695.
61. The Stroke Prevention by Aggressive Reduction in Cholesterol Levels (SPARCL) Investigators: High-dose atorvastatin after stroke or transient ischemic attack. *N Engl J Med* 2006;355:549–559.
62. Kinlay S, Schwartz GG, Olsson AG, et al: High-dose atorvastatin enhances the decline in inflammatory markers in patients with acute coronary syndromes in the MIRACL study. *Circulation* 2003;108:1560–1566.
63. Kinlay S, Schwartz GG, Olsson AG, et al: Effect of atorvastatin on risk of recurrent cardiovascular events after an acute coronary syndrome associated with high soluble CD40 ligand in the

Myocardial Ischemia Reduction with Aggressive Cholesterol Lowering (MIRACL) study. *Circulation* 2004;110:386–391.

64. Tsimikas S, Witztum JL, Miller ER, et al: High-dose atorvastatin reduces plasma levels of oxidized LDL in patients with acute coronary syndromes in the MIRACL trial. *Circulation* 2004;110: 1406–1412.
65. Ridker PM, Cannon CP, Morrow D, et al: C-reactive protein levels and outcomes after statin therapy. *N Engl J Med* 2005;352:20–28.
66. Wiviott SD, Cannon CP, Morrow DA, et al: Can low-density lipoprotein be too low? The safety and efficacy of achieving very low low-density lipoprotein with intensive statin therapy. *J Am Coll Cardiol* 2005;46:1411–1416.
67. Kleemann R, Verschuren L, de Rooij BJ, et al: Evidence for anti-inflammatory activity of statins and PPARalpha activators in human C-reactive protein transgenic mice *in vivo* and in cultured human hepatocytes *in vitro*. *Blood* 2004;103:4188–4194.
68. Voleti B, Agrawal A: Statins and nitric oxide reduce C-reactive protein production while inflammatory conditions persist. *Mol Immunol* 2006;43:891–896.
69. Verma S, Yeh ETH: C-reactive protein and atherothrombosis—Beyond a biomarker: an actual partaker of lesion formation. *Am J Physiol Regul Integr Comp Physiol* 2003;285:R1253–R1256.
70. LaRosa JC, Grundy SM, Waters DD, et al: Intensive lipid lowering with atorvastatin in patients with stable coronary disease. *N Engl J Med* 2005;352:1425–1435.
71. Pedersen TR, Faergeman O, Kastelein JJ, et al: High-dose atorvastatin vs usual-dose simvastatin for secondary prevention after myocardial infarction: The IDEAL study: a randomized controlled trial. *JAMA* 2005;294:2437–2445.
72. Grundy SM, Cleeman JI, Merz CN, et al: Implications of recent clinical trials for the National Cholesterol Education Program Adult Treatment Panel III Guidelines. *J Am Coll Cardiol* 2004;44:720–732.
73. Taneva E, Borucki K, Wiens L, et al: Early effects on endothelial function of atorvastatin 40 mg twice daily and its withdrawal. *Am J Cardiol* 2006;97:1002–1006.
74. Chu CS, Lee KT, Lee MY, et al: Effects of atorvastatin and atorvastatin withdrawal on soluble CD40L and adipocytokines in patients with hypercholesterolemia. *Acta Cardiol* 2006;61: 263–269.
75. Li JJ, Chu JM, Zhang CY, et al: Changes in plasma inflammatory markers after withdrawal of statin therapy in patients with hyperlipidemia. *Clin Chem Acta* 2006;366:269–273.
76. Lee KT, Lai WT, Chu CS, et al: Effect of withdrawal of statin on C-reactive protein. Clin Cardiol 2004;102:166–170.
77. Puccetti A, Pasqui AL, Pastorelli M, et al: Platelet hyperactivity after statin treatment discontinuation. *Thromb Haemost* 2003;90:476–482.
78. Vecchione C, Brandes RP: Withdrawal of 3-hydroxy–3-methylglutaryl coenzyme A reductase inhibitors elicits oxidative stress and induces endothelial dysfunction in mice. *Circ Res* 2002;91:173–179.
79. Endres M, Laufs U: Effects of statins on endothelium and signaling mechanisms. *Stroke* 2004;35(suppl 1):2708–2711.
80. McGowan MP, Treating to New Target (TNT) Study Group: There is no evidence for an increase in acute coronary syndromes after short-term abrupt discontinuation of statins in stable cardiac patients. *Circulation* 2004;110:2333–2335.
81. Heeschen C, Hamm CW, Laufs U, et al: Withdrawal of statins increases event rates in patients with acute coronary syndromes. *Circulation* 2002;105:1446–1452.
82. Heeschen C, Hamm CW, Laufs U, et al: Withdrawal of statins in patients with acute coronary syndromes. *Circulation* 2003; 107:e27.
83. Schwartz GG, Olsson AG: The case for intensive statin therapy after acute coronary syndromes. *Am J Cardiol* 2005;96(suppl): 45F–53F.

CHAPTER 40

Special Patient Populations: Transplant Recipients

Hallvard Holdaas, Jon A. Kobashigawa, Bengt Fellstrøm, and Alan G. Jardine

INTRODUCTION

Solid organ transplantation has become the treatment of choice for many patients with end-stage organ failure. Kidney, heart, liver, and to some extent, pancreas and lung transplantation are now firmly established management options. In recent decades, improved handling of acute rejection episodes and infection, coupled with advances in surgical procedures, has resulted in higher graft and patient survival in both the short and long term. The 2006 annual report of the U.S. Health Resources and Service Administration on organ procurement and transplantation shows that 1-year survival rates were highest for kidney and pancreas recipients, ranging from about 95% to 98%, while the corresponding survival rates for liver and heart recipients were 87% and 85%.[1]

However, premature cardiovascular disease remains a major limitation to long-term survival following kidney or heart transplantation.[2–4] Many transplant recipients have pre-existing cardiovascular disease or multiple cardiovascular risk factors at the time of transplantation. Heart recipients are at risk of developing a particularly aggressive form of coronary artery disease called cardiac allograft vasculopathy (CAV).[4] Cardiovascular risk factors in liver transplant recipients differ from those in heart or kidney transplantation, primarily because of the hemodynamic and metabolic changes associated with chronic liver disease.[5] Nevertheless, cardiovascular disease is also an important factor restricting long-term survival following liver transplantation.[6,7]

Evidence relating to the role of dyslipidemia as a risk factor for cardiovascular disease in solid organ transplantation is somewhat limited. Most information has been derived from observational studies and/or registry analyses in renal graft recipients and, to a lesser degree, from heart transplant patients. Data showing an association between dyslipidemia and cardiovascular events are more indicative in nature following liver transplantation and lung transplantation.

In contrast to the accumulated experience from large intervention trials in the general population over the last 10 to 15 years that has demonstrated the benefits of lipid lowering using statin therapy,[8] large controlled trials investigating the effect of dyslipidemia treatment on cardiovascular disease in solid organ recipients are scarce.

In renal transplant recipients, lipid lowering with a statin has been shown to reduce cardiac morbidity and mortality in a large randomized controlled trial.[9,10] There are also indications from two randomized trials in heart transplant patients that lipid lowering with statin therapy has a preventive cardiovascular effect,[11–13] although benefits were largely focused on pleiotrophic effects (inflammatory and immune modulating). In liver, lung, and pancreas transplant recipients, no randomized controlled trials have been undertaken regarding the effect of lipid-lowering therapy on cardiovascular risk.

RENAL TRANSPLANTATION

The causes of hyperlipidemia in transplant patients are more complex than in the general population. Immunosuppressive agents and concomitant drugs such as diuretics and β-blockers can have a negative effect on the lipid profile, while impaired renal function with or without proteinuria can also contribute.[14–17] Known risk factors for raised total cholesterol and low-density lipoprotein (LDL) cholesterol following transplantation include obesity, male gender, and ethnicity.[18,19]

The lipoprotein profile following renal transplantation is characterized by an increase in both total cholesterol and LDL cholesterol levels.[20–24] An increase of around 25% to 30% in total cholesterol is typical.[20,25] The peak incidence of hypercholesterolemia occurs 3 to 6 months post-transplant and remains stable at an elevated level from 12 months after transplantation.[26–28] It is estimated that 60% of the renal transplant population has a total cholesterol level above 240 mg/dL (6.2 mmol/L) and LDL cholesterol level above 132 mg/dL (3.4 mmol/L).[29] Changes in high-density lipoprotein (HDL) cholesterol after transplantation are more variable, with studies reporting unchanged, increased, or decreased levels.[17,30,31] These differences may be partly due to variations in the dose of corticosteroids used in each trial. Increases in triglyceride concentration are also observed after transplantation.[21,23,29] In addition, levels of apolipoprotein B and lipoprotein(a) are elevated, and LDL oxidation may increase following transplantation.[32,33] Finally, there are also indications that renal transplant patients exhibit an increased cholesterol absorption rate.[34]

A problem that is specific to the transplant population is the impact of immunosuppressive medication. Corticosteroids promote insulin resistance, leading to secondary hyperinsulinemia, with a reduction in lipoprotein lipase activity, overproduction of triglycerides, and secretion of very-low-density lipoproteins (VLDLs).[35] A significant correlation between corticosteroid dose and hyperlipidemia has been observed in renal transplant patients,[28,36,37] and the contribution of corticosteroids to hypercholesterolemia has been demonstrated in corticosteroid-eliminating studies in which withdrawal was associated with a significant decrease in cholesterol and LDL cholesterol.[38,39] Hyperlipidemia is also related to use of calcineurin inhibitor (CNI) therapy, that is, cyclosporine and tacrolimus.[28,40–42] Total cholesterol levels might be 30 to 36 mg/dL (0.8–0.9 mmol/L) higher in renal transplant patients treated with cyclosporine, prednisolone, and azathioprine than in those who received prednisolone and azathioprine alone,[43] and trough concentrations of cyclosporine appear to correlate with LDL cholesterol levels.[43] Cyclosporine interferes with lipid metabolism in several ways. Cholesterol clearance is reduced, probably via decreased LDL receptor synthesis and binding.[44,45] Lipoprotein lipase activity is inhibited, which could explain the increase in triglycerides.[46] Cyclosporine also interferes with the bile acid biosynthetic pathway, leading to hypercholesterolemia.[47]

For tacrolimus, the prevailing view has been that the incidence and severity of hyperlipidemia is reduced compared to cyclosporine therapy, and in general, cyclosporine has a more detrimental effect on total cholesterol, LDL cholesterol, and triglycerides than tacrolimus.[40,48] A reduction of 20% to 25% in LDL cholesterol has been reported after conversion from cyclosporine to tacrolimus,[49,50] and Wissing et al.[50] reported that switching to tacrolimus was associated with a significant reduction in LDL cholesterol. However, the same authors observed that addition of statin therapy to the cyclosporine regimen was a more efficient way to manage dyslipidemia.[51]

The proliferation-signal inhibitors (PSI), everolimus and sirolimus, are stronger inducers of hyperlipidemia than CNI agents.[52–54] The mechanisms by which PSIs affect lipid levels may be related to changes in lipoprotein lipase[55] and an increased production of triglycerides with increased secretion of VLDL.[56] Interference with an insulin-dependent signaling pathway has also been suggested as a means by which PSI therapy may disturb lipid metabolism.[56] Regardless of the mechanisms involved, alterations in blood lipid levels appear to be related to the trough level of PSIs and decrease over time post-transplant as PSI blood concentrations are reduced.[48,52,57] Lipid data from two large controlled studies in which renal transplant patients were converted to sirolimus have been analyzed by Blum.[58] Sirolimus-treated patients had higher lipid levels than controls, but the difference diminished over time. At 1 year post-transplant, mean total cholesterol was 30 mg/dL (0.8 mmol/L) higher in patients randomized to sirolimus 5 mg/day than in controls, partly driven by increased used of statins.

In contrast, azathioprine and mycophenolic acid (MPA), the active metabolite of mycophenolic mofetil (MMF), or enteric-coated mycophenolate sodium (EC-MPS), are not associated with an adverse effect on lipid profile in transplant recipients.[59] The incidence of hypercholesterolemia is significantly higher in patients treated with cyclosporine and prednisolone versus cyclosporine and MMF,[60] and converting renal transplant recipients from cyclosporine/azathioprine to MMF leads to an improvement in levels of total cholesterol and triglycerides.[61]

ASSOCIATION OF DYSLIPIDEMIA AND CARDIOVASCULAR EVENTS IN RENAL TRANSPLANT RECIPIENTS

Despite advances in immunosuppressive therapy and improved graft survival rates, renal transplant recipients have a significantly reduced life expectancy compared to the nontransplant population.[62,63] This is due largely to premature cardiovascular disease, which is the leading cause of death in patients with a functioning renal graft.[62,64–67] A study by Lindholm et al. has confirmed that death with a functioning graft is the major cause of graft loss in long-term transplant survivors, predominantly caused by ischemic heart disease,[65] and the European Dialysis and Transplant Association (EDTA) registry shows that approximately 40% to 45% of deaths in kidney graft recipients result from cardiovascular causes.[62] In the placebo arm of the Assessment of Lescol in Renal Transplantation (ALERT) core study and extension trial, approximately 50% of deaths were attributable to cardiovascular causes[9,10] (Fig. 40-1). Although one recent study showed that kidney transplant patients have a 17% lower risk of acute myocardial infarction than patients awaiting a transplant,[68] the risk of a cardiac event remains several-fold higher than in the general population.[63]

A number of analyses have attempted to link dyslipidemia and the risk of cardiovascular events in the renal transplant population; most were small observational studies based on registry data.[3,17,22,28,64,69–75] Kasiske et al. compared the observed cardiovascular risk in a cohort of renal transplant

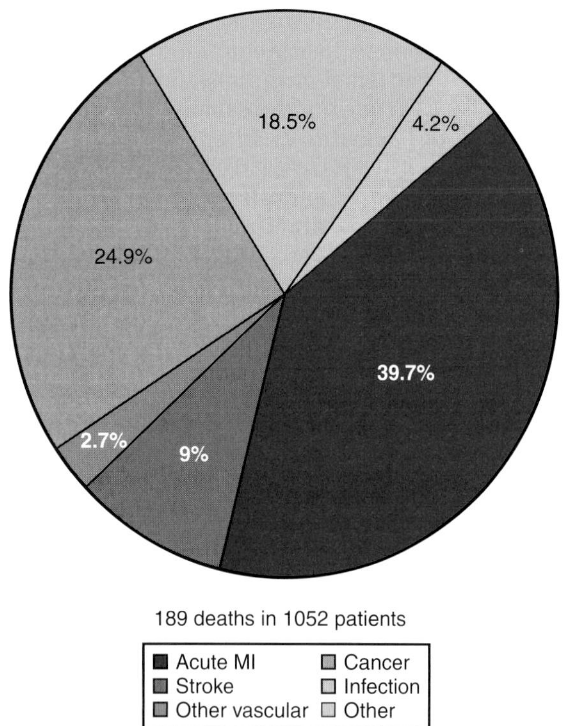

FIGURE 40-1 Causes of death in renal transplant recipients in the placebo arm in the ALERT trial. (Adapted from Ref. 9.)

recipients with that predicted from the Framingham cardiovascular risk factor data.[3] The results indicated that smoking, diabetes, total cholesterol, LDL cholesterol, and blood pressure were all associated with adverse outcome.[3] Although the Framingham risk score predicted ischemic heart disease after renal transplantation, it tended to underestimate the risk, particularly that associated with diabetes mellitus.[3] In renal transplant patients, the relationship between atherogenic lipids and cardiovascular outcome is not as clear as in the general population.

The prospective, randomized ALERT trial examined the association between lipids and cardiovascular events (myocardial infarction or cardiac death) in renal transplant patients.[10,76] The baseline characteristics of the study population have been reported previously.[77] In the placebo arm (n = 1052), LDL cholesterol was found to be a major risk factor for the occurrence of a coronary event. An increment in LDL cholesterol of 38 mg/dL (1 mmol/L) was associated with a 41% increase in risk of a coronary event,[10,76] while doubling the increment in LDL cholesterol to 76 mg/dL (2 mmol/L) resulted in a twofold increase in events.[78] Moreover, the authors could demonstrate a clear association between all lipid subfractions and myocardial infarction or cardiac death. The event rate was increased by 31% by an increase of 38 mg/dL (1 mmol/L) in total cholesterol, and by 11% for an increase of 88 mg/dL (1 mmol/L) in triglycerides. High triglycerides or low HDL cholesterol showed a similar, but lesser impact. Increasing HDL cholesterol by 38 mg/dL (1 mmol/L) resulted in a 45% reduction in the risk of a cardiac event.[10,76] The association between an atherogenic profile and cardiovascular risk has thus been established in renal transplant patients.

In addition to lipid risk factors, renal function per se after transplantation may have an impact on the cardiovascular event rate. Impaired renal function and renal graft loss are associated with increased mortality.[79–82] In an analysis of data from the ALERT trial, Fellstrøm et al. demonstrated that loss of graft function was associated with near doubling of the risk for an acute cardiac event, noncardiovascular death, or all-cause mortality.[14] Reduced renal function without graft loss was also a risk factor for cardiovascular events.[14,15] In the same analysis, conventional risk factors such as age, diabetes, history of coronary disease, blood pressure, smoking, and male gender were also risk factors: The event rate in diabetic patients was approximately twice that of nondiabetics, patients with a past history of coronary heart disease had three times as many events as patients without such a history, and older patients had more events.[14,78] Cigarette smoking was associated with an increased risk,[14] consistent with previous reports.[3,83] To summarize, data from the placebo arm of the ALERT trial established an association between an atherogenic lipid profile and cardiac outcome in renal transplant patients, as has been shown previously in large trials undertaken in diverse populations.[76]

TREATING DYSLIPIDEMIA IN THE RENAL TRANSPLANT POPULATION

Lipid-lowering therapy in renal transplant recipients poses certain challenges. Dietary restrictions[84–86] or lifestyle interventions such as exercise[87] alone do not appear to offer adequate control of hyperlipidemia following renal transplantation. Pharmacotherapy is therefore required in addition to standard dietary modifications. Until a few years ago, however, there was uncertainty whether lipid-lowering agents could be used safely and effectively in renal transplant patients as well as showing minimal or predictable interactions with the patient's immunosuppressive therapy. As a result, the transplant community has been reluctant to prescribe lipid-lowering agents other than statins, mostly due to the complex drug–drug interaction in immunosuppressed patients and fear of rhabdomyolysis. In the case of bile acid sequestrants (resins), for example, it is well established that cholestyramine may alter the absorption of cyclosporine.[88] However, by separating the intake of cholestyramine from the cyclosporine dose by 4 hours, no significant decrease is observed in the cyclosporine peak concentration or in the area under the exposure-time curve.[89] Additionally, bile acid resins should not be used when triglyceride levels are elevated since these agents have a tendency to increase triglyceride concentration.[48] Moreover, compliance has been reported to be very low with resins.[72] Bezafibrate, clofibrate, fenofibrate, and gemfibrozil all stimulate lipoprotein lipase activity, which promotes breakdown of triglyceride-rich lipids and inhibits hepatic VLDL cholesterol production.[48] The dose of fibrates must be reduced to minimize the risk of myositis/rhabdomyolysis. Fibrates should not be used in combination with statin therapy in solid organ transplant patients because of additive toxicity.[90] The poor tolerability profile of nicotinic acid precludes its general use in transplant patients,[91] and the sustained-release formulation of niacin, developed to correct low HDL cholesterol, should be avoided because of an increased propensity to cause hepatotoxicity.[92,93] Experience with probucol is limited in solid organ transplantation.[48]

Landmark trials performed in the general population have established statin therapy as the preferred medical treatment of both primary and secondary dyslipidemic disorders.[8] Similarly, statin treatment is an important tool in management of hyperlipidemia in renal transplant recipients. There are currently six statins available—simvastatin, lovastatin, pravastatin, atorvastatin, fluvastatin, and rosuvastatin—all of which lower LDL cholesterol. These have each been used widely in recipients of solid organ transplantation, with the exception of rosuvastatin, for which the experience in organ transplantation is limited.[94,95]

With adequate dosing, statins effectively lower total cholesterol and LDL cholesterol in the renal transplant population.[85,96–109] However, the lipid concentration targets recommended by the American Heart Association[112] and the National Cholesterol Education Program[110,111] for the general population, and the specific targets established for renal graft recipients[113] are difficult to attain in all patients. Ezetimibe is a new agent that acts through a novel mechanism, blocing absorption of dietary and biliary cholesterol by the small-intestine enterocyte brush border.[114] Ezetimibe 10 mg daily appears to reduce LDL cholesterol levels by approximately 20% when used alone or in combination with statin therapy. Although ezetimibe has not been used extensively in solid organ transplantation, small series in renal and heart transplant recipients have indicated that it may be effective and safe either as monotherapy or as a supplement to statin treatment in order to lower atherogenic lipids further.[115–124]

The omega-3 fatty acids, eicosapentaenoic acid (EPA) and docosahexaenoic acid (DHA), that are found in fish oil extracts have been shown to reduce VLDL cholesterol and triglyceride levels.[125] However, a recent meta-analysis of randomized controlled trials in renal transplant patients could not confirm any benefits except for a modest decrease in triglyceride levels.[126]

POTENTIAL PHARMACOKINETIC STATIN INTERACTIONS IN TRANSPLANT RECIPIENTS

In general, drug–drug interaction involving statins occurs most frequently when potent cytochrome P450 (CYP)3A4 inhibitors, such as macrolide antibiotics, azole antifungals, and protease inhibitors, among others, are combined with CYP3A4-metabolized statins (lovastatin, simvastatin, and atorvastatin). In transplant recipients, however, interactions between statins and immunosuppressive medication comprise an additional complication. Several of the most widely used immunosuppressive drugs, including cyclosporine, tacrolimus, sirolimus, and everolimus, are metabolized via CYP3A4.[127] The pharmacokinetic interaction between cyclosporine and tacrolimus has been studied extensively, particularly since this can lead to elevated blood concentrations of statins.

All statins, with the exception of pravastatin and rosuvastatin, are almost completely metabolized before elimination. The metabolism of atorvastatin, lovastatin, and simvastatin is primarily mediated by CYP3A4. Pravastatin is also partly metabolized by CYP3A4, but is mainly subjected to a variety of conjugation reactions so that unlike the other statins, approximately 10% of an oral dose of pravastatin is excreted unchanged via the kidneys.[128] Fluvastatin is also a CYP3A4 substrate, but it is primarily metabolized by CYP2C9.[128]

For many drugs, there is an overlap between their affinity to CYP3A4 and their affinity to P-glycoprotein,[129] and many of the drugs that are metabolized via CYP3A4 are also transported via other molecules such as organic anion transporting polypeptides (OATP).[130] Increased systemic exposure of statins when coadministered with cyclosporine may, therefore, be due either to transport interactions or to inhibition of CYP3A4 metabolism, or to a combination of both. In this regard, it is noteworthy that cyclosporine is highly bound to plasma lipoproteins, and a general lipid-lowering effect therefore has the potential to increase the free fraction. Akhlaghi et al. have investigated the effect of simvastatin on the free fraction of cyclosporine and observed an increase of approximately one-third.[131]

Concomitant administration of cyclosporine and atorvastatin leads to approximately a sixfold increase in the plasma exposure of atorvastatin.[96] In contrast, tacrolimus does not influence the pharmacokinetics of atorvastatin in renal transplant patients, indicating that tacrolimus should be the CNI of choice in transplant patients requiring statin treatment.[106] Similar results have been found with other statins. Plasma exposure of lovastatin increases up to 20-fold when administered with cyclosporine,[132] and there are reports of 5- to 23-fold increases in plasma levels of pravastatin during concomitant treatment with cyclosporine.[132,133] Plasma exposure of simvastatin following a single 20-mg dose is increased almost threefold in the presence of cyclosporine,[134] and plasma levels of fluvastatin increase by around twofold.[135] The area under the curve for the extended-release formulation of fluvastatin (fluvastatin 80 mg XL) was also approximately twofold higher in the presence of cyclosporine.[101] Finally, with rosuvastatin, cyclosporine increased the area under the curve by between 7- and 11-fold in heart transplant recipients compared to healthy subjects, although cyclosporine pharmacokinetics remained unaltered.[94] In general, the effect of statins on the pharmacokinetics of cyclosporine and tacrolimus is of less clinical importance than changes in statin exposure.[90]

For all the statins other than fluvastatin and pravastatin, single cases of rhabdomyolysis in transplant patients have been reported.[136–148] Generally, however, statins are well tolerated, although clinicians should be alert to the potential for drug–drug interactions in order to minimize the risk of myopathy during long-term statin therapy in transplanted patients.

EFFECT OF LIPID LOWERING IN RENAL TRANSPLANT RECIPIENTS

Prior to the ALERT trial, no prospective randomized trial of statin therapy in solid organ transplant patients had been performed, although an observational study by Cosio et al. indicated that statin treatment could be beneficial.[149] In their initial crude analysis, Cosio et al. showed no statistically significant relationship between statin use and survival, but after correction for recipient age, transplant year, and serum cholesterol, the correlation did indeed become significant.[149]

In the ALERT trial, treatment with fluvastatin significantly reduced levels of total and LDL cholesterol. From a mean baseline LDL cholesterol level of 4.1 mmol/L (159 mg/dL), fluvastatin-treated patients showed a sustained reduction throughout the study: The mean LDL cholesterol level was 3.1 mmol/L (120 mg/dL) prior to dose doubling and 2.7 mmol/L (104 mg/dL) at the end of the study.[9,10] There was a 19% nonsignificant reduction in the primary composite endpoint, the occurrence of major adverse cardiovascular events (MACE), defined as cardiac death, nonfatal myocardial infarction, and coronary intervention procedures. The core study was followed by the ALERT extension trial, which was a 2-year open-label extension during which all patients were offered fluvastatin treatment. LDL cholesterol was lowered by 36% compared to baseline. Moreover, in the extension trial, the risk of MACE was 29% lower in patients who had been initially randomized to fluvastatin, and cardiac death or nonfatal myocardial infarction was reduced by 36%.[9]

In the core ALERT trial, investigators observed 35% risk reduction for cardiac death and nonfatal myocardial infarction and an absolute net reduction in LDL cholesterol of 39 mg/dL (1 mmol/L). Fluvastatin significantly reduced the risk of cardiac death by 38% and the risk of cardiac death or first definite nonfatal myocardial infarction by 35% versus placebo. The effect of statin therapy on cardiac events is probably an underestimate due to a 14% dropout rate in the placebo arm. However, the data indicate that statin treatment of 31 renal transplant patients for 5 years would prevent one cardiac death or nonfatal myocardial infarction, representing a relatively small management cost for this population.

The 1-mmol/L (38-mg/dL) reduction in LDL cholesterol by fluvastatin and the 35% reduction in cardiac events observed in the ALERT study are similar to the results seen in all large statin trials in nontransplant populations.[76]

These data from the ALERT core study[10] and the extension trial[9] have established the benefit of fluvastatin treatment for the prevention of cardiac morbidity and mortality in renal transplant recipients (Fig. 40-2). It should be noted that over the total duration of follow-up in the ALERT study, 95% of patients in both the placebo and fluvastatin arms were receiving cardiovascular medication, demonstrating the cardiovascular complexity of this population.

One remaining question is the optimal time at which to initiate statin therapy after renal transplantation. Our recommendation is that statin treatment should be initiated early post-transplant, that is, within days or a few weeks. This is based on safety data from the Study of Lescol in Acute Rejection (SOLAR), a randomized, placebo-controlled trial of renal transplant patients in which fluvastatin treatment was initiated within 2 days after transplantation.[103] There was no difference between the treatment and placebo arms in terms of musculoskeletal symptoms, liver enzymes, creatine kinase, or other side effects. Furthermore, a post hoc analysis of data from the ALERT trial demonstrated that starting statin treatment early after transplantation, as compared to later (i.e., more than 2 years) was associated with no difference in side effect profile. Patients who started fluvastatin therapy less than 2 years post-transplant, however, had a 59% reduction in cardiac death and nonfatal myocardial infarction compared to those who began treatment more than 6 years after transplantation.[150]

Hypercholesterolemia has also been linked to accelerated atherosclerotic vascular disease in the transplanted graft.[21,75,151,152] It has been claimed that statin treatment might have a protective effect for both acute and chronic rejection, and delay the histologic deterioration usually observed in renal grafts.[153–155] These putative effects of statins have been linked to an immunomodulatory mechanism beyond their cholesterol-lowering action,[11,156,157] which may also help to prevent CAV, a form of chronic rejection in heart transplant patients (see following Heart Transplantation section). The immunomodulatory effects of statins in renal transplant are reviewed elsewhere.[158] However, three large short-term, randomized, controlled trials[103,159,160] and one long-term trial (ALERT) have failed to detect any significant difference in the risk of rejection between patients treated with a statin or placebo.[9,81] A systematic review of 13 randomized, controlled intervention trials in renal transplant recipients concluded that statins do not decrease the risk of rejection, although results confirmed their effectiveness in improving cardiovascular risk and reducing cardiac events.[161]

HEART TRANSPLANTATION

Lipid levels are usually elevated following heart transplantation.[162] The International Society for Heart and Lung Transplantation registry reveals that 68% of heart transplant patients have hyperlipidemia, defined as high levels of any class of lipoproteins, by 1 year after transplantation, and that 86% of patients are hyperlipidemic by 5 years post-transplant.[163] Approximately half of all heart transplant procedures are undertaken in patients with ischemic cardiomyopathy, and a substantial portion of these patients have a history of hyperlipidemia. Both clinical and experimental observations suggest that hyperlipidemia may be important in the development of CAV,[4] one of the major factors that limits long-term survival following heart transplantation. It is characterized by concentric intimal proliferation and diffuse narrowing along the entire length of the vessel, which can lead to obliteration of the graft vessels and, ultimately, to graft failure. Both immunologic and nonimmunologic risk factors have been associated with the development of CAV, but among the nonimmunologic factors, cholesterol and triglycerides have been the most widely reported.[164]

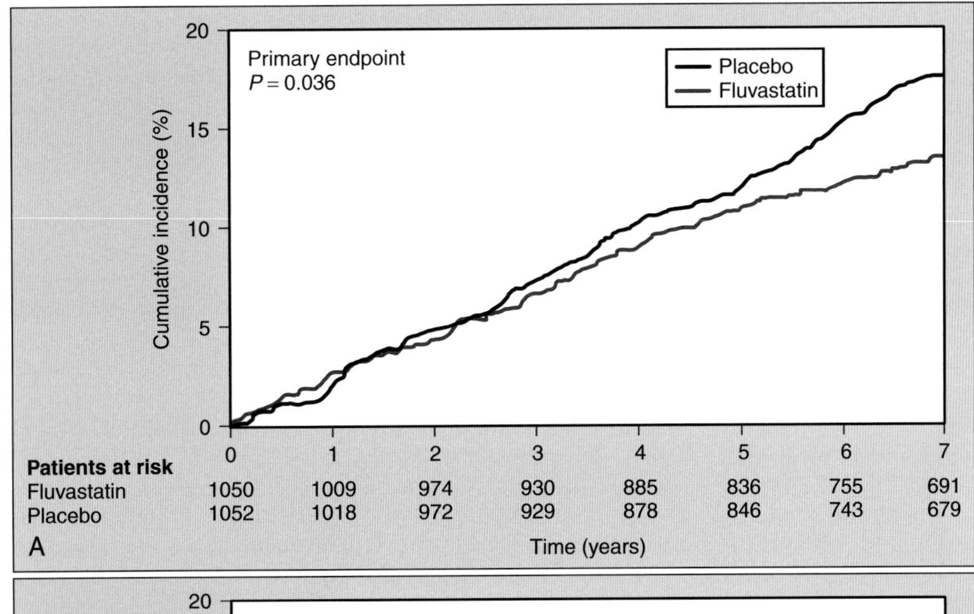

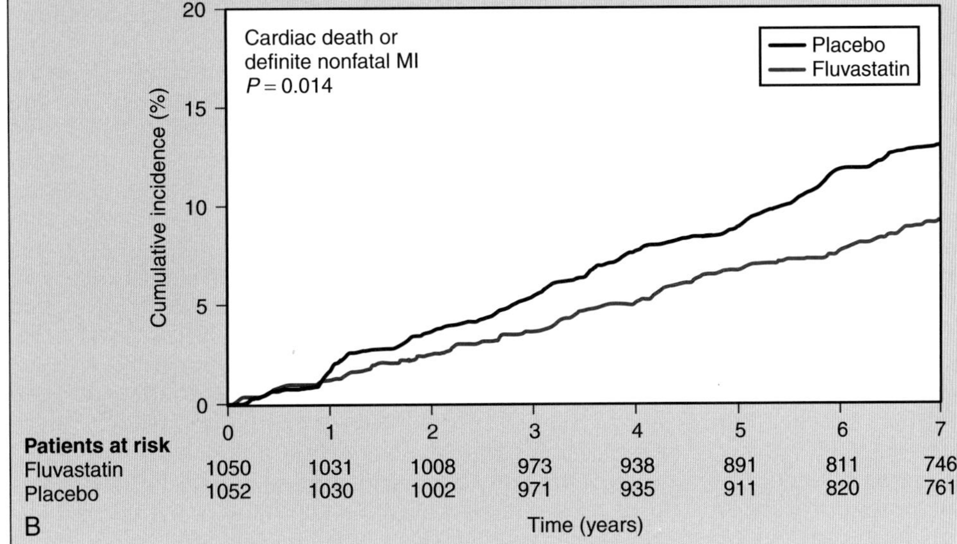

FIGURE 40-2 Cumulative rates for **(A)** primary endpoint (major adverse cardiovascular events [MACE]), and **(B)** composite endpoint of cardiac death or definite nonfatal myocardial infarction (MI), by original treatment group (Kaplan–Meier estimates), based on intention to treat. (Adapted from Ref. 9.)

In a retrospective study, elevated lipid values at 6 months after transplantation had a strong predictive value for the development of CAV at 3 years.[165] In another trial, raised LDL cholesterol at 1 year post-transplant was the only predictor of the development or progression of CAV detected by intravascular ultrasound (IVUS).[166] IVUS is an invasive procedure performed at the time of coronary angiography, whereby an ultrasound catheter is placed into the coronary artery to obtain an image of the thickness of the arterial wall. A multicenter study has reported that IVUS-identified intimal thickness at 1 year after heart transplantation is predictive for CAV and survival at 5 years.[167] Finally, in a recent multicenter assessment of ongoing post-transplant risk factors in 280 heart transplant patients who survived for at least 1 year after transplantation, multivariate Cox regression analysis showed that patients with high levels of total cholesterol experienced a greater incidence of nonfatal MACE (relative risk 4.34, $P = 0.01$). Nonfatal MACE included myocardial infarction, congestive heart failure, need for percutaneous cardiac intervention, permanent pacemaker, peripheral vascular disease, and cerebrovascular accident. The authors concluded that risk factor modification, such as cholesterol lowering, should be considered to improve outcome following heart transplantation.[168]

Dyslipidemia varies according to the immunosuppressive regimen. Lipid profiles in renal and liver transplant recipients are improved with tacrolimus therapy compared to cyclosporine. In a large randomized study, 129 stable heart transplant recipients who had undergone transplantation more than 12 months previously and were receiving cyclosporine, all of whom had mild dyslipidemia that persisted despite treatment, were switched to tacrolimus or maintained on cyclosporine.[169] At 6 months, patients who had converted to tacrolimus showed a greater decrease in total cholesterol (from 5.5 to 4.9 mmol/L) than those who continued to receive cyclosporine (5.6 to 5.4 mmol/L; $P = 0.008$). There were no changes in HDL cholesterol and triglyceride levels, but apolipoprotein B levels were reduced in the tacrolimus cohort versus the cyclosporine group ($P < 0.001$).[169] The newer PSI agents (sirolimus and everolimus) have been shown to increase triglyceride levels in heart transplant recipients, although total cholesterol levels are maintained in the normal range when cholesterol-lowering medication is given, and the development of IVUS-defined CAV is reduced in patients receiving PSI therapy.[170,171]

Clinical trials of statin therapy have demonstrated outcome benefits in nontransplant patients in both primary and secondary prevention settings.[8] Kobashigawa et al. evaluated the use of pravastatin for the primary prevention of hyperlipidemia in heart transplant recipients.[11] Ninety-seven heart transplant patients were randomized to pravastatin or no treatment within the first 2 weeks post-transplant. Twelve months after transplantation, the pravastatin group had significantly lower mean cholesterol levels than the control group (193 ± 36 mg/dL vs. 248 ± 49 mg/dL, $P < 0.001$). This, surprisingly, was accompanied by a lower frequency of graft rejection accompanied by hemodynamic compromise (3 vs. 14 patients, $P = 0.005$), and by improved survival (94% vs. 78%, $P = 0.025$) and a lower incidence of CAV as determined by angiography and at autopsy (3 vs. 10 patients, $P = 0.049$). In a subgroup of patients, IVUS measurements at baseline and at 1 year after transplantation showed significantly reduced progression of coronary artery intimal thickening in the pravastatin group compared to the control group ($P < 0.04$). In another subgroup, the cytotoxicity of natural killer cells was significantly lower in the pravastatin group than in control patients (9.8% vs. 22.2% specific lysis, $P = 0.014$). These findings suggest that the role of pravastatin in reducing CAV may relate not only to cholesterol lowering but also to an unexpected cholesterol-independent immunosuppressive effect. Ten-year follow-up data from this study demonstrate continued survival benefit (68% vs. 48% in the control group, $P = 0.026$) and a significantly lower incidence of angiographic CAV and/or death in the pravastatin group (57% vs. 80% in the control group, $P = 0.009$).[12]

Other studies have also demonstrated a beneficial effect of statin therapy on the development of CAV. In another single-center randomized trial, in which 72 heart transplant patients were randomized to simvastatin or no statin, there was a lower incidence of CAV in the simvastatin-treated patients.[172] IVUS performed at baseline and at 1 year post-transplant revealed intimal thickening to be less progressed in the simvastatin group. Eight-year follow-up also demonstrated persistence of survival benefit (88.6% vs. 59.5% among controls, $P < 0.006$) and a lower incidence of angiographic CAV (24.4% vs. 54.7%, $P < 0.02$).[13]

As in nontransplant patients, simvastatin has been found to have protective effects on coronary vasomotor function and the coronary release of interleukin-6 (IL-6) and tumor necrosis factor–α (TNF-α) in heart transplant recipients without angiographically detectable disease, suggesting that endothelial cell function is improved and inflammatory cytokine release is inhibited.[173] The association between statin therapy and death or fatal graft rejection has been assessed using Heart Transplant Lipid Registry data from 12 centers.[174] The study included 1186 patients with a mean follow-up of 580 days, of whom 937 patients (79%) received statin therapy (pravastatin, simvastatin, lovastatin, or fluvastatin). The statin-treated group had a lower frequency of death (4.0% vs. 13.7%, $P < 0.001$) and fatal rejection (2.4% vs. 7.2%, $P < 0.001$). This study represented the largest population of heart transplant recipients that has been analyzed to determine the relationship between statin therapy and clinical outcomes in actual practice. The authors concluded that statin therapy was significantly associated with a reduced risk of death and fatal rejection, benefits that were independent of lipid values.

Other, nonstatin cholesterol-lowering agents have been used to treat heart transplant patients. Fibric acid derivatives have been reported to decrease lipid levels to a moderate extent (15%–20%) and to reduce inflammation, as well as lowering proinflammatory activity in endothelial cells. Use of fibric acid derivatives has been limited by gastrointestinal adverse effects, elevated urea and creatinine levels, and reduced intestinal absorption of cyclosporine.[116,175] Niacin reduces LDL cholesterol and triglyceride levels in heart transplant patients, and raises HDL cholesterol concentration,[116] but adverse effects such as flushing and pruritis have restricted its use. Cholestyramine binds to bile acids and inhibits reabsorption,[175] but it is less effective than statins in lowering LDL cholesterol levels and can influence cyclosporine absorption.[116,175] Ezetimibe inhibits the absorption of dietary and biliary cholesterol, without affecting the absorption of triglycerides or fat-soluble vitamins, but coadministration with cyclosporine results in a 12-fold increase in ezetimibe concentration.[116] In one report, however, ezetimibe was reported to be effective and safe in heart transplant patients who were intolerant of statins or unable to reach target lipid levels with statin therapy.[123] In severe familial hypercholesterolemia, which is rarely observed in heart transplant recipients, treatment with statins can be combined with extracorporeal cholesterol elimination procedures such as heparin-induced extracorporeal LDL cholesterol precipitation (HELP). HELP precipitates LDL cholesterol from the plasma and eliminates it via an extracorporeal filter system. HELP enables total cholesterol levels to be kept within any desired target range, and has been used successfully and without adverse effects in heart transplant patients. However, it is costly and time consuming.[175]

It is not clear whether the clinical benefits of statins in transplant recipients are due to their powerful cholesterol-lowering effects alone or whether they are partly due to their cholesterol-independent effects on vascular function, plaque growth, plaque rupture, or thrombosis. There are several clinical findings in heart transplant patients that may suggest a potential mechanism for an immunosuppressive property of statins. It has been reported that a marked decrease in lipoprotein concentration is associated with an increase in the unbound fraction of cyclosporine,[131] which may in turn increase the biologic activity of cyclosporine. Additionally, Regazzi et al. have observed markedly elevated serum levels of pravastatin in patients receiving cyclosporine.[176] Such supranormal serum levels of pravastatin may be necessary for the immunosuppressive properties of this drug to be exhibited, and may explain why clinically adverse immune responses (such as those associated with opportunistic infections) are not observed in nontransplant patients treated with pravastatin.[177]

There have been two reports revealing direct and previously unknown immunologic effects of statins.

The first was published by Kwak and colleagues.[156] Based on a series of elegant experiments monitoring cell surface expression of major histocompatibility complex class II (MHC-II) assayed by fluorescence-activated cell sorting and immunoflourescence and by mRNA levels, the authors concluded that statins effectively repress the induction of MHC-II expression by interferon-γ in a dose-dependent manner. They also reported that in the presence of L-mevalonate, the effect of statins on MHC-II expression is abolished, indicating that it is indeed the effect of statins as HMG-CoA reductase inhibitors that mediates repression of MHC-II. It was noted that repression of MHC-II expression by statins is highly specific for the inducible form of MHC-II expression, and does not affect constitutive expression of MHC-II in highly specialized antigen-presenting cells, such as dendritic cells and B-lymphocytes. Moreover, this effect of statins appears specific for MHC-II and does not influence MHC class I (MHC-I) expression. Through mixed-lymphocyte reactions, T-lymphocyte proliferation could be blocked by monoclonal antibodies against MHC-II. Pretreatment of endothelial cells or macrophages with statins reduces subsequent T-lymphocyte proliferation. This previously unknown effect of statins as MHC-II repressors was also observed in other cell types including primary human smooth muscle cells and fibroblasts. Through mRNA experiments, the authors established that the specific mechanism whereby statins inhibit MHC-II induction is a selective repressive effect on the induction of expression of promoter IV of the MHC-II transactivator *CIITA* gene.

The second recently discovered immunosuppressive action of statins was reported by Weitz-Schmidt et al.,[157] who demonstrated that this class of drug selectively blocks the β_2 integrin, leukocyte function antigen–1 (LFA-1). LFA-1 is a costimulator of T cells that is expressed on the surface of leukocytes. When activated, it binds to intercellular adhesion molecule–1 (ICAM-1). Weitz-Schmidt and colleagues demonstrated that lovastatin and, subsequently, other statins bind selectively to LFA-1 and prevent LFA-1–mediated adhesion and lymphocyte costimulation. This effect was unrelated to statin-related inhibition of HMG-CoA. These two reports suggest that immunomodulation by statins may be beneficial in solid organ transplant recipients, not only in conventional atherosclerosis, which involves chronic inflammatory processes, but also in CAV in heart transplant recipients. However, inhibition of inducible expression of MHC-II molecules and selective blocking of LFA-1 have not yet been shown to lead to reduced immunologic recognition at the clinical level.

Statins also appear to play a role in reducing oxidation-sensitive signaling pathways.[178] There is extensive evidence linking hypercholesterolemia with increased lipid peroxidation and increased oxidative stress.[179] Several of the cholesterol-independent actions of statins have been traced to prenylation of regulatory proteins, such as G proteins, Ras, Rho, and Rab, while other effects have been linked to geranyl-geranylation, such as inhibition of proliferation and induction of apoptosis in smooth muscle cells,[180] inhibition of integrin-dependent leukocyte adhesion[181] and increased fibrinolytic activity.[182] Detection of improved vascular function in the absence of hypercholesterolemia,[183] supports the hypothesis that these effects are cholesterol independent.[184] Unequivocal evidence that many of these effects are due to protein prenylation has been provided by the fact that they are reversible by addition of geranylgeranyl-pyrophosphate (PP) (or farnesyl-PP), which does not restore cholesterol synthesis, while they are not reversed by the addition of squalene or cholesterol.[182,185]

Other compounds exist that can act as a site downstream from the HMG-CoA reductase inhibitors, and which block isoprenylation more effectively, but do not influence cholesterol production. In a recent paper, Si and Imagawa evaluated a potent farnesyltransferase inhibitor, A-228839,[186] and showed that it inhibited lectin-induced lymphocyte proliferation, and that this effect was additive to cyclosporine. A-228839 also significantly disrupted the polarized shape of 1E5 T cells at physiologic concentrations. Finally, A-228839 inhibited lymphocyte Th-1 cytokine production at submicromolar levels and promoted apoptosis in lectin-activated lymphocytes. The authors believe this new agent has potent immunomodulatory properties *in vitro* and that *in vivo* trials are warranted.

In conclusion, hyperlipidemia after heart transplantation is common. CAV, the major factor limiting long-term survival, appears to be aggravated by the presence of hyperlipidemia, which has been reported to cause inflammation. Statins appear to reduce inflammation and atherogenesis by lowering cholesterol levels, but additionally, several recent papers have established a mechanism by which statins may exert a cholesterol-independent immunosuppressive effect. Clinical studies have demonstrated that statin therapy in heart transplant patients is associated with benefits in terms of survival, severity of rejection, and CAV through 10 years of follow-up. The clinical and experimental reports that indicate an immunomodulatory effect of statins support the routine use of statin treatment in heart transplant patients.

LIVER TRANSPLANTATION

Dyslipidemia is estimated to affect 40% to 60% of liver transplant patients, depending on the definition used and the era.[187–191] Hyperlipidemia may occur either as hypercholesterolemia or hypertriglyceridemia in the liver transplant population, but more frequently as mixed hyperlipidemia.[192,193] One study has claimed that long-term cardiovascular risk following liver transplantation is more than three times the expected risk in an age- and gender-matched control group.[7] Liver transplant recipients share the same causes of dyslipidemia as recipients of other type of solid organ grafts: genetic disposition, obesity, renal dysfunction, metabolic syndrome, and diabetes mellitus.[191,194] Diabetes mellitus may also be a contributing factor in liver transplant patients.[192] The immunosuppressive regimens used in liver transplant patients are, in principle, similar to those employed in kidney and heart transplant recipients, and thus in broad terms, the impact of immunosuppressive medication on lipid profiles is the same as discussed in the Renal Transplantation and Heart Transplantation sections. Historically, however, prednisolone has often been tapered more quickly in liver transplant patients, and discontinued earlier and more frequently than in the other solid organ programs, leading to more favorable lipid profile.[191]

ASSOCIATION BETWEEN DYSLIPIDEMIA AND CARDIOVASCULAR EVENTS IN LIVER TRANSPLANT RECIPIENTS

In contrast to kidney and heart transplantation, relatively few studies have examined the relationship between lipids and cardiovascular events in liver transplant recipients.[6,188,189,192,194–198] Abbasoglu et al. reported that death with a functioning graft occurred in 61% of liver transplant patients in their population, and that cardiovascular and cerebrovascular events were second only to recurrent disease as a cause of graft loss.[194] In a more recent paper, Guckelberger et al.[195] followed 483 primary liver transplants for 10 years. Univariate analysis indicated that age, gender, body mass index, cholesterol, creatinine, diabetes mellitus, glucose, and systolic blood pressure were significantly associated with fatal or nonfatal cardiovascular events. In a multivariate analysis, however, only age, gender, and cholesterol were found to be independent predictors of cardiovascular events.[6] It is reasonable to conclude that dyslipidemia is probably a modifiable risk factor for cardiovascular events in liver transplant recipients, as in other types of solid organ transplantation.

TREATING DYSLIPIDEMIA IN THE LIVER TRANSPLANT POPULATION

There has been a relatively modest focus on dyslipidemia and its consequences in liver transplantation. No randomized, placebo-controlled, lipid-lowering trials with cardiovascular endpoints have been conducted to date in liver transplant recipients, and only a small number of studies have examined the effect of statins in liver transplantation.[199–201] All three published studies of statin therapy in liver transplantation,[199–201] however, have confirmed that atherogenic lipids are lowered safely. Imagawa et al. studied liver transplant patients receiving cyclosporine-based (n = 65) or tacrolimus-based (n = 17) immunosuppression, and concluded that pravastatin was safe and effective in reducing cholesterol levels.[199] In terms of drug–drug interactions, Taylor et al. have assessed the effect of atorvastatin on the pharmacokinetic profile of cyclosporine.[200] The area under the curve for cyclosporine was found to increase by 9% in the presence of atorvastatin, but this is of questionable clinical significance. The impact of cyclosporine on the pharmacokinetics of atorvastatin was not investigated, although in renal transplant recipients, cyclosporine has been shown to increase the area under curve for atorvastatin by sixfold.[96]

One therapeutic option in liver transplant recipients who do not respond adequately to statin monotherapy may be ezetimibe, which appears to have a negligible risk of hepatotoxicity.[117,121]

Hypertriglyceridemia is not infrequent in liver transplant recipients.[191] Fish oil has been proposed as a first-line treatment for a moderate increase in triglyceride concentration, while fibrates (gemfibrozil or fenofibrate) are recommended for more refractory cases.[193] The sustained-release form of niacin, used to correct low HDL cholesterol, should be avoided because of an increased propensity for hepatotoxicity.[92,93]

PEDIATRIC AND ADOLESCENT TRANSPLANT RECIPIENTS

Dyslipidemia is not uncommon in pediatric and adolescent transplant recipients. Singh et al. compared lipid values 1 year after heart transplantation among children participating in the North America Pediatric Transplant study against those of nontransplant children in the United States.[202] The median values of total and LDL cholesterol were similar to those of controls, but 39% of the transplant patients had an LDL cholesterol level above 100 mg/dL (2.6 mmol/L). The authors concluded that lipid levels considered to be within the intervention range in adults at high risk of coronary artery disease are common after cardiac transplantation in children. Independent risk factors for elevated total cholesterol and LDL cholesterol were patient age and administration of cyclosporine or prednisone.[202]

The problem of hyperlipidemia is not unique to pediatric or adolescent heart transplant recipients. The incidence of hyperlipidemia in pediatric renal transplant recipients is generally 30% to 75%,[203–206] and pediatric liver transplant recipients are also susceptible to hyperlipidemia.[207,208] The immunosuppressive regimens used in pediatric and adolescent transplant patients are generally in accordance with those followed in adult transplantation, and thus the impact of immunosuppressive medication on dyslipidemia will in principle be the same as discussed in the Renal Transplantation and Heart Transplantation sections.

No epidemiologic data exist that show an association between dyslipidemia and cardiovascular outcome in pediatric or adolescent transplant recipients. That lipids could be a risk factor for cardiovascular events in these age groups is inferred from the general population and from randomized trials in adult solid organ transplantation.[8,9] Furthermore, there are relatively few studies examining the use of lipid-lowering agents in young transplant recipients, and those that have been undertaken are characterized by small numbers of patients and short follow-up, both in renal[209–212] and heart[213–218] transplantation. In general, statin treatment has been well tolerated in pediatric and adolescent transplant patients, although in one study of atorvastatin in 38 pediatric heart transplant recipients, two patients developed rhabdomyolysis and four developed myalgia.[213] A retrospective review of 129 pediatric heart recipients has indicated an association between pravastatin therapy and a reduced incidence of CAV.[216] The known interaction between cyclosporine and pravastatin, which leads to a several-fold increase in pravastatin exposure, has also been observed in pediatric heart transplant recipients.[215]

Although all statins except rosuvastatin have pediatric use labeling in their FDA-approved prescribing information, this is based on studies of children and adolescents with familial hypercholesterolemia, not after organ transplantation. However, the available preliminary data suggest that statin therapy is relatively safe. Statin treatment should therefore be considered in adolescent solid organ transplant recipients who have elevated LDL cholesterol. Despite the apparent safety of statins in children with regards to growth and development,[219] additional data on long-term safety are required before statin therapy can be recommended in pediatric transplant populations.

CONCLUSION

Atherogenic lipids increase the risk of cardiovascular disease in solid organ transplant recipients, and lipid-lowering intervention is warranted following transplantation. It appears worthwhile to offer routine statin therapy to solid organ transplant patients as secondary prevention, and statins should also be considered for primary prevention. Because of complex pharmacokinetic interactions with immunosuppressive agents, a low starting dose of statins, with the exception of fluvastatin in renal transplantation, should be used. Other strategies, including addition of ezetimibe or other lipid-modifying agents, may be used cautiously to enhance the effectiveness of lipid lowering in organ transplant recipients.

REFERENCES

1. Collins AJ, Kasiske B, Herzog C, et al: Excerpts from the United States Renal Data System 2006 Annual Data Report. *Am J Kidney Dis* 2007;49:S1–S296.
2. Holdaas H: Preventing cardiovascular outcome in patients with renal impairment: Is there a role for lipid-lowering therapy? *Am J Cardiovasc Drugs* 2005;5:255–269.
3. Kasiske BL, Chakkera HA, Roel J: Explained and unexplained ischemic heart disease risk after renal transplantation. *J Am Soc Nephrol* 2000;11:1735–1743.
4. Kobashigawa JA, Kasiske BL: Hyperlipidemia in solid organ transplàntation. *Transplantation* 1997;63:331–338.
5. Bostom AD, Brown RS Jr., Chavers BM, et al: Prevention of post-transplant cardiovascular disease—report and recommendations of an ad hoc group. *Am J Transpl* 2002;2:491–500.
6. Guckelberger O, Byram A, Klupp J, et al: Coronary event rates in liver transplant recipients reflect the increased prevalence of cardiovascular risk-factors. *Transpl Int* 2005;18:967–974.
7. Johnston SD, Morris JK, Cramb R, et al: Cardiovascular morbidity and mortality after orthotopic liver transplantation. *Transplantation* 2002;73:901–906.
8. Baigent C, Keech A, Kearney PM, et al: Efficacy and safety of cholesterol-lowering treatment: prospective meta-analysis of data from 90,056 participants in 14 randomised trials of statins. *Lancet* 2005;366:1267–1278.
9. Holdaas H, Fellstrom B, Cole E, et al: Long-term cardiac outcomes in renal transplant recipients receiving fluvastatin: the ALERT extension study. *Am J Transpl* 2005;5:2929–2936.
10. Holdaas H, Fellstrom B, Jardine AG, et al: Effect of fluvastatin on cardiac outcomes in renal transplant recipients: a multicentre, randomised, placebo-controlled trial. *Lancet* 2003;361:2024–2031.
11. Kobashigawa JA, Katznelson S, Laks H, et al: Effect of pravastatin on outcomes after cardiac transplantation. *N Engl J Med* 1995;333:621–627.
12. Kobashigawa JA, Moriguchi JD, Laks H, et al: Ten-year followup of a randomized trial of pravastatin in heart transplant patients. *J Heart Lung Transpl* 2005;24:1736–1740.
13. Wenke K, Meiser B, Thiery J, et al: Simvastatin initiated early after heart transplantation: 8-year prospective experience. *Circulation* 2003;107:93–97.
14. Fellstrom B, Jardine AG, Soveri I, et al: Renal dysfunction as a risk factor for mortality and cardiovascular disease in renal transplantation: experience from the Assessment of Lescol in Renal Transplantation trial. *Transplantation* 2005;79:1160–1163.
15. Fellstrom B, Jardine AG, Soveri I, et al: Renal dysfunction is a strong and independent risk factor for mortality and cardiovascular complications in renal transplantation. *Am J Transpl* 2005;5:1986–1991.
16. Fernandez-Fresnedo G, Escallada R, Rodrigo E, et al: The risk of cardiovascular disease associated with proteinuria in renal transplant patients. *Transplantation* 2002;73:1345–1348.
17. Kasiske BL, Umen AJ: Persistent hyperlipidemia in renal transplant patients. *Medicine (Baltimore)* 1987;66:309–316.
18. Burrell DE, Antignani A, Goldwasser P, et al: Lipid abnormalities in black renal patients. *N Y State J Med* 1991;91:192–196.
19. Kasiske BL: Risk factors for cardiovascular disease after renal transplantation. *Miner Electrolyte Metab* 1993;19:186–195.
20. Aakhus S, Dahl K, Wideroe TE: Hyperlipidaemia in renal transplant patients. *J Intern Med* 1996;239:407–415.
21. Dimeny E, Wahlberg J, Lithell H, et al: Hyperlipidaemia in renal transplantation—risk factor for long-term graft outcome. *Eur J Clin Invest* 1995;25:574–583.
22. Drueke TB, Abdulmassih Z, Lacour B, et al: Atherosclerosis and lipid disorders after renal transplantation. *Kidney Int Suppl* 1991;31:S24–S28.
23. Moore R, Thomas D, Morgan E, et al: Abnormal lipid and lipoprotein profiles following renal transplantation. *Transpl Proc* 1993;25:1060–1061.
24. Pannu HS, Singh D, Sandhu JS: Lipid profile before and after renal transplantation—a longitudinal study. *Ren Fail* 2003;25:411–417.
25. Appel G: Lipid abnormalities in renal disease. *Kidney Int* 1991;39:169–183.
26. Rao VK: Posttransplant medical complications. *Surg Clin North Am* 1998;78:113–132.
27. Tse KC, Lam MF, Yip PS, et al: A long-term study on hyperlipidemia in stable renal transplant recipients. *Clin Transpl* 2004;18:274–280.
28. Vathsala A, Weinberg RB, Schoenberg L, et al: Lipid abnormalities in cyclosporine-prednisone-treated renal transplant recipients. *Transplantation* 1989;48:37–43.
29. Coresh J, Longenecker JC, Miller ER, III, et al: Epidemiology of cardiovascular risk factors in chronic renal disease. *J Am Soc Nephrol* 1998;9:S24–S30.
30. Hilbrands LB, Demacker PN, Hoitsma AJ, et al: The effects of cyclosporine and prednisone on serum lipid and (apo)lipoprotein levels in renal transplant recipients. *J Am Soc Nephrol* 1995;5:2073–2081.
31. Jung K, Scheifler A, Blank W, et al: Changed composition of high-density lipoprotein subclasses HDL2 and HDL3 after renal transplantation. *Transplantation* 1988;46:407–409.
32. Fellstrom B: Impact and management of hyperlipidemia posttransplantation. *Transplantation* 2000;70:SS51–SS57.
33. Ghanem H, van den Dorpel MA, Weimar W, et al: Increased low-density lipoprotein oxidation in stable kidney transplant recipients. *Kidney Int* 1996;49:488–493.
34. Siirtola A, Ketomaki A, Miettinen TA, et al: Cholesterol absorption and synthesis in pediatric kidney, liver, and heart transplant recipients. *Transplantation* 2006;81:327–334.
35. Kasiske BL: Hyperlipidemia in patients with chronic renal disease. *Am J Kidney Dis* 1998;32:S142–S156.
36. Cattran DC, Steiner G, Wilson DR, et al: Hyperlipidemia after renal transplantation: natural history and pathophysiology. *Ann Intern Med* 1979;91:554–559.
37. Ponticelli C, Barbi GL, Cantaluppi A, et al: Lipid disorders in renal transplant recipients. *Nephron* 1978;20:189–195.
38. Pascual J, van Hooff JP, Salmela K, et al: Three-year observational follow-up of a multicenter, randomized trial on tacrolimus-based therapy with withdrawal of steroids or mycophenolate mofetil after renal transplant. *Transplantation* 2006;82:55–61.
39. Vanrenterghem Y, van Hooff JP, Squifflet JP, et al: Minimization of immunosuppressive therapy after renal transplantation: results of a randomized controlled trial. *Am J Transpl* 2005;5:87–95.

40. Jardine AG: Assessing the relative risk of cardiovascular disease among renal transplant patients receiving tacrolimus or cyclosporine. *Transpl Int* 2005;18:379–384
41. Kirk JK, Dupuis RE: Approaches to the treatment of hyperlipidemia in the solid organ transplant recipient. *Ann Pharmacother* 1995;29:879–891.
42. Ligtenberg G, Hene RJ, Blankestijn PJ, et al: Cardiovascular risk factors in renal transplant patients: cyclosporin A versus tacrolimus. *J Am Soc Nephrol* 2001;12:368–373.
43. Kasiske BL, Tortorice KL, Heim-Duthoy KL, et al: The adverse impact of cyclosporine on serum lipids in renal transplant recipients. *Am J Kidney Dis* 1991;17:700–707.
44. Al Rayyes O, Wallmark A, Florén CH: Additive inhibitory effect of hydrocortisone and cyclosporine on low-density lipoprotein eceptor activity in cultured HepG2 cells. *Hepatology* 1997;26:967–971.
45. Rayyes OA, Wallmark A, Floren CH: Cyclosporine inhibits catabolism of low-density lipoproteins in HepG2 cells by about 25%. *Hepatology* 1996;24:613–619.
46. Vaziri ND, Liang K, Azad H: Effect of cyclosporine on HMG-CoA reductase, cholesterol 7alpha-hydroxylase, LDL receptor, HDL receptor, VLDL receptor, and lipoprotein lipase expressions. *J Pharmacol Exp Ther* 2000;294:778–783.
47. McCashland TM, Donovan JP, Amelsberg A, et al: Bile acid metabolism and biliary secretion in patients receiving orthotopic liver transplants: differing effects of cyclosporine and FK 506. *Hepatology* 1994;19:1381–1389.
48. Mathis AS, Dave N, Knipp GT, et al: Drug-related dyslipidemia after renal transplantation. *Am J Health Syst Pharm* 2004;61: 565–585.
49. McCune TR, Thacker LR II, Peters TG, et al: Effects of tacrolimus on hyperlipidemia after successful renal transplantation: a Southeastern Organ Procurement Foundation multicenter clinical study. *Transplantation* 1998;65:87–92.
50. Urbizu JM, Amenabar JJ, Gomez-Ullate P, et al: Immunosuppression using tacrolimus/mycophenolate versus neoral/ mycophenolate following kidney transplantation: a single-center experience. *Transpl Proc* 2002;34:87–88.
51. Wissing KM, Unger P, Ghisdal L, et al: Effect of atorvastatin therapy and conversion to tacrolimus on hypercholesterolemia and endothelial dysfunction after renal transplantation. *Transplantation* 2006;82:771–778.
52. MacDonald AS: A worldwide, phase III, randomized, controlled, safety and efficacy study of a sirolimus/cyclosporine regimen for prevention of acute rejection in recipients of primary mismatched renal allografts. *Transplantation* 2001;71:271–280.
53. Neumayer HH, Paradis K, Korn A, et al: Entry-into-human study with the novel immunosuppressant SDZ RAD in stable renal transplant recipients. *Br J Clin Pharmacol* 1999;48:694–703.
54. Vitko S, Tedesco H, Eris J, et al: Everolimus with optimized cyclosporine dosing in renal transplant recipients: 6-month safety and efficacy results of two randomized studies. *Am J Transpl* 2004;4:626–635.
55. Hoogeveen RC, Ballantyne CM, Pownall HJ, et al: Effect of sirolimus on the metabolism of apo. *Transplantation* 2001;72:1244–1250.
56. Morrisett JD, bdel-Fattah G, Hoogeveen R, et al: Effects of sirolimus on plasma lipids, lipoprotein levels, and fatty acid metabolism in renal transplant patients. *J Lipid Res* 2002;43:1170–1180.
57. Groth CG, Backman L, Morales JM, et al: Sirolimus (rapamycin)-based therapy in human renal transplantation: Similar efficacy and different toxicity compared with cyclosporine. Sirolimus European Renal Transplant Study Group. *Transplantation* 1999;67:1036–1042.
58. Blum CB: Effects of sirolimus on lipids in renal allograft recipients: an analysis using the Framingham risk model. *Am J Transpl* 2002;2:551–559.
59. Miller LW: Cardiovascular toxicities of immunosuppressive agents. *Am J Transpl* 2002;2:807–818.
60. Stegall MD, Wachs ME, Everson G, et al: Prednisone withdrawal 14 days after liver transplantation with mycophenolate: a prospective trial of cyclosporine and tacrolimus. *Transplantation* 1997;64:1755–1760.
61. Ducloux D, Fournier V, Bresson-Vautrin C, et al: Mycophenolate mofetil in renal transplant recipients with cyclosporineassociated nephrotoxicity: a preliminary report. *Transplantation* 1998;65:1504–1506.
62. Briggs JD: Causes of death after renal transplantation. *Nephrol Dial Transpl* 2001;16:1545–1549.
63. Foley RN, Parfrey PS, Sarnak MJ: Clinical epidemiology of cardiovascular disease in chronic renal disease. *Am J Kidney Dis* 1998;32:S112–S119.
64. Aakhus S, Dahl K, Wideroe TE: Cardiovascular disease in stable renal transplant patients in Norway: morbidity and mortality during a 5-yr follow-up. *Clin Transpl* 2004;18:596–604.
65. Lindholm A, Albrechtsen D, Frodin L, et al: Ischemic heart disease—major cause of death and graft loss after renal transplantation in Scandinavia. *Transplantation* 1995;60:451–457.
66. Madsen M, Jespersen B, Lokkegaard H, et al: Kidney transplantation activity and outcome in Denmark 1990–1999. *Clin Transpl* 2000;357–358.
67. Ojo AO, Hanson JA, Wolfe RA, et al: Long-term survival in renal transplant recipients with graft function. *Kidney Int* 2000;57: 307–313.
68. Kasiske BL, Maclean JR, Snyder JJ: Acute myocardial infarction and kidney transplantation. *J Am Soc Nephrol* 2006;17: 900–907.
69. Aker S, Ivens K, Guo Z, et al: Cardiovascular complications after renal transplantation. *Transpl Proc* 1998;30:2039–2042.
70. Bumgardner GL, Wilson GA, Tso PL, et al: Impact of serum lipids on long-term graft and patient survival after renal transplantation. *Transplantation* 1995;60:1418–1421.
71. Hillebrand GF, Schlosser S, Schneeberger H, et al: No clinical evidence of hyperlipidemia as a risk factor for chronic renal allograft failure. *Transpl Proc* 1999;31:1391–1392.
72. Kasiske BL, Guijarro C, Massy ZA, et al: Cardiovascular disease after renal transplantation. *J Am Soc Nephrol* 1996;7:158–165.
73. Ong CS, Pollock CA, Caterson RJ, et al: Hyperlipidemia in renal transplant recipients: natural history and response to treatment. *Medicine (Baltimore)* 1994;73:215–223.
74. Pollock CA, Mahony JF, Ong CS, et al: Hyperlipidemia in renal transplant recipients: does it matter and can we treat it? *Transpl Proc* 1995;27:2152–2153.
75. Roodnat JI, Mulder PG, Zietse R, et al: Cholesterol as an independent predictor of outcome after renal transplantation. *Transplantation* 2000;69:1704–1710.
76. Jardine AG, Holdaas H, Fellstrom B, et al: Fluvastatin prevents cardiac death and myocardial infarction in renal transplant recipients: post-hoc subgroup analyses of the ALERT Study. *Am J Transpl* 2004;4:988–995.
77. Holdaas H, Fellstrom B, Holme I, et al: Effects of fluvastatin on cardiac events in renal transplant patients: ALERT (Assessment of Lescol in Renal Transplantation) study design and baseline data. *J Cardiovasc Risk* 2001;8:63–71.
78. Soveri I, Holdaas H, Jardine A, et al: Renal transplant dysfunction—importance quantified in comparison with traditional risk factors for cardiovascular disease and mortality. *Nephrol Dial Transpl* 2006;21:2282–2289.
79. Abbott KC, Bucci JR, Cruess D, et al: Graft loss and acute coronary syndromes after renal transplantation in the United States. *J Am Soc Nephrol* 2002;13:2560–2569.
80. Abbott KC, Yuan CM, Taylor AJ, et al: Early renal insufficiency and hospitalized heart disease after renal transplantation in the era of modern immunosuppression. *J Am Soc Nephrol* 2003;14:2358–2365.
81. Fellstrom B, Holdaas H, Jardine AG, et al: Effect of fluvastatin on renal end points in the Assessment of Lescol in Renal Transplant (ALERT) trial. *Kidney Int* 2004;66:1549–1555.
82. Gill JS, Abichandani R, Kausz AT, et al: Mortality after kidney transplant failure: the impact of non-immunologic factors. *Kidney Int* 2002;62:1875–1883.
83. Woo YM, McLean D, Kavanagh D, et al: The influence of preoperative electrocardiographic abnormalities and cardiovascular risk factors on patient and graft survival following renal transplantation. *J Nephrol* 2002;15:380–386.
84. Foldes K, Maklary E, Vargha P, et al: Effect of diet and fluvastatin treatment on the serum lipid profile of kidney transplant, diabetic recipients: a 1-year follow up. *Transpl Int* 1998;11(suppl 1): S65–S68.
85. Massy ZA, Ma JZ, Louis TA, et al: Lipid-lowering therapy in patients with renal disease. *Kidney Int* 1995;48:188–198.
86. Tonstad S, Holdaas H, Gorbitz C, et al: Is dietary intervention effective in post-transplant hyperlipidaemia? *Nephrol Dial Transpl* 1995;10:82–85.
87. Painter PL, Hector L, Ray K, et al: Effects of exercise training on coronary heart disease risk factors in renal transplant recipients. *Am J Kidney Dis* 2003;42:362–369.

88. Keogh A, Day R, Critchley L, et al: The effect of food and cholestyramine on the absorption of cyclosporine in cardiac transplant recipients. *Transpl Proc* 1988;20:27–30.
89. Jensen RA, Lal SM, az-Arias A, et al: Does cholestyramine interfere with cyclosporine absorption? A prospective study in renal transplant patients. *ASAIO J* 1995;41:M704–M706.
90. Ballantyne CM, Corsini A, Davidson MH, et al: Risk for myopathy with statin therapy in high-risk patients. *Arch Intern Med* 2003;163:553–564.
91. Lal SM, Hewett JE, Petroski GF, et al: Effects of nicotinic acid and lovastatin in renal transplant patients: a prospective, randomized, open-labeled crossover trial. *Am J Kidney Dis* 1995;25:616–622.
92. Parra JL, Reddy KR: Hepatotoxicity of hypolipidemic drugs. *Clin Liver Dis* 2003;7:415–433.
93. Vogt A, Kassner U, Hostalek U, et al: Evaluation of the safety and tolerability of prolonged-release nicotinic acid in a usual care setting: The NAUTILUS study. *Curr Med Res Opin* 2006;22:417–425.
94. Launay-Vacher V, Izzedine H, Deray G: Statins' dosage in patients with renal failure and cyclosporine drug–drug interactions in transplant recipient patients. *Int J Cardiol* 2005;101:9–17.
95. Samman A, Imai C, Straatman L, et al: Safety and efficacy of rosuvastatin therapy for the prevention of hyperlipidemia in adult cardiac transplant recipients. *J Heart Lung Transpl* 2005;24:1008–1013.
96. Asberg A, Hartmann A, Fjeldsa E, et al: Bilateral pharmacokinetic interaction between cyclosporine A and atorvastatin in renal transplant recipients. *Am J Transpl* 2001;1:382–386.
97. Asberg A, Holdaas H, Jardine AG, et al: Fluvastatin reduces atherogenic lipids without any effect on native endothelial function early after kidney transplantation. *Clin Transpl* 2003;17:385–390.
98. Gullestad L, Nordal KP, Berg KJ, et al: Interaction between lovastatin and cyclosporine A after heart and kidney transplantation. *Transpl Proc* 1999;31:2163–2165.
99. Hermann M, Asberg A, Christensen H, et al: Substantially elevated levels of atorvastatin and metabolites in cyclosporine-treated renal transplant recipients. *Clin Pharmacol Ther* 2004;76:388–391.
100. Hermann M, Asberg A, Christensen H, et al: Atorvastatin does not affect the pharmacokinetics of cyclosporine in renal transplant recipients. *Eur J Clin Pharmacol* 2005;61:59–62.
101. Holdaas H, Hagen E, Asberg A, et al: Evaluation of the pharmacokinetic interaction between fluvastatin XL and cyclosporine in renal transplant recipients. *Int J Clin Pharmacol Ther* 2006;44:163–171.
102. Holdaas H, Hartmann A, Stenstrom J, et al: Effect of fluvastatin for safely lowering atherogenic lipids in renal transplant patients receiving cyclosporine. *Am J Cardiol* 1995;76:102A–106A.
103. Holdaas H, Jardine AG, Wheeler DC, et al: Effect of fluvastatin on acute renal allograft rejection: a randomized multicenter trial. *Kidney Int* 2001;60:1990–1997.
104. Imamura R, Ichimaru N, Moriyama T, et al: Long term efficacy of simvastatin in renal transplant recipients treated with cyclosporine or tacrolimus. *Clin Transpl* 2005;19:616–621.
105. Kobashigawa JA, Murphy FL, Stevenson LW, et al: Low-dose lovastatin safely lowers cholesterol after cardiac transplantation. *Circulation* 1990;82:IV281–IV283.
106. Lemahieu WP, Hermann M, Asberg A, et al: Combined therapy with atorvastatin and calcineurin inhibitors: no interactions with tacrolimus. *Am J Transpl* 2005;5:2236–2243.
107. Martinez-Castelao A, Grinyo JM, Gil-Vernet S, et al: Lipidlowering long-term effects of six different statins in hypercholesterolemic renal transplant patients under cyclosporine immunosuppression. *Transpl Proc* 2002;34:398–400.
108. Rehman MA, al-Sulaiman MH, Mousa DH, et al: Effects of simvastatin in hyperlipidemic renal transplant patients receiving cyclosporine. *Transplantation* 1995;60:397–399.
109. Yoshimura N, Oka T, Okamoto M, et al: The effects of pravastatin on hyperlipidemia in renal transplant recipients. *Transplantation* 1992;53:94–99.
110. Third Report of the National Cholesterol Education Program (NCEP) Expert Panel on Detection, Evaluation, and Treatment of High Blood Cholesterol in Adults (Adult Treatment Panel III): Final report. *Circulation* 2002;106:3143–3421.
111. Grundy SM, Cleeman JI, Merz CN, et al: Implications of recent clinical trials for the National Cholesterol Education Program Adult Treatment Panel III guidelines. *Circulation* 2004;110:227–239.
112. Smith SC Jr, Allen J, Blair SN, et al: AHA/ACC guidelines for secondary prevention for patients with coronary and other atherosclerotic vascular disease: 2006 update endorsed by the National Heart, Lung, and Blood Institute. *J Am Coll Cardiol* 2006;47:2130–2139.
113. Kasiske B, Cosio FG, Beto J, et al: Clinical practice guidelines for managing dyslipidemias in kidney transplant patients: a report from the Managing Dyslipidemias in Chronic Kidney Disease Work Group of the National Kidney Foundation Kidney Disease Outcomes Quality Initiative. *Am J Transpl* 2004;4(suppl 7):13–53.
114. Sudhop T, Lutjohann D, Kodal A, et al: Inhibition of intestinal cholesterol absorption by ezetimibe in humans. *Circulation* 2002;106:1943–1948.
115. Bergman AJ, Burke J, Larson P, et al: Interaction of single-dose ezetimibe and steady-state cyclosporine in renal transplant patients. *J Clin Pharmacol* 2006;46:328–336.
116. Bilchick KC, Henrikson CA, Skojec D, et al: Treatment of hyperlipidemia in cardiac transplant recipients. *Am Heart J* 2004;148:200–210.
117. Buchanan C, Smith L, Corbett J, et al: A retrospective analysis of ezetimibe treatment in renal transplant recipients. *Am J Transpl* 2006;6:770–774.
118. Gazi IF, Liberopoulos EN, Athyros VG, et al: Statins and solid organ transplantation. *Curr Pharm Des* 2006;12:4771–4783.
119. Kohnle M, Pietruck F, Kribben A, et al: Ezetimibe for the treatment of uncontrolled hypercholesterolemia in patients with high-dose statin therapy after renal transplantation. *Am J Transpl* 2006;6:205–208.
120. Koshman SL, Lalonde LD, Burton I, et al: Supratherapeutic response to ezetimibe administered with cyclosporine. *Ann Pharmacother* 2005;39:1561–1565.
121. Langone AJ, Chuang P: Ezetimibe in renal transplant patients with hyperlipidemia resistant to HMG-CoA reductase inhibitors. *Transplantation* 2006;81:804–807.
122. Panichi V, Manca-Rizza G, Paoletti S, et al: Safety and effects on the lipid and C-reactive protein plasma concentration of the association of ezetimibe plus atorvastatin in renal transplant patients treated by cyclosporine-A: a pilot study. *Biomed Pharmacother* 2006;60:249–252.
123. Patel AR, Ambrose MS, Duffy GA, et al: Treatment of hypercholesterolemia with ezetimibe in cardiac transplant recipients. *J Heart Lung Transpl* 2007;26:281–284.
124. Puthenparumpil JJ, Keough-Ryan T, Kiberd M, et al: Treatment of hypercholesterolemia with ezetimibe in the kidney transplant population. *Transpl Proc* 2005;37:1033–1035.
125. Bays HE, Dujovne CA: Drugs for treatment of patients with high cholesterol blood levels and other dyslipidemias. *Prog Drug Res* 1994;43:9–41.
126. Tatsioni A, Chung M, Sun Y, et al: Effects of fish oil supplementation on kidney transplantation: a systematic review and meta-analysis of randomized, controlled trials. *J Am Soc Nephrol* 2005;16:2462–2470.
127. Thervet E, Legendre C, Beaune P, et al: Cytochrome P450 3A polymorphisms and immunosuppressive drugs. *Pharmacogenomics* 2005;6:37–47.
128. Asberg A: Interactions between cyclosporin and lipid-lowering drugs: implications for organ transplant recipients. Drugs 2003;63:367–378.
129. Zhang Y, Benet LZ: The gut as a barrier to drug absorption: Combined role of cytochrome P450 3A and P-glycoprotein. *Clin Pharmacokinet* 2001;40:159–168.
130. Bramow S, Ott P, Thomsen NF, et al: Cholestasis and regulation of genes related to drug metabolism and biliary transport in rat liver following treatment with cyclosporine A and sirolimus (Rapamycin). *Pharmacol Toxicol* 2001;89:133–139.
131. Akhlaghi F, McLachlan AJ, Keogh AM, et al: Effect of simvastatin on cyclosporine unbound fraction and apparent blood clearance in heart transplant recipients. *Br J Clin Pharmacol* 1997;44:537–542.
132. Olbricht C, Wanner C, Eisenhauer T, et al: Accumulation of lovastatin, but not pravastatin, in the blood of cyclosporinetreated kidney graft patients after multiple doses. *Clin Pharmacol Ther* 1997;62:311–321.

133. Regazzi MB, Iacona I, Campana C, et al: Altered disposition of pravastatin following concomitant drug therapy with cyclosporin A in transplant recipients. *Transpl Proc* 1993;25:2732–2734.
134. Arnadottir M, Eriksson LO, Thysell H, et al: Plasma concentration profiles of simvastatin 3-hydroxy–3-methyl-glutaryl-coenzyme A reductase inhibitory activity in kidney transplant recipients with and without ciclosporin. *Nephron* 1993;65:410–413.
135. Goldberg R, Roth D: Evaluation of fluvastatin in the treatment of hypercholesterolemia in renal transplant recipients taking cyclosporine. *Transplantation* 1996;62:1559–1564.
136. Corpier CL, Jones PH, Suki WN, et al: Rhabdomyolysis and renal injury with lovastatin use. Report of two cases in cardiac transplant recipients. *JAMA* 1988;260:239–241.
137. Corsini A, Holdaas H: Fluvastatin in the treatment of dyslipidemia associated with chronic kidney failure and renal transplantation. *Ren Fail* 2005;27:259–273.
138. East C, Alivizatos PA, Grundy SM, et al: Rhabdomyolysis in patients receiving lovastatin after cardiac transplantation. *N Engl J Med* 1988;318:47–48
139. Grekas D, Kassimatis E, Makedou A, et al: Combined treatment with low-dose pravastatin and fish oil in post-renal transplantation dislipidemia. *Nephron* 2001;88:329–333.
140. Gumprecht J, Zychma M, Grzeszczak W, et al: Simvastatinin-duced rhabdomyolysis in a CsA-treated renal transplant recipient. *Med Sci Monit* 2003;9:CS89–CS91.
141. Kotanko P, Kirisits W, Skrabal F: Rhabdomyolysis and acute renal graft impairment in a patient treated with simvastatin, tacrolimus, and fusidic acid. *Nephron* 2002;90:234–235.
142. Kusus M, Stapleton DD, Lertora JJ, et al: Rhabdomyolysis and acute renal failure in a cardiac transplant recipient due to multiple drug interactions. *Am J Med Sci* 2000;320:394–397.
143. Maltz HC, Balog DL, Cheigh JS: Rhabdomyolysis associated with concomitant use of atorvastatin and cyclosporine. *Ann Pharmacother* 1999;33:1176–1179.
144. Rodriguez JA, Crespo-Leiro MG, Paniagua MJ, et al: Rhabdomyolysis in heart transplant patients on HMG-CoA reductase inhibitors and cyclosporine. *Transpl Proc* 1999;31:2522–2523.
145. Rodriguez ML, Mora C, Navarro JF: Cerivastatin-induced rhabdomyolysis. *Ann Intern Med* 2000;132:598.
146. Segaert MF, De SC, Vandewiele I, et al: Drug-interaction-induced rhabdomyolysis. *Nephrol Dial Transpl* 1996;11:1846–1847. Stirling CM, Isles CG: Rhabdomyolysis due to simvastatin in a transplant patient: are some statins safer than others? *Nephrol Dial Transpl* 2001;16:873–874.
147. Stirling CM, Isles CG: Rhabdomyolysis due to simvastatin in a transplant patient: are some statins safer than others? *Nephrol Dial Transpl* 2001;16:873–874.
148. Weise WJ, Possidente CJ: Fatal rhabdomyolysis associated with simvastatin in a renal transplant patient. *Am J Med* 2000;108:351–352.
149. Cosio FG, Pesavento TE, Pelletier RP, et al: Patient survival after renal transplantation III: the effects of statins. *Am J Kidney Dis* 2002;40:638–643.
150. Holdaas H, Fellstrom B, Jardine AG, et al: Beneficial effect of early initiation of lipid-lowering therapy following renal transplantation. *Nephrol Dial Transpl* 2005;20:974–980.
151. Hamar P, Muller V, Kohnle M, et al: Metabolic factors have a major impact on kidney allograft survival. *Transplantation* 1997;64:1135–1139.
152. Isoniemi H, Nurminen M, Tikkanen MJ, et al: Risk factors predicting chronic rejection of renal allografts. *Transplantation* 1994;57:68–72.
153. Katznelson S, Wilkinson AH, Kobashigawa JA, et al: The effect of pravastatin on acute rejection after kidney transplantation—a pilot study. *Transplantation* 1996;61:1469–1474.
154. Masterson R, Hewitson T, Leikis M, et al: Impact of statin treatment on 1-year functional and histologic renal allograft outcome. *Transplantation* 2005;80:332–338.
155. Tuncer M, Suleymanlar G, Ersoy FF, et al: Comparison of the effects of simvastatin and pravastatin on acute rejection episodes in renal transplant patients. *Transpl Proc* 2000;32:622–625.
156. Kwak B, Mulhaupt F, Myit S, et al: Statins as a newly recognized type of immunomodulator. *Nat Med* 2000;6:1399–1402.
157. Weitz-Schmidt G, Welzenbach K, Brinkmann V, et al: Statins selectively inhibit leukocyte function antigen-1 by binding to a novel regulatory integrin site. *Nat Med* 2001;7:687–692.
158. Holdaas H, Jardine A: Acute renal allograft rejections, a role for statins? *Minerva Urol Nefrol* 2003;55:111–119.
159. Kasiske BL, Heim-Duthoy KL, Singer GG, et al: The effects of lipid-lowering agents on acute renal allograft rejection. *Transplantation* 2001;72:223–227.
160. Sahu K, Sharma R, Gupta A, et al: Effect of lovastatin, an HMG CoA reductase inhibitor, on acute renal allograft rejection. *Clin Transpl* 2001;15:173–175.
161. Lentine KL, Brennan DC: Statin use after renal transplantation: a systematic quality review of trial-based evidence. *Nephrol Dial Transpl* 2004;19:2378–2386.
162. Stamler JS, Vaughan DE, Rudd MA, et al: Frequency of hypercholesterolemia after cardiac transplantation. *Am J Cardiol* 1988;62:1268–1272.
163. Taylor DO, Edwards LB, Boucek MM, et al: Registry of the International Society for Heart and Lung Transplantation: twenty-third official adult heart transplantation report–2006. *J Heart Lung Transpl* 2006;25:869–879.
164. Valantine HA: Role of lipids in allograft vascular disease: a multicenter study of intimal thickening detected by intravascular ultrasound. *J Heart Lung Transpl* 1995;14:S234–S237.
165. Eich D, Thompson JA, Ko DJ, et al: Hypercholesterolemia in long-term survivors of heart transplantation: an early marker of accelerated coronary artery disease. *J Heart Lung Transpl* 1991;10:45–49.
166. Kapadia SR, Nissen SE, Ziada KM, et al: Impact of lipid abnormalities in development and progression of transplant coronary disease: a serial intravascular ultrasound study. *J Am Coll Cardiol* 2001;38:206–213.
167. Kobashigawa JA, Tobis JM, Starling RC, et al: Multicenter intravascular ultrasound validation study among heart transplant recipients: outcomes after five years. *J Am Coll Cardiol* 2005;45:1532–1537.
168. Kobashigawa JA, Starling RC, Mehra MR, et al: Multicenter retrospective analysis of cardiovascular risk factors affecting long-term outcome of *de novo* cardiac transplant recipients. *J Heart Lung Transpl* 2006;25:1063–1069.
169. White M, Haddad H, Leblanc MH, et al: Conversion from cyclosporine microemulsion to tacrolimus-based immunoprophylaxis improves cholesterol profile in heart transplant recipients with treated but persistent dyslipidemia: the Canadian multicentre randomized trial of tacrolimus vs cyclosporine microemulsion. *J Heart Lung Transpl* 2005;24:798–809.
170. Eisen HJ, Tuzcu EM, Dorent R, et al: Everolimus for the prevention of allograft rejection and vasculopathy in cardiactransplant recipients. *N Engl J Med* 2003;349:847–858.
171. Keogh A, Richardson M, Ruygrok P, et al: Sirolimus in *de novo* heart transplant recipients reduces acute rejection and prevents coronary artery disease at 2 years: a randomized clinical trial. *Circulation* 2004;110:2694–2700.
172. Wenke K, Meiser B, Thiery J, et al: Simvastatin reduces graft vessel disease and mortality after heart transplantation: four-year randomized trial. *Circulation* 1997;96:1398–1402.
173. Weis M, Pehlivanli S, Meiser BM, et al: Simvastatin treatment is associated with improvement in coronary endothelial function and decreased cytokine activation in patients after heart transplantation. *J Am Coll Cardiol* 2001;38:814–818.
174. Wu AH, Ballantyne CM, Short BC, et al: Statin use and risks of death or fatal rejection in the Heart Transplant Lipid Registry. *Am J Cardiol* 2005;95:367–372.
175. Wenke K: Management of hyperlipidaemia associated with heart transplantation. *Drugs* 2004;64:1053–1068.
176. Regazzi MB, Iacona I, Campana C, et al: Clinical efficacy and pharmacokinetics of HMG-CoA reductase inhibitors in heart transplant patients treated with cyclosporin A. *Transpl Proc* 1994;26:2644–2645.
177. McPherson R, Tsoukas C, Baines MG, et al: Effects of lovastatin on natural killer cell function and other immunological parameters in man. *J Clin Immunol* 1993;13:439–444.
178. Palinski W, Tsimikas S: Immunomodulatory effects of statins: mechanisms and potential impact on arteriosclerosis. *J Am Soc Nephrol* 2002;13:1673–1681.
179. Napoli C, de Nigris F, Palinski W: Multiple role of reactive oxygen species in the arterial wall. *J Cell Biochem* 2001;82: 674–682.
180. Laufs U, Liao JK: Direct vascular effects of HMG-CoA reductase inhibitors. *Trends Cardiovasc Med* 2000;10:143–148.
181. Liu L, Moesner P, Kovach NL, et al: Integrin-dependent leukocyte adhesion involves geranylgeranylated protein(s). *J Biol Chem* 1999;274:33334–33340.

182. Essig M, Nguyen G, Prie D, et al: 3-Hydroxy–3-methylglutaryl coenzyme A reductase inhibitors increase fibrinolytic activity in rat aortic endothelial cells. Role of geranylgeranylation and Rho proteins. *Circ Res* 1998;83:683–690.
183. Wassmann S, Laufs U, Baumer AT, et al: HMG-CoA reductase inhibitors improve endothelial dysfunction in normocholesterolemic hypertension via reduced production of reactive oxygen species. *Hypertension* 2001;37:1450–1457.
184. Endres M, Laufs U, Huang Z, et al: Stroke protection by 3-hydroxy–3-methylglutaryl (HMG)-CoA reductase inhibitors mediated by endothelial nitric oxide synthase. *Proc Natl Acad Sci U S A* 1998;95:8880–8885.
185. Guijarro C, Blanco-Colio LM, Ortego M, et al: 3-Hydroxy–3-methylglutaryl coenzyme a reductase and isoprenylation inhibitors induce apoptosis of vascular smooth muscle cells in culture. *Circ Res* 1998;83:490–500.
186. Si MS, Ji P, Tromberg BJ, et al: Farnesyltransferase inhibition: a novel method of immunomodulation. *Int Immunopharmacol* 2003;3:475–483.
187. Gisbert C, Prieto M, Berenguer M, et al: Hyperlipidemia in liver transplant recipients: prevalence and risk factors. *Liver Transpl Surg* 1997;3:416–422.
188. Guckelberger O, Bechstein WO, Neuhaus R, et al: Cardiovascular risk factors in long-term follow-up after orthotopic liver transplantation. *Clin Transpl* 1997;11:60–65.
189. Guckelberger O, Mutzke F, Glanemann M, et al: Validation of cardiovascular risk scores in a liver transplant population. *Liver Transpl* 2006;12:394–401.
190. Mathe D, Adam R, Malmendier C, et al: Prevalence of dyslipidemia in liver transplant recipients. *Transplantation* 1992;54:167–170.
191. Neal DA, Alexander GJ: Can the potential benefits of statins in general medical practice be extrapolated to liver transplantation? *Liver Transpl* 2001;7:1009–1014.
192. Reuben A: Long-term management of the liver transplant patient: diabetes, hyperlipidemia, and obesity. *Liver Transpl* 2001;7:S13–S21.
193. Sethi A, Stravitz RT: Review article: medical management of the liver transplant recipient—a primer for non-transplant doctors. *Aliment Pharmacol Ther* 2007;25:229–245.
194. Munoz SJ: Hyperlipidemia and other coronary risk factors after orthotopic liver transplantation: pathogenesis, diagnosis, and management. *Liver Transpl Surg* 1995;1:29–38.
195. Abbasoglu O, Levy MF, Brkic BB, et al: Ten years of liver transplantation: an evolving understanding of late graft loss. *Transplantation* 1997;64:1801–1807.
196. Appleton CP, Hurst RT, Lee KS, et al: Long-term cardiovascular risk in the orthotopic liver transplant population. *Liver Transpl* 2006;12:352–355.
197. Fernandez-Miranda C, de la CA, Morales JM, et al: Lipoprotein abnormalities in long-term stable liver and renal transplanted patients. A comparative study. *Clin Transpl* 1998;12:136–141.
198. Neuberger J: Liver transplantation. *J Hepatol* 2000;32:198–207.
199. Imagawa DK, Dawson S III, Holt CD, et al: Hyperlipidemia after liver transplantation: natural history and treatment with the hydroxy-methylglutaryl-coenzyme A reductase inhibitor pravastatin. *Transplantation* 1996;62:934–942.
200. Taylor PJ, Kubler PA, Lynch SV, et al: Effect of atorvastatin on cyclosporine pharmacokinetics in liver transplant recipients. *Ann Pharmacother* 2004;38:205–208.
201. Zachoval R, Gerbes AL, Schwandt P, et al: Short-term effects of statin therapy in patients with hyperlipoproteinemia after liver transplantation: results of a randomized cross-over trial. *J Hepatol* 2001;35:86–91.
202. Singh TP, Naftel DC, Webber S, et al: Hyperlipidemia in children after heart transplantation. *J Heart Lung Transpl* 2006;25:1199–1205.
203. Goldstein S, Duhamel G, Laudat MH, et al: Plasma lipids, lipoproteins and apolipoproteins AI, AII, and B in renal transplanted children: what risk for accelerated atherosclerosis? *Nephron* 1984;38:87–92.
204. Saland JM, Ginsberg H, Fisher EA: Dyslipidemia in pediatric renal disease: epidemiology, pathophysiology, and management. *Curr Opin Pediatr* 2002;14:197–204.
205. Silverstein DM: Indications and outcome of treatment of hyperlipidemia in pediatric allograft recipients. *Pediatr Transpl* 2003;7:7–10.
206. Silverstein DM, Palmer J, Polinsky MS, et al: Risk factors for hyperlipidemia in long-term pediatric renal transplant recipients. *Pediatr Nephrol* 2000;14:105–110.
207. Hyams JS, Treem WR, Andrews WS, et al: Lipid abnormalities in pediatric hepatic allograft recipients. *J Pediatr Gastroenterol Nutr* 1989;9:441–444.
208. McDiarmid SV, Gornbein JA, Fortunat M, et al: Serum lipid abnormalities in pediatric liver transplant patients. *Transplantation* 1992;53:109–115.
209. Argent E, Kainer G, Aitken M, et al: Atorvastatin treatment for hyperlipidemia in pediatric renal transplant recipients. *Pediatr Transpl* 2003;7:38–42.
210. Butani L: Prospective monitoring of lipid profiles in children receiving pravastatin preemptively after renal transplantation. *Pediatr Transpl* 2005;9:746–753.
211. Butani L, Pai MV, Makker SP: Pilot study describing the use of pravastatin in pediatric renal transplant recipients. *Pediatr Transpl* 2003;7:179–184.
212. Krmar RT, Ferraris JR, Ramirez JA, et al: Use of atorvastatin in hyperlipidemic hypertensive renal transplant recipients. *Pediatr Nephrol* 2002;17:540–543.
213. Chin C, Gamberg P, Miller J, et al: Efficacy and safety of atorvastatin after pediatric heart transplantation. *J Heart Lung Transpl* 2002;21:1213–1217.
214. Chin C, Rosenthal D, Bernstein D: Lipoprotein abnormalities are highly prevalent in pediatric heart transplant recipients. *Pediatr Transpl* 2000;4:193–199.
215. Hedman M, Neuvonen PJ, Neuvonen M, et al: Pharmacokinetics and pharmacodynamics of pravastatin in pediatric and adolescent cardiac transplant recipients on a regimen of triple immunosuppression. *Clin Pharmacol Ther* 2004;75:101–109.
216. Mahle WT, Vincent RN, Berg AM, et al: Pravastatin therapy is associated with reduction in coronary allograft vasculopathy in pediatric heart transplantation. *J Heart Lung Transpl* 2005;24:63–66.
217. Penson MG, Fricker FJ, Thompson JR, et al: Safety and efficacy of pravastatin therapy for the prevention of hyperlipidemia in pediatric and adolescent cardiac transplant recipients. *J Heart Lung Transpl* 2001;20:611–618.
218. Seipelt IM, Crawford SE, Rodgers S, et al: Hypercholesterolemia is common after pediatric heart transplantation: initial experience with pravastatin. *J Heart Lung Transpl* 2004;23:317–322.
219. Stefanutti C, Lucani G, Vivenzio A, et al: Diet only and diet plus simvastatin in the treatment of heterozygous familial hypercholesterolemia in childhood. *Drugs Exp Clin Res* 1999;25:23–28.

CHAPTER 41

Special Patient Populations: Chronic Renal Disease

Alan G. Jardine, Patrick B. Mark, Hallvard Holdaas, and Bengt Fellstrøm

INTRODUCTION

Chronic kidney disease (CKD) is associated with increased incidence of dyslipidemia and of premature cardiovascular disease (CVD).[1–3] However, the relationship is not as clear as that seen in the general population.[1–3] The pattern and magnitude of dyslipidemia are dependent on the degree of renal impairment, proteinuria, treatment, and the primary renal disease (PRD) (e.g., diabetes). The nature of CVD in patients with progressive PRD may also differ from the general population, with a disproportionate increase in fatal cardiac events, arrhythmias, and heart failure rather than typical coronary artery disease (CAD).[2,3] Despite these caveats, the National Kidney Foundation Task Force[3,4] and other national clinical guidelines recommend that patients with CKD be treated as patients at the highest risk for CVD, based on the reclassification of CKD by estimated glomerular filtration rate (eGFR) rather than serum creatinine.[4]

PRD causes progressive loss of renal excretory function (GFR) that is dependent on the underlying disease, genetic and environmental factors, and associated risk factors such as hypertension, hyperlipidemia, and proteinuria.[1–3] The rate of loss of renal function varies, and the proportion of patients who ultimately reach end-stage renal disease (ESRD) (with the requirement for dialysis and transplantation) is relatively small, although the associated human and economic costs of ESRD are considerable.[5] As GFR declines, the pattern of cardiovascular (CV) risk factors—including dyslipidemia—changes, reflecting both the impact of renal function and the indirect effects of undernutrition and chronic inflammation.[1,2,6,7] ESRD is associated with the need for dialysis (and/or transplantation), of which there are two forms—hemodialysis and peritoneal dialysis—that have different effects on CV risk factors, including dyslipidemia.[1,6,7] An appreciation of the variable nature of CV risk factors through the natural history of PRD is central to understanding the impact and treatment of hyperlipidemia in this population (Table 41-1; Fig. 41-1).

CHRONIC KIDNEY DISEASE AND LIPID METABOLISM

The characteristic features of the dyslipidemia associated with CKD are high triglycerides (TG), low high-density lipoprotein (HDL) cholesterol (see Table 41-1; Fig. 41-1), elevated intermediate-density lipoprotein (IDL) cholesterol, and a variable (often neutral) effect on low-density lipoproteins (LDL) and total plasma cholesterol.[1,2,6–9] There are also a variety of qualitative changes in lipoproteins, specifically failure of maturation and an excess of TG-rich, more-atherogenic lipoproteins.[8,9] Contributory factors include the direct effect of reduced GFR, the effects of proteinuria, the impact of treatment, and malnutrition in patients with more advanced renal failure.

Mechanisms of Dyslipidemia

The observed changes in lipoproteins reflect alterations in enzyme and receptor function. The enzymatic defects associated with uremic dyslipidemia have been extensively investigated, and expertly reviewed by Vaziri.[10] The key effects are listed in Table 41-1 and Figure 41-1. A central effect is reduced function of lipoprotein lipase (LPL), due to reduced gene expression,[10,11] reduced endothelial expression (compounded in patients on hemodialysis by displacement of endothelial LPL by heparin[12]), and reduced LPL activity.[13] In addition to heparin, there are circulating factors

TABLE 41-1 Patterns and Determinants of Dyslipidemia in Renal Failure

Lipid Subclass	Patient Population				Mechanisms and Observed Effects
	CRF/CKD	CKD Plus Proteinuria	Peritoneal Dialysis	Hemodialysis	
Total cholesterol	↔	↑	↑	↔	Malnutrition, inflammation, and reduced food intake are major effects balancing the direct effect of CKD on plasma lipids.
LDL cholesterol	↔	↑	↑	↔	Malnutrition, inflammation, and reduced food intake are major effects balancing the direct effect of CKD on plasma lipids. Increased HMG-CoA activity in proteinuric states. Reduced LDL receptor function.
HDL cholesterol	↓	↓	↓	↓	Reduced apoA-I, LCAT, and hepatic lipase; increased CETP and ACAT contribute to reduced HDL cholesterol and increased HDL TG content.
TG	↑	↑	↑	↑	Reduced lipoprotein lipase and VLDL receptor function.
Other lipoproteins	↑ IDL ↑ Small dense LDL (LDL III) ↑ VLDL ↑ Lp(a) ↑ Oxidized LDL	↑ IDL ↑ Small dense LDL (LDL III) ↑ VLDL ↑ Lp(a) ↑ Oxidized LDL	↑ IDL	↑ IDL	Reduced hepatic lipase and LRP. Reduced VLDL receptor.

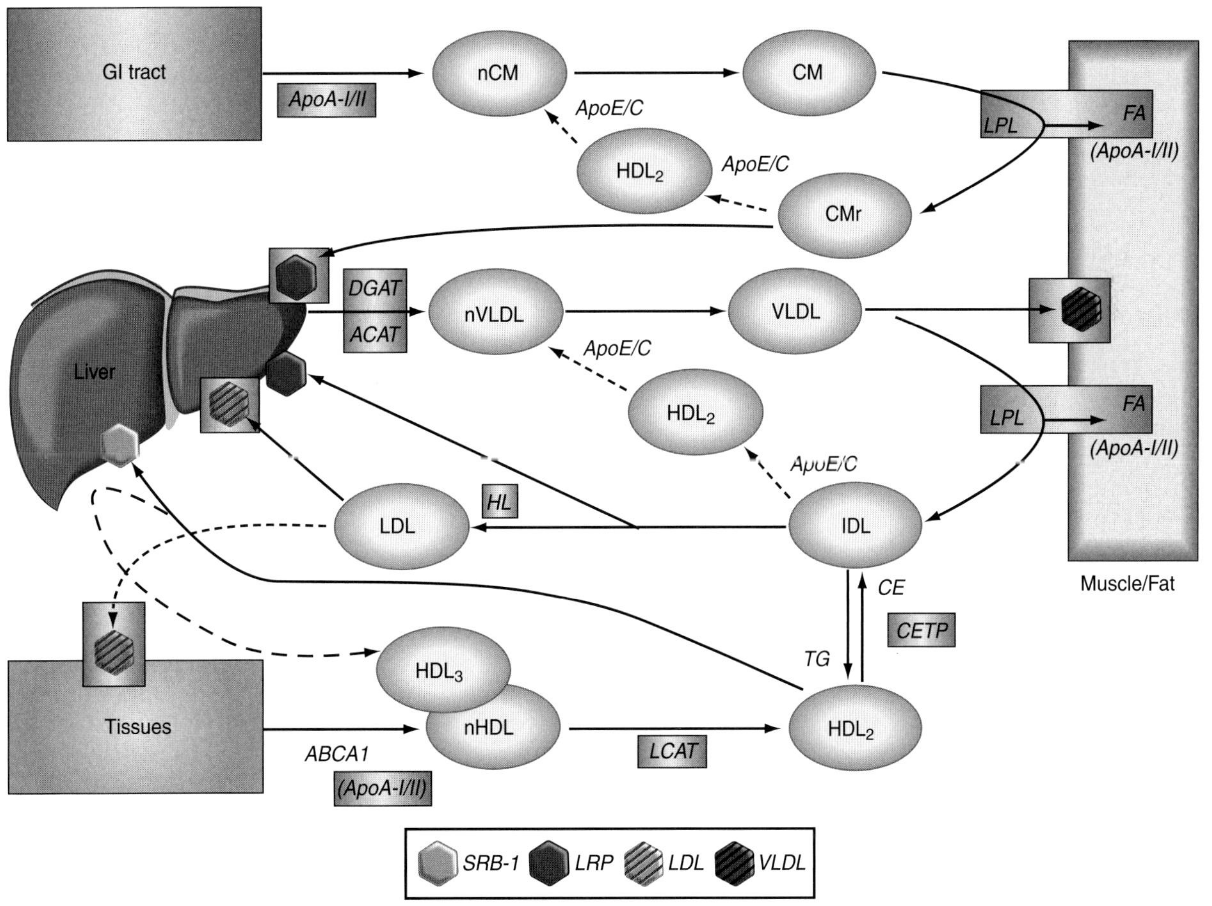

FIGURE 41-1 Key abnormalities in lipid metabolism associated with renal failure, and their effects on circulating lipids. The main defects are shaded. Hexagonal markers indicate receptors (see text). Lipid subfractions are circled (n = nascent). Enzymes, transporters, and apoproteins are marked (see text for details). Major defects are as follows. (1) *High TG:* Reduced activity of LPL and HL are the principal defects that lead to impaired removal of TG from CM and VLDL. (2) *Increased IDL:* Reduced HL and impaired LRP are the major contributors to impaired CM remnant and IDL clearance, and hence elevated IDL levels. (3) *Low HDL:* Reduced apoA-I, reduced cholesterol esterification by LCAT, and increased CETP exchange of CE for TG lead to low HDL levels, increased HDL-TG, and reduced HDL cholesterol. (4) *Elevated chylomicron and VLDL concentrations* are largely a consequence of reduced LPL activity. For additional detail and abbreviations, see text. (Adapted from Ref. 10.)

in renal failure that impair LPL function. These include increased pre-β-HDL and reduced apolipoprotein (apo) C-II, which inhibits LPL activity, and reduced apoE, which in turn reduces substrate binding to endothelial LPL.[10,14] Elevated parathyroid hormone and insulin resistance may also reduce LPL function in CKD.[10,15] The impact of reduced LPL function is to reduce lipolysis of very-low-density lipoproteins (VLDL) and chylomicrons (CM), resulting in increased plasma levels. Hepatic lipase activity[16] is also impaired and contributes to the observed pattern of dyslipidemia,[1,2,6,7,16] specifically the impaired clearance of IDL and increased TG concentration in IDL, LDL, HDL, and CM.

3-Hydroxy-3-methylglutaryl–coenzyme A (HMG-CoA) reductase is the major rate-limiting enzyme for cholesterol biosynthesis. In experimental models of CKD,[17] most evidence suggests that reduced GFR does not affect cholesterol synthesis, although heavy proteinuria in the nephrotic range does increase HMG-CoA reductase expression.[18,19] In experimental animals, renal failure is associated with reduced lecithin: cholesterol acyltransferase (LCAT) gene expression in the liver,[20] and thus impaired cholesterol esterification. Functional LCAT deficiency is consistently observed in animal models of CKD[10,20] and in patients with ESRD,[21] and is a major factor that contributes to reduced HDL cholesterol uptake from peripheral tissue, failure of HDL maturation, and low levels of plasma HDL cholesterol in CKD. Cholesteryl ester is exchanged for TG, between HDL and IDL, under the influence of cholesteryl ester transfer protein (CETP) (see Fig. 41-1).

The activity of CETP appears to be increased by approximately one-third[22] in patients receiving hemodialysis and is increased in the presence of proteinuria. Increased CETP may thus contribute to the higher levels of HDL TG seen in renal failure (see Table 41-1) (see Fig. 41-1). HDL contains apoA-I and apoA-II, which activate LCAT and hepatic lipase, respectively. Both apoA-I and apoA-II are reduced in models of renal failure, a consequence of reduced hepatic gene expression[23] that contributes to reduced synthesis and maturation of HDL. ApoA-II also serves as the ligand for scavenger receptor class B type I (SR-BI), an HDL-binding protein that targets HDL cholesteryl ester and TG for disposal[24] (see below).

Acyl–coenzyme A cholesterol acyltransferase (ACAT) limits de-esterification of cholesteryl esters and release of free cholesterol from extrahepatic tissues.[10] ACAT gene expression and activity is increased in CKD, which further impairs HDL-mediated cholesterol uptake and maturation.[25] Hypertriglyceridemia is a characteristic component of uremic dyslipidemia.[1,2,6,7,10] Hepatic acyl–coenzyme A:diacylglycerol acyltransferase (DGAT) is the final step in TG biosynthesis.[10] Although DGAT activity is reduced in experimental CKD,[26,27] with the implication that clearance of TG—rather than increased production—is the mechanism of hypertriglyceridemia, DGAT activity is greatly increased in proteinuric states,[27] contributing to the hypertriglyceridemia that characterizes the nephrotic syndrome.

In addition to enzymatic defects, changes in receptors and other proteins contribute to dyslipidemia. LDL receptor–related protein (LRP) clears plasma IDL and CM (targeted by apoE and apoB)[10] remnants in the liver. In experimental models of CKD, LRP expression is reduced, contributing to elevated levels of CM and IDL.[10,28] The VLDL receptor mediates apoE-dependent VLDL clearance in skeletal and cardiac muscle, fat, and brain. Impaired expression of the VLDL receptor[29,30] may contribute to elevated VLDL in uremia. The LDL receptor mediates the uptake of LDL cholesterol by the liver. Low GFR does not alter LDL receptor expression in the liver, although it is substantially reduced in the presence of proteinuria.[10,31,32] Reduced LDL receptor expression thus contributes to the pattern of dyslipidemia seen in proteinuric states and the nephrotic syndrome (see Table 41-1; see Fig. 41-1). ApoA-I and apoA-II are the major protein constituents of HDL; reduced levels of apoA-I and apoA-II are a consistent finding in patients with ESRD[10,23,31] and contribute to low HDL levels. ApoA-I is the ligand for ATP-binding cassette transporter (ABCA1) and SR-BI, which are responsible for the translocation of cholesterol to HDL in peripheral tissues and the unloading of cholesterol in the liver, respectively.[10,31] The HDL receptor SR-BI is reduced in the presence of nephrotic-range proteinuria, although not by renal impairment per se,[24,32] thus contributing to failure of reverse cholesterol transport in CKD associated with proteinuria.

Patterns of Dyslipidemia

The typical patterns of dyslipidemia in CKD are shown in Fig. 41-1 and Table 41-1. The major abnormalities are an increase in TG-rich particles and failure of maturation of individual particles. Reduced activity of LPL and hepatic lipase results in reduced clearance of CM and VLDL (and hence release of apoA-I and apoA-II), resulting in increased levels of TG (and TG-rich particles) in the plasma. The reduced apoA-I and apoA-II, which form the substrate for nascent HDL, contribute to reduced HDL that, in turn, contributes to impaired TG/cholesteryl ester exchange with IDL and the subsequent predominance of atherogenic, small dense LDL. In addition, there are major increases in oxidized LDL and lipoprotein(a) (Lp[a]) in patients with advanced chronic renal failure and in patients receiving chronic hemodialysis and peritoneal dialysis.[1,10,33,34]

RELATIONSHIP TO OUTCOMES

Cardiovascular Outcomes

In patients with early CKD, several studies have shown increased CV mortality. An analysis of more than 1 million patients from the Kaiser-Permanente database showed a progressive increase in CV and all-cause mortality associated with reduced eGFR.[35] Several other post hoc analyses of CV interventional trials, including those of lipid-lowering therapy,[36–38] have shown a similar inverse relationship between eGFR and outcome. Although these may provide evidence supporting the role of renal dysfunction as a CV risk factor, interpretation is confounded by the strong association of CV risk factors with renal impairment.[36–38] In ESRF, the relationship between total or

LDL cholesterol and CV (or all-cause) mortality typically reveals a "J-" or "U-"shaped relationship that contrasts with the progressive, linear relationship seen in other populations.[39] This relationship has led to reluctance to employ CV protection strategies identified in the general population. However, it is an example of reverse epidemiology,[39,40] in which CKD and its associated comorbid disease, malnutrition, and inflammation contribute to (and are associated with) low serum lipids (Fig. 41-2). When inflammatory markers, such as interleukin-6 (IL-6) and C-reactive protein (CRP), are corrected for, the underlying relationship between lipids and CV events is similar to that in the general population,[39] lending support to the use of lipid-lowering therapy in this population.

Renal Outcomes

Glomerulosclerosis is the histologic lesion that characterizes advanced stages of most forms of PRD. It shares similarities with atherosclerosis[41]; the glomerulus is replaced by extracellular matrix, produced by mesangial cells (which have phenotypic similarities with vascular smooth muscle cells). *In vitro*, the exposure of mesangial cells to LDL cholesterol and oxidized LDL is associated with increased matrix production; both lipoprotein and oxidized lipids have been identified in biopsy specimens from human kidneys.[42,43] Similarly, in experimental models, hypercholesterolemia is associated with the development of glomerulosclerosis[41,44,45] and lipid-lowering therapy with the attenuation of histologic changes.[41,45] An additional pathophysiologic mechanism may involve the direct effects of filtered lipoproteins on renal tubular cell function leading to tubulo-interstitial fibrosis. Statin therapy may interfere with this mechanism by reducing tubular protein uptake.[10,45,46] In patients with CKD,[43,47,48] including transplant recipients with impaired renal function, hyperlipidemia has been associated with glomerulosclerosis and with more rapid loss of renal function. Moreover, although proteinuria contributes to hyperlipidemia, the contributions of hyperlipidemia and proteinuria are independent and additive.[48]

IMPACT OF LIPID-LOWERING AGENTS ON LIPID MARKERS

Statins

Several small-scale studies have addressed the lipid-lowering efficacy and safety of statins in CKD. The United Kingdom Heart and Renal Protection (UK- HARP) study,[49] a prelude to the Study of Heart and Renal Protection (SHARP) (below), examined the effect of simvastatin 20 mg/day versus placebo in 448 patients with CKD (serum creatinine >1.7 mg/dL [150 μmol/L], including 73 patients on dialysis and 133 renal transplant recipients). The study had a 2×2 factorial design with aspirin. After 3 months, in the simvastatin arm total cholesterol fell from 202 to 163 mg/dL (–18%), LDL cholesterol from 124 to 84 mg/dL (–30%), non-HDL cholesterol from 164 to 116 (–28%), and TG from 189 to 162 (–15%), and there was a 5% increase in HDL cholesterol from 38 to 40 mg/dL. There was no impact on apoA-I levels, but statin therapy reduced apoB from 0.99 to 0.75 g/L (–23%). Lesser effects were observed at 12 months, a reflection of 80% compliance. The impact and pattern of changes resulting from statin use in the predialysis patients were similar to those observed in the general population; the effects in the subgroup receiving dialysis were qualitatively similar but proportionately around 25% of that the nondialysis group.

In a follow-up study, UK-HARP-II,[50] 203 nontransplant patients with CKD (152 predialysis, 51 dialysis recipients) were randomized to simvastatin

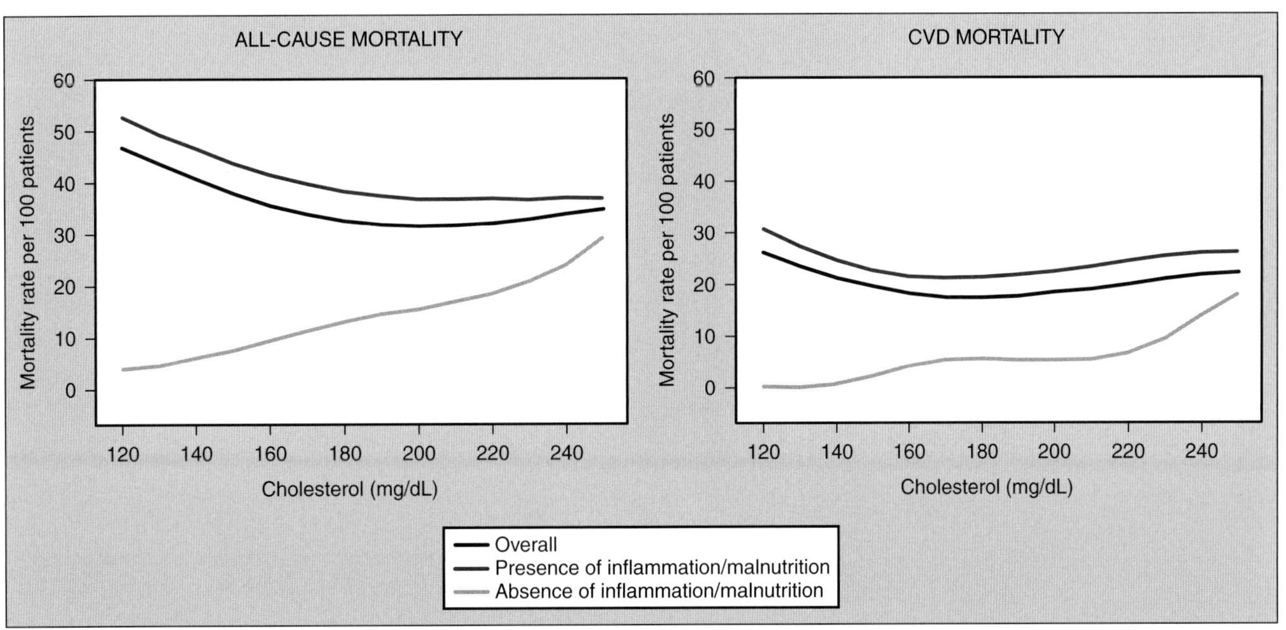

FIGURE 41–2 Relationship between total cholesterol and all-cause or CVD mortality in dialysis patients. The curves show an inverse relationship with total cholesterol that masks the underlying progressive relationship in patients without markers of inflammation. (From Ref. 39.)

with or without ezetimibe 10 mg/day. At 3 months in all patients, addition of ezetimibe resulted in a substantial benefit compared to simvastatin alone, without any significant increase in adverse events. Total cholesterol was reduced relatively by a further 25% (198 to 130 mg/dL vs. 195 to 151 mg/dL), LDL cholesterol by 21% (121 to 64 mg/dL vs. 117 to 81 mg/dL), and non-HDL cholesterol by 27% (158 to 87 mg/dL vs. 155 to 111 mg/dL). The simvastatin-dependent reduction in TG and apoB was further increased by approximately 10%, and there was no effect on HDL cholesterol or apoA-I.[50]

In Die Deutsche Diabetes Dialyse (4D) study, in type 2 diabetic hemodialysis patients receiving atorvastatin 10 mg/day, LDL cholesterol fell from 121 to 72 mg/dL,[51] although other lipid subfractions have not yet been reported (Fig. 41-3). An earlier study of atorvastatin 10 mg daily versus placebo in patients receiving peritoneal dialysis showed a 29% reduction in total cholesterol, a 40% reduction in LDL cholesterol, a 14.3% reduction in TG, and a 7.4% increase in HDL cholesterol in 59 patients who completed 16 weeks of treatment.[52] Overall, the treatment was well tolerated with a small increase in minor gastrointestinal side effects.

Fibrates

Fibrates are typically used in patients with hypertriglyceridemia—as seen in renal disease. However, their use in renal disease has been associated with an increased incidence of myositis, rhabdomyolysis and increased serum creatinine,[10,53] particularly when used in combination with statins.[10,53,54] A detailed comparison of cerivastatin and fenofibrate[54] in 12 patients with the nephrotic syndrome demonstrated comparable reductions in total cholesterol (21% vs. 19%, respectively), apoB (21% vs. 27%), and apoE (20% vs. 32%). Cerivastatin had a greater impact on LDL cholesterol (23% vs. 8% reduction) and IDL cholesterol (20% vs. 8%), but an inferior effect on TG (14% vs. 41%), VLDL cholesterol (16% vs. 52%), apoC-II and apoC-III, and $VLDL_1$ and $VLDL_2$. HDL was increased by 19% by fenofibrate. As discussed above, the tendency toward small dense LDL in CKD is atherogenic. Fenofibrate increased LDL_1 and LDL_2, but reduced LDL_3, statin therapy reduced LDL_1 and LDL_3, but had no effect on LDL_2. The overall effect of fibrate on LDL cholesterol was neutral. Atherogenic, cholesterol, and TG-rich remnants were also reduced by fibrate but not by statin therapy.

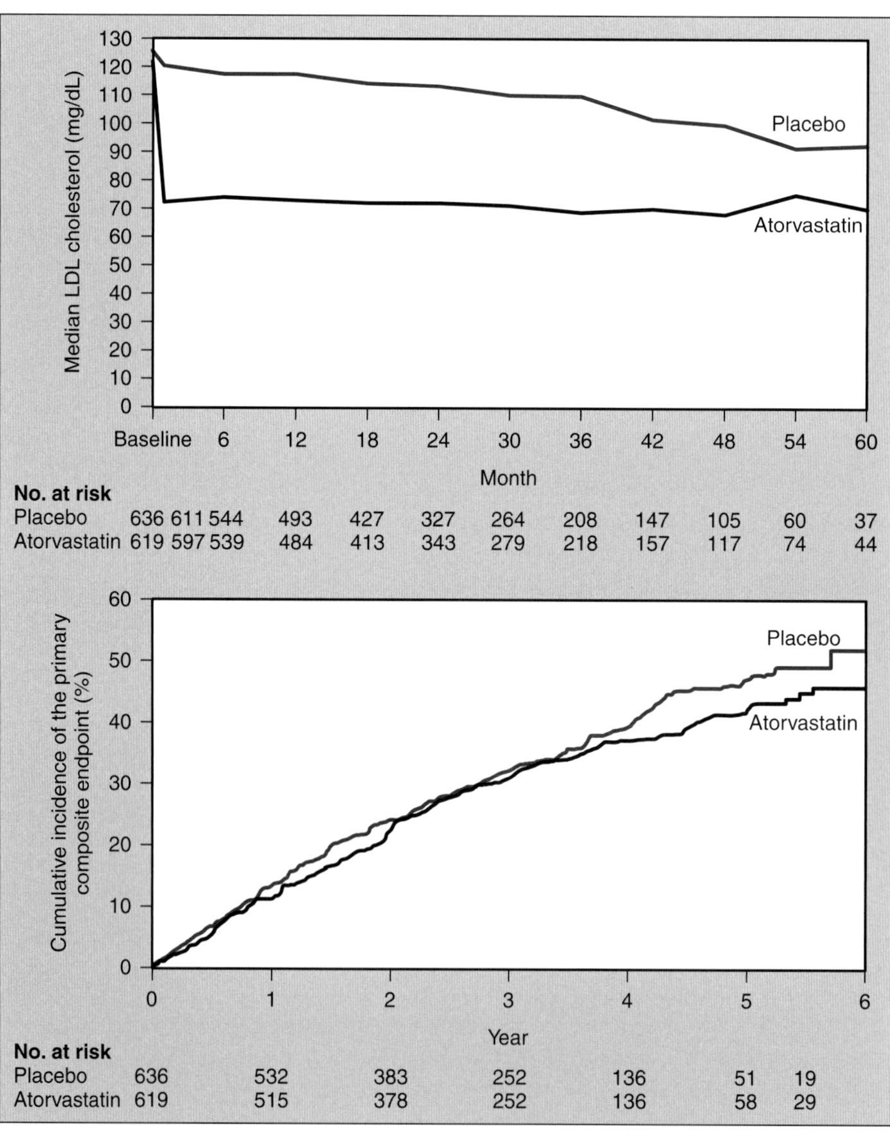

FIGURE 41-3 The 4D study showed the impact of atorvastatin on plasma lipids and absence of a significant impact on the composite CV endpoint in patients with type 2 diabetes receiving hemodialysis therapy. (From Ref. 41.)

Nicotinic Acid Derivatives

Niacin and related compounds may have beneficial effects on HDL cholesterol and hypertriglyceridemia in renal disease. However, there are limited data on their effect in kidney disease.[55] Bile acid sequestrants have not proved popular and have a side effect profile that is unlikely to be well tolerated in CKD.[10] One additional therapeutic approach in patients with advanced renal failure is the effect of phosphate binders, specifically sevelamer and related compounds. In addition to binding phosphate, these agents bind lipids in the gut, reducing total cholesterol by approximately 20% and LDL cholesterol by around 20%, but without appreciable effects on HDL cholesterol or TG.[56]

Side Effects

Statin therapy is most commonly associated with gastrointestinal side effects. These do not appear to be particularly increased in patients with mild CKD. However, there is a small increased risk of rhabdomyolysis, which is further increased by the concomitant use of statins and fibrates in CKD.[53] Fibrates have been associated with acute renal failure.[53] Thus, although there are potentially favorable effects of fibrates, statins have been favored in clinical use, and the combination of statin and fibrate is discouraged in published guidelines.

Statins are the most commonly used first-line agents. They differ in their metabolism and, specifically, metabolism by the microsomal enzymes CYP3A4 and CYP2C9. Recommendations about dosage reduction for individual agents according to the degree of renal impairment vary, but in general it is not necessary to reduce dosage more than 50%, unless agents are used in combination with cyclosporin A.[1,10,53,56,57] Plasma levels of statins metabolized by CYP3A4 (e.g., simvastatin, lovastatin) are greatly increased in the presence of cyclosporine or tacrolimus and should be avoided or used at low dose.

TREATMENT GUIDELINES AND TARGETS

The National Kidney Foundation KDOQI guidelines have generally adopted the applicability of guidelines (and the recommended targets) established for other populations[1,3,4,57] for patients with CKD stages 1 to 4 (normal renal function to predialysis). They have further recommended that patients with CKD 1 to 4 be treated as high CV risk and acknowledged that further clinical trials are required. A similar approach has been adopted in the guidelines for treatment in other countries including the United Kingdom, although most guidelines acknowledge the absence of specific outcome trial data.

INTERVENTION: CLINICAL TRIALS

There have been numerous studies on the impact of individual lipid-lowering therapies in patients at different stages of PRD, with varying degrees of renal impairment and proteinuria, including nephrotic syndrome. In general, the pattern and proportional effects on lipid subtypes are similar to those seen in other patient populations.

Tonelli and colleagues have used the Pravastatin Pooling Project (PPP), which combined data on 19,700 patients from the major CV intervention trials using pravastatin (Long-Term Intervention with Pravastatin in Ischaemic Disease [LIPID], West of Scotland Coronary Prevention Study [WOSCOPS], and Cholesterol and Recurrent Events [CARE]),[58–61] as well as data from the individual trials. Post hoc analyses using eGFR compared 2876 patients (14.6%) with eGFR greater than 90 mL/min ("normal renal function"), 12,333 (62.6%) with eGFR 60 to 90 mL/min ("mild renal insufficiency"), and 4491 (22.8%) with eGFR less than 60 mL/min ("moderate renal failure"). The eGFR was lower in patients in secondary prevention trials[58,62–65] compared with primary prevention. There was a strong association of low eGFR with pre-existing coronary disease and established risk factors for CAD such as age and hypertension, and with adverse outcome. Post hoc analysis showed that patients with moderate renal dysfunction randomized to pravastatin had a hazard ratio of 0.77 for the composite CV endpoint of cardiac death, nonfatal myocardial infarction (MI), and coronary revascularization, and 0.79 for an extended composite endpoint that included stroke.[58,62] There was no difference in all-cause mortality unless primary prevention studies were excluded, a reflection of the fact that patients with pre-existing CV disease are more likely to die of CVD than other causes. However, it reinforces the view that post hoc analyses inform us of the impact of statins in patients with primary CHD (and associated risk factors) and coexistent CKD, rather than the effects on CV outcomes in patients with primary CKD. Nevertheless, it is widely thought that these analyses support the use of statins in CKD.[57]

In a subsequent study using the PPP database, Tonelli and colleagues examined the effects of pravastatin in patients with CKD (eGFR <60 mL/min or <90 mL/min plus proteinuria) and diabetes.[65] This study demonstrated an additive risk for CKD associated with diabetes, and statin therapy reduced the frequency of composite CV endpoints (including MI, cardiac death, and coronary intervention). Again, statin therapy did not reduce all-cause mortality, nor did it have a significant reduction on composite cardiac endpoints in patients with both CKD and diabetes. While this may reflect the futility of a single intervention in patients with complex CVD, it may also reflect the disproportionate increase in sudden death rather than MI in this population. A subgroup analysis of the Lipid-Lowering Arm Anglo-Scandinavian Cardiac Outcomes Trial–(ASCOT-LLA),[62] a large-scale study in patients with at least three conventional CV risk factors, showed a benefit of statin therapy in patients with undefined renal dysfunction on CV endpoints that was comparable with that in the overall population. In a subgroup analysis of the Heart Protection Study (HPS),[64] 450 of 20,500 patients had mild chronic renal failure (serum creatinine 1.5–2.3 mg/dL). The proportional risk reduction with simvastatin (40 mg/day) in this subgroup was comparable to that in the overall study population, as was a post hoc analysis of the 4D study.[65] A pooled analysis of the 30 fluvastatin studies[66] subdivided patients by an eGFR of 50 mL/min (approximately 10% had a GFR of <50 mL/min). Overall, fluvastatin (20–80 mg) therapy reduced CV events by 41% compared to placebo. Renal function did not influence either the therapeutic benefit or the observed effects, with a comparable overall reduction in LDL cholesterol of up to 34.4% in patients with eGFR less than 50 mL/min and 32.2% in those with eGFR greater than 50 mL/min.

In patients with ESRD receiving hemodialysis therapy, there is only a single interventional trial. The 4D trial,[51] perhaps unexpectedly, failed to show a significant reduction in CV events in hemodialysis patients given atorvastatin for a median of 4 years. It was a randomized, placebo-controlled study in 1255 type 2 diabetic patients on chronic hemodialysis who had been on dialysis for less than 2 years. Atorvastatin (20 mg/day) lowered mean LDL cholesterol levels by 42%, to 72 mg/dL, without a significant reduction in the primary endpoint (a composite of cardiac death, nonfatal MI, and fatal or nonfatal stroke). While the investigators speculated that the results reflect a different pathogenesis of vascular events in diabetic patients with ESRD or that the intervention was too late in the natural history of such complex disease, atorvastatin therapy did reduce the incidence of MI. Thus, an alternative explanation is that in the complex mixture of CVD that affects patients with ESRD, the relationship between cholesterol and MI is present (and lipid-lowering reduces this endpoint) but that MI is not the dominant CV endpoint.

Another interventional trial relevant to this area is the Assessment of Lescol in Renal Transplantation (ALERT) study[67,68] in renal transplant recipients who, even with a single functioning transplanted kidney, had a degree of renal impairment. In this related population in which patients were randomized to fluvastatin or placebo, all lipid parameters were associated strongly with the development of MI, but much less so with cardiac death, which is more dependent on left ventricle hypertrophy and hypertension.

Finally, although there are limited data on interventional studies of nonstatin therapy, in a post hoc analysis of the Veterans Affairs HDL Intervention Trial (VA-HIT)[69] in patients with CHD, low HDL cholesterol, and LDL cholesterol below 140 mg/dL who were treated with gemfibrozil or placebo, approximately 40% had a creatinine clearance below 75 mL/min; patients with a serum creatinine in excess of 2 mg/dL were excluded. The proportional reduction in the composite cardiac endpoint of MI cardiac death, or stroke was reduced by 25% overall and in the patients with relatively low eGFR. Gemfibrozil use was associated with a 35% reduction in TG, a 5% increase in HDL cholesterol, but no significant reduction in LDL cholesterol. This study lends support to the view that fibrates have comparable efficacy to statins in patients with pre-existing CHD who have low HDL cholesterol but not elevated LDL cholesterol.

Renal Endpoints

The parallels between atherosclerosis and the evidence linking hyperlipidemia and progression of renal disease have led to the expectation that statins may protect against progression of PRD. Small-scale studies using simvastatin, pravastatin, and fluvastatin have provided evidence to support this notion. A study by Bianchi and colleagues in 56 patients with proteinuric, progressive renal disease demonstrated that atorvastatin (in combination with blockade of the renin–angiotensin system) reduced proteinuria and the rate of loss of GFR by approximately 50%.[70] A pooled analysis of nearly 4000 patients included in clinical trials of rosuvastatin noted a progressive increase (1 to 3 mL/min) in eGFR in patients receiving rosuvastatin therapy.[71] The rosuvastatin development program identified a small increase in proteinuria in patients receiving statin therapy. This is likely to be common to other statins and does not compromise renal function. Moreover, the mechanism is unresolved and may be due to (potentially beneficial) impaired tubular uptake of protein, rather than increased glomerular proteinuria.[46,71] Clinical trials to investigate the renal mechanism and benefits of statin therapy are ongoing.

Future Trials

From the above, it remains uncertain whether it is appropriate to treat CV risk across the spectrum of renal failure using paradigms adopted from the general population. The nature of dyslipidemia in renal patients is different from that in the general population, as is the pattern of CV outcomes and their relationship with lipid levels. Data from patients with primary CV disease and concomitant mild CKD suggest that statin therapy should be effective in patients with mild renal impairment, but whether this observation holds in patients with PRD is unresolved. Patients with advanced CKD receiving statin therapy do benefit from the therapy. Thus, one pragmatic approach is to assume that all intervening stages of CKD will enjoy similar benefits.[64] This has been the approach of most guidelines, with the caveat that patients with CKD are at increased risk of adverse events. Two ongoing trials will report shortly in this area. A Study to Evaluate the Use of Rosuvastatin in Subjects on Regular Haemodiolysis: an Assessment of Survival and Cardiovascular Events (AURORA) randomized 2800 patients receiving hospital hemodialysis to rosuvastatin 10 mg or placebo, with a composite CV endpoint.[72,73] This study differs from the 4D study in size and the fact that only a small proportion are diabetic. The SHARP study[74] recruited 9000 patients (stratified to include 3000 dialysis and 6000 predialysis patients), randomized to receive simvastatin 40 mg/day and ezetimibe 10 mg daily or placebo. This should answer the question of efficacy of lipid lowering in patients with primary CKD and, in addition to supplying data on the safety and efficacy of simvastatin and ezetimibe, will provide data on a more potent regimen. In the meantime, while waiting for trial results, many physicians and patients have taken the view that statins are likely to have benefits on CAD similar to those in the general population, resulting in a progressive increase in statin use in many groups of patients with advanced and ESRD.

REFERENCES

1. Pritchard SS: Impact of dyslipidaemia in end-stage renal disease. *J Am Soc Nephrol* 2003;14:S315–S320.
2. Tonelli M, Pfeffer MA: Kidney disease and cardiovascular risk. *Ann Rev Med* 2007;58:123–139.
3. Sarnak MJ, Levey AS, Schoolwerth AC, et al: Kidney disease as a risk factor for the development of cardiovascular disease: a statement from the American Heart Association Councils on Kidney in Cardiovascular Disease, High Blood Pressure Research, Clinical Cardiology and Epidemiology and Prevention. *Circulation* 2003;108:2154–2169.
4. National Kidney Foundation: K/DOQI Clinical Practice Guidelines for managing dyslipidemias in chronic kidney disease. *Am J Kidney Dis* 2003;41:S1–S92.
5. Remuzzi G, Benigni A, Remuzzi A: Mechanisms of progression and regression of renal lesions of chronic glomerulopathies and diabetes. *J Clin Invest* 2006;116:288–296.
6. Keane WF: Lipids and progressive renal failure. *Wien Klin Wochenschrift* 1996;108:420–424.
7. Cases A, Coll E: Dyslipidemia and the progression of renal disease in chronic renal failure patients. *Kidney Int Suppl* 2005;99: S87–S93.
8. Deighan CJ, Caslake MJ, McConnell M, Boulton-Jones JM, Packard CJ: Atherogenic lipoprotein phenotype in end-stage renal failure: origin and extent of small dense low-density lipoprotein formation. *Am J Kidney Dis* 2000;35:852–862.
9. Deighan CJ, Caslake MJ, McConnell M, Boulton-Jones JM, Packard CJ: The atherogenic lipoprotein phenotype: small dense LDL and lipoprotein remnants in nephrotic range proteinuria. *Atherosclerosis* 2001;157:211–220.
10. Vaziri ND: Dyslipidaemia of chronic renal failure: the nature, mechanisms and potential consequences. *Am J Physiol Renal Physiol* 2006;290:F262–F272.
11. Vaziri ND, Liang K: Down-regulation of tissue lipoprotein lipase expression in experimental chronic renal failure. *Kidney Int* 1996;50:1928–1935.
12. Chan MK, Persaud J, Varghese Z, Moorhead JF: Pathogenic roles of post-heparin lipases in lipid abnormalities in hemodialysis patients. *Kidney Int* 1984;25:812–818.
13. Goldberg A, Sherrard DJ, Brunzell JD: Adipose tissue lipoprotein lipase in chronic haemodialysis: role in plasma triglyceride metabolism. *J Clin Endocrinol Metab* 1978;47:1173–1182.
14. Attman PO, Samuelsson O, Alaupovic P: Lipoprotein metabolism and renal failure. *Am J Kidney Dis* 1993;21:573–592.
15. Roullet JB, Lacour B, Yvert JP, Drueke T: Correction by insulin of disturbed TG-rich lipoprotein metabolism in rats with chronic renal failure. *Am J Physiol* 1986;250:E373–E376.
16. Klin M, Smogorzewski M, Ni Z, Zhang G, Massry SG: Abnormalities in hepatic lipase in chronic renal failure: role of excess parathyroid hormone. *J Clin Invest* 1996;97:2197–2173.
17. Pandak WM, Vlahcevic ZR, Heuman DM, Krieg RJ, Hanna JD, Chan JC: Post-transcriptional regulation of 3-hydroxy–3-methylglutaryl coenzyme A reductase and cholesterol 7 alpha hydroxylase in rats with sub-total nephrectomy. *Kidney Int* 1994;46:358–364.
18. Vaziri ND, Liang K, Parks JS: Acquired Lecithen-cholesterol-acyl-transferase deficiency in the nephrotic syndrome. *Am J Physiol Renal Physiol* 2001;280:F823–F828.
19. Vaziri ND, Sato T, Liang K: Molecular mechanism of altered cholesterol synthesis in focal glomerulosclerosis. *Kidney Int* 2003;63:1756–1763.
20. Vaziri ND, Liang K, Parks JS: Downregulation of lecithin-cholesterol acyl transferase (LCAT) in chronic renal failure. *Kidney Int* 2001;59:2192–2196.
21. Guarnieri GF, Moracchiello M, Campanacci L, et al: Lecithin: cholesterol acyltransferase (LCAT) activity in chronic uremia. *Kidney Int* 1978;13:S26–S30.
22. Kimura H, Miyazaki R, Imura T, et al: Hepatic lipase mutation may reduce vascular disease prevalence in hemodialysis patients with high CETP levels. *Kidney Int* 2003;64:1829–1837.
23. Vaziri ND, Deng G, Liang K: Hepatic HDL receptor, SR-B1 and Apo A-I expression in chronic renal failure. *Nephrol Dial Transpl* 1999;14:1462–1466.
24. Acton S, Rigotti A, Landschulz KT, Xu S, Hobbs HH, Krieger M: Identification of scavenger receptor SRB-1 as a high-density lipoprotein receptor. *Science* 1996;271:518–520.
25. Liang K, Vaziri ND: Upregulation of acyl-CoA: cholesterol acyltransferase in chronic renal failure. *Am J Physiol* 2002;283: E676–E681.
26. Vaziri ND, Dang B, Zhan CD, Liang K: Downregulation of hepatic acyl-CoA: diglycerol acyltransferase in chronic renal failure. *Am J Physiol* 2004;287:F90–F94.
27. Vaziri ND, Kim CH, Phan D, Kim S, Liang K: Upregulation of acyl-CoA: diglycerol acyltransferase in chronic renal failure. *Kidney Int* 2004;66:262–267.
28. Kim C, Vaziri ND: Downregulation of hepatic LDL receptor related protein in chronic renal failure. *Kidney Int* 2005;67:1028–1032.
29. Liang K, Oveisi F, Vaziri ND: Role of secondary hyperparathyroidism in the genesis of hypertriglyceridaemia and VLDL receptor deficiency in chronic renal failure. *Kidney Int* 1998;53: 626–630.
30. Vaziri ND, Liang K: Down-regulation of VLDL receptor in experimental chronic renal failure. *Kidney Int* 1996;50:1928–1935.
31. Fielding CJ, Fielding PE: Cellular cholesterol efflux. *Biochim Biophys Acta* 2001;1533:175–189.
32. Liang K, Vaziri ND: Downregulation of hepatic high-density lipoprotein receptor, SR-B1 in nephrotic syndrome. *Kidney Int* 1999;56:621–626.
33. Maggi E, Bellazzi R, Falaschi F, et al: Enhanced LDL oxidation in uraemic patients: an additional mechanism for accelerated atherosclerosis. *Kidney Int* 1994;45:876–883.
34. Navab M, Berliner JA, Subbanagounder G, et al: HDL and the inflammatory response induced by LDL-derived oxidized phospholipids. *Arterioscler Thromb Vasc Biol* 2001;21:481–488.
35. Go AS, Chertow GM, Fan D, McCulloch CE, Hsu C: Chronic kidney disease and the risks of death, cardiovascular events, and hospitalisation. *N Engl J Med* 2004;351:1296–1305.
36. Anavekar NS, McMurray JJ, Velazquez EJ, et al: Relation between renal dysfunction and cardiovascular outcomes after myocardial infarction. *N Engl J Med* 2004;351:1285–1295.
37. Tonelli M, Jose P, Curhan G, et al: Cholesterol and Recurrent Events (CARE) Trial Investigators. Proteinuria, impaired kidney function, and adverse outcomes in people with coronary disease: analysis of a previously conducted randomised trial. *BMJ* 2006;17:332(7555).
38. Tonelli M, Isles C, Curhan GC, et al: Effect of pravastatin on cardiovascular events in people with chronic kidney disease. *Circulation* 2004;110:1557–1563.
39. Liu Y, Coresh J, Eustace JA, : Association between cholesterol level and mortality in dialysis patients. *JAMA* 2004;291: 451–459.
40. Kalantar-Zadeh K, Fouque D, Kopple JD: Outcome research, nutrition and reverse epidemiology in maintenance dialysis patients. *J Ren Nutr* 2004;14:64–71.
41. Border WA, Ruoslahti E: Transforming growth factor-beta in disease: the dark side of tissue repair. *J Clin Invest* 1992;90:1–7.
42. Abrass CK: Cellular lipid metabolism and the role of lipids in progressive renal disease. *Am J Nephrol* 2004;24:46–53.
43. Takemura T, Yoshioka K, Aya N: Apolipoproteins and lipoprotein receptors in glomeruli in human kidney diseases. *Kidney Int* 1993;43:918–927.
44. Marsh JB: Lipoprotein metabolism in experimental nephrosis. *Proc Soc Exp Biol Med* 1996;213:178–186.
45. Yoshimura A, Nemoto T, Sugenoya Y, et al: Effect of simvastatin on proliferative nephritis and cell-cycle protein expression. *Kidney Int Suppl* 1999;71:S84–S87.
46. Verhulst A, D'Haese PC, De Broe ME: Inhibitors of HMG-CoA reductase reduce receptor-mediated endocytosis in human kidney proximal tubular cells. *J Am Soc Nephrol* 2004;15: 2249–2257.
47. Attman PO, Samuelsson O, Alaupovic P: Progression of renal failure: role of apolipoprotein B–containing lipoproteins. *Kidney Int* 1997;63:S98–S101.
48. Samuelsson O, Mulec H, Knight-Gibson C, et al: Lipoprotein abnormalities are associated with increased rate of progression of human chronic renal insufficiency. *Nephrol Dial Transpl* 1997;12(9):1908–1915.
49. Baigent C, Landray M, Leaper C, et al: First United Kingdom Heart and Renal Protection (UK-HARP-1) study: biochemical efficacy and safety of simvastatin and safety of low dose aspirin in chronic kidney disease. *Am J Kidney Dis* 2005;45:473–484.

50. Landray M, Baigent C, Leaper C, et al: The Seecond United Kingdom Heart and Renal Protection (UK-HARP-II) study: a randomized controlled study of the safety and efficacy of adding ezetimibe to simvastatin as initial therapy among patients with CKD. *Am J Kidney Dis* 2005;45:385–395.
51. Wanner C, Krane V, Marz W, et al: Atorvastatin in patients with type 2 diabetes mellitus undergoing hemodialysis. German Diabetes and Dialysis Study Investigators. *N Engl J Med* 2005;353:238–248.
52. Harris KP, Wheeler DC, Chong CC: A placebo-controlled trial examining atorvastatin in dyslipidaemic patients undergoing CAPD. *Kidney Int* 2002;61:81469–81474.
53. Broeders N, Knoop C, Antoine M, Tielemans C: Fibrate-induced increase in blood urea and creatinine: is Gemfibrozil an innocuous agent? *Nephrol Dial Transplant* 2000;15:1993–1999.
54. Deighan CJ, Caslake MJ, McConnell M, Boulton-Jones JM, Packard CJ: Comparative effects of cerivastatin and fenofibrate on the atherogenic lipoprotein phenotype in proteinuric renal disease. *J Am Soc Nephrol* 2001;12:341–348.
55. Owada A, Suda S, Hata T: Antiproteinuric effect of niceritol a nicotinic acid derivative in chronic renal disease with proteinuria. *Am J Med* 2003;114:347–353.
56. Chertow GM, Burke SK, Raggi P: Sevelamer attenuates the progression of coronary and aortic calcification in haemodialysis patients. *Kidney Int* 2002;62:245–252.
57. Campese VM, Park J: HMG-CoA reductase inhibitors and the kidney. *Kidney Int* 2007;71:1215–1222.
58. Tonelli M, Isles C, Curhan GC, et al: Effect of pravastatin on cardiovascular events in people with chronic kidney disease. *Circulation* 2004;110:1557–1563.
59. Sacks FM, Pfeffer MA, Moye LA, et al: The effect of pravastatin on coronary events after myocardial infarction in patients with average cholesterol levels. Cholesterol and Recurrent Events Trial investigators. *N Engl J Med* 1996;335:1001–1009.
60. The Long-Term Intervention with Pravastatin in Ischaemic Disease (LIPID) Study Group: Prevention of cardiovascular events and death with pravastatin in patients with coronary heart disease and a broad range of initial cholesterol levels. *N Engl J Med* 1998;339:1349–1357.
61. Shepherd J, Cobbe SM, Ford I, et al: Prevention of coronary heart disease with pravastatin in men with hypercholesterolemia. West of Scotland Coronary Prevention Study Group. *N Engl J Med* 1995;333:1301–1307.
62. Tonelli M, Keech A, Shepherd J, et al: Effect of pravastatin in people with diabetes and chronic kidney disease. *J Am Soc Nephrol* 2005;16:3748–3754.
63. Sever PS, Dahlof B, Poulter NR, et al: Prevention of coronary and stroke events in patients who have average or lower than average cholesterol concentrations, in the Anglo-Scandanavian Cardiac Outcomes Trial–Lipid Lowering Arm (ASCOTT-LLA): a multicentre randomized clinical trial. *Lancet* 2003;361:1149–1158.
64. Heart Protection Study Collaborative Group: MRC/BHF Heart Protection Study of cholesterol lowering with simvastatin in 20,536 high-risk individuals: a randomised placebo-controlled trial. *Lancet* 2002;360:7–22.
65. Chonchoi M, Cook M, Kjekshus J, Pedersen TR, Lindenfeld J: Simvastatin for secondary prevention of all-cause mortality and major coronary events in patients with mild chronic renal insufficiency. *Am J Kidney Dis* 2007;49:373–382.
66. Holdaas H, Wanner C, Ablethauser C, Gimpelewicz C, Isaacsohn J: The effect of fluvastatin on cardiac outcomes in patients with moderate to severe renal insufficiency: a pooled analysis of double-blind, randomized trials. *Int J Cardiol* 2007;117:64–74.
67. Jardine AG, Holdaas H, Fellstrom B, et al: Fluvastatin prevents cardiac death and myocardial infarction in renal transplant recipients: post-hoc subgroup analyses of the ALERT Study. *Am J Transpl* 2004;4:988–995.
68. Holdaas H, Fellstrom B, Cole E, et al: Long-term cardiac outcomes in renal transplant recipients receiving fluvastatin: The ALERT Extension Study. Assessment of Lescol in Renal Transplantation (ALERT) Study Investigators. *Am J Transpl* 2005;5: 2929–2936.
69. Tonelli M, Collins D, Robins S, Bloomfield H, Curhan GC: Veterans' Affairs High-Density Lipoprotein Intervention Trial (VA-HIT) Investigators. Gemfibrozil for secondary prevention of cardiovascular events in mild to moderate chronic renal insuffiency. *Kidney Int* 2004;66:1123–1130.
70. Bianchi S, Bigazzi R, Caiazza A, Campese VM: A controlled, prospective study of the effects of atorvastatin on proteinuria and progression of kidney disease. *Am J Kidney Dis* 2003;41: 565–570.
71. Vidt DG, Harris S, McTaggart F, Ditmarsch M, Sager PT, Sorof JM. Effect of short-term rosuvastatin treatment on estimated glomerular filtration rate. *Am J Cardiol* 2006;97:1602–1606.
72. Fellstrom B, Zannad F, Schmieder R, et al: Effect of rosuvastatin on outcomes in chronic haemodialysis patients—design and rationale of the AURORA study. *Curr Control Trials Cardiovasc Med* 2005;23:6–9.
73. Fellstrom B, Holdaas H, Jardine AG, et al: Effect of Rosuvastatin on outcomes in chronic haemodialysis patients: baseline data from the AURORA Study. *Kidney Blood Press Res* 2007;30(5):314–322.
74. Baigent C, Landry M: Study of Heart and Renal Protection (SHARP). *Kidney Int Suppl* 2003;84:S207–S210.

CHAPTER 42

Special Patient Populations: Lipid Abnormalities in High-Risk Ethnic Groups

Krishnaswami Vijayaraghavan and Prakash C. Deedwania

INTRODUCTION

Current information on risks of cardiovascular disease (CVD) is obtained mainly from studies of Caucasians of European origin. Nonetheless, people of other ethnic groups experience an excessive load of CVD, including coronary heart disease (CHD) and stroke.[1,2] It has been postulated that urbanization or embracing a Westernized lifestyle has different effects on metabolic and vascular dysfunction across populations; for instance, South Asians have a higher prevalence of CHD and cardiovascular mortality compared with Europeans. African Americans demonstrate higher rates of CHD and stroke, while Africans in the United Kingdom have lower CHD rates and higher stroke rates than Britons of European descent.[3,4] The Chinese and Japanese demonstrate consistently high rates of stroke but not CHD. North American indigenous peoples have high rates of CHD, while Mexican Americans have a higher prevalence of both stroke and CHD.

Despite the fact that conventional cardiovascular risk factors such as smoking, blood pressure, and total cholesterol predict risk *within* these ethnic groups, they do not fully account for the differences in risk *between* ethnic groups, signifying that alternative explanations might exist. Ethnic groups show differences in abdominal obesity, insulin resistance, and C-reactive protein (CRP), adiponectin, and plasma homocysteine levels. The striking differences in CVD risk across racial and ethnic groups are likely due in part to genetic, biological, and environmental factors, and can provide valuable clues to causation in patterns of disease presentation, therapeutic needs, and response to treatment. In addition, dyslipidemia requiring drug treatment is common in the middle-aged and older adult population of the United States who demonstrate no evidence of clinical CVD. Suboptimal treatment and control of dyslipidemia have been a major point of concern among the intermediate- and high-risk groups, and provide evidence of gender- and ethnicity-related disparities. The impact of CVD as a public health problem in the United States and the proven benefits of lipid-lowering therapy for primary prevention are such that efforts to improve the treatment and control of dyslipidemia and to eradicate disparities in dyslipidemia management should be considered among our highest national healthcare quality improvement priorities.[5,6] Ongoing studies should increase understanding of ethnicity as a potential independent risk factor, thus enabling better identification of treatment targets and selection of therapy in specific populations. This review describes the prevalence of cardiovascular risk factors, mainly focusing on lipid abnormalities in high-risk ethnic groups, differences among the groups, probable causative factors for the disparities, and potential for future research opportunities.

HISPANICS AND LATINOS

CVD is the leading cause of death among Hispanics. CVD accounted for 27.3% of deaths among Hispanic men and 33.1% of deaths among women. In a recent U.S. Outcomes Research–Population Study, data collected from Mexican American and non-Hispanic white (NHW) adults aged 20 years and over who participated in the 1999–2002 National Health and Nutrition Examination Survey (NHANES), type 2 diabetes was significantly more prevalent in Mexican Americans (13%, age- and gender-adjusted) than in NHW (8%); however, Mexican Americans compared to NHW were more likely to be both diagnosed (77% vs. 65%) and treated (63% vs. 47%). Mexican Americans had a slightly lower adjusted prevalence of dyslipidemia, at 31% versus 35%. Awareness of hypertension and dyslipidemia were significantly lower in Mexican Americans (57% vs. 71% for hypertension, and 33% vs. 56% for dyslipidemia). Treatment rates for hypertension and dyslipidemia were also significantly lower in Mexican Americans (42% vs. 61% for hypertension, 14% vs. 30% for dyslipidemia). Adjusting for age, gender, education, and access to care indicated that Mexican Americans were significantly more likely than NHW to be aware of and treated for their diabetes, but significantly less likely to be aware of and treated for their hypertension or dyslipidemia.[7–9] The prevalence of dyslipidemia in ethnic populations is shown in Table 42-1.

Data from the NHANES 1999–2002 showed that overall, 63.3% of participants whose test results indicated high blood cholesterol or who were taking a cholesterol-lowering medication had been told by a professional that they had high cholesterol.[10] Women were less likely than men to be aware of their condition; blacks and Mexican Americans were less likely to be aware of their condition than were whites. Fewer than half of Mexican Americans with high cholesterol were aware of their condition.[11,12]

The Multi-Ethnic Study of Atherosclerosis (MESA) is a National Heart, Lung, and Blood Institute (NHLBI)–sponsored, multicenter study designed to investigate the prevalence, correlates, and progression of subclinical CVD in multiple ethnicities. Six field centers recruited a population-based sample of 6814 men (47%) and women free from symptomatic CVD.[13] Sample participants were 45 to 84 years old at baseline (2000–2002) and 38% white, 28% black, 22% Hispanic, and 12% Chinese. Control of dyslipidemia to the NHLBI's National Cholesterol Education Program Adult Treatment Panel III (NCEP ATP III) goal was observed in 75.2% (797/1060) of participants with treated dyslipidemia and 40.6% (797/1964) of all participants with dyslipidemia (Tables 42-2 and 42-3). Men were more likely than women to qualify for drug therapy and less likely to be treated and controlled. Relative to NHW, Chinese Americans were less likely to qualify for drug treatment, but no differences in treatment and control rates were observed. African and Hispanics had prevalence of dyslipidemia that was comparable to that of NHW but their dyslipidemia was less likely to be treated and controlled. Ethnic disparities were attenuated substantially by adjustment for healthcare access variables; however, the gender disparities persisted despite adjustment for risk factors, socioeconomic characteristics, and healthcare access variables. Control of dyslipidemia was achieved less commonly in the high– and intermediate– CVD risk groups than in the low-risk group. Among high-risk individuals, 19.7% of those who did not qualify for lipid-lowering drug treatment had coronary artery calcium (CAC) greater than 400. The proportion of drug treatment–qualifying persons who were not treated differed by presence and severity of CAC, with 48.0%, 46.8%, and 39.6% of eligible persons with no CAC, with CAC more than 0 and less than 400, and with CAC greater than 400 not receiving treatment, respectively (P for difference = 0.04).

The multicenter Study Assessing Rosuvastatin in the Hispanic Population (STARSHIP)[14] was designed to assess the efficacy of rosuvastatin and atorvastatin in lowering low-density lipoprotein (LDL) cholesterol. In an open-label trial, 696 Hispanic patients with LDL cholesterol levels of 130 to 300 mg/dL and triglyceride levels of less than 400 mg/dL (at medium or high risk of CHD) were randomized to receive 10 or 20 mg of rosuvastatin or 10 or 20 mg of atorvastatin for 6 weeks. At week 6, LDL cholesterol was decreased more by 10 mg of rosuvastatin than by 10 mg of atorvastatin (45% vs. 36%, $P < 0.0001$) and more by 20 mg of rosuvastatin than by 20 mg of atorvastatin (50% vs. 42%, $P < 0.0001$). Significantly greater decreases were also observed with rosuvastatin for total cholesterol, non–high-density lipoprotein (non-HDL) cholesterol, apolipoprotein (Apo) B, and lipid ratios compared with milligram-equivalent doses of atorvastatin.

There are sufficient data that describe the Latino population as high risk for CVD. Multiple studies have suggested that there was a disproportionately higher prevalence of CHD in these subjects.[1,9,13,15,16] Hence, there is a need to identify and treat these individuals to decrease the overall burden of CVD.

AFRICAN AMERICANS

Multiple published reports have addressed the disparities in risk factors in the African American population.[17–19] A 10% population-wide decrease in total cholesterol levels may result in an estimated 30% reduction in the incidence of CHD. Data from NHANES 1999–2002 showed that overall, 63.3% of participants

TABLE 42-1 Prevalence (%) of Lipid Abnormalities in High-Risk Ethnic Populations

Group	Men	Women	Men	Women	Men	Women
	LDL >130 mg/dL	LDL >130 mg/dL	HDL <40 mg/dL	HDL <40 mg/dL	TG >150 mg/dL	TG >150 mg/dL
Non-Hispanic whites	49.6	43.7	40.5	14.5	36.9	25
African Americans	46.3	41.6	24.3	13	21.4	14.4
Mexican Americans	43.6	41.6	40.1	18.4	39.7	35.2
			HDL <35 mg/dL	HDL <35 mg/dL		
American Indians	46	27	19	11	28	21
	LDL >160 mg/dL	LDL >160 mg/dL				
Pacific Islanders	5.5	NA	6.4	NA	18.7	NA

LDL, low-density lipoprotein; HDL, high-density lipoprotein; NA, not available; TG, triglycerides.

TABLE 42-2 Observed Lipid and Lipoprotein Concentrations in MESA Study Participants, 2000–2002

	Non-Hispanic Whites Mean (SD)		Chinese Mean (SD)		Blacks Mean (SD)		Hispanics Mean (SD)		
	Men	Women	Men	Women	Men	Women	Men	Women	Total Mean (SD)
Cholesterol (mg/dL)	188.1 (32.8)	201.3 (32.6)	189.7 (31.2)	194.6 (31.4)	181.4 (34.2)	195.8 (36.1)	192.8 (36.8)	200.9 (36.0)	193.5 (34.7)
LDL cholesterol (mg/dL)	117.3 (29.5)	116.9 (30.6)	116.5 (28.5)	113.9 (29.2)	113.5 (32.1)	118.8 (33.5)	119.3 (33.2)	119.6 (32.8)	117.2 (31.5)
HDL cholesterol (mg/dL)	45.4 (12.1)	59.0 (15.7)	46.0 (10.8)	53.4 (13.1)	46.8 (12.5)	57.1 (15.7)	42.7 (10.0)	52.7 (13.7)	51.2 (14.8)
Triglycerides (mg/dL)	127.4 (65.5)	127.0 (64.9)	135.7 (68.3)	136.4 (65.7)	106.2 (56.5)	99.2 (47.8)	154.1 (75.0)	143.1 (66.3)	125.9 (65.5)

LDL, low-density lipoprotein; HDL, high-density lipoprotein; SD, standard deviation.

TABLE 42-3 Estimated 10-Year Risk of Coronary Heart Disease and Dyslipidemia Prevalence, Treatment, and Control among MESA Study Participants, 2000–2002

		Non-Hispanic Whites		Chinese		Blacks		Hispanics		
Characteristic	N	Men	Women	Men	Women	Men	Women	Men	Women	Total
10-Year risk of coronary heart disease, %	6704	13	3.8	12.5	4	13.4	4.6	13.3	4.5	8.4
Prevalence of dyslipidemia, %	6704	36.9	24.4	26.9	21	31.2	29.1	32.1	26.8	29.3
Prevalence of lipid-lowering drug therapy, %										
All MESA participants	6704	19.2	16.3	12.5	15.6	14.9	17.2	12.7	13.4	15.8
Participants with dyslipidemia	1964	52	66.7	46.6	74.1	47.7	58.9	39.4	50	54
Control of dyslipidemia										
LDL cholesterol <ATP III drug initiation level, %	6704	80.3	91.6	83.8	93.3	81.8	86	78.5	85.7	85
LDL cholesterol <ATP III drug treatment goal, %										
· All MESA participants	6704	62.9	75.6	66.3	79.5	62.1	67.4	58.6	68	67.4
· Participants with dyslipidemia	1964	39.7	57.5	35.9	61.2	32.7	38.7	27	37.3	40.6
· On drug therapy	1060	76.4	86.2	77.1	82.5	68.5	65.7	68.5	74.5	75.3

whose test results indicated high blood cholesterol or who were taking a cholesterol-lowering medication had been told by a professional that they had high cholesterol. Blacks and Mexican Americans were less likely to be aware of their condition than were whites. Fewer than half of Mexican Americans with high cholesterol were aware of their condition.[20] Between 1988–1994 and 1999–2002, the age-adjusted mean total serum cholesterol level of adults age 20 and older decreased from 206 mg/dL to 203 mg/dL, and LDL cholesterol levels decreased from 129 mg/dL to 123 mg/dL. The mean level of LDL cholesterol for American adults age 20 and older is 123 mg/dL. According to NHANES 1999–2002, among NHW, mean LDL cholesterol levels were 126 mg/dL for men and 121 mg/dL for women.[10] Among non-Hispanic blacks, the mean LDL cholesterol level was 121 mg/dL for both men and women, and among Mexican Americans, mean LDL cholesterol levels were 125 mg/dL for men and 117 mg/dL for women. The mean level of high-density lipoprotein (HDL) cholesterol for American adults age 20 and older is 51.3 mg/dL.[21] According to NHANES 1999–2002, among NHW, mean high-density lipoprotein (HDL) cholesterol levels were 45.5 mg/dL for men and 52.9 for women, and among non-Hispanic blacks, mean HDL cholesterol levels were 51.0 mg/dL for men and 57.3 for women. Among Mexican Americans, mean HDL cholesterol levels were 45.0 mg/dL for men and 52.9 for women. American Heart Association (AHA) data suggest that 45% of African Americans demonstrate elevated LDL cholesterol. However, CHD risk appears to be similar between African Americans and the general population.[22] The increase in cardiovascular morbidity in this population may be due to clustering of risk with hypertension and its consequences of end-organ damage.[15,16,23]

In the African-American Rosuvastatin Investigation of Efficacy and Safety (ARIES) trial,[24] 774 African American adults with LDL cholesterol 160 to 300 mg/dL and triglycerides less than 400 mg/dL were randomized to receive open-label rosuvastatin 10 or 20 mg or atorvastatin 10 or 20 mg for 6 weeks. At week 6, significantly greater reductions in low-density lipoprotein cholesterol, total cholesterol, non-HDL cholesterol, and apolB concentrations, as well as lipoprotein and apolipoprotein ratios, were seen with rosuvastatin versus milligram-equivalent atorvastatin doses ($P < 0.017$ for all comparisons). Rosuvastatin 10 mg also increased HDL cholesterol significantly more than atorvastatin 20 mg ($P < 0.017$). Although statistical comparisons were not performed, larger proportions of rosuvastatin-treated patients than atorvastatin-treated patients achieved NCEP ATP III LDL cholesterol goals.[5,24] The median high-sensitivity CRP (hsCRP) levels were significantly reduced from baseline with rosuvastatin 20 mg and atorvastatin 20 mg among all patients, and with rosuvastatin 10 and 20 mg and atorvastatin 20 mg in those patients with a baseline CRP level greater than 2.0 mg/L. The two study medications were well tolerated during the 6-week study period. This study exemplifies the effectiveness of lipid therapy in the African American population and suggests that if barriers to access and coverage of prescription medications caused by socioeconomic status are eliminated, benefits will be equal.

The Atherosclerosis Risk in Communities (ARIC) study found that LDL cholesterol was highly predictive of cardiovascular risk in African Americans.[25–27] In a cross-sectional study of multiethnic population in New York City,[18] the distribution and predictors of lipids and lipoproteins was examined in 1118 elderly subjects (≥65 years of age), in a multiethnic urban community (22% NHW, 34% African American, and 44% Hispanic). Mean levels of total cholesterol, total/cholesterol HDL cholesterol ratio, and triglycerides decreased with increasing age ($P < 0.001$). LDL cholesterol and total cholesterol were lower among men, whereas women had higher levels of HDL cholesterol ($P < 0.001$). Hispanics had lower LDL cholesterol, total cholesterol, and HDL cholesterol levels, whereas African Americans had a lower total cholesterol/HDL cholesterol ratio and triglyceride levels along with higher HDL cholesterol levels ($P < 0.001$). Diabetes was more prevalent among Hispanics and African Americans ($P = 0.002$), and body mass index was higher in African Americans ($P = 0.009$).

Age-adjusted prevalence of dyslipidemia in various ethnic groups is shown in Fig. 42-1, 42-2, and 42-3. In multiple-point prevalence studies assessing lipoprotein subclasses among African Americans, there was evidence for higher frequency of the 514T allele of the gene for hepatic lipase *(LIPC)* in Afro-Caribbean men,[28,29] compared to Caucasians or African Americans associated with high HDL cholesterol and contributing to a favorable outcome. In the Bogalusa Heart Study,[30]

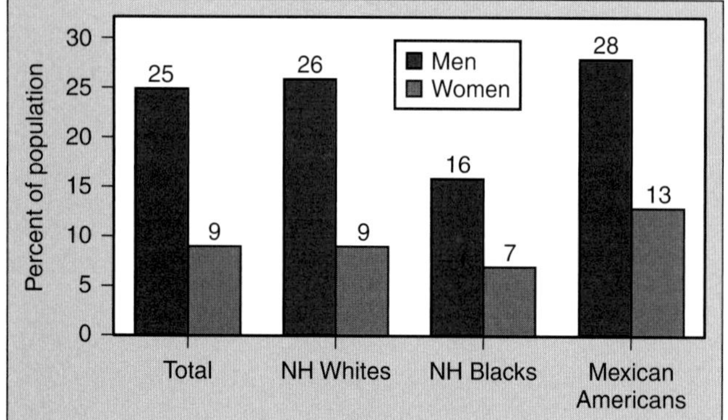

FIGURE 42-1 Age-adjusted prevalence of adults age 20 and older with HDL cholesterol under 40 mg/dL by race/ethnicity and gender (NHANES, 2003–2004). (From National Center for Health Statistics and National Heart, Lung, and Blood Institute.)

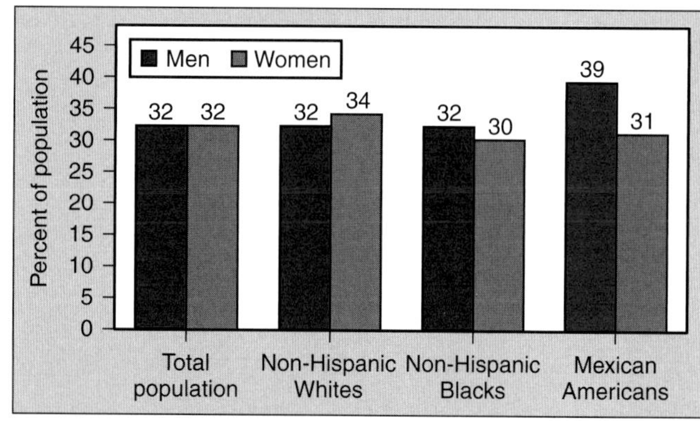

FIGURE 42-2 Age-adjusted prevalence of adults age 20 and older with LDL cholesterol of 130 mg/dL or higher by race/ethnicity and gender (National Health and Nutrition Examination Survey, 2003–2004). (From National Center for Health Statistics and National Heart, Lung, and Blood Institute.)

Caucasians had significantly higher very-low-density lipoprotein (VLDL) and small dense LDL compared to African Americans. Lipoprotein(a) [Lp(a)] has been shown to be significantly higher in the African American population compared to Caucasians, which could partially explain the higher rate of CHD in spite of having higher levels of HDL cholesterol.[31] To identify genes for lipid-related traits, a genomewide linkage analyses for levels of triglycerides and HDL, LDL, and total cholesterol in Caucasian, Hispanic, and African American families from the Genetics of NIDDM (GENNID) study was performed at Translational Genomics Research Institute.[32] Most lipid traits showed significant estimates of heritability ($P < 0.001$), with the exception of triglycerides and the triglyceride/HDL cholesterol ratio in African Americans. Variance components analysis identified linkage on chromosome 3p12.1–3q13.31 for the triglyceride/HDL cholesterol ratio (logarithm of odds [LOD] = 3.36) and triglyceride (LOD = 3.27) in Caucasian families. Statistically significant evidence for linkage was identified for the triglyceride/HDL cholesterol ratio (LOD = 2.45) on 11p in Hispanic families in a region that showed possible evidence of linkage (LOD = 2.26) for triglycerides in this population. In African Americans, the strongest evidence for linkage (LOD = 2.26) was found on 19p13.2–19q13.42 for total cholesterol. These findings provide strong support for previous reports of linkage for lipid-related traits, suggesting the presence of genes on 3p12.1–3q13.31, 11p15.4–11p11.3, and 19p13.2–19q13.42 that may influence traits underlying lipid abnormalities associated with type 2 diabetes.[33]

NATIVE AMERICANS

Critical data for CVD among Native Americans have been imperfect because of classification bias caused by race as well as events. For example, people who died from alcohol or unknown causes were more likely to be identified as American Indian on their death certificates than were people who died from other causes. Both forms of misclassification led to an underestimation of CVD mortality rates, and the inadequate

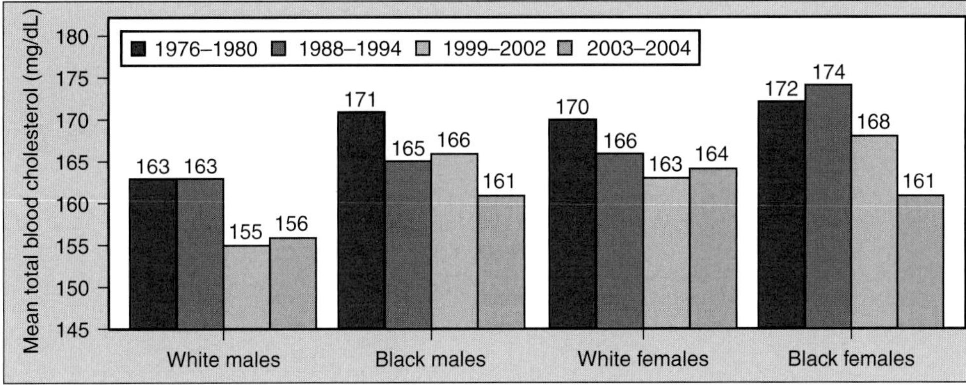

FIGURE 42-3 Trends in mean total serum cholesterol among adolescents between the ages of 12 and 17 years by race/ethnicity, gender, and survey (National Health and Nutrition Examination Survey, 1976–1980, 1988–1994, 1999–2002, and 2003–2004). (From National Center for Health Statistics and National Heart, Lung, and Blood Institute.)

data collection contributed to the flawed appearance of a CVD mortality advantage for American Indians, in spite of a documented high prevalence of CVD risk factors. Logistic barriers such as multiple tribes, heterogeneity of culture, and widespread language groups led to inadequate representation of Native Americans. The Strong Heart Study (SHS) was designed to address the deficiency in data on CVD and its associated risk factors in American Indians.[34,35] The largest epidemiological study of American Indians supported by the NHLBI, it includes 13 tribes and communities in three culturally and geographically diverse areas of Arizona, North and South Dakota, and Oklahoma, and uses standardized methods to assess risk factors in longitudinal analyses. Racial/ethnic misclassification bias was essentially eliminated by this study. The SHS data have revealed that American Indian CHD mortality rates either exceed or nearly equal the rates in the general U.S. populations, thus suggesting further evidence of ethnic disparity in CVD burden. Incidence of fatal CHD is increasing in American Indians in contrast to declining rates in the U.S. population overall. Native Americans seem to have gradually decreased their total cholesterol levels, improved hypertension treatment rates, and decreased smoking rates; and yet, prevalence of hypertension and dyslipidemia have significantly increased. In addition, the burden of diabetes has markedly increased. Although the general U.S. population is also experiencing an increase in diabetes, the diabetes prevalence in this group is dramatically higher than it is in the general population.[36]

In the Navajo Health and Nutritional Survey (NHNS), 40% of adults had cholesterol greater than 200 mg/dL and 10% had cholesterol greater than 240 mg/dL. In addition, 46% of men and 27% of women cholesterol high LDL cholesterol (>130 mg/dL), 19% of men and 11% of women had low HDL cholesterol (<40 mg/dL), and triglyceride levels were high in 28% of men and 21% of women.[37] An elevated triglyceride level was a significant predictor of CVD in Native American women in the SHS.[34]

PACIFIC ISLANDERS

It has been observed that men of Japanese ancestry residing in the United States appeared to have higher rates of CHD and lower rates of stroke than did their counterparts living in Japan. The Honolulu Heart Program (HHP) was initiated to study 8006 men of Japanese ancestry who were 45 to 68 years old in 1965 and lived on the Hawaiian island of Oahu.[38] Prevalence of high LDL cholesterol (>160 mg/dL) was only 5.5%, low HDL cholesterol (<40 mg/dL) was 6.4%, and high triglyceride (>150 mg/dL) was 18.7%. The study also revealed a continuum of risk by glucose tolerance status, with increasingly unfavorable CVD risk factors as subjects progressed from normal to impaired glucose tolerance to overt diabetes. In addition, glucose intolerance and overt diabetes were risk factors for thromboembolic and hemorrhagic stroke, CHD, sudden death, and all-cause mortality, independent of coexistent risk factors. In 1997, the American Diabetes Association (ADA) lowered the diagnostic cutoff point for diabetes from a fasting glucose of more than 140 to more than 126 mg/dL and suggested that the oral glucose tolerance test was not needed in epidemiologic studies. The World Health Organization (WHO) also lowered the threshold for fasting glucose in 1998, but it maintained use of the 2-hour postload glucose. When the WHO and ADA criteria for diabetes were applied to the HHP older adult cohort, the investigators observed that 66% of the individuals who had diabetes according to the WHO criteria were missed by the ADA criteria. When the fasting and postload glucose measures were analyzed as continuous variables, the 2-hour measurement was a superior predictor of total mortality independent of fasting glucose. The study also revealed that the mean body mass index (BMI) of older Japanese men with diabetes, 24 kg/m^2, was in the range that is considered normal by anthropometric standards for whites. The observation that diabetes frequently occurs in the normal weight range (BMI 18.5–25 kg/m^2) in older Japanese men suggests that the BMI thresholds for elevated diabetes risk may be different and need to be revised for different ethnicities, as recommended by the WHO.

SOUTH ASIANS

South Asians, Asian Indians, and Indian Americans are terms that have been used interchangeably for a population that mainly hails from the Indian subcontinent (India, Pakistan, Bangladesh, Nepal, Bhutan, and Sri Lanka). This is a unique ethnic group in whom multiple risk factors seem to be responsible for the increasingly high rates of CHD. Published scientific studies suggest that high levels of small dense LDL, triglycerides, homocysteine, Lp(a) and low levels of HDL (especially of the HDL_{2b} subfraction), with or without diabetes, may be the major contributors of risk.[39–45] However, most of the studies have included only a small number of subjects, and have tested only a small number of risk factors. Insulin resistance syndrome, or metabolic syndrome, appears to be more common among Asian Indians than among Caucasians in the United States and appears to be a common underlying etiology uniting most of the above risk factors.[46] Unfortunately, relatively little is known about how the metabolic syndrome relates to atherosclerosis risk in U.S. Asian Indians.

Burden of CVD in Asian Indians

Of the 1 billion Asian Indians, about 15 million live outside India and about 2.2 million live in North America. The estimated prevalence of CHD varies from 7.2% to 11%.[47,48] The age-adjusted prevalence of myocardial infarction (MI) or angina was three times greater in Asian Indian men compared to the Framingham Offspring Study. Compared to the Framingham Offspring Study,[49] Asian Indian men had higher prevalence of diabetes (9% vs. 1.1%). Of all deaths in 1990, WHO reports that 25% were attributable to CVD. Asian Indians who migrated to the United Kingdom, South Africa, Singapore, and North America have a 1.5- to 4-fold higher risk of CVD compared to the local population.[50,51]

Dyslipidemia as a Risk Factor

South Asians have a higher rate of CVD than Europeans and yet have lower rates of elevated cholesterol, smoking, and hypertension.[2,52] High triglycerides, low HDL, and high levels of small dense LDL are more prevalent in Asian Indian men than high levels of LDL.[52] In a case–control study assessing risk factors for acute MI, there was no association of lipid profile with acute myocardial infarction.[53] Miller and McKeigue[54] have shown in independent studies a low level of total cholesterol, primarily due to low HDL cholesterol, in Asian Indians in the United Kingdom. South Asians in Canada presenting to the hospital with acute MI also had low rates of hyperlipidemia compared to controls (36% vs. 42%). In the Study of Health Assessment and Risk in Ethnic Groups (SHARE),[17] triglycerides was higher and HDL cholesterol lower in South Asians compared to Chinese and Europeans. However, there were no differences in LDL cholesterol levels compared to Europeans. Only 14% of Asian Indian men and 5% of Asian Indian women had optimal HDL cholesterol levels in the Coronary Artery Disease in Asian Indians (CADI) study.[55] In contrast, two studies in the United Kingdom found total cholesterol to be closely correlated to the extent of coronary atheroma or angioplasty. Asian Indians in multiple cross-sectional studies appear to have abnormal subfractions of the lipid profile.[56] It is possible that the threshold at which total cholesterol and LDL cholesterol levels become important may have to be set lower and HDL set higher and that small variations in these may have long-term effects in South Asians.

A large lipid-lowering trial among South Asians, the Investigation of Rosuvastatin in South Asians (IRIS),[57] showed that statins were effective and safe in decreasing total cholesterol, LDL cholesterol, and non-HDL cholesterol, with a high percentage of the population reaching their target goal according to NCEP ATP III guidelines. This was a randomized study of 740 patients in the United States and Canada receiving 10 or 20 mg of rosuvastatin compared to 10 or 20 mg of atorvastatin. Rosuvastatin 10 and 20 mg decreased LDL cholesterol by 45% and 50%, respectively, and atorvastatin 10 mg and 20 mg decreased LDL by 40% and 47%, respectively. Target goals were achieved in 79% and 89% of patients with rosuvastatin 10 mg and 20 mg, respectively, and in 76% and 85% of patients with atorvastatin 10 mg and 20 mg, respectively. This was the first intervention study of lipid-lowering agents in North America among South Asians.[57]

Insulin Resistance as a Risk Factor

Multiple studies have suggested that insulin resistance is highly prevalent in Asian Indians.[58–63] Many studies performed in urban and rural settings in India confirm the high prevalence of risk factors in the urban population, in whom parameters comprising insulin resistance are clustered.[59–63] McKeigue et al.,[53,54,64–66] in the Study of Distributions of CHD Risk, compared South Asians in the United Kingdom and Europeans living in the United Kingdom. Prevalence of diabetes was 4.3 times higher in South Asians with higher levels of abdominal obesity, triglycerides, and fasting insulin, and lower HDL cholesterol.[61]

Ramachandran et al., in their assessment of risk variables for CHD, noted significant association with hemoglobin A1c, fasting blood sugar, and abdominal obesity, suggesting that insulin resistance may play a significant role.[68,69] There is a high prevalence (10%–19%) of impaired glucose tolerance, central obesity, high triglycerides, and low HDL in South Asians in Canada.[17] The rate of diabetes is higher in South Asians in the United Kingdom and in Trinidad (19%–21%).[41] Misra et al. studied the cluster of factors associated with insulin resistance and CHD, and demonstrated significantly high prevalence of hypertension, obesity, impaired glucose tolerance, hyperinsulinemia, high LDL cholesterol, triglycerides, and low HDL cholesterol in young North Indians with manifest CHD.[47,67,70] Also, South Asians were more likely than controls to have diabetes (43.4% vs. 28.2%), despite lower BMI, and lower levels of dyslipidemia and smoking history in a Canadian study.[17] Clustering of cardiovascular risk factors in urban Asian Indians occurred in a study from Tamil Nada, India.[71–74] The components of insulin resistance syndrome, that is, primarily abdominal obesity, dyslipidemia, and impaired glucose tolerance, seemed to have the greatest significance.[75–77] Reaven has suggested that type 2 diabetes may be just one of the features of the insulin resistance complex, and insulin resistance itself is an independent risk factor for CVD.[78] Asian Indians appear to have a high prevalence of abdominal obesity and diabetes in cross-sectional studies. However, Afro-Caribbean and Pima Indians, in spite of a high incidence of obesity and diabetes, do not seem to fit in with the insulin resistance complex, as the prevalence of CVD is low. An interesting finding in a few studies of increased coronary disease in spite of lower levels of cholesterol and body fat percent/obesity has been suggested as the Indian paradox.[79,80] It is plausible that independent or cluster effects of fasting insulin, C peptide, leptin, abdominal obesity without increase in BMI, and plasminogen activator inhibitor–1 (PAI-1) levels may have causal relationships to development of diabetes or CVD.[55,81–87]

Other Emerging Risk Factors

Elevated levels of Lp(a) have been shown to be strong predictors of CHD.[88,89] Lp(a) has also been shown to be an independent risk factor for CAD in type 2 diabetic patients from South India compared to North American whites.[89] South Asians living in North America have elevated levels of Lp(a) as demonstrated in three different studies.[17] The CADI study showed a trend of elevated Lp(a) in South Asians (25%, compared to 19% of Euro-Americans).[90–93] In the NHW in the Churchgoer Study from Chicago, Lp(a) was 16.3 mg/dL, compared to 20.2 mg/dL among South Asian Indians ($P < 0.002$). In the third study from Canada, South Asians had a significantly higher mean Lp(a) compared to Canadians (34.1 vs. 17.3 mg/dL, $P < 0.013$), and was associated with increased risk of atherothrombotic events.[17]

Apo(a) has homology to plasminogen, competing with the substrate, thus allowing apoB to be actively taken up by foam cells. Lp(a) levels were 3 to 10 times higher in Asian Indians, and there was a threefold excess risk of instability compared to Chinese individuals in Singapore.[94,95] South Asians also had higher plasma homocysteine level and a higher rate of CVD, suggesting a possible association between elevated homocysteine levels and CHD.[96] In assessing the risk of CHD in Asian Indian men in the United Kingdom,[97] two case–control studies found that Asian Indians had a 6% higher concentration of homocysteine compared to Europeans. In a study from Canada, South Asian Indians had higher homocysteine levels compared to Chinese and Europeans (11.22, 10, and 9.2 mg/L, respectively; $P < 0.001$).[17] South Asians also had a higher prevalence of insulin resistance and diabetes, and there was a strong association between PAI-1 levels[98] and diabetes, suggesting that PAI-1 may be an indirect marker of insulin resistance syndrome.

In SHARE,[17] Anand and colleagues noted that South Asians had elevated PAI-1 levels compared to Europeans and Chinese, and being of South Asian ethnicity was an independent determinant of cardiovascular events.[98] Lipoprotein-associated phospholipase A_2 may also be elevated in Asian Indians.[99] Atheromatous plaque reflected serum total cholesterol levels in a comparative morphologic study of endarterectomy of coronary atherosclerotic plaques removed from patients from the southern part of India and Caucasians from Ottawa, Canada.[100] As BMI greater than 23 kg/m^2 appears to be a marker of risk in Asian Indians, and obesity is related to high leptin levels, there may be a direct association of risk between CVD and leptin, and an inverse association with adiponectin.[101,102] HsCRP has been shown to be a significant marker of risk for CVD in multiple studies.[103,104] In addition, elevated hsCRP appears to be highly prevalent (60%) in asymptomatic Asian Indians[70]; PAI-1 levels, factor VIII activity,[105] and platelet–endothelial cell adhesion molecule seem to be elevated in this population.[106]

The Asian Indian diet is high in carbohydrates and low in proteins. With nutritional transition in recent years, fat consumption seems to have increased with the availability of inexpensive vegetable oils. There has been a shift in consumption from a diet low in fats and high in carbohydrates to high-fat, less–complex carbohydrate, and increased energy-rich foods. To determine the association between saturated fat intake and prevalence of CHD and risk factor, Singh et al. studied 1806 subjects who were divided into three groups based on fat consumption.[79,80] The prevalence of CHD and risk factors was higher in urban populations with high–saturated fat intake and moderate intake, compared to saturated fat consumption of less than 7% per day. In a study exploring the link between carbohydrates and Asian diet, Ahmad[107] suggested high carbohydrates and moderate fat intake increased the risk of insulin resistance, diabetes, and high cholesterol leading to CHD. In a study of Asian Indian physicians in the United States, Yagalla showed abdominal obesity and altered lipoprotein levels to be associated with high CHD and saturated fat consumption to be associated with physical inactivity.[101]

Hence, there are multiple concerns that center around dietary transitions with altered vegetarian status, meal patterns, increased use of fast and convenience foods, changes in the frequency of using traditional Indian foods, and inclusion of other ethnic and Westernized foods as substitutes. This has led to a nutritional transition from a low-fat, high–complex carbohydrate diet to one rich in saturated fat and animal protein, and low in fiber and trace elements. Associated with physical inactivity, this nutritional transition appears to confer increased CVD risk.[108] INTERHEART is a case–control study of acute MI in 52 countries, enrolling 15,152 cases and 14,820 controls.[109,110] The relation of smoking, history of hypertension or diabetes, waist/hip ratio, dietary patterns, physical activity, consumption of alcohol, blood apolipoproteins, and psychosocial factors to MI were reported. Abnormal lipids, smoking, hypertension, diabetes, abdominal obesity, psychosocial factors, consumption of fruits, vegetables, and alcohol, and regular physical activity were all significantly related to acute MI ($P < 0.0001$ for all risk factors, except $P = 0.03$ for alcohol). These associations were noted in men and women, old and young, and all regions of the world. Collectively, these nine risk factors accounted for 90% of the population-attributable risk in men and 94% in women, suggesting that risk factor modification has the potential to prevent most premature cases of MI. In certain smaller studies, there are suggestions of specific genetic markers analyzed by quantitative trait linkage that may predispose the exponential risk noticed in this subgroup.[111,112]

SUMMARY

Individuals from ethnic minorities are increasing in number in the United States and comprise a rising proportion of the population. Epidemiologic and cross-sectional studies in minorities in the United States and other countries suggest an increasing prevalence of CHD. Along with this rise, there is evidence for a positive correlation with lipid abnormalities. Traditional risk factors appear to confer most of the risk for CHD. In addition, other risks such as low HDL cholesterol, high triglyceride levels, insulin resistance, diabetes, Lp(a), dietary indiscretion, and physical inactivity seem to be playing an important role in escalating the risk. Urbanization with adoption of a Westernized lifestyle in terms of nutritional transition, mixed with a genetic predisposition to CHD, may be contributing to the mounting prevalence of CHD among certain ethnic groups. Even though there are differences in risk factors by ethnic group, it is not clear whether there are differences in treatment strategies. A few interventional studies have shown efficacy and safety of statins in cholesterol reduction. However, whether there is cardiovascular event reduction is not clear, as minority populations have not been included in sufficient numbers in large-scale interventional studies. Nonetheless, identification of risk factors and aggressive risk factor modification with optimization of medical therapies should be the cornerstone of management in all ethnic groups. While such an approach underscores the importance of reducing the odds of a cardiovascular event and death on a continuum, there is an ongoing need to explore the differences in ethnic minorities that could explain the disparity in CHD risk. Future research should focus on multiple issues that include a consensual and conceptual definition of race, policies for CHD prevention, and better quantification of cultural factors, socioeconomic conditions, and environmental aspects. Lower cutpoints for cardiovascular risk factors and genetic susceptibility for differences in risk should be addressed a part of large prospective cohort studies. Interventions at the socioeconomic and political levels to alter health behavior models to decrease risk should also be undertaken. Better understanding and cognizance of the disparities of CHD risks will help healthcare professionals to cultivate culturally sensitive prevention and intervention programs targeted toward quelling the epidemic of CVD in high-risk ethnic groups.

REFERENCES

1. National Heart, Lung, and Blood Institute: Morbidity and Mortality: 2002 Chart Book on Cardiovascular, Lung, and Blood Diseases. http://www.nhlbi.nih.gov/resources/docs/02_chtbk.pdf.
2. Singh RB: Coronary artery disease in South Asians. *Indian Heart J* 1997;49(2):222–223.
3. Yusuf S, Reddy S, Ounpuu S, Anand S: Global burden of cardiovascular diseases. Part I: General considerations, the epidemiologic transition, risk factors, and impact of urbanization. *Circulation* 2001;104:2746–2753.
4. Yusuf S, Reddy S, Ounpuu S, Anand S: Global burden of cardiovascular diseases. Part II: variations in cardiovascular disease by specific ethnic groups and geographic regions and prevention strategies. *Circulation* 2001;104:2855–2864.
5. Expert Panel on Detection, Evaluation and Treatment of High Blood Cholesterol in Adults (ATP III): Executive summary of the third report of the NCEP. *JAMA* 2000;285:2486.
6. Sharma S, Malarcher AM, Giles WH, Myers G: Racial, ethnic and socioeconomic disparities in the clustering of cardiovascular disease risk factors. *Ethn Dis* 2004;14(1):43–48.
7. Kurian AK, Cardarelli KM. Racial and ethnic differences in cardiovascular disease risk factors: a systemic review. *Ethn Dis* 2007;17(1):143–152.
8. LaRosa JC, Brown CD: Cardiovascular risk factors in minorities. *Am J Med* 2005;118(12):1314–1322.
9. Rodriguez C, Pablos-Mendez A, Palmas W, Lantigua R, Mayeux R, Berglund L: Comparison of modifiable determinants of lipids and lipoprotein levels among African-American, Hispanics, and non-Hispanic Caucasians ≥65 years of age living in New York City. *Am J Cardiol* 2002;89(2):178–183.
10. Keevil JG, Cullen MW, Gangnon R, et al: Implications of cardiac risk and low-density lipoprotein cholesterol distributions in the United States for the diagnosis and treatment of dyslipidemia: data from National Health and Nutrition Examination Survey 1999 to 2002. *Circulation* 2007;115(11): 363–1370.
11. Sundquist J, Winkleby MA: Cardiovascular risk factors in Mexican American adults: a transcultural analysis of NHANES III 1988–1994. *Am J Public Health* 1999;89(5):723–730.
12. Winkleby MA, Kraemer HC, Ahn DK, Varady AN: Ethnic and socioeconomic differences in cardiovascular disease risk factors: findings for women from the Third National Health and Nutrition Examination Survey, 1988–1994. *JAMA* 1998;280: 356–362.
13. Goff DC Jr, Bertoni AG, Kramer H, et al: Dyslipidemia prevalence, treatment, and control in the Multi-Ethnic Study of Atherosclerosis (MESA). *Circulation* 2006;113:647–656.
14. Lloret R, Ycas J, Stein M, for the STARSHIP Study Group: comparison of rosuvastatin versus atorvastatin in Hispanic-Americans with hypercholesterolemia from the STARSHIP trial. *Am J Cardiol* 2006;98(6):768–773.
15. Centers for Disease Control and Prevention: Disparities in screening for and awareness of high blood cholesterol: United States, 1999–2002. *MMWR Morb Mortal Wkly Rep* 2005;54: 117–119.
16. Centers for Disease Control and Prevention: Behavioral Risk Factor Surveillance System: Prevalence Data. Atlanta, GA: U.S. Department of Health and Human Services, 2006. http://apps.nccd.cdc.gov/brfss/index.asp.
17. Hall WD, Clark LT, Wenger NK, et al: The metabolic syndrome in African Americans: a review. African-American Lipid and Cardiovascular Council. *Ethn Dis* 2003;13(4):414–428.
18. Harris-Hooker S, Sanford GL: Lipids, lipoproteins and coronary heart disease in minority populations. *Atherosclerosis* 1994;108(Suppl)S83–S104.
19. American Heart Association Statistics Committee and Stroke Statistics Subcommittee: Heart Disease and Stroke Statistics—2007 Update. A Report from the American Heart Association Statistics Committee and Stroke Statistics Subcommittee. *Circulation* 2007;115:e69–e171.
20. Anand SS, Yusuf S, Vuksan V, et al: Differences in risk factors, atherosclerosis, and cardiovascular disease between ethnic groups in Canada: The Study of Health Assessment and Risk in Ethnic Groups (SHARE). *Lancet* 2000;356:279–284.
21. Morrison JA, Barton BA, Biro FM, Sprecher DL: The conjoint trait of low high-density lipoprotein cholesterol and high triglycerides in adolescent black and white males. *Metabolism* 1998;47(5):514–521.
22. Rubins HB, Robins SJ, Collins J, et al: Distribution of lipids in 8,500 men with coronary artery disease, Department of Veterans Affairs HDL Intervention Trial Study Group. *Am J Cardiol* 1995;75(17):1196–1201.
23. Carnethon MR, Lynch, EB, Dyer AR, et al: Comparison of risk factors for cardiovascular mortality in black and white adults. *Arch Intern Med* 2006;166(11):1196–1202.
24. Ferdinand KC, Watson KE, Neal RC et al: Comparison of efficacy and safety of rosuvastatin versus atorvastatin in African American patients in a six week trial. ARIES Study Group. *Am J Cardiol* 2006;97(2):229–235.
25. Jones DW, Chambless LE, Folsom AR et al: Risk factors for coronary disease in African Americans: The Atherosclerosis Risk in Communities Study, 1987–1997. *Arch Intern Med* 2002;162: 2565–2571.
26. Metcalf PA, Sharrett AR, Folsom AR, et al: African American–white differences in lipids, lipoproteins, and apolipoproteins, by educational attainment, among middle-aged adults: The Atherosclerosis Risk in Communities Study. *Am J Epidemiol* 1998;148(8):750–760.
27. Sorlie PD, Sharrett AR, Patsch W, et al: The relationship between lipids/lipoproteins and atherosclerosis in African Americans and whites: The Atherosclerosis Risk in Communities Study. *Ann Epidemiol* 1999;9(3):149–158.

28. Miljkovic-Gacie I, Bunker CH, Ferrell RE, et al: Lipoprotein subclass and particle size differences in Afro-Caribbeans, African Americans, and white Americans: associations with hepatic lipase gene variation. *Metabolism* 2006;55(1):96–102.
29. Miller GJ, Beckles BLA, Maude GD, et al: Ethnicity and other characteristics predictive of CHD in a developing community: principal results of the St. James survey, Trinidad. *Int J Epidemiol* 1989;18:808–817.
30. Srinivasan SR, Segrest JP, Elkasabany AM, Berenson GS: Distribution and correlates of lipoproteins and their subclass in black and white young adults. The Bogalusa Heart Study. *Atherosclerosis* 2001;159(2);391–397.
31. Zoratti R: A review on ethnic differences in plasma triglycerides and high-density–lipoprotein cholesterol: Is the lipid pattern the key factor for the low coronary heart disease rate in people of African origin? *Eur J Epidemiol* 1998;14(1):9–21.
32. Malhotra A, Wolford JK, American Diabetes Association GENNID Study Group: Analysis of quantitive lipid traits in the genetics of NIDDM (GENNID) study. *Diabetes* 2005;54(10):3007–3014.
33. Adeyemo AA, Johnson T, Acheampong J, et al: A genome wide quantitative trait linkage analysis for serum lipids in type 2 diabetes in an African population. *Atherosclerosis* 2005;181(2):389–397.
34. Lee ET, Cowan LD, Welty TK, et al: All-cause mortality and cardiovascular disease mortality in three American Indian populations, aged 45–74 years, 1984–1988. The Strong Heart Study. *Am J Epidemiol* 1998;147:995–1008.
35. Welty TK, Rhoades DA, Yeh F, et al: Changes in cardiovascular disease risk factors among American Indians. The Strong Heart Study. *Ann Epidemiol* 2002;12:97–106.
36. Aronoff SL, Bennett PH, Gorden P, Rushforth N, Miller M: Unexplained hyperinsulinemia in normal and prediabetic Pima Indians compared with normal Caucasians. An example of racial differences in insulin secretion. *Diabetes* 1977;26:827–840.
37. Mendlein JM, Freedman DS, Peter DG, et al: Risk factors for coronary disease among Navajo Indians: findings from the Navajo Health and Nutritional Survey. *J Nutr* 1997;127:2099s–2105s.
38. Rodriguez BL, Curb JD, Burchfiel CM, et al: Impaired glucose tolerance, diabetes, and cardiovascular disease risk factor profiles in the elderly. The Honolulu Heart Program. *Diabetes Care* 1996;19:587–590.
39. Balarajan R, Bulusu L, Adelstein AM, et al: Patterns of mortality among migrants to England and Wales from the Indian subcontinent. *BMJ (Clin Res Ed)* 1984;289:1185.
40. Ballantyne CM, Hoogeveen RC, Bang H, Coresh J, Folsom AR, Heiss G, Sharrett AR: Lipoprotein-associated phospholipase A2, high-sensitivity C-reactive protein, and risk for incident coronary heart disease in middle-aged men and women in the Atherosclerosis Risk in Communities (ARIC) Study. *Circulation* 200424;109(7):837–842.
41. Beckles GL, Miller GJ, Kirkwood BR, Alexis SD, Carson DC: High total and cardiovascular disease mortality in adults of Indian descent in Trinidad, unexplained by major coronary risk factors. *Lancet* 1986;1:1298–1301.
42. Bhalodkar NC, Blum S, Enas EA: Accuracy of the ratio of triglycerides to high-density lipoprotein cholesterol for predicting low-density lipoprotein cholesterol particle sizes, phenotype B, and particle concentrations among Asian Indians. *Am J Cardiol* 2006;97(7):1007–1009.
43. Bhalodkar NC, Blum S, Rana T, Bhalodkar A, Kitchappa R, Kim KS, Enas E: Comparison of levels of large and small high-density lipoprotein cholesterol in Asian Indian men compared with Caucasian men in the Framingham Offspring Study. *Am J Cardiol* 2004;94(12);1561–1563.
44. Bhatnagar D, Anand IS, Durrington PN, et al: Coronary risk factors in people from the indian subcontinent living in West London and their siblings in India. *Lancet* 1995;345:405–409.
45. Bhopal R, Unwin N, White M, et al: Heterogeneity of coronary heart disease risk factors in Indian, Pakistani, Bangladeshi, and European origin populations: cross-sectional study. *BMJ* 1999;319(7204):215–220.
46. Pais P, Pogue J, Gerstein H, et al: Risk factors for acute myocardial infarction in Indians: a case–control study. *Lancet* 1996;348:358–363.
47. Misra J, Girinath M, Viswanathan V: Risk variables for coronary artery disease in Asian Indians. *Am J Cardiol* 2001;87:267–271.
48. Reddy KS, Yusuf S: Emerging epidemic of CVD in the developing countries. *Circulation* 1998;97:596–601.
49. Wilson PWF, Christiansen JC, Anderson KM, Kannel WB: Impact of national guidelines for cholesterol risk factor screening: The Framingham Offspring Study. *JAMA* 1989;262:41–44.
50. Singh Bedi U, Sing S, Syed A, Aryafar H, Arora R: Coronary artery disease in South Asians, an emergent risk group. *Cardiol Rev* 2006;14:74–80.
51. Uppaluri CR: Heart disease and its related risk factors in Asian Indians. *Ethn Dis* 2002;12(1):45–53.
52. Singh V, Deedwania P: Dyslipidemia in special populations: Asian Indians, African Americans, and Hispanics. *Curr Atheroscler Rep* 2006;8(1):32–40.
53. McKeigue PM, Shah B, Marmot MG: Relation of central obesity and insulin resistance with high diabetes prevalence and cardiovascular risk in South Asians. *Lancet* 1991;337:382–386.
54. McKeigue PM, Miller GJ, Marmot MG: Coronary heart disease in South Asians overseas: a review. *J Clin Epidemiol* 1989;42:597.
55. Enas EA, Garg A, Davidson MA, et al: Coronary heart disease and its risk factors in first-generation immigrant Asian Indians to the United States of America. *Indian Heart J* 1996;48:343–352.
56. Kulkarni KR, Markovitz JH, Nanda NC, Segrest JP: Increased prevalence of smaller and denser LDL particles in Asian Indians. *Arterioscler Throm Vasc Biol* 1999;19(11):2749–2755.
57. Deedwania PC, Gupta M, et al: Comparison of rosuvastatin and atorvastatin in South Asian patients at risk of coronary artery disease (from the IRIS trial). *Am J Cardiol* 2007;99:1538–1543.
58. Festa A, Hanley AJ, Tracy RP, D'Agostino R Jr, Haffner SM: PAI-1, obesity, insulin resistance and risk of cardiovascular events. *Thomb Haemost* 1997;78(1):656–660.
59. Gupta M, Brister S: Is South Asian ethnicity and independent cardiovascular risk factor? *Can J Cardiol* 2006;22(3):193–197.
60. Gupta R, Gupta HP, Kumar N, Joshi AK, Gupta VP: Lipoprotein, lipids and the prevalence of hyperlipidemia in rural India. *J Cardiovasc Risk* 1994;1(2):179–184.
61. Gupta R, Gupta VP, Sarna M, et al: Prevalence of coronary heart disease and risk factors in an urban Indian population: Jaipur Heart Watch-2. *Indian Heart J* 2002;54(1):59–66.
62. Gupta R, Gupta VP: Meta-analysis of coronary heart disease prevalence in India. *Indian Heart J* 1996;48:241–245.
63. Gupta R, Sarna M, Thanvi J, Rastogi P, Kaul V, Gupta VP: High prevalence of multiple coronary risk factor in Punjabi Bhatia community: Jaipur Heart Watch-3. *Indian Heart J* 2004;56(6):646–652.
64. McKeigue PM, Ferrie JE, Pierpoint T, et al: Association of early-onset coronary heart disease in South Asian Men with glucose intolerance and hyperinsulinemia. *Circulation* 1993;87:152–161.
65. McKeigue PM, Marmot MG, Adelstein AN, et al: Diet and risk factors for coronary heart disease in Asians in northwest London. *Lancet* 1985;ii:1086–1089.
66. McKeigue PM: Coronary heart disease in Indians, Pakistanis, and Bangladeshis: aetiology and possibilities for prevention. *Br Heart J* 1992;67:341–342.
67. Misra A, Reddy RB, Reddy KS, Mohan A, Baja JS: Clustering of impaired glucose tolerance, hyperinsulinemia and dyslipidemia in young North Indian Patients with coronary heart disease: a preliminary case–control study. *Indian Heart J* 1999;51(3):275–280.
68. Ramachandran A, Sathyamurthy I, Snehalatha C, et al: Risk variables for coronary artery disease in Asian Indians. *Am J Cardiol* 2001;87:267–271.
69. Ramachandran A, Snehalata C, Latha E, Satyavani K, Vijay V: Clustering of cardiovascular risk factors in Urban Asian Indians. *Diabetes Care* 1998;21:967–971.
70. Misra A: C-reactive protein in young individuals: problems and implications for Asian Indians. *Nutrition* 2004;20(5):478–481.
71. Mohan V, Deepa R, Rani SS, Premalatha G: Prevalence of coronary artery disease and its relationship to lipids in a selected population in South India: The Chennai Urban Population Study (CUPS No. 5). *J Am Coll Cardiol* 2001;38:682–687.
72. Mohan V, Deepa R, Velmurugan K, Gokulakrishnan K: Association of small dense LDL with coronary artery disease and diabetes in urban Asian Indians—the Chennai Urban Rural Epidemiology Study (CURES-8). *J Assoc Physicians India* 2005;53:95–100.

73. Mohan V, Deepa R, Velmurugan K, Premalatha G: Association of C-reactive protein with body fat, diabetes and coronary artery disease in Asian Indians: The Chennai Urban Rural Epidemiology Study (CURES-6). *Diabet Med* 2005;22(7):863–870.
74. Shanthi Rani CS, Rema M, Deepa R, et al: The Chennai Urban Population Study (CUPS): methodological details (CUPS paper no. 1). *Int J Diabetes Dev Countries* 1999;19:149–155.
75. Jadhav UM: Association of small dense LDL with a coronary artery disease and diabetes in urban Asian Indians—the Chennai urban Asian Indians—The Chennai Urban Rural Epidemiology Study (CURES 8). *J Assoc Physicians India* 2005;53:492–493 (author reply 493).
76. Jafar TH, Jafary FH, Jessani S, Chaturvedi N: Heart disease epidemic in Pakistan: women and men at equal risk. *Am Heart J* 2005;150(2):221–226.
77. Jolly KS, Pais P, Rihal CS: Coronary artery disease among South Asians: identification of a high risk population. *Can J Cardiol* 1996;12(6):569–571.
78. Reaven GM: Role of insulin resistance in human disease. *Diabetes* 1988;37:1595–1607.
79. Singh RB, Niaz MA, Beegom R, Wander GS, Thakur AS, Rissam HS: Body fat percent by bioelectrical impedance analysis and risk of coronary artery disease among urban men with low rates of obesity: the Indian paradox. *J Am Coll Nutr* 1999;18(3):268–273.
80. Singh RB, Rastogi V, Niaz MA, Ghosh S, Sy RG, Janus ED: Serum cholesterol and coronary artery disease in populations with low cholesterol levels: the Indian paradox. *Int J Cardiol* 1998;65(1):81–91.
81. Chambers JC, Obeid OA, Refsum H, et al: Plasma homocysteine concentrations and risk of coronary heart disease in United Kingdom Indian Asian and European men. *Lancet* 2000;355(9203):523–527.
82. Cruickshank JK, Clark PM, Riste LK, Cooper J, Hales CN: Insulin deficiency but excess proinsulin secretion during glucose challenge of British AfroCaribbean and Indo-origin populations with high rates of diabetes. *Diab Med* 1993;10:524.
83. Deedwania P, Singh V: Coronary artery disease in South Asians: evolving strategies for treatment and prevention. *Indian Heart J* 2005;57:617–631.
84. Deepa R, Velmurugan K, Saravanan G, Dwarakanath V, Agarwal S, Mohan V: Relationship of tissue plasminogen activator, plasminogen activator inhibitor-1 and fibrinogen with coronary artery disease in South Indian male subjects. *J Assoc Physicians India* 2002;50:901–906.
85. Dhawan J, Bray CL, Warburton R, Ghambhir DS, Morris J: Insulin resistance, high prevalence of diabetes, and cardiovascular risk in immigrant Asians: genetic or environmental effect? *Br Heart J* 1994;72(5):413–421.
86. Dhawan J: Coronary heart disease risks in Asian Indians. *Curr Opin Lipidol* 1996;7:196–198.
87. Drewnowski A, Popkin BM: The nutrition transition: new trends in the global diet. *Nutr Rev* 1997;55:31–43.
88. Anand SS, Enas EA, Pogue J, Haffner S, Pearson T, Yusuf S: Elevated lipoprotein(a) levels in South Asians in North America. *Metabolism* 1998;47:182–184.
89. Mohan V, Deepa R, Haranath SP, et al: Lipoprotein(a) is an independent risk factor for coronary artery disease in NIDDM patients in South India. *Diabetes Care* 1998;21:1819–1823.
90. Enas EA, Mehta J: Malignant coronary artery disease in young Asian Indians, thoughts on pathogenesis, prevention and therapy. Coronary Artery Disease in Asian Indians (CADI) Study. *Clin Cardiol* 1995;18(3):131–135.
91. Enas EA, Yusuf S, Mehta JL: Prevalence of coronary artery disease in Asian Indians. *Am J of Cardiol* 1992;70:945–949.
92. Enas EA, Yusuf S: Third meeting of the International Working Group on Coronary Artery Disease in South Asians, 29 March 1998, Atlanta, USA. *Indian Heart J* 1999;51(1):99–103.
93. Thomas I, Gupta S, Sempos C, Cooper R: Serum lipids in Indian physicians living in the US compared to US born physicians. *Atherosclerosis* 1986;61:99–106.
94. Hughes K, Aw TC, Kuperan P, Choo M: Central obesity, insulin resistance, syndrome X, lipoprotein(a), and cardiovascular risk in Indians, Malays, and Chinese in Singapore. *J Epidemiol Community Health* 1997;51(4):394–399.
95. Tan CE, Tai ES, Tan CS, et al: APOE polymorphism and lipid profile in three ethnic groups in the Singapore population. *Atherosclerosis* 2003;170(2):253–260.
96. Senaratne MP, MacDonald K, DeSilva D: Possible ethnic differences in plasma homocysteine levels associated with coronary artery disease between South Asian and East Asian immigrants. *Clin Cardiol* 2001;24(11):730–734.
97. Martyn CN: Serum homocysteine and risk of coronary heart disease in United Kingdom Indian Asians. Lancet 2000;355(9203):512–513.
98. Nagi DK, Knowler WC, Hanson RL, Ali VM, Yudkin JS: Plasminogen activator inhibitor (PAI-1) and non–insulin-dependent diabetes in Pima Indians, south Asians and Europeans. Populations at varying risk of NIDDM and coronary artery disease. *Thromb Haemost* 1996;75(6):921–927.
99. Tselepsis AD, John Chapman M: Inflammation, bioactive lipids and atherosclerosis: potential roles of a lipoprotein-associated phospholipase A2, platelet activating factor-acetylhydrolase. *Atheroscler Suppl* 2002;3(4):57–68.
100. Varghese PJ, Arumugam SB, Cherian KM, Walley V, Farb A, Virmani R: Atheromatous plaque reflects serum total cholesterol levels: a comparative morphologic study of endarterectomy coronary atherosclerotic plaques removed from patients from the southern part of India and Caucasians from Ottawa, Canada. *Clin Cardiol* 1998;21(5):335–340.
101. Yagalla MV, Hoerr SL, Song WO, et al: Relationship of diet, abdominal obesity and physical activity to plasma lipoprotein level in Asian Indian physicians residing in the U.S. *J Am Diet Assoc* 1996;96(3):257–261.
102. Yudkin JS, Jajnik CS, Mohamed-Ali V, Bulmer K: High levels of circulating proinflammatory cytokines and leptin in urban, but not rural, Indians. A potential explanation for increased risk of diabetes and coronary heart disease. *Diabetes Care* 1999;22(2):363–364.
103. Ridker PM, Wilson PW, Grundy SM. Should C-reactive protein be added to metabolic syndrome and to assessment of global cardiovascular risk? *Circulation* 2004;109(23):2818–2825.
104. Ridker PM: High-sensitivity C-reactive protein: potential adjunct for global risk assessment in the primary prevention of cardiovascular disease. *Circulation* 2001;103(13):1813–1818.
105. Saha N, Heng CK, Mozoomdar BP, et al: Racial variation of factor VII activity and antigen levels and their correlates in healthy Chinese and Indians at low and high risk for coronary artery disease. *Atherosclerosis* 1995;117(1):33–42.
106. Fang L, Wei H, Chowdhury SH, et al: Association of Leu 125Val polymorphism of platelet endothelial cell adhesion molecule-1 (PECAM-1) gene and soluble level of PECAM-1 with coronary artery disease in Asian Indians. *Indian J Med Res* 2005;121(2):92–99.
107. Ahmad U, Frossard PM: Coronary heart disease in South Asia: need to redefine risk. *Int J Cardiol 2006*;107(2):289–290.
108. Williams B: Westernized Asians and cardiovascular disease: nature or nurture? *Lancet* 1995;345:401.
109. Ounpuu S, Negassa A, Yusuf S, for the INTER-HEART Investigators: INTER-HEART: a global study of risk factors for acute myocardial infarction. *Am Heart J* 2001;141:711–721.
110. Yusuf S, Hawken S, Onpuu S, et al: Effect of potentially modifiable risk factors associated with myocardial infarction in 52 countries (the INTERHEART study): case–control study. *Lancet* 2004;364:937–952.
111. Pati N, Pati U: Paraoxonase gene polymorphism and coronary artery disease in Indian subjects. *Int J Cardiol* 1998;66(2): 165–168.
112. Sarkar PD, TMS, Madhusudhan B: Association between paraoxonase activity and lipid levels in patients with premature coronary artery disease. *Clin Chim Acta* 2006;373:77–81.

CHAPTER 43

Special Patient Populations: HIV Patients

Rajagopal V. Sekhar and Ashok Balasubramanyam

INTRODUCTION

The introduction of highly active antiretroviral therapy (HAART) has increased survival, decreased morbidity, and improved the nutritional status of patients infected with human immunodeficiency virus–1 (HIV-1). However, these benefits have been accompanied in a very high proportion of patients by unusual body composition alterations (often described as "lipodystrophy") and lipid metabolic abnormalities. Lipodystrophy manifests as fat accumulation in the truncal or dorsocervical regions, loss of fat in the limbs and face, or a combination of central fat accumulation and peripheral fat loss. The lipid metabolic abnormalities are characteristically manifested by moderate to severe hypertriglyceridemia with increases in low-density lipoprotein (LDL) cholesterol and modest decreases in high-density lipoprotein (HDL) cholesterol. Insulin resistance is a very frequent concomitant of these alterations, and is associated with a modest increase in the prevalence of diabetes (particularly among patients receiving certain protease inhibitor drugs). The Data Collection on Adverse Events of Anti-HIV Drugs (DAD) study group noted a diabetes prevalence of 3.1% among 23,347 patients in that cohort.

The combination of lipodystrophy and dyslipidemia in HIV patients is most aptly described as "HIV-associated dyslipidemic lipodystrophy" (HADL).[1] HADL is associated with a striking increase in the risk of developing cardiovascular disease. While there is clearly an urgent need for appropriate therapy, current approaches to treat both the dyslipidemia and the lipodystrophy have been problematic and at best partially effective. Barriers to effective therapy include limited understanding of the pathogenesis of HADL, the need for persisting with some antiretroviral agents despite their propensity to induce dyslipidemia or insulin resistance in patients who have achieved excellent HIV control, adverse interactions between lipid-lowering agents and antiretroviral drugs, ineffective therapeutic responses to standard lipid-lowering drugs, a high prevalence of liver dysfunction that limits the pharmacologic options, and issues of medication compliance associated with polypharmacy. There is limited consensus on approaches to treat the dyslipidemia, but as yet there are no consistently effective or approved therapies for the lipodystrophy associated with HADL.

COMPONENTS OF HIV-ASSOCIATED DYSLIPIDEMIC LIPODYSTROPHY

There is currently no widely accepted and practical case definition of HADL.[2] Lipodystrophy has been identified by clinicians and researchers based on varying descriptions of anthropomorphic changes in HIV patients, using different methods to measure total and regional body fat, self-reports of body shape changes, or less than objective criteria.[3] The HIV Lipodystrophy Case Definition Study Group has developed a multifactorial statistical model to improve diagnostic accuracy, incorporating the parameters of age, sex, duration of HIV infection, HIV disease stage, waist/hip ratio, anion gap, serum HDL cholesterol concentration, and anthropometry.[4] This model is reportedly 79% sensitive and 80% specific for the diagnosis of lipodystrophy in HIV patients. However, its practicability in the clinical setting has been limited by its emphasis on detecting lipoatrophy rather than fat accumulation, and by the need for imaging techniques to quantify fat gain or loss in varying body depots.

A practical approach to HADL is to begin with the understanding that it includes a combination of metabolic abnormalities and changes in body morphology. The metabolic changes include distinctive dyslipidemia and insulin resistance. Changes in body morphology include a varying combination of central fat accumulation and peripheral (including facial) fat loss. The most significant risks to developing lipodystrophy appear to be increased duration of HIV infection, high viral load, low CD4 nadir prior to HAART treatment, and prolonged survival and duration of HAART, as observed in the longitudinal HIV Out-Patient Study (HOPS).[5,6] Antiretroviral drugs have also been implicated in the evolution of lipodystrophy. The use of the nucleoside reverse transcriptase inhibitor (NRTI) stavudine[7,8] or combination therapy employing two NRTIs such as stavudine and didanosine has been associated with severe lipoatrophy.[9]

Dyslipidemia

Abnormalities in serum lipid levels (Table 43-1) were described in HIV patients prior to the advent of HAART.[10–12] These abnormalities took the form of hypertriglyceridemia[10] and elevated free fatty acid (FFA) levels,[11] together with decreased plasma total cholesterol,[12] HDL cholesterol, apolipoprotein (apo) A-I, LDL cholesterol, and apoB-100 levels.[11] The elevated triglyceride levels were due to increased triglyceride content of very-low-density lipoprotein (VLDL), LDL, and HDL, coupled with decreased triglyceride clearance.[11]

Since the widespread use of HAART, triglyceride levels in HIV patients have risen even more significantly. Multiple studies have noted a strong link between the use of protease inhibitor (PI) drugs and the development of dyslipidemia in patients with HADL.[13–17] Dyslipidemia associated with PI drugs is characterized by both hypercholesterolemia and in hypertriglyceridemia. In a 5-year historical cohort analysis of 221 HIV-infected patients, the cumulative incidence of new-onset hypercholesterolemia, hypertriglyceridemia, and lipodystrophy was 24%, 19%, and 13%, respectively, and was associated with PI therapy.[18] The incidence of hypercholesterolemia and hypertriglyceridemia was significantly elevated in 1160 HIV patients in a Swiss cohort study, of whom 60% received a single PI–based regime, and 15% were on a dual PI–based regimen.[19]

Individual PI agents differ in their capacity to induce lipid changes, especially hypertriglyceridemia. Ritonavir, nelfinavir, and saquinavir have been significantly associated with hypertriglyceridemia, while amprenavir is less strongly associated. Switching to atazanavir resulted in a 46% decrease in hypertriglyceridemia in one study.[20] Periard et al.[14] found that ritonavir conferred the highest risk of hypercholesterolemia (20-fold increase), followed by nelfinavir (ninefold), and indinavir (fourfold). Furthermore, healthy, non–HIV-infected adults given ritonavir for 2 weeks experienced significant elevations in plasma triglycerides, VLDL cholesterol, intermediate-density lipoprotein (IDL) cholesterol, apoB, and lipoprotein(a), together with a decrease in HDL cholesterol levels.[18] The mechanism underlying these changes is not clear.

There is also indirect evidence of the inimical effects of PI drugs in the form of partial reversal of dyslipidemia when they are discontinued in so-called "switch" studies,[21] and worsening of the lipid profile when PI and NRTI drugs are combined.[22] NRTIs have also been implicated in the development of HIV-associated dyslipidemia. In one study, combinations of a dual NRTI–based regime with either a PI or a non-NRTI (NNRTI) agent were significantly associated with hypercholesterolemia.[23]

The duration of exposure to HAART appears to be an important factor in the development of lipid changes.[24] The Swiss cohort study noted increased non-HDL cholesterol levels with longer exposure to either PI- or NNRTI-based therapy.[23] Longer exposure to PI-based therapy was also associated with increased triglyceride concentrations. NNRTI agents were associated with variable effects on triglyceride levels, which rose slightly in patients exposed to efavirenz, but declined in patients exposed to nevirapine, whereas with increased exposure to NRTI therapy, HDL cholesterol concentrations increase and triglyceride concentrations decrease. Comparison of three common PI-based therapies revealed that nelfinavir was associated with little change in the lipid profile upon increasing exposure, the combination of indinavir and ritonavir was associated with the worst lipid profile, and the combination of lopinavir with ritonavir was intermediate. Increasing exposure to abacavir was associated with a decrease in triglyceride levels.[25] Additional factors associated with increased risk of developing hypertriglyceridemia include CD4 counts and HIV RNA levels, but the association with CD4 cell count and HIV viral load differed between regimens. In patients who were naive to antiretroviral therapy, in patients having prior exposure to antiretroviral therapy but not currently receiving any antiretroviral therapy, or in patients currently receiving NRTI alone, the risk of having elevated triglycerides rose with increasing HIV RNA, but not with CD4 cell count, whereas in patients treated with protease inhibitors, NRTIs, or both, the risk of elevations in triglycerides increased with both increasing HIV viral titers and increasing CD4 counts.[24]

Insulin Resistance

Insulin resistance in patients with HADL[26] is likely mediated by both direct effects of HAART drugs and lipotoxicity resulting from serious dysregulation of adipocyte function and intermediary metabolism of fatty acids. About 35% of HIV patients treated with PI drugs develop insulin resistance, and a smaller proportion develop glucose intolerance; the reported incidence of diabetes is considerably lower at around 7%.[27] PI agents may induce insulin resistance in skeletal muscle by inhibiting the function of the insulin-sensitive glucose transporter Glut4, even at therapeutic concentrations.[28] Nondiabetic HIV-positive patients receiving PI-based HAART have abnormal responses to an oral glucose challenge, with increased levels of fasting insulin, 2-hour insulin, and 2-hour glucose.[27] NRTI drugs, especially the thymidine analogues, may also induce insulin resistance in muscle and liver. The mechanism underlying this effect is unclear, but could involve lipotoxicity resulting from the known ability of these agents to disrupt mitochondrial oxidative phosphorylation and induce a defect in fatty acid oxidation. Thus, a combination of the direct effects of PI and NRTI drugs, together with the indirect effects of dysregulated adipocyte lipolysis resulting in ectopic deposition of fat in viscera (e.g., liver and skeletal muscle)

TABLE 43-1 Cardiovascular Risk Factors in Data Collection on Adverse Events of Anti-HIV Drugs Study Population at Baseline According to Current Use of Antiretroviral Therapy

	Total	Naive	No Current ART	NRTI Only	Combination with NNRTI	Combination with PI	Combination with PI Plus NNRTI	P[a]	Missing Data (%)
Number of patients	17,852	2315	1082	1898	3493	7749	1315		
Age >45 years male, >55 years female (%)	24.7	13.1	18.8	23.7	27.6	26.2	34.8	<0.001	0.1
Body mass index (kg/m^2) [median (IQR)]	23 (21–25)	23 (21–25)	23 (20–25)	23 (21–25)	23 (21–25)	23 (21–25)	22 (21–24)	<0.0001	13.9
Body mass index >30 kg/m^2 [% (95% CI)]	3.5 (3.2–3.8)	4.8 (3.9–5.8)	3.7 (2.5–4.9)	3.0 (2.1–3.8)	3.9 (3.2–4.6)	3.1 (2.8–3.7)	2.3 (1.5–3.4)	<0.001	
Current smoker [% (95% CI)]	51.5 (50.3–52.7)	55.1 (51.9–58.4)	59.0 (54.1–63.9)	52.7 (49.0–56.5)	47.5 (44.9–50.1)	51.6 (49.8–53.3)	45.9 (41.7–50.1)	<0.001	18.5
Family history of CHD [% (95% CI)]	11.4 (10.8–12.0)	11.4 (9.8–13.1)	9.0 (6.9–11.1)	12.5 (10.3–14.6)	12.6 (11.1–14.1)	10.8 (9.9–11.8)	13.1 (10.5–15.8)	<0.09	37.2
Previous CVD [% (95% CI)]	1.4 (1.2–1.6)	0.6 (0.3–0.9)	1.3 (0.6–2.0)	1.8 (1.2–2.5)	1.9 (1.3–2.2)	1.3 (1.1–1.6)	1.9 (1.1–2.6)	<0.002	2.1
Hypertension [% (95% CI)]	8.5 (8.1–8.9)	6.1 (5.0–7.1)	8.7 (6.8–10.5)	7.0 (5.8–8.3)	9.6 (8.5–10.6)	8.9 (8.2–9.5)	10.1 (8.3–12.0)	<0.001	8.0
Diabetes mellitus [% (95% CI)]	2.5 (2.2–2.7)	1.2 (0.7–1.7)	1.1 (0.4–1.7)	2.4 (1.7–3.1)	3.5 (2.9–4.2)	2.3 (2.0–2.6)	4.2 (3.1–5.3)	<0.001	3.3
Total cholesterol (mmol/L) [median (IQR)]	5.1 (4.2–6.0)	4.4 (3.7–5.2)	4.4 (3.7–5.2)	4.6 (3.9–5.4)	5.3 (4.5–6.1)	5.3 (4.5–6.3)	5.9 (4.9–7.1)	<0.0001	17.6
Total cholesterol ≥6.2 mmol/L) [% (95% CI)]	22.2 (21.4–22.9)	7.7 (6.4–8.9)	9.5 (7.3–11.4)	9.8 (8.2–11.3)	22.8 (21.0–24.6)	27.0 (25.7–28.2)	44.1 (40.1–47.9)	<0.001	
HDL cholesterol (mmol/L) [median (IQR)]	1.1 (0.9–1.4)	1.1 (0.9–1.4)	1.1 (0.8–1.3)	1.1 (0.9–1.5)	1.2 (1.0–1.5)	1.1 (0.9–1.4)	1.1 (0.9–1.4)	<0.0001	54.2
HDL cholesterol ≤0.9 mmol/L [% (95% CI)]	25.7 (24.6–26.8)	25.5 (22.6–28.5)	35.0 (30.0–39.9)	24.8 (21.5–28.6)	19.1 (16.7–21.5)	27.1 (25.5–28.8)	23.8 (20.0–27.7)	<0.001	
Triglycerides (mmol/L) [median (IQR)]	1.7 (1.1–2.8)	1.3 (0.9–1.9)	1.5 (1.1–2.3)	1.4 (0.9–2.2)	1.6 (1.0–2.7)	1.9 (1.2–3.1)	2.5 (1.6–4.2)	<0.0001	17.6
Triglycerides ≥2.3 mmol/L [% (95% CI)]	33.8 (32.7–34.6)	15.2 (13.8–17.3)	25.9 (22.5–29.3)	22.7 (20.3–25.0)	31.8 (29.7–33.9)	40.0 (38.5–41.5)	54.3 (49.9–58.7)	<0.001	
Lipodystrophy [% (95% CI)]	25.4 (24.6–26.1)	2.2 (1.6–2.8)	20.6 (17.9–23.3)	20.8 (18.7–22.8)	31.2 (29.3–33.1)	29.7 (28.5–31.0)	35.1 (31.9–38.3)	<0.001	1.1

[a] Chi-square for comparison of frequencies, Kruskal-Wallis for comparison of distributions.

IQR, interquartile range; PI, protease inhibitor; NNRTI, non-nucleoside reverse transcriptase inhibitor; NRTI, nucleoside reverse transcriptase inhibitor; CHD, coronary heart disease; CI, confidence interval; CVD, cardiovascular disease; NA: not applicable. (From Ref. 24.)

may cause the insulin resistance that develops in HIV patients.[29–31] Again, individual agents may have varying effects; the PI atazanavir did not affect insulin sensitivity in healthy subjects, while both lopinavir and ritonavir induced insulin resistance.[32]

Fat Redistribution

The lipodystrophy or "fat redistribution" characteristic of HADL is manifested by varying degrees of fat loss and fat accumulation in a depot-specific pattern.[13,33] The reported prevalence of lipodystrophy varies widely because of the lack of clearly defined and practicable clinical criteria, ranging from 13% to 84%. This abnormal fat distribution generally presents in one of three forms: (1) generalized or localized lipoatrophy usually involving the extremities, buttocks, and face; (2) lipohypertrophy with generalized or local fat deposition involving the abdomen, breasts, dorsocervical region, and supraclavicular area; and (3) a mixed pattern with central adiposity and peripheral lipoatrophy.[34] Several studies have noted that a significant proportion of HIV patients develop increased abdominal fat following initiation of HAART.[13,34–36] The Fat Redistribution and Metabolic Changes in HIV Infection (FRAM) Study examined the contributions of peripheral lipoatrophy and central fat accumulation to the phenotype of HIV-associated lipodystrophy and found that HIV-infected men had peripheral fat loss, but that there were no differences between HIV-infected men and HIV-negative controls in the degree of increase in central fat.[37] In addition, there were no correlations between changes in central fat accumulation and peripheral fat loss in the HIV-infected men, suggesting that the peripheral fat loss and central fat deposition may not be causally linked.

PI drugs were initially implicated as the main cause of lipodystrophy,[18] but similar body fat changes were later noted in association with the use of NRTI and NNRTI drugs as well.[38] There is some suggestion that the PI agents are associated more with visceral fat accumulation and the NRTI agents more with peripheral lipoatrophy, although the distinction is by no means absolute. The molecular effects of these different agents on adipocyte function and metabolism suggest that a combination of effects of different classes of HAART drugs could underlie some of the body fat changes. For example PI drugs have been described *in vitro* to increase lipolysis[39] and reduce expression of the adipocyte-specific transcription factor sterol regulatory element–binding protein–1c (SREBP1c), SREBP1c-dependent lipoprotein lipase (LPL), and fatty acid synthase,[40] while NRTI agents have been shown to promote adipocyte apoptosis.[41] These effects could synergize to produce "lipoatrophy" *in vivo*. However the drug concentrations used in these *in vitro* studies significantly exceeded the therapeutic concentrations generally achieved in patients, suggesting that other factors may be involved in the pathogenesis of HADL.

PATHOPHYSIOLOGY

Although pathophysiologic investigations of HADL have focused on the role of HAART drugs, the underlying etiologic factors are likely to be multifactorial. Factors intrinsic to the virus, host immune responses and disease status, as well as treatment duration and type, may play key roles.[42] Data from HOPS[43] suggest that the risk factors for lipoatrophy include drugs (especially exposure to and duration of NRTI thymidine analogues such as stavudine and zidovudine), age, immunologic parameters such as the CD4 T-cell count, viral factors such as HIV load, and Caucasian ethnicity. Risk factors for fat accumulation include duration of therapy, age, CD4 T-cell count, HIV load, exposure to PIs, and female gender. While such epidemiologic risk factor assessments are helpful in understanding the heterogeneity of possible causes of HADL, they cannot define etiologies or mechanisms. To understand how abnormal fat distribution develops and how this is related to dyslipidemia, insulin resistance, and atherosclerosis, it is important to test mechanistic hypotheses.

Increased intra-abdominal fat is linked to the development of metabolic syndrome, which predisposes to cardiovascular disease (Fig. 43-1). Intra-abdominal fat accumulation is also associated with lipid deposition in skeletal muscle and the liver, leading to insulin resistance. This is accompanied by increases in circulating prothrombotic and proatherogenic factors such as FFAs, tumor necrosis factor–α (TNF-α), interleukin-6 (IL-6), and plasminogen activator inhibitor–1 (PAI-1), and declines in circulating factors linked to insulin sensitivity (e.g., adiponectin, leptin). Since a characteristic feature of HADL is peripheral lipoatrophy, fundamental questions to ask regarding its pathophysiology are whether and how this is linked to the development of insulin resistance, visceral fat accumulation, and dyslipidemia.

Metabolic Defects

Data from recent metabolic studies[44,45] reveal specific defects that could underlie the complex lipid abnormalities, anthropomorphic changes, and insulin resistance[46] in HADL. Sekhar et al. used stable isotopes, mass spectrometry, and indirect calorimetry to study lipid kinetics in HADL patients with dyslipidemia and centripetal fat redistribution, in both fasted[44] and fed[47] states. Compared to non-HIV subjects matched for age, gender, and body mass index, HADL subjects had specific defects in lipid turnover that could explain key features of the phenotype. Total lipolysis was a significantly increased in the fasted state, and although this was accompanied by a modest increase in intra-adipocyte recycling of fatty acids, there was a net increase in FFA release into the plasma. There was no proportionate increase in plasma fatty acid oxidation, causing increased delivery of FFAs to the liver for re-esterification and VLDL triglyceride synthesis. Concomitantly, fasting serum concentrations of both FFAs and VLDL triglycerides were profoundly elevated and HDL cholesterol concentrations were low in the HADL patients. The fundamental defect in the regulation of fasting lipolysis has been corroborated by other investigators.[45,48] Despite wide variation in other etiological factors linked to HADL such as age, duration and composition of HAART therapy, and duration of disease and viral and immune factors,

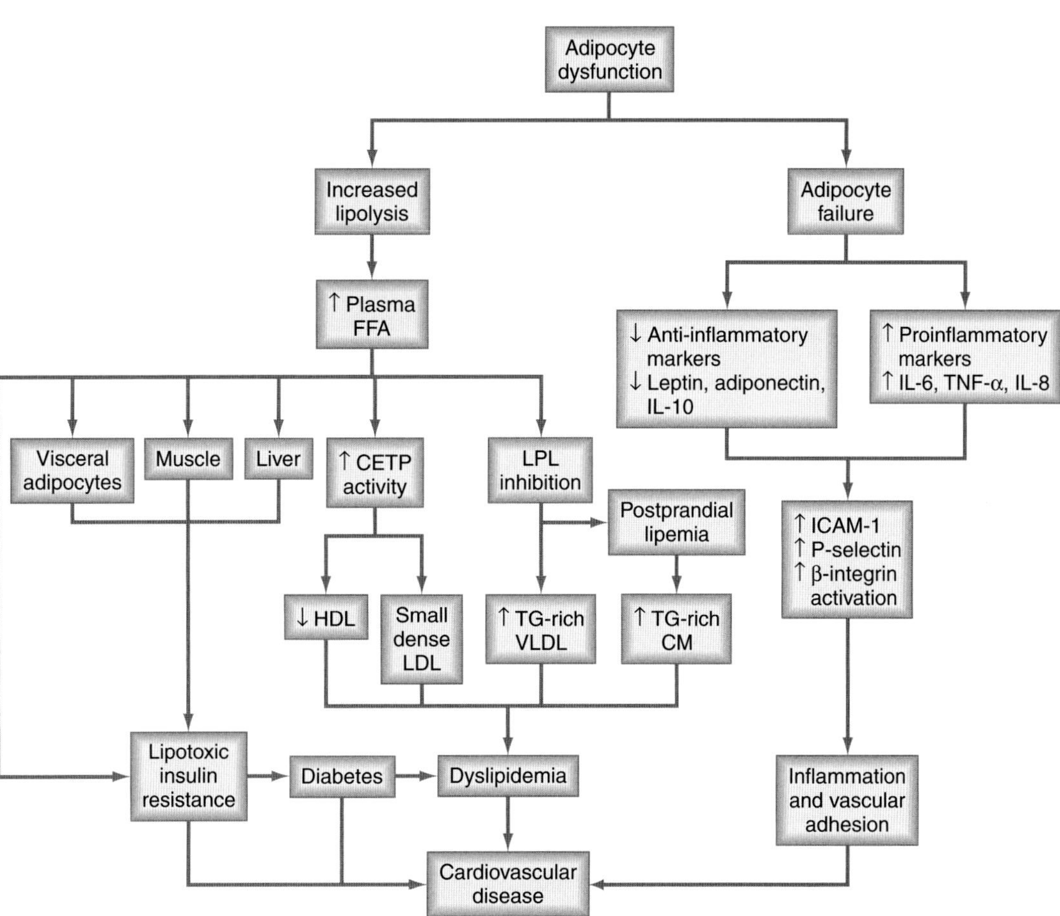

FIGURE 43-1 Algorithm for adipocyte dysfunction in HIV-associated dyslipidemic lypodystrophy (HADL). CETP, cholesteryl ester transfer protein; CM, chylomicron; FFA, free fatty acid; HDL, high-density lipoprotein; ICAM, intercellular adhesion molecule; IL, interleukin; LDL, low-density lipoprotein; LPL, lipoprotein lipase; TG, triglyceride; TNF-α, tumor necrosis factor–α; VLDL, very-low-density lipoprotein. Source: Sekhar RV et al. *Curr Atheroscler Rep* 2004;6:173–179.

patients with HADL seem to have a consistent pattern of increased total lipolysis, which could be a mechanistic common pathway leading to both the metabolic and anthropomorphic defects.

To identify defects in the disposal of dietary fat, chylomicron triglyceride concentrations were measured. After a 14-hour fast, HADL patients had fivefold higher plasma chylomicron triglyceride concentrations compared to non-HIV controls, indicating a severe defect in dietary lipid clearance. This was associated with marked retardation in postprandial nonoxidative disposal of orally administered labeled triglyceride from the chylomicron pool.[47]

How Could These Metabolic Defects Result in HADL Phenotype?

The specific defects in lipid kinetics in both fasted and fed states appear necessary and perhaps sufficient to explain the severe hypertriglyceridemia, as well as the tendency to develop intrahepatic and intramyocellular fat accumulation, and (at least in part) the insulin resistance in HADL. Additional mechanisms would be required to explain the visceral adiposity and localized fat accumulation in other depots.

These defects could lead to the HADL phenotype as follows. If lipolysis were elevated most markedly in peripheral adipose depots such as in the femoral–gluteal region, the result would be peripheral lipoatrophy. With blunted plasma fatty acid oxidation, there would be increased fatty acid flux to the liver resulting in increased production and secretion of triglyceride-rich VLDLs, as well as "ectopic" deposition of fat in metabolically active tissues such as muscle and visceral adipocytes, resulting in lipotoxic insulin resistance[30,31] and central adiposity.[49] Despite blunted plasma fatty acid oxidation, HADL patients also appear to have increased oxidation of fat derived from nonplasma sources such as intramyocellular and intrahepatic lipid depots. Abnormal oxidative products of intravisceral lipid deposits have been strongly associated with both insulin resistance and impaired glucose metabolism,[50] due to impaired insulin signaling.[51] Increased plasma FFA concentrations would also inhibit the activity of adipocyte LPL,[52] and defective LPL function would impair clearance of both the triglyceride-rich VLDL particles hypersecreted by the liver and triglyceride-rich chylomicrons transporting dietary fat, exacerbating hypertriglyceridemia. The molecular mechanisms responsible for the lipid kinetic defects and the putative metabolic outcomes are likely to be heterogeneous, including various HAART agents, factors expressed by HIV per se,[53,54] and factors related to the immune response.

Hormonal and Cytokine Defects

Proinflammatory adipocytokines are increased in fat depots of HIV patients, likely as a concomitant of the fundamental adipocyte dysfunction, and these may influence the development of HADL. Elevated levels of TNF-α and IL-6 have been reported in abdominal subcutaneous fat in patients with HADL,[55] compared to HIV patients without lipodystrophy. Plasma levels of soluble TNF receptor type 1 are also elevated, and are correlated with both insulin resistance and cardiovascular risk.[56]

Adiponectin is an important mediator of insulin sensitivity. HADL patients are uniformly deficient in adiponectin, and this deficiency is correlated with hypertriglyceridemia, central obesity, low HDL cholesterol, and decreased peripheral fat mass.[57,58] HIV infection per se may contribute to an abnormal regulation of adiponectin secretion.[59] HADL patients with lipoatrophy also have low plasma leptin concentrations. Leptin deficiency predisposes to increased lipid accumulation in nonadipose sites,[60] and leptin resistance has been described in other forms of lipodystrophy.[60] Hence, hypoleptinemia in lipoatrophic HADL patients may lead to lipotoxicity and exacerbate insulin resistance.

Partial or complete growth hormone (GH) deficiency is present in about one-third of patients with HADL.[61] Functional assessment of the growth hormone axis showed diminished GH pulse amplitude and GH concentrations despite apparently normal insulin-like growth factor–1 (IGF-1) levels in these patients; these manifestations of GH deficiency were associated with increased visceral fat.[61] Of note, when HADL subjects with GH deficiency received physiologic replacement with GH, they responded with a decrease in lipolytic activity, a key defect in lipid turnover in subjects with HADL.[62] Consistent with this finding are the salutary effects on both lipid levels and visceral fat of a growth hormone–releasing hormone (GHRH) agonist that raises circulating levels of GH to physiologic concentrations.[63]

COMPLICATIONS AND CARDIOVASCULAR RISK

Patients with HADL have multiple risk factors for accelerated cardiovascular disease, including elevated plasma levels of insulin, total, LDL, and non-HDL cholesterol, and triglycerides, and decreased HDL cholesterol. Other traditional risk factors such as smoking, hypertension, and diabetes also further increase the risk for cardiovascular disease. The DAD study group reported an increased incidence of myocardial infarction (adjusted relative risk 1.16/year of exposure) in patients exposed to combination antiretroviral therapy, with no effect of age or gender.[64] The adjusted relative risk was 1.16/year of exposure to PI drugs and 1.05/year of exposure to NNRTI drugs.[65] Other studies have also found an association between the use of PI drugs and myocardial infarction.[66–68]

Patients with HADL are also at increased risk of cerebrovascular disease, as suggested by a study that measured increased carotid intima–media thickness in HADL compared to HIV patients without lipodystrophy.[69]

THERAPEUTIC STRATEGIES

Interventions Targeting Dyslipidemia

The severe dyslipidemia of HADL patients requires urgent and effective therapy, but this has not been realized due to several important obstacles. Many classes of lipid-lowering drugs are contraindicated in the presence of liver dysfunction, which is highly prevalent in HIV patients because of the adverse effects of antiretroviral agents, high frequency of drug or alcohol abuse, and coinfection with hepatitis C virus (HCV). HCV coinfection rates in HIV patients are as high as 80% among urban intravenous drug users[70,71] and 16% to 25% among patients at risk of infection from sexual contact.[72] In one series of "all comers" with HIV, the prevalence of HCV coinfection was 45.7%.[73] Furthermore, patients with HCV–HIV coinfection have higher serum and liver concentrations of HCV than non-HIV patients with HCV.[72] The high prevalence of HCV infection and liver dysfunction in HADL patients restricts the use of potent antilipid medications such as statins and fibrates.

Treating dyslipidemia in HADL patients is challenging because our limited understanding of the pathogenesis precludes firm recommendations based on rational approaches. Completed clinical trials have shown only partial effects or equivocal results, and some major clinical trials are still ongoing. At the present time, it would be prudent to recommend that HADL patients undergo careful evaluation and management of dyslipidemia using Adult Treatment Panel III guidelines established by the National Cholesterol Education Program (NCEP ATP III).

Lifestyle Modifications

NCEP ATP III dietary recommendations should be prescribed through individualized dietary counseling by a qualified dietitian, reinforcement of dietary principles at subsequent clinical visits, and encouraging motivation to achieve these goals. NCEP ATP III guidelines identify hypertriglyceridemia as a contributor to cardiac risk and specify dietary fat reduction as a means of lowering both LDL cholesterol and triglycerides. Hypertriglyceridemia in HADL patients is due in part to severe impairment of dietary triglyceride disposal.[47] This suggests that restriction of dietary fat intake may have a significant impact on triglyceride reduction in HADL subjects.

Additional cardiac risk equivalents should also be addressed as a part of lifestyle interventions, including active encouragement and support for smoking cessation, improving physical activity based on the underlying cardiac status, age, and other limitations, and addressing adequate control of hypertension. While there is a lack of carefully controlled studies evaluating lifestyle changes alone, the effect of diet and exercise on lipid levels in HADL patients may be available in the near future through ongoing studies such as Heart Positive.[74]

Pharmacotherapy

The choice of lipid-lowering drugs is guided by the type of dyslipidemia and includes the following classes.

HMG-CoA Inhibitors. Statins inhibit 3-hydroxy-3-methylglutaryl–coenzyme A (HMG-CoA), the rate-limiting step in endogenous cholesterol synthesis, and are the first line of therapy for patient with elevated LDL cholesterol, or elevated non-HDL cholesterol when triglyceride concentrations range from 200 to 499 mg/dL. However, as some statins share the cytochrome P450 (CYP)3A4 hepatic isoenzyme pathway for excretion with numerous antiretroviral agents used by HADL patients, there is potential for severe increases in the serum concentrations of these drugs, leading to increased risk of rhabdomyolysis and renal failure. In a study evaluating pharmacokinetic interactions between the PI agents and statins, nelfinavir increased the steady-state area under the plasma-concentration time curve of atorvastatin by 122% and that of simvastatin by 517%.[75] For these reasons, there are special recommendations for the use of statins in patients with HADL. Simvastatin is contraindicated in patients taking PI drugs, and atorvastatin is restricted to a daily dose of 10 mg. Other statins are excreted by a different cytochrome P450 isoenzyme pathway, and include pravastatin, fluvastatin (CYP2C9, and a smaller contribution through CYP3A4), and rosuvastatin (CYP2C9, CYP2C19).[76–78] Pravastatin can be used at a starting dose of 20 to 40 mg/day, and titrated up to a maximal dose of 80 mg daily. Studies evaluating pravastatin therapy have found a fairly consistent reduction in total cholesterol concentrations of 17% to 19%, with 19% reduction in LDL cholesterol, no change in HDL cholesterol,[79–81] and a modest (9%) fall in triglycerides. Similar changes in total cholesterol levels were noted with fluvastatin.[82] In an open-label, single-arm extension study, atorvastatin (10 mg/day) induced a more robust change in total cholesterol (–27%), LDL cholesterol (–37%), and triglycerides (–41%).[83] HADL patients receiving statins should be monitored with liver and renal function tests and measurements of muscle enzymes at follow-up visits.

Fibric Acid Derivatives. Fibrates have been used to treat hypertriglyceridemia associated with HADL. In a retrospective study, Rao et al. noted a 37% drop in plasma triglyceride concentrations when fenofibrate was titrated up to a maximal dose of 162 mg/day.[84] Other studies have found a similar improvement in triglycerides with associated elevations in both HDL cholesterol (12%) and LDL cholesterol (8%).[81] Fenofibrate therapy also improved the atherogenic lipid profile in HIV subjects with hypertriglyceridemia. In addition to beneficial changes in plasma concentrations of triglycerides (–40%), there were also improvements in the levels of apoC-III (–21%), total cholesterol (–14%), apoB (–17%), non–HDL cholesterol (–17%), HDL cholesterol (+15%), and apoA-I (+11%). Fenofibrate increased LDL particle size and enhanced LDL resistance to oxidation.[85] Fibrates have also been noted to improve hypercholesterolemia (21.9%) in HADL patients.[86]

Ezetimibe. This cholesterol absorption inhibitor has been found to lower LDL cholesterol by up to 20% in HIV-infected patients with dyslipidemia.[87] As with non-HIV patients with hypercholesterolemia,[88,89] incremental LDL cholesterol lowering may be achieved by the addition of ezetimibe to statin therapy in HADL patients. In one study of HADL patients unable to achieve LDL cholesterol goals with pravastatin, 61.5% achieved plasma LDL cholesterol levels of less than 130 mg/dL when ezetimibe was added.[90]

Niacin. The effect of niacin on HADL has been examined in 33 nondiabetic patients with well-controlled HIV infection on antiretroviral therapy and fasting hypertriglyceridemia who were treated with 2000 mg of extended-release niacin for up to 44 weeks. There were significant improvements in triglycerides, total cholesterol, HDL cholesterol, and non-HDL cholesterol. Additional improvements were also found in large HDL and large VLDL particle concentrations by nuclear magnetic resonance spectroscopy. There was an initial worsening of glycemic parameters, but these increases in glycemia and insulin resistance tended to be transient.[91]

Other Treatment Approaches

In a small randomized, placebo-controlled study examining the roles of diet (6-week duration) and omega-3 fatty acids (8-week duration) in 11 patients with HIV-associated hypertriglyceridemia, the responses to dietary control were similar in both groups, but the patients treated with omega-3 fatty acids showed a fourfold greater fall in triglycerides compared to placebo (14.5%).[92] These metabolic effects were confirmed in a larger randomized, placebo-controlled study in 142 subjects with HIV and hypertriglyceridemia treated with omega-3 fatty acids (18% eicosapentaenoic acid and 12% docosahexaenoic acid) for 8 weeks; in 22.4% of patients on omega-3 fatty acids, serum triglycerides, normalized, were compared to 6.5% in the placebo group. In an open-label extension for an additional 8-week period in the same study, the omega-3 fatty acid group maintained the decrease in triglyceride levels, whereas the original placebo group, which was now treated with omega-3 fatty acids, showed a further 21.2% decrease.[93] Wohl et al. compared the effects of omega-3 fatty acids to lifestyle modifications (diet and exercise) for 16 weeks in 53 HIV patients with hypertriglyceridemia, and found that while the omega-3 fatty acid group showed an initially significant fall in triglycerides at the fourth week (25%), which was sustained at 16 weeks (19.5%), the differences between the two study arms at 16 weeks were not statistically significant.[94] These studies suggest that while omega-3 fatty acids appear to play a beneficial role in lowering triglycerides in HIV patients with hypertriglyceridemia, their specific contributions need further evaluation.

Another antilipolytic drug acipimox has also been evaluated in HIV patients with dyslipidemia. In a randomized, placebo-controlled study using acipimox (250 mg TID) in 23 patients for 3 months, there was a significant fall in the lipolytic rate in the acipimox-treated group, accompanied by significant lowering of triglyceride and fatty acid concentrations.[95]

Interventions Aimed at Insulin Resistance

Insulin resistance is an important component of HIV lipodystrophy, and targeted interventions to improve insulin sensitivity have been tested. Metformin was studied in a placebo-controlled study in 26 nondiabetic HIV patients using a dose of 500 mg twice daily for 3 months, and patients in the metformin arm showed significant improvement in insulin sensitivity with reductions in mean insulin area under the curve (AUC) 120 minutes after a glucose tolerance test.[96] In addition, metformin also appears to improve cardiovascular risk factors such as PAI-1 and tissue plasminogen activator (tPA) levels.[97] In another study evaluating the effects of metformin or rosiglitazone alone or in combination, the addition of rosiglitazone (with placebo or with metformin) resulted in a significant decrease in the insulin AUC, while the use of metformin alone resulted in a nonsignificant reduction in insulin AUCs.[98] Similar improvement in insulin sensitivity have been noted in other studies of thiazolidinedione drugs, including both pioglitazone[99] and rosiglitazone[100,101]; rosiglitazone has also been noted to improve adiponectin levels.[101] Overall, both metformin and the thiazolidinediones appear to have a favorable impact on insulin sensitivity in patients with HIV-associated insulin resistance. Lowering fatty acid and triglyceride levels with acipimox was also associated with modest improvement in insulin sensitivity, presumably as a result of improving lipotoxic insulin resistance.[95]

Interventions Aimed at Improving Body Morphology

Reversal of lipoatrophy and lipohypertrophy is challenging, because of limitations in our understanding of underlying mechanisms. The current approaches involved in improving body morphology are aimed at manipulation of antiretroviral therapy, pharmacologic therapy, and surgical interventions.

Modifying HAART regimes with substitution of implicated drugs (e.g., stavudine) has been shown to have an impact in arresting lipoatrophy,[102,103] but the results are not consistent, and such approaches carry the potential complication of losing virologic control. Experimental approaches with L-carnitine and anabolic steroids have met with limited success in reversing lipoatrophy.[104,105] Surgical approaches include the placement of implants to reverse facial lipoatrophy, or the injection of fillers including polylactic acid and polyacrylamide gel,[106,107] liquid injectable silicone,[108,109] lipo-filling, and bilateral malar silicone implants.[110]

Therapy of fat accumulation in HADL is equally complex, and approaches include lifestyle modification including diet and exercise, as well as pharmacotherapy. One important target has been visceral fat accumulation, and trials have examined the role of GH, GH–releasing factor, and metformin. Pharmacological doses of GH are effective in improving visceral adiposity, but at the expense of increased glucose intolerance and arthralgias. A randomized, double-blinded placebo-controlled trial used a GH–releasing factor that led to dose-dependent physiologic increases in IGF-1, and resulted in increased lean body mass and reduced truncal and visceral fat.[111] In another placebo-controlled trial, treating 412 HIV subjects with a synthetic GH–releasing factor for 26 weeks led to significantly decreased visceral fat (15.2% reduction), increased lean mass, decreased triglyceride concentrations, and increased HDL cholesterol levels.[112] In a placebo-controlled trial in patients with HIV lipodystrophy, metformin decreased visceral abdominal fat as well as subcutaneous abdominal fat.[96] While these studies are encouraging, further research is needed to recommend effective pharmacologic strategies targeting specific mechanistic defects. Surgical approaches to improve lipohypertrophy, such as liposuction, have met with short-term gains, but long-term results are disappointing, as there is a tendency for the fat deposition to reappear.[113]

CONCLUSIONS

The precise pathophysiologic mechanisms underlying the heterogeneous manifestations of HADL remain unclear. Many data have been acquired from human epidemiologic and metabolic studies, but these now need to be translated into mechanistic studies in animal or cellular models. Meanwhile, there is a pressing need to diagnose and treat patients for lipodystrophic changes and the attendant dyslipidemia to alleviate the metabolic syndrome and its associated cardiovascular risks.

Important future developments should include a more thorough understanding of the molecular pathogenesis of HADL, as well as availability of rational treatment options. Until then, clinicians should continue to use best-practice guidelines for the treatment of metabolic syndrome and reduction of cardiovascular risk factors, using both lifestyle and pharmacologic approaches. The latter must be based on a good understanding of their interactions with HAART agents and effects on other medical conditions that are common in patients with HIV infection.

REFERENCES

1. Balasubramanyam A, Sekhar RV, Jahoor F, Jones PH, Pownall HJ: Pathophysiology of dyslipidemia and increased cardiovascular risk in HIV lipodystrophy: a model of "systemic steatosis." *Curr Opin Lipidol* 2004;15:59–67.
2. Wanke C: Editorial comment: a case definition for HIV lipodystrophy—a work in progress. *AIDS Read* 2003;13:492–493.
3. Belloso WH, Quiros RE, Ivalo SA, et al: Agreement analysis of variables involved in lipodystrophy syndrome definition in HIV-infected patients. *J Acquir Immune Defic Syndr* 2003;32:104–111.
4. Carr A, Emery S, Law M, Puls R, Lundgren JD, Powderly WG: An objective case definition of lipodystrophy in HIV-infected adults: a case–control study. *Lancet* 2003;361:726–735.
5. Mauss S, Corzillius M, Wolf E, et al: Risk factors for the HIV-associated lipodystrophy syndrome in a closed cohort of patients after 3 years of antiretroviral treatment. *HIV Med* 2002;3:49–55.
6. Lichtenstein KA, Ward DJ, Moorman AC, et al: Clinical assessment of HIV-associated lipodystrophy in an ambulatory population. *AIDS* 2001;15:1389–1398.
7. van der Valk M, Casula M, Weverlingz GJ, et al: Prevalence of lipoatrophy and mitochondrial DNA content of blood and subcutaneous fat in HIV-1–infected patients randomly allocated to zidovudine- or stavudine-based therapy. *Antivir Ther* 2004;9:385–393.
8. Nolan D, Hammond E, James I, McKinnon E, Mallal S: Contribution of nucleoside-analogue reverse transcriptase inhibitor therapy to lipoatrophy from the population to the cellular level. *Antivir Ther* 2003;8:617–626.
9. Dube MP, Parker RA, Tebas P, et al: Glucose metabolism, lipid, and body fat changes in antiretroviral-naive subjects randomized to nelfinavir or efavirenz plus dual nucleosides. *AIDS* 2005;19:1807–1818.
10. Grunfeld C, Kotler DP, Hamadeh R, Tierney A, Wang J, Pierson RN: Hypertriglyceridemia in the acquired immunodeficiency syndrome. *Am J Med* 1989;86:27–31.

11. Grunfeld C, Pang M, Doerrler W, Shigenaga JK, Jensen P, Feingold KR: Lipids, lipoproteins, triglyceride clearance, and cytokines in human immunodeficiency virus infection and the acquired immunodeficiency syndrome. *J Clin Endocrinol Metab* 1992;74: 1045–1052.
12. Constans J, Pellegrin JL, Peuchant E, et al: Plasma lipids in HIV-infected patients: a prospective study in 95 patients. *Eur J Clin Invest* 1994;24:416–420.
13. Carr A, Samaras K, Burton S, et al: A syndrome of peripheral lipodystrophy, hyperlipidaemia and insulin resistance in patients receiving HIV protease inhibitors. *AIDS* 1998;12:F51–F58.
14. Periard D, Telenti A, Sudre P, et al: Atherogenic dyslipidemia in HIV-infected individuals treated with protease inhibitors. The Swiss HIV Cohort Study. *Circulation* 1999;100:700–705.
15. Mulligan K, Grunfeld C, Tai VW, et al: Hyperlipidemia and insulin resistance are induced by protease inhibitors independent of changes in body composition in patients with HIV infection. *J Acquir Immune Defic Syndr* 2003;23:35–43.
16. Behrens G, Dejam A, Schmidt H, et al: Impaired glucose tolerance, beta cell function and lipid metabolism in HIV patients under treatment with protease inhibitors. *AIDS* 1999;13: F63–F70.
17. Carr A, Samaras K, Thorisdottir A, Kaufmann GR, Chisholm DJ, Cooper DA: Diagnosis, prediction, and natural course of HIV-1 protease-inhibitor–associated lipodystrophy, hyperlipidaemia, and diabetes mellitus: a cohort study. *Lancet* 1999;353: 2093–2099.
18. Tsiodras S, Mantzoros C, Hammer S, Samore M: Effects of protease inhibitors on hyperglycemia, hyperlipidemia, and lipodystrophy: a 5-year cohort study. *Arch Intern Med* 2000;160: 2050–2056.
19. Fellay J, Boubaker K, Ledergerber B, et al: Prevalence of adverse events associated with potent antiretroviral treatment: Swiss HIV Cohort Study. *Lancet* 2001;358:1322–1327.
20. Mobius U, Lubach-Ruitman M, Castro-Frenzel B, et al: Switching to atazanavir improves metabolic disorders in antiretroviral-experienced patients with severe hyperlipidemia. *J Acquir Immune Defic Syndr* 2005;39:174–180.
21. Hatano H, Miller KD, Yoder CP, et al: Metabolic and anthropometric consequences of interruption of highly active antiretroviral therapy. *AIDS* 2000;14:1935–1942.
22. van der Valk M, Gisolf EH, Reiss P, et al: Increased risk of lipodystrophy when nucleoside analogue reverse transcriptase inhibitors are included with protease inhibitors in the treatment of HIV-1 infection. *AIDS* 2001;15:847–855.
23. Jones R, Sawleshwarkar S, Michailidis C, et al: Impact of antiretroviral choice on hypercholesterolaemia events: the role of the nucleoside reverse transcriptase inhibitor backbone. *HIV Med* 2005;6:396–402.
24. Friis-Moller N, Weber R, Reiss P, et al: Cardiovascular disease risk factors in HIV patients—association with antiretroviral therapy. Results from the DAD study. *AIDS* 2003;17: 1179–1193.
25. Young J, Weber R, Rickenbach M, et al: Lipid profiles for antiretroviral-naive patients starting PI- and NNRTI-based therapy in the Swiss HIV cohort study. *Antivir Ther* 2005;10:585–591.
26. van der Valk M, Bisschop PH, Romijn JA, et al: Lipodystrophy in HIV-1-positive patients is associated with insulin resistance in multiple metabolic pathways. *AIDS* 2001;15:2093–2100.
27. Hadigan C, Meigs JB, Corcoran C, et al: Metabolic abnormalities and cardiovascular disease risk factors in adults with human immunodeficiency virus infection and lipodystrophy. *Clin Infect Dis* 2001;32:130–139.
28. Murata H, Hruz PW, Mueckler M: Indinavir inhibits the glucose transporter isoform Glut4 at physiologic concentrations. *AIDS* 2002;16:859–863.
29. Shikuma CM, Day LJ, Gerschenson M: Insulin resistance in the HIV-infected population: the potential role of mitochondrial dysfunction. *Curr Drug Targets Infect Disord* 2005;5:255–262.
30. Gan SK, Samaras K, Thompson CH, et al: Altered myocellular and abdominal fat partitioning predict disturbance in insulin action in HIV protease inhibitor–related lipodystrophy. *Diabetes* 2002;51:3163–3169.
31. Sutinen J, Hakkinen AM, Westerbacka J, et al: Increased fat accumulation in the liver in HIV-infected patients with antiretroviral therapy-associated lipodystrophy. *AIDS* 2002;16: 2183–2193.
32. Noor MA, Parker RA, O'Mara E, et al: The effects of HIV protease inhibitors atazanavir and lopinavir/ritonavir on insulin sensitivity in HIV-seronegative healthy adults. *AIDS* 2004;18: 2137–2144.
33. Lo JC, Mulligan K, Tai VW, Algren H, Schambelan M: "Buffalo hump" in men with HIV-1 infection. *Lancet* 1998;351:867–870.
34. Saint-Marc T, Partisani M, Poizot-Martin I, et al: Fat distribution evaluated by computed tomography and metabolic abnormalities in patients undergoing antiretroviral therapy: preliminary results of the LIPOCO study. *AIDS* 2000;14:37–49.
35. Bernasconi E, Boubaker K, Junghans C, et al: Abnormalities of body fat distribution in HIV-infected persons treated with antiretroviral drugs: The Swiss HIV Cohort Study. *J Acquir Immune Defic Syndr* 2002;31:50–55.
36. Miller J, Carr A, Smith D, et al: Lipodystrophy following antiretroviral therapy of primary HIV infection. *AIDS* 2000;14:2406–2407.
37. Bacchetti P, Gripshover B, Grunfeld C, et al: Fat distribution in men with HIV infection. *J Acquir Immune Defic Syndr* 2005;40: 121–131.
38. Saint-Marc T, Partisani M, Poizot-Martin I, et al: A syndrome of peripheral fat wasting (lipodystrophy) in patients receiving long-term nucleoside analogue therapy. *AIDS* 1999;13:1659–1667.
39. Lenhard JM, Furfine ES, Jain RG, et al: HIV protease inhibitors block adipogenesis and increase lipolysis i*n vitro*. *Antiviral Res* 2000;47:121–129.
40. Miserez AR, Muller PY, Spaniol V: Indinavir inhibits sterol-regulatory element-binding protein-1c–dependent lipoprotein lipase and fatty acid synthase gene activations. *AIDS* 2002;16: 1587–1594.
41. Nolan D, John M, Mallal S: Antiretoviral therapy and the lipodystrophy syndrome, part 2: concepts in aetiopathogenesis. *Antivir Ther* 2001;6:145–160.
42. Nolan D, Pace C: Potential roles for uncoupling proteins in HIV lipodystrophy. *Mitochondrion* 2004;4:185–191.
43. Lichtenstein KA: Redefining lipodystrophy syndrome: risks and impact on clinical decision making. *J Acquir Immune Defic Syndr* 2005;39:395–400.
44. Sekhar RV, Jahoor F, White AC, et al: Metabolic basis of HIV-lipodystrophy syndrome. *Am J Physiol Endocrinol Metab* 2002;283:E332–E337.
45. Reeds DN, Mittendorfer B, Patterson BW, Powderly WG, Yarasheski KE, Klein S: Alterations in lipid kinetics in men with HIV-dyslipidemia. *Am J Physiol Endocrinol Metab* 2003;285:E490–E497.
46. Behrens GM, Boerner AR, Weber K, et al: Impaired glucose phosphorylation and transport in skeletal muscle cause insulin resistance in HIV-1-infected patients with lipodystrophy. *J Clin Invest* 2002;110:1319–1327.
47. Sekhar RV, Jahoor F, Pownall HJ, et al: Severely dysregulated disposal of postprandial triacylglycerols exacerbates hypertriacylglycerolemia in HIV lipodystrophy syndrome. *Am J Clin Nutr* 2005;81:1405–1410.
48. Hadigan C, Borgonha S, Rabe J, Young V, Grinspoon S: Increased rates of lipolysis among human immunodeficiency virus-infected men receiving highly active antiretroviral therapy. *Metabolism* 2002;51:1143–1147.
49. Bjorntorp P: The regulation of adipose tissue distribution in humans. *Int J Obes Relat Metab Disord* 1996;20:291–302.
50. Dobbins RL, Szczepaniak LS, Bentley B, Esser V, Myhill J, McGarry JD: Prolonged inhibition of muscle carnitine palmitoyltransferase-1 promotes intramyocellular lipid accumulation and insulin resistance in rats. *Diabetes* 2001;50:123–130.
51. Griffin ME, Marcucci MJ, Cline GW, et al: Free fatty acid-induced insulin resistance is associated with activation of protein kinase C theta and alterations in the insulin signaling cascade. *Diabetes* 1999;48:1270–1274.
52. Saxena U, Goldberg IJ: Interaction of lipoprotein lipase with glycosaminoglycans and apolipoprotein C-II: effects of free-fatty-acids. *Biochim Biophys Acta* 1990;1043:161–168.
53. Kino T, Gragerov A, Kopp JB, Stauber RH, Pavlakis GN, Chrousos GP: The HIV-1 virion-associated protein vpr is a coactivator of the human glucocorticoid receptor. *J Exp Med* 1999;189:51–62.
54. Kino T, Gragerov A, Slobodskaya O, Tsopanomichalou M, Chrousos GP, Pavlakis GN: Human immunodeficiency virus

type 1 (HIV-1) accessory protein Vpr induces transcription of the HIV-1 and glucocorticoid-responsive promoters by binding directly to p300/CBP coactivators. *J Virol* 2002;76:9724–9734.

55. Johnson JA, Albu JB, Engelson ES, et al: Increased systemic and adipose tissue cytokines in patients with HIV-associated lipodystrophy. *Am J Physiol Endocrinol Metab* 2004;286: E261–E271.
56. Vigouroux C, Maachi M, Nguyen TH, et al: Serum adipocytokines are related to lipodystrophy and metabolic disorders in HIV-infected men under antiretroviral therapy. *AIDS* 2003;17: 1503–1511.
57. Addy CL, Gavrila A, Tsiodras S, Brodovicz K, Karchmer AW, Mantzoros CS: Hypoadiponectinemia is associated with insulin resistance, hypertriglyceridemia, and fat redistribution in human immunodeficiency virus-infected patients treated with highly active antiretroviral therapy. *J Clin Endocrinol Metab* 2003;88:627–636.
58. Tong Q, Sankale JL, Hadigan CM, et al: Regulation of adiponectin in human immunodeficiency virus-infected patients: relationship to body composition and metabolic indices. *J Clin Endocrinol Metab* 2003;88:1559–1564.
59. Sankale JL, Tong Q, Hadigan CM, et al: Regulation of adiponectin in adipocytes upon exposure to HIV-1. *HIV Med* 2006;7: 268–274.
60. Unger RH: The physiology of cellular liporegulation. *Annu Rev Physiol* 2003;65:333–347.
61. Rietschel P, Hadigan C, Corcoran C, et al: Assessment of growth hormone dynamics in human immunodeficiency virus-related lipodystrophy. *J Clin Endocrinol Metab* 2001;86:504–510.
62. D'Amico S, Shi J, Sekhar RV, et al: Physiologic growth hormone replacement improves fasting lipid kinetics in patients with HIV lipodystrophy syndrome. *Am J Clin Nutr* 2006;84:204–211.
63. Koutkia P, Canavan B, Breu J, Torriani M, Kissko J, Grinspoon S: Growth hormone-releasing hormone in HIV-infected men with lipodystrophy: a randomized controlled trial. *JAMA* 292:210–218.
64. Friis-Moller N, Sabin CA, Weber R, et al: Combination antiretroviral therapy and the risk of myocardial infarction. *N Engl J Med* 2003;349:1993–2003.
65. Friis-Moller N, Reiss P, Sabin CA, et al: Class of antiretroviral drugs and the risk of myocardial infarction. *N Engl J Med* 2007;356:1723–1735.
66. Mary-Krause M, Cotte L, Simon A, Partisani M, Costagliola D: Increased risk of myocardial infarction with duration of protease inhibitor therapy in HIV-infected men. *AIDS* 2003;17:2479–2486.
67. Holmberg SD, Moorman AC, Williamson JM, et al: Protease inhibitors and cardiovascular outcomes in patients with HIV-1. *Lancet* 2002;360:1747–1748.
68. Varriale P, Saravi G, Hernandez E, Carbon F: Acute myocardial infarction in patients infected with human immunodeficiency virus. *Am Heart J* 2004;147:55–59.
69. Coll B, Parra S, Alonso-Villaverde C, et al: HIV-infected patients with lipodystrophy have higher rates of carotid atherosclerosis: the role of monocyte chemoattractant protein-1. *Cytokine* 2006;34:51–55.
70. Strasfeld L, Lo Y, Netski D, Thomas DL, Klein RS: The association of hepatitis C prevalence, activity, and genotype with HIV infection in a cohort of New York City drug users. *J Acquir Immune Defic Syndr* 2003;33:356–364.
71. Thio CL, Nolt KR, Astemborski J, Vlahov D, Nelson KE, Thomas DL: Screening for hepatitis C virus in human immunodeficiency virus-infected individuals. *J Clin Microbiol* 2000;38:575–577.
72. Sherman KE, Rouster SD, Chung RT, Rajicic N: Hepatitis C Virus prevalence among patients infected with Human Immunodeficiency Virus: a cross-sectional analysis of the US adult AIDS Clinical Trials Group. *Clin Infect Dis* 2002;34:831–837.
73. Gonzalez Cerrajero M PGA, de los Santos Gil I, Sanz Sanz J: Prevalence of hepatitis C virus among HIV-infected patients in Area 2 of Madrid. *An Med Interna* 2006;23:111–114.
74. Samson SL, Pownall HJ, Scott LW, et al: Heart positive: design of a randomized controlled clinical trial of intensive lifestyle intervention, niacin and fenofibrate for HIV lipodystrophy/dyslipidemia. *Contemp Clin Trials* 2006;27:518–530.
75. Hsyu PH, Schultz-Smith MD, Lillibridge JH, Lewis RH, Kerr BM: Pharmacokinetic interactions between nelfinavir and 3-hydroxy–3-methylglutaryl coenzyme A reductase inhibitors atorvastatin and simvastatin. *Antimicrob Agents Chemother* 2001;45:3445–3450.
76. Benesic A, Zilly M, Kluge F, et al: Lipid lowering therapy with fluvastatin and pravastatin in patients with HIV infection and antiretroviral therapy: comparison of efficacy and interaction with indinavir. *Infection* 2004;32:229–233.
77. Calza L, Colangeli V, Manfredi R, et al: Rosuvastatin for the treatment of hyperlipidaemia in HIV-infected patients receiving protease inhibitors: a pilot study. *AIDS* 2005;19:1103–1105.
78. Johns KW, Bennett MT, Bondy GP: Are HIV+ patients resistant to statin therapy? *Lipids Health Dis* 2007;6:27.
79. Baldini F, Di Giambenedetto S, Cingolani A, Murri R, Ammassari A, De Luca A: Efficacy and tolerability of pravastatin for the treatment of HIV-1 protease inhibitor–associated hyperlipidaemia: a pilot study. *AIDS* 2000;14:1660–1662.
80. Moyle GJ, Lloyd M, Reynolds B, Baldwin C, Mandalia S, Gazzard BG: Dietary advice with or without pravastatin for the management of hypercholesterolaemia associated with protease inhibitor therapy. *AIDS* 2001;15:1503–1508.
81. Aberg JA, Zackin RA, Brobst SW, et al: A randomized trial of the efficacy and safety of fenofibrate versus pravastatin in HIV-infected subjects with lipid abnormalities: AIDS Clinical Trials Group Study 5087. *AIDS Res Hum Retroviruses* 2005;21:757–767.
82. Doser N, Kubli S, Telenti A, et al: Efficacy and safety of fluvastatin in hyperlipidemic protease inhibitor-treated HIV-infected patients. *AIDS* 2002;16:1982–1983.
83. Palacios R, Santos J, Gonzalez M, et al: Efficacy and safety of atorvastatin in the treatment of hypercholesterolemia associated with antiretroviral therapy. *J Acquir Immune Defic Syndr* 2002;30:536–537.
84. Rao A, D'Amico S, Balasubramanyam A, Maldonado M: Fenofibrate is effective in treating hypertriglyceridemia associated with HIV lipodystrophy. *Am J Med Sci* 2004;327:315–318.
85. Badiou S, Merle De Boever C, Dupuy AM, Baillat V, Cristol JP, Reynes J: Fenofibrate improves the atherogenic lipid profile and enhances LDL resistance to oxidation in HIV-positive adults. *Atherosclerosis* 2004;172:273–279.
86. Calza L, Manfredi R, Chiodo F: Statins and fibrates for the treatment of hyperlipidaemia in HIV-infected patients receiving HAART. *AIDS* 2003;17:851–859.
87. Coll B, Aragones G, Parra S, Alonso-Villaverde C, Masana L: Ezetimibe effectively decreases LDL cholesterol in HIV-infected patients. *AIDS* 2006;20:1675–1677.
88. Gagne C, Bays HE, Weiss SR, et al: Efficacy and safety of ezetimibe added to ongoing statin therapy for treatment of patients with primary hypercholesterolemia. *Am J Cardiol* 2002;90:1084–1091.
89. Pearson TA, Denke MA, McBride PE, Battisti WP, Brady WE, Palmisano J: A community-based, randomized trial of ezetimibe added to statin therapy to attain NCEP ATP III goals for LDL cholesterol in hypercholesterolemic patients: the ezetimibe add-on to statin for effectiveness (EASE) trial. *Mayo Clin Proc* 2005;80:587–595.
90. Negredo E, Molto J, Puig J, et al: Ezetimibe, a promising lipid-lowering agent for the treatment of dyslipidaemia in HIV-infected patients with poor response to statins. *AIDS* 2006;20: 2159–2164.
91. Dube MP, Wu JW, Aberg JA, et al: Safety and efficacy of extended-release niacin for the treatment of dyslipidaemia in patients with HIV infection: AIDS Clinical Trials Group Study A5148. *Antivir Ther* 2006;11:1081–1089.
92. Carter VM, Woolley I, Jolley D, Nyulasi I, Mijch A, Dart A: A randomised controlled trial of omega-3 fatty acid supplementation for the treatment of hypertriglyceridemia in HIV-infected males on highly active antiretroviral therapy. *Sex Health* 2006;3:287–290.
93. De Truchis P, Kirstetter M, Perier A, et al: Reduction in triglyceride level with N–3 polyunsaturated fatty acids in HIV-infected patients taking potent antiretroviral therapy: a randomized prospective study. *J Acquir Immune Defic Syndr* 2007;44:278–285.
94. Wohl DA, Tien HC, Busby M, et al: Randomized study of the safety and efficacy of fish oil (omega-3 fatty acid) supplementation with dietary and exercise counseling for the treatment of antiretroviral therapy-associated hypertriglyceridemia. *Clin Infect Dis* 2005;41:1498–1504.
95. Hadigan C, Liebau J, Torriani M, Andersen R, Grinspoon S: Improved triglycerides and insulin sensitivity with 3 months of acipimox in human immunodeficiency virus-infected patients with hypertriglyceridemia. *J Clin Endocrinol Metab* 2006;91: 4438–4444.

96. Hadigan C, Corcoran C, Basgoz N, Davis B, Sax P, Grinspoon S: Metformin in the treatment of HIV lipodystrophy syndrome: a randomized controlled trial. *JAMA* 2000;284:472–477.
97. Hadigan C, Meigs JB, Rabe J, et al: Increased PAI-1 and tPA antigen levels are reduced with metformin therapy in HIV-infected patients with fat redistribution and insulin resistance. *J Clin Endocrinol Metab* 2001;86:939–943.
98. Mulligan K, Yang Y, Wininger DA, et al: Effects of metformin and rosiglitazone in HIV-infected patients with hyperinsulinemia and elevated waist/hip ratio. *AIDS* 2007;21:47–57.
99. Gavrila A, Hsu W, Tsiodras S, et al: Improvement in highly active antiretroviral therapy-induced metabolic syndrome by treatment with pioglitazone but not with fenofibrate: A 2 × 2 factorial, randomized, double-blinded, placebo-controlled trial. *Clin Infect Dis* 2005;40:745–749.
100. Tomazic J, Karner P, Vidmar L, Maticic M, Sharma PM, Janez A: Effect of metformin and rosiglitazone on lipid metabolism in HIV infected patients receiving protease inhibitor containing HAART. *Acta Dermatovenerol Alp Panonica Adriat* 2005;14:99–105.
101. van Wijk JP, de Koning EJ, Cabezas MC, et al: Comparison of rosiglitazone and metformin for treating HIV lipodystrophy: a randomized trial. *Ann Intern Med* 2005;143:337–346.
102. John M, McKinnon EJ, James IR, et al: Randomized, controlled, 48-week study of switching stavudine and/or protease inhibitors to combivir/abacavir to prevent or reverse lipoatrophy in HIV-infected patients. *J Acquir Immune Defic Syndr* 2003;33:29–33.
103. McComsey GA, Paulsen DM, Lonergan JT, et al: Improvements in lipoatrophy, mitochondrial DNA levels and fat apoptosis after replacing stavudine with abacavir or zidovudine. *AIDS* 2005;19:15–23.
104. Mauss S, Schmutz G: L-Carnitine in the treatment of HIV-associated lipodystrophy syndrome. *HIV Med* 2001;2:59–60.
105. Day L, Shikuma C, Gerschenson M: Acetyl-L-carnitine for the treatment of HIV lipoatrophy. *Ann N Y Acad Sci* 2004;1033:139–146.
106. Negredo E, Higueras C, Adell X, et al: Reconstructive treatment for antiretroviral-associated facial lipoatrophy: a prospective study comparing autologous fat and synthetic substances. AIDS Patient Care STDS 2006;20:829–837.
107. El-Beyrouty C, Huang V, Darnold CJ, Clay PG: Poly-L-lactic acid for facial lipoatrophy in HIV. *Ann Pharmacother* 2006;40:1602–1606.
108. Orentreich D, Leone AS: A case of HIV-associated facial lipoatrophy treated with 1000-cs liquid injectable silicone. *Dermatol Surg* 2004;30:548–551.
109. Jones DH, Carruthers A, Orentreich D, et al: Highly purified 1000-cSt silicone oil for treatment of human immunodeficiency virus-associated facial lipoatrophy: an open pilot trial. *Dermatol Surg* 2004;30:1279–1286.
110. Mori A, Lo Russo G, Agostini T, Pattarino J, Vichi F, Dini M: Treatment of human immunodeficiency virus-associated facial lipoatrophy with lipofilling and submalar silicone implants. *J Plast Reconstr Aesthet Surg* 2006;59:1209–1216.
111. Falutz J, Allas S, Kotler D, et al: A placebo-controlled, dose-ranging study of a growth hormone releasing factor in HIV-infected patients with abdominal fat accumulation. *AIDS* 2005;19:1279–1287.
112. Falutz J, Allas S, Blot K, et al: Metabolic effects of a growth hormone–releasing factor in patients with HIV. *N Engl J Med* 2007;357:2359–2370.
113. Hultman CS, McPhail LE, Donaldson JH, Wohl DA: Surgical management of HIV-associated lipodystrophy: role of ultrasonic-assisted liposuction and suction-assisted lipectomy in the treatment of lipohypertrophy. *Ann Plast Surg* 2007;58:255–263.

CHAPTER 44

Investigational Agents Affecting Atherogenic Lipoproteins

Harold Bays

SQUALENE SYNTHASE INHIBITORS

3-Hydroxy-3-methylglutaryl–coenzyme A (HMG-CoA) reductase is the enzyme that converts HMG-CoA to mevalonic acid (mevalonate), and is the rate-limiting step in cholesterol synthesis and the production of cholesterol intermediaries. Inhibitors of HMG-CoA are commonly referred to as "statins," which are the most widely studied and most commonly administered cholesterol-lowering agents. Further down from the actions of HMG-CoA reductase, and before the end product of cholesterol synthesis, is the production of squalene, which is generated by the enzyme squalene synthase (SS)[1] (Fig. 44-1).

Various SS inhibitors (SSI) have been evaluated over the years as cholesterol-lowering agents, with TAK 475 (lapaquistat) advancing furthest in development. One of the justifications for the development of these drugs is the suggestion that statin intolerances may be related to statin-induced reductions in downstream mevalonate-derived products[2] (see Fig. 44-1). Because SSIs do not impair the synthesis of many of these mevalonate-derived products, SSIs may have theoretical tolerability advantages in statin-intolerant patients, or in patients at risk for statin intolerance.[3]

For example, a reduction in mevalonate with statins impairs downstream protein prenylation processes, which otherwise occur through the enzymes farnesyltransferase, geranylgeranyltransferase-I, and Rab geranylgeranyl transferase. Prenylation (or isoprenylation/lipidation) is the addition of specific carbon chains to proteins, which helps facilitate protein attachment to cellular membranes (Fig. 44-2). These added prenyl moieties are derived from enzymatic products such as farnesyl or geranyl geranyl, which are downstream from HMG-CoA reductase. By regulating the location of intracellular proteins through influencing their potential for attachment to cell membranes (many of which are often involved in electron or ion transfer), alterations in prenylation processes may affect various cellular signaling cascades.[4] Examples of prenyl substrates whose concentration is reduced by statin-induced inhibition of HMG CoA include nonsterol, prenylated products such as heme A, ubiquinone, dolichol, and Δ^2-isopentenyl tRNA.

The porphyrin core of heme A is formed from farnesyl-pyrophosphate (PP), and is an important component of the electron transport chain and oxidative phosphorylation.[5] Ubiquinone (coenzyme Q10) is a prenylated protein whose production is also an important component of the electron transport chain and functions as an antioxidant in mitochondrial and other lipid membranes—all of which are important in the normal functioning of muscle.[6] (Note: Although not always consistent in clinical trials [or in clinical practice], coenzyme Q10 administration reportedly may improve pain in some patients with statin-induced myalgias.[7,8]) Other isoprenoids include dolichol (which is an isoprenoid required for glycoprotein synthesis), and isopentyl adenosine (which is required for RNA synthesis)[6]—both of which play important roles in normal muscle physiology. Finally, other proteins that are activated by prenylation include Rho, Rac, and Ras, which are guanosine triphosphate (GTP) binders that promote cell maintenance, and attenuate apoptosis. Impaired activation of these GTP-binding proteins through impaired prenylation may promote muscle apoptosis.[6,9]

A theoretical advantage of SSIs is that they avoid the blockade of protein prenylation induced by statins. Thus, if these processes do play a role in statin intolerances, then SSIs may be a use-ful therapeutic alternative in patients intolerant to statins. Furthermore, when SSIs are administered in combination with statins, then this may help "replenish"

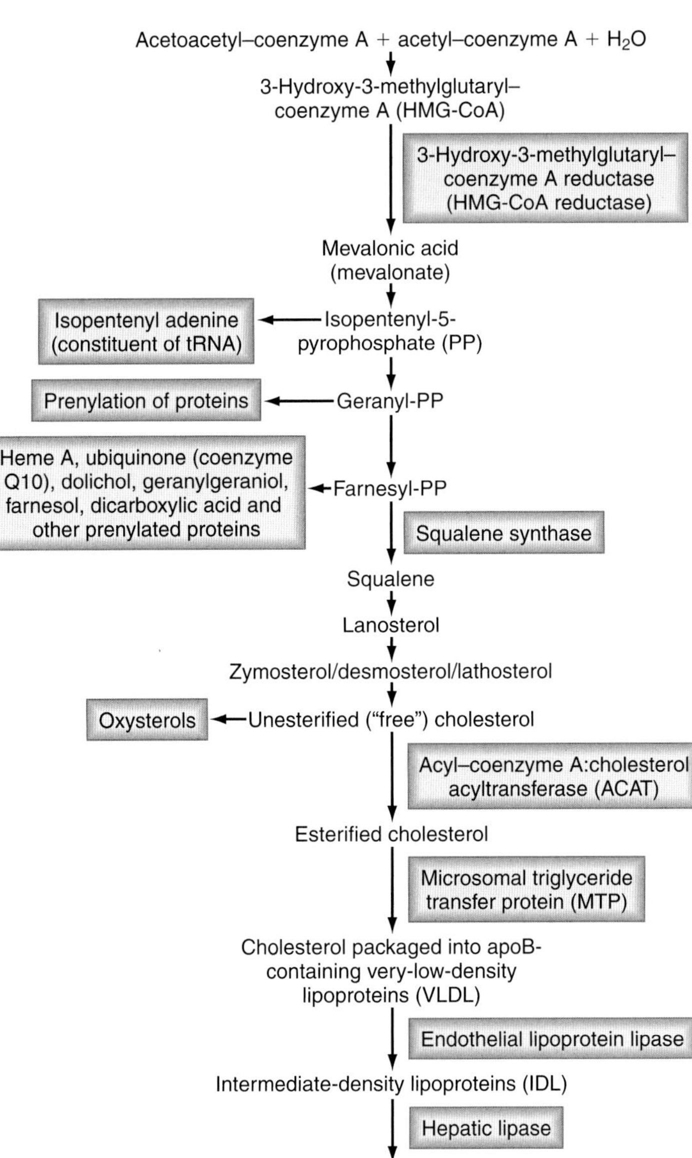

FIGURE 44-1 Hepatic cholesterol synthesis and lipoprotein packaging. The hepatic synthesis of cholesterol involves multiple enzymatic steps, including the rate-limiting step of HMG-CoA reductase, as well as other important enzymes such as squalene synthase. Afterward, "free" cholesterol is esterified and incorporated into VLDL particles and released into the circulation. VLDL particles are then subject to further enzymatic processes in the circulation that generate other atherogenic lipoproteins, such as LDLs.

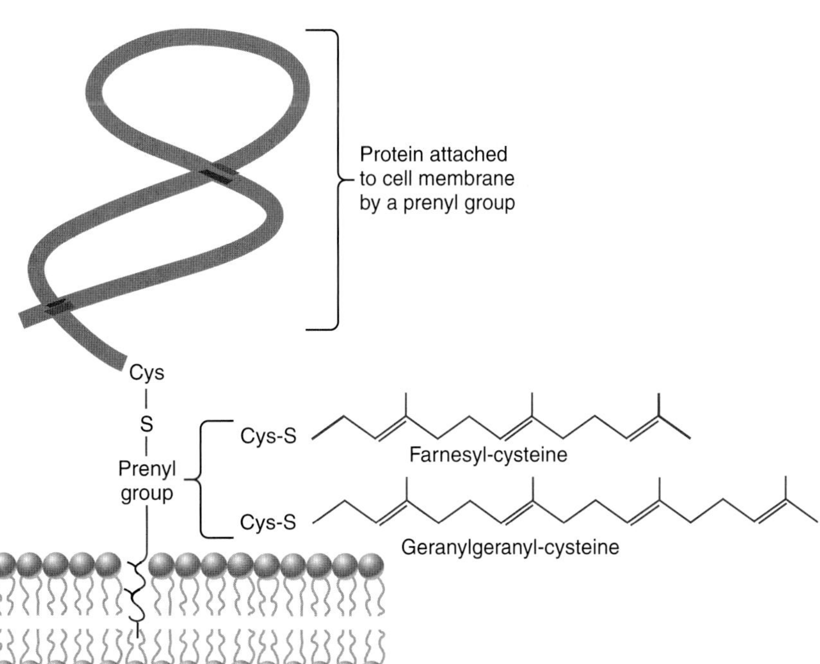

FIGURE 44-2 Protein anchoring to a cellular membrane by the process of lipidation/prenylation. Prenylation (or isoprenylation) is the addition of hydrophobic, lipophilic carbon chains to proteins, which promotes protein attachment to cellular membranes. In this illustration, the amino acid cysteine portion of the protein is attached to the (iso)prenoids farnesyl and/or geranylgeranyl anchor via a thioether linage (R-S-R).[45]

protein prenylation (by blocking the enzymatic step that converts farnesyl-PP to squalene), and thus represents another theoretical, use in patients intolerant to higher-dose statins. In other words, patients with muscle intolerance to high-dose statins may theoretically benefit from adding a SSI agent (such as lapaquistat) to a lower, more tolerated dose of statin. This approach would have the added advantage of achieving similar, if not greater low-density lipoprotein (LDL) cholesterol lowering than using higher statin doses.

But just as inhibition of SS may have theoretical benefits, theoretical disadvantages may also exist. For example, the increased generation of isoprenyl products by SSIs may not always be favorable. Farnesol-derived dicarboxylic acids (FDDCAs) may be increased with SSIs. Animal studies have shown that some SSIs increase urinary levels of these FDDCAs and increase the risk of toxic acidosis,[10] which has contributed to the abandonment of other SSI development programs.[11] Animal studies specific to lapaquistat have shown some increase in urinary levels of FDDCAs, but this apparently did not result in toxic acidosis.[11] Human data do not support urine or blood evidence of acidosis with lapaquistat.[12]

Finally, other theoretical effects of SSIs are uncertain, such as the potential effects on cellular nuclear receptors. Liver X receptors (LXRs) may be either negatively or positively affected by various applicable metabolites found within the pathway between the enzymes HMG-CoA and SS,[13] which may in turn affect both lipid and glucose metabolism. From a clinical perspective, activation of LXR is one potential mechanism proposed as to how and why another cholesterol-lowering drug class, bile acid sequestrants, may lower glucose levels.[14] Human studies have not supported any effect of lapaquistat on glucose levels.[12]

Early evidence supports that inhibiting SS may have tolerability/safety benefits regarding statins, at least for muscle. Evaluation of human skeletal myocytes (through a human rhabdomyosarcoma cell line) has suggested that lapaquistat may decrease statin-induced myotoxicity.[15] However, despite these promising findings, any potential muscle safety or tolerability advantages of lapaquistat compared to statins, or when added to statins, will be dependent on the results of clinical trials and will present challenges.

Muscle-related adverse experiences are among the most common reported reasons for statin intolerance,[16] and perhaps the most common adverse experience resulting in patient discontinuation. Unfortunately, statin clinical trial data do not provide an accurate, objective assessment of the frequency of statin intolerance or muscle adverse experiences. This is because most statin clinical trials were not designed to specifically assess muscle-related complaints. Statin clinical trials have not routinely employed a formalized, exhaustive diagnostic evaluation of all cases of emergent myalgias or increased muscle enzymes occurring during the conduct of such trials, and no accepted validated scale exists that is specific for statin-induced muscle adverse experiences.[16] Investigators and protocols have often excluded patients with prior intolerance to statins, and patients with prior intolerance to statins often have chosen not to participate in statin clinical trials.[17] In fact, if the clinical trial data were used as the exclusive source to assess myalgias, then the published data would suggest that statin administration results in no statistical increase in myalgias beyond that of placebo, with nonspecific muscle aches, joint pains, or muscle weakness unassociated with elevations in creatine kinase (CK) levels being reported in only about 5% of study participants,[18] with a range as wide as 0.3% to 33%.[19] Nonetheless, while true that many cases of myalgias found in statin-treated patients are often unrelated to statin use, statin-induced myalgia is a reality faced by many clinicians even when, and many might say most often when, muscle enzymes are not elevated. Finally, statins have been described to result in potential neurologic or rheumatologic adverse experiences.[16] Thus, it is possible that some patients who complain of profound muscle pain and profound muscle weakness may not be having muscle problems at all; instead, body pain or muscle weakness may actually be related to other body systems. This would be clinically supported by the fact that statin-induced myalgias are rarely accompanied by objective physical examination findings reflective of muscle damage, such as fasciculations or muscle wasting.[16]

As opposed to myalgias, statin-induced increases in CK levels are well-established. But the terms used to describe this finding, such as myopathy and rhabdomyolysis, have varying definitions,[16] which again complicates the objective and comparative assessment of these adverse experiences. Furthermore, when significant statin-induced CK levels do occur, they occur rarely, making muscle safety comparisons between individual statins and between statins other lipid-altering drugs even more difficult. Finally, in the rare cases when CK levels are significantly increased in statin clinical trials, the etiology is not always clear, even with the most extreme elevations as is found with rhabdomyolysis. This is because rhabdomyolysis has numerous potential causes, even when it occurs in statin-treated patients (Table 44-1). Until SSIs have been shown in head-to-head, definitive clinical trials to have tolerability and/or safety benefits over statins (whether as monotherapy or when added to lower-dose statins), they may best be viewed as simply a new class of lipid-altering drugs. Hence, both the efficacy and safety/tolerability of an SSI such as lapaquistat should be judged based on its known pharmacokinetics/pharmacodynamics and the results of its monotherapy and combination clinical trials.

When oral drug has been administered to healthy males, lapaquistat has been shown to undergo rapid gastrointestinal absorption (T_{max} = 3.5 hours), and is converted to active metabolites with the major route of excretion being biliary, and thus feces (only 0.2% renal excretion).[20] Although significantly metabolized through the cytochrome P450 (CYP) 3A4 system, lapaquistat does not have significant drug interactions with statins metabolized through this same enzyme system, such as atorvastatin.[21] From a lipid standpoint, lapaquistat monotherapy significantly lowers LDL cholesterol, apolipoprotein (apo B), and triglyceride (TG) levels as monotherapy[22] (although less than the starting doses of some statins), with similar lipid-altering effects when added to stable statin therapy[23] (Fig. 44-3 and 44-4).

TABLE 44-1	Examples of Non statin Causes of Rhabdomyolysis
Increased muscular activity Acute psychosis	
Severe dystonia	
Sporadic, extreme sport activity (especially in untrained individuals)	
Status asthmaticus	
Status epilepticus	
Muscle injury Blunt trauma or crush injuries	
Burns	
Electric shock	
Lightning	
Near drowning	
Prolonged immobilization due to drug effect, orthopedic injuries/ limitations, or neurologic diseases such as stroke or Guillain-Barré syndrome	
Shaken baby syndrome	
Drugs 3,4-methylenedioxymethamphetamine (MDMA, ecstasy)	
Aminocapric acid	
Amphetamine	
Amphotericin B	
Anesthetic and paralytic agents (malignant hyperthermia syndrome)	
Antibiotics	
Antihistamines	
Antipsychotics	
Barbiturates	
Caffeine	
Cocaine	
Corticosteroids	
Cyclosporine	
Ethanol	
Ethylene glycol	
Fibrates/fibric acid derivatives	
Hallucinogens	
Heroin	
Iron-dextran	
Isopropanol	
Ketamine hydrochloride	
Lysergic acid diethylamide (LSD)	
Methamphetamine	
Methanol	
Neuroleptics (neuroleptic malignant syndrome)	
Opiates (including methadone)	
Phencyclidine	
Phenylpropanolamine	
Propofol	
Quinine	
Salicylates	
Sedative hypnotics	
Selective serotonin reuptake inhibitors (the serotonin syndrome)	
Theophylline	
Tricyclic antidepressants	
Ischemia Compression	
Hypovolemia or severe dehydration	
Sickle trait	
Vascular injury	
Toxins Bee (massive) envenomations	
Carbon monoxide	
Ethanol	
Etyhylene glycol	
Haff's fish	
Hornet venom	
Isopropyl alcohol	
Mercuric chloride	
Quail (hemlock herbs)	
Snake envenomations	
Spider envenomations (widow)	
Staphylococcal	
Tetanus toxin	
Toluene	
Inflammatory myopathies Polymyositis	
Dermatomyositis	
Infections ***1. Bacterial*** Bacillus	
Borrelia burgdorferi	
Brucella	
Clostridium (perfringens and tetani)	
Escherichi coli	
Herbicola lathyri	
Legionella	
Leptospirosis	
Listeria	
Mycoplasma	
Plasmodium	
Rickettsia	
Salmonella	
Shigella	
Staphylococcus epidermiditis	
Streptococcus (Group B, pneumoniae, and pyogenes)	

Continued

TABLE 44-1 Examples of Non statin Causes of Rhabdomyolysis—cont'd
Tularemia *(Francisella tularensis)*
Vibrio
Viridans streptococci
2. Viral Adenovirus
Coxsackievirus
Cytomegalovirus
Echovirus
Epstein Barr virus
Herpes family viruses (including varicella)
Human immunodeficiency virus
Influenza A and B
Parainfluenza
3. Parasites Malaria *(Plasmodium falciparum)*
4. Fungus Candida
Asperigillus
Metabolic disorders Diabetic hyperosmolar coma
Diabetic ketoacidosis
Hypokalemia
Hyponatremia
Hypophosphatemia
Hyperthyroidism
Hypothyroidism
Hereditary Metabolic Myopathies ***1. Abnormal Carbohydrate Metabolism*** Lactate dehydrogenase deficiency
Mitochondrial respiratory chain enzyme deficiencies
Myoadenylate deaminase deficiency
Myophosphorylase deficiency (McArdle disease or glycogen phosphorylase deficiency type V)
Phosphofructokinase deficiency (Tarui's disease)
Phosphoglycerate kinase deficiency
Phosphoglycerate mutase deficiency
2. Abnormal Lipid Metabolism Carnitine deficiency
Carnitine palmityl transferase deficiency
Short-chain and long-chain acyl-coenzyme A dehydrogenase deficiency
3. Abnormalities of Purine Metabolism Myoadenylate deaminase deficiency
Duchenne's muscular dystrophy
Others Anticholinergic syndrome
Hyperthermia
Hypothermia
Idiopathic
Serotonin syndrome
Withdrawal of L-dopa

From Refs. 46–48.

Lapaquistat lowers C-reactive protein as monotherapy and in combination with statins.[12,24] Regarding safety, while individual lapaquistat monotherapy[12] and individual combination trials with statins[24] have not definitively demonstrated significant safety concerns, in a broader analysis of multiple trials, occurrences of transaminase elevations with the lapaquistat 100-mg dose appear to be greater than when compared to control groups. Lapaquistat development has been discontinued, and decisions regarding further development will likely depend on the efficacy and further safety assessments of doses of less than 100 mg/day[12] (see Fig. 44-3).

MICROSOMAL TRIGLYCERIDE TRANSFER PROTEIN INHIBITORS

Microsomal triglyceride transfer protein (MTP) transfers lipids (TGs, cholesteryl esters, and phosphatidylcholine) into apoB-containing lipoproteins such as very-low-density lipoprotein (VLDL) particles originating from the liver. MTP also transfers lipids to chylomicrons originating from the intestine (Fig. 44-5). Increased chylomicron production contributes to postprandial hypertriglyceridemia (Fig. 44-6). Increased VLDL production increases fasting TG, increases other atherogenic lipoproteins, and increases non–high-density lipoprotein (HDL) cholesterol levels, which in turn increases coronary heart disease (CHD) risk. Given the associated metabolic environment that often accompanies excessive body weight due to positive caloric balance,[25–27] hypertriglyceridemia is often associated with a constellation of CHD risk factors currently termed "metabolic syndrome," which often manifests a lipid pattern consisting of hypertriglyceridemia, low HDL cholesterol levels, and increased presence of small dense LDL particles (Fig. 44-7). Because LDL particles and the cholesterol carried by LDL particles are derived from VLDL (Fig. 44-8), then a decrease in VLDL production through impairment of the transfer of lipids into VLDL particles (such as through an inhibition of MTP) would be expected to reduce both cholesterol and TG blood levels.

Virtual absence of MTP is found in abetalipoproteinemia, which is an autosomal recessive genetic disorder whose signs and symptoms appear in the first few months of life, and results from defective MTP production. Patients typically have very low total cholesterol (~40 mg/dL) and TG (<10 mg/dL) levels, and are not able to transport lipid-soluble vitamins to peripheral tissues, which may necessitate water-soluble vitamin E to help prevent neurological disorders (movement disorders such as ataxia, tremors dysmetria, and dysarthria).[28] Patients may also have steatorrhea and malnutrition (due to intestinal fat malabsorption), ophthalmologic problems

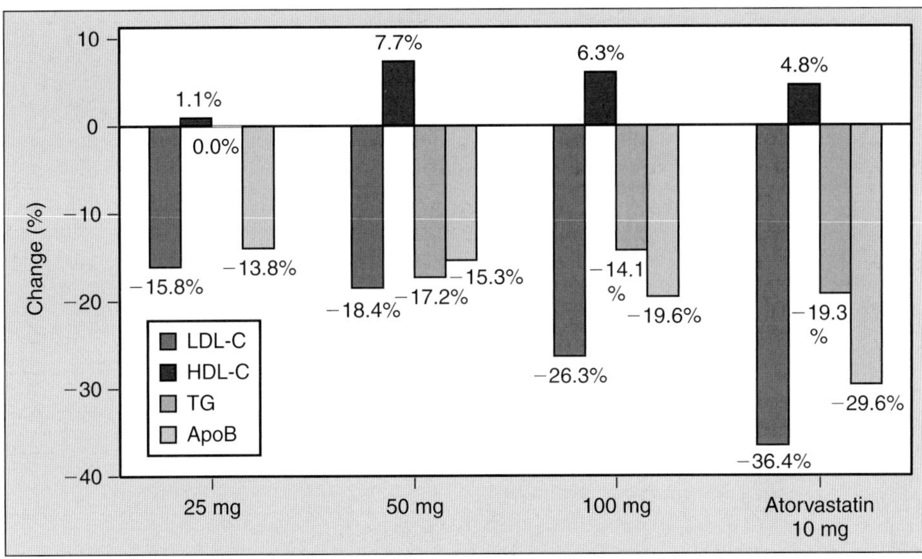

FIGURE 44-3 Placebo-corrected lipid effects of lapaquistat 25-, 50-, and 100-mg monotherapy. LDL-C, low-density lipoprotein cholesterol; HDL-C, hgih-density lipoprotein cholesterol; TG, triglycerides; Apo, apolipoprotein. (From Ref. 22.)

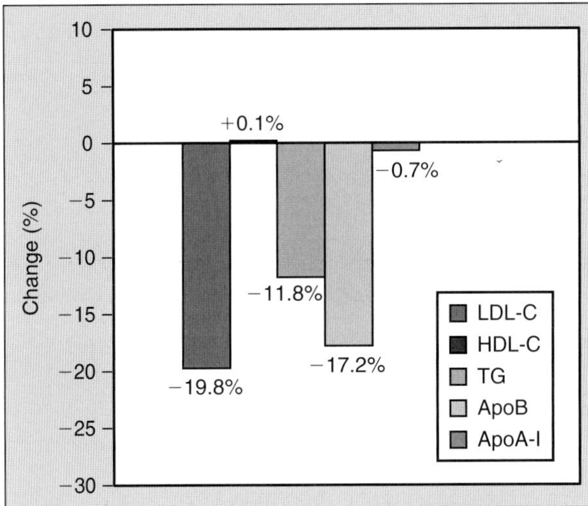

FIGURE 44-4 Placebo-corrected lipid effects of lapaquistat 100 mg added to atorvastatin 10 or 20 mg. LDL-C, low-density lipoprotein cholesterol; HDL-C, high-density lipoprotein cholesterol; TG, triglycerides; Apo, apolipoprotein. (From Ref. 23.)

(night blindness, poor eyesight, retinitis pigmentosa—possibly related to vitamin A deficiency—cataracts, and ophthalmoplegia); muscle abnormalities (weakness and contractures leading to kyphoscoliosis); and hematological disorders (iron and folate deficiency anemia, clotting disorders, and acanthocytosis).[29] Abetalipoproteinemia is also associated with "fatty liver" (hepatosteatosis),[30] which may lead to cirrhosis.[31] Partial MTP deficiency is found in patients with familial hypobetalipoproteinemia (FHBL), which is an autosomal dominant disorder typically resulting in fasting total cholesterol of about 90 mg/dL, LDL cholesterol around 20 mg/dL, and TG close to 35 mg/dL.[32] Postprandial lipemia (including apoB-48–containing chylomicronemia) is decreased as well.[32] Many patients with FHBL have mild liver enzyme elevations due to hepatosteatosis.[33]

Due to the profound potential to reduce lipid levels through impairment of this enzyme, various MTP inhibitors have been evaluated in clinical trials. Unfortunately, because they impair the transfer of TG out of both the liver and the intestine as part of their intrinsic mechanism of action, MTP inhibitor drug development has been hampered by unacceptable hepatosteatosis ("fatty liver") with elevated liver enzymes, and intestinal fat malabsorption (diarrhea). These adverse experiences have essentially negated the possibility of marketing the highest dose of MTP inhibitors. However, an alternative approach is developing MTP inhibitors at lower, more tolerable doses, with the intent of using them in statin-intolerant patients, or in combination with other lipid-altering drugs (including statins) for which they may provide complementary lipid benefits. Examples of MTP inhibitors in development include AEGR-733 (BMS-201038) and AEGR-427 (implitapide or Bay 13-9952).[34]

AEGR-733 is an MTP inhibitor being developed as an oral, once-daily treatment for dyslipidemia. From a drug interaction standpoint, earlier *in vitro* studies had suggested that AEGR-733 may modestly inhibit CYP 3A4. However, studies of AEGR-733 have revealed no significant increases in lipid-altering drugs metabolized through this enzyme system, such as atorvastatin and simvastatin. Furthermore, AEGR-733 does not appear to have significant drug interactions with other lipid-altering drugs such as rosuvastatin, ezetimibe, and fenofibrate.[34] From an efficacy standpoint, earlier clinical trials of doses of 25 to 100 mg/day administered over 7 days demonstrated dramatic LDL cholesterol reductions of 54% to 86%. However, these doses were accompanied by a high rate of hepatosteatosis and gastrointestinal adverse experiences. Similarly, a study of AEGR-733 administered as monotherapy and titrated to its highest dose in this study (1.0 mg/kg/day) for 4 weeks to six patients with homozygous familial hypercholesterolemia demonstrated that LDL cholesterol levels were reduced by 51%, apoB by 56%, TG by 65%, non-HDL cholesterol by 60%; HDL cholesterol by 2%, and apoA-I by 6%. This study also described elevations in liver enzymes in four of six study subjects, as well as increases in hepatic fat (as assessed by magnetic resonance imaging of the liver) ranging from less than 10% to more than 40%.[35] Hence, while higher AEGR-733 doses (up to 60–80 mg/day) continue to be

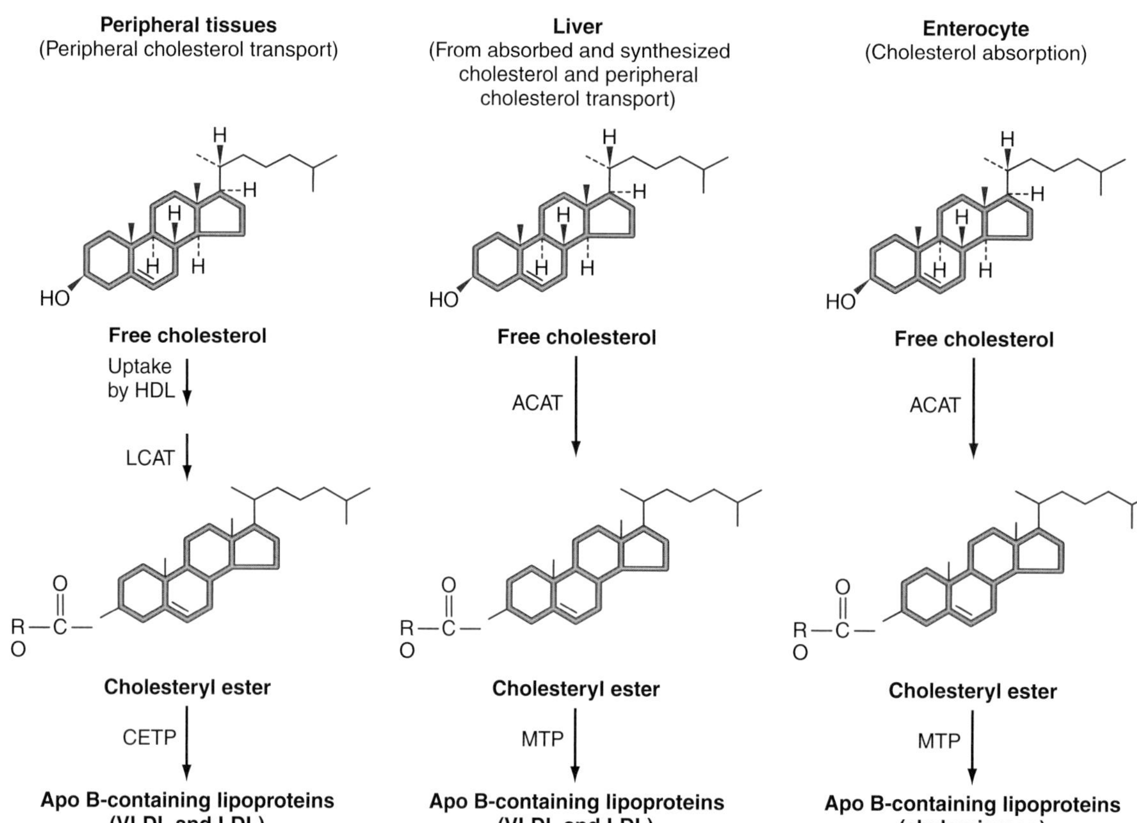

FIGURE 44-5 Analogy of free cholesterol packaging into apoB-containing lipoproteins in peripheral tissues, liver, and intestine. Free (unesterified) cholesterol undergoes esterification, and is then is packaged into atherogenic, apoB-containing lipoproteins. In the circulation, the transfer of cholesterol from HDLs to apoB-containing lipoproteins occurs through cholesteryl ester transfer protein (CETP). In the liver and enterocyte, the transfer of cholesterol to apoB-containing lipoproteins occurs through microsomal triglyceride transfer protein (MTP). (Adapted from Ref. 49.)

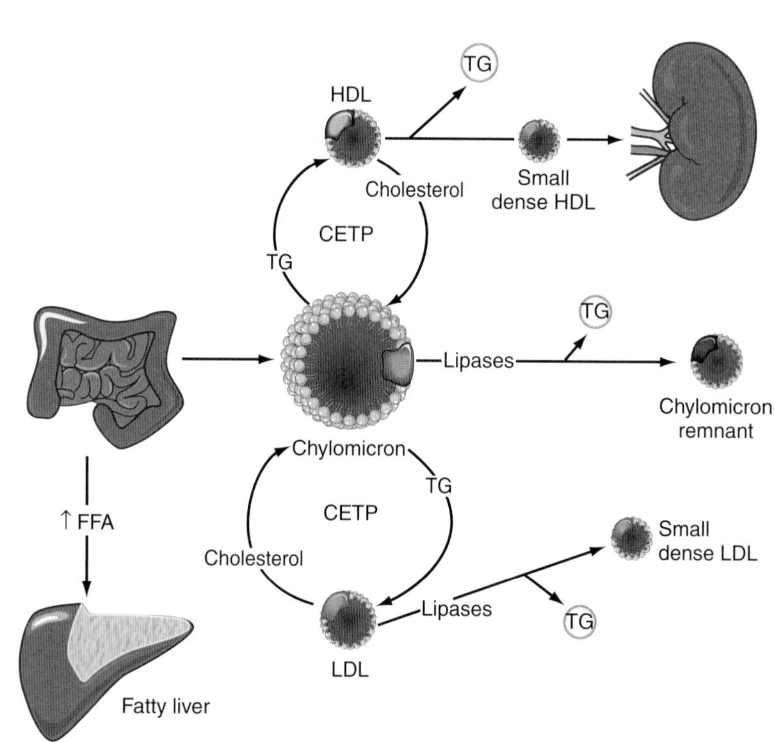

FIGURE 44-6 Generation of postprandial hypertrigiyceridemia and other lipid abnormalities. Intestinal lipids are carried by triglyceride-rich, apoB-48–containing chylomicrons that through lipases, result in chylomicron remnant formation that may be atherogenic. Other enzymatic exchanges may result in the lipid pattern often seen with the "metabolic syndrome," such as hypertriglyceridemia, reduced HDL cholesterol levels, and small dense LDL cholesterol levels. (Adapted from Ref. 50.)

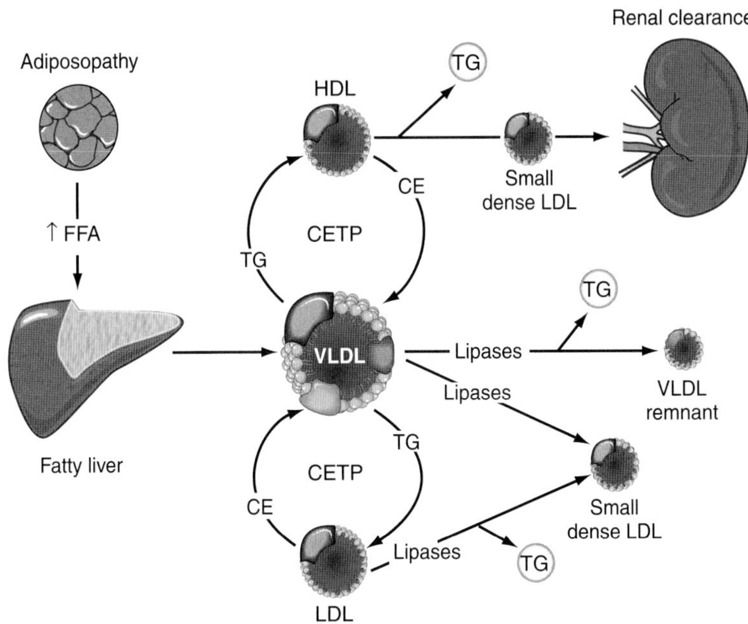

FIGURE 44-7 Generation of fasting hypertriglyceridemia and other lipid abnormalities. Hepatic triglycerides are incorporated into apoB-100–containing VLDL particles that through lipases, result in VLDL remnant formation. Both VLDL particles and their remnants are considered atherogenic. Other enzymatic exchanges may result in the lipid pattern often seen with the "metabolic syndrome," such as hypertriglyceridemia, reduced HDL cholesterol levels, and small dense LDL. CE, cholesteryl esters; CETP, cholesteryl ester transfer protein; FFA, free fatty acids; HDL, high-density lipoprotein; LDL, low-density lipoprotein; TG, triglycerides; VLDC, very-low-density lipoprotein. (Adapted from Ref. 51.)

evaluated for the rare patients with severe dyslipidemia (such as homozygous familial hypercholesterolemia), a lower-dose (2.5–10 mg) strategy has been implemented for potential therapy in a broader population of less severe dyslipidemia, with the intent of a more tolerable monotherapy agent (Fig. 44-9), and/or agent that might be combined with other lipid-altering drugs. One example would be AEGR-733 5 to 10 mg in combination with ezetimibe, which may prove to be a useful therapeutic option in patients intolerant to statins, or in patients in whom statin use is not indicated. In a 12-week trial to evaluate this combination, AEGR-733 5 to 10 mg/day lowered LDL cholesterol by 19% to 30%, ezetimibe 10 mg/day lowered LDL cholesterol by about 20%, and the combination of AEGR-733 5 to 10 mg/day plus ezetimibe 10 mg/day lowered LDL cholesterol by 35% to 46%[36] (Fig. 44-10). Interestingly, patients administered AEGR-733 experience weight loss, which may be beneficial in many overweight, dyslipidemic patients.[37]

The primary reason for AEGR-733 therapy discontinuation was due to hepatic enzyme elevation (Table 44-2). Ongoing studies include AEGR-733 hepatic imaging studies and those of AEGR-733 in combination with atorvastatin.[34]

AEGR-427, or implitapide, is also an MTP inhibitor whose earlier clinical trials at high doses demonstrated dramatic reductions in LDL cholesterol levels (Fig. 44-11). However, implitapide doses of 80 mg resulted in a high rate (14%) of discontinuations due to the adverse experiences of gastrointestinal intolerance and elevations in liver enzymes. Implitapide 160 mg had an especially high and unacceptable rate of discontinuation (42%). As with AEGR-733, future development of implitapide will be focused on lower doses (30–50 mg) in hopes of achieving sufficient lipid-lowering effects with an acceptable safety/tolerability profile.[34]

ANTISENSE OLIGONUCLEOTIDES TO APOLIPOPROTEIN B

Statins, SSIs and MTP inhibitors represent therapeutic approaches wherein lipid enzymes are inhibited for the purpose of altering cholesterol production and/or its incorporation into lipoproteins. Another approach to reduce elevated cholesterol levels is to impair the gene expression of apolipoprotein components of atherogenic lipoproteins, thus reducing their production.

The information carried by the nuclear genetic helix molecule, DNA (Fig. 44-12), encodes the "blueprint" for constructing cellular components, and these instructions are carried by genes. Genes are sequences of DNA nucleotides containing regulatory regions which determine when and how proteins are produced. DNA nucleotides are typically composed of a sugar (pentose), phosphate groups, and a nitrogen-containing heterocylic base (purine or pyrimidine), and when bound together in sequence, form nucleic acids.

DNA is dual stranded, and one strand represents the "sense" genetic code sequence, while the other paired strand (containing complementary purine/pyrimidine bases) has "antisense" genetic coding. During transcription when the sense and antisense DNA strands separate,

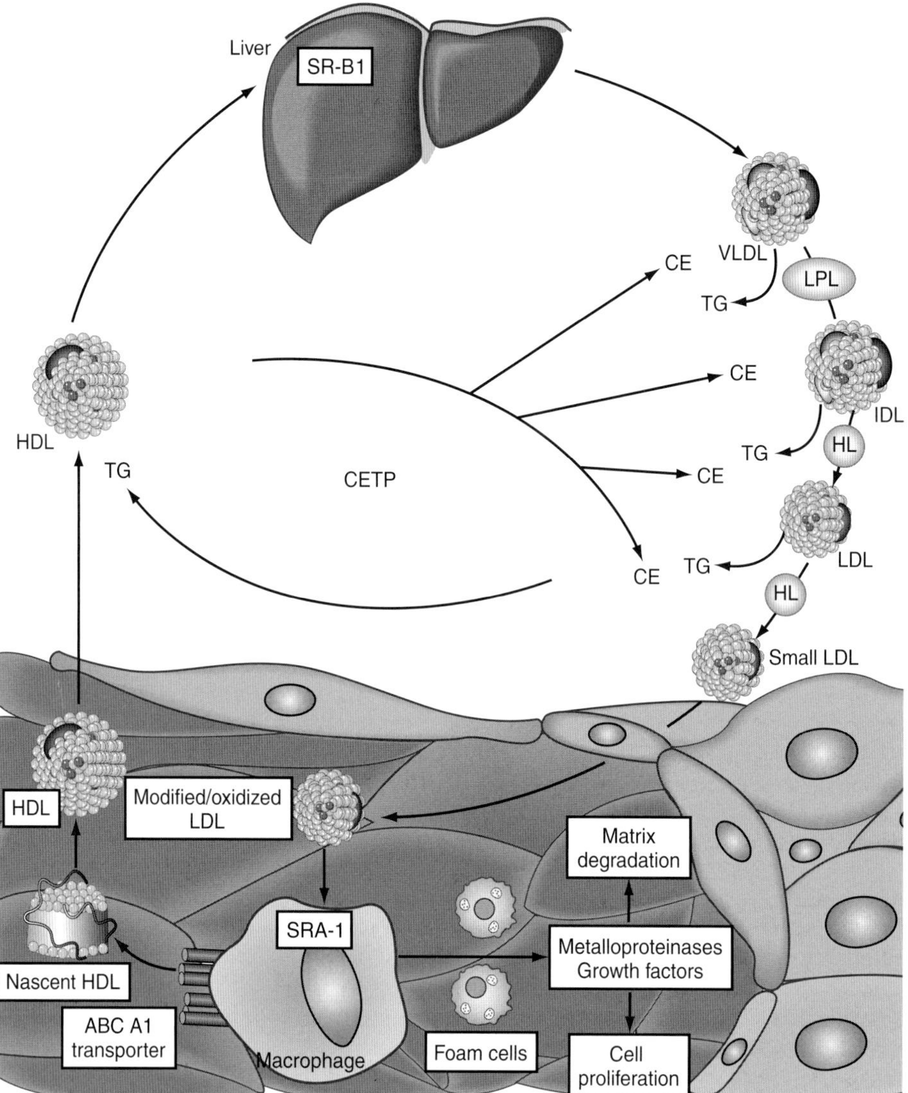

FIGURE 44-8 Conversion of very-low-density lipoprotein (VCDL) particles to low-density lipoprotein (LDL) particles and other enzyme-mediated lipid exchanges. Once triglyceride-rich apoB-100–containing VLDL particles are released by the liver into the circulation, various lipases promote the formation of intermediate-density lipoproteins (IDLs) and LDLs. Further lipase activity contributes to the formation of small dense LDL particles, which may enhance their atherogenecity. Cholesterol from peripheral tissues is carried back to the liver via high-density lipoproteins (HDLs). One of the peripheral tissues of clinical importance includes the vasculature. Cholesterol carried by HDL particles can undergo uptake by the liver, or can be transferred to atherogenic lipoproteins. (Adapted from Ref. 51.)

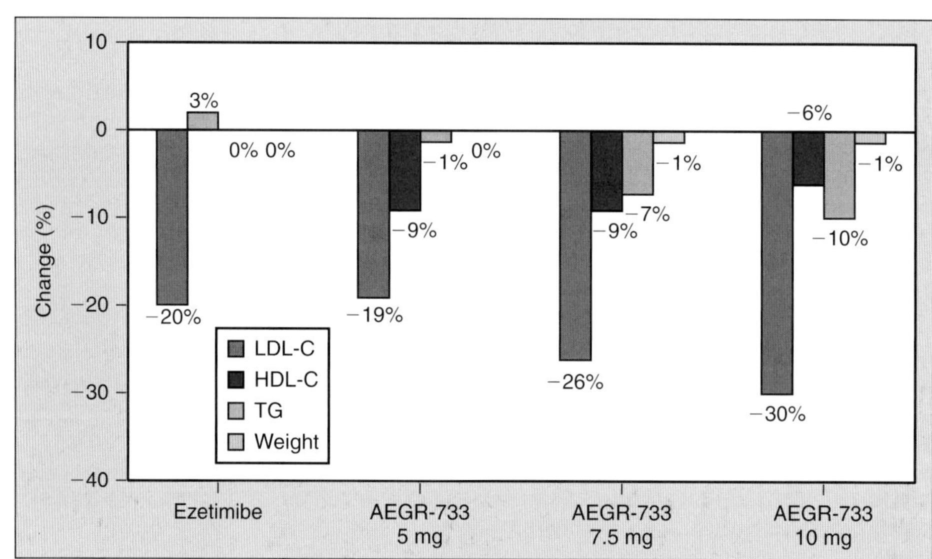

FIGURE 44-9 Lipid efficacy of the Microsomal triglyceride transfer protein (MTP) inhibitor AEGR-733 monotherapy compared to ezetimibe. The ezetimibe effects on lipid parameters were generalized, based on the data derived from multiple treatment arms at 4, 8, and 12 weeks. LDL-C, low-density lipoprotein cholesterol; HDL-C, high-density lipoprotein cholesterol; TG, triglycerides. (From Ref. 34.)

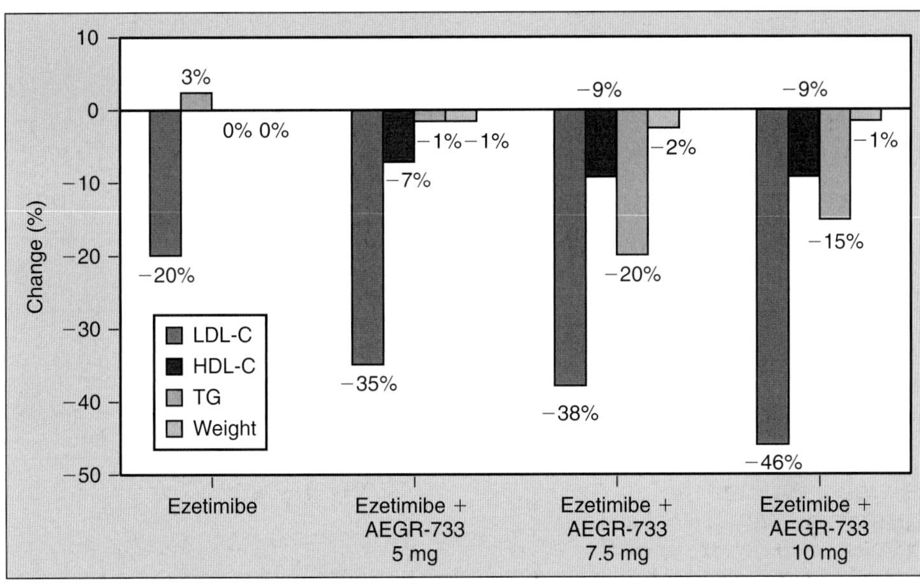

FIGURE 44-10 Lipid efficacy of the MTP inhibitor AEGR-733 when combined with ezetimibe. The ezetimibe effects on lipid parameters were generalized, based on the data derived from multiple treatment arms at 4, 8, and 12 weeks. LDL-C, low-density lipoprotein cholesterol; HDL-C, hgih-density lipoprotein cholesterol; TG, triglycerides. (From Ref. 34.)

TABLE 44-2 Discontinuation Rate of Subjects in AEGR-733/Ezetimibe Clinical Trial

		Adverse Events				
Drugs Evaluated	**Total Number of Subjects Discontinuing Treatment**	**Hepatic**	**Gastrointestinal**	**Muscle**	**Neurologic**	**Vascular**
Ezetimibe	4	ø	2	1	1	0
AEGR-733	9	6	2	0	0	1
AEGR-733 + Ezetimibe	4	3	1	1	0	0

Notes: One subject involved in the trial suffered a severe adverse event that was determined to be a fatal myocardial infarction. This event occurred 7 days after the patient had completed the trial and was deemed by the investigator and the medical monitor to be unrelated to drug therapy. Some subjects had more than one reason for study discontinuation.

From Ref. 34.

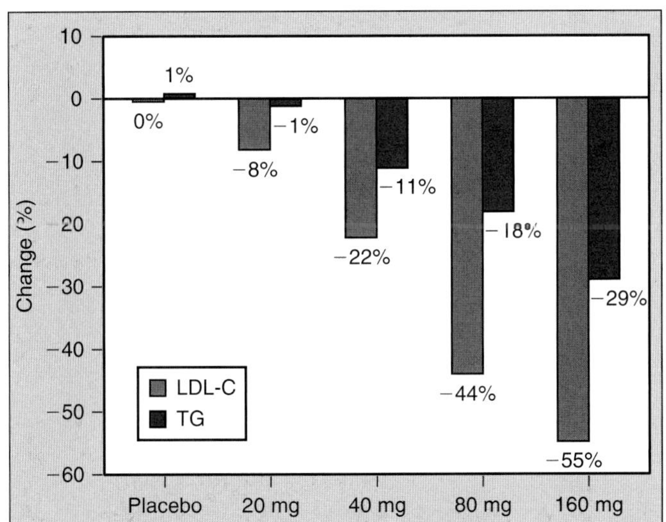

FIGURE 44-11 Percent reduction in low-density lipoprotein cholesterol (LDL-C) and triglyceride (TG) levels with implitapide after 4 weeks.[1,34]

the antisense DNA strand serves as a template for the formation of single-stranded mRNA, which is synthesized with complementary base pairings and is termed *sense*. These sense mRNA then migrate from the nucleus into the cytosol where ribosomes "translate" the genetic information for the purpose of producing proteins. Through this protein translational process, therapeutic agents are being investigated that are enzyme-dependent antisense (e.g., agents with RNase-like activity that degrades the target mRNA, single-stranded DNA, RNA, and phosphorothioate modified oligonucleotides) or steric-blocking antisense (which bind to target mRNA, impairing its translation) (Fig. 44-13). Obstacles to overcome in the development of antisense agents include specificity, drug distribution, therapeutic effects, potential toxicities, administration, and clinical applicability.

If antisense agents can be developed that specifically impair pathologic or pathogenic proteins that cause or significantly contribute to human disease, then antisense agents have the potential to be highly specific in their therapeutic effects. Theoretically, such specificity may improve efficacy and reduce "collateral" adverse side effects of less selective approaches and agents. By impairing "sense" mRNA prior to translation, the formation of an unfavorable protein is impaired before it has the potential to cause disease. This is in contrast to many other therapeutic approaches wherein the target is the clinical consequence of the production of a pathological or pathogenic protein. Furthermore, it is possible that the universe of antisense agents is greater than existing, traditional therapeutic agents because of potential to discriminate treatment targets based on genetic sequencing.

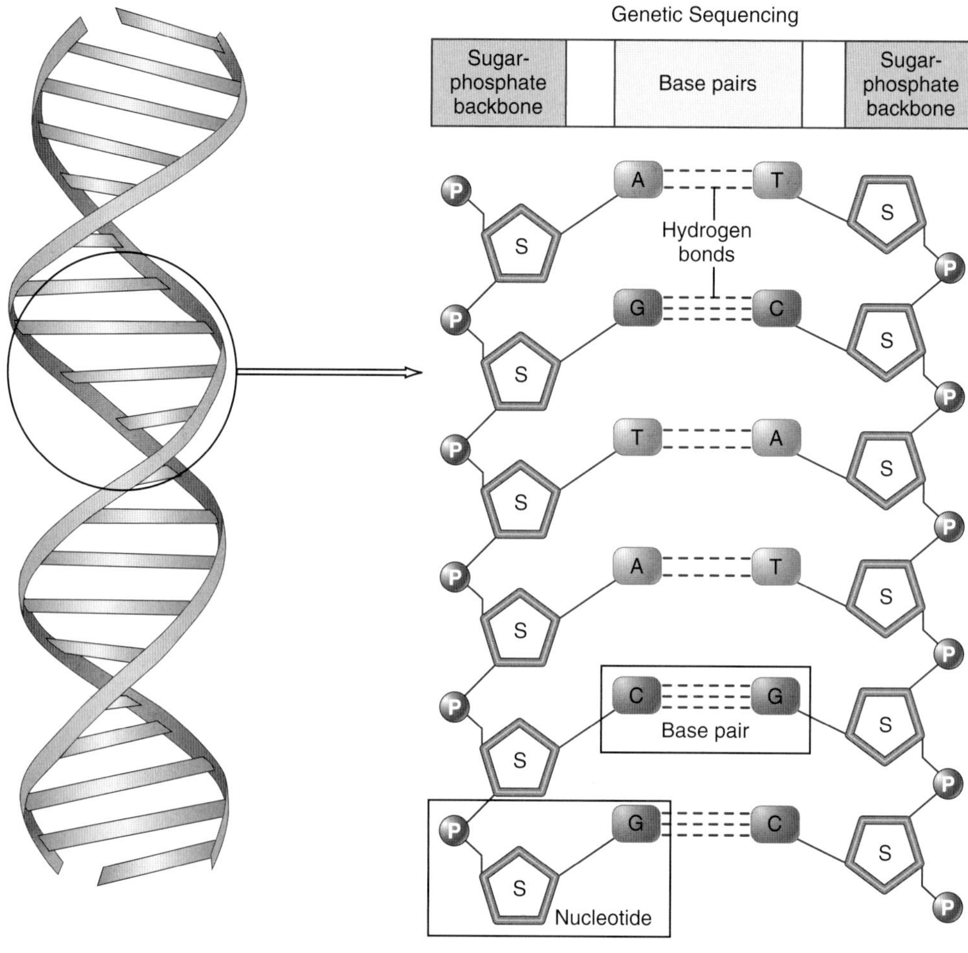

FIGURE 44-12 Simplified figure of deoxyribonucieic acid (DNA) sequencing which constitutes a gene. DNA is a nuclear genetic helix molecule that encodes the "blueprint" information for constructing cellular components. A nucleotide is composed of a sugar (pentose), phosphate backbone, and a nitrogen-containing heterocylic base (purine or pyrimidine). Sequences of nucleotides forming nucleic acids are illustrated by DNA. Genes are strands of DNA that contain coding sequences which determine what and when functional proteins are translated, and thus determine what and when in herited traits are expressed.

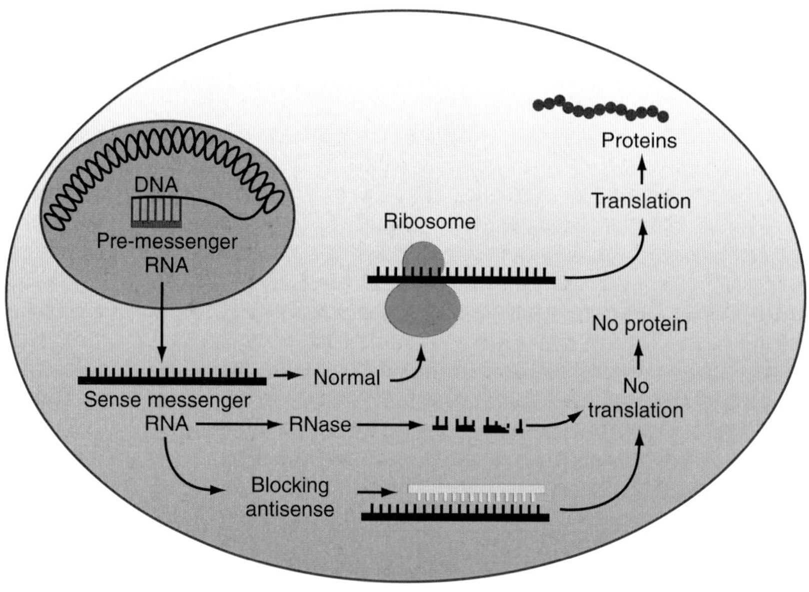

FIGURE 44-13 Antisense disruption of protein translation. One strand of the dual-stranded DNA represents the "sense" genetic code sequence, while the other paired strand represents "antisense" genetic coding. During transcription, the antisense DNA strand serves as a template for the formation of single-stranded messenger ribonucleic acids (mRNA), which is termed "sense." Sense mRNA migrate from the nucleus into the cytosol where ribosomes "translate" the genetic information for protein production. Antisense agents block target sense mRNA, impairing its associated protein translation and production.

Antisense agents are in development toward treating metabolic (diabetes mellitus and dyslipidemia), cardiovascular (including vascular inflammation), asthma/rhinitis, inflammatory bowel, ocular, viral, neurodegenerative, acromegaly, and oncological diseases. Antisense agents have been studied in various formulations, such as through aerosol, enema, intrathecal, intravenous, subcutaneous, intravitreal, oral, and topical administrations. The most common methodology has been the use of antisense oligonucleotides (ASOs), which are typically comprised of 20 or fewer base components that collectively constitute a single-strand antisense nucleotide sequence complementary to mRNA. These ASOs impair the specific protein produced through the translation of the sense mRNA. In addition, ASOs most often accumulate in organs and tissues such as the liver, kidney, spleen, bone marrow, and fat cells, much less so in skeletal muscle and heart, and do not appear to accumulate in the brain; are typically metabolized by endonucleases and exonucleases and then excreted in the urine; and quickly equilibrate tissue levels with blood levels.

Early clinical trials suggested that the toxicities of ASOs were mostly attributable to their structure and potential mechanisms of action and not to any particular ASO or target mRNA sequence. Preclinical and clinical adverse experiences have included injection site reactions (sometimes severe), mild thrombocytopenia, hyperglycemia, disruption of the complement and coagulation cascades, hypotension, and dose-limiting hepatocellular degeneration.[38] An example of such a drug in clinical use is the intravitreal administration of fomivirsen,[39] which is a 21-nucleotide antisense agent that is complementary to cytomegalovirus (CMV) mRNA,[40] and which is approved for local treatment for CMV retinitis in patients with acquired immunodeficiency syndrome who are intolerant, or who have not responded, to other CMV treatments. Fomivirsen administration has been associated with ocular and systemic adverse experiences, although as with many drugs used in chronically or severely ill patients, it is unclear how many are directly due to the drug. The most frequently reported adverse experiences involve ocular inflammation (iritis and vitritis). However, because fomivirsen is administered intravitreally, and not orally, subcutaneously, or intravenously, then this is likely not to be an illustrative example of what adverse experiences might be expected from an oligonucleotide antisense agents that are administered in a more systemic manner.

ISIS 301012 (mipomersen) is an ASO that selectively targets apoB-100, which is a critical protein in the synthesis of atherogenic lipoproteins such as LDL and VLDL. Preclinical animal studies have reported that mipomersen reduces apoB-100, reduces circulating inflammatory cytokines, and reduces atherosclerotic plaques.[41] A subcutaneous formulation is furthest in development.[42] Although not in current development, an oral formulation was evaluated with 1-month oral capsule administration of mipomersen in normal volunteers resulting in an average of 6% bioavailability and a reduction in apoB-100 of approximately 13%. Drug–drug interaction studies suggested no interactions with simvastatin or ezetimibe.[41]

In the first in-human study, a short-term (4-week) administration of a single 50- to 400-mg subcutaneous dose of mipomersen in 36 volunteers with mild dyslipidemia (median baseline LDL cholesterol levels among treatment groups ranging from 118 to 136 mg/dL) demonstrated up to a 50% reduction in apoB, up to a 35% reduction in LDL cholesterol, and up to a 27% reduction in TG levels with the 200-mg dose. Further reductions in these lipoproteins were seen with the 400-mg dose. Interestingly, apoB and LDL cholesterol levels remained significantly below baseline up to 3 months after the last dose, at least in part potentially related to prolonged tissue levels. No drug-related serious adverse experiences were reported in the study. The most common adverse experience was erythema at the injection site (21 of 29 subjects). Four (14%) of the 29 treated subjects had elevated alanine aminotransferase (ALT) levels related to the study drug that were asymptomatic and not associated with elevated bilirubin levels or prothrombin time prolongation. One subject had ALT elevations more than three times the upper limit of normal, which returned to normal after 2 weeks off the study drug. A direct correlation was found between the maximum ALT and maximum apoB reduction, both of which occurred at the highest doses of mipomersen.[43]

In a phase II clinical trial,[44] mipomersen at 50 to 400 mg/week in patients with moderate hypercholesterolemia (median baseline LDL cholesterol levels among treatment groups ranging from 154 to 206 mg/dL), administered as subcutaneous monotherapy for 13 weeks, reduced LDL cholesterol levels by 12% to 70%, with apoB levels in some patients being so low as to be undetectable (Table 44-3). HDL cholesterol levels were decreased, which may have been an assay-specific finding. Otherwise, TG and non–HDL cholesterol levels were also substantially reduced. When added to ongoing stable statin therapy, mipomersen 30 to 400 mg/week in patients with persistent hypercholesterolemia (median baseline LDL cholesterol levels among treatment groups ranging from 107 to 168 mg/dL), administered as subcutaneous combination therapy for 5 weeks, reduced LDL cholesterol by 4% to 47%. No significant changes were found in HDL cholesterol levels. Mipomersen also lowered apoB, non-HDL cholesterol, and TG levels (Table 44-4). In both of these phase II studies, (whose final reported results are pending), the most common adverse experiences were injection-site reactions in as much as 90% of study participants. Several patients developed elevated liver enzymes. After evaluation of these data, it was decided that the 400 mg/week dose would not advance into registration studies, with induction doses to be 200 to 300 mg/week, and maintenance doses of 100 to 200 mg/week.[44]

Finally, other studies have examined the relative efficacy and safety in patients with homozygous and heterozygous familial hypercholesterolemia special population. In June 2006, the U.S. Food and Drug

TABLE 44-3 Mipomersen Monotherapy and Mediam Percent Change in Lipid Levels Compared to Baseline

		Mipomersen (mg/wk)				
Lipid	**Placebo**	**50**	**100**	**200**	**300**	**400**
ApoB	7%	-22%	-23%	-47%	-61%	>-70%
LDL cholesterol	2%	12%	-22%	-42%	-62%	-70%
VLDL cholesterol	-17%	-14%	14%	-54%	-52%	-63%
Non-HDL cholesterol	4%	-17%	-21%	-44%	-54%	-65%
HDL cholesterol	2%	9%	-5%	-1%	-15%	-18%
ApoA-I	0%	8%	-2%	-2%	-14%	-9%
Total cholesterol	6%	-12%	-34%	-34%	-46%	-56%
Triglycerides	-13%	-7%	-46%	-46%	-43%	-53%
ApoB:apoA-I	11%	-22%	-46%	-46%	-51%	-69%
Total cholesterol: HDL cholesterol	-4%	-14%	-34%	-34%	-35%	-53%

From Ref. 44.

apo, apolipoprotein HDL, high-density lipoprotein; LDL, low-density lipoprotein; VLDL, very-low-density lipoprotein.

TABLE 44-4 Mipomersen Added to Stable Statin Therapy and Median Percent Change in Lipid Levels Compared to Baseline

		Mipomersen (mg/wk)				
Lipid	Placebo	30	100	200	300	400
ApoB	-1%	0%	-20%	-24%	-52%	-51%
LDL cholesterol	-4%	4%	-22%	-30%	-51%	-47%
VLDL cholesterol	7%	8%	10%	-25%	-63%	-69%
Non-HDL cholesterol	-1%	8%	-20%	-22%	-51%	-49%
HDL cholesterol	9%	1%	-4%	6%	5%	6%
ApoA-I	0%	0%	-6%	1%	2%	-6%
Total cholesterol	2%	5%	-15%	-13%	-42%	-34%
Triglycerides	0%	4%	4%	-25%	-41%	-35%

From Ref. 44.
apo, apolipoprotein; HDL, high-density lipoprotein; LDL, low-density lipoprotein; VLDL, very-low-density lipoprotein.

Administration granted orphan drug status to mipomersen for the treatment of patients with homozygous familial hypercholesterolemia.[41]

Thus, the biggest challenge regarding this agent and this approach to treating dyslipidemia is establishing a short- and long-term acceptable safety profile. Development of an efficacious and safe oral preparation may enhance its tolerability, by avoiding acute injection site reactions. The clinical significance of elevated liver enzyme elevations found with mipomersen is unclear. It may represent true liver toxicity; human liver biopsy studies with mipomersen administration have not been done. It may also represent promotion of "fatty liver" through blocking the production of VLDL particles, and thus impairing the transport of TG from the liver to the circulation. Finally, elevations in liver enzymes with mipomersen could represent a normal hepatic reaction to reductions in hepatic levels of available apoB. It is likely that these short and long-term safety/tolerability concerns will need to be clarified prior to approval for broad clinical use in patients.

REFERENCES

1. Bays H, Stein EA: Pharmacotherapy for dyslipidaemia—current therapies and future agents. *Expert Opin Pharmacother* 2003;4:1901–1938.
2. Charlton-Menys V, Durrington PN: Squalene synthase inhibitors: clinical pharmacology and cholesterol-lowering potential. *Drugs* 2007;67:11–16.
3. Amano Y, Nishimoto T, Tozawa R, et al: Lipid-lowering effects of Tak-475, a squalene synthase inhibitor, in animal models of familial hypercholesterolemia. *Eur J Pharmacol* 2003;466:155–161.
4. Menys VC, Durrington PN: Squalene synthase inhibitors. *Br J Pharmacol* 2003;139:881–882.
5. Manoukian AA, Bhagavan NV, Hayashi T, et al: Rhabdomyolysis secondary to lovastatin therapy. *Clin Chem* 1990;36:2145–2147.
6. Wortmann RL: Dose-related statin myopathy: is it an issue? *Cleve Clin J Med* 2005;72:751–3, 756.
7. Nawarskas JJ: HMG-COA reductase inhibitors and coenzyme Q10. *Cardiol Rev* 2005;13:76–79.
8. Caso G, Kelly P, Mcnurlan MA, et al: Effect of coenzyme Q10 on myopathic symptoms in patients treated with statins. *Am J Cardiol* 2007;99:1409–1412.
9. Thompson PD, Clarkson P, Karas RH: Statin-associated myopathy. *JAMA* 2003;289:1681–1690.
10. Bostedor RG, Karkas JD, Arison BH, et al: Farnesol-derived dicarboxylic acids in the urine of animals treated with zaragozic acid A or with farnesol. *J Biol Chem* 1997;272:9197–9203.
11. Nishimoto T, Amano Y, Tozawa R, et al: Lipid-lowering properties of Tak-475, a squalene synthase inhibitor, *in vivo* and *in vitro*. *Br J Pharmacol* 2003;139:911–918.
12. Bays HE, Weiss RJ, Rhyne JM, Chen Y, Lopez C, Spezzi AH: Lapaquistat acetate monotherapy: effects of a novel squalene synthase inhibitor on LDL cholesterol Levels and other lipid parameters in patients with primary hypercholesterolemia. Presented at American Heart Association conference, Orlando, FL, November 4–7, 2007 (abstract 682).
13. Forman BM, Ruan B, Chen J, et al: The orphan nuclear receptor Lxralpha is positively and negatively regulated by distinct products of mevalonate metabolism. *Proc Natl Acad Sci U S A* 1997;94:10588–10593.
14. Bays HE, Goldberg RB. The forgotton Bile Acid Sequestrants: Is Now a Good Time to Remember? American Journal of Therapeutics 2007;14:567–580.
15. Nishimoto T, Tozawa R, Amano Y, et al: Comparing myotoxic effects of squalene synthase inhibitor, T-91485, and 3-hydroxy-3-methylglutaryl coenzyme a (HMG-COA) reductase inhibitors in human myocytes. *Biochem Pharmacol* 2003;66:2133–2139.
16. Bays H: Statin safety: an overview and assessment of the data—2005. *Am J Cardiol* 2006;97:6c–26c.
17. Ballantyne CM, Corsini A, Davidson MH, et al: Risk for myopathy with statin therapy in high-risk patients. *Arch Intern Med* 2003;163:553–564.
18. Pasternak RC, Smith SC, Jr, Bairey-Merz CN, et al: ACC/AHA/NHLBI clinical advisory on the use and safety of statins. *Circulation* 2002;106:1024–1028.
19. Daugird AJ, Crowell K, Saseen J: Clinical inquiries. Do statins cause myopathy? *J Fam Pract* 2003;52:973–977.
20. Karim A, Abeyrantne A, Siebert F, Hetman L, Teshima K, Kondo T: Tak-475, a squalene synthase inhibitor: mass balance and excretion study. *Clin Pharmacol Ther* 2007;91(Suppl 1):S114 (abstract).
21. Piper E, Price G, Munsaka M, Karim A: Tak-475, a squalene synthase inhibitor, coadministered with atorvastatin: a pharmacokinetic study. *Clin Pharmacol Ther* 2007;91(Suppl 1):S37 (abstract).
22. Piper E, Price G, Chen Y: Tak-475, a squalene synthase inhibitor improves lipid profle in hyperlipidemic subjects. *Circulation* 2006;114(Suppl 18):II-288 (abstract 1493).
23. Perez A, Kupfer S, Chen Y: Addition of Tak-475 to atorvastatin provides incremental lipid benefits. *Circulation* 2006;114(Suppl 18):II-113 (abstract 675).
24. Davidson MH, Maki KC, Zavoral JH, Yu S, Popovici C, Price GD: Lapaquistat acetate, a novel squalene synthase inhibitor, co-administered with atorvastatin reduces plasma lipids and C-reactive protein levels in subjects with primary hypercholesterolemia. Presented at American Heart Association conference, Orlando, FL, November 4–7, 2007 (abstract 193).
25. Bays H, Ballantyne C: Adiposopathy: why do adiposity and obesity cause metabolic disease? *Future Lipidol* 2006;1:389–420.
26. Bays H, Blonde L, Rosenson R: Adiposopathy: How do diet, exercise, weight loss and drug therapies improve metabolic disease? *Expert Rev Cardiovasc Ther* 2006;4:871–895.
27. Bays H, Dujovne CA: Adiposopathy is a more rational treatment target for metabolic disease than obesity alone. *Curr Atheroscler Rep* 2006;8:144–156.
28. Wetterau JR, Gregg RE, Harrity TW, et al: An MTP inhibitor that normalizes atherogenic lipoprotein levels in WHHL rabbits. *Science* 1998;282:751–754.
29. Berriot-Varoqueaux N, Aggerbeck LP, Samson-Bouma M, et al: The role of the microsomal triglygeride transfer protein in abetalipoproteinemia. *Annu Rev Nutr* 2000;20:663–697.
30. Avigan MI, Ishak KG, Gregg RE, et al: Morphologic features of the liver in abetalipoproteinemia. *Hepatology* 1984;4:1223–1226.
31. Partin JS, Partin JC, Schubert WK, et al: Liver ultrastructure in abetalipoproteinemia: evolution of micronodular cirrhosis. *Gastroenterology* 1974;67:107–118.
32. Hooper AJ, Robertson K, Barrett PH, et al: Postprandial lipoprotein metabolism in familial hypobetalipoproteinemia. *J Clin Endocrinol Metab* 2007;92:1474–1478.

33. Sen D, Dagdelen S, Erbas T: Hepatosteatosis with hypobetalipoproteinemia. *J Natl Med Assoc* 2007;99:284–286.
34. Aegerion Pharmaceuticals, Inc. Common stock registration statement. Amendment no. 3 to Form S-1. Washington, DC: U.S. Securities Exchange Commission, 2007.
35. Cuchel M, Bloedon LT, Szapary PO, et al: Inhibition of microsomal triglyceride transfer protein in familial hypercholesterolemia. *N Engl J Med* 2007;356:148–156.
36. Samaha FF, Mckenney J, Bloedon LT, Sasiela WJ, Rader DJ: Efficacy and safety of the MTP-inhibitor AEGR-733, as monotherapy and in combination with ezetimibe. Presented at Drugs Affecting Lipid Metabolism Conference, New York, October 4–7, 2007 (abstract 330)
37. Samaha FF, Mckenney J, Bloedon LT, Sasiela WJ, Rader DJ: MTP-inhibitor, AEGR-733, reduces body weight in patients with hypercholesterolemia. Presented at Drugs Affecting Lipid Metabolism Conference, New York, October 4–7, 2007 (abstract 345).
38. Jason TL, Koropatnick J, Berg RW: Toxicology of antisense therapeutics. *Toxicol Appl Pharmacol* 2004;201:66–83.
39. The Vitravene Study Group: Safety Of intravitreous fomivirsen for treatment of cytomegalovirus retinitis in patients with AIDS. *Am J Ophthalmol* 2002;133:484–498.
40. Grillone LR, Lanz R: Fomivirsen. *Drugs Today (Barc)* 2001;37: 245–255.
41. http://www.isispharm.com/product pipeline.html#301012. Isis Pharmaceuticals Product Pipeline. Accessed June 11, 2007.
42. Burnett JR: Drug evaluation: Isis-301012, an antisense oligonucleotide for the treatment of hypercholesterolemia. *Curr Opin Mol Ther* 2006;8:461–467.
43. Kastelein JJ, Wedel MK, Baker BF, et al: Potent reduction of apolipoprotein B and low-density lipoprotein cholesterol by short-term administration of an antisense inhibitor of apolipoprotein B. *Circulation* 114:1729–1735.
44. Brookes L: Antisense drug Isis 301012 lowers LDL cholesterol alone and in combination with statins. Medscape Cardiology, June 12, 2007.
45. Casey PJ: Biochemistry of protein prenylation. *J Lipid Res* 1992;33:1731–1740.
46. Craig S: Rhabdomyolysis. http://www.emedicine.com/emerg/topic508.htm. Last accessed May 21, 2007.
47. Muscal E. Rhabdomyolysis. http://www. emedicine.com/ped/topic2003.htm. Last accessed May 21, 2007.
48. Sauret JM, Marinides G, Wang GK: Rhabdomyolysis. *Am Fam Physician* 2002;65:907–912.
49. Bays HE. Ezetimibe. Expert Opin Investig Drugs 2002;11:1587–604.
50. Bays H, Ballantyne C. Adiposopathy: why do adiposity and obesity cause metabolic disease? Future Lipidol 2006;1:389–420.
51. Bays H, McKenney J, Davidson M: Torcetrapib/atorvastatin combination therapy. Expert Rev Cardiovasc Ther 2005;3:789–820.

CHAPTER 45

Therapeutic Targeting of High-Density Lipoprotein Metabolism

Daniel J. Rader

INTRODUCTION

As discussed in Chapter 10, plasma concentrations of high-density lipoprotein (HDL) cholesterol and its major protein apolipoprotein (apo) A-I are inversely associated with risk of atherosclerotic cardiovascular disease.[1] The National Cholesterol Education Program Adult Treatment Panel III (NCEP ATP III) guidelines recognized low HDL cholesterol (<40 mg/dL) as a potential target for therapeutic intervention.[2,3] However, even in patients treated to very aggressive low-density lipoprotein (LDL) cholesterol goals, coronary events still occur at a high rate, and low HDL cholesterol remains a major risk factor.[4–6] While therapeutic lifestyle changes can modestly raise HDL cholesterol levels, as discussed in Chapters 20 and 21, and drugs such as niacin and fibrates have HDL-raising effects, also discussed in Chapters 25 and 26, low HDL cholesterol remains prevalent and represents a major unmet medical need. Thus, therapies targeted toward HDL are of obvious interest as a potential strategy to further reduce morbidity and mortality due to atherosclerotic cardiovascular disease. A great deal has been learned in the last two decades regarding the physiology and pathophysiology of HDL metabolism (see Chapter 4) and human genetics affecting HDL levels (see Chapter 7).[7,8] While much remains to be learned, this explosion in our knowledge base has given rise to new therapeutic targets for HDL. The goal of this chapter is to review the progress being made in the development of new therapeutic approaches to HDL metabolism and reverse cholesterol transport (RCT).

BASIC CONCEPTS IN THERAPEUTIC TARGETING OF HIGH-DENSITY LIPOPROTEIN METABOLISM, REVERSE CHOLESTEROL TRANSPORT, AND HIGH-DENSITY LIPOPROTEIN FUNCTION

The physiology of HDL metabolism[7,8] is described in detail in Chapter 4 and reviewed briefly here (Fig. 45-1). Nascent HDL is produced by both the intestine and the liver. Based on studies in mice, apoA-I is secreted by enterocytes and hepatocytes in a lipid-poor state and then in the extracellular state rapidly acquires free cholesterol and phospholipids via the ATP-binding cassette A1 (ABCA1) transporter from the same cells. These nascent HDL particles acquire additional cholesterol from other tissues, including from cholesterol-loaded macrophages (foam cells) in the atherosclerotic plaque. The enzyme lecithin: cholesterol acyltransferase (LCAT) converts free cholesterol to cholesteryl ester (CE) on HDL, resulting in the formation of mature HDL particles. HDL cholesterol can be directly taken up by the liver, in a process that involves at least in part the scavenger receptor class B type I (SR-BI). In addition, the cholesteryl ester transfer protein (CETP) can transfer CEs out of HDL to apoB-containing lipoproteins in exchange for triglycerides, thus depleting HDL of cholesterol and enriching it in triglycerides. Triglyceride enrichment makes the HDL a better substrate for hepatic lipase (HL), which hydrolyzes HDL triglycerides and generates smaller

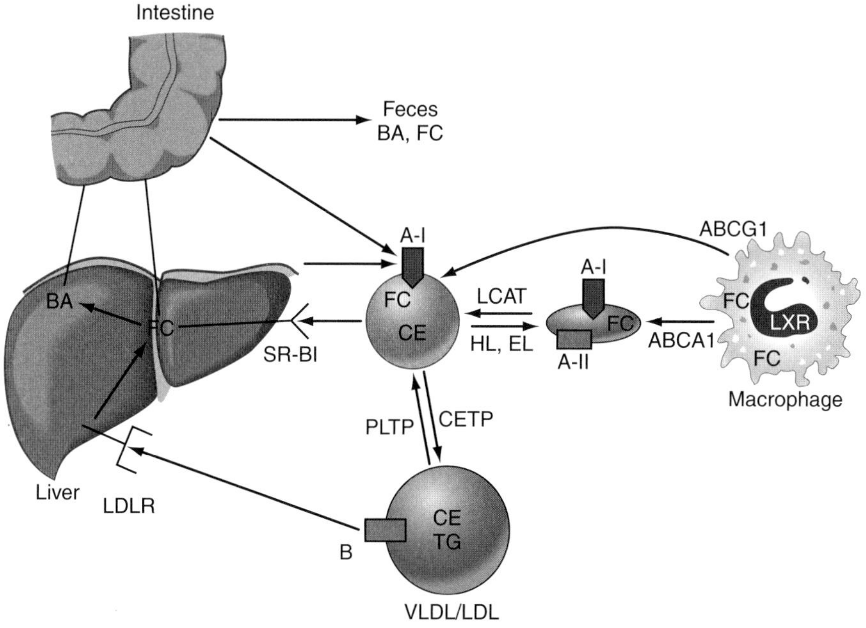

FIGURE 45-1 HDL metabolism and reverse cholesterol transport.

HDL particles. A related enzyme, endothelial lipase (EL), hydrolyzes HDL phospholipids and accelerates HDL catabolism. ApoA-I itself is catabolized by both the kidneys and the liver through processes that are not completely understood.

HDL and apoA-I promote a process known as *reverse cholesterol transport* (RCT) in which they serve as acceptors for the efflux of free cholesterol from peripheral tissues (Fig. 45-1). The full RCT pathway is completed when peripheral cholesterol is returned to the liver for excretion in bile and ultimately feces. It is likely that this process is atheroprotective when applied specifically to the lipid-loaded macrophage in the atherosclerotic plaque. The best-known pathway for cholesterol efflux from the lipid-loaded macrophage is the ABCA1 transporter, which promotes efflux of cholesterol to lipid-poor apoA-I.[9] ABCG1 is another member of this gene family that promotes cholesterol efflux from macrophages to mature HDL particles.[10,11] ABCA1 and ABCG1 are both important and are complementary in their ability to promote macrophage RCT *in vivo*[12] and protect against atherosclerosis in mouse models.[13] The expression of macrophage ABCA1 and ABCG1 are up-regulated by natural and synthetic agonists of the liver X receptor (LXR).[14] The importance of the fate of the cholesterol after it effluxes from the macrophage is uncertain, but some data suggest that events distal to cholesterol efflux may regulate the rate of RCT. For example, hepatic SR-BI expression is a positive regulator of RCT in mice.[15] The physiologic importance of hepatic SR-BI in humans remains to be determined.[16] It is possible that HDL protects against atherosclerosis by properties other than promoting RCT. For example, HDL has been shown to have antioxidant and anti-inflammatory properties,[17] as well as endothelial nitric oxide–promoting and antithrombotic effects[18] (Fig. 45-2).

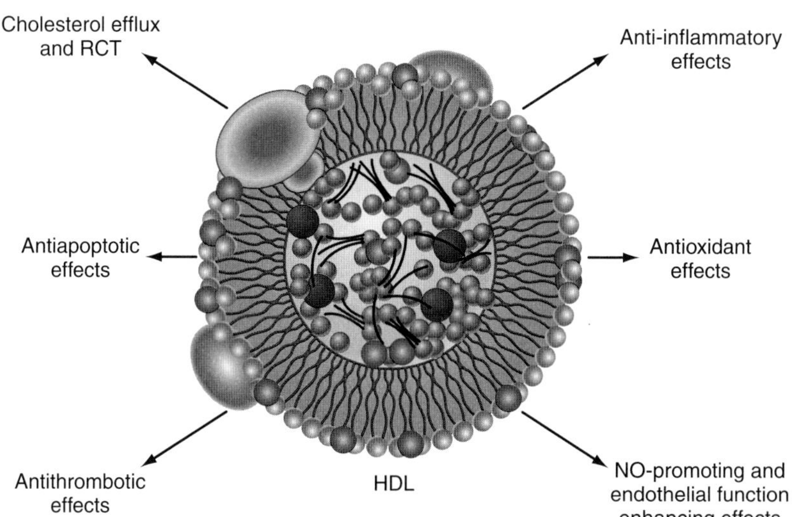

FIGURE 45-2 Mechanisms by which HDL may be antiatherogenic.

RAISING HIGH-DENSITY LIPOPROTEIN CHOLESTEROL THROUGH INHIBITION OF CHOLESTERYL ESTER TRANSFER PROTEIN

CETP transfers CE from HDL to apoB-containing lipoproteins in exchange for triglycerides, thus resulting in CE depletion of HDL and CE enrichment of apoB-containing lipoproteins. Humans genetically deficient in CETP have markedly increased plasma HDL cholesterol levels,[19,20] an observation that identified CETP as a potential therapeutic target. Several CETP inhibitors were developed and advanced into clinical development. The CETP inhibitor JTT-705 (now called dalcetrapib) was the first to be reported on in the peer-reviewed literature. In subjects with mild dyslipidemia, JTT-705 at 900 mg daily for 4 weeks resulted in a 34% increase in HDL cholesterol.[21] A phase II trial in dyslipidemic subjects demonstrated that 600 mg of JTT-705 in combination with pravastatin 40 mg for 4 weeks resulted in a 28% increase in HDL cholesterol levels.[22]

Another CETP inhibitor, torcetrapib, was shown to increase HDL cholesterol in healthy volunteers with normal lipid levels in a dose-dependent fashion, with a 91% increase at the 240-mg dose.[23] A small crossover trial in subjects with low HDL cholesterol levels designed to study the metabolic effects of CETP inhibition involved administration of 120 mg of torcetrapib either as monotherapy or added to stable atorvastatin therapy.[24] Administration of torcetrapib 120 mg increased HDL cholesterol by 46% as monotherapy and by 61% in the combination with atorvastatin. A subgroup that then received 240 mg of torcetrapib monotherapy had a mean increase in HDL cholesterol of 106%. In phase II trials in patients with low HDL cholesterol, torcetrapib resulted in substantial, dose-dependent increases in HDL cholesterol as monotherapy[25] as well as in combination with atorvastatin.[26]

However, the approach of CETP inhibition as a therapeutic strategy suffered a severe blow with the early termination in December 2006[27] of a large phase III clinical event outcome trial of torcetrapib 60 mg plus atorvastatin compared with atorvastatin alone, called the Investigation of Lipid Level Management to Understand Its Impact in Atherosclerotic Events (ILLUMINATE) trial.[28] The Data Safety Monitoring Board overseeing the ILLUMINATE trial reported an adverse imbalance of mortality in the torcetrapib arm, and as a consequence, the study was terminated and the development of torcetrapib was stopped. Even major cardiovascular events, the primary endpoint of the trial, were significantly increased in the torcetrapib group despite an increase in HDL cholesterol of more than 70% and a decrease in LDL cholesterol of 25%. Subsequently, the results of phase III atherosclerosis imaging trials were presented. The major conclusion of these three studies, one using intravascular ultrasound (IVUS) of the coronaries[29] and two using ultrasound of the carotids to assess carotid intima–media thickness,[30,31] was that torcetrapib 60 mg failed to slow progression of atherosclerosis despite increases in HDL cholesterol of greater than 50% and reductions of LDL cholesterol of about 20%. However, torcetrapib causes variable increases in blood pressure in some individuals,[28–31] an effect specific to the molecule and not based on the mechanism of CETP inhibition.[32,33] Indeed, in the ILLUMINATE trial there was evidence that torcetrapib therapy resulted in increased aldosterone levels.[28] Another potent CETP inhibitor, anacetrapib, has been shown to substantially influence plasma lipids without causing elevation in blood pressure.[34] At this time, it remains uncertain whether the adverse events in the ILLUMINATE trial and the lack of efficacy in the atherosclerosis imaging trials were related to the mechanism of CETP inhibition or unique to the torcetrapib molecule.[32,33]

There are legitimate concerns about the mechanism of CETP inhibition as a therapeutic strategy for atherosclerosis. Most of these concerns revolve around the concept that CETP inhibition, while it raises HDL cholesterol levels, may retard the process of RCT, by which HDL cholesterol is returned to the liver for excretion (Fig. 45-3). With regard to cholesterol efflux, a recent study indicated that HDL from CETP-deficient subjects is more effective than

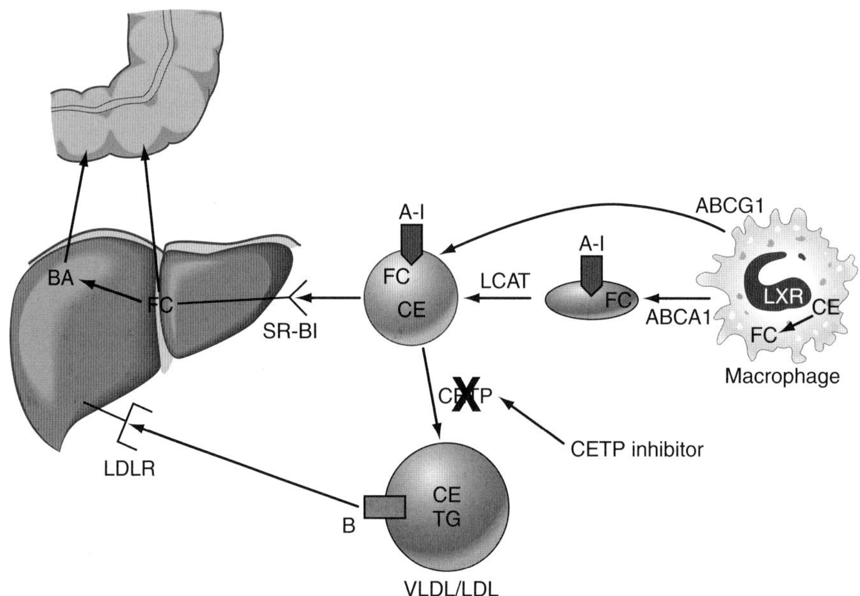

FIGURE 45-3 CETP inhibition and relationship to macrophage cholesterol efflux and reverse cholesterol transport.

control HDL in promoting macrophage cholesterol efflux via the ABCG1 pathway,[35] and that HDL from subjects receiving torcetrapib was more effective in promoting cholesterol efflux from macrophages.[36] However, CETP-deficient persons have significantly slower turnover of apoA-I,[37] and treatment with torcetrapib was demonstrated to reduce the turnover of apoA-I.[38] Administration of torcetrapib to subjects with low HDL cholesterol resulted in no significant effect on fecal neutral sterol excretion, despite the substantial increase in HDL cholesterol levels.[38] Evidence that CETP mediates the targeting of HDL cholesterol to bile was provided by studies performed by Schwartz and colleagues. Injection of HDL labeled with a CE tracer in humans demonstrated that the labeled cholesterol that was excreted into bile was mostly first transferred to apoB-containing lipoproteins,[16] suggesting a role for CETP in RCT. Conversely, when CETP is expressed in mice (which naturally lack it), RCT from macrophages to feces is substantially increased.[39] However, in mice lacking the LDL receptor, CETP expression resulted in a trend toward reduced macrophage RCT,[39] suggesting the possibility that the effect of CETP on RCT may depend in part on the efficiency of hepatic clearance of apoB-containing lipoproteins.

Ultimately, the most important issue is the effect of reduced CETP activity on atherosclerosis. Unfortunately, the question of whether homozygous CETP deficiency causes reduced, or increased, risk of CHD is not definitively established.[40] Individuals heterozygous for CETP mutations have only a modest increase in HDL cholesterol levels and have no major difference in cardiovascular risk.[41] Additional genetic studies of CETP polymorphisms in other populations[42] and measurement of CETP in large prospective observational studies[43] are conflicting. Animal studies are generally supportive of the concept that CETP inhibition reduces atherosclerosis. While mice lack CETP, rabbits have very abundant CETP and have thus been used for CETP inhibition atherosclerosis studies. JTT-705 was found to markedly reduce atherosclerosis in rabbits, but also substantially reduced atherogenic apoB-lipoproteins in this model.[44] A more recent study with torcetrapib attempted to "clamp" the levels of atherogenic lipoproteins and determined that CETP inhibition with torcetrapib significantly reduced the progression of atherosclerosis.[45] Overall, the status of CETP inhibition as a therapeutic strategy is uncertain at this time. It is possible that a "clean" CETP inhibitor such as dalcetrapib or anacetrapib will be antiatherogenic in humans, but this question has become considerably more complicated to address given the clinical outcome results with torcetrapib.[33]

PROMOTING MACROPHAGE CHOLESTEROL EFFLUX THROUGH LIVER X RECEPTOR AGONISM

Promotion of macrophage RCT is considered one of the "holy grails" for the treatment of atherosclerosis.[46] Therapy to promote the first step of this process relevant to atherosclerosis, namely cholesterol efflux from macrophages, is of obvious interest. The best-understood pathway for macrophage cholesterol efflux is the ABCA1 transporter, which promotes cholesterol efflux to lipid-poor apoA-I.[47] Mature HDL is also capable of promoting cholesterol efflux from macrophages via the transporter ABCG1.[10,11] The major regulators of ABCA1 and ABCG1 gene expression are the nuclear receptors LXR-α and LXR-β, which act as heterodimers with their partner the retinoid X receptor (RXR).[14] Synthetic LXR agonists up-regulate ABCA1 and ABCG1 expression and result in increased cholesterol efflux to both lipid-poor apoA-I and mature HDL. A synthetic LXR agonist substantially promoted macrophage cholesterol efflux and RCT *in vivo* despite having only a modest effect in raising plasma HDL cholesterol levels[48] (Fig. 45-4). Synthetic LXR agonists have been shown to inhibit atherosclerosis progression[49,50] and even promote atherosclerosis regression[51] in mice despite having little effect on plasma HDL cholesterol levels. These combined data support the concept of LXR agonists as effective antiatherosclerotic agents.

However, some LXR agonists have been found to cause hepatic steatosis and hypertriglyceridemia in animals, believed to be due to inducing the hepatic expression of sterol regulatory element–binding protein 1c (SREBP1c), which in turn induces expression of fatty acid synthetic genes.[52] Furthermore, in animals that express CETP, some LXR agonists have been shown to increase LDL cholesterol levels.[53] These issues have slowed the development of LXR agonists. Ideally, LXR

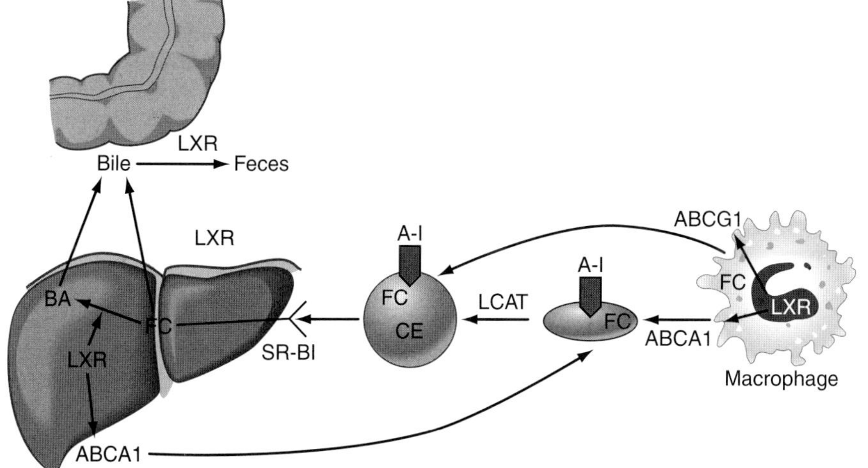

FIGURE 45-4 The role of LXR agonism in promoting macrophage reverse cholesterol transport.

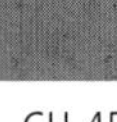

modulators would be developed that are relatively selective for either specific tissues (i.e., macrophages over liver) or for specific genes (i.e., ABCA1/G1 over SREBP1c). One LXR agonist has been reported to be partially selective and to induce less hepatic steatosis.[54] Alternatively, a selective modulator of LXR-β (which is less abundant in liver), but not LXR-α, might have less adverse effects on steatosis and plasma lipids. Given the abundance of preclinical data indicating promotion of macrophage RCT and reduction in atherosclerosis, there remains substantial interest in LXR agonism as a therapeutic approach. Hopefully, LXR agonists will advance in clinical development and it will be possible to assess their effects on plasma and liver lipids.

PEROXISOME PROLIFERATOR-ACTIVATED RECEPTOR-α AGONISTS MAY BOTH PROMOTE MACROPHAGE CHOLESTEROL EFFLUX AND UP-REGULATE APOLIPOPROTEIN A-I TRANSCRIPTION

Peroxisome proliferator–activated receptor–α (PPAR-α) is a nuclear receptor involved in the regulation of lipid metabolism. Fibrates are relatively weak PPAR-α agonists that are currently clinically available for the treatment of hypertriglyceridemia. PPAR-α agonists have at least two metabolic effects on HDL metabolism that may be antiatherogenic: up-regulation of apoA-I transcription and promotion of macrophage cholesterol efflux. PPAR-α agonists have been shown to up-regulate transcription of the human *APOA1* gene *in vitro* and in mice.[55–57] Studies addressing the effect of PPAR-α agonists on apoA-I production in humans have generally been small, but are consistent with increased apoA-I production.[58,59] Based on overexpression studies in animals,[60–62] it is generally regarded that up-regulation of apoA-I transcription is one of the most desirable approaches to targeting HDL metabolism. Thus, this effect of PPAR-α agonists would be expected to be antiatherogenic. In addition, macrophages express PPAR-α, and treatment of macrophages *in vitro* with fibrates has been shown to up-regulate ABCA1 and increase cholesterol efflux,[63] possibly via up-regulation of LXR itself. While it has not been directly demonstrated that PPAR-α agonists promote RCT *in vivo,* administration of a synthetic PPAR-α agonist to mice reduced atherosclerosis and inhibited foam cell formation in an ABCA1-independent but LXR-dependent manner.[64] The concept that PPAR-α agonists may both up-regulate apoA-I transcription and promote macrophage cholesterol efflux suggests that they should be potent antiatherogenic agents. While fibrates do generally reduce cardiovascular risk in appropriate patient populations,[65] their effects are not as profound as might be predicted based on the above. However, fibrates are relatively weak PPAR-α agonists, and new, more potent PPAR-α agonists could theoretically have greater effects. One such compound was reported to have disappointing effects on plasma HDL cholesterol levels,[66] but these studies did not assess the kinetics of HDL turnover or RCT. There remains a need to explore the potential of newer, more potent PPAR-α agonists to promote RCT.

PEROXISOME PROLIFERATOR-ACTIVATED RECEPTOR-β/δ AGONISTS MAY RAISE HIGH-DENSITY LIPOPROTEIN CHOLESTEROL LEVELS THROUGH UNCERTAIN MECHANISMS

PPAR-β/δ is another nuclear receptor involved in regulating lipid and energy metabolism. A synthetic PPAR-β/δ agonist was shown to raise HDL cholesterol levels in a rhesus monkey model of the metabolic syndrome.[67] While this study suggested that it was able to promote macrophage cholesterol efflux,[67] there remains controversy about whether PPAR-β/δ agonists promote macrophage cholesterol efflux. Administration of a synthetic PPAR-β/δ agonist to mice had no effect on macrophage foam cell formation.[64] Early human studies suggest relatively modest effects of a PPAR-β/δ agonist on HDL cholesterol levels.[68] Whether PPAR-β/δ agonists promote RCT or have any role in modulation of plasma lipids or prevention of atherosclerotic disease remains to be determined.

INHIBITING APOLIPOPROTEIN A-I CATABOLISM THROUGH INHIBITION OF ENDOTHELIAL LIPASE

The catabolism of apoA-I is an important determinant of plasma apoA-I concentrations.[7] Studies in animals using trapped ligands[69] established that approximately one-third of apoA-I is catabolized by the kidneys and two-thirds by the liver. Lipid-poor apoA-I is glomerularly filtered and then catabolized by proximal renal tubular epithelial cells, where it is internalized and degraded by cubilin.[70,71] Because only lipid-poor apoA-I can be glomerularly filtered, there is interest in the factors that regulate the generation of lipid-poor apoA-I through remodeling of HDL by hydrolysis of HDL triglycerides and phospholipids. HL has the ability to hydrolyze especially HDL triglycerides, which increase in HDL after exchange of its CE for triglyceride by CETP.[7] Hydrolysis of HDL triglycerides by HL results in the shedding of lipid-poor apoA-I from HDL, increased apoA-I filtration and renal catabolism, and significantly faster catabolism.[72] However, while pharmacologic inhibition of HL would be expected to slow apoA-I catabolism and increase apoA-I levels, HL also plays a role in the lipolysis of atherogenic, apoB-containing remnant particles. Thus, HL has not been a major focus of drug development.

However, a close relative of HL is EL, which may provide a more attractive target for slowing apoA-I catabolism and raising HDL cholesterol (Fig. 45-5). First reported in 1999,[73,74] EL has relatively more phospholipase activity and is even more active in hydrolyzing HDL phospholipids than HL.[75] Overexpression of EL in mice results in reduction in HDL cholesterol and apoA-I levels,[73,76] due to increased catabolism primarily via the kidneys.[77] Conversely, antibody inhibition[78] or gene deletion[76,79] of EL results in increased HDL cholesterol and apoA-I levels. Subjects with high HDL cholesterol levels have potentially functional mutations in the EL gene *(LIPG)*,[80]

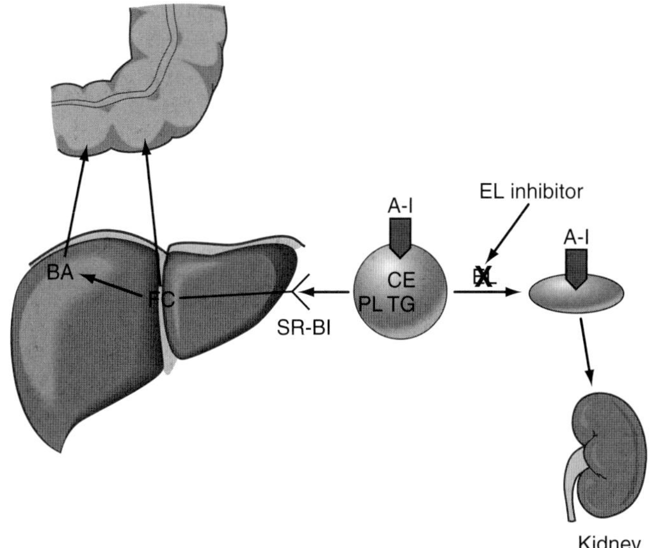

FIGURE 45-5 The effect of inhibition of endothelial lipase on HDL metabolism.

and plasma EL levels in humans are significantly inversely associated with HDL cholesterol levels and strongly correlated with other components of the metabolic syndrome, such as waist and insulin resistance,[81] as well as with markers of inflammation.[82] Atherosclerosis studies in EL-knockout mice have been conflicting,[83,84] but plasma EL levels in humans are significantly associated with coronary atherosclerosis.[81] Thus, pharmacologic inhibition of EL would be expected to slow apoA-I catabolism and increase apoA-I and HDL cholesterol levels, and is therefore a good target for the development of small-molecule inhibitors for raising apoA-I and HDL cholesterol.

PARENTERAL ADMINISTRATION OF FULL-LENGTH APOLIPOPROTEINA-I OR APOLIPOPROTEINA-I MIMETIC PEPTIDES

ApoA-I overexpression is highly antiatherogenic, so in concept, repeated parenteral infusions of full-length apoA-I might be expected to have antiatherogenic effects. Acute bolus intravenous infusion of apoA-I in humans demonstrates relatively little increase in HDL cholesterol levels but measurable increases in apoA-I and phospholipids.[85] Four subjects with heterozygous familial hypercholesterolemia infused with a single bolus of proapoA-I had a 39% increase in fecal sterol excretion, suggesting promotion of reverse cholesterol transport.[86] ApoA-I_{Milano} is a rare, naturally occurring point mutation in apoA-I that causes low HDL cholesterol levels but not increased cardiovascular risk.[87] Studies in animals have shown that apoA-I_{Milano} expression is associated with reduced atherosclerosis.[87] In a small clinical trial, five weekly infusions of recombinant apoA-I_{Milano} complexed with phospholipids resulted in no change in HDL cholesterol or apoA-I levels but a significant reduction from baseline in coronary atheroma volume as measured by IVUS.[88] While this small study carried with it some important caveats, such as the lack of a significant difference with the placebo group,[89] it provided some degree of proof of concept that parenteral infusion of apoA-I can impact atherosclerosis and in a relatively short time. Interestingly, there is little evidence that apoA-I_{Milano} is more effective at protecting against atherosclerosis than wild-type apoA-I. In fact, a head-to-head comparison of the two in a mouse atherosclerosis model suggested that both reduced atherosclerosis to a similar extent.[90] A clinical trial of wild-type apoA-I complexed with phospholipids (similar to apoA-I_{Milano}) was carried out using IVUS to assess coronary atheroma. Similar to the apoA-I_{Milano} study, this study showed significant regression compared to baseline but not to the placebo group.[91] Overall, this pair of studies involving intravenous infusion of apoA-I support the idea of targeting HDL through a parenteral approach. Another approach under development is that of selective delipidation of autologous HDL *ex vivo* with reinfusion of the resultant lipid-poor apoA-I.[92]

ApoA-I mimetic peptides are also of substantial therapeutic interest.[93] ApoA-I has 10 amphipathic helices that are adapted to bind lipids on one face and interact with the aqueous environment on the other. Small amphipathic peptides of 18 to 22 amino acids based loosely on the apoA-I amphipathic helical sequence have similar properties to apoA-I, including the ability to promote cellular cholesterol efflux as well as to activate LCAT. Repeated injection of the peptide L-5F reduced the progression of atherosclerosis in mice.[94] The apoA-I mimetic peptide ETC-642 (also known as RLT peptide) promotes LCAT activation and is also in clinical development. Several other apoA-I mimetic peptides have been developed and tested in cell and animal models.[93] There is some hope that parenterally adminisistered apoA-I mimetic peptides may prove to be an effective method of treating acute coronary syndromes in humans.

One oral apoA-I mimetic peptide that is in clinical development is called D-4F. D-4F is an 18–amino acid peptide almost identical in sequence to L-5F mentioned above, but differs in that it is has one less phenylalanine residue on the hydrophobic face and is composed of all D–amino acids. As a result, it is not recognized by gut peptidases as are naturally occurring proteins containing L–amino acids, and is therefore not degraded in the gut and is orally bioavailable. Oral administration of D-4F has been shown to reduce atherosclerosis in mice without raising levels of HDL cholesterol.[95] Although its mechanism remains uncertain, some data suggest that its major effect may be to enhance the anti-inflammatory function of HDL.[96] D-4F has also been shown to promote macrophage RCT *in vivo* in mice.[97] A phase I single-dose study of D-4F in humans with coronary disease or risk equivalent showed that even a single oral dose improved HDL anti-inflammatory function.[98] D-4F may provide a test of the hypothesis that enhancing HDL function without increasing plasma HDL cholesterol levels can reduce atherosclerosis or cardiovascular risk.

SUMMARY

Low HDL cholesterol levels are an unmet medical need, and there is major interest in developing new HDL-targeted therapeutics. There are relatively few validated targets for HDL. CETP inhibition had advanced the furthest in clinical development, but is now in question as a result of the increased mortality with the CETP inhibitor torcetrapib. Additional current targets for small-molecule development, such as LXR agonists and EL inhibitors, are promising, but data in humans are needed to assess their potential. Previously unsuspected genes involved in HDL metabolism are being identified by genomewide studies, and some of these will likely become therapeutic targets. We will likely witness over the next decade the clinical development of several novel HDL-targeted therapies.

REFERENCES

1. Boden WE: High-density lipoprotein cholesterol as an independent risk factor in cardiovascular disease: assessing the data from Framingham to the Veterans Affairs High—Density Lipoprotein Intervention Trial. *Am J Cardiol* 2000;86:19L-22L.
2. Expert Panel on Detection, Evaluation, and Treatment of High Blood Cholesterol in Adults: Executive summary of the third report of the National Cholesterol Education Program (NCEP) Expert Panel on Detection, Evaluation, and Treatment of High Blood Cholesterol in Adults (Adult Treatment Panel III). *JAMA* 2001;285:2486–2497.
3. Grundy SM, Cleeman JI, Merz CN, et al: Implications of recent clinical trials for the National Cholesterol Education Program Adult Treatment Panel III guidelines. *Circulation* 2004;110: 227–239.
4. Cannon CP, Braunwald E, McCabe CH, et al: Intensive versus moderate lipid lowering with statins after acute coronary syndromes. *N Engl J Med* 2004;350:1495–1504.
5. LaRosa JC, Grundy SM, Waters DD, et al: Intensive lipid lowering with atorvastatin in patients with stable coronary disease. *N Engl J Med* 2005;352:1425–1435.
6. Ashen MD, Blumenthal RS: Clinical practice. Low HDL cholesterol levels. *N Engl J Med* 2005;353:1252–1260.
7. Lewis GF, Rader DJ: New insights into the regulation of HDL metabolism and reverse cholesterol transport. *Circ Res* 2005;96:1221–1232.
8. Rader DJ: Molecular regulation of HDL metabolism and function: implications for novel therapies. *J Clin Invest* 2006;116: 3090–3100.
9. Tall AR: Role of ABCA1 in cellular cholesterol efflux and reverse cholesterol transport. *Arterioscler Thromb Vasc Biol* 2003;23:710–711.
10. Wang N, Lan D, Chen W, Matsuura F, and Tall AR: ATP-binding cassette transporters G1 and G4 mediate cellular cholesterol efflux to high-density lipoproteins. *Proc Natl Acad Sci U S A* 2004;101:9774–9779.
11. Kennedy MA, Barrera GC, Nakamura K, et al: ABCG1 has a critical role in mediating cholesterol efflux to HDL and preventing cellular lipid accumulation. *Cell Metab* 2005;1:121–131.
12. Wang X, Collins HL, Ranalletta M, et al: Macrophage ABCA1 and ABCG1, but not SR-BI, promote macrophage reverse cholesterol transport *in vivo*. *J Clin Invest* 2007;117:2216–2224.
13. Yvan-Charvet L, Ranalletta M, Wang N, et al: Combined deficiency of ABCA1 and ABCG1 promotes foam cell accumulation and accelerates atherosclerosis in mice. *J Clin Invest* 2007;117: 3900–3908.
14. Repa JJ, Mangelsdorf DJ: The liver X receptor gene team: potential new players in atherosclerosis. *Nat Med* 2002;8:1243–1248.
15. Zhang Y, Da Silva JR, Reilly M, Billheimer JT, Rothblat GH, Rader DJ: Hepatic expression of scavenger receptor class B type I (SR-BI) is a positive regulator of macrophage reverse cholesterol transport *in vivo*. *J Clin Invest* 2005;115:2870–2874.
16. Schwartz CC, VandenBroek JM,Cooper PS: Lipoprotein cholesteryl ester production, transfer, and output *in vivo* in humans. *J Lipid Res* 2004;45:1594–1607.
17. Barter PJ, Nicholls S, Rye KA, Anantharamaiah GM, Navab M, Fogelman AM: Antiinflammatory properties of HDL. *Circ Res* 2004;95:764–772.
18. Mineo C, Deguchi H, Griffin JH, Shaul PW: Endothelial and antithrombotic actions of HDL. *Circ Res* 2006;98:1352–1364.
19. Brown ML, Inazu A, Hesler CB, et al: Molecular basis of lipid transfer protein deficiency in a family with increased high-density lipoproteins. *Nature* 1989;342:448–451.
20. Inazu A, Brown ML, Hesler CB, et al: Increased high-density lipoprotein levels caused by a common cholesteryl-ester transfer protein gene mutation. *N Engl J Med* 1990;323:1234–1238.
21. de Grooth GJ, Kuivenhoven JA, Stalenhoef AF, et al: Efficacy and safety of a novel cholesteryl ester transfer protein inhibitor, JTT-705, in humans: a randomized phase II dose-response study. *Circulation* 2002;105:2159–2165.
22. Kuivenhoven JA, de Grooth GJ, Kawamura H, et al: Effectiveness of inhibition of cholesteryl ester transfer protein by JTT-705 in combination with pravastatin in type II dyslipidemia. *Am J Cardiol* 2005;95:1085–1088.
23. Clark RW, Sutfin TA, Ruggeri RB, et al: Raising high-density lipoprotein in humans through inhibition of cholesteryl ester transfer protein: an initial multidose study of torcetrapib. *Arterioscler Thromb Vasc Biol* 2004;24:490–497.
24. Brousseau ME, Schaefer EJ, Wolfe ML, et al: Effects of an inhibitor of cholesteryl ester transfer protein on HDL cholesterol. *N Engl J Med* 2004;350:1505–1515.
25. Davidson MH, McKenney JM, Shear CL, Revkin JH: Efficacy and safety of torcetrapib, a novel cholesteryl ester transfer protein inhibitor, in individuals with below-average high-density lipoprotein cholesterol levels. *J Am Coll Cardiol* 2006;48:1774–1781.
26. McKenney JM, Davidson MH, Shear CL, Revkin JH: Efficacy and safety of torcetrapib, a novel cholesteryl ester transfer protein inhibitor, in individuals with below-average high-density lipoprotein cholesterol levels on a background of atorvastatin. *J Am Coll Cardiol* 2006;48:1782–1790.
27. Cholesterol: The good, the bad, and the stopped trials. *Lancet* 2006;368:2034 (editorial).
28. Barter PJ, Caulfield M, Eriksson M, et al: Effects of torcetrapib in patients at high risk for coronary events. *N Engl J Med* 2007;357:2109–2122.
29. Nissen SE, Tardif JC, Nicholls SJ, et al: Effect of torcetrapib on the progression of coronary atherosclerosis. *N Engl J Med* 2007;356:1304–1316.
30. Kastelein JJ, van Leuven SI, Burgess L, et al: Effect of torcetrapib on carotid atherosclerosis in familial hypercholesterolemia. *N Engl J Med* 2007;356:1620–1630.
31. Bots ML, Visseren FL, Evans GW, et al: Torcetrapib and carotid intima–media thickness in mixed dyslipidaemia (RADIANCE 2 study): a randomised, double-blind trial. *Lancet* 2007;370: 153–160.
32. Tall AR, Yvan-Charvet L, Wang N: The failure of torcetrapib: was it the molecule or the mechanism? *Arterioscler Thromb Vasc Biol* 2007;27:257–260.
33. Rader DJ: Illuminating HDL—is it still a viable therapeutic target? *N Engl J Med* 2007;357:2180–2183.
34. Krishna R, Anderson MS, Bergman AJ, et al: Effect of the cholesteryl ester transfer protein inhibitor, anacetrapib, on lipoproteins in patients with dyslipidaemia and on 24-h ambulatory blood pressure in healthy individuals: two double-blind, randomised placebo-controlled phase I studies. *Lancet* 2007;370: 1907–1914.
35. Matsuura F, Wang N, Chen W, Jiang XC, Tall AR: HDL from CETP-deficient subjects shows enhanced ability to promote cholesterol efflux from macrophages in an apoE- and ABCG1-dependent pathway. *J Clin Invest* 2006;116:1435–1442.
36. Yvan-Charvet L, Matsuura F, Wang N, et al: Inhibition of cholesteryl ester transfer protein by torcetrapib modestly increases macrophage cholesterol efflux to HDL. *Arterioscler Thromb Vasc Biol* 2007;27:1132–1138.
37. Ikewaki K, Rader DJ, Sakamoto T, et al: Delayed catabolism of high-density lipoprotein apolipoproteins A-I and A-II in human cholesteryl ester transfer protein deficiency. *J Clin Invest* 1993;92:1650–1658.
38. Brousseau ME, Diffenderfer MR, Millar JS, et al: Effects of cholesteryl ester transfer protein inhibition on high-density lipoprotein subspecies, apolipoprotein A-I metabolism, and fecal sterol excretion. *Arterioscler Thromb Vasc Biol* 2005;25:1057–1064.
39. Tanigawa H, Billheimer JT, Tohyama J, Zhang Y, Rothblat G, Rader DJ: Expression of cholesteryl ester transfer protein in mice promotes macrophage reverse cholesterol transport. *Circulation* 2007;116:1267–1273.
40. Qasim A, Rader DJ: Human genetics of variation in high-density lipoprotein cholesterol. *Curr Atheroscler Rep* 2006;8:198–205.
41. Curb JD, Abbott RD, Rodriguez BL, et al: A prospective study of HDL cholesterol and cholesteryl ester transfer protein gene

mutations and the risk of coronary heart disease in the elderly. *J Lipid Res* 2004;45:948–953.

42. Boekholdt SM, Thompson JF: Natural genetic variation as a tool in understanding the role of CETP in lipid levels and disease. *J Lipid Res* 2003;44:1080–1093.
43. Boekholdt SM, Kuivenhoven JA, Wareham NJ, et al: Plasma levels of cholesteryl ester transfer protein and the risk of future coronary artery disease in apparently healthy men and women: the prospective EPIC (European Prospective Investigation into Cancer and Nutrition)—Norfolk population study. *Circulation* 2004;110:1418–1423.
44. Okamoto H, Yonemori F, Wakitani K, Minowa T, Maeda K, Shinkai H: A cholesteryl ester transfer protein inhibitor attenuates atherosclerosis in rabbits. *Nature* 2000;406:203–207.
45. Morehouse LA, Sugarman ED, Bourassa PA, et al: Inhibition of CETP activity by torcetrapib reduces susceptibility to diet-induced atherosclerosis in New Zealand White rabbits. *J Lipid Res* 2007;48:1263–1272.
46. Cuchel M, Rader DJ: Macrophage reverse cholesterol transport: key to the regression of atherosclerosis? *Circulation* 2006;113: 2548–2555.
47. Wang N, Tall AR: Regulation and mechanisms of ATP-binding cassette transporter A1–mediated cellular cholesterol efflux. *Arterioscler Thromb Vasc Biol* 2003;23:1178–1184.
48. Naik SU, Wang X, Da Silva JS, et al: Pharmacological activation of liver X receptors promotes reverse cholesterol transport *in vivo*. *Circulation* 2006;113:90–97.
49. Terasaka N, Hiroshima A, Koieyama T, et al: T-0901317, a synthetic liver X receptor ligand, inhibits development of atherosclerosis in LDL receptor-deficient mice. *FEBS Lett* 2003;536: 6–11.
50. Joseph SB, McKilligin E, Pei L, et al: Synthetic LXR ligand inhibits the development of atherosclerosis in mice. *Proc Natl Acad Sci U S A* 2002;99:7604–7609.
51. Levin N, Bischoff ED, Daige CL, et al: Macrophage liver X receptor is required for antiatherogenic activity of LXR agonists. *Arterioscler Thromb Vasc Biol* 2005;25:135–142.
52. Li AC, Glass CK: PPAR- and LXR-dependent pathways controlling lipid metabolism and the development of atherosclerosis. *J Lipid Res* 2004;45:2161–2173.
53. Groot PH, Pearce NJ, Yates JW, et al: Synthetic LXR agonists increase LDL in CETP species. *J Lipid Res* 2005;46:2182–2191.
54. Miao B, Zondlo S, Gibbs S, et al: Raising HDL cholesterol without inducing hepatic steatosis and hypertriglyceridemia by a selective LXR modulator. *J Lipid Res* 2004;45:1410–1417.
55. Berthou L, Duverger N, Emmanuel F, et al: Opposite regulation of human versus mouse apolipoprotein A-I by fibrates in human apolipoprotein A-I transgenic mice. *J.Clin.Invest* 1996;97:2408–2416.
56. Staels B, Auwerx J: Regulation of apo A-I gene expression by fibrates. *Atherosclerosis* 1998;137(Suppl):S19–S23.
57. Vu-Dac N, Chopin-Delannoy S, Gervois P, et al: The nuclear receptors peroxisome proliferator-activated receptor alpha and Rev-erbalpha mediate the species-specific regulation of apolipoprotein A-I expression by fibrates. *J Biol Chem* 1998;273:25713–25720.
58. Watts GF, Barrett PH, Ji J, et al: Differential regulation of lipoprotein kinetics by atorvastatin and fenofibrate in subjects with the metabolic syndrome. *Diabetes* 2003;52:803–811.
59. Bilz S, Wagner S, Schmitz M, Bedynek A, Keller U, Demant T, et al: Effects of atorvastatin versus fenofibrate on apoB-100 and apoA-I kinetics in mixed hyperlipidemia. *J Lipid Res* 2004;45: 174–185.
60. Rubin E, Krauss R, Spangler E, Verstuyft J, Clift S: Inhibition of early atherogenesis in transgenic mice by human apolipoprotein AI. *Nature* 1991;353:265–267.
61. Plump A, Scott C, Breslow J: Human apolipoprotein A-I gene expression increases high-density lipoprotein and suppresses atherosclerosis in the apolipoprotein E-deficient mouse. *Proc Natl Acad Sci U S A* 1994;91:9607–9611.
62. Tangirala RK, Tsukamoto K, Chun SH, Usher D, Pure E, Rader DJ: Regression of atherosclerosis induced by liver-directed gene transfer of apolipoprotein A-I in mice [see comments]. *Circulation* 1999;100:1816–1822.
63. Chinetti G, Lestavel S, Bocher V, et al: PPAR-alpha and PPAR-gamma activators induce cholesterol removal from human macrophage foam cells through stimulation of the ABCA1 pathway. *Nat.Med* 2001;7:53–58.
64. Li AC, Binder CJ, Gutierrez A, et al: Differential inhibition of macrophage foam-cell formation and atherosclerosis in mice by PPARalpha, beta/delta, and gamma. *J Clin Invest* 2004;114:1564–1576.
65. Despres JP, Lemieux I, Robins SJ: Role of fibric acid derivatives in the management of risk factors for coronary heart disease. *Drugs* 2004;64:2177–2198.
66. Nissen SE, Nicholls SJ, Wolski K, et al: Effects of a potent and selective PPAR-alpha agonist in patients with atherogenic dyslipidemia or hypercholesterolemia: Two randomized controlled trials. *JAMA* 2007;297:1362–1373.
67. Oliver WR, Jr, Shenk JL, Snaith MR, et al: A selective peroxisome proliferator-activated receptor delta agonist promotes reverse cholesterol transport. *Proc Natl Acad Sci U S A* 2001;98: 5306–5311.
68. Sprecher DL, Massien C, Pearce G, et al: Triglyceride:high-density lipoprotein cholesterol effects in healthy subjects administered a peroxisome proliferator activated receptor delta agonist. *Arterioscler Thromb Vasc Biol* 2007;27:359–365.
69. Glass C, Pittman RC, Weinstein DB, Steinberg D: Dissociation of tissue uptake of cholesterol ester from that of apoprotein A-I of rat plamsa high-density lipoprotein: selective delivery of cholesterol ester to liver, adrenal, and gonad. *Proc Natl Acad Sci U S A* 1983;80:5435–5439.
70. Hammad SM, Stefansson S, Twal WO: Cubilin, the endocytic receptor for intrinsic factor-vitamin B12 complex, mediates high-density lipoprotein holoparticle endocytosis. *Proc Natl Acad Sci U S A* 1999;96:10158–10163.
71. Barth JL, Argraves WS: Cubilin and megalin: partners in lipoprotein and vitamin metabolism. *Trends Cardiovasc Med* 2001;11:26–31.
72. Lamarche B, Uffelman KD, Carpentier A, et al: Triglyceride enrichment of HDL enhances *in vivo* metabolic clearance of HDL apo A-I in healthy men. *J Clin Invest* 1999;103:1191–1199.
73. Jaye M, Lynch KJ, Krawiec J, et al: A novel endothelial-derived lipase that modulates HDL metabolism. *Nat Genet* 1999;21: 424–428.
74. Hirata K, Diechek HL, Cioffi JA, et al: Cloning of a unique lipase from endothelial cells extends the lipase gene family. *J Biol Chem* 1999;274:14170–14175.
75. McCoy MG, Sun GS, Marchadier D, Maugeais C, Glick JM, Rader DJ: Characterization of the lipolytic activity of endothelial lipase. *J Lipid Res* 2002;43:921–929.
76. Ishida T, Choi S, Kundu RK, et al: Endothelial lipase is a major determinant of HDL level. *J Clin Invest* 2003;111:347–355.
77. Maugeais C, Tietge UJ, Broedl UC, et al: Dose-dependent acceleration of high-density lipoprotein catabolism by endothelial lipase. *Circulation* 2003;108:2121–2126.
78. Jin W, Millar JS, Broedl U, Glick JM, Rader DJ: Inhibition of endothelial lipase causes increased HDL cholesterol levels *in vivo*. *J Clin Invest* 2003;111:357–362.
79. Ma K, Cilingiroglu M, Otvos JD, Ballantyne CM, Marian AJ, Chan L: Endothelial lipase is a major genetic determinant for high-density lipoprotein concentration, structure, and metabolism. *Proc Natl Acad Sci U S A* 2003;100:2748–2753.
80. deLemos AS, Wolfe ML, Long CJ, Sivapackianathan R, Rader DJ: Identification of genetic variants in endothelial lipase in persons with elevated high-density lipoprotein cholesterol. *Circulation* 2002;106:1321–1326.
81. Badellino KO, Wolfe ML, Reilly MP, Rader DJ: Endothelial lipase concentrations are increased in metabolic syndrome and associated with coronary atherosclerosis. *PLoS Med* 2006;3:e22.
82. Badellino KO, Wolfe ML, Reilly MP, Rader DJ: Endothelial lipase is increased *in vivo* by inflammation in humans. *Circulation* 2008;117:678–685.
83. Ishida T, Choi SY, Kundu RK, et al: Endothelial lipase modulates susceptibility to atherosclerosis in apolipoprotein-E-deficient mice. *J Biol Chem* 2004;279:45085–45092.
84. Ko KW, Paul A, Ma K, Li L, Chan L: Endothelial lipase modulates HDL but has no effect on atherosclerosis development in apoE-/- and LDLR-/- mice. *J Lipid Res* 2005;46:2586–2594.
85. Nanje MN, Crouse JR, King JM, et al: Effects of intravenous infusion of lipid-free apo A-I in humans. *Arterioscler Thromb Vasc Biol* 1996;16:1203–1214.
86. Eriksson M, Carlson LA, Miettinen TA, Angelin B: Stimulation of fecal steroid excretion after infusion of recombinant proapolipoprotein A-I: potential reverse cholesterol transport in humans. *Circulation* 1999;100:594–598.

87. Chiesa G, Sirtori CR: Apolipoprotein A-IMilano: current perspectives. *Curr Opin Lipidol* 2003;14:159–163.
88. Nissen SE, Tsunoda T, Tuzcu EM, et al: Effect of recombinant ApoA-I_{Milano} on coronary atherosclerosis in patients with acute coronary syndromes: a randomized controlled trial. *JAMA* 2003;290:2292–2300.
89. Rader DJ: High-density lipoproteins as an emerging therapeutic target for atherosclerosis. *JAMA* 2003;290:2322–2324.
90. Lebherz C, Sanmiguel J, Wilson JM, Rader DJ: Gene transfer of wild-type ApoA-I and ApoA-I_{Milano} reduce atherosclerosis to a similar extent. *Cardiovasc Diabetol* 2007;6:15.
91. Tardif JC, Gregoire J, L'Allier PL, et al: Effects of reconstituted high-density lipoprotein infusions on coronary atherosclerosis: a randomized controlled trial. *JAMA* 2007;297:1675–1682.
92. Sacks F , Alaupovic P, Kostner G, et al: Selective plasma HDL delipidation and reinfusion: a unique new approach for acute HDL therapy in the treatment of cardiovascular disease. Presented at American Heart Association Scientific Sessions, New Orleans, LA, November 7, 2004.
93. Navab M, Anantharamaiah GM, Reddy ST, Fogelman AM: Apolipoprotein A-I mimetic peptides and their role in atherosclerosis prevention. *Nat Clin Pract Cardiovasc Med* 2006;3: 540–547.
94. Garber DW, Datta G, Chaddha M, et al: A new synthetic class A amphipathic peptide analogue protects mice from diet-induced atherosclerosis. *J Lipid Res* 2001;42:545–552.
95. Navab M, Anantharamaiah GM, Hama S, et al: Oral administration of an Apo A-I mimetic peptide synthesized from D-amino acids dramatically reduces atherosclerosis in mice independent of plasma cholesterol. *Circulation* 2002;105:290–292.
96. Anantharamaiah GM, Mishra VK, Garber DW, et al: Structural requirements for antioxidative and anti-inflammatory properties of apolipoprotein A-I mimetic peptides. *J Lipid Res* 2007;48:1915–1923.
97. Navab M, Anantharamaiah GM, Reddy ST, et al: Oral D-4F causes formation of pre-beta high-density lipoprotein and improves high-density lipoprotein-mediated cholesterol efflux and reverse cholesterol transport from macrophages in apolipoprotein E-null mice. *Circulation* 2004;109:3215–3220.
98. Bloedon LT, Dunbar R, Duffy D, et al: Safety, pharmacokinetics, and pharmacodynamics of oral apoA-I mimetic peptide D-4F in high-risk cardiovascular patients. *J Lipid Res* 2008;49:1344–1352.

CHAPTER 46

Experimental Therapies of the Vessel Wall

Robert S. Rosenson

Strategies for preventing complications of atherosclerotic vascular disease have emphasized risk factor modification using treatment approaches supported by an abundance of evidence—aspirin and/or clopidogrel, β-adrenergic blockers, angiotensin-converting enzyme inhibitors (ACE-I), and 3-hydroxy-3-methylglutaryl–coenzyme A (HMG-CoA) reductase inhibitors (statins).[1] Among outpatients with established atherosclerotic vascular disease or with multiple risk factors for atherothrombosis and treated with multiple classes of evidence-based therapies, the 1-year risk for cardiovascular events (cardiovascular death, myocardial infarction, stroke, or hospitalization for atherothrombotic event) ranges from 5.31% for patients with multiple risk factors to 12.58% for patients with symptomatic arterial disease in one vascular bed, 21.14% for patients with two affected vascular beds, and 26.27% for patients with three symptomatic arterial beds.[2] In patients with acute coronary syndromes, the rate of subsequent cardiovascular events has ranged from 14.7% to 22.4% at 2 to 2.5 years after the inciting event, despite intensive treatment with statins.[3,4] The high risk of recurrent cardiovascular events—even among those receiving standard-of-care therapies based on evidence—has prompted investigations into novel approaches directed at reducing vascular inflammation and improving stability of vulnerable plaques in an effort to further reduce the risk of cardiovascular events. The various experimental approaches discussed in this chapter—and the underlying rationale for each—are shown in Figure 46-1.

This chapter will review novel experimental therapies that target the vessel wall. An overview of specific inflammatory pathways in atherothrombosis will be discussed to foster an understanding regarding their potential role as vascular-specific therapeutic targets. The antiatherothrombotic effects of currently available therapies on the vessel wall will not be discussed, as this topic has been extensively reviewed.[5–8]

OXIDATIVE STRESS AND THE INFLAMMATORY BASIS OF ATHEROSCLEROSIS

Oxidative stress represents an imbalance between the production and degradation of reactive oxygen species (ROS). ROS activate the redox-sensitive transcription nuclear factors, which, in turn, activate the transcription of genes encoding chemokines, cytokines and endothelium-localized adhesion molecules (products involved in mediating inflammatory and immune responses), and proteolytic enzymes that impair the structural integrity of the fibrous caps of advanced, complex atheroma.[6] Oxidative modification of low-density lipoprotein (LDL) is required for cholesterol loading of tissue macrophages—one of the hallmark histopathologic features of early atheromatous lesions. Further, oxidized lipids promote thrombogenesis by increasing platelet aggregation through activation of phospholipase A_2 (PLA_2) and increased thromboxane A_2 production from platelets.[9]

Various enzymes identified in atherosclerotic lesions contribute to the oxidative modification of phospholipids comprising LDL.[6] These enzymes include lipoxygenases, members of the PLA_2 superfamily, nicotinamide adenine dinucleotide (NADPH) oxidases, xanthine oxidase, nitric oxide synthases, and myeloperoxidase.

Beyond its role in LDL oxidation, myeloperoxidase fosters instability of atherosclerotic plaques.[10] High numbers of myeloperoxidase-expressing macrophages have been observed in advanced atherosclerotic lesions in the region in which the fibrous cap has ruptured.[11] One endproduct of myeloperoxidase-catalyzed reactions is the pro-oxidant

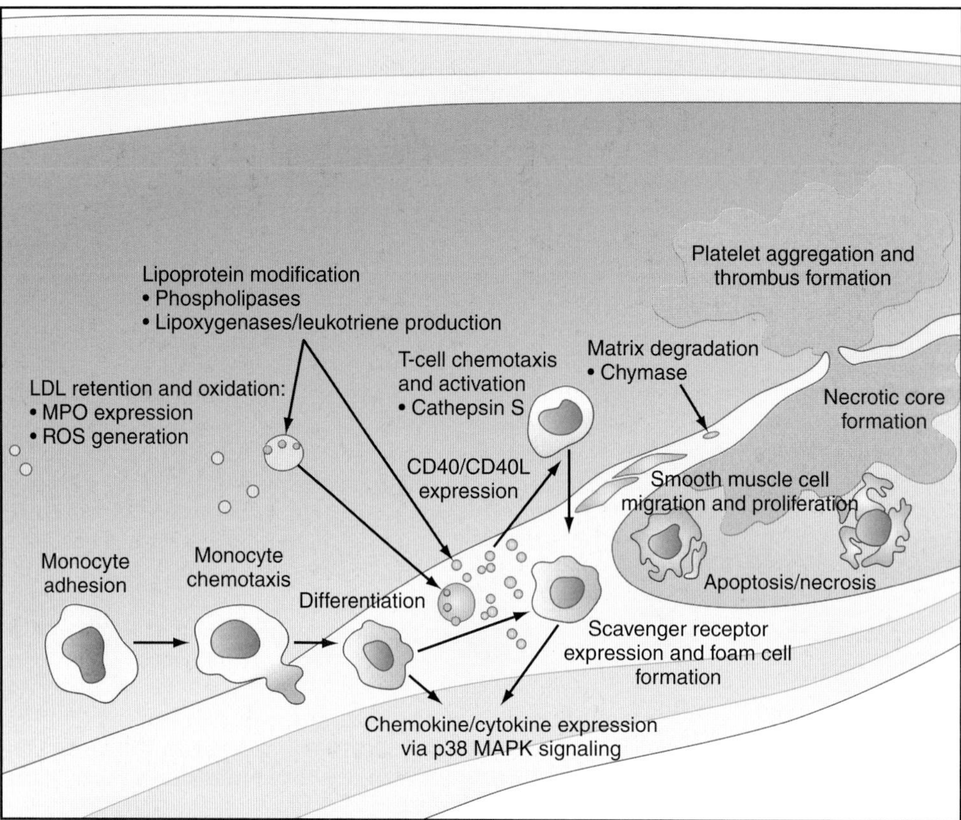

FIGURE 46-1 Key steps in atherogenesis and the progression of atherosclerosis. Many of the novel experimental approaches discussed in this chapter are highlighted. CD40, cluster designation 40; CD40L, cluster designation 40 ligand; MAPK, mitogen-activated protein kinase; MPO, myeloperoxidase; ROS, reactive oxygen species.

species hypochlorous acid. Proteins modified by hypochlorous acid accumulate at eroded or ruptured sites of human coronary atheroma. Hypochlorous acid can activate matrix metalloproteinases (MMPs) and inactivate inhibitors of metalloproteinase (TIMPs), and, thereby, contribute to structural weakening of the fibrous cap within atherosclerotic plaques.

The production of MMP-2 and MMP-9 by macrophages occurs through a prostaglandin E_2–mediated pathway.[12] In human atherosclerotic plaques, MMP expression is regulated, in part, by the cyclooxygenase-2 (COX-2)/prostaglandin E_2 synthase (mPGES) pathway. COX-2/mPGES is an inducible enzyme complex that responds to several inflammatory stimuli that activate nuclear factor (NF)–κB. NF-κB is a redox-sensitive transcription factor that is activated by many stimuli including ROS, angiotensin II, and the receptor for advanced glycosylation endproducts (RAGE). In mast cells, activation of MMP-1 and MMP-3 is mediated by the protease chymase.[13]

Vascular Antioxidants

Endogenous antioxidant defense mechanisms are mediated by glutathione peroxidase, superoxide dismutase, and catalase. The principal antioxidant mechanism in human cells involves glutathione and glutathione peroxidases.[14] Glutathione peroxidases contain selenocysteine at their active sites. Glutathione peroxidase–1 is a key intracellular enzyme that uses glutathione to reduce hydrogen peroxide to water and lipid peroxides to alcohol. This enzyme inhibits 5-lipoxygenase in mononuclear cells and macrophages in atherosclerotic lesions.

The efficacy of vitamin C, vitamin E, and beta-carotene has been evaluated in the primary and secondary prevention of cardiovascular events.[15] Although observational trials of vitamin E have been encouraging, clinical benefit in primary prevention with vitamin E or beta-carotene supplementation (alone or in combination) has not been demonstrated in randomized controlled trials. For secondary prevention, all but one study with vitamin E observed little or no benefit. The exception was one trial involving patients on hemodialysis.[16]

Synthetic vascular antioxidants include probucol and its succinic acid derivative succinobucol (Atherogenics, Inc., Alpharetta, GA). Both probucol and succinobucol produce favorable antiatherosclerotic effects in animals[17,18] and humans.[19–22] The reduction in intimal thickening after balloon injury may be attributable to the effects of probucol on promoting endothelial cell growth and inhibiting vascular smooth muscle cell proliferation, which may be mediated through the induction of heme oxygenase–1 activity.[23] This antiproliferative effect is independent of both the cholesterol-lowering and antioxidant effects of probucol.[17,18]

The Canadian Antioxidant Restenosis Trial (CART-1) studied the effects of probucol (500 mg twice daily) and succinobucol (70, 140, or 280 mg daily) on restenosis assessed by intravascular ultrasonography (IVUS) 2 weeks before and 4 weeks after percutaneous coronary interventions (PCI).[19] At follow-up, the luminal area at the PCI site was 2.66 ± 1.58 mm^2 for placebo, 3.69 ± 2.69 mm^2 for probucol, 2.75 ± 1.76 mm^2 for succinobucol 70 mg, 3.17 ± 2.26 mm^2 for succinobucol 140 mg, and 3.36 ± 2.12 mm^2 for succinobucol 280 mg ($P \leq 0.05$ for probucol vs. placebo and succinobucol 280 mg vs. placebo). The differences in restenosis rates between the treatment groups were not statistically significant (37.5% in the placebo group, 25.5% in the probucol group, and 26% in the succinobucol treatment groups).

Probucol therapy was accompanied by a 35.1% reduction in high-density lipoprotein (HDL) cholesterol levels at 1 month compared with a 0.2% decrease in the placebo group and 4.4%, 9.0%, and 18.7% decreases in the succinobucol treatment groups ($P < 0.01$ for placebo vs. probucol and for succinobucol 140 mg vs. 280 mg). Safety concerns with probucol treatment included an increase in the QTc interval greater than 60 ms in 17.4% of probucol-treated patients compared with 4.8% of placebo-treated patients, whereas the increased frequency of QTc prolongation was observed in 2.5% to 4.8% of succinobucol-treated patients. CART-1 demonstrated reduced restenosis with probucol and succinobucol; however, the reduction in HDL cholesterol and the QTc prolongation was less with the succinic acid derivative.

CART-2 was a randomized placebo-controlled trial that investigated the effects of succinobucol on coronary atheroma in 232 PCI patients as assessed by coronary IVUS.[24] After 12 months of therapy, succinobucol reduced plaque volume by 4.0 mm^3 ($P = 0.001$ vs. baseline), but a similar reduction also was observed in the placebo group, and the difference was not statistically significant ($P = 0.12$). Further, succinobucol therapy was accompanied by unfavorable changes in LDL cholesterol (+4% vs. –9% with placebo) and HDL cholesterol (–14% vs. –1% with placebo).

The Aggressive Reduction of Inflammation Stops Events (ARISE) trial was a double-blind, placebo-controlled trial designed to compare the effect of treatment with succinobucol (300 mg daily) on the time to first incident of a major cardiovascular event in 6100 patients with a recent acute coronary syndrome.[25] Following a 14-day placebo run-in phase, patients were randomly assigned, in a double-blind manner, to treatment with succinobucol 300 mg daily (two tablets with a meal) (n = 3078) or placebo (n = 3066). At study completion, investigators observed no difference in the primary endpoint, which comprised cardiovascular death, resuscitated cardiac arrest, myocardial infarction, stroke, unstable angina, and revascularization procedures. However, the secondary composite endpoint of cardiovascular death, myocardial infarction, cardiac arrest, and stroke was lower with succinobucol than with placebo (6.7% vs. 8.2%, hazard ratio [HR], 0.81; $P = 0.028$). Despite fewer myocardial infarctions, heart failure occurred more often in succinobucol-treated patients (n = 107) than in those receiving placebo (n = 83). Consistent with other succinobucol trials, LDL cholesterol increased by 10 mg/dL, HDL cholesterol fell by 5 mg/dL, and C-reactive protein (CRP) did not change. Even though succinobucol had adverse effects on plasma LDL cholesterol and HDL cholesterol, it was not unreasonable to expect a favorable outcome from an agent that effectively blocked oxidative modification of LDL and reduced expression of vascular cell adhesion molecule–1 (VCAM-1).

Although multiple clinical trials of antioxidant vitamin therapy have failed to demonstrate a reduction in incident cardiovascular events,[26] the findings reported from ARISE with the powerful antioxidant succinobucol are particularly disappointing because succinobucol therapy reduced major cardiovascular events. This trial emphasizes the importance of trial design and selection of an appropriate primary endpoint.

In the next section, the rationale for inhibiting or blocking the effects of downstream effectors of oxidative stress will be discussed. This section will review leukotriene antagonists and phospholipase inhibitors.

LIPOXYGENASE PATHWAYS: CONTRIBUTION OF LEUKOTRIENES AND LEUKOTRIENE RECEPTORS TO ATHEROTHROMBOSIS

Lipoxygenases are an important source of reactive oxygen species that contribute to the oxidative modification of LDL. The 5-lipoxygenase (5-LO) enzyme and the 5-LO-activating protein (FLAP) results in the formation of the unstable precursor leukotriene A_4 (LTA_4), which is subsequently hydrolyzed into LTB_4 or conjugated with glutathione to form cysteinyl leukotrienes that include LTC_4, LTD_4, and LTE_4 (Fig. 46-2).

Variants in the FLAP[27–30] and LTA_4 hydrolase gene[31] have been previously associated with an increased risk of myocardial infarction and stroke. A variant 5-lipoxygenase genotype (ALOX5) promoter was detected in 6.0% of 470 healthy middle-aged men and women enrolled in the Los Angeles Atherosclerosis Study.[29] In multivariate analyses, the intima–media thickness was increased in carriers of two variant alleles compared with carriers of the common allele (odds ratio, 4.1; 95% confidence interval [CI], 2.1 to 8.2; $P < 0.001$). In a genomewide scan in two populations, a four-marker single-nucleotide polymorphism haplotype in the locus spanning the gene ALOX5AP, which encodes the FLAP, was associated with an increased risk of myocardial infarction and stroke.[29] In 713 Icelandic individuals with myocardial infarction, haplotype A had a frequency of 15.8% versus 9.5% in 837 population-based controls. Haplotype A was associated with a 1.8-fold (population-attributable risk, 0.135) increased risk of myocardial infarction and stroke. The population-attributable risk associated with haplotype A was 3.5%. In a British cohort that included 753 individuals with myocardial infarction and 730 controls, a nonsignificant increase in the prevalence of haplotype A was observed among myocardial infarction survivors. In contrast, haplotype B, a distinct and mutually exclusive haplotype, was detected in 7.5% of individuals with myocardial infarction compared with 4.0% of controls (relative risk, 1.95; population-attributable risk, 0.072).

The haplotype for the LTA_4 hydrolase (LTA4H) pathway is associated with a 1.2-fold increased relative risk for myocardial infarction and 1.4-fold relative risk for myocardial infarction and stroke in Caucasians in the United States in models that adjusted for conventional risk factors including LDL cholesterol, hypertension,

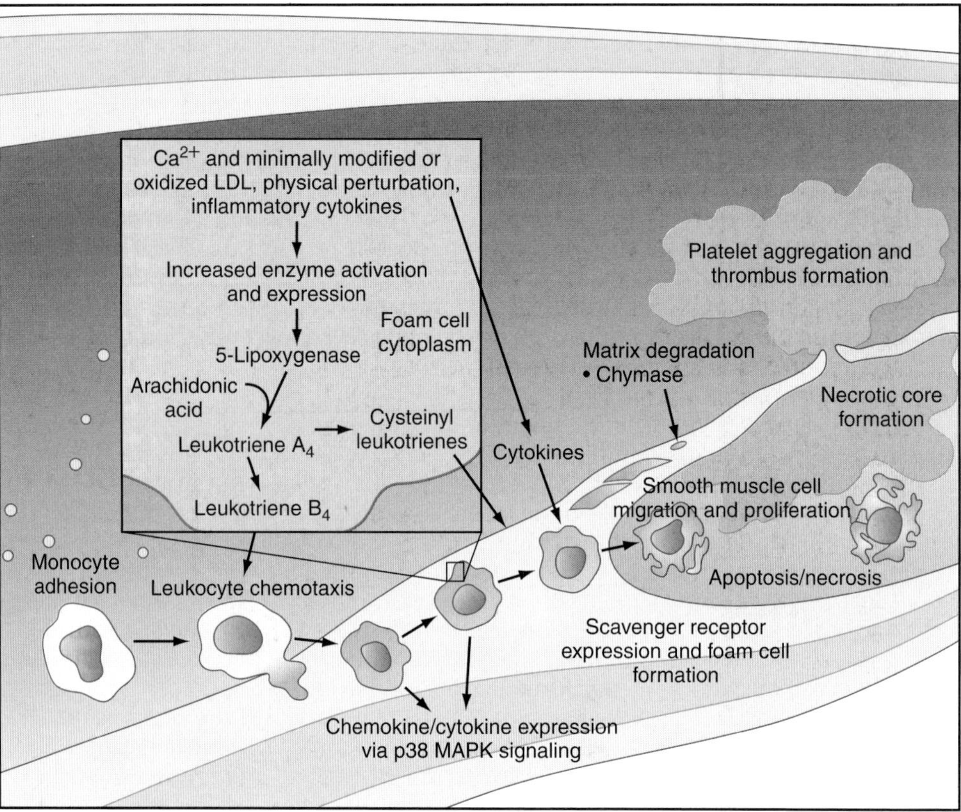

FIGURE 46-2 5-Lipoxygenase activity contributes to atherosclerosis through oxidation of low-density lipoprotein (LDL) and the generation of leukotrienes. MAPK, mitogen-activated protein kinase.

and diabetes.[30] However, the LTAH4 haplotype has a much higher relative risk of 3.5 for myocardial infarction in African Americans ($P < 0.001$).

Leukotrienes

Leukotrienes exert proinflammatory actions within the vessel wall by their interactions with 7-transmembrane, G-protein–coupled cell surface receptors.[31] The four subclasses of receptors include BLT_1 and BLT_2, which are high- and low-affinity receptors for LTB_4, and $CysLT_1$ and $CysLT_2$ (cysteinyl-leukotriene receptors).

Large numbers of 5-LO–expressing cells are found in advanced atherosclerotic lesions in the regions that are most prone to rupture.[32] In human atherosclerotic lesions, 5-LO is expressed by a subset of CD68-positive macrophages.[33] In the region of 5-LO positive macrophages, LTB_4 increase the expression of the BLT_1 receptor and mediates human effector T-cell recruitment.[34] Unexpectedly, interferon-γ (IFN-γ) down-regulates BLT_1 expression in monocytes.[35]

LTB_4 promotes monocyte chemotaxis and adhesion. It is a potent chemoattractant for mononuclear cells through the induction of monocyte chemoattractant protein–1 (MCP-1) and CD36,[36,37] and it mediates monocyte adhesion by increased expression of the β_2 integrin CD11b.[38]

Complex vulnerable vascular plaques contain abundant activated neutrophils that produce LTB_4, which induces the expression and activation of myeloperoxidase. Myeloperoxidase generates hypochlorous acid that further enhances the oxidative modification of LDL,[39] and it inactivates inhibitors of MMPs, thereby increasing the susceptibility of plaques to rupture.[40]

Leukotriene Receptors

Leukotrienes mediate their vascular effects through binding to high-affinity leukotriene receptors. The LT B_4 receptor is present on macrophages, neutrophils, and eosinophils. Early stages of atherosclerosis involve monocyte recruitment to the atherosclerotic lesion mediated by BLT_1 receptor–induced MCP-1 production and integrin-mediated adhesion. In contrast, in later stages of atherosclerosis, BLT_2 receptor mRNA expression is increased in macrophage-rich regions relative to BLT_1 expression.[41] LTB_4 interactions with the BLT_1 receptor on T cells increases their secretion of MMP-2, -3, and -9.[42] This pathway provides a link between innate immunity and plaque instability.

In addition to leukocytes, vascular cells express BLT receptors. LTB_4-triggered BLT_1 activation in endothelial cells induces vasoconstriction and migration and proliferation of vascular smooth muscle cells,[43] which is a crucial process involved in intimal hyperplasia. In vascular smooth muscle cells, activation of BLT_1 receptors involves pathways mediated by NF-κB.[44]

CysLTs activate $CysLT_1$ and $CysLT_2$ receptors that are expressed on human monocytes, macrophages, and mast cells.[45] In human blood monocytes and monocyte-derived macrophages, $CysLT_1$ receptor expression is increased by interleukin-4 (IL-4) or IL-13.[46]

The augmented expression of $CysLT_4$ by inflammatory cytokines increased LTD_4-mediated monocyte migration. $CysLT_2$ receptor signaling in endothelial cells increases expression of the chemokine macrophage inflammatory protein–2 (MIP-2), which may promote leukocyte recruitment.[47]

Leukotriene Inhibitors

The effects of a FLAP inhibitor (DG-031, deCode genetics, Reykjavik, Iceland) on inflammatory biomarkers were examined in a short-term, randomized, placebo-controlled crossover trial in 268 patients with genetic variants in the leukotriene pathway.[48] The study population included 191 carriers of the FLAP gene and 77 carriers of the LTA_4 hydrolase gene in whom 85% were treated with statins. Enrolled subjects in this trial were randomly assigned to treatment with DG-031 250 mg, DG-031 500 mg, DG-031 750 mg, or placebo. After 2 weeks, treatment with DG-031 750 mg reduced ionomycin-activated neutrophil production of LTB_4 by 26% (95% CI, 10% to 39%, $P = 0.003$) and myeloperoxidase release from neutrophils by 12% (95% CI, 2% to 21%; $P = 0.02$). At 2 weeks, there was a nonsignificant reduction in CRP levels (16%; 95% CI, –2% to 31%; $P = 0.07$); however, a larger carryover effect was observed at 4 weeks (25% [95% CI, 5% to 40%]; $P = 0.02$). These data illustrate that inhibition of FLAP reduces several biomarkers that identify patients at increased risk for cardiovascular events among patients with specific genetic variants in the lipoxygenase pathway.

The LTCAD Study was designed to investigate the effects of veliflapon (DG-051), a LTA_4 hydrolase inhibitor, on cardiovascular events among 3450 African American patients with a positive LTA4H HapK genetic variant and established coronary artery disease.[48] As discussed earlier, the LTA4H haplotype is more strongly associated with myocardial infarction among African Americans than among Caucasian Americans. Eligible patients were randomly assigned to treatment with veliflapon or placebo within 5 to 30 days of their acute coronary syndrome event. The primary outcome measure was the time to first occurrence of the composite endpoint including hospitalization for unstable angina or urgent revascularization, fatal or nonfatal myocardial infarction, fatal or nonfatal stroke, or cardiovascular-related death. However, this study was suspended within 6 months of enrollment because of a formulation problem with the product.

The LTB_4 synthesis inhibitor, 2,4,6-triiodophenol (AM-24, Industrial Farmaceutica Catabria, S.A., Spain) acts, in part, through inhibiting 5-LO.[49] In healthy volunteers, dose-dependent inhibition of LTB_4 synthesis has been demonstrated, in which 75% of maximal LTB_4 synthesis inhibition is achieved with oral administration at 3 days and 90% of maximal LTB_4 synthesis inhibition is achieved after 3 weeks of treatment.

Experimental studies indicate that LTB_4 is involved in early atherosclerotic processes that involve monocyte chemotaxis and smooth muscle cell migration and proliferation as well as in later stages of atherosclerosis through stimulatory effects on myeloperoxidase and inactivation of inhibitors of MMPs. Future trials that investigate the effects of leukotriene inhibition should include studies involving subjects with early stages of atherosclerosis.

Leukotriene Receptor Antagonism

The LTB_4 receptor antagonist, CP-105,696, has been investigated for its effects on lesion progression in murine models of atherosclerosis.[50] In apolipoprotien (apo) E−/− and fat-fed LDL receptor (LDLR)−/− mice, treatment with LTB_4 receptor antagonist reduced lipid accumulation, surface expression of the β_2 integrin CD11b, and macrophage infiltration in lesions.

Antagonists of the $CysLT_1$ receptor have been used clinically in the treatment of asthma. These compounds include zafirlukast, montelukast, and pranlukast. The calcium signal induced by LTD_4 in macrophages is inhibited by montelukast.[51] A cardiovascular biomarker study has been initiated with montelukast in which subjects at high risk for coronary heart disease will be randomized to treatment with montelukast or placebo in a crossover design.[52] The primary outcome measure with leukotriene receptor antagonism is the change from baseline in various cardiovascular biomarkers, including CRP, LTB_4, LTD_4, LTE_4, and lipid levels. Secondary outcome measures include other inflammatory mediators such as cytokines, chemokines, adhesion molecules, and myeloperoxidase.

PHOSPHOLIPASES

PLA_2 enzymes hydrolyze fatty acids from the sn-2 position of glycophospholipids to generate lysophospholipids and nonesterified fatty acid.[53] These products may act intracellularly, or they may be further metabolized into proinflammatory mediators. Lysophosphatidylcholine triggers a panoply of cellular proinflammatory responses (Table 46-1). Arachidonic acid is a common fatty acid product released by cellular and extracellular PLA_2, resulting in the generation of oxidation products, including prostaglandins, thromboxanes, and leukotrienes[54] (Fig. 46-3).

The PLA_2 superfamily consists of enzymes that are largely calcium dependent, with lipoprotein-associated PLA_2 (Lp-PLA_2) representing a calcium-independent member.[55] This particular enzyme also differs from other phospholipases, such as secretory PLA_2 ($sPLA_2$), in that it is a serine protease. Serine proteases are characterized by an active-sites serine residue that form a catalytic triad with a histidine residue and an aspartic residue.[56]

Secretory Phospholipase$_2$

The secretory phospholipases are a family of enzymes that hydrolyze fatty acids in a calcium-dependent process. The $sPLA_2$ family contains more than 10 enzymes; like all phospholipases, these are responsible for

TABLE 46-1 Biological Effects of Putative Inflammatory and Proatherogenic Products Derived from Enzymatic Hydrolysis of LDL-Associated Oxidized Phospholipids

Mediator	Cellular Target	Effects
LysoPC	Endothelial cells	Homing of inflammatory cells: up-regulation of adhesive molecules (VCAM-1, ICAM-1) and MCP-1 Formation of inflammatory mediators: activation of Ca^{2+}-dependent PLA_2 enzymes and arachidonic acid release Functional responses: impaired proliferation/migration and reduced NO-dependent vasodilation Cytotoxicity: apoptosis
	Smooth muscle cells	Homing of inflammatory cells: up-regulation of MCP-1 Oxidative stress: NADPH oxidase activation and ROS-dependent ERK1/2 phosphorylation Functional responses: increased growth factor gene expression, proliferation, and migration LDL retention: up-regulation of biglycan core protein and elongation of GAG chains Cytotoxicity: apoptosis
	Monocytes/macrophages	Formation of inflammatory mediators: up-regulation of cytokines (IL-1β Ca^{2+}-dependent PLA_2 enzymes and arachidonic acid release Functional responses: increased chemotaxis Cytotoxicity: increased cellular permeability and apoptosis
	T cells	Functional responses: increased chemotaxis Immune response: interferon-γ up-regulation
	Neutrophils	Oxidative stress: NADPH oxidase activation and myeloperoxidase release Functional responses: increased chemotaxis, elastase release
oxNEFA	Monocytes/macrophages	Cytotoxicity: increased cellular permeability and apoptosis

From Ref. 64, with permission.

GAG, glycosaminoglycan; ICAM-1, intercellular adhesive molecule-1; IL-1β, interleukin-1β; lysoPC, lysophosphatidylcholine; oxNEFA, oxidized nonesterified fatty acids; MCP-1, monocyte chemoattractant protein-1; NO, nitric oxide; PLA_2, phospholipase A_2; ROS, reactive oxygen species; VCAM-1, vascular cell adhesive molecule-1.

hydrolyzing phospholipids. These enzymes are produced and secreted in the walls of human blood vessels,[57,58] and may contribute to the development of atherosclerosis locally through mechanisms that are lipoprotein dependent[59] and lipoprotein independent.

The most notable isoforms implicated in the pathogenesis of atherosclerosis belong to groups IIa, V, and X. Group IIa $sPLA_2$, the best-studied $sPLA_2$, is an acute-phase protein that is induced in many tissues during inflammation. In contrast, group V $sPLA_2$ is not an acute phase reactant, but its production is augmented by inflammatory stimuli.[60]

$sPLA_2$ enzymes also modulate the atherogenicity of LDL and atheroprotective properties of HDL. For example, group V and X $sPLA_2$ hydrolyze LDL and increase the binding of LDL to cell-surface proteoglycans.[60,62] This step is crucial because it facilitates the uptake of cholesteryl esters into macrophages. Macrophage-specific expression of $sPLA_2$ increases intracellular oxidative stress and increases foam cell formation.[54] Furthermore, group IIa $sPLA_2$ stimulates LDL oxidation by lipoxygenase.[54] Group IIa and group V $sPLA_2$ associate with HDL and accelerate atherosclerosis by decreasing the capacity of HDL to mediate cholesterol efflux from lipid-laden macrophages, and depleting the antioxidant paraoxonase activity on HDL particles.[62a] Groups V and X $sPLA_2$ are more potent in hydrolyzing HDL than group IIa $sPLA_2$.

Group IIa $sPLA_2$ binds to ischemic myocardium in regions adjacent to infarcted areas in patients with myocardial infarction.[61] Localization of $sPLA_2$ in the ischemic myocardium was detected 12 to 24 hours after the onset of symptoms. As the time course for acute-phase changes in plasma $sPLA_2$ precedes CRP, it is possible that products of $sPLA_2$ activity, namely lysophospholipids, serve as ligands for CRP in reversibly injured membranes of myocytes. Ischemia induces a loss of membrane stability resulting in a flip-flop of the cardiomyocyte plasma membrane and translocation of phosphatidylserine and phosphatidylethanolamine to the outer leaflet. These phospholipids provide a substrate to which CRP binds, and together, the CRP–ligand complex activates complement (Fig. 46-4). Complement activation, in turn, triggers inflammation in the ischemic myocardium.[93]

PLA_2 enzymes hydrolyze phospholipids from the inner leaflet of cell membranes that have been exposed by reversible or irreversible injury. Lysophosphatidylcholine generated by the action of PLA_2 enzymes ($sPLA_2$ and $cPLA_2$) serve as a ligand for CRP.[63] After CRP binds to lysophosphatidylcholine, it is able to activate complement.[61,63]

Selective Secretory Phospholipase A_2 Inhibitors

Substituted indoles, 6,7-benzoindoles and indolizines are potent inhibitors of $sPLA_2$.[64a] Varespladib sodium (sodium 2-(1-benzyl-2-ethyl-3-oxamoylindol-4-ly) oxyacetate; A-001, Anthera Pharmaceuticals, San Mateo, CA; or previously LY315920, Eli Lilly & Co., Indianapolis, IN; or S5920, Shionogi & Company, Ltd., Osaka, Japan) and varespladib methy (1-H-indole-3-glyoxamide; A-002, Anthera Pharmaceuticals, San Mateo, CA; or previously LY333013, Eli Lilly & Co., Indianapolis, IN; or S3013, Shionogi & Company, Ltd., Osaka, Japan) are small molecule inhibitors of $sPLA_2$ with specificity towards group IIA (IC_{50}: 9–14 nM), group V (IC_{50}: 77 nM), and group X (IC_{50}: 15 nM) $sPLA_2$. LY311727 (3-[1-bennzyl-3-carbamoylmethyl)-2-ethly-indol-5-yl]oxypropylphosphonic acid; Eli Lilly & Co., Indianapolis, IN), an analogue of A-001, is another $sPLA_2$ that has been tested in experimental animal studies and *ex vivo* experiments.

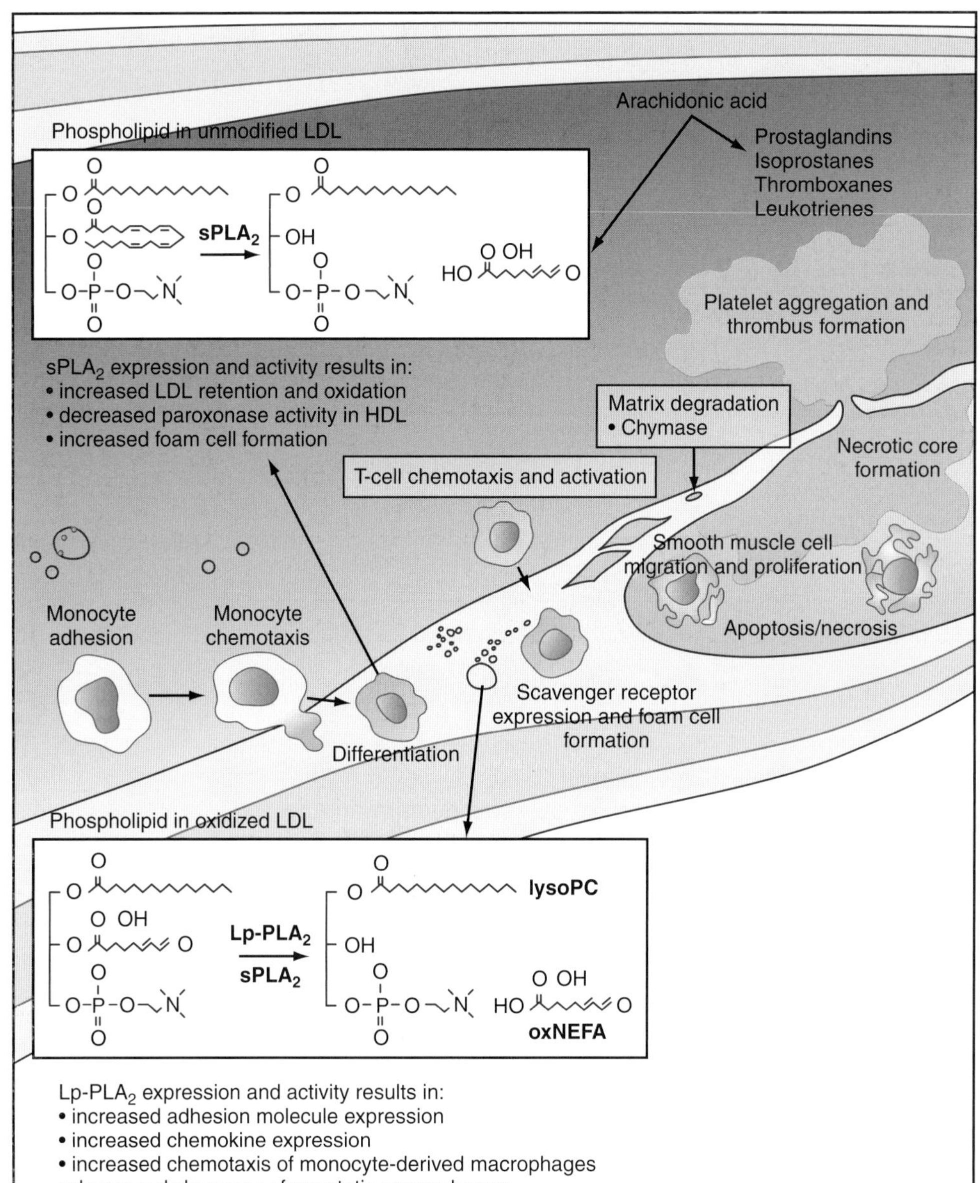

FIGURE 46-3 Phospholipases contribute to atherosclerosis through the production of lipid mediators of inflammation (e.g., lysophosphatidylcholine, eicosanoids). HDL, high-density lipoprotein; LDL, low-density lipoprotein; Lp-PLA_2, lipoprotein-associated phospholipase A_2; $sPLA_2$, secretory phospholipase A_2; lysoPC, lysophosphatidylcholine; oxNEFA, oxidized nonesterified fatty acids.

Selective $sPLA_2$ inhibition produces anti-inflammatory effects indirectly by reducing proinflammatory lipid mediators,[57,65] and directly by inhibiting transcriptional activation of inflammatory mediators.[66] Human atherosclerotic arteries incubated with specific inhibitors for group IIa $sPLA_2$, the monoclonal antibody 187 (Hoffmann-La Roche Inc., Nutley, NJ) and selective synthetic $sPLA_2$ inhibitor LY311727, reduced enzymatic activity of $sPLA_2$ as measured by the release of fatty acids from phospholipid liposomes or LDL.[57] In murine macrophages, LY311727 inhibits $sPLA_2$-mediated release of arachidonic acid.[66] In an oleic acid–induced acute lung injury model, pretreatment with the selective $sPLA_2$ inhibitor S-5920 or varespladib sodium reduced plasma concentrations of MCP-1.[67]

The transcription factor NF-κB belongs to the Rel family of transcription factors and is involved in the regulation of genes encoding cytokines, cytokine receptors, and adhesion molecules.[68] TNF-signaling pathways are involved in the activation of NF-κB, which remains inactive in the cytoplasm bound to the inhibitor inhibitory NF κB (IκB) until it is released and translocated to the nucleus upon phosphorylation and degradation of IκB. Two different TNF receptors mediate signal transduction of TNF, but TNF receptor p55 is the main signaling receptor in most cells.

TNF induces activation of cytosolic group IV PLA_2 and groups IIa and V $sPLA_2$.[69,70] In the human keratinocyte cell line HaCaT, the presence of the $sPLA_2$ inhibitors 12-epi-scalaradial and LY311727 (A002 analogue) reduced TNFR receptor p55–induced activation of NF-κB and expression of ICAM-1.[66] LY311727 (A002 analogue) inhibited TNF activation of NF-κB in a dose-dependent manner, with a 10-μM concentration of LY311727 inhibiting activation by 50%.

In atherosclerosis models, selective inhibition of $sPLA_2$ reduces plaque area. Angiotensin II stimulates macrophage uptake of oxidized LDL, leading to foam-cell formation, and it induces aortic aneurysms. Selective $sPLA_2$ inhibition reduced plaque area by more than 50%

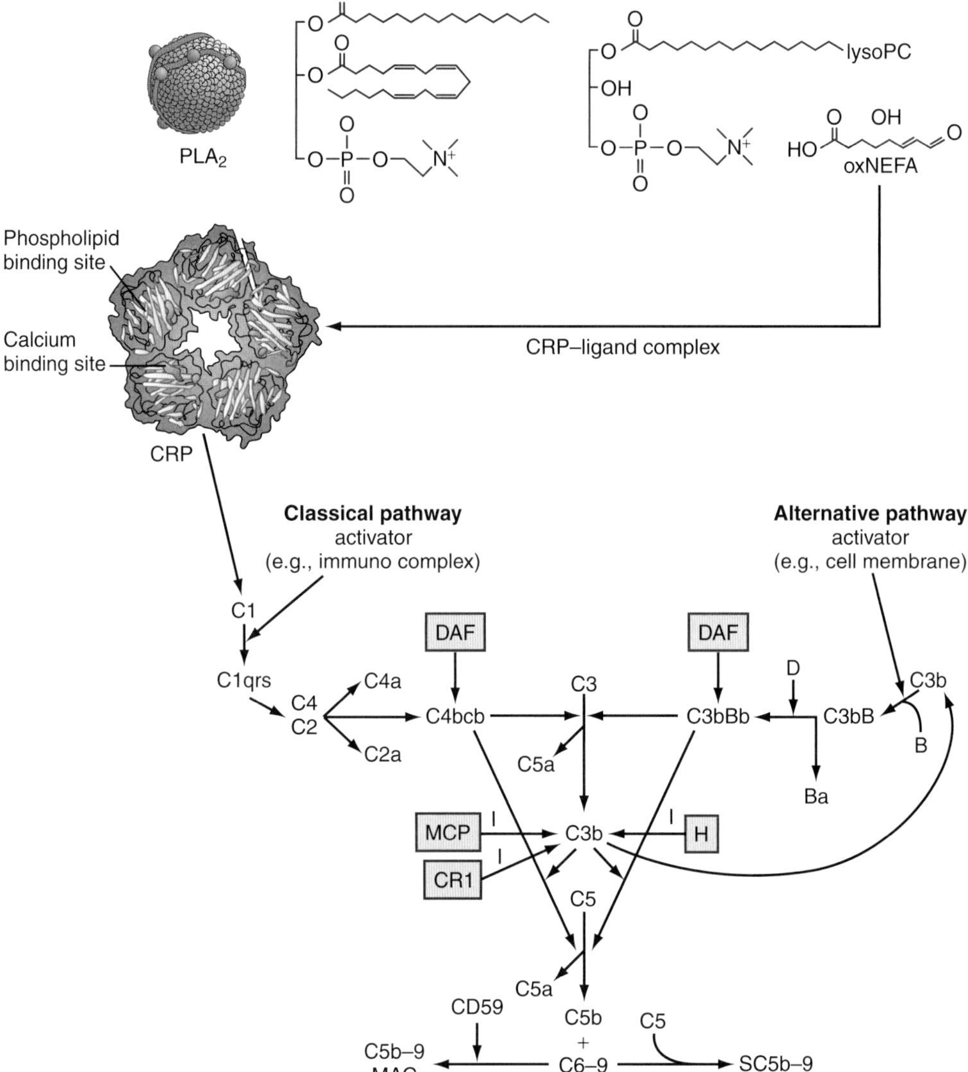

FIGURE 46-4 Phospholipase activity on lipoproteins generates lysophospholipids and oxidized nonesterified fatty acids. The binding of lysophospholipids to CRP activates the complement cascade, thereby triggering inflammation in ischemic myocardium. CRP, C-reactive protein; DAF, decay-accelerating factor; lysoPC, lysophosphatidylcholine; PLA_2, phospholipase A_2; MCP, membrane cofactor protein; oxNEFA, oxidized nonesterified fatty acids.

and reduced aneurysm formation.[71] In apo E-/- mice, $sPLA_2$ inhibition reduced plaque area.

An ischemia–reperfusion injury model was used to investigate the effects of cytotoxic neutrophil responses in group X $sPLA_2$–deficient mice. The neutrophils from group-X–deficient mice had 20% to 50% lower respiratory burst activity, lower elastase release, and a reduced migratory response.[72] The abnormal neutrophil response was reversed by the addition of arachidonic acid or exogenous $sPLA_2$-X protein. In wild-type mice, the addition of LY374388 reduced infarct size and improved left ventricular ejection fraction in the ischemia–reperfusion injury model.

Phospholipase Levels and Serological Markers of Atherosclerosis (PLASMA) was a Phase II, randomized, double-blind, placebo-controlled, parallel-arm, dose-ranging clinical pharmacology study of four doses of the selective $sPLA_2$ inhibitor, 1-H-indole-3-glyoxamide, or varespladib methyl (Anthera Pharmaceuticals, San Mateo, CA).[73] The primary outcome measure following 8 weeks of treatment was the change in plasma $sPLA_2$ level and activity from baseline. Secondary outcome measures included change in inflammatory biomarkers and lipoprotein particles. Published findings from the PLASMA trial are expected by the end of 2008.[73a] The $sPLA_2$ Inhibition to Decrease Enzyme Release after PCI (SPIDER-PCI) trial will investigate the effects of treatment with varespladib on peripercutaneous coronary intervention myocardial infarction incidence in patients undergoing elective PCI. A Study of the Safety and Efficacy of A-002 in Subjects with Acute Coronary Syndromes (FRANCIS-ACS) is an ongoing randomized, placebo-controlled trial designed to investigate the effect of varespladib methyl 500 mg daily in addition to atorvastatin 80 mg daily on major acute cardiovascular events in patients with acute coronary syndrome.

Lipoprotein-Associated Phospholipase A_2

Lp-PLA_2 is a predominantly macrophage-synthesized lipase that is up-regulated in the intima of atherosclerotic lesions and co-localizes with macrophages (and macrophage apoptosis). In plasma, Lp-PLA_2 is bound to lipoproteins, with a greater affinity for the polar surface of LDL particles, particularly electronegative small LDL particles. Lp-PLA_2 hydrolyzes oxidatively modified phosphatidylcholine on LDL, generating lysophosphatidylcholine and oxidized nonesterified fatty acids. Lp-PLA_2 activity increases the release of F2-isoprostanes *in vivo*,[74] and these products of lipid peroxidation exert several proinflammatory effects.

Lysophosphatidylcholine and oxidized nonesterified fatty acids are chemoattractants for monocytes[64] and elicit proatherogenic effects in endothelial cells, T cells, neutrophils, and smooth-muscle cells.[75] These proatherogenic effects include increased expression of adhesion molecules and chemokines, increased chemotaxis, induction of inflammatory cytokines and activation of proteolytic enzymes that impair the structural integrity of the fibrous plaque.

Selective Lipoprotein-Associated Phospholipase A_2 Inhibitors

Azetidinones represent the class of selective Lp-PLA_2 inhibitors that target the active-site serine residue of the enzyme.[76] Several selective and highly potent azetidinone inhibitors have been developed as pharmacological tools. In healthy volunteers, several oral inhibitors of Lp-PLA_2 reduce circulating enzyme activity by more than 95% in a dose-dependent manner.

In vitro experiments demonstrate that selective Lp-PLA_2 inhibition (SB-677116, SB-222657; GlaxoSmithKline, Philadelphia, PA) can reduce the generation of lysophosphatidylcholine and oxidized nonesterified fatty acids, and abrogate some of the inflammatory and proatherogenic effects of these inflammatory mediators.[53,77,78] Specifically, selective Lp-PLA_2 inhibition with SB-222657 inhibits monocyte chemotaxis and protects monocyte/macrophage cell death.[77,78] In *ex vivo* experiments, the selective Lp-PLA_2 inhibitor SB-677116 blocked lipopolysaccharide-stimulated production of oxidized fatty acids.[78a]

In patients undergoing elective carotid endarterectomy, Lp-PLA_2 inhibition with SB-480848 (darapladib) was accompanied by a dose-dependent inhibition of Lp-PLA_2 activity in plasma and atherosclerotic plaque.[79] After 14 days of therapy, Lp-PLA_2 activity was reduced by 80% in plaque and in plasma. The Integrated Biomarkers and Imaging Study (IBIS-2) was a randomized, double-blind, placebo-controlled trial designed to explore the effects of darapladib on coronary plaque deformability, composition, and volume and several biomarkers.[80] After 12 months of treatment, there was no difference in the primary endpoints of plaque deformability and CRP. Expansion of necrotic core volume was halted in darapladib-treated patients, whereas it increased in placebo-treated patients, resulting in a significant treatment difference. These intraplaque compositional changes were not accompanied by a difference in total atheroma volume. The reduction in necrotic core volume is consistent with the antiapoptotic mechanisms of action for selective Lp-PLA_2 inhibitors that have been shown to reduce Iysophosphatidyl choline that contributes to oxidized LDL–mediated cell death of human monocytes/macrophages[77] and inhibited intracellular protease (caspase-3 and caspase-8) activity involved in carotid atheroma cell death.[81]

NOVEL IMMUNOMODULATORS

T Cell–Mediated Immune Responses

CD40 signaling involves interactions with TNF receptor–associated factors (TRAFs).[82] Signaling by TRAFs activates cell signaling pathways that include extracellular signal–regulated kinases (ERK), p38 mitogen–activated protein kinases (MAPK), and c-Jun N-terminal kinase (JNK). Oxidized LDL is one of the initial triggers of CD40 and CD40 ligand (CD40L) expression by T lymphocytes, macrophages, endothelial cells, and smooth muscle cells in atheroma.

CD40–CD40L (recently named CD154) interactions promote T cell–dependent B-cell activation, and induction of inflammatory pathways mediate atherosclerosis progression (through effects on cytokine, chemokine, and adhesion molecule expression), plaque instability (through effects on metalloproteinase expression), and thrombogenesis (through effects on tissue factor expression and on the platelet IIa/IIIb receptor). The proinflammatory mediator CD40L can be cleaved from cell membranes to form a biologically active soluble fragment (sCD40L).

CD4+ T cell–mediated immune responses are triggered by major histocompatibility complex (MHC) class II molecules/peptide complexes. Antigen-presenting cells (dendritic cells, B cells, and macrophages) internalize extracellular antigens that are processed by endosomal or lysosomal proteases to form peptides that associate with MHC-II. MHC-II/peptide complexes activate CD4+ T cells that activate other immune cells that include B cells, CD8+ T cells, and macrophages.

The immune response may be inhibited by interfering with antigen presentation to MHC-II. A requisite initiating process in peptide loading of MHC-II involves proteolysis of the invariant chain molecules by cysteine proteases. Cathepsin S is a cysteine protease expressed in many antigen-presenting cells, and it is responsible for the final proteolytic step that generates the class II–associated, invariant chain peptide (CLIP) that occupies the MHC II peptide–binding groove.

In addition to antigen presentation to MHC-II, cathepsin S is involved in cross presentation of exogenous antigens by MHC-I to CD8+ T cells via the independent presentation of antigenic peptides to CD8+ T cells.[83] Cross-presentation involves a cytosolic transporter associated with antigen processing (TAP)–dependent pathway and a vacuolar TAP–independent pathway. The vacuolar TAP–independent pathway is susceptible to inhibition by cysteine protease inhibitors.

Further, cathepsin S is expressed by plaque microvessels, where it contributes to neovascularization of atherosclerotic plaque, a central process to plaque growth and thrombotic complications. The formation of neovessels requires degradation of the extracellular matrix.

Inhibitors of Cathepsin S

Cathepsin S inhibition has been considered a potential therapeutic approach for atherosclerosis. Cathepsin S inhibitors prevent presentation of antigen from different MHC-II haplotypes,[84] and they may be considered as therapeutic targets to reduce the inflammatory response in atherosclerosis.

Experimental models have shown that LDL receptor–deficient mice develop atherosclerosis on a high-fat diet, but mice deficient in both LDL receptor and cathepsin S develop less atherosclerosis.[85] At this time, no clinical trials in humans are under way to investigate the effects of cathepsin S inhibition on cardiovascular outcomes.

Chemokine Receptor Antagonists

Chemokines or chemotactic cytokines are small molecules that mediate leukocyte migration and activation. Chemokines are classified into one of two major subfamilies based on the position of the cysteine residues in their sequence. The CC family contains adjacent cysteines, and the CXC family is characterized by cysteines that are separated by a single intervening amino acid. MCP-1 (CCL2) mediates chemotaxis of monocytes to inflammatory sites through specific binding to the cell surface CC chemokine receptor–2 (CCR2).[86] CCR2 is a G-protein–coupled, seven-transmembrane receptor superfamily that is abundantly expressed on monocytes. The interaction of MCP-1 with CCR2 activates the MAPK signal transduction pathway that is a key component of cellular events that lead to integrin activation and chemotaxis.[87,88]

Selective absence of MCP-1 and CCR2 in atherosclerosis-prone mice that were fed high-fat diets reduced monocyte infiltration and atherosclerotic lesion formation.[89,90] These data demonstrate a critical role for MCP-1 in the initiation and progression of atherosclerosis, and suggest that chemokine receptor antagonism may serve as a target of preventive therapies.

Several orally bioavailable, small molecule, glycinamide-based CCR2 antagonists have been developed. These agents have a γ-aminoamide core that has been modified to inhibit MCP-1–induced monocyte chemotaxis.[91] One compound, (2S)-N-[3, 5-bis(trifluoromethyl) benzyl]-2-(4-fluorophenyl)-4-(4-phenylpiperidin-1-γl)butanamide (Merck Research Laboratories, Rahway, NJ USA)[92], has a CCR2 IC_{50} of 59 nM and a functional inhibition of MCP-1 for monocyte chemotaxis of 41 nM. Replacing the 2-aryl moiety on the butyramide core with a cyclopentane scaffold improved the potency of this compound for CCR2 binding (1.3 nM) and functional chemotaxis (0.45 nM).[92]

Another selective small molecule antagonist of the CCR2 receptor, INCP3344 (Incyte Corporation, Wilmington, DE USA),[93,94] has been studied in inflammatory disease models. INCP3344 inhibits *in vitro* binding of CCL2 to mouse monocytes (IC_{50}=10 nM).[94] This compound exhibits a dose-dependent inhibition of CCL2-mediated functional responses such as ERK phosphorylation that is induced by MCP-5 ligand-specific binding to CCR2, monocyte chemotaxis, and macrophage infiltration into a thioglycolate-induced peritonitis model.

Mitogen-Activated Protein Kinase

MAPKs represent an intracellular signaling pathway that integrates and processes various extracellular signals mediated through ERK, JNK, and p38.[94] Among these signaling peptides, the p38 subfamily of MAPK is considered the central regulator of inflammation. The p38 subfamily of the MAPK superfamily comprises four isoforms: p38α, p38β, p38δ, and p38γ. The p38α isoform is involved in the inflammatory response of monocytes, whereas the function of the other isoforms has not been elucidated.

The p38 MAPK has a central role in inflammation that is mediated by transcription-dependent mechanisms and post-translational regulation. Many inflammatory response proteins depend on the p38 signaling cascade for their production.[95] The inflammatory mediators that depend on p38 signaling for their production include proinflammatory cytokines, chemokines, degradative enzymes, growth factors, and adhesion molecules and COX-2.

The p38 pathway mediates CCR1 and CCR2 expression, and transduces the chemotaxis signal pathway induced by chemokines.[96] The p38 MAPK signaling cascade increases endothelial expression of VCAM-1 at the post-transcriptional level.[97]

Activation of the p38 pathway is mediated by sequential protein phosphorylation through a MAPK module that involves MAPK kinase (MAP3K) to MAPK kinase (MAP2K) to MAPK[98] (Fig. 46-5). This classical p38 activation pathway is activated by stressful and inflammatory stimuli. The principal MAP2Ks responsible for dual phosphorylation of p38 are MAPK kinase (MKK)3 and MKK6. Phosphorylation of p38 by G-protein–coupled receptor kinase-2 (GRK2) at a residue on the docking groove (Thr123) impairs binding to upstream MKKs or downstream substrates.

MAPK-activated protein kinase–2 (MK2) is a major substrate of p38. MK2 has a specific docking site for p38α that resides predominantly in the nucleus of resting cells. Stress or inflammatory stimulation activates p38 and phosphorylates MK2 in the nucleus. The phosphorylation of MK2 unmasks the MK2 nuclear export signal resulting in translocation of the MK2–p38α complex into the cytoplasm. The MK2–p38α complex regulates the stability and efficient translation of short-lived mRNAs of inflammatory mediator genes, and it is involved in post-translational regulation of cytokine expression.

Mitogen-Activated Protein Kinase Inhibitors

Several p38 MAPK inhibitors have been shown to reduce inflammation in experimental animals; however, these inhibitors have failed in clinical trials.[95] The first generation of p38 inhibitors had a common mechanism of action that involved competitive inhibition of the adenosine-binding pocket (ATP-binding site) of p38. These pyridinyl imidazole inhibitors were found to be hepatotoxic and potentially carcinogenic, as they were potent inducers of some cytochrome P450 isoenzymes

Structurally diverse new inhibitors were designed to occupy the less-conserved surrounding hydrophobic areas of p38 binding site that induce conformational reorganization in the protein that does not involve ATP binding. These compounds—BIRB796 (1-5-*tert*-butyl-2-p-tolyl-2H-pyrazol-3-yl)-3-[4-(2-morpholin-4-yl-ethoxy)naphthalen-1-yl]urea), SCIO469, and VX702 (2-(2,4-difluorophenylthio)-5-(2,6-dichlorophenyl)-6Hpyrimido[1,6-b]pyridazin-6-1e)—were accompanied

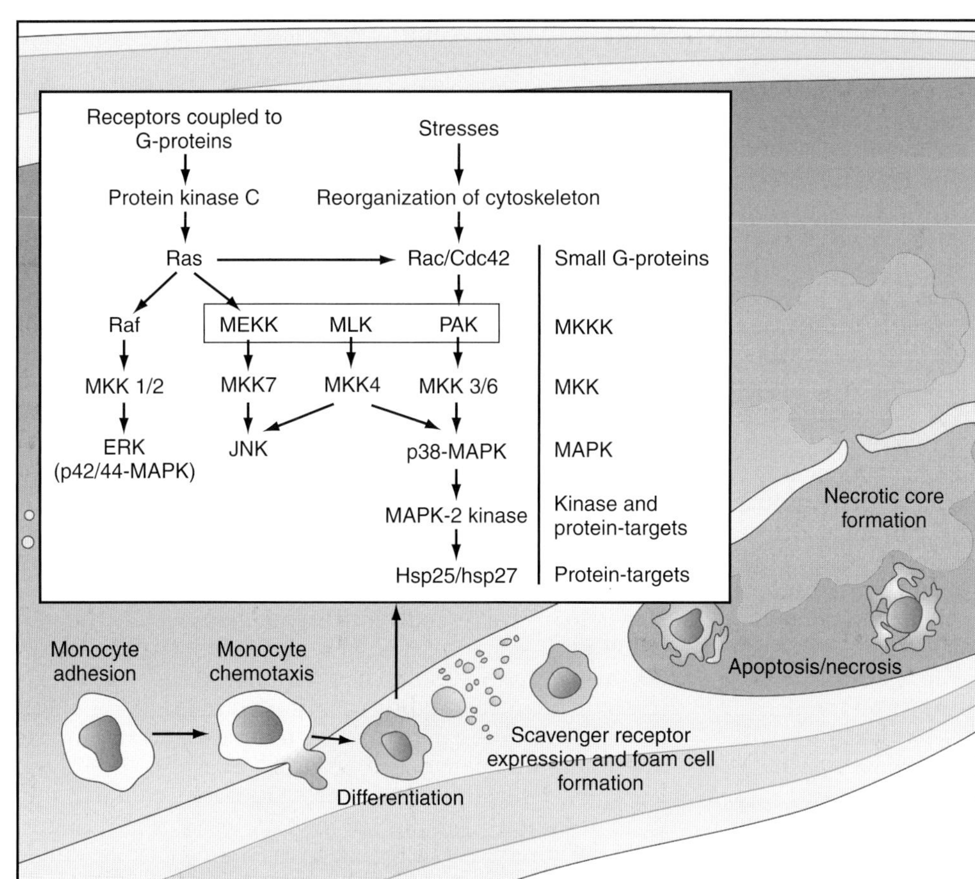

FIGURE 46-5 Activation of the p38 MAP kinase signaling pathway increases the expression of inflammatory cytokines, chemokines, and other mediators of vascular inflammation. ERK, extracellular signal–regulated kinase; JNK, Jun N-terminal kinase; MAPK, mitogen-activated protein kinase; MEKK, MAP/ERK kinase; MKK, kinase of MAP kinase; MKKK, kinase of MKK; MLK, mixed lineage kinase; PAK, p21-activated kinase.

by serious adverse hepatic and central nervous system effects.[98] Later, it was determined that these compounds inhibited other closely related kinases.[99]

Strategies that are not involved in ATP competition involve inhibition of other molecules that inhibit the p38 MAPK pathway. Potential novel targets for inhibition of the p38 pathway include direct activation of p38 autophosphorylation or, alternatively, inhibition of upstream kinases or downstream effectors (see Fig. 46-5). Small molecules that interfere with the MK2–p38α interaction or translocation of the complex may serve as useful targets for MK2 inhibition.

Serine Protease Inhibitors

Chymase is a mast cell serine protease that is stored in a macromolecular complex with heparin proteoglycan.[100] Prior to secretion, chymase is activated intracellularly by dipeptidyl peptidase I. Chymase is secreted from mast cells, and it remains bound to heparin proteoglycans of mast cell granule remnants. The proteoglycan–bound chymase is resistant to endogenous protease inhibitors, and this prolongs its activity for several weeks.

Chymase is localized in the adventitial layer of the vessel, and plays a role in converting angiotensin I to angiotensin II; however, it differs from ACE, which is a carboxypeptidase primarily localized in the endothelium. The angiotensin II formed by chymase is involved in vascular remodeling. Chymase induces apoptosis of vascular smooth muscle cells by degrading fibronectin and consequent disruption of focal adhesions.[101] It also degrades the extracellular matrix through activation of MMP-1 and MMP-3 and transforming growth factor–β1 (TGF-β1). TGF-β1 can inhibit smooth muscle cell differentiation, migration, and proliferation, which, in turn, reduces the synthesis and secretion of extracellular matrix.

Mast Cell Stabilizers and Chymase Inhibitors

The effects of chymase may be attenuated either by reduced mast cell secretion of chymase or through the use of specific chymase inhibitors. Mast cell stabilizers prevent the secretion of chymase and, in addition, other mast cell contents such as chemotaxins, cytokines, growth factors, and other serine proteases.[100]

Tranilast, N-(3,5-dimethyoxycinnamoyl) anthranilic acid, is the mast cell stabilizer that has been studied most extensively. In experimental animal models, tranilast administered 2 weeks before and 4 weeks after balloon injury to the carotid artery of dogs eliminated the increase in mast cell content, chymase production and activity, and intimal thickening in the injured vessel.[102] Similarly, tranilast given 3 days before and 14 days after balloon injury to the rat carotid injury reduced neointimal thickening.[103]

Clinical trial data from the second Tranilast Restenosis Following Angioplasty Trial (TREAT-2) demonstrated reduced rates of restenosis after percutaneous transluminal coronary angioplasty.[104] In TREAT-2, a total of 297 patients were given tranilast or placebo for 3 months from the day after the angioplasty. The rate of restenosis, defined as a loss of 50% or more of the intimal gain, was reduced in the tranilast group versus the placebo group (26% vs. 42%, $P = 0.012$). The differences in restenosis at 3 months were not maintained at 12 months. The Prevention of REStenosis with Tranilast and its Outcomes (PRESTO) trial randomized 1184 patients within 4 hours of PCI to tranilast or placebo for 3 months.[105] Tranilast therapy did not change intimal hyperplasia quantified by IVUS, or restenosis by arteriography or IVUS. Further, there were no differences in clinical outcomes that included the composite of death, myocardial infarction, or ischemia-directed vessel revascularization.

In contrast to favorable effects of tranilast in experimental models, TREAT-2, and PRESTO involved the administration of tranilast after the angioplasty procedure. It is possible that mast cell stabilization may be ineffective after the mast cell has released its contents. Future studies should consider pretreatment with tranilast before PCI.

Other chymase inhibitors also have been studied in balloon-mediated injury in experimental animal models. In these studies, chymase inhibition with 2-(5-formylamino-6-oxo-2 phenyl-1,6-dihydropyrimidine-1-yl-N-[2-hepatyl]acetamide (NK3201) reduced the increase in chymase activity in the injured arteries and diminished neointimal proliferation.[100] Another chymase inhibitor—BCEAB—inhibited basic fibroblast growth factor–mediated angiogenesis and local blood flow in hamster sponge granulomas.[106] It also reduced basic fibroblast growth factor–mediated increase in chymase activity and vascular endothelial growth factor (VEGF) mRNA.

The clinical benefits of chymase inhibition in humans remains uncertain; however, data from experimental animal models in reducing intimal thickening (when mast cell stabilizers are administered before balloon-mediated vascular injury) and angiogenesis (with chymase inhibitors) are encouraging.

Complement Activation, Inflammation, and Thrombogenesis

The complement system is part of plasma cascade systems that are activated by the classical, alternative, or lectin pathway. The complement activation products C3a and C5a are involved in various aspects of the inflammatory process that include activation of leukocytes and endothelial cells, induction of genes involved in cytokine production, inducible nitric oxide, and apoptosis. Other components of the complement cascade, the C5b-9 membrane attack complex (MAC), perpetuate the inflammatory response through increased production of reactive oxygen species and LTB_4 generation in polymorphonuclear leukocytes[107] and increased adhesion of neutrophils to the endothelium. MAC influences neutrophil adhesion through the translocation of P-selectin from Weibel-Palade bodies to the endothelium.[108] Further complement activation promotes coagulation. MAC insertion into cell membranes is accompanied by cell surface membrane vesicles that express binding sites for factor Va, which is necessary for assembly of the prothrombinase complex. Complement activation and consequent MAC formation activates tissue factor.

Complement Inhibition

The complement system has been designated a therapeutic target to reduce myocardial necrosis and adverse clinical outcomes after ischemic injury. MAC is present in animal and human infarcted myocardial tissue.[109,110] Complement inhibition reduced infarct size and improved cardiac function in several animal models, and decreased neutrophil infiltration and apoptosis.[110] The cardioprotective effects of a C1 esterase inhibitor were investigated in an experimental model of myocardial ischemia and reperfusion injury.[110]

Several human trials have investigated the effect of pexelizumab, a single-change anti-C5 complement antibody, on infarct size (primary outcome) and total mortality and myocardial infarction (secondary outcome) after fibrinolysis,[111] primary PCI in patients with acute ST segment–elevation myocardial infarction,[112] and in surgical patients undergoing cardiopulmonary bypass.[113] In these trials, patients were randomly assigned to receive placebo or pexelizumab 2.0 mg/kg bolus with or without a 0.05 mg/kg/hour infusion for 20 hours. Pexelizumab had no measurable effect on infarct size (measured by creatinine kinase MB fraction or troponin concentrations); however, a significant reduction was observed in 90-day mortality (1.8% vs. 5.9% with placebo, $P = 0.014$ with pexelizumab bolus plus infusion) among acute myocardial infarction patients undergoing primary PCI. Among cardiac surgical patients, post hoc analysis showed a reduction in the composite endpoint of death or myocardial infarction for the isolated–coronary artery bypass graft patient groups treated with bolus plus infusion (3% vs. 8%, $P = 0.007$) on postoperative day 4 (3% vs. 9%, $P = 0.004$) and on postoperative day 30.

At this time, no further clinical trials with pexelizumab have been registered. In two published clinical trials, pexelizumab did not reduce infarct size, the primary outcome measure, but did reduce cardiovascular events. It is possible that complement inhibition reduces inflammatory pathways that contribute to cardiovascular events beyond its effect on limiting infarct size.

CONCLUSIONS

Looking to the future, the possibility of novel therapies that affect inflammatory processes within the vessel wall requires support from randomized clinical trials that investigate whether cardiovascular outcomes differ between individuals with high and low levels of a specific biomarker and how these differences in clinical events are related to a change in these markers.

Antioxidant therapy for the prevention of initial and recurrent cardiovascular events has failed in multiple studies using multiple therapies, including vitamins and more powerful synthetic antioxidants. The inflammatory response in atherosclerosis may be mitigated by interrupting pathways that trigger inflammatory genes or block the downstream effectors. The LO pathway is a key regulator involved in inflammation, endothelial dysfunction, smooth muscle cell proliferation, and thrombogenesis. Despite the success of leukotriene antagonists in asthma, one clinical trial with a 5-LO inhibitor has been terminated. The most promising novel therapies are the PLA_2 inhibitors. Several clinical trials with selective inhibitors of $sPLA_2$ and $Lp\text{-}PLA_2$ have been initiated. Small molecules that block chemotaxis represent another approach to diminishing proinflammatory effects.

Complement inhibition reduces infarct size in experimental animals, but similar findings have not been observed in trials involving patients. Nevertheless, complement inhibition has been shown to reduce clinical cardiovascular events.

With the high burden of cardiovascular disease despite the use of multiple evidence-based therapies, there is the prospect that novel therapies that target the vessel wall will provide incremental benefit for the high-risk cardiovascular disease patient.

REFERENCES

1. National Heart, Lung, and Blood Institute, Smith SC, Allen J, Blair SN, et al: AHA/ACC guidelines for secondary prevention for patients with coronary and other atherosclerotic vascular disease: 2006 update endorsed by the National Heart, Lung, and Blood Institute. *J Am Coll Cardiol* 2006;47:2130–2139.
2. Steg PG, Bhatt DL, Wilson PW, et al: One-year cardiovascular event rates in outpatients with atherothrombosis. *JAMA* 2007;297:1197–206.
3. Cannon CP, Braunwald E, McCabe CH, et al: Intensive versus moderate lipid lowering with statins after acute coronary syndromes. *N Engl J Med* 2004;350:1495–1504.
4. de Lemos JA, Blazing MA, Wiviot SD, et al: Early intensive vs a delayed conservative simvastatin strategy in patients with acute coronary syndromes: phase Z of the A to Z trial. *JAMA* 2004;292:1307–1316.
5. Rosenson RS, Tangney CC: Antiatherothrombotic properties of statins: implications for cardiovascular event reduction. *JAMA* 1998;279:1643–1650.
6. Rosenson RS: Statins in atherosclerosis: lipid-lowering agents with antioxidant capabilities. *Atherosclerosis* 2004;173:1–12.
7. Liao J: Clinical implications for statin pleiotropy. *Curr Opin Lipidol* 2005;16:624–629.
8. Dandona P, Dhindsa, Ghanim H, Chaudhuri A: Angiotensin II and inflammation: the effect of angiotensin-converting enzyme inhibition and angiotensin II receptor blockade. *J Hum Hypertens* 2007;21:20–27.
9. Ferroni P, Basili S, Falco A, Davi G: Oxidant stress and platelet activation in hypercholesterolemia. *Antioxid Redox Signal* 2004;6:747–56.
10. Nicholls SJ, Hazen SL: Myeloperoxidase and cardiovascular disease. *Arterioscler Thromb Vasc Biol* 2005;25:1102–1111.
11. Sugiyama S, Okada Y, Sukhova GK, et al: Macrophages myeloperoxidase regulation by granulocyte macrophage colony-stimulating factor in human atherosclerosis and implications in acute coronary syndromes. *Am J Pathol* 2001;158:879–891.
12. Cipollone F, Fazia ML: Cyclooxygenase-2 inhibition: vascular inflammation and cardiovascular risk. *Curr Atheroscler Rep* 2006;8:245–251.
13. Leskinen MJ, Lindstedt KA, Wang Y, Kovanen PT: Mast cell chymase induces smooth muscle cell apoptosis by a mechanism involving fibronectin degradation and disruption of focal adhesions. *Arterioscler Thromb Vasc Biol* 2003;23:238–243.
14. Blankenberg S, Rupprecht HJ, Bickel C, et al: Glutathione peroxidase 1 activity and cardiovascular events in patients with coronary artery disease. *N Engl J Med* 2003;349:1605–1613.
15. Vivekananthan DP, Penn MS, Sapp SK, et al: Use of antioxidant vitamins for the prevention of cardiovascular disease: meta-analysis of randomised trials. *Lancet* 2003;361:2017–2023.
16. Boaz M, Smetana S, Weinstein T, et al: Secondary prevention with antioxidants of cardiovascular disease in endstage renal disease (SPACE): randomised placebo-controlled trial. *Lancet* 2000;356:1213–1218.
17. Shinomiya M, Shirai K, Saito Y, Yoshida S: Inhibition of intimal thickening of the carotid artery of rabbits and of outgrowth of explants of aorta by probucol. *Atherosclerosis* 1992;97:143–148.
18. Ishizaka N, Kurokawa k, Taguchi J, et al: Inhibitory effect of a single local probucol administration on neointimal formation in balloon-injured rat carotid artery. *Atherosclerosis* 1995;118: 53–56.
19. Tardif JC, Cote G, Lesperance J, et al: Probucol and multivitamins in the prevention of restenosis after coronary angioplasty. Multivitamins and Probucol Study Group. *N Engl J Med* 1997;337:365–372.
20. Yokoi H, Daida H, Kuwabara Y, et al: Effectiveness of an antioxidant in preventing restenosis after percutaneous transluminal coronary angioplasty: The Probucol Angioplasty Restenosis Trial. *J Am Coll Cardiol* 1997;30:855–862.
21. Sawayama Y, Shimizu C, Maeda N, et al: Effects of probucol and pravastatin on common carotid atherosclerosis in patients with asymptomatic hypercholesterolemia. Fukuoka Atherosclerosis Trial (FAST). *J Am Coll Cardiol* 2002;39:610–616.
22. Tardif J, Gregoire J, Schwartz L, et al: Effects of AGI-1067 and probucol after percutaneous coronary interventions. *Circulation* 2003;107:552–558.
23. Deng YM, Wu BJ, Witting PK, Stocker R: Probucol protects against smooth muscle cell proliferation by upregulating heme oxygenase-1. *Circulation* 2004;110:1855–1860.
24. Tardif JC, Gregoire J, L'Allier PL, et al: Effects of the antioxidant succinobucol (AGI-1067) on human atherosclerosis in a randomized clinical trial. Atherosclerosis 2008;197:480–486.
25. Tardif JC, McMurray JJ, Klug E, et al: Effects of succinobucol (AGI-1067) after an acute coronary syndrome: a randomised, double-blind, placebo-controlled trial. *Lancet* 2008;371:176–1768.
26. Steinberg D, Witztum JL: Is the oxidative modification hypothesis relevant to human atherosclerosis? Do the antioxidant trials conducted to date refute the hypothesis? *Circulation* 2002;105:2107–2111.
27. Helgadottir A, Gretarsdottir S, St Clair D, et al: Association between the gene encoding 5-lipoxygenase-activating protein and stroke replicated in a Scottish population. *Am J Hum Genet* 2005;76:505–509.
28. Helgadottir A, Manolescu A, Thorleifsson G, et al: The gene encoding 5-lipoxygenase activating protein confers risk of myocardial infarction and stroke. *Nat Genet* 2004;36:233–239.
29. Dwyer JH, Allayee H, Dwyer KM, et al: Arachidonate 5-lipoxygenase promoter genotype, dietary arachidonic acid, and atherosclerosis. *N Engl J Med* 2004;350:29–37.
30. Helgadottir A, Manolescu A, Helgason A, et al: A variant of the gene encoding leukotriene A4 hydrolase confers ethnicity-specific risk of myocardial infarction. *Nat Genet* 2006;38:68–74.
31. Back M, Hansson GK: Leukotriene receptors in atherosclerosis. *Ann Med* 2006;38:493–502.
32. Cipollone F, Mezzetti A, Fazia ML, et al: Association between 5-lipoxygenase expression and plaque instability in humans. *Arterioscler Thromb Vasc Biol* 2005;25:1665–1670.
33. Spanbroek R, Grabner R, Lotzer K, et al: Expanding expression of the 5-lipoxygenase pathway within the arterial wall during human atherogenesis. *Proc Natl Acad Sci U S A* 2003;100: 1238–1243.
34. Tager AM, Bromley SK, Medoff BD, et al: Leukotriene B4 receptor BLT1 mediates early effector T cell recruitment. *Nat Immunol* 2003;4:937–939.
35. Pettersson A, Sabirsh A, Bristulf J, et al: Pro- and anti-inflammatory substances modulate expression of the leukotriene B4 receptor, BLT1, in human monocytes. *J Leukoc Biol* 2005;77:1018–1025.
36. Subbarao K, Jala VR, Mathis S, et al: Role of leukotriene B4 receptors in the development of atherosclerosis: potential mechanisms. *Arterioscler Thromb Vasc Biol* 2004;24:369–375.
37. Huang L, Zhao A, Wong F, et al: Leukotriene B4 strongly increases monocyte chemoattractant protein-1 in human monocytes. *Arterioscler Thromb Vasc Biol* 2004;24:1748–1749.
38. Friedrich EB, Tager AM, Liu E, et al: Mechanisms of leukotriene B4-triggered monocyte adhesion. *Arterioscler Thromb Vasc Biol* 2003;23:1761–1767.
39. Schmitt D, Shen Z, Zhang R, et al: Leukocytes utilize myeloperoxidase-generated nitrating intermediates as physiological catalysts for the generation of biologically active oxidized lipids and sterols in serum. *Biochemistry* 1999;38:16904–16915.
40. Eiserich JP, Baldus S, Brennan ML, et al: Myeloperoxidase, a leukocyte-derived vascular NO oxidase. *Science* 2002;296: 2391–2394.
41. Yokomizo T, Izumi T, Shimizu T: Co-expression of two LTB4 receptors in human mononuclear cells. *Life Sci* 2001;68: 2207–2212.

42. Leppert D, Hauser SL, Kishiyama JL, et al: Stimulation of matrix metalloproteinase-dependent migration of T cells by eicosanoids. *FASEB J* 2005;9:1473–1481.
43. Allen S, Dashwood M, Morrison K, Yacoub M: Differential leukotriene constrictor responses in human atherosclerotic coronary arteries. *Circulation* 1998;97:2406–2413.
44. Back M, Bu DX, Branstrom R, et al: Leukotriene B4 signaling through NF-kappaB–dependent BLT1 receptors on vascular smooth muscle cells in atherosclerosis and intimal hyperplasia. *Proc Natl Acad Sci U S A* 2005;102:17501–17506.
45. Lotzer K, Spanbroek R, Hildner M, et al: Differential leukotriene receptor expression and calcium responses in endothelial cells and macrophages indicate 5-lipoxygenases-dependent circuits of inflammation and atherogenesis. *Arterioscler Thromb Vasc Biol* 2003;23:e32–36.
46. Thivierge M, Stankova J, Rola-Pleszczynski M: IL-13 and IL-4 up-regulate cysteinyl leukotriene 1 receptor expression in human monocytes and macrophages. *J Immunol* 2001;167:2855–2860.
47. Uzonyi B, Lotzer K, Jahn S, et al: Cysteinyl leukotriene 2 receptor and protease-activated receptor 1 activate strongly correlated early genes in human endothelial cells. *Proc Natl Acad Sci U S A* 2006;103:6326–6231.
48. Hakonarson H, Thorvaldsson S, Helgadottir A, et al: Effects of a 5-lipoxygenase–activating protein inhibitor on biomarkers associated with risk of myocardial infarction. *JAMA 2005;*293: 2245–2256.
49. Troconiz IF, Zsolt I, Garrido MJ, et al: Dealing with time-dependent pharmacokinetics during the early clinical development of a new leukotriene B4 synthesis inhibitor. *Pharm Res* 2006;23:1533–1542.
50. Aiello R, Bourassa PA, Lindsey S, et al: Leukotriene B4 receptor antagonism reduces monocytic foam cells in mice. *Arterioscler Thromb Vasc Biol* 2002;22:443–449.
51. Lotzer K, Spanbroek R, Hildner M, et al: Differential leukotriene receptor expression and calcium responses in endothelial cells and macrophages indicate 5-lipoxygenase–dependent circuits of inflammation and atherogenesis. *Arterioscler Thromb Vasc Biol* 2003;23:e32–36.
52. University of Florida: Role of the arachidonate 5-lipoxygenase pathway in coronary heart disease. Clinicaltrials.gov. http://www.clinicaltrials.gov/ct/show/NCT00379808?order=1.
53. MacPhee CH, Moores KE, Boyd HF, et al: Lipoprotein-associated phospholipase A2, platelet-activating factor acetylhydrolase, generates two bioactive products during the oxidation of low-density lipoprotein: use of a novel inhibitor. *Biochem J* 1999;338:479–487.
54. Tietge UJ, Practico D, Ding T, et al: Macrophage-specific expression of group IIA sPLA2 results in accelerated atherogenesis by increasing oxidative stress. *J Lipid Res* 2005;46:1604–1614.
55. Burke JE, Dennis EA: Phospholipase A_2 Biochemistry. *Cardiovasc Drugs Ther* 2008 (in press).
56. Tjoelker LW, Eberhardt C, Unger J, et al: Plasma platelet-activating factor acetylhydrolase is a secreted phospholipase A(2) with a catalytic triad. *J Biol Chem* 1995;270:25481–25487.
57. Hurt-Camejo E, Andersen S, Standal R, et al: Localization of nonpancreatic secretory phospholipase A2 in normal and atherosclerotic arteries: activity of the isolated enzyme on low-density lipoproteins. *Arterioscler Thromb Vasc Biol* 1997;17:300–309.
58. Menschikowski M, Kasper M, Lattke P, et al: Secretory group II phospholipase A2 in human atherosclerotic plaques. *Atherosclerosis* 1995;118:173–181.
59. Ivandic B, Castellani LW, Wang XP, et al: Role of group II secretory phospholipase A2 in atherosclerosis: 1. Increased atherogenesis and altered lipoproteins in transgenic mice expressing group IIa phospholipase A2. *Arterioscler Thromb Vasc Biol* 1999;19:1284–1290.
60. Rosengren B, Peilot H, Umaerus M, et al: Secretory phospholipase A2 group V: lesion distribution, activation by arterial proteoglycans, and induction in aorta by a Western diet. *Arterioscler Thromb Vasc Biol* 2006;26:1579–1585.
61. Nijmeijer R, Lagrand WK, Vissner CA, et al: CRP, a major culprit in complement-mediated tissue damage in acute myocardial infarction? *Int Immunopharmacol* 2001;1:403–414.
62. Hanasaki K, Yamada K, Yamamoto S, et al: Potent modification of low-density lipoprotein by group X secretory phospholipase A2 is linked to macrophage foam cell formation. *J Biol Chem* 2002;277:29116–29124.
62a. Leitinger N, Watson AD, Hama Sy, et al: Role of Group II secretory phospholipase A_2 in atherosclerosis: 2. Potential involvement of biologically active oxidized phospholipids. *Arterioscler Thromb Vasc Biol* 1999,19:1291–1298.
63. Nijmeijer R, Lagrand WK, Baidoshvili A, et al: Secretory type II phospholipase A(2) binds to ischemic myocardium during myocardial infarction in humans. *Cardiovasc Res* 2002;53:138–146.
64. Zalewski A, Macphee C: Role of lipoprotein-associated phospholipase A2 in atherosclerosis: biology, epidemiology, and possible therapeutic target. *Arterioscler Thromb Vasc Biol* 2005;25:923–931.
64a. Oslund RC, Cermak N, Gelb MH: Highly specific and broadly potent inhibtors of mammmalian secreted phospholipases A2. *J Med Chem* 2008;51:4708–4714.
65. Balboa MA, Balsinde J, Winstead MV, et al: Novel group V phospholipase A2 involved in arachidonic acid mobilization in murine P388D1 macrophages. *J Biol Chem* 1996;271:32381–32384.
66. Thommesen L, Sjursen W, Gasvik K, et al: Selective inhibitors of cytosolic or secretory phospholipase A2 block TNF-induced activation of transcription factor nuclear factor-kappa B and expression of ICAM-1. *J Immunol* 1998;161:3421–3430.
67. Data on File. Anthera.
68. Kumar A, Takada Y, Boriek AM, Aggarwal BB: Nuclear factor-kappaB: its role in health and disease. *J Mol Med* 2004;82: 434–448.
69. Dennis EA: The growing phospholipase A2 superfamily of signal transduction enzymes. *Trends Biochem Sci* 1997;22:1–2.
70. Baeuerle PA, Henkel T: Function and activation of NF-kappa B in the immune system. *Annu Rev Immunol* 1994;12:141–179.
71. Trias J, Personal Communication.
72. Fujioka D, Kawabata K, Salto Y, Kobayashi T, et al: Reduction in myocardial ischemia/reperfusion injury in group X secretory phospholipase A_2-deficient mice. Circulation 2008;117:2977–2985.
73. Anthera Pharmaceuticals: PLASMA Trial. Phospholipase Levels and Serological Markers of Atherosclerosis: a dose-ranging clinical pharmacology study of A-002 in subjects with stable coronary artery disease. Clinicaltrials.gov. http://www.clinicaltrials.gov/ct/show/NCT00455546?order=1.
73a. Rosenson RS, Hislop, C, McConnell D, et al: Effects of a selective inhibitor of secretory phospholipase A_2 on low density lipoproteins and inflammatory pathways. *Lancet* 2008 (in press).
74. Stafforini DM, Sheller JR, Blackwell TS, et al: Release of free F2-isoprostanes from esterified phospholipids is catalyzed by intracellular and plasma platelet-activating factor acetylhydrolases. *J Biol Chem* 2006;281:4616–4623.
75. Mangin EL, Kugiyama K, Nguy JH, et al: Effects of lysolipids and oxidatively modified low-density lipoprotein on endothelium-dependent relaxation of rabbit aorta. *Circ Res* 1993;72:161–166.
76. Tew DG, Boyd HF, Ashman S, et al: Mechanism of inhibition of LDL phospholipase A2 by monocyclic-beta-lactams. Burst kinetics and the effect of stereochemistry. *Biochemistry* 1998;37:10087–10093.
77. Carpenter KL, Dennis IF, Challis IR, et al: Inhibition of lipoprotein-associated phospholipase A2 diminishes the death-inducing effects of oxidised LDL on human monocyte-macrophages. *FEBS Lett* 2001;505:357–363.
78. Shi Y, Zhang P, Zhang L, et al: Role of lipoprotein-associated phospholipase A2 in leukocyte activation and inflammatory responses. *Atherosclerosis* 2007;191:54–62.
78a. Rosenson RS, Vracar-Graber M, Helenowaski I: Lipoprotein associated phospholipase A_2 inhibition reduces generation of oxidized fatty acids. *Cardiovasc Drugs Ther* 2008;22:55–58.
79. Johnson A, Zalewski A, Janmohamed S, et al: Lipoprotein-associated phospholipase A2 (lp-PLA2) activity, an emerging CV risk marker, can be inhibited in atherosclerotic lesions and plasma by novel pharmacologic intervention: the results of a multicenter clinical study. Presented at American Heart Association Scientific Sessions 2004, poster 2745, New Orleans, LA, November 7–10, 2004.
80. Serruys PW, García-García HM, Buszman P, et al: Effects of the direct lipoprotein-associated phospholipase A_2 inhibitor darapladib on human coronary atherosclerotic plaque. *Circulation* 2008;118:1172–1182.
81. Shi Y, Zalewski A, Macphee C, Dawson M: Selective inhibitor of lipoprotein-associated phospholipase A_2 attenuates markers of plaque vulnerability in humans. *Circulation* 2007;116:11–108.
82. Schonbeck U, Libby P: CD40 signaling and plaque instability. *Circ Res* 2001;89:1092–1103.

83. Shen L, Sigal LJ, Boes M, Rock KL: Important role of cathepsin S in generating peptides for TAP-independent MHC class I crosspresentation *in vivo*. *Immunity* 2004;21:155–165.
84. Thurmand RL, Sun S, Sehon CA, et al: Identification of a potent and selective noncovalent cathepsin S inhibitor. *J Pharmacol Exp Ther* 2004;308:268–276.
85. Sukhova GK, Zhang Y, Pan JH, et al: Deficiency of cathepsin S reduces atherosclerosis in LDL receptor-deficient mice. *J Clin Invest* 2003;11:897–906.
86. Charo IF, Myers SJ, Herman A, et al: Molecular cloning and functional expression of two monocyte chemoattractant protein 1 receptors reveals alternative splicing of the carboxyl-terminal tails. *Proc Natl Acad Sci U S A* 2004;91:2752–2756.
87. Wain JH, Kirby JA, Ali S: Leucocyte chemotaxis: examination of mitogen-activated protein kinase and phosphoinositide 3-kinase activation by monocyte chemoattractant proteins-1, -2, -3 and -4. *Clin Exp Immunol* 2002;127:436–444.
88. Ashida N, Arai H, Yamasaki M, Kita T: Distinct signaling pathways for MCP-1-dependent integrin activation and chemotaxis. *J Biol Chem* 2001;276:16555–16560.
89. Boring L, Gosling J, Cleary M, Charo IF: Decreased lesion formation in CCR2-/- mice reveals a role for chemokines in the initiation of atherosclerosis. *Nature* 1998;394:894–897.
90. Gosling J, Slaymaker S, Gu L, et al: MCP-1 deficiency reduces susceptibility to atherosclerosis in mice that overexpress human apolipoprotein B. *J Clin Invest* 1999;103:773–778.
91. Pasternak A, Marino D, Vicario PP, et al: Novel, orally bioavailable gamma-aminoamide CC chemokine receptor 2 (CCR2) antagonists. *J Med Chem* 2006;49:4801–2804.
92. Yang L, Butora G, Jiao RX, et al: Discovery of 3-piperidinyl–1-cyclopentanecarboxamide as a novel scaffold for highly potent CC chemokine receptor 2 antagonists. *J Med Chem* 2007;50: 2609–2611.
93. Nijmeijer R, Lagrand WK, Vissner CA, et al: CRP, a major culprit in complement-mediated tissue damage in acute myocardial infarction? *International Immunopharmacol* 2001;1:403–414.
94. Brodmerkel CM, Huber R, Covington M, et al: Discovery and pharmacological characterization of a novel rodent-active CCR2 antagonist, INCB3344. *J Immunol* 2005;175:5370–5378.
95. Zhang J, Shen B, Lin A: Novel strategies for inhibition of the p38 MAPK pathway. Trends Pharmacol Sci 2007;28:286–295.
96. Ko J, Yun CY, Lee JS, et al: p38 MAPK and ERK activation by 9-cis-retinoic acid induces chemokine receptors CCR1 and CCR2 expression in human monocytic THP-1 cells. *Exp Mol Med* 2007;39:129–138.
97. Pietersma A, Tilly BC, Gaestel M, et al: p38 mitogen activated protein kinase regulates endothelial VCAM-1 expression at the post-transcriptional level. *Biochem Biophys Res Commun* 1997;230:44–48.
98. Lee M, Dominguez C: MAP kinase p38 inhibitors: clinical results and an intimate look at their interactions with p38alpha protein. *Curr Med Chem* 2005;12:2979–2994.
99. Fabian MA, Biggs WH, Treiber DK, et al: A small molecule-kinase interaction map for clinical kinase inhibitors. *Nat Biotechnol* 2005;23:329–336.
100. Doggrel SA, Wanstall JC: Vascular chymase: pathophysiological role and therapeutic potential of inhibition. *Cardiovasc Res* 2004;61:653–662.
101. Leskinen MJ, Lindstedt KA, Wang Y, Kovanen PT: Mast cell chymase induces smooth muscle cell apoptosis by a mechanism involving fibronectin degradation and disruption of focal adhesions. *Arterioscler Thromb Vasc Biol* 2003;23:238–243.
102. Shiota N, Okunishi H, Takai S, et al: Tranilast suppresses vascular chymase expression and neointima formation in balloon-injured dog carotid artery. Circulation 1999;99:1084–1090.
103. Takahashi A, Taniguchi T, Ishikawa Y, et al: Tranilast inhibits vascular smooth muscle cell growth and intimal hyperplasia by induction of p21(waf1/cip1/sdi1) and p53. *Circ Res* 1999;84:543–550.
104. Tamai H, Katoh K, Yamaguchi T, et al: The impact of tranilast on restenosis after coronary angioplasty: the second tranilast restenosis following angioplasty trial (TREAT-2). *Am Heart J* 2004;143:506–513.
105. Holmes DR, Savage M, LaBlanche JM, et al: Results of Prevention of REStenosis with Tranilast and its Outcomes (PRESTO) trial. *Circulation* 2002;106:1243–1250.
106. Muramatsu M, Yamada M, Takai S, Miyazaki M: Suppression of basic fibroblast growth factor-induced angiogenesis by a specific chymase inhibitor, BCEAB, through the chymase-angiotensin-dependent pathway in hamster sponge granulomas. *Br J Pharmacol* 2002;137:554–560.
107. Seeger W, Suttorp N, Hellwig A, Bhakdi S: Noncytolytic terminal complement complexes may serve as calcium gates to elicit leukotriene B4 generation in human polymorphonuclear leukocytes. *J Immunol* 1986;137:1286–1293.
108. Hattori R, Hamilton KK, McEver RP, Sims PJ: Complement proteins C5b-9 induce secretion of high molecular weight multimers of endothelial von Willebrand factor and translocation of granule membrane protein GMP-140 to the cell surface. *J Biol Chem* 1989;264:9053–9060.
109. Pinckard RN, O'Rourke RA, Crawford MH, et al: Complement localization and mediation of ischemic injury in baboon myocardium. *J Clin Invest* 1980;66:1050–1056.
110. Horstick G, Heimann A, Gotze O, et al: Intracoronary application of C1 esterase inhibitor improves cardiac function and reduces myocardial necrosis in an experimental model of ischemia and reperfusion. *Circulation* 1997;95:701–708.
111. Mahaffey KW, Granger CB, Nicolau JC, et al: Effect of pexelizumab, an anti-C5 complement antibody, as adjunctive therapy to fibrinolysis in acute myocardial infarction: the COMPlement inhibition in myocardial infarction treated with thromboLYtics (COMPLY) trial. *Circulation* 2003;108: 1176–1183.
112. Granger CB, Mahaffrey KW, Weaver WD, et al: Pexelizumab, an anti-C5 complement antibody, as adjunctive therapy to primary percutaneous coronary intervention in acute myocardial infarction: The COMplement inhibition in Myocardial infarction treated with Angioplasty (COMMA) trial. *Circulation* 2003;108:1184–1190.
113. Shernan SK, Fitch JC, Nussmeier NA, et al: Impact of pexelizumab, an anti-C5 complement antibody, on total mortality and adverse cardiovascular outcomes in cardiac surgical patients undergoing cardiopulmonary bypass. *Ann Thorac Surg* 2004;77:942–950.

Index

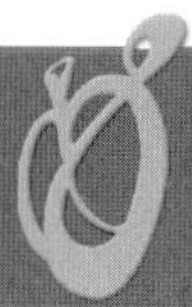